PATHOBIOLOGY OF OCULAR DISEASE

A DYNAMIC APPROACH

Second Edition

Part B

To Catherine and Felicity

PATHOBIOLOGY OF OCULAR DISEASE

A DYNAMIC APPROACH

Second Edition

Part B

edited by

Alec Garner
Institute of Ophthalmology
University of London
London, England

Gordon K. Klintworth
Duke University Medical Center
Durham, North Carolina

Marcel Dekker, Inc.   New York•Basel•Hong Kong

Library of Congress Cataloging-in-Publication Data

Pathobiology of occular disease : a dynamic approach / edited by Alec
  Garner, Gordon K. Klintworth. — 2nd ed.
        p.   cm.
    Includes bibliographical references and index.
    ISBN 0-8247-9136-3 (v. A : alk. paper). — ISBN 0-8247-9137-1 (v.
B : alk. paper)
    1. Eye—Pathophysiology. I. Garner, Alec. II. Klintworth,
Gordon K.
    [DNLM: 1. Eye Diseases—pathology. 2. Eye Diseases-
-physiopathology.   WW 140 P297 1994]
RE67.P38 1994
617.7'1—dc20
DNLM/DLC
for Library of Congress   93-46485
                                                                            CIP

The publisher offers discounts on this book when ordered in bulk quantities. For more information, write to Special Sales/Professional Marketing at the address below.

This book is printed on acid-free paper.

MARCEL DEKKER, INC.
270 Madison Avenue, New York, New York 10016

Current printing (last digit):
10 9 8 7 6 5 4 3 2 1

PRINTED IN THE UNITED STATES OF AMERICA

Foreword to the Second Edition

Over a decade has passed since I contributed a foreword to the first edition of this scholarly work, and in that short time biomedical research has advanced further than could have been imagined. This second edition is accordingly expanded, and the fifty-four chapters, covering a wide range of disciplines, illustrate in a striking way the influence of this progress in the field of ophthalmology. The advances derive in the main from highly sophisticated developments in research technology, providing new concepts rather than etiological revelations. Thus, many blinding diseases, as from cataract, glaucoma, diabetes, and age-related maculopathy, still await definitive explanations of their cause, but our increasing appreciation of the many factors apparently playing a role in their pathogenesis, so well expounded here, provide a sure foundation for tomorrow's achievements in rational therapy.

Whether the authors are clinicians, pathologists, or other scientists, they are all authorities in their subjects and together present, to a standard equal to the best in medical literature, our latest knowledge of eye disease, within the context of cognate progress in general pathology. It is a most impressive work and surely unequalled in its particular approach to diseases of the eye, not as an organ sequestered in the orbit, but as one vulnerable to diseases of the body as a whole.

In congratulating the authors I express my hope that this second edition will continue to provide both pleasure and profit to the wide readership it will undoubtedly attract.

Norman Ashton, CBE, FRS
Emeritus Professor of Pathology
University of London and
The Royal College of Surgeons of England

Foreword to the First Edition

No systematized presentation of the pathology of the eye existed in any language until 1808 when James Wardrop, a Scotsman then aged 26, published his first edition of *Essays on the Morbid Anatomy of the Human Eye*, followed the next year by *Fungus Haemotodes or Soft Cancer* which established retinoblastoma as a recognized entity. Although these books were not the first to describe or illustrate specimens or ocular disease, and in fact contained little morbid anatomy as now defined, they introduced, by dissections and macroscopical studies, an area of investigation eventually to become the specialty of ophthalmic pathology.

The subsequent development of microscopy in the late nineteenth century and early twentieth century and its wider use throughout all aspects of laboratory science led to an immense and still expanding increase in knowledge. The revelations of histology and histopathology had as dramatic an impact as those of electron microscopy in modern times, and ophthalmic pathology in its turn became largely concerned with the documentation of macroscopical and microscopical features of diseased ocular tissues. There followed many textbooks dealing excusively or predominantly with these aspects; the most widely admired are beautifully illustrated first with superb paintings and drawings and later by photographic reproductions, which in the last two decades reached the highest quality. These remain classic textbooks in ophthalmology and are of inestimable value, but curiously ophthalmic pathology continued to be confined to morbid anatomy long after pathology itself had branched out to found the present main disciplines of histopathology, chemical pathology, hematology, medical microbiology, and immunopathology. Even today ophthalmic pathology is usually equated with histopathology of the eye; that is certainly the main interest of American, Canadian, and European ophthalmic pathology societies. This has been at least partly due to the fact that for many years opthalmic pathology was a part-time pursuit of ophthalmologists engaged in exacting clinical practice, and perhaps it would be as reasonable to expect them to have had the time to become conversant with the many developments in pathology as it would be to expect a general pathologist to be skilled, for instance, in the latest methods of cataract extraction or the management of glaucoma. Thus while freely acknowledging that the present sum of knowledge in ophthalmic pathology is much indebted to them, I have always been convinced that future progress must be more widely based. In 1957 I wrote

> If in the future, eye pathology is to be taught and practised in the traditional way, as an elaborate recording of histologic minutiae, then the subject is not too demanding and may well be undertaken as a part-time pursuit, and probably best by the ophthalmologist who is most able to extract the greatest clinical value from the findings. But if the study of ocular pathology is to have its full meaning, the eye must be regarded as a unit of an entire organism, and its behavior in disease must as far as possible be related to that of the whole. Research in this field, in common with the general tendency, should concern itself with disease mechanisms rather than with disease patterns, and for this purpose the widest possible knowledge of pathologic processes is desirable and the whole armamentarium of modern scientific method should be

available. To establish ocular pathology on this broad basis will demand the full and concentrated attention of workers trained and experienced in the appropriate disciplines.*

Nearly a quarter of a century later I have nothing to add to these convictions and I warmly welcome this monumental work in two volumes planned and executed on the lines I had so hopefully visualized, and I am proud that such a notable work should have been assembled by Professor Alec Garner, my successor as director of the Department of Pathology at the Institute of Ophthalmology in London, and Professor Gordon Klintworth some-time visiting professor there. With their able collaborators they present in these comprehensive volumes exactly the approach to ocular disease that is essential both for its immediate elucidation and for the whole future development of the subject, not in isolation but within the context of pathology as a whole.

With this conviction I warmly commend this book to everyone interested and involved in this fascinating field of learning, and wish all those concerned in its production the success so richly deserved.

> *Norman Ashton, CBE, FRS*
> *Emeritus Professor of Pathology*
> *University of London and*
> *The Royal College of Surgeons of England*

---

*Am. J. Ophthalmol. 44:5–6, 1957.

Preface to the Second Edition

A knowledge of pathology is the basis of sound medicine, and the thinking ophthalmologist is keen to understand, as well as may be, the forces responsible for the clinical manifestations of eye disease. Only then can management be pursued in a rational manner. The descriptive elements of ophthalmic pathology are fundamental and need to be precisely defined in the interests of accurate diagnosis. But beyond that utilitarian function is their importance as building blocks in comprehending the nature of the disease processes per se, and it is to this second objective in particular that the present text is directed. Correspondingly, we have not sought to provide a detailed manual of diagnostic pathology—there are now a number of excellent texts and atlases available that achieve this purpose far better than we could ever have hoped to do. Instead, where possible, we have tried to interpret the facts and to provide a feeling for the dynamic aspects of ophthalmic pathology.

As noted in the preface to the first edition, laudable though such a purpose may be, it is difficult to succeed. Firstly, depending on the particular disease state under consideration, it requires a sound knowledge of a range of complementary disciplines such as molecular biology, biochemistry, immunology, and genetics. In this regard, we have been fortunate in having the services of many recognized experts in these various fields capable of writing with authority. Secondly, not all the necessary building blocks are yet identified, let alone in position. Nevertheless, an incredible body of new information has accrued in almost every field in the twelve years since the first edition, especially in the understanding of disease at the molecular level, and an update of our text had become imperative if it was to remain relevant. We were encouraged to take up the challenge by the favorable reception of the first edition and because, despite the welcome increase in textbooks related to the pathology of eye disease, ours remains the only reasonably comprehensive attempt to address the functional aspects of the subject.

As with the first edition, this has been a daunting task, and we are more than grateful to our contributors, who have responded to their briefs quite magnificently. For one reason or another, we have had to enlist the help of a number of new authors, and such has been the enormous volume of new material to be covered that even existing authors have had to engage in extensive revision of their chapters, amounting in some cases to a complete rewrite.

Again, we very much hope that the attraction of the book will extend beyond the precious but small number of practicing ophthalmic pathologists to pathologists working in other fields, because study of the eye has relevance far beyond its own orbit. Clinical ophthalmologists too will, we trust, find much to assist them in the evaluation and treatment of their patients. We hope that others outside the medical community—those employed in related disciplines of biology, immunology, and genetics—will also discover something of value.

We are very conscious of and more than happy to acknowledge the enormous assistance provided by our secretaries, Pat Goodwin, Carmen Quarrie, Wanda Dietze, Elizabeth Barnard, Karen Alliume, and

Kristina Boewe. We are also indebted to Allan T. Summers for his painstaking role in verifying and completing countless references. Finally, as before, we want to thank our wives, Catherine and Felicity, who have been most supportive, and we hope they will find pleasure in the outcome which we take great delight in dedicating to them.

Alec Garner
Gordon K. Klintworth

Preface to the First Edition

Such is the volume of ophthalmologic and pathological writing that only by stepping aside completely from one's commitment to engage actively in these disciplines would it be possible to absorb all that might profitably be read. It would be irresponsible of any potential author or editor to unleash on the busy student yet more reading matter should it not fill a real need. There are in existence already several excellent treatises relating to the pathological anatomy of the eye, and it would have been redundant for us to seek to emulate them; rather we have sought to direct attention to dynamic considerations and disease mechanisms, and so complement the emphasis on descriptive pathology to be found in other writings on the subject. Hence the title *Pathobiology of Ocular Disease: A Dynamic Approach.*

It is our belief that knowing the appearance of a lesion and being able to recognize it is only the beginning of the story. If appropriate and rational treatment is to be instituted, it is also necessary to understand what is happening and, where possible, why. For instance, from the practicing clinician's standpoint, more important than to recognize granulomatous inflammation when seen in a microscopical preparation is to have some idea of what that means in terms of causative factors and likely behavior. That is not to say we decry descriptive pathology—far from it, for morphology and function are but the two sides of the same coin and are patently interdependent. But the job of the pathologist is both to identify disease processes and to interpret them in behavioral terms. It was with this dual role of pathology in mind that we invited the various contributors to compose their chapters.

However, success is an elusive goal when the brief is so demanding. To state what and where is one thing; to ask how and why is quite another. Nevertheless, as editors, we feel that our contributors have responded magnificently and it is our fervent hope that the result will meet the needs of serious students of ophthalmology, be they trainees or more experienced practitioners, who are keen to understand the nature of the disorders they are called on to treat. The emphasis on dynamic disease processes inevitably encompasses the whole gamut of pathological disciplines—microbiology, immunology, and biochemistry, as well as histopathology, and this all-embracing interpretation of pathology serves further to distinguish our book from existing texts.

For a variety of reasons, which need not be spelt out here, ophthalmic pathology is commonly viewed with suspicion by other pathologists. Trained as general pathologists ourselves, we as editors hope that, by relating the specific matters of ocular pathology to the basic and more general aspects of disease processes, we will have gone some way towards persuading our colleagues that study of the eye is both fascinating and rewarding.

Inevitably, to assemble a multiauthor compendium of the sort we have compiled, such that there is not too much diversity of approach, has involved a great deal of effort, not only for the editors, but also for the gallant contributors who have had to contend with a seemingly endless stream of queries and comments. We want to thank them for their cooperation and forbearance.

Other people whose assistance has been invaluable are acknowledged elsewhere but we would also put on record our appreciation of the unstinting advice and practical help provided by the staff of our publisher, Marcel Dekker, Inc., and of the colossal support we have received from our secretaries, Catherine Thornton, Pat Goodwin, Louise Hart, Frances Slocum, Candiss Weaver, Pat Burks, Bonnie Lynch, Diane Evans, Linda Brogan, Marge Penny, and Virginia Hotelling. Lastly, if for no other reason than that they are the ones who at the end of the day have had to bear with us when the task of preparing the book weighed overheavily on our shoulders, we want to thank our wives and children for their tolerance and encouragement.

This book would not have been possible without the assistance of many individuals. Aside from the vital role of the authors and the editorial staff of Marcel Dekker, Inc., numerous individuals provided critical reviews of chapters. In this regard, we wish to thank the following:

Mathea R. Allansmith	D. Doniach	John F. R. Kuck, Jr.
Douglas R. Anderson	Roberta Meyers Elliot	Robert Machemer
Norman Ashton	Bernard F. Fetter	Kenneth S. McCarty, Jr.
Elaine R. Berman	Ben S. Fine	Don Minckler
Stanley Braverman	Ramon L. Font	Ralph Muller
Robert P. Burns	Robert Y. Foos	G. Richard O'Connor
R. Jean Campbell	Doyle G. Graham	M. Bruce Shields
Leo T. Chylack	Donald B. Hackel	James Tiedeman
David G. Cogan	Hal K. Hawkins	Robert Trelstad
Byron P. Croker, Jr.	Hannah Kinney	F. Stephen Vogel
Anthony J. Dark	Jin H. Kinoshita	Lorenz E. Zimmerman

Allan Summers, Susan Feinglos, Ginger Reeves, Betty Adams, Mary Ann Brown, and Janet Shields were most helpful in checking and completing the innumerable references.

The following assisted authors with specific chapters: Nancy L. Robinson, Glenn P. Kimball, and Karen A. Pelletier (Chapter 49), David Andrews (Chapter 48), Joseph Hackett (Chapter 40).

Alec Garner
Gordon K. Klintworth

Contributors

Daniel M. Albert, M.D.   Professor and Chairman, Department of Ophthalmology, University of Wisconsin—Madison, Madison, Wisconsin

Elaine R. Berman, Ph.D.   Professor of Experimental Ophthalmology and Head, Eye Biochemistry Unit, Hadassah-Hebrew University Medical School, Jerusalem, Israel

Alan C. Bird, M.D., F.R.C.S., F.C.Ophth.   Professor, Department of Clinical Ophthalmology, Institute of Ophthalmology, University of London, London, England

Edward H. Bossen, M.D.   Professor, Department of Pathology, Duke University Medical Center, Durham, North Carolina

R. Jean Campbell, M.B., Ch.B.   Consultant, Departments of Pathology and Ophthalmology, Mayo Clinic and Mayo Foundation, and Professor of Pathology, Mayo Medical School, Rochester, Minnesota

Anthony J. Dark, M.D., F.R.C.S.Ed.   Associate Professor, Department of Ophthalmology, State University of New York Health Science Center at Syracuse, Syracuse, New York

Sohrab Darougar, M.D., D.T.M.Ph., F.R.C.Path., D.Sc.*   Professor, Public Health Ophthalmology, Department of Preventive Ophthalmology, Institute of Ophthalmology, University of London, London, England

Gordon N. Dutton, M.D., F.R.C.S., F.C.Ophth.   Consultant Ophthalmologist, Department of Ophthalmology, Tennent Institute of Ophthalmology, Glasgow, Scotland

David L. Easty, M.D., F.R.C.S., F.C.Ophth.   Professor, Department of Ophthalmology, Bristol Eye Hospital, Bristol, England

C. Stephen Foster, M.D., F.A.C.S.   Director, Immunology and Uveitis Service, Department of Ophthalmology, Harvard Medical School and Massachusetts Eye and Ear Infirmary, Boston, Massachusetts

Alec Garner, M.D., Ph.D., F.R.C.P., F.C.Ophth.   Professor and Director, Department of Pathology, Institute of Ophthalmology, University of London, London, England

W. Richard Green, M.D.   Professor of Ophthalmology and Associate Professor of Pathology, Departments of Ophthalmology and Pathology, The Johns Hopkins University School of Medicine, Baltimore, Maryland

---

Present affiliation: Professor, Preventive Medicine Research Unit, Royal Veterinary College, University of London, London, England.

Ian Grierson, B.Sc., Ph.D.   Littlewoods Professor of Ophthalmology, Unit of Ophthalmology, Department of Medicine, The University of Liverpool and Royal Liverpool University Hospital, Liverpool, England

Hans E. Grossniklaus, M.D.   Associate Professor, Departments of Ophthalmology and Pathology, and Director, L. F. Montgomery Eye Pathology Laboratory, Emory University School of Medicine, Atlanta, Georgia

Kim Neal Hakin, F.R.C.S., F.C.Ophth.   Senior Registrar in Ophthalmology, Moorfields Eye Hospital, London, England

J. Godfrey Heathcote, M.A., M.B., B.Ch., Ph.D., F.R.C.P.C.   Chief of Pathology, St. Joseph's Health Centre, and Associate Professor, Departments of Pathology and Ophthalmology, The University of Western Ontario, London, Ontario, Canada

Paul Hiscott, M.B.B.S., Ph.D., F.R.C.S., F.C.O.Path.   Lecturer, Unit of Ophthalmology, Department of Medicine, The University of Liverpool and Royal Liverpool University Hospital, Liverpool, England

Ali Aijaz Hussain, B.Sc., Ph.D.   Senior Research Lecturer, Department of Ophthalmology, United Medical and Dental Schools of Guy's and St. Thomas's Hospitals, London, England

Barrie Jay, M.D., F.R.C.S., F.C.Ophth.   Emeritus Professor of Clinical Ophthalmology, Institute of Ophthalmology, University of London, London, England

Kelly A. Jones, H.T.(A.S.C.P.)   Senior Histotechnician/Electron Microtechnician, Department of Ophthalmic Pathology, University of Maryland at Baltimore, Baltimore, Maryland

Jeremy Joseph, M.D., F.R.C.S., F.C.Ophth.   Senior Registrar, Ophthalmic Department, The Royal Free Hospital, London, England

Gordon K. Klintworth, M.D., Ph.D.   Professor, Department of Pathology, and Joseph A. C. Wadsworth Research Professor and Director of Research, Department of Ophthalmology, Duke University Medical Center, Durham, North Carolina

James G. Lewis, Ph.D.   Assistant Professor, Department of Pathology, Duke University Medical Center, Durham, North Carolina

Susan Lightman, M.B., B.S., Ph.D., F.C.Ophth., F.R.C.P.   Professor, Department of Clinical Science, Institute of Ophthalmology, Moorfields Eye Hospital, London, England

Curtis E. Margo, M.D.   Professor, Departments of Ophthalmology and Pathology, University of South Florida College of Medicine, Tampa, Florida

John Marshall, B.Sc., Ph.D.   Frost Professor of Ophthalmology, Department of Ophthalmology, United Medical and Dental Schools of Guy's and St. Thomas's Hospitals, London, England

Alison C. E. McCartney, M.A., M.D., F.R.C.Path., F.R.C.Ophth.   Senior Lecturer in Ophthalmic Pathology, Departments of Pathology and Ophthalmology, United Medical and Dental Schools of Guy's and St. Thomas's Hospitals, London, England

Donald S. Minckler, M.D.   Professor, Department of Ophthalmology, Doheny Eye Institute, University of Southern California School of Medicine, Los Angeles, California

Donald A. Morris, M.D.   Associate Clinical Professor, Department of Ophthalmology, Montefiore Hospital and Medical Center, Albert Einstein College of Medicine, Bronx, New York

Terrence P. O'Brien, M.D.   Assistant Professor, Department of Ophthalmology, The Johns Hopkins University School of Medicine, Baltimore, Maryland

Alan D. Proia, M.D., Ph.D.   Associate Professor, Departments of Ophthalmology and Pathology, Duke University Medical Center, Durham, North Carolina

Amjad H. S. Rahi, M.D., Ph.D., F.C.Ophth., F.R.C.Path.   Chief of Immunology and Histopathology Services, Regional Laboratories and Blood Bank, Ministry of Health, Dammam, Saudi Arabia; and Reader Emeritus in Immunopathology, University of London, London, England

Sankaran Rajagopalan, M.D.   Faculty Research Associate, Division of Ophthalmic Pathology, Department of Ophthalmology, University of Maryland at Baltimore, Baltimore, Maryland

Merlyn M. Rodrigues, M.D., Ph.D.   Professor and Director, Division of Ophthalmic Pathology, Department of Ophthalmology, University of Maryland at Baltimore, Baltimore, Maryland

José A. Sahel, M.D.   Professeur des Universités—Praticien Hospitalier, Clinique Ophtalmologique, Hôpitaux Universitaires, Strasbourg, France

John Peter Sarks, F.R.C.S., F.R.A.C.O.   Honorary Consultant, Prince of Wales Hospital, Sydney, New South Wales, Australia

Shirley Sarks, F.R.C.S., F.R.A.C.O., M.D.   Head, Ophthalmology Department, Lidcombe Hospital, Sydney, New South Wales, Australia

Mark W. Scroggs, M.D.   Resident in Ophthalmology, Department of Ophthalmology, Duke University School of Medicine, Durham, North Carolina

John D. Shelburne, M.D., Ph.D.   Professor, Department of Pathology, Duke University School of Medicine, Durham, North Carolina

Brian S. F. Shine, M.Sc., M.D., M.R.C.Path.   Consultant Chemical Pathologist, Stoke Mandeville Hospital, Aylesbury, England

Barbara A. Wiard Streeten, M.D.   Professor, Departments of Ophthalmology and Pathology, State University of New York Health Science Center at Syracuse, Syracuse, New York

Elise Torczynski, M.D.   Professor, Departments of Ophthalmology and Pathology, Rush Medical Center, Chicago, Illinois

John D. Treharne, B.Sc., Ph.D., F.R.C.Path.   Reader in Virology, Section of Virology, Department of Pathology, Institute of Ophthalmology, University of London, London, England

Catherine Williams, F.C.Ophth.   Research Fellow, Department of Ophthalmology, Bristol Eye Hospital, Bristol, England

David J. Wilson, M.D.   Associate Professor, Department of Ophthalmology, and Director of Ophthalmic Pathology, Casey Eye Institute, The Oregon Health Sciences University, Portland, Oregon

Anthony F. Winder, D.M., Ph.D., F.R.C.Path., M.R.C.P.   Professor and Head, Department of Chemical Pathology and Human Metabolism, Royal Free Hospital and School of Medicine, University of London; and Institute of Ophthalmology and Moorfields Eye Hospital, London, England

Fulton Wong, Ph.D.   Associate Professor of Ophthalmology and Neurobiology, Departments of Ophthalmology and Neurobiology, Duke University Medical Center, Durham, North Carolina

Contents of Part B

Contents of Part A

Basic Principles

Immunological Principles

Abbreviations

A   adenine
AA   amyloid protein A
ACAID   anterior chamber-associated immune deviation
ACE   angiotensin-converting enzyme
ACL   acromegaloid features, cutis verticis gyrata, and leukoma syndrome
ACR   acetylcholine receptor
ACTH   adrenocorticotropin
AD   autosomal dominant
ADCC   antibody-dependent cell-mediated cytotoxicity
ADH   aldehyde dehydrogenase
ADP   adenosine diphosphate
adRP   autosomal dominant retinitis pigmentosa
ADVIRC   autosomal dominant vitreoretinochoroidopathy
AEF   amyloid enhancing factor
aFGF   acid fibroblast growth factor
AIDS   acquired immunodeficiency syndrome
AKC   acute keratoconjunctivitis
AL   amyloid protein L (amyloid light-chain protein)
Ala   alanine
ALV   avian leukosis virus
AMD   age-related macular degeneration
ANA   antinuclear antibodies
ANCA   antineutrophil cytoplasmic antibody
AP   amyloid p-component

APECE   autoimmune, polyendocrinopathy, candidiasis, and ectodermal dystrophy
AP sites   apurinic/pyrimidinic sites
APUD cells   amine precursor uptake and decarboxylation cells
AR   aldose reductase
AR   autosomal recessive
arRP   autosomal recessive retinitis pigmentosa
Arg   arginine
AS   ankylosing spondylitis
ASA   ascorbic acid
Asn   asparagine
Asp   aspartate
ATP   adenosine triphosphate
ATPase   adenosine triphosphatase
ATV   acute transforming viruses
B   B lymphocytes
BALT   bronchus-associated lymphoid tissue
BCG   Bacillus Calmette-Guérin
BCNU   bis(chloroethyl)-1-nitrosourea
BD   Behçet's disease
BE   receptors binding apo E lipoprotein
bFGF   basic fibroblast growth factor
BLD   basal laminar deposit (basal linear deposit)
BP   benzo[a]pyrene
bp   base pairs
β-TG   β-thromboglobulin
C   cytosine

In the interest of editorial consistency, abbreviations that sometimes appear in the scientific literature in the plural form, e.g., GAGs, PGs, PMNs, have been standardized in this volume to appear without the "s." The singular or plural usage can be inferred according to context.

C1 first component of complement

C1q q subfraction of first component of complement

C1r r subfraction of first component of complement

C1s s subfraction of first component of complement

C2 second component of complement

C2a a fragment of second component of complement

C2b b fragment of second component of complement

C3 third component of complement

C3a a fragment of third component of complement

C3b b fragment of third component of complement

C3d d fragment of third component of complement

C4 fourth component of complement

C4b b fragment of fourth component of complement

C4b2a C3 convertase

C4b2a3b C5 convertase

C5 fifth component of complement

C5a a fragment of fifth component of complement

C5b b fragment of fifth component of complement

C5b67 complex of C5b with C6 and C7

C6 sixth component of complement

C7 seventh component of complement

C8 eighth component of complement

C9 ninth component of complement

Ca²⁺ calcium ion

Ca²⁺-stimulated ATPase calcium-stimulated adenosine triphosphatase

CA cytosine-adenine dinucleotide

CALLA common acute lymphoblastic antigen

CALT conjunctiva-associated lymphoid tissue

CAMAK cataract, microcephaly, arthrogryposis, and kyphosis

CAMFAK cataract, microcephaly, failure to thrive, arthrogryposis, and kyphosis

cAMP cyclic adenosine monophosphate

CAM cell adhesion molecules

C-ANCA cytoplasmic staining antineutrophil cytoplasmic antibody

CATT cytosine-adenine-thymine-thymine

CBH cutaneous basophil hypersensitivity

CCRG cooperative cataract research group

CD cluster of differentiation antigen

CD4 marker for helper T lymphocytes

CD8 marker for suppressor T lymphocytes

CD11b receptor for C3bi (also known as CR3)

CD11c receptor for C3bi and C3dg (also known as CR4)

Cd21 receptor for C3d (also known as CR2)

CD35 receptor for C3b (also known as CR1)

CAK chronic actinic keratopathy

CDK climatic droplet keratopathy

cDNA complementary deoxyribonucleic acid

CETP cholesterol ester transfer protein

CG cytosine-guanine dinucleotide

cGMP cyclic guanosine monophosphate

CGRP calcitonin gene-related peptide

CHED congenital hereditary endothelial dystrophy

CHRPE congenital hypertrophy of the retinal pigment epithelium

CI-MPR cation-independent mannose-phosphate receptor

cm centimeter

CME cystoid macular edema

CNBr cyanogen bromide

CNS central nervous system

CO₂ carbon dioxide

CoA coenzyme A

ConA concanavalin-A

CoQ ubiquinone (coenzyme Q)

CP cicatricial pemphigoid

CpG cytosine phosphate guanine dinucleotide

C/PL cholesterol-phospholipid ratio

CR1 receptor for C3b (also known as CD35)

CR2 receptor for C3d (also known as CD21)

CR3 receptor for C3bi (also known as CD11b)

CR4 receptor for C3bi and C3dg (also known as CD11c)

CRALBP intracellular retinaldehyde binding proteins

CSF cerebrospinal fluid

CSNB congenital stationary night blindness

CT computed tomography

CTAP connective tissue activating protein

Cu²⁺ cupric ion

cw cataract webbed (a mutant deer mouse)

Da Dalton

DAF decay-accelerating factor

DAG diaminoglycol

DG diacylglycerol

DH delayed hypersensitivity

DHS dehydroascorbic acid

DIDMOAD diabetes insipidus, diabetes mellitus, optic atrophy, and deafness

DMN dimethylnitrosamine

DMS   dimethylsulfate
DNA   deoxyribonucleic acid
DTT   dithiothreitol
ECF-A   eosinophilic chemotactic factor of anaphylaxis
ECM   extracellular matrix
ECP   eosinophil cationic protein
EDN   eosinophil-derived neurotoxin
EDS   Ehlers-Danlos syndrome
EDTA   ethylenediaminetetraacetic acid
EEP   EDTA-extractable proteins
EETs   epoxyeicosatrienoic acid
EGF   epidermal growth factor
EKG   electrocardiogram
ELAM-1   endothelial leukocyte adhesion molecule 1
ELISA   enzyme-linked immunosorbent assay
EM   erythema multiforme; electron microscopy
Endo   endothelial cells
Eo   eosinophils
EOG   electrooculography
Epi   epithelial cells
ER   endoplasmic reticulum
ERG   electroretinogram
ERP   early receptor potential
ESAF   endothelial cell angiogenesis factor
ESR   erythrocyte sedimentation rate
Fab   fragment antigen binding
FACS   fluorescence-activated cell sorter
FAD   flavin adenine dinucleotide
FAP   familial amyloid polyneuropathy
Fb   fibroblasts
F_c constant fragment of immunoglobulin; crystallizable fragment of immunoglobulin
Fe^{2+} ferrous ion
Fe^{3+} ferric ion
FEV   familial exudative vitreoretinopathy
FGF   fibroblast growth factor
FH   familial hypercholesterolemia
FHI   Fuchs' heterochromic iridocyclitis
FMN   flavin mononucleotide
Fuc   fucose
G   guanine
g   gram
G3P   glyceraldehyde 3-phosphate
G3PD   glyceraldehyde 3-phosphate dehydrogenase
GAG   codon for glutamic acid
GAG   glycosaminoglycan
Gal   galactose
GALT   gut-associated lymphoid tissue
GAPO   growth retardation, alopecia, pseudoanodontia, and optic atrophy syndrome

GCA   giant cell arteritis
GCD   granular corneal dystrophy
GBM   glomerular basement membrane
GDP   guanosine diphosphate
GIT   gastrointestinal tract
Glu   glutamate
Gly   glycine
GM-CSF   granulocyte-macrophage colony-stimulating factor
GMP-140   granule membrane protein
GRO (MGSA)   a cytokine
GSH   glutathione reduced form
GSSG   oxidized form of glutathione
GTP   guanosine triphosphate
GUG   codon for valine
h   hour
5-HT   5-hydroxytryptamine
HbA   adult hemoglobin
HbC   hemoglobin C
HbF   fetal hemoglobin
HbS   hemoglobin S (sickle cell hemoglobin)
HbSC   hemoglobin SC
HDL   high-density lipoprotein
HDL-1   high-density lipoprotein fraction 1
HDL-2   high-density lipoprotein fraction 2
HDL-3   high-density lipoprotein fraction 3
5-HETE   5-hydroxyeicosatetraenoic acid
12-HETE   12-hydroxyeicosatetraenoic acid
12(R)-HETE   12(R)-hydroxyeicosatetraenoic acid
15-HETE   15-hydroxyeicosatetraenoic acid
HETE   hydroxyeicosatetraenoic acids
His   histidine
HIV   human immunodeficiency virus
HLA   human leukocyte antigen
HLA-DR   a class II histocompatibility antigen
HMG   hydroxymethylglutaryl
HMW kininogen   high-molecular-weight kininogen
HPETE   hydroperoxyeicosatetraenoic acids
HPLC   high-performance liquid chromatography
HPV   human papillomavirus
HSP   heat-shock protein
HTGL   hepatic triglyceride lipase
HTLV I   human T cell leukemia virus I
HTLV II   human T cell leukemia virus II
ICAM-1   intercellular adhesion molecules 1
ICAM-2   intercellular adhesion molecules 2
IDL   intermediate-density lipoproteins
IFN-α   interferon-α
IFN-β   interferon-β
IFN-γ   interferon-γ
Ig   immunoglobulin
IgA   immunoglobulin A

IgD   immunogobulin D
IgE   immunoglobulin E
IGF   insulin-like growth factors
IgG   immunoglobulin G
IgM   immunoglobulin M
IOL   intraocular lens
IL   interleukin
IL-1   interleukin-1
IL-1α   interleukin-1α
IL-1β   interleukin-1β
IL-2   interleukin-2
IL-3   interleukin-3
IL-4   interleukin-4
IL-5   interleukin-5
IL-6   interleukin-6
IL-7   interleukin-7
IL-8   interleukin-8
IL-9   interleukin-9
IL-10   interleukin-10
ILGF-1   insulin-like growth factor 1
ILGF-2   insulin-like growth factor 2
ILM   inner limiting membrane of retina
Ile   isoleucine
IOP   intraocular pressure
IP$_3$ inositol trisphosphate
IPM   interphotoreceptor matrix
IRBP   interphotoreceptor cell binding protein
IRMA   intraretinal microvascular abnormality
ISCOM   immunostimulatory complexes
JA   juvenile rheumatoid arthritis
JCT   juxtacanalicular connective tissue
K+   potassium ion
kb   kilobase
KC   keratoconus
K cells   killer T lymphocyte
KCS   keratoconjunctivitis sicca
kD   kilodalton
Ker   keratinocyte
KID   keratitis, ichthyosis, deafness syndrome
K_m Michaelis constant
KS   keratan sulfate
KSPG   keratan sulfate proteoglycan (lumican)
LAK   lymphokine-activated killer cell
LAM-1   leukocyte adhesion molecule 1
LCA   leukocyte common antigen
LCAT   lecithin-cholesterol-acyltransferase
LCD   lattice corneal dystrophy
LDH   lactic dehydrogenase
LDL   low-density lipoprotein
LE   lupus erythematosus
LEC CAM   lectin-epithelial growth factor-complement binding adhesion molecules
LECAM-1   lectin-EGF-complement adhesion molecule

Leu   leucine
LFA-1   synonym for CD18
LGL   large granular lymphocyte
L-GP   lactosaminoglycan-glycoprotein
LHON   Leber's hereditary optic neuropathy
LMW kininogens   low-molecular-weight kininogens
LOCS   lens opacities case-control classification system
lop   lens opacities (a mutant mouse)
LPL   lipoprotein lipase
LPS   lipopolysaccharide
LTB$_4$ leukotriene B$_4$
LTC$_4$ leukotriene C$_4$ (previously known as SRS-A)
LTD$_4$ leukotriene D$_4$
LTE$_4$ leukotriene E$_4$
LTR   long terminal repeat
Lys   lysine
M   molar
MAC   membrane attack complex
MALT   mucosa-associated lymphoid tissue
Man   mannose
Man-6-P   mannose 6-phosphate
MBP   major basic protein
MBP   myelin basic protein
MC   mast cells
5mc   5-methylcytosine
MCAF   macrophage chemotactic factor
MCD   macular corneal dystrophy
MDP   muramyl dipeptide
MELAS   myoclonic epilepsy, lactic acidosis, and stroke-like episodes
MERRF   myoclonic epilepsy with red ragged fibers
Mg   magnesium
Mg^{2+} magnesium ion
7MG   methylation of guanine on nitrogen in 7th position
MGSA (GRO)   a cytokine
MHC   major histocompatibility complex
MIF   macrophage inhibition factor
MLD   metachromatic leukodystrophy
mM   millimolar
mm   millimeter
Mn   manganese
MO   macrophages/monocytes
Moab   monoclonal antibody
MPS   mucopolysaccharidosis
M_r molecular radius
MRI   magnetic resonance imaging
mRNA   messenger ribonucleic acid
MS   multiple sclerosis
MtDNA   mitochondrial DNA

MW molecular weight
Na⁺ sodium ion
Na⁺,K⁺ATPase sodium-potassium adenosine triphosphatase
NaCl sodium chloride
NAD⁺ nicotinamide adenine dinucleotide (oxidized form)
NADH nicotinamide adenine dinucleotide (reduced form)
NADP⁺ nicotinamide adenine dinucleotide phosphate (oxidized form)
NADPH nicotinamide adenine dinucleotide phosphate (reduced form)
NARP neurogenic muscle weakness, ataxia and retinitis pigmentosa
N-CAM neural cell adhesion molecule
NCL neuronal ceroid lipofuscinosis
nDNA nuclear DNA
Nd:YAG neodymium:yttrium-aluminum-garnet
N-FKyn 3-hydroxykynurenine
NK natural killer (cells)
nm nanometer
NMR nuclear magnetic resonance
nop nuclear opacification (a mutant mouse)
NSE neuron-specific enolase
O₂⁻ oxygen radical
OH· hydroxyl radical
O⁴MT methylation of thymine on oxygen in 4th position
O⁶MG methylation of guanine on oxygen in 6th position
OCSS oculocraniosomatic syndromes
3-OH Kyn *N*-formylkynurenine
OLM outer limiting membrane of retina
OPMD oculopharyngeal muscular dystrophy
ORF open reading frame
P platelets
p short arm of a chromosome
P53 a suppressor gene
PAF platelet-activating factor
PADGEM platelet activation-dependent granule external membrane protein
P-ANCA perinuclear staining antineutrophil cytoplasmic antibody
PC phosphatidylcholine
PCR polymerase chain reaction
PD polyol dehydrogenase
PDGF platelet-derived growth factor
PDE phosphodiesterase
PE phosphatidylethanolamine
PF-4 platelet factor 4
PG proteoglycan; prostaglandin
PGD₂ prostaglandin D₂
PGE₂ prostaglandin E₂
PGF₂α prostaglandin F₂α

PGI₂ prostacyclin
PHA phytohemaglutinin
PHPV persistent hyperplastic primary vitreous
Pᵢ inorganic phosphate
PI phosphatidylinositol
PIP₂ phosphatidylinositol 4,5-bisphosphate
PMMA polymethylmethacrylate
PML progressive multifocal leukoencephalopathy
PMN polymorphonuclear leukocyte
POAG primary open-angle glaucoma
PPD purified protein derivative of tuberculin
pRb retinoblastoma gene product
PS phosphatidylserine
PUFA polyunsaturated fatty acids
PUK peripheral ulcerative keratitis
PVD posterior vitreous detachment
PVR proliferative vitreoretinopathy
³¹P-NMR phosphorous 31-nuclear magnetic resonance
q long arm of a chromosome
R rad
RA rheumatoid arthritis
RANTES a cytokine (regulated on activation, normal T expressed and secreted)
RAR retinoic acid receptor
RARE retinoic acid-response element
Rb retinoblastoma gene
⁸⁶Rb rubidium 86
RBC red blood cell
RBP retinal binding protein
RCS Royal College of Surgeons
ROI reactive oxygen intermediates
ROP retinopathy of prematurity
RP retinitis pigmentosa
RPE retinal pigment epithelium
RSV Rous sarcoma virus
S sulfur
³⁵S sulfur isotope 35
s second
SAA serum amyloid protein A
SAC seasonal allergic conjunctivitis
SALT skin-associated lymphoid tissue
SAM senescence accelerated mouse
SAP serum amyloid protein
SDS-PAGE sodium dodecyl sulfate–polyacrylamide gel electrophoresis
Se selenium
SED spondyloepiphyseal dysplasia with dwarfism
SEER Surveillance, Epidemiology, and End Results
SEM scanning electron microscopy
SEM standard error of the mean
Ser serine

SIgA   secretory component of immunoglobulin A
sIL-2R   soluble interleukin-2 receptor
SLE   systemic lupus erythematosus
SLS   segment long spacing
SO   sympathetic ophthalmia
SOD   superoxide dismutase
sp.   species
SPK   superficial punctate keratitis
SRBC   sheep red blood cell
SRP   signal recognition particle
SRS-A   slow-reacting substance of
    anaphylaxis (currently known as leukotriene
    C_4)
SS   Sjögren's syndrome
SSCP   single-stranded conformational
    polymorphism
SSPE   subacute sclerosing panencephalitis
SV40   simian virus 40
T   thymine, T lymphocyte
TATA   thymine-adenine-thymine-adenine
T_c phase separation temperature
Tc   cytotoxic T cell
TCR   T cell receptor
TCR V$_b$ variable region of the T cell receptor
    b chain
TEM   transmission electron microscopy
TG   thymine-guanine dinucleotide
TGF-β   transforming growth factor β
TH   helper T cell
TH1   helper T cell involved in cell-mediated
    immunity

TH2   helper T cell that stimulates antibody
    production by B cells
Thr   threonine
TIMP   tissue inhibitor of metalloproteinase
TNF   tumor necrosis factor
TNF-α   tumor necrosis factor α
TNF-β   tumor necrosis factor β
TPA   12-O-tetradecanoylphobol-13-acetate
TRIC   trachoma and inclusion conjunctivitis
tRNA   transfer RNA
Ts   suppressor T-cell
TSTA   tumor-specific transplantation antigen
TXA$_2$ thromboxane A$_2$
Tyr   tyrosine
UDP   uridine diphosphate
UV   ultraviolet
UV-A   ultraviolet band A (320–400 nm)
UV-A1   ultraviolet band A1 (320–340 nm)
UV-A2   ultraviolet band A2 (340–400 nm)
UV-B   ultraviolet band B (290–320 nm)
Val   valine
VCAM-1   vascular cell adhesion molecule 1
VEP   visual evoked potential
VIP   vasoactive intestinal peptide
VKC   vernal keratoconjunctivitis
VKH   Vogt-Koyanagi-Hirada syndrome
VLCFA   very long chain fatty acids
VLDL   very low density lipoprotein
WTV   weak transforming virus
XR   X-linked recessive
xRP   X-linked recessive retinitis pigmentosa

29

Sphingolipidoses and Neuronal Ceroid Lipofuscinosis

Elaine R. Berman

Hadassah-Hebrew University Medical School, Jerusalem, Israel

I. INTRODUCTION

The importance of the sphingolipidoses to the ophthalmologist has long been appreciated, and an early review of this subject by Cogan and Kuwabara [10] is highly recommended not only for its historical perspective but also as a general background for appreciating the enormous advances made in this field during the past 25 years. The disorders in this group are caused by inherited defects—either an absence or malfunction—of a specific lysosomal enzyme, resulting in the accumulation of undegraded substrate within the lysosome (see Chap. 26). In the sphingolipidoses the damaging effects are especially pronounced in the central nervous system (CNS); visceral tissues are secondarily affected only in some of these disorders. Although the individual disorders were initially described as single disease entities, it soon became apparent that without exception they all display considerable heterogeneity in age of onset as well as progression and severity of clinical expression. Over the years these observations led to the establishment of subgroups, usually designated infantile, juvenile, or adult onset. Heterogeneity also became apparent when measuring residual activities of mutant enzymes, which in nearly all cases varied considerably from one patient to the next.

Of the eight groups of inborn errors of sphingolipid metabolism now recognized, all are inherited as autosomal recessive traits with the exception of Fabry's disease, which is an X-linked disorder. Nearly all the sphingolipidoses are associated with grayness or a cherry-red spot at the macula and optic atrophy, whereas corneal clouding is found consistently only in Fabry's disease and in some cases of GM_1 gangliosidosis. The cherry-red spot is due to the deposition of opaque sphingolipids in the ganglion cell layer. This obscures the choroidal vessels everywhere but the macula, where the normal color of the choroidal vessels appears as a cherry-red spot [46]. Tay-Sachs is the most common metabolic disease causing cherry-red spots, but although the basic cause is similar in all sphingolipidoses—accumulation of undegraded sphingolipids—the appearance of the macular lesion and the severity of visual loss varies considerably in the different sphingolipidoses.

Sphingolipids derive their name from sphingosine, an 18-carbon amino alcohol whose structural formula is shown in Figure 1. Although widely distributed in nature, sphingosine is never present in the free state in animal cells: instead, the amino group is substituted in amide linkage to a long-chain fatty acid of 16 carbon atoms or more. This N-acyl fatty acid derivative of sphingosine is called ceramide and is the basic structural unit of all mammalian sphingolipids. The distinguishing feature of the individual members of this group is the moiety esterified to the carbon-1 hydroxyl group of ceramide. In all cases except sphingomyelin, the carbon-1 atom of ceramide is joined in glycosidic linkage to carbohydrates, either simple or complex. As shown in Figure 2, a monosaccharide, glucose or galactose, results in the formation of glucocerebroside or galactocerebroside, respectively. Oligosaccharide substitution, without sialic acid,

SPHINGOSINE

$$\overset{1}{\text{HOCH}_2}-\overset{2}{\text{CH}}-\overset{3}{\text{CH}}-\overset{4}{\text{CH}}=\overset{5}{\text{CH}}-(\text{CH}_2)_{12}\,\text{CH}_3$$
$$\text{NH}\quad\text{OH}$$
$$\text{H}$$

+

FATTY ACID

$$\text{OH}$$
$$\text{C}=\text{O}$$
$$\text{CH}_2$$
$$\text{R}$$

CERAMIDE

[Cer]

$$\text{HOCH}_2-\text{CH}-\text{CH}-\text{CH}=\text{CH}-(\text{CH}_2)_{12}\,\text{CH}_3$$
$$\text{NH}\quad\text{OH}$$
$$\text{C}=\text{O}$$
$$\text{CH}_2$$
$$\text{R}$$

Figure 1 Chemical structures of sphingosine and ceramide. The major fatty acids are palmitate and stearate, containing 16 and 18 carbon atoms, respectively. Small amounts of longer chain fatty acids, saturated or unsaturated, are also present. The overall fatty acid composition varies with the tissue source and the individual sphingolipid.

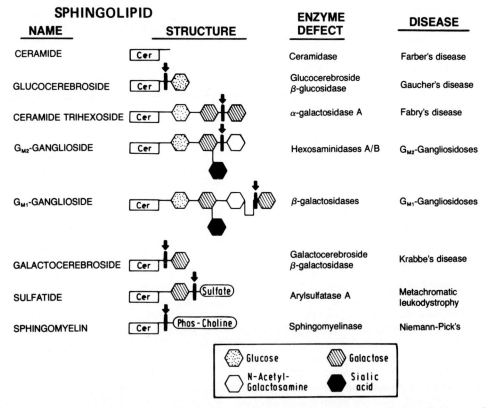

SPHINGOLIPID NAME	ENZYME DEFECT	DISEASE
CERAMIDE	Ceramidase	Farber's disease
GLUCOCEREBROSIDE	Glucocerebroside β-glucosidase	Gaucher's disease
CERAMIDE TRIHEXOSIDE	α-galactosidase A	Fabry's disease
G_{M2}-GANGLIOSIDE	Hexosaminidases A/B	G_{M2}-Gangliosidoses
G_{M1}-GANGLIOSIDE	β-galactosidases	G_{M1}-Gangliosidoses
GALACTOCEREBROSIDE	Galactocerebroside β-galactosidase	Krabbe's disease
SULFATIDE	Arylsulfatase A	Metachromatic leukodystrophy
SPHINGOMYELIN	Sphingomyelinase	Niemann-Pick's

Glucose   Galactose
N-Acetyl-Galactosamine   Sialic acid

Figure 2 Structural formulas of the sphingolipids stored in the eight known groups of sphingolipidoses, with enzyme defects and the location of the metabolic blocks shown for each disorder.

894

results in ceramide di- or trihexosides; if the oligosaccharide contains amino sugars and sialic acid, the sphingolipid is classified as a ganglioside. Substitution of ceramide with galactose-3-sulfate or phosphoryl-choline results in the formation of sulfatides or sphingomyelin, respectively. In recent years, greatly improved analytical techniques have enabled these closely related complex lipids to be isolated and identified in nearly all tissues containing them.

II. SPHINGOLIPIDOSES

A. Farber's Disease

This disorder, originally known as lipogranulomatosis, is inherited as an autosomal recessive trait. It is recognized in infancy by painful and progressively deformed joints, multiple subcutaneous nodules, progressive hoarseness, and nutritional failure. The illness usually leads to death within a few months or years. Of the 40 known cases of Farber's disease, about half are the classic type, with onset in infants ranging in age from 2 weeks to 4 months [64]. The phenotype is now subdivided into six subtypes, and there may be some correlation between the age of onset of subcutaneous nodules and life expectancy. Older patients are more mildly affected, and patients diagnosed as having mild, type 3, Farber's disease survive until 16–18 years of age.

The basic lesion is a granuloma containing variable numbers of foamy histiocytes [64]. Lymph nodes, lung, and visceral tissues contain great excesses of ceramide (Figs. 1 and 2), a substance normally found only in trace amounts in these or other tissues. A marked deficiency of ceramidase, which catalyses the hydrolysis of ceramide to sphingosine and fatty acid, is the basic enzymatic defect in this disorder. The diagnosis can be made by analyzing the activity of this enzyme in tissue biopsies or, more simply, in cultured skin fibroblasts or circulating leukocytes. Deficiency of this enzyme leads to ceramide accumulation in neural, visceral, and subcutaneous tissues. It is thought that ceramide accumulation is responsible for granuloma formation and histiocytic response, since subcutaneous injection of ceramide in rats causes lesions similar to those seen in Farber's disease [64].

Ocular abnormalities have been reported in several patients. An early report of an 8-month-old girl described a diffuse gray opacification with a faint cherry-red center in the macular region, whereas the peripheral retina showed peppery granulations considered essentially normal [12]. Light microscopic examination of postmortem tissue from this patient revealed an accumulation of glycolipid in the retinal ganglion cells. This was confirmed in another patient, and further electron microscopic studies revealed intracellular inclusion bodies of varying morphology and density in retinal ganglion cells, neurons, and glia [100,102]. The accumulated material was extracted and identified by high-pressure liquid chromatography as ceramide [101]. Thus it is reasonable to assume that the ceramidase deficiency in Farber's disease is present in the retina as well as in the other tissues just described.

The grayish opacification of the retina in the foveola with a cherry-red center causes no visual disturbances and is similar to the abnormality seen in metachromatic leukodystrophy [79]. However, the clinical course and enzymatic defects of the two disorders are strikingly different.

B. Gaucher's Disease

Clinical Features. Gaucher's disease is the most common of the lysosomal storage disorders [3]. Three autosomal recessive phenotypes of Gaucher's disease are now recognized: type 1 (chronic non-neuronopathic), type 2 (infantile, acute neuronopathic), and type 3 (juvenile, subacute neuronopathic).

Type 1, the classic or benign adult form, is the most common. Although Gaucher's disease is panethnic, it is especially prevalent among Ashkenazi Jews, in whom the incidence has been estimated as between 1 in 600 and 1 in 2500 [3]; carrier frequency may be as high as 1:50 to 1:70. Its onset can be at any age but is most often during childhood, and clinical progression is usually slow. There is no neurological involvement, and affected individuals may have a normal life span. A slowly progressive splenomegaly with moderate hepatomegaly are caused by deposition of glycolipid in the reticuloendo-thelial system. These early signs may go unrecognized for many years. Bone pain and degenerative changes in the skeleton are a leading cause of discomfort and disability in 50–70% of type 1 patients [24]. Nevertheless, the extent of bone disease is highly variable among patients. Type 2 (acute neuronopathic) Gaucher's disease is a rare disorder characterized by extensive neurovisceral storage. It is rapidly progressive, resulting in death before 2 years of age. Type 3 (subacute neuronopathic) Gaucher's disease is also rare and panethnic. Similar to type 2, it is classified as a neurovisceral storage disorder; patients develop ataxia, myoclonus, seizures, and dementia. Death occurs in early childhood.

Ocular Manifestations.   The cherry-red spots or other fundus abnormalities seen in the macula of so many other disorders of sphingolipid metabolism are not found in Gaucher's disease. Many patients with the type 1 adult form have brown, wedge-shaped conjunctival pingueculae [24,77]. Light and electron microscopy of the conjunctiva has not revealed Gaucher's cells [95]. Other studies report the presence of lipid-laden macrophages in the ciliary body [86] and in the inner layers of the retina [77]. Fundus abnormalities, such as perimacular grayness, have been documented [13], but this is controversial because they appear to be present in only a limited number of cases.

Biochemistry and Molecular Genetics.   Much of the pioneering work several decades ago on the abnormal biochemistry in sphingolipid storage diseases dealt with the pathogenesis of Gaucher's disease. The presence of lipid-laden cells throughout the reticuloendothelial system was noted before the turn of the century. Known as Gaucher's cells, they are 20–100 μm in diameter and are filled with massive deposits of glucocerebroside, which accumulates because of a deficiency of glucocerebrosidase, an enzyme that normally catalyzes the hydrolysis of glucocerebroside to ceramide and glucose (Fig. 2). Electron microscopy of Gaucher's cells shows the cytoplasm filled with distended lysosomes containing tubular structures composed of glucocerebroside strands [3]. They are present throughout the reticuloendothelial system. Gaucher's disease homozygotes can be diagnosed by measuring glucocerebrosidase activity in leukocytes using a variety of natural and synthetic substrates. Detection of heterozygotes is somewhat less certain because of overlapping enzyme activities in heterozygotes and controls. For example, 5–20% of known carriers have enzyme activities in the normal range instead of the expected 50% activity [3]. Moreover, the marked clinical heterogeneity among type 1 patients does not correlate with the levels of residual enzyme activity of individual patients.

Recent studies of the glucocerebrosidase gene and its mutations provided more accurate methods for resolving these problems. The gene for glucocerebrosidase has been cloned and mapped to chromosome 1 (1q21) [3]. A molecular weight of 58,000 for glucocerebrosidase was calculated from the 516 amino acid residues deduced from cDNA sequencing. The structural gene for glucocerebrosidase has at least 11 exons and 10 introns contained within approximately 7 kb, and sequencing of the genomic DNA has provided considerable information on the mutations in type 1 and type 2 Gaucher's disease. Four different point mutations have been described in the glucocerebrosidase gene of Gaucher's patients, two of which are being extensively studied [68]. One, resulting from an A→G transition, occurs at amino acid residue 370 and produces a substitution of serine for asparagine. This is a major mutation in the nonneuronopathic form and accounts for three-quarters of the Gaucher's alleles among patients who are Ashkenazi Jews [68]; the mutation results in the synthesis of an enzyme with abnormal properties including reduced specific activity. The second most common mutation is a T→C transition at amino acid residue 444, resulting in the substitution of proline for leucine. This mutation is found in all three disease types and is located directly at the catalytic site of the enzyme. The third mutation is a G→C transversion that results in the substitution of a proline residue for arginine at amino acid residue 415, and the fourth is a G→A transition that substitutes glycine for arginine at amino acid residue 120. A newly developed chain reaction technique has been used to amplify the portion of the glucocerebrosidase gene containing the first three mutations [25]. The results obtained from examining 27 Gaucher's cell lines indicate the feasibility of using this method for distinguishing between homozygous patients, carriers, and normal genotypes. Using a similar technique, several mutant alleles were found in uncharacterized Gaucher's disease patients.

The availability of both cDNA and genomic DNA for human glucocerebrosidase raises the possibility of somatic cell gene therapy for patients with Gaucher's disease [3]. This disorder is considered an important candidate for human gene transfer because the phenotypic cellular defect is manifested only in cells of macrophage lineage. The observations that both type 1 and type 2 Gaucher's fibroblasts transfected with a human-mouse cDNA chimeric retroviral vector in vitro expressed active glucocerebrosidase activity are highly encouraging [3]. Nevertheless, even though some cell lines expressed this enzyme for as long as 24 months after retrovirally mediated gene transfer, long-term expression in whole animals is still uncertain.

C. Fabry's Disease

Clinical Features. Fabry's disease was first described at the turn of the century as a dermatological entity because of the cutaneous vascular lesions (angiokeratoma corporis diffusum). Other major clinical signs associated with this X-linked disorder include burning pains in the extremities, fever, and renal dysfunction, most of them developing in childhood or early adolescence. Angiokeratomas, the characteristic skin lesions in Fabry's disease, appear early in life. They develop slowly as clusters of individual punctate spots, dark red to blue-black in color, in the superficial layers of the skin [15]. With increasing age, burning pains throughout the body become more frequent and severe, and there is a progressively increased deposition of glycosphingolipids throughout the vascular system. Death of affected hemizygous males usually occurs during the third or fourth decade of life as a result of renal failure or cardiac disease. The disorder is panethnic, and over 400 cases have been reported, most of them occurring in whites.

A characteristic feature of this disorder is the massive accumulation of ceramide trihexoside and related neutral glycosphingolipids with terminal α-galactosyl moieties throughout the cardiovascular and renal systems [19]. These sphingolipids are deposited in the endothelial and epithelial cells of the renal glomerulus, in the endothelial and smooth muscle cells of blood vessels, in most viscera, and in many ocular tissues, including the corneal epithelium and lens. Fabry's disease is one of the few inborn errors of metabolism in which alleviation of some of the symptoms by enzyme replacement therapy has been attempted [16]. Multiple injections over a period of 4 months of purified splenic and plasma forms of α-galactosidase into two brothers with Fabry's disease resulted in a dramatic, albeit transient, lowering of the levels of blood glycosphingolipids; however, the long-term benefits of such therapy are still uncertain.

Ocular Manifestations. The ocular signs in Fabry's disease are well known and consist of a keratopathy and star-shaped opacities in the posterior region of the lens. Storage of ceramide trihexoside in the blood vessels of the retina and conjunctiva presumably causes the tortuosity, dilatations, and aneurysms found in this disease [63,87]. Vision is usually not impaired, but one case report described a 16-year-old boy with Fabry's disease who suffered sudden visual loss secondary to a central retinal artery occlusion [88]. The corneal changes, designated cornea verticillata, are especially striking and occur in virtually all affected males [87]. As seen ophthalmoscopically, the lesion is localized in the epithelial or subepithelial layers and resembles a series of spokes radiating from a central hub. Heterozygous females may be either asymptomatic or, in some cases, have some of the clinical manifestations in attenuated form; skin lesions and corneal opacities are the most common sign in some, but not all, of such carriers. Whorllike corneal deposits were observed in 22 of the 25 heterozygotes studied by Sher and coworkers [87], and in many cases these depositions were found to be more severe in carriers than in affected hemizygous males. It has been suggested that the unusual corneal dystrophic pattern results from the formation of a series of subepithelial ridges or possibly from duplication of the basement membrane [26].

Electron microscopic studies have shown numerous lamellar osmiophilic deposits in the basal cells of the corneal epithelium, which probably represent ceramide trihexoside deposits (Fig. 3). Ultrastructural changes are not confined to this tissue, however, but are also present in the lens epithelium, iris pigment epithelium, smooth muscle cells of the choroidal arterioles, and the endothelial cells and pericytes of all ocular blood vessels [26]. Dense osmiophilic inclusion bodies are present in stromal fibrocytes, in the endothelial cells of the blood capillaries, and in the epithelial cells of the conjunctiva.

Studies of conjunctival ultrastructure provide an important tool in the diagnosis of Fabry's disease, lamellar inclusions similar to those found in the cornea being present in more than 70% of the conjunctival cells of hemizygotes beyond the age of 7 years [59]. The conjunctival abnormalities frequently precede both the corneal changes and the systemic clinical signs, and hence biopsy of this tissue provides a convenient and reliable procedure for the early diagnosis of Fabry's disease.

Biochemistry and Molecular Genetics. Fabry's disease is caused by a deficiency of the lysosomal enzyme α-galactosidase (Fig. 2). This enzyme is one of a family of exoglycosidases that effect the sequential breakdown of glycosphingolipids throughout the body. In some Fabry's hemizygotes, there is no detectable enzyme activity in blood or tissues; in others the activity of α-galactosidase is about 10–25% of that found in similar sources from normal individuals. Recent studies of the kinetic properties of α-galactosidase and its differential activity toward synthetic and natural substrates have shown that the breakdown of glycosphingolipids and gangliosides is mediated by nonenzymatic lysosomal proteins called sphingolipid activator proteins [15] or saposins [68]. Four such proteins have been cloned and sequenced,

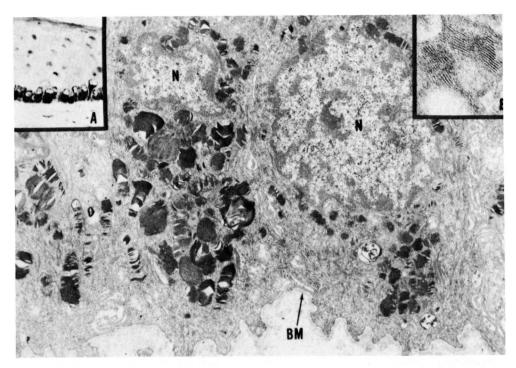

Figure 3   Lamellar inclusion bodies accumulating in the basal cells of the corneal epithelium in Fabry's disease. N, nuclei; BM, basal membrane. (×7000) Inset A: the same region of the epithelium at lower magnification. (×275) Dense staining with Sudan black B and oil red O is observed mainly in the basal cells and rarely in the superficial cells. Inset B: the lamellar deposits at high magnification. (×80,000) (Reproduced with permission from R.L. Font and B.S. Fine. Ocular pathology in Fabry's disease: Histochemical and electron microscopic observations. *Am. J. Ophthalmol. 73*:419–430, 1972.)

and the possibility that one of them, designated SAP-1 [15], may play a role in the pathogenesis of some forms of Fabry's disease is now under investigation.

A clinical diagnosis of hemizygotes and heterozygotes can be confirmed by examining the activity of α-galactosidase in plasma or leukocytes. Since the biochemical defect is also expressed in lacrimal fluid, tears offer the most convenient tissue source for analysis (see Chap. 26). Heterozygous females usually have about half the activity of unaffected individuals. However, more accurate methods of detection based on analyses of gene structure are now available.

Somatic cell and in situ hybridization studies have localized the α-galactosidase gene to a region on the long arm of the X chromosome, specifically at the Xq22.33 locus [15,45]. Both the full-length cDNA and genomic sequences coding this lysosomal enzyme have been isolated and characterized. The gene is approximately 12 kb and contains seven exons. Biochemical studies of the defective α-galactosidase enzyme in Fabry's hemizygotes suggest three major categories of enzyme deficiency [15]:

1. Patients with no detectable enzyme activity and no immunologically reactive enzyme protein. The mutations in this group include partial or complete gene deletions, as well as partial gene duplications, point mutations that alter transcription or mRNA processing, and point mutations that lead to defective enzyme conformation.
2. Patients with no detectable enzyme deficiency but with essentially normal levels of immunologically reactive enzyme protein. The genetic lesions in this group are mainly point mutations that lead to the synthesis of a kinetically defective enzyme.
3. Atypical hemizygotes with some residual enzyme activity. The lesions in these patients consist of exonic point mutations that alter either kinetic or stability properties of the enzyme; nevertheless,

the enzyme retains sufficient catalytic activity to hydrolyze, albeit to a limited extent, synthetic substrates as well as glycosphingolipids.

A number of point mutations have been characterized in Fabry's hemizygotes [15,68]. These include two amino acid substitutions; one is at amino acid residue 356 in which tryptophan is replaced for arginine, and the other at amino acid residue 301 in which glycine replaces arginine. Southern hybridization studies on DNA isolated from over 120 Fabry's cell lines resulted in the detection of six gene rearrangements consisting of five partial gene deletions and one partial duplication. Cell lines from other affected hemizygotes show alterations in restriction endonuclease cleavage sites, and several patients had transcript abnormalities. Another cDNA for α-galactosidase has been isolated in Nova Scotia and used as a probe for identifying Fabry's carriers in a large kindred living in this area [45]. In this case, the major mutation in several carriers, as well as in some affected hemizygotes, was in the allele of the polymorphic NcoI site located 3′ to the gene. Thus, as in other inherited disorders, the wide variety of molecular lesions at the genetic level finds its expression in the clinical variability of the disorder. Fabry's disease results from a heterogeneous group of mutations that affect the synthesis, processing, or stability of α-galactosidase.

D. GM$_2$ Gangliosidoses

This group of heritable disorders is characterized by excessive deposition of GM$_2$ ganglioside (and a few related glycolipids) in neuronal cells. The accumulation of this sphingolipid is the consequence of defects in two lysosomal isoenzymes, hexosaminidase A and B (Fig. 4). In addition, recent investigations showed that the same clinical picture can be caused by an inherited defect in a nonenzymatic lysosomal protein called GM$_2$ activator. As a result of extensive investigations during the past decade, three nonallelic enzymic variants of GM$_2$ gangliosidosis are now recognized [68,83]: (1) Tay-Sach disease (variant B, hexosaminidase α-subunit deficiency); (2) Sandhoff's disease (variant O, hexosaminidase β-subunit deficiency), and (3) GM$_2$ activator deficiency (variant AB). Some but not all of these disorders are heterogeneous in age of onset as well as in severity and progression of the clinical symptoms. Thus the three major subtypes of GM$_2$ gangliosidosis are further classified according to age of onset into infantile, late infantile, juvenile, and adult cases. For the ophthalmologist, both Tay-Sachs and Sandhoff's disease are

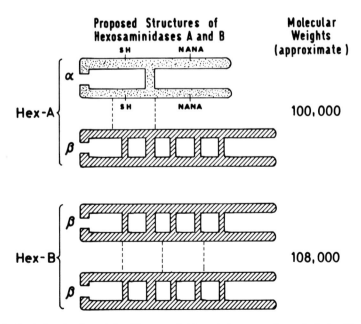

Figure 4 Hypothetical structural models of hexosaminidase A (one α and one β chain, Hex-A) and hexosaminidase B (two β chains, Hex-B). Cross-linking is probably by S-S linkage. The α chains contain sulfhydryl groups (SH) and sialic acid (NANA, N-acetylneuraminic acid).

associated with cherry-red spots in the macula [46], but their presence in the GM_2 activator disorder is uncertain owing to the limited number of cases examined [83].

Tay-Sachs Disease (Hexosaminidase α-Subunit Deficiency, Variant B)

This prototype of storage disorders is probably the best known and most extensively studied of any in this group. It provides a classic example of the sequential elucidation of a genetic disease, beginning with the earliest clinical description and progressing to the chromosomal mapping of the defective gene and elucidation of multiple mutations at the hexosaminidase locus.

Clinical Features.   The phenotype of this disorder was described independently, before the turn of the century by a British ophthalmologist, Tay [92], and an American neurologist, Sachs [81]. Onset is before the age of 6 months and is recognized by retarded development, hypotonia, general apathy, and an exaggerated response to sharp sounds that causes rapid extension of both arms and a startled facial expression (the "startle reaction"). Ophthalmoscopic examination at this time reveals pale optic disks and cherry-red spots at both maculae. Progressive neurological deterioration ensues until death in the second or third year of life.

A remarkable predilection for children of Ashkenazi (eastern European) Jewish ancestry has been noted from the earliest description. We now know that the carrier frequency in this ethnic group is 1 in 30, the highest of any known inborn error of metabolism [83]. This estimate is based on the results of several large-scale screening programs carried out during the last two decades, after discovery of the basic enzymatic defect in hexosaminidase A [73]. With accurate methods for detecting heterozygotes, genetic counseling, and prenatal monitoring, the birth of affected Tay-Sachs phenotypes has been reduced dramatically.

Postmortem studies reveal a diffuse atrophy of the brain, with cerebral cortical and other neurons in the CNS filled with material reacting to some, but not all, lipid stains. The retinal ganglion cell layer is affected similarly.

Ocular Pathology.   The macular cherry-red spot is the hallmark of both Tay-Sachs and Sandhoff's disease; it usually appears by 6 months of age. Optic atrophy is invariably present by the second year. Ganglion cells of the retina are filled with concentric or parallel lamellar whorls representing undegraded lipid material (Fig. 5). These are undoubtedly gangliosides, which in the normal eye are present in only trace amounts [8], but in most, if not all, of the gangliosidoses their accumulation in ganglion cell layer is appreciable. Since these abnormal inclusion bodies are usually surrounded by a single limiting membrane and are acid phosphatase positive, they are of lysosomal origin [94]. They are almost indistinguishable from the multilamellar cytoplasmic bodies in cerebral ganglion cells of Tay-Sachs patients.

Biochemistry and Molecular Genetics.   The accumulation of gangliosides in the cerebral cortex of patients with Tay-Sachs disease in amounts 10 times greater than normal was noted by Klenk [47] in Germany more than five decades ago. Dramatic advances in lipid chemistry and technology led subsequently to the isolation and identification of a family of gangliosides, distinguishable from one another by minor chemical and structural differences. Only one of the gangliosides in this group accumulates in Tay-Sachs disease, the GM_2 type (Fig. 2).

The breakthrough in our understanding of the pathogenesis of Tay-Sachs disease came with the observation by Okada and O'Brien [73] that two isoenzymes of hexosaminidase, designated A and B, are present in normal human tissues and can be separated by starch gel electrophoresis. One of them, the A component, was absent in extracts of tissues from patients with Tay-Sachs disease.

This observation opened two decades of research that has led not only to the elucidation of the molecular pathology of Tay-Sachs disease but also to an understanding of a closely related disorder, Sandhoff's disease, in which there is a deficiency of both the heat-labile isoenzyme, hexosaminidase A, and the heat-stable form, hexosaminidase B [28]. The hexosaminidase isoenzymes act in vivo by hydrolyzing the terminal N-acetylgalactosaminyl residues from GM_2 gangliosides (Fig. 2). Their absence is consistent with the accumulation of this specific ganglioside, as well as its asialo derivative, in neural tissues of Tay-Sachs disease.

Although gangliosides do not accumulate outside the CNS in Tay-Sachs disease, the enzymatic defect is expressed in all tissues of the body, as well as in serum. Hexosaminidase activity can be easily assayed in serum, leukocytes, fibroblasts, and tears using a variety of synthetic substrates [35]. Whereas Tay-Sachs patients have virtually undetectable activity, heterozygotes display about 50% of the activity of normal

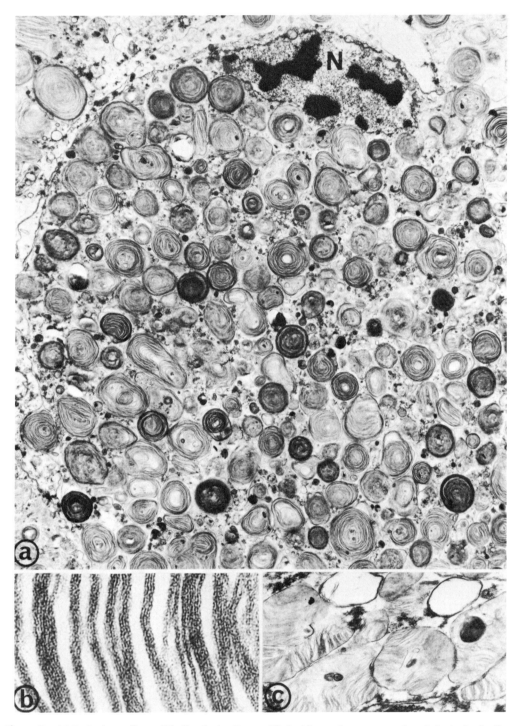

Figure 5   (a) Retinal ganglion cell in Tay-Sachs disease filled with membranous cytoplasmic inclusion bodies. The accumulation of round or oval-shaped lamellar bodies has caused displacement of the nucleus peripherally. (×8850) (b) Membranous lamellae at higher magnification. (×174,000) (c) Cytoplasmic lamellar inclusions in the inner nuclear layer of the retina in Tay-Sachs disease. (×23,000) (Reproduced with permission from R.C. Tripathi and N. Ashton. Application of electron microscopy to the study of ocular inborn errors of metabolism. *Birth Defects* 12(3):69–104, 1976.)

individuals. These findings led to the development of simple and inexpensive screening programs for many populations, especially those at greatest risk, the Jewish communities. A recently improved method utilizes a centrifugal analyzer for automation of enzyme assays in screening programs of Jewish populations in England [51]. Thus genetic counseling combined with prenatal diagnosis, amniocentesis for detecting affected fetuses, and termination of pregnancy when necessary have reduced the incidence of Tay-Sachs disease by 90% [83].

The molecular defects in the GM_2 gangliosidoses are complex because a three-loci, three-polypeptide system is required to degrade this ganglioside [61,67,83]. A mutation at the α-chain locus gives rise to a deficiency of hexosaminidase A, but at the β-chain locus this causes deficiencies of both hexosaminidase A and B. A deficiency at the activator locus gives rise to a deficiency in activator protein.

The primary defect in Tay-Sachs disease is mutation of the α-chain gene, which is encoded in chromosome 15 [31]; this results in the synthesis of an inactive, immunologically undetectable hexosaminidase A enzyme. The disease is very heterogeneous at the molecular level, at least 13 known allelic mutations having been described to date [61,67,68]. As shown by analyses of DNA in Tay-Sachs carriers [36,67,68,75], 2 of these mutations have a high frequency in the Ashkenazi Jewish population. One is a four-nucleotide insertion in exon 11 that causes premature termination and unstable mRNA. This mutation accounts for about 70% of the Tay-Sachs alleles in the American Jewish population. Another mutation in the splice site of intron 12 has been found in another 20% of this population group. Thus, 2 mutations, for brevity termed the insertion and the splice, account for about 90% of the mutations in Ashkenazi Jewish carriers in the United States and England [52]. Another large Jewish population originating from Morocco also has a high carrier frequency for Tay-Sachs disease, estimated at about 1 in 60 [65]. However, the molecular defects in the two subpopulations are different. The mutation found in a Moroccan Jewish patient was an in-frame phenylalanine codon deletion in the α-subunit chain of hexosaminidase A. This mutation impairs the folding and assembly of the α-subunit. A rare enzymatic variant of Tay-Sachs disease, called "B_1" or chronic GM_2 gangliosidosis [68], was shown to have an arginine-to-cystine mutation at amino acid residue 504 together with a glycine-to-serine mutation at amino acid residue 269 [76]; this caused the secretion of the α-subunit of hexosaminidase A as an enzymatically inactive α-monomer instead of the normal $\alpha\alpha$-dimer.

Sandhoff's Disease (Hexosaminidase β-Subunit Deficiency, Variant O)

Clinical Features. First described as "an exceptional case of Tay-Sachs disease" [82], the clinical course and ocular manifestations of Sandhoff's disease are nearly indistinguishable from those of classic Tay-Sachs disease. However, this disorder occurs mainly, if not entirely, in non-Jewish families, and, visceral involvement, particularly in the kidney, is a prominent feature.

Sandhoff's disease is characterized biochemically by the neuronal and visceral deposition of GM_2 ganglioside (Fig. 2) and its asialo derivative, as well as GM_2 globoside, a sphingolipid composed of ceramide-glucose-galactose-galactose-N-acetylgalactosamine [71,83]. This globoside is a normal constituent, albeit in trace amounts, of erythrocytes and other nonneural tissues. It does not accumulate in tissues of Tay-Sachs disease, but in Sandhoff's disease it is found at levels 15 times higher than normal, especially in the kidney. The enzymatic defect in Sandhoff's disease it is found at levels 15 times higher than normal, especially in the kidney. The enzymatic defect in Sandhoff's disease is the absence of both the A and B isoenzymes of hexosaminidase (Fig. 4). The structural relationship of these enzymes to one another, and the role of each in the pathogenesis of two different genetic disorders having the same phenotypic expression, is best appreciated at the molecular level, as described here.

Ocular Manifestations. As in Tay-Sachs disease, a cherry-red spot in the macula is one of the most distinguishing features of this disorder. Electron microscopic studies have revealed somewhat different abnormalities, however. For example, the membranous bodies in the retina are not completely identical in the two disorders. In Tay-Sachs disease (Fig. 5), the lamellae are mainly concentric, and the particles, which are fairly homogeneous in size, are round or oval. In Sandhoff's disease (Fig. 6), the deposits are more pleomorphic and often confluent [27].

Biochemistry and Molecular Genetics. Patients with a defect or absence of the β-subunit of hexosaminidase, encoded on chromosome 5 [31], lack activity of both major hexosaminidase isoenzymes, A and B [83]. This explains why globosides and oligosaccharides, in addition to GM_2 ganglioside, accumulate in visceral and neural tissues, respectively, of Sandhoff patients.

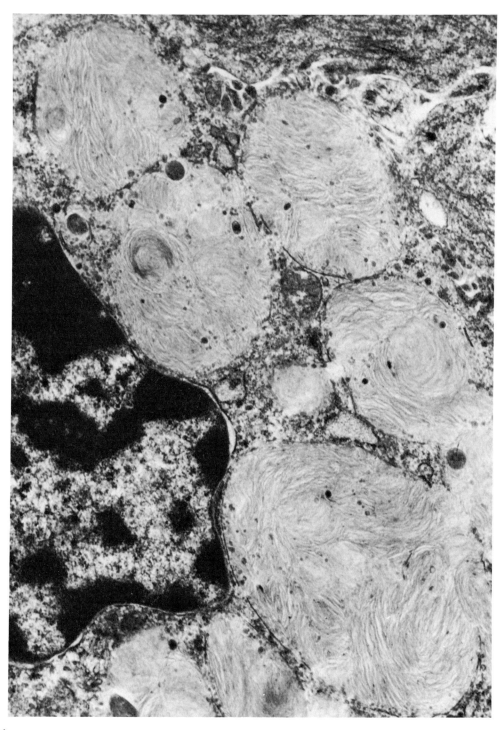

Figure 6   Retinal ganglion cell in Sandhoff's disease filled with pleomorphic membranous cytoplasmic bodies varying in size from 0.5 to 6 μm in diameter. Some of the smaller bodies appear to be fused. (×29,000) (Reproduced with permission from A. Garner. Ocular pathology of GM_2-gangliosidosis-type 2 (Sandhoff's disease). *Br. J. Ophthalmol. 57*:514–520, 1973.)

Similar to the mutations of the α-subunit, those of the β-subunit are a heterogeneous group. To date, however, only four mutations have been characterized in the hexosaminidase B gene [61,68]. One of the more common mutations is a 16 kb deletion of exons 1–5 that precludes the production of hexosaminidase B mRNA. This was found at relatively high frequency (8 of 30) among Sandhoff alleles. Two others involve a G→A transition at intron 12 and duplication of a sequence located between intron 13 and exon 14. These mutations were found in milder (juvenile) forms of Sandhoff's disease.

GM$_2$ Activator Deficiency (Variant AB)

A severe deficiency of lysosomal activator protein results in the accumulation of GM$_2$ gangliosides exactly as in α- or β-subunit deficiency disorders [83]. Accordingly, the clinical signs, in the few cases studied, are identical to Tay-Sachs and Sandhoff's diseases.

The GM$_2$ activator is a small acid 24 kD lysosomal protein [83]. It specifically promotes the hydrolysis of GM$_2$ ganglioside by hexosaminidase isoenzymes, probably by forming 1:1 water-soluble complexes with ganglioside substrate. The activator functions primarily as a cosubstrate with the ganglioside but does not really "activate" it. This protein has recently been purified and its mechanism of action studied intensively. The gene for GM$_2$ activator protein has been mapped to chromosome 5 in the human genome. This variant of GM$_2$ gangliosidosis is rare, with only five known cases described. Recently, the cDNA encoding the GM$_2$ activator protein has been cloned, but there are as yet no data on mutation analyses [68].

E. GM$_1$ Gangliosidoses

Clinical Features. The infantile form of GM$_1$ gangliosidosis (type 1) manifests itself from birth onward; the clinical features combine neurological and skeletal abnormalities [72]. Among the former are progressive psychomotor retardation, frequent convulsions, and ultimate decerebrate rigidity. Features resembling certain mucopolysaccharidoses, such as mucopolysaccharidosis type 1-H (Hurler), include coarse facial features with frontal bossing and depressed nasal ridge, hepatosplenomegaly, and other features of dysostosis multiplex. This disease is invariably fatal by the second year of life.

Juvenile GM$_1$ gangliosidosis (type 2) has a later onset, slower progression, and milder bony abnormalities and fewer severe neurological and psychomotor changes than the infantile GM$_1$ gangliosidosis type 1 [70]. Visceromegaly is absent, but subtle skeletal abnormalities can be detected by careful roentgenographic examination. Slow neurological deterioration leads to death during the first decade.

Adult GM$_1$ gangliosidosis has been recognized as a clinical entity only during the past 5 years owing to an increased number of cases diagnosed in adult neurology clinics [72]. Clinical signs include gait disturbance, dysarthria, and a slowly progressive dystonia affecting the face and limbs. There is little intellectual or visual impairment.

Ocular Manifestations. Ocular changes in the GM$_1$ gangliosidoses are varied and are not present in all cases. Thus, mild corneal clouding has been noted in two cases [1,17], and esotropia and nystagmus are occasionally observed. Cherry-red spots in a creamy white macula occur in about 50% of infantile type 1 cases but have not been observed in either the juvenile or adult form [72]. Optic atrophy has been reported in one case of juvenile GM$_1$ gangliosidosis [32], and retinal hemorrhages have been reported occasionally. Blindness occurs early in the infantile form and late in the juvenile form. There may be mild corneal clouding in some cases. The neuronal involvement has its counterpart in the retinal ganglion cells, which are filled with membranous cytoplasmic bodies [17]. These laminated bodies, composed of thin concentric and/or parallel lamellae, are surrounded by single membranes, and represent aggregates of undegraded ganglioside accumulated within the lysosomes (Figs. 7 and 8). The corneal epithelial cells and the corneal fibroblasts, however, contain single-membrane–bound vesicles filled with finely granular material that probably represents undegraded oligosaccharides or glycosaminoglycans.

Biochemistry and Molecular Genetics. The primary storage substance throughout the nervous system is GM$_1$ ganglioside; chemical analyses show that it has the same sugar and fatty acid composition as that found in normal tissue (Fig. 2). The quantity formed in the infantile form is massive, and it is deposited throughout the body. Only moderate amounts of stored ganglioside are found in the juvenile form; if present in the adult forms, it is localized to specific neural tissues, such as cortex and white matter in the brain [72]. Appreciable amounts of galactose-containing oligosaccharides are also stored in these

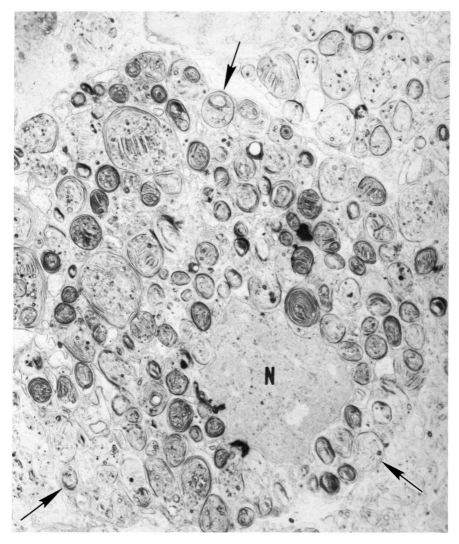

Figure 7   Retinal ganglion cell in GM_1 gangliosidosis type 2 contains scattered storage vesicles surrounded by single membranes (arrows). Some of the cytosomes have prominent lamellar membranes; others have vesicles only. ($\times$12,000) (Reproduced with permission from H.H. Goebel, J.D. Fix, and W. Zeman. Retinal pathology in GM_1-gangliosidosis, type II. *Am. J. Ophthalmol.* 75:434–441, 1973.)

disorders; they are found exclusively in visceral tissues and accumulate as a result of incomplete degradation of cellular glycoproteins. Excess oligosaccharides are also excreted in the urine, where the amounts generally correlate with the severity of the disease [72]. Because there are both neurological and visceral involvements, with storage of lipids and complex carbohydrates, respectively, this disorder may in fact be classified among the mucolipidoses [44].

The enzymatic defect in the GM_1 gangliosidoses is a nearly complete absence of lysosomal acid β-galactosidase activity [71,72]. This enzyme hydrolyzes the nonreducing terminal galactose from a variety of substrates, including GM_1 ganglioside, asialo ganglioside, galactose-containing oligosaccharides, and keratan sulfate. Diagnosis of GM_1 gangliosidosis can be made by measuring the activity of this enzyme in leukocytes, cultured skin fibroblasts, and amnionic cells.

Structural studies of this enzyme in normal tissues have given considerable insight into the nature

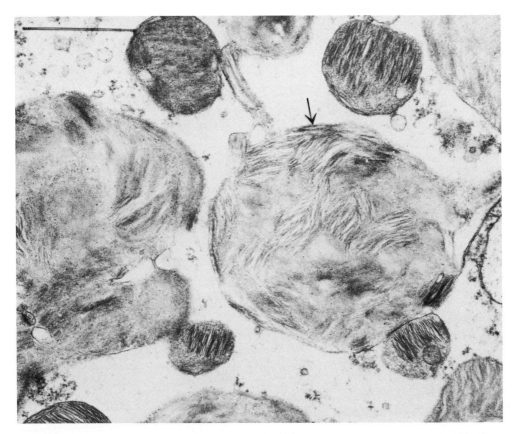

Figure 8 Membranous cytoplasmic bodies (arrow) in the ganglion cell layer of the retina in GM_1 gangliosidosis, type 2. The abnormal storage bodies contain lamellar membranes embedded in an amorphous matrix.
($\times 31,000$) (Reproduced by courtesy of Dr. H.H. Goebel.)

of the defect in GM_1 gangliosidosis. This lysosomal enzyme is synthesized as an 88 kD precursor coded
by a structural locus on chromosome 3 [72]. Processing in the endoplasmic reticulum and maturation in the
Golgi apparatus (see Chap. 28) result in the production of the mature 64 kD monomeric form of acid
β-galactosidase. Normally this monomer aggregates to a large 700 kD polymer, a step mediated by a 32 kD
protein coded by a separate locus on chromosome 22. This association is thought to protect the enzyme
from intralysosomal proteolytic degradation. All 16 GM_1 gangliosidosis patients studied produced normal
quantities of immunoreactive acid β-galactosidase, but when tested on either synthetic or naturally
occurring substrates, it showed little or no activity [72]. An absence of 32 kD protective protein has been
noted in some cases of GM_1 gangliosidosis, which may explain its lack of catalytic activity.

Recently, cDNA clones coding the human acid β-galactosidase were used as probes for examining
genetic abnormalities in 12 Japanese patients with various forms of GM_1 gangliosidosis [69]. Four distinct
mutations were found, all of them causing inactivation of the catalytic site of the enzyme. In 1 patient
with the infantile form, a point mutation at amino acid residue 49 resulted in the substitution of cystine for
arginine, and in another, a mutation was found in residue 457, resulting in a substitution of threonine for
arginine; 4 juvenile patients had point mutations at amino acid residue 201, resulting in substitution of
cystine for arginine, and 6 adult patients were homozygous for a point mutation at residue 51, resulting in
isoleucine-threonine substitution. These and other studies in Japan showed no crossover between the
identified mutations and the three clinical phenotypes, suggesting that, for the first time, clinical subtypes
may be identified using this cDNA clone.

F. Krabbe's Disease

Clinical Features.   Also known as globoid cell leukodystrophy, this severe neurodegenerative disorder has its onset before 6 months of age. Spasticity, generalized weakness, and progressive psychomotor degeneration are found in all cases; the disorder is rapidly progressive, leading to death by the second year. Although the infantile form was the first type recognized, juvenile and late-onset or adult forms are also known [2,91]. The presence of multinucleated globoid cells in the white matter provides a morphological basis for diagnosing this disorder. The cerebral atrophy that characterizes Krabbe's disease is a consequence of complete demyelination of cerebral white matter.

Optic atrophy [40] and sluggish pupillary reactions are found in virtually all cases [22,91]. Blindness occurs early in the disorder and may precede the loss of pupillary reflexes. Electron microscopic examination of an autopsy specimen from a case of infantile Krabbe's disease revealed characteristic tubular inclusions and globoid cells in the extensively demyelinated optic nerve (Fig. 9) [9,18].

Biochemistry.   The enzymatic defect in Krabbe's disease is a generalized deficiency of lysosomal galactocerebroside β-galactosidase (Fig. 2). Not only neural tissues but also others, such as liver, spleen, kidney, leukocytes, and cultured fibroblasts, show a similar defect in this enzyme. The last two are convenient sources of tissue for diagnosis of both affected individuals and carriers. It should be noted that two human lysosomal storage disorders are caused by deficiencies in lysosomal β-galactosidases. They can be distinguished on the basis of substrate specificity: in GM_1 gangliosidosis, the enzyme is inactive toward ganglioside substrate, whereas in Krabbe's disease, the enzyme is inactive toward galactocerebroside. In the latter case, there is a failure to degrade galactocerebroside to ceramide and galactose. It is thought that the accumulation of another closely related glycolipid, psychosine, which is also a substrate for the defective enzyme, is the principal cause for destruction of oligodendroglia [91].

The gene for galactocerebroside β-galactosidase has not yet been isolated and cloned because the enzyme is not sufficiently pure either for amino acid sequencing or for production of monospecific antibodies. Hence the location on the chromosome of the gene is not known. To circumvent this problem, genetic linkage analysis has been used to study polymorphic DNA probes in a large number of Krabbe's patients and their families [103]. These studies localized the mutant allele to chromosome 14.

G.   Metachromatic Leukodystrophy

Clinical Features.   Several phenotypes of metachromatic leukodystrophy (MLD) are now recognized, the most severe type having its onset during the second year of life [48]. Demyelination and accumulation of metachromatic sulfatides (cerebroside sulfate) in the white matter of the CNS, peripheral nerves, and certain viscera, including the liver, gallbladder, and kidney, are characteristic of most forms. Juvenile forms presenting between ages 4 and 12, as well as adult forms, have also been described. In most cases the earliest signs are gait disturbances and mental regression; weakness, loss of speech, mental confusion, and other neurological signs are also present to varying degrees in all forms of MLD. Seven disorders, classified according to age of onset and biochemical defect, are now thought to comprise the MLD family [48]. Five of the forms are called MLD, and they are classified only according to age of onset. Two additional types have been delineated rather recently and are named according to the biochemical defect: one is multiple sulfatase deficiency, and the other is cerebroside sulfate sulfatase activator deficiency.

Ocular Manifestations.   Many of the ocular features of MLD are similar to those found in multiple sulfatase deficiency [23]. Optic atrophy resulting from retrograde degeneration has been reported in a case of adult-onset MLD [79]. This may occur late in the disease. Abnormal foveal grayness has also been reported in some cases of the late infantile type [11], but cherry-red spots are not a common feature of MLD [5,46]. Histopathological and ultrastructural studies of the adult form have shown an extensive loss of ganglion cells, but the rest of the retina is normal [79]. Demyelination of the optic nerve and concomitant accumulation of abnormal neuroglia containing dense membrane-limited inclusion bodies are the most striking findings (Fig. 10). Quigley and Green [79] suggested that the abnormalities in sulfatide metabolism leading to the degeneration of optic nerve myelin also cause retrograde ganglion cell degeneration, an hypothesis supported by the finding of relatively large amounts of metachromatic material (cerebroside sulfate) in the optic nerve compared with the retina. Electron microscopic examination of conjunctival biopsies from several forms of MLD revealed osmiophilic inclusion bodies containing fibrillogranular

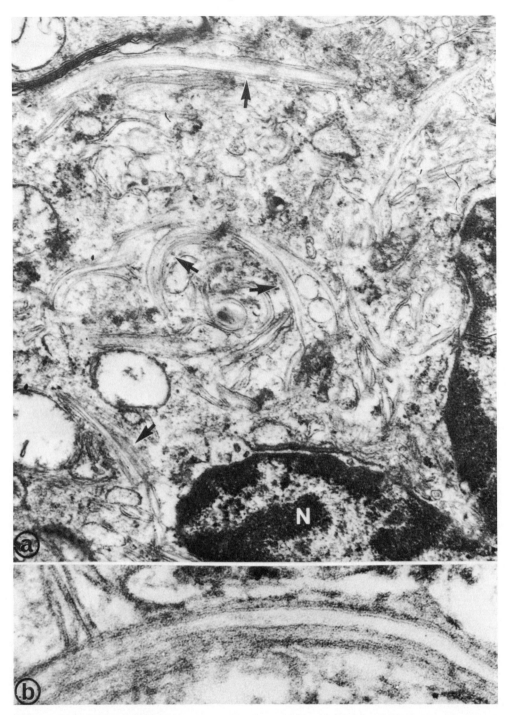

Figure 9   (a) Optic nerve in Krabbe's disease, showing extensive demyelination. Globoid cells with indented nuclei (N) contain straight or gently curved paracrystalline filaments (arrows) similar to the helical tubules accumulating in neural tissue of Krabbe's disease. (×40,000) (b) The lamellar structure of the tubules at higher magnification. (×172,000) (Reproduced with permission from R.C. Tripathi and N. Ashton. Applications of electron microscopy to the study of ocular inborn errors of metabolism. *Birth Defects 12*(3):69–104, 1976.)

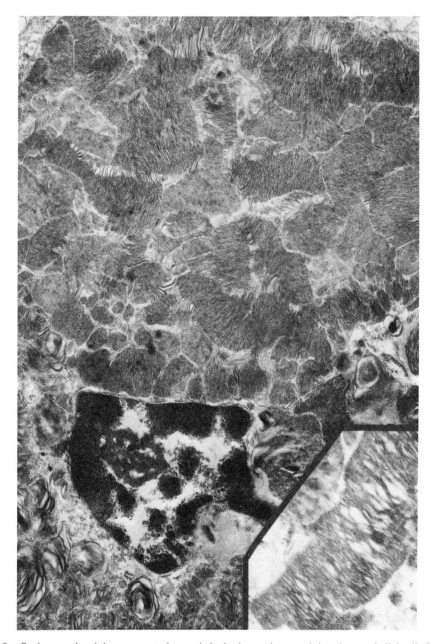

Figure 10   Optic nerve in adult-onset metachromatic leukodystrophy containing abnormal glial cells filled with single-membrane–limited lamellar inclusion bodies. The cells are larger than normal glia and are devoid of cellular processes. (×17,200) Inset: lamellar inclusion body at higher magnification. (×47,800) (Reproduced with permission from H.A. Quigley and W.R. Green. Clinical and ultrastructural ocular histopathological studies of adult-onset metachromatic leukodystrophy. *Am. J. Ophthalmol. 82*:472–479, 1975.)

material similar to that found in most mucopolysaccharidoses [60]. Pigmentary retinal degeneration also appears to be associated with some cases of arylsulfatase A deficiency [97].

Biochemistry and Molecular Genetics. Although long known to be caused by a deficiency of arylsulfatase A (Fig. 2), the precise biochemical abnormalities have been difficult to establish because of anomalous kinetic behavior displayed by both the normal and the mutant forms of the enzyme. However, it is now established that the functional impairment of arylsulfatase A, the heat-labile component of cerebroside sulfatase, is the primary enzymatic abnormality in the late infantile, juvenile, and adult forms of MLD [48]. There is a generalized deficiency of this enzyme in kidney, liver, brain, leukocytes, cultured skin fibroblasts, cultured bone marrow cells, and body fluids, such as serum and tears. Some residual activity can often be detected, however, especially in the adult form of MLD. Patients with multiple sulfatase deficiency have, in addition to arylsulfatase A deficiency, defects in other sulfatases (steroid sulfatase and mucopolysaccharide sulfatases). In this case, a defect in the posttranslational glycosylation of multiple sulfatases leads to the production of unstable inactive enzymes [48]. Another form of MLD is caused by a deficiency of an activator protein, saposin B, that is essential for the hydrolysis of cerebroside sulfate in cultured skin fibroblasts.

Although most MLD patients can be diagnosed by enzyme analyses using either leukocytes or cultured skin fibroblasts, a phenomenon termed pseudodeficiency is frequently encountered. Many individuals have only 20–30% of normal activity yet do not develop clinical signs of MLD. The enzyme in such cases has a structural alteration affecting the glycosylation site [48,68]; as a result, only one of two possible sites is glycosylated. This affects the catalytic function of the enzyme to the extent that only 20–30% of normal activity is expressed; however, this is sufficient to prevent accumulation of sulfatides in the tissues, and hence these individuals do not develop clinical signs of MLD.

All forms of MLD are transmitted as autosomal recessive traits, and all of them appear to be genetically distinct [48]. The locus for arylsulfatase A has been mapped to the long arm of chromosome 22 in the q13 band [14]. Two mutations have been found in several cases of late juvenile MLD: one is a point mutation in the codon for amino acid residue 193 that substitutes cystine for tryptophan; the other is a nucleotide substitution in the splice site of intron 2 [68]. Another mutation in adult forms of MLD occurs at amino acid residue 426 that results in a substitution of leucine for proline. A second point mutation reported in a Japanese patient with adult-onset MLD occurs in exon 2 at amino acid residue 99, and results in a substitution of aspartic acid for glycine [49]. In a recent study of 68 patients with late infantile, juvenile, and adult MLD, two alleles, 1 and A, were identified and found to account for over half of all the arylsulfatase alleles in this group of patients [78]. The most severe form of MLD, the late infantile type, was associated with homozygosity for allele 1, which does not encode catalytically functional arylsulfatase A enzyme. Other mutations were associated with less severe forms of MLD, and these individuals had larger amounts of residual enzyme activity. This is the first example of how molecular genetic techniques can be used to establish reasonably direct relationships between clinical heterogeneity and severity of an inherited disease.

The gene for sphingolipid activator protein (saposin B) has been mapped to chromosome 10 [48]. Cloning and sequencing studies led to the detection of two mutations affecting this protein: one is the substitution of isoleucine for threonine, and the other is a 33-nucleotide insertion into RNA between nucleotides 777 and 778 [68].

The gene for pseudodeficiency has been cloned, and two mutations have so far been detected in these individuals. One of them leads to loss of one of the two N-glycosylation sites in the enzyme, and the second leads to loss of a polyadenylation signal that is used for termination of the major arylsulfatase A mRNA species [29,30]. The presence of large numbers of individuals carrying the pseudodeficiency allele makes genetic counseling difficult since they are often misdiagnosed as MLD carriers. A rapid screening procedure now available, based on primer amplification of either the pseudodeficiency allele or the arylsulfatase A gene, should help to distinguish between individuals carrying mutations on these genes [29].

H. Niemann-Pick Disease

Clinical Features. This disorder is now more appropriately termed the Niemann-Pick group of diseases, or sphingomyelin-cholesterol lipidoses [90]. A newly proposed classification takes into account the wide variability in clinical phenotype, including patients with only mild sphingomyelinase deficiencies

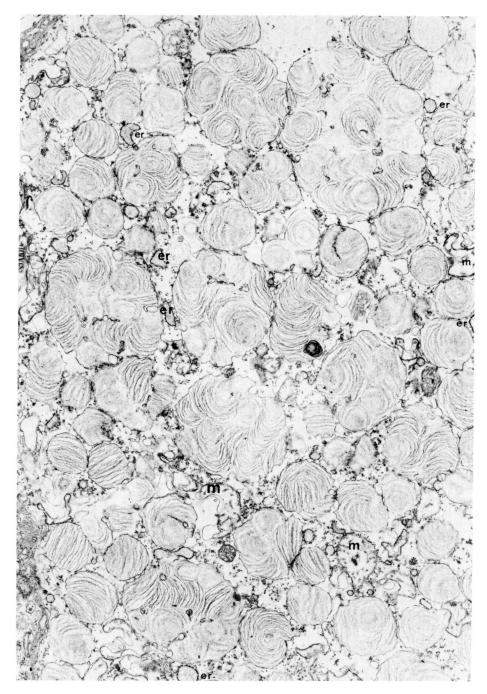

Figure 11 Retinal ganglion cell in type A Niemann-Pick disease, showing abundance of round inclusion bodies containing parallel or concentrically laminated membranes. Some appear to be compressed and in the process of fusing. Mitochondria (m) and endoplasmic reticulum (er) are also seen. (×17,100) (Reproduced with permission from J. Libert, D. Toussaint, and R. Guiselings. Ocular findings in Niemann-Pick disease. *Am. J. Ophthalmol.* *80*:991–1002, 1975.)

or even normal activities. The characteristic foam cell is found in macrophages of spleen, bone marrow, lungs, and lymph nodes in all or most forms of Niemann-Pick disease. The Niemann-Pick group of diseases can be divided into two broad groups, each with three clinical forms [90].

Type I.   Lipidoses with sphingomyelinase deficiency and primary sphingomyelin storage
  A.   Acute form is characterized by massive visceromegaly, nervous system involvement from early infancy, and rapid neurological deterioration resulting in death before the age of 5 years. Sphingomyelinase activity is less than 5% of normal. This form accounts for about 75% of cases reported in world literature.
  B.   In the subacute form, formerly type B in the Crocker classification, patients have severe sphingomyelinase deficiency and develop visceral changes early in life. However, unlike those in the first group, there is marked phenotypic heterogeneity in nervous system involvement.
  C.   In the chronic form, often called the adult form, patients have low levels of sphingo-myelinase activity, but clinical signs do not appear until adulthood. Splenomegaly or hepatomegaly is present but not extensive.
Type II. Lipidoses with uncertain primary defect and secondary sphingomyelin storage
  A.   Acute form patients have hepatosplenomegaly as an early sign in infancy, and psychomotor disturbances appear during the next few years. Death occurs during the first decade, usually from respiratory infection. Sphingomyelinase activity is often normal, but several lipids are nevertheless stored in spleen and liver; these include varying amounts of sphingomyelin as well as cholesterol and other glycolipids.
  B.   In the subacute form, formerly classified as type C or type D Niemann-Pick disease, patients show progressive motor retardation, foam cells, hepatosplenomegaly, and the presence of sea-blue histiocytes in the bone marrow. Age of onset varies from infancy to 18 years, and age of death is also highly variable. Deposition of sphingomyelin is minimal, and there is some evidence supporting the view that both the subacute and the chronic forms are associated with a defect in either the intracellular transport of cholesterol or its esterification [90].
  C.   In the chronic form, patients may have normal or even higher than normal levels of sphingomyelinase activity. Onset is in adulthood and is characterized by progressive dementia, cerebellar ataxia, and foam cells in bone marrow, spleen, and liver.

Ocular Manifestations.   In view of this new proposed classification, it may not always be possible to correlate previously published eye findings based on the Crocker classification of four types of Niemann-Pick disease (A–D). In general, however, group I disease bears close resemblance to types A and B, and group II disorders are for the most part similar to types C and D.

Ocular changes have been reported in nearly all forms of Niemann-Pick disease [96,98]. They appear in some patients with the infantile (type A) form during the first year of life and consist of macular cherry-red spots as well as corneal opacification and brown discoloration of the anterior lens capsule. In enzymatically proven type B patients, bilateral reddish brown (not cherry-red) spots at the macula surrounded by punctate white deposits or macular halo have been observed [39,62]. An opaque appearance of the perimacular area with minimum optic nerve pallor has been observed in type C Niemann-Pick disease [74].

Widespread ocular involvement is evident from electron microscopic studies that show abundant multilamellar cytoplasmic bodies in a variety of ocular tissues. These lamellar inclusions, varying in size from 0.2 to 3.0 μm and surrounded by single membranes, accumulate in retinal ganglion cells (Fig. 11), amacrine and pigment epithelial cells, Müller cells, corneal fibroblasts, endothelium, and epithelium, as well as in lens epithelium [58,80]. The multilamellar cytoplasmic bodies may vary slightly in morphology from one tissue to the next, but the lamellae are rather similar, with periodicities ranging from 5.5 to 6.5 nm. The abnormal inclusions in the lens epithelium are particularly striking (Fig. 12). A

Figure 12   (A) Lens epithelium in type A Niemann-Pick disease, showing single-membrane–bound cytoplasmic bodies with predominantly lamellar architecture. They are round or oval in shape, are surrounded by a single trilamellar membrane, and contain alternating osmiophilic and osmiophobic strands with periodicities of

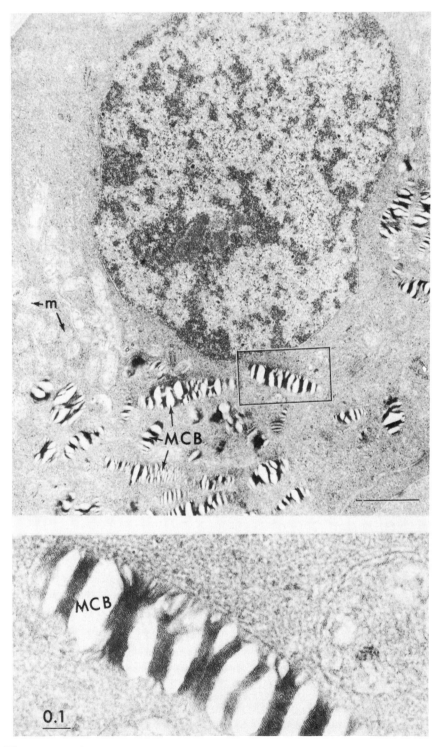

5.5–6 nm. They contrast sharply with the mitochondria (m). (×17,000) (B) The structural details of the membrane-bound cytoplasmic bodies (MCB) enclosed in the rectangular area of A are shown in greater detail at higher magnification. (×75,000) (Reproduced with permission from R.M. Robb and T. Kuwabara. The ocular pathology of type A Niemann-Pick disease. *Invest. Ophthalmol. 12*:366–377, 1973.)

second pleomorphic type of inclusion body, with dense lamellar structures alternating with granular, vacuolar, or whorled masses, is widespread throughout the eye, being found in Müller cells of the retina, conjunctival, and corneal epithelial cells, keratocytes, ciliary muscles, choroidal fibroblasts, and other tissues [58]. The birefringency observed under polarized light appears to parallel the specific sites of lamellar deposition. This is best explained in terms of the chemical composition and structure of the lamellae, which consist of "head-and-tail" orientation of the polar (phosphocholine) and nonpolar (ceramide) moieties of sphingomyelin.

Conjunctival changes that appear to be unique to Niemann-Pick disease have been described [56,57]. This tissue reflects the generalized storage of sphingomyelin and/or cholesterol; in type A, lamellar inclusions are present in the fibrocytes and epithelium, as well as in the pericytes and endothelial cells of the blood capillaries. The Schwann cells are particularly engorged with myelinlike whorls. By contrast, ultrastructural changes in these cell types are far less severe in type B patients, and in type C Niemann-Pick disease, only the conjunctival fibroblasts show an accumulation of multivesicular inclusions. Thus, once the disorder has been diagnosed by assay of sphingomyelinase in leukocytes or other suitable tissue, a conjunctival biopsy may add another parameter (in addition to clinical signs and enzyme analyses) for distinguishing among the three types of Niemann-Pick disease.

Biochemistry and Metabolic Abnormalities.   The metabolic defect in the three forms of type I Niemann-Pick disease is a deficiency of the lysosomal enzyme sphingomyelinase, which degrades sphingomyelin to ceramide and phosphocholine [90]. Diagnosis of type I disease can be made by measuring the activity of this enzyme in cultured skin fibroblasts, leukocytes, or tissue biopsy specimens. There is considerable heterogeneity in these disorders, however, since the degree of deficiency varies considerably among patients. Type I disease (formerly designated types A and B) is about 10 times more frequent among individuals of Ashkenazi Jewish ancestry than in the general population. The molecular basis of these disorders in the Ashkenazi Jewish community were recently examined using two partial cDNA encoding human sphingomyelinase [55]. These studies uncovered a substitution of arginine for leucine at amino acid residue 496 in 32% of Niemann-Pick type A (probably type IA in the new classification) patients of Ashkenazi Jewish descent that occurred in only 5.6% of non-Jewish patients. This allele was not present in 180 unaffected individuals of Jewish descent who were examined. Further studies using this clone will add greatly to our understanding of the molecular basis of this complex group of disorders.

The primary defects in type II forms of Niemann-Pick disease are unknown [90]. Sphingomyelin storage is less marked than in type I disease. Sphingomyelinase activity in tissue biopsy specimens is often normal, but in cultured fibroblasts its activity varies from normal to only 20% of normal. A decrease in cholesterol esterification has been noted in some patients. Diagnosis of type II forms by enzyme analyses is therefore uncertain.

III. NEURONAL CEROID LIPOFUSCINOSIS (BATTEN DISEASE)

Clinical Features.   Neuronal ceroid lipofuscinosis (NCL) is the term now applied to a group of severe neurodegenerative disorders first described by Batten at the turn of the century. In the years that followed, similar syndromes were described by Mayou, Vogt, Jansky, Bielschowsky, Spielmeyer, Sjögren, Hagberg, Haltia, Santavuori, and Kufs, all of whose names became associated with this heterogeneous group of disorders. Since the biochemical defect was not (and still is not) known, they have been classified mainly according to age of onset and description of the abnormal storage substances. The name neuronal ceroid lipofuscinosis defines the two types of autofluorescent lipopigments, ceroid and lipofuscin, that accumulate in the neuronal perikarya and other cells. No excess of gangliosides or other sphingolipids is found in this group of disorders. However, this nomenclature has recently been questioned on two grounds: (1) the term "neuronal" is misleading since in addition to brain, many other cell types (smooth muscles, Schwann cells, glands, skin, conjunctiva, and leukocytes) also have storage substances, and (2) the pigments do not precisely resemble either ceroid or lipofuscin [4].

The four clinical phenotypes of NCL now recognized are (1) the infantile form (Hagberg-Santavuori-Haltia) [38,84] with clinical onset before the second year of life; (2) the late infantile form (Jansky-Bielschowsky), with onset at 2–4 years of age and rapid deterioration until death within about 5 years; (3) the juvenile form (Batten-Spielmeyer-Vogt-Sjögren), which is the most common type, with onset at 4–8 years of age and slowly progressive neurological deterioration until death after about 10 years; and (4) the adult (Kufs) form, which is relatively rare and poorly defined clinically. All these disorders are inherited as autosomal recessive traits. Visual disturbances are present in the first three forms but are not found in the adult type [54]. There is considerable clinical variability in all forms of NCL, making early diagnosis difficult. Presenting signs are often nonspecific, consisting of seizures with concomitant speech, motor, and visual impairment; these are followed by progressive intellectual regression, blindness, and cerebellar dysfunction. The presenting signs in the infantile (Hagberg-Santavuori-Haltia) form consist of rapid psychomotor deterioration, ataxia, muscular hypotonia, myoclonic jerks, and generalized convulsions [84]. All patients reported so far were considered blind by the age of 2 years. Optic atrophy as well as macular and retinal dystrophy were usually present; pigmentary changes were not reported. Early extinction of the electroretinogram (ERG) has been noted in most cases. Visual disturbances often appear later in the Jansky-Bielschowsky form and sometimes are not observed at all, especially in cases of early death. Recent studies show that the Jansky-Bielschowsky form of neuronal ceroid lipofuscinosis is far more heterogeneous than previously thought [85]. The juvenile (Batten-Spielmeyer-Sjögren) type of neuronal ceroid lipofuscinosis has insidious intellectual and behavioral deterioration, with onset between 4 and 8 years of age. It is always accompanied by retinal atrophy and macular pigmentary degeneration at an early stage [6,33].

Ocular Manifestations.   Visual disturbances are well documented and are usually among the earliest presenting signs in all but the adult form of NCL. The macular cherry-red spots characteristic of ganglioside (and other sphingolipid) storage diseases are not seen in any of the NCL types. Instead, there is a granular pigmentary macular degeneration as well as a peripheral pigmentary retinopathy, with formation of "bony spicules" and narrowing of retinal vessels. Optic atrophy is variable. The widespread degeneration of the neuroepithelium and the pigment epithelium is reflected in profound ultrastructural changes in the retina.

Infantile type (Hagberg-Santavuori).   Visual deterioration is recognizable by 1 year of age, and pupillary reflexes are diminished or absent by the second year of life [54]. There is progressive hypopigmentation of the fundus, as well as optic atrophy with attenuated retinal vessels [4]. Mild retinal epithelial clumping was observed in a 7-year-old patient, and by 15 years of age, this patient had nystagmus and exotropia. The eyelids, conjunctivae, and corneas were normal, but posterior stellar cataracts were present in both eyes. A second patient manifested pale optic disks by 2 years of age and was blind by 7 years. Other findings were similar to those in the first patient. Both patients had retinal degeneration with hyperpigmented "bone spicules." The ERG was extinguished in these cases, as well as in other cases examined previously [4].

Late infantile type (Jansky-Bielschowsky-Haltia).   Visual impairment appears relatively late (between 28 months and 5 years) in this form of NCL [54]. Most cases examined showed macular pigment mottling and optic atrophy with attenuation of retinal vessels by 3–5 years of age. The ERG signal is small at first and afterward is unrecordable. Electron microscopic studies in the late infantile (Jansky-Bielschowsky) form reveal a complex pathomorphological pattern of retinal deterioration [34,93]. There is a loss of photoreceptors in the central region of the retina, and only remnants remain in the equatorial areas. Curvilinear bodies similar to those found in neural tissue (Fig. 13) are also present throughout the retina (Fig. 14). Melanin granules are frequently associated with these residual bodies. Later studies [93] also revealed extensive degeneration of the photoreceptors and loss of ganglion cell layer. Curvilinear profiles were observed in retinal ganglion cells, macrophages, and retinal pigment epithelial (RPE) cells and in pericytes and endothelial cells of retinal and choroidal blood vessels.

Juvenile type (Batten-Vogt-Spielmeyer-Sjögren).   Early reduction of central vision and fine mottling of the macular pigment are usually apparent even before visual impairment is demonstrable [6,41,54]. An early ERG change is reduction in the B wave, and later the ERG is unrecordable. Optic atrophy with attenuation of retinal vessels is observed, and later peripheral clumped aggregates are seen [54]. These visual changes usually precede neurological signs in the juvenile type of NCL. The retinopathy in this form of NCL, although bearing a general resemblance to that found in the late infantile form, is more severe [33,34,93].

Consequent to the complete loss of inner and outer segments, the resulting space is occupied by villous processes probably deriving from the RPE. Melanin-containing cells that resemble pigment epithelia but are devoid of basal lamina and villous processes fill the outer layers. Many of the cellular membranes

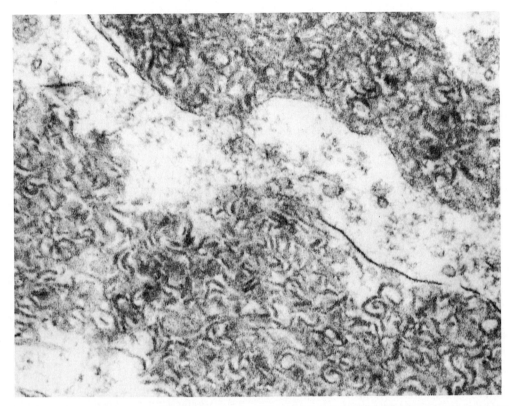

Figure 13   Ultrastructure of neural tissue in late infantile neuronal ceroid lipofuscinosis. The cell is filled with cytosomes containing curvilinear inclusion bodies. (×97,000) (Reproduced by courtesy of Dr. B.D. Lake.)

are disrupted, and melanosomes are embedded in the matrices of the residual bodies, whereas other areas of the RPE are devoid of melanin. There is uncertainty about whether the accumulation of lipopigments is the cause or result of the degenerative changes in the RPE.

There is a marked accumulation of curvilinear and fingerprint bodies in ganglion cells, Müller cells, and astrocytes and in blood vessel pericytes and mural cells. The general picture in this form of neuronal ceroid lipofuscinosis is one of complete disorganization and degeneration of the retinal architecture, especially the outer half.

Adult Type (Kufs').   There are usually no ocular symptoms in Kufs' disease; unlike the other three forms, there is neither loss of vision nor pigmentary degeneration. Although skin or muscle biopsies may be used to confirm a clinical diagnosis of Kufs' disease based on the presence of curvilinear and/or multilaminated profiles, conjunctival biopsies may be much more informative because of the variety of cells that can be examined [93].

Biochemistry and Molecular Genetics.   The biochemical basis of NCL is complex and ambiguous, mainly because of uncertainties in the chemical definition of the lysosome-derived autofluorescent granules. Whereas the stored substances have been identified and the enzyme defects characterized in other lysosomal disorders, the chemical nature of the storage substance(s) comprising the lipopigments that accumulate in NCL remain unknown; the formation of lipopigments may in fact be secondary to the primary defect [89]. These autofluorescent granules are recognizable morphologically as osmiophilic membrane-bound cytoplasmic deposits; electron microscopic examination reveals curvilinear, fingerprint, or granule patterns. Present knowledge suggests that ceroid, although not found normally in tissues, may accumulate in certain disease states. In contrast, lipofuscin has a fairly ubiquitous distribution in normal tissues and is especially abundant in brain, liver, heart, and the retinal pigment epithelium [20,21]. One view on the biogenesis of the autofluorescent granules is that the fluorogenic component is derived from the

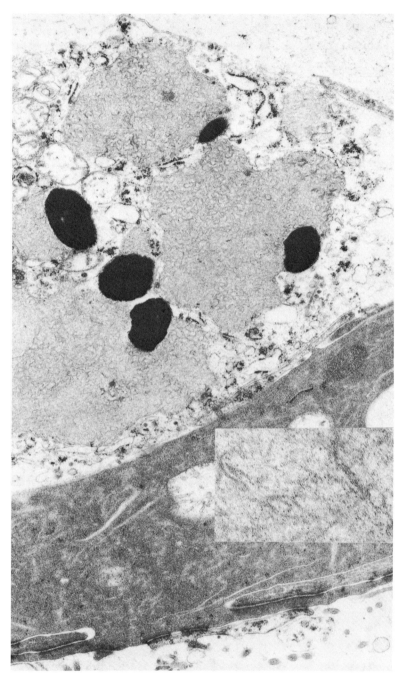

Figure 14 Equatorial region of the retina in late infantile neuronal ceroid lipofuscinosis. In the pigment epithelial cells, melanin granules are fused with curvilinear bodies. (×21,500) Inset: substructure of the curvilinear bodies at higher magnification, showing alternating dark and light unordered membranous sheets. (×109,500) (Reproduced with permission from H.H. Goebel, W. Zeman, and E. Damaske. An ultrastructural study of the retina in the Jansky-Bielschowsky type of neuronal ceroid-lipofuscinosis. *Am. J. Ophthalmol. 83*: 70–73, 1977.

nonenzymatic peroxidation of polyunsaturated fatty acids. Such fragments as malonaldehyde, thought to be released in this process, form Schiff-base complexes with amino groups residing in various cellular membranes. The resulting cross-linked polymeric substances are sequestered into autophagic vacuoles that are not catabolized further [20]. Thus, lipofuscin probably represents a special kind of lysosome-derived organelle or residual body that is not released from the cell once it is formed; rather, it accumulates slowly during the lifetime of the individual and for this reason is often called age pigment. Autofluorescent granules are present in amounts far higher than expected for the age group in patients with NCL.

Electron microscopic studies have shed some light on the classification of the principal forms of NCL since distinct ultrastructural abnormalities appear to be associated with at least three of them. The infantile form is characterized by massive infiltration of phagocytic cells, many of them bi- or even trinucleated, having coarse granular cytoplasm and small hyperchromatic nuclei [38]. In the late infantile form, densely packed curvilinear bodies occur throughout the cytoplasm (Fig. 13); in the juvenile type, characteristic "fingerprint" patterns are consistently observed. It is reasonable to assume that in most cases the abnormal accumulations represent the same autofluorescent lipopigments as those observed by light microscopy. Although tentatively characterized as ceroid and lipofuscin by their characteristic fluorescence spectra in chloroform-methanol extracts of brain tissue from NCL patients, this is not the complete answer.

Studies undertaken to elucidate the chemical nature of the curvilinear bodies in the late infantile form of neuronal ceroid lipofuscinosis showed that the accumulating fluorescent substances are not extractable with chloroform-methanol but can be solubilized using a mixture of dimethyl sulfoxide and water [99]. The principal fluorescent substance isolated was not lipofuscin but, rather unexpectedly, a metabolite of either retinol or retinoic acid complexed to a peptide or, possibly, to cholesterol [66].

More recently, entirely new approaches to the chemical pathology of NCL were undertaken [89]. One important observation is that dolichol and dolichol pyrophosphoryl-oligosaccharides accumulate in tissues and are excreted in the urine in all forms of the disease. The specificity of this biochemical abnormality has been questioned, however, since dolichols also accumulate in aging brain and in patients with Alzheimer's disease. Other investigators have found excessive urinary excretion of low-molecular-weight peptides, a finding that may provide a marker for identifying the juvenile subtype [50]. In yet another approach, storage material from postmortem specimens of brain from the four forms of NCL was isolated, purified, and analyzed by gel electrophoresis [37]. Although many components were present, one of them, subunit c of mitochondrial ATP synthetase, was present in greatly elevated levels in patients with late infantile, juvenile, and adult subtypes but was found at normal levels in the infantile form of this disease. Further studies of abnormal proteins in this group of diseases revealed large amounts of methylated lysine residues in the juvenile form of NCL [43]. The specific protein(s) carrying the excess trimethyllysine could not be identified, but a possible relationship to mitochondrial synthetase cannot be excluded. In other investigations, a generalized decrease in phospholipids and fatty acids in erythrocytes and platelets of the juvenile subtype has been reported [7]. Thus, despite several decades of intensive investigation, the chemical nature of the autofluorescent lipopigments that accumulate in NCL remains unknown.

The genetic defects in these autosomal recessive disorders are also unknown, precluding the use of usual genomic or cDNA cloning procedures for the detection of mutant alleles. This problem has been circumvented through the use of recently improved linkage analysis techniques combined with molecular genetic approaches that allow approximate localization of the defective gene(s). Using these techniques, the infantile and juvenile forms have been localized to chromosomes 1 and 16, respectively [42,89]. These findings provide the first direct evidence that the different forms of NCL are caused by nonallelic mutations, thus opening the way to more precise definitions of the mutations causing these disorders.

REFERENCES

1. Babarick, A., Benson, P.F., Fensom, A.H., and Barrie, H. Corneal clouding in GM_1-generalized gangliosidosis. *Br. J. Ophthalmol. 60*:565–576, 1976.
2. Baker, R.L., Trautmann, J.C., Younge, B.R., Nelson, K.D., and Zimmerman, D. Late juvenile-onset Krabbe's disease. *Ophthalmology 97*:1176–1180, 1990.
3. Barranger, J.A., and Ginns, E.I. Glucosylceramide lipidoses: Gaucher disease. In *The Metabolic Basis of Inherited Disease*, 6th ed., C.R. Scriver, A.L. Beaudet, W.S. Sly, and D. Valle (Eds.), McGraw-Hill, New York, pp. 1677–1698, 1989.

4. Bateman, J.B., and Philippart, M. Ocular features of the Hagberg-Santavuori syndrome. *Am. J. Ophthalmol.* *102*:262–271, 1986.

5. Bateman, J.B., Philippart, M., and Isenberg, S. Ocular features of multiple sulfatase deficiencies and a new variant of metachromatic leukodystrophy. *J. Pediatr. Ophthalmol. Strabismus.* *21*:133–139, 1984.

6. Beckerman, B.L., and Rapin, I. Ceroid lipofuscinosis. *Am. J. Ophthalmol.* *80*:73–77, 1975.

7. Bennett, M.J., Galloway, J.H., Cartwright, I.J., Gillis, W.S., and Hosking, G.P. Decreased erythrocyte and platelet phospholipids and fatty acids in juvenile neuronal ceroid-lipofuscinosis (Batten disease). *Neuropediatrics 21*:202–205, 1990.

8. Berman, E.R., *Biochemistry of the Eye*, Plenum Press, New York, 1991.

9. Brownstein, S., Meagher-Villemure, K., Polomeno, R.C., and Little, J.M. Optic nerve in globoid leukodystrophy (Krabbe's disease). *Arch. Ophthalmol. 96*:864–870, 1978.

10. Cogan, D.G., and Kuwabara, T. The sphingolipidoses and the eye. *Arch. Ophthalmol. 79*:437–452, 1968.

11. Cogan, D.G., Kuwabara, T., and Moser, H. Metachromatic leukodystrophy. *Ophthalmologica 160*:2–17, 1970.

12. Cogan, D.G., Kuwabara, T., Moser, H., and Hazard, G.W. Retinopathy in a case of Farber's lipogranulomatosis. *Arch. Ophthalmol. 75*:752–757, 1966.

13. Cogan, D., Chu, F., Gittinger, J., and Tychsen, L.: Fundus abnormalities in Gaucher's disease. *Arch. Ophthalmol. 98*:2202–2203, 1980.

14. DeLuca, C., Brown, J.A., and Shows, T.B. Lysosomal arylsulfatase deficiencies in humans: Chromosome assignments for arylsulfatase A and B. *Proc. Natl. Acad. Sci. USA 76*:1957–1961, 1979.

15. Desnick, R.J., and Bishop, D.F. Fabry disease: α-galactosidase deficiency; Schindler disease: α-N-Acetylgalactosaminidase deficiency. In *The Metabolic Basis of Inherited Disease*, 6th ed., C.R. Scriver, A.L. Beaudet, W.S. Sly, and D. Valle (Eds.), McGraw-Hill, New York, pp. 1751–1796, 1989.

16. Desnick, R.J., Dean, K.J., Grabowski, G., Bishop, D.F., and Sweeley, C.C. Enzyme therapy in Fabry disease: Differential in vivo plasma clearance and metabolic effectiveness of plasma and splenic α-galactosidase A isoenzymes. *Proc. Natl. Acad. Sci. USA 76*:5326–5330, 1979.

17. Emery, J.M., Green, W.R., Wyllie, R.G., and Howell, R.R. GM$_1$-gangliosidosis: Ocular and pathological manifestations. *Arch. Ophthalmol. 85*:177–187, 1971.

18. Emery, J.M., Green, W.R., and Hubb, D.S. Krabbe's disease: Histopathology and ultrastructure of the eye. *Am. J. Ophthalmol. 74*:400–406, 1972.

19. Faraggiona, T., Churg, J., Grishman, E., Strauss, L., Predo, A., Bishop, D.F., Schuchman, E., and Desnick, R.J. Light and electron-microscopic histochemistry of Fabry's disease. *Am. J. Pathol. 103*:247–262, 1981.

20. Feeney, L. Lipofuscin and melanin of human retinal pigment epithelium: Fluorescence, enzyme cytochemical and ultrastructural studies. *Invest. Ophthalmol. Vis. Sci. 17*:583–600, 1978.

21. Feeney-Burns, L. The pigments of the retinal pigment epithelium. In *Current topics in Eye Research*, Vol. 2, J.A. Zadunaisky and H. Davson (Eds.), Academic Press, New York, pp. 119–178, 1980.

22. Filling-Katz, M.R., Barton, N.W., and Katz, N.N.K. Krabbe's disease. In *The Eye in Systemic Disease*, D.H. Gold and T.A. Weingeist (Eds.), J. B. Lippincott, Philadelphia, pp. 360–362, 1990.

23. Filling-Katz, M.R., Barton, N.W., and Katz, N.N.K. Metachromatic leukodystrophies. In *The Eye in Systemic Disease*, D.H. Gold and T.A. Weingeist (Eds.), J. B. Lippincott, Philadelphia, pp. 381–384, 1990.

24. Filling-Katz, M.R., Barton, N.W., and Katz, N.N.K. Gaucher's disease. In *The Eye in Systemic Disease*, D.H. Gold and T.A. Weingeist (Eds.), J. B. Lippincott, Philadelphia, pp. 365–368, 1990.

25. Firon, N., Eyal, N., Kolodny, E.H., and Horowitz, M. Genotype assignment in Gaucher disease by selective amplification of the active glucocerebrosidase gene. *Am. J. Hum. Genet. 46*:527–532, 1990.

26. Font, R.L., and Fine, B.S. Ocular pathology in Fabry's disease: Histochemical and electron microscopic observations. *Am. J. Ophthalmol. 73*:419–430, 1972.

27. Garner, A. Ocular pathology of GM$_2$-gangliosidosis type 2. (Sandhoff's disease). *Br. J. Ophthalmol. 57*:514–520, 1973.

28. Geiger, B., and Arnon, R. Chemical characterization and subunit structure of human N-acetylhexosaminidases A and B. *Biochemistry 15*:3484–3493, 1976.

29. Gieselmann, V. An assay for the rapid detection of the arylsulfatase A pseudodeficiency allele facilitates diagnosis and genetic counseling for metachromatic leukodystrophy. *Hum. Genet. 86*:251–255, 1991.

30. Gieselmann, V., Fluharty, A.L., Tonnesen, T., and von Figura, K. Mutations in the arylsulfatase A pseudodeficiency allele causing metachromatic leukodystrophy. *Am. J. Hum. Genet. 49*:407–413, 1991.

31. Gilbert, G., Kucherlapati, R., Creagan, R.P., Murnane, M.J., Darlington, G.S., and Ruddle, F.H. Tay-Sachs and Sandhoff's disease: The assignment of genes for hexosaminidase A and B to individual human chromosomes. *Proc. Natl. Acad. Sci. USA 72*:263–267, 1975.

32. Goebel, H.H., Fix, J.D., and Zeman, W. Retinal pathology in GM$_1$-gangliosidosis, type II. *Am. J. Ophthalmol. 75*:434–441, 1973.

33. Goebel, H.H., Fix, J.D., and Zeman, W. The fine structure of the retina in neuronal ceroid-lipofuscinosis. *Am. J. Ophthalmol. 77*:25–39, 1974.

34. Goebel, H.H., Zeman, W., and Damaske, E. An ultrastructural study of the retina in the Jansky-Bielschowsky type of neuronal ceroid-lipofuscinosis. *Am. J. Ophthalmol. 83*:70–79, 1977.

35. Goldberg, J.D., Truex, J.H., and Desnick, R.J. Tay-Sachs disease: An improved, fully-automated method of heterozygote identification by tear β-hexosaminidase assay. *Clin. Chim. Acta 77*:43–52, 1977.

36. Grebner, E.E., and Tomczak, J. Distribution of three α-chain β-hexosaminidase A mutations among Tay-Sachs carriers. *Am. J. Hum. Genet. 48*:604–607, 1991.

37. Hall, N.A., Lake, B.D., Dewji, N.N., and Patrick, A.D. Lysosomal storage of subunit c of mitochondrial ATP synthase in Batten disease (ceroid-lipofuscinosis). *Biochem. J. 275*:269–272, 1991.

38. Haltia, M., Rapola, J., Santavuori, P., and Keranen, A. Infantile type of so-called neuronal ceroid-lipofuscinosis. Part 2. Morphological and biochemical studies. *J. Neurol. Sci. 18*:269–285, 1973.

39. Hammersen, G., Oppermann, H.C., Harms, E., Blassmann, K., and Harzer, K. Oculoneural involvement in an enzymatically proven case of Niemann-Pick disease type B. *Eur. J. Pediatr. 132*:77–84, 1979.

40. Harcourt, B., and Ashton, N. Ultrastructure of the optic nerve in Krabbe's leukodystrophy. *Br. J. Ophthalmol. 57*:885–891, 1973.

41. Hittner, H.M., and Zeller, R.S. Ceroid-lipofuscinosis (Batten's disease). *Arch. Ophthalmol. 93*:178–183, 1975.

42. Jarvela, I., Haataja, L., Puhakka, L., Palotie, A., Renlund, M., Aula, P., and Peltonen, L. Infantile form of neuronal ceroid lipofiscinosis (NCL1) maps to the short arm of chromosome 1. *Genomics 9*:170–173, 1991.

43. Katz, M.L., and Rodgigues, M. Juvenile ceroid lipofuscinosis. Evidence for methylated lysine in neural storage body protein. *Am. J. Pathol. 138*:323–332, 1991.

44. Kenyon, K.R. Ocular ultrastructure of inherited metabolic disease. In *Genetic and Metabolic Eye Disease*, M.F. Goldberg (Ed.), Little, Brown, Boston, pp. 139–185, 1974.

45. Kirkilionis, A.J., Riddell, D.C., Spence, M.W., and Fenwick, R.G. Fabry disease in a large Nova Scotia kindred: Carrier detection using leukocyte α-galactosidase activity and an NcoI polymorphism, detected by an α-galactosidase cDNA clone. *J. Med Genet. 28*:232–240, 1991.

46. Kivlin, J., Sanborn, G., and Myers, G. The cherry red spot in Tay-Sachs and other storage disorders. *Ann. Neurol. 17*:356–360, 1985.

47. Klenk, E. Beitrage zur Chemie der Lipoidosen Niemann-Pick'sch Krankheit und amaurotische Idiotie. *Hoppe Seylers Z. Physiol. Chem. 262*:128–143, 1939–1940.

48. Kolodny, E.H. Metachromatic leukodystrophy and multiple sulfatase deficiency: Sulfatide lipidosis. In *The Metabolic Basis of Inherited Disease*, 6th ed., C.S. Scriver, A.L. Beaudet, W.S. Sly, and D. Valle (Eds.), McGraw-Hill, New York, pp. 1721–1750, 1989.

49. Kondo, R., Wakamatsu, N., Fukuhara, N., Miyatake, T., and Tsuji, S. Identification of a mutation in the arylsulfatase A gene of a patient with adult-onset metachromatic leukodystrophy. *Am. J. Hum. Genet. 48*:971–978, 1991.

50. LaBadie, G.U., and Pullarkat, R.K. Low molecular weight urinary peptides in ceroid-lipofuscinoses: Potential biochemical markers for the juvenile subtype. *Am. J. Med. Genet. 37*:592–599, 1990.

51. Landels, E.C., Ellis, I.H., Bobrow, M., and Fensom, A.H. Tay-Sachs disease heterozyote detection: Use of a centrifugal analyser for automation of hexosaminidase assays with two different artificial substrates. *J. Med. Genet. 28*:101–109, 1991.

52. Landels, E.C., Ellis, I.H., Fenson, A.H., Green, P.M., and Bobrow, M. Frequency of the Tay-Sachs disease splice and insertion mutations in the UK Ashkenazi Jewish population. *J. Med. Genet. 28*:177–180, 1991.

53. Latham, T.E., Theophilus, B.D.M., Grabowski, G.A., and Smith, F.I. Hetergeneity of mutations in the β-glucosidase gene of Gaucher disease patients. *DNA Cell Biol. 10*:15–21, 1991.

54. Lavery, M.A. Batten's disease. In *The Eye in Systemic Disease*, D.H. Gold and T.A. Weingeist (Eds.), J. B. Lippincott, Philadelphia, pp. 350–352, 1990.

55. Levran, O., Desnick, R.L., and Schuchman, E.H. Niemann-Pick disease: A frequent missense mutation in the acid sphingomyelinase gene of Ashkenazi Jewish type A and B patients. *Proc. Natl. Acad. Sci. USA 88*:3748–3752, 1991.

56. Libert, J., and Danis, P. Diagnosis of type A Niemann-Pick's disease by conjunctival biopsy. *Pathol. Eur. 10*:233–239, 1975.

57. Libert, J., and Danis, P. Differential diagnosis of type A, B and C Niemann-Pick disease by conjunctival biopsy. *J. Submicrosc. Cytol. 11*:143–157, 1979.

58. Libert, J., Toussaint, D., and Guiselings, R. Ocular findings in Niemann-Pick disease. *Am. J. Ophthalmol. 80*:991–1002, 1975.

59. Libert, J., Tondeur, M., and van Hoof, F. The use of conjunctival biopsy and enzyme analysis in tears for the diagnosis of homozygotes and heterozygotes with Fabry disease. *Birth Defects 12*(3):221–239, 1976.

60. Libert, J., van Hoof, F., Toussaint, D., Roozitalab, H., Kenyon, K.R., and Green, W.R. Ocular findings in metachromatic leukodystrophy: An electron microscopic and enzyme study in different clinical and genetic variants. *Arch. Ophthalmol. 97*:1496–1504, 1979.

61. Mahuran, D.J. The biochemistry of Hex A and Hex B gene mutations causing GM$_2$ gangliosidosis. *Biochim. Biophys. Acta 1096*:87–94, 1991.

62. Matthews, J.D., Weiter, J.J., and Kolodny, E.H. Macular halos associated with Niemann-Pick type B disease. *Ophthalmology 93*:933–937, 1986.

63. McCulloch, C. Fabry's disease. In *The Eye in Systemic Disease*, D.H. Gold and T.A. Weingeist (Eds.), J. B. Lippincott, Philadelphia, pp. 355–358, 1990.

64. Moser, H.W., Moser, A.B., Chen, W.W., and Schram, A.W. Ceramidase deficiency: Farber lipogranulomatosis, In *The Metabolic Basis of Inherited Disease*, 6th ed., McGraw-Hill, New York, pp. 1645–1654, 1989.

65. Navon, R., and Proia, R.L. Tay Sachs disease in Moroccan Jews: Deletion of a phenylalanine in the α-subunit of β-hexosaminidase. *Am. J. Hum. Genet.* 48:412–419, 1991.

66. Nelson, E.C., and Halley, B.A. Retinoyl complexes in Batten disease. *Science* 198:527–528, 1977.

67. Neufeld, E.F. Natural history and inherited disorders of a lysosomal enzyme, β-hexosaminidase. *J. Biol. Chem.* 264:10927–10930, 1989.

68. Neufeld, E.F. Lysosomal storage diseases. *Annu. Rev. Biochem.* 60:257–280, 1991.

69. Nishimoto, J., Nanba, E., Inui, K., Okada, S., and Suzuki, K. GM_1-gangliosidosis (genetic β-galactosidase deficiency): Identification of four mutations in different clinical phenotypes among Japanese patients. *Am. J. Hum. Genet.* 49:566–574, 1991.

70. O'Brien, J.S., Ho, M.W., Veath, M.L., Wilson, J.F., Myers, G., Opitz, J.M., Zurhein, G.M., Spranger, J.W., Hartmann, H.A., Haneberg, B., and Grosse, F.R. Juvenile GM_1-gangliosidosis: Clinical, pathological, chemical, and enzymatic studies. *Clin. Genet.* 3:411–434, 1972.

71. O'Brien, J.S. Molecular genetics of GM_1 β-galactosidase. *Clin. Genet.* 8:303–313, 1975.

72. O'Brien, J.S. β-Galactosidase deficiency (GM_1 gangliosidosis, galactosialidosis, and Morquio syndrome type B): Ganglioside sialidase deficiency (mucolipidosis IV). In *The Metabolic Basis of Inherited Disease*, 6th ed., C.R. Scriver, A.L. Beaudet, W.S. Sly, and D. Valle (Eds.), McGraw-Hill, New York, pp. 1797–1806, 1989.

73. Okada, S., and O'Brien, J.S. Tay-Sachs disease: generalized absence of a beta D-N-acetylhexosaminidase component. *Science* 165:698–700, 1969.

74. Palmer, M., Green, W.R., Maumenee, I.H., Valle, D.L., Singer, H.S., Morton, S.J., and Moser, H.W. Niemann-Pick disease-type C. Ocular histopathologic and electron microscopic studies. *Arch. Ophthalmol.* 103:817–822, 1985.

75. Paw, B.H., Tieu, P.T., Kaback, M.M., Lim, J., and Neufeld, E.F. Frequency of three Hex A mutant alleles among Jewish and non-Jewish carriers identified in a Tay-Sachs screening program. *Am. J. Hum. Genet.* 47:698–703, 1990.

76. Paw, B.H., Wood, L.C., and Neufeld, E.F. A third mutation at the CpG dinucleotide of codon 504 and a silent mutation at codon 506 of the Hex A gene. *Am. J. Hum. Genet.* 48:1139–1146, 1991.

77. Petrohelos, M., Tricoulis, D., Kotsiras, I., and Vouzoukos, A. Ocular manifestations of Gaucher's disease. *Am. J. Ophthalmol.* 80:1006–1010, 1975.

78. Polten, A., Fluharty, A.L., Fluharty, C.B., Kappler, J., von Figura, K., and Gieselmann, V. Molecular basis of different forms of metachromatic leukodystrophy. *N. Engl. J. Med.* 324:18–22, 1991.

79. Quigley, H.A., and Green, W.R. Clinical and ultrastructural ocular histopathologic studies of adult-onset metachromatic leukodystrophy. *Am. J. Ophthalmol.* 82:472–479, 1975.

80. Robb, R.M., and Kuwabara, T. The ocular pathology of type A Niemann-Pick disease. *Invest. Ophthalmol.* 12:366–377, 1973.

81. Sachs, B. A family form of idiocy, generally fatal, associated with early blindness. *J. Nerv. Ment. Dis.* 23:475–479, 1896.

82. Sandhoff, K., Andreae, U., and Jatzkewitz, H. Deficient hexosaminidase activity in an exceptional case of Tay-Sachs disease with additional storage of kidney globoside in visceral organs. *Life Sci.* 7:283–288, 1968.

83. Sandhoff, K., Conzelmann, E., Neufeld, E.F., Kaback, M., and Suzuki, K. The GM_2 gangliosidases. In *The Metabolic Basis of Inherited Disease*, 6th ed., C.R. Scriver, A.L. Beaudet, W.S. Sly, and D. Valle (Eds.), McGraw-Hill, New York, pp. 1807–1839, 1989.

84. Santavuori, P., Haltia, M., Rapola, J., and Raitta, C. Infantile type of so-called neuronal ceroid-lipofuscinosis. Part I. A clinical study of 15 patients. *J. Neurol. Sci.* 18:257–267, 1973.

85. Santavuori, P., Rapola, J., Nuutila, A., Raininko, R., Launes, J., and Herva, R. The spectrum of Jansky-Bielschowsky disease. *Neuropediatrics* 22:92–96, 1991.

86. Sasaki, T., and Tsukahara, S. A new ocular finding in Gaucher's disease: A report of two brothers. *Ophthalmologica* 191:206–209, 1985.

87. Sher, N.A., Letson, R.D., and Desnick, R.J. The ocular manifestations in Fabry's disease. *Arch. Ophthalmol.* 97:671–676, 1979.

88. Sher, N.A., Reiff, W., Letson, R.D., and Desnick, R.J. Central artery occlusion complicating Fabry's disease. *Arch. Ophthalmol.* 96:815–817, 1978.

89. Siakotos, A., Haines, J., and Dawson, G. Conference Report. Third International Symposium on the Neuronal Ceroid-Lipofuscinoses (Batten's disease). *J. Med. Genet.* 28:284–285, 1991.

90. Spence, M.W., and Callahan, J.W. Sphingomyelin-cholesterol lipidoses: The Niemann-Pick group of diseases. In *The Metabolic Basis of Inherited Disease*, 6th ed., C.R. Scriver, A.L. Beaudet, W.S. Sly, and D. Valle (Eds.), McGraw-Hill, New York, pp. 1655–1676, 1989.

91. Suzuki, K., and Suzuki, Y. Galactosylceramide lipidosis: Globoid-cell leukodystrophy (Krabbe disease). In *The Metabolic Basis of Inherited Disease*, 6th ed., C.R. Scriver, A.L. Beaudet, W.S. Sly, and D. Valle (Eds.), McGraw-Hill, New York, pp. 1699–1720, 1989.

92. Tay, W. Symmetrical changes in the region of the yellow spot in each eye of an infant. *Trans. Ophthalmol. Soc. U.K.* 1:155–157, 1881.

93. Traboulsi, E.I., Green, W.R., Luckenbach, M.W., and de la Cruz, Z.C. Neuronal ceroid lipofuscinosis: Ocular histopathologic and electron microscopic studies in the late infantile, juvenile, and adult forms. *Graefes Arch. Clin. Exp. Ophthalmol. 225*:391–402, 1987.

94. Tripathi, R.C., and Ashton, N. Application of electron microscopy to the study of ocular inborn errors of metabolism. *Birth Defects 12*(3):69–104, 1976.

95. Ueno, H., Ueno, S., and Matsuo, N. Electron microscopic study of Gaucher cells in the eye. *Jpn. J. Ophthalmol. 24*:75–81, 1980.

96. Walton, D.S., Robb, R.M., and Crocker, A.C. Ocular manifestations of group A Niemann-Pick disease. *Am. J. Ophthalmol. 85*:174–180, 1978.

97. Weiter, J.J., Feingold, M., Kolodny, E.H., and Raghaven, S.S. Retinal pigment epithelial degeneration associated with leukocyte arylsulfatase A deficiency. *Am. J. Ophthalmol. 90*:768–772, 1978.

98. Weiter, J.J., and Matthews, J.D. Niemann-Pick disease. In *The Eye in Systemic Disease*, D.H. Gold and T.A. Weingeist (Eds.), J. B. Lippincott, Philadelphia, pp. 378–381, 1990.

99. Wolfe, L.S., Ng Ying Kin, N.M.K., Baker, R.R., Carpenter, S., and Andermann, F. Identification of retinoyl complexes as the autofluorescent component of the neuronal storage material in Batten disease. *Science 195*: 1360–1362, 1977.

100. Zarbin, M.A., Green, W.R., Moser, H.W., and Morton, S.J. Farber's disease: Light and electron microscopic study of the eye. *Arch. Ophthalmol. 103*:73–80, 1985.

101. Zarbin, M.A., Green, W.R., Moser, H.W., and Tiffany, C. Increased levels of ceramide in the retina of a patient with Farber's disease. *Arch. Ophthalmol. 106*:1163, 1988.

102. Zarbin, M., and Green, W.R. Farber's disease. In *The Eye in Systemic Disease*, D.H. Gold and T.A. Weingeist (Eds.), J. B. Lippincott, Philadelphia, pp. 353–355, 1990.

103. Zlotogora, J., Chakraborty, S., Knowlton, R.G., and Wenger, D.A. Krabbe disease locus mapped to chromosome 14 by genetic linkage. *Am. J. Hum. Genet. 47*:37–44, 1990.

30
Mucolipidoses

Elaine R. Berman
Hadassah-Hebrew University Medical School, Jerusalem, Israel

I. INTRODUCTION

First delineated by Spranger and Wiedemann [38] in 1970, the nosological position of this heterogeneous group of genetic disorders is still being revised as new biochemical and molecular genetic data become available. The seven or eight entities originally described shared clinical and radiographical features of both the mucopolysaccharidoses (MPS; see Chap. 28) and the sphingolipidoses (see Chap. 29); hence, the name *mucolipidosis* was proposed. Excessive storage of lipids as well as complex carbohydrates in many of the mucolipidoses finds its expression in profound ultrastructural changes at the cellular level in both neural and visceral tissues; in the eye, both cornea and neural retina are affected to varying degrees in all these disorders.

The inherited diseases originally classified as mucolipidoses (MLS) are now subdivided according to the specific enzymatic defect (Table 1). Rapid progress has been made during the past few years in identifying the abnormal metabolites in all these disorders, one of the most important being the α-neuraminidase deficiency in mucolipidosis I (ML-I). Hence this disorder has been named *sialidosis*. Two major subtypes of sialidosis are now recognized [26] and designated types I and II [9,15]. The only other disorder still classified according to the general terminology, MLS, is mucolipidosis IV (ML-IV). As shown in Table 1, two other groups of inherited lysosomal disorders have also been reclassified. The first are known as disorders of glycoprotein degradation and include mannosidosis, fucosidosis, and galactosialidosis. The second group consists of disorders of lysosomal enzyme phosphorylation and localization: I-cell disease (mucolipidosis II; ML-II) and pseudo-Hurler polydystrophy (mucolipidosis III; ML-III).

II. SIALIDOSIS (MUCOLIPIDOSIS I AND MUCOLIPIDOSIS IV)

A. Sialidosis (Mucolipidosis I)

This disorder has been known for more than two decades [38]. Additional cases reported in the world literature during the ensuing years provided sufficient evidence to distinguish two phenotypic variants, types I and II.

Sialidosis Type I

Known as the cherry-red spot–myoclonus syndrome [33], the age of onset is variable but usually appears during the second decade. At least 15 confirmed cases are now known [9], all of them presenting with myoclonus or gait abnormalities. There are no skeletal changes or Hurler-like facies, and all patients are of normal intellect.

Apart from myoclonus, which is usually severe, the major presenting complaint is decreased visual acuity, which may be associated with impaired color vision or night blindness [9]. Cherry-red macular

Table 1 Mucolipidoses and Other Inherited Lysosomal Storage Disorders

Disorder	Enzymatic and other protein deficiency	Ocular signs
Mucolipidoses with a deficiency of a single lysosomal enzyme		
Sialidosis (mucolipidosis I)		
Type I[a]	α-Neuraminidase	Cherry-red spots, loss of visual acuity, punctate corneal opacities
Type II[b]	α-Neuraminidase	Cherry-red spots, fine corneal opacities
Mucolipidosis IV	Ganglioside sialidase	Corneal clouding, retinal degeneraton
Disorders of glycoprotein degradation		
Mannosidosis	α-D-Mannosidase	Spoke-shaped lens opacities
Fucosidosis	α-L-Fucosidase	Venous tortousities
Galactosialidosis	34 kD protein[c]	Cherry-red spots, corneal clouding[c]
Disorders of lysosomal enzyme phosphorylation and localization		
I-cell disease (mucolipidosis II, ML-II)	Lysosomal phosphotransferase[d]	Corneal opacities
Pseudo-Hurler polydystrophy (mucolipidosis III, ML-III)	Lysosomal phosphotransferase[d]	Corneal opacities

[a]Cherry-red spot–myoclonus phenotype; onset in second decade of life; normal somatic features.
[b]Onset early in life; dysostosis multiplex and visceromegaly; mental retardation; cherry-red spot in older children.
[c]Mutation at a locus on chromosome 22 that leads to deficiencies of both β-galactosidase and neuraminidase; corneal clouding is found only in the late infantile form.
[d]Defect in one of two enzymes required for synthesis of mannose-6-phosphate recognition marker that is essential for targeting of lysosomal enzymes.

spots are present in all cases examined [37]; in addition, mild corneal clouding and lens opacities have been reported [15,16].

The biochemical defect is a generalized deficiency of α-neuraminidase, an enzyme that cleaves terminal sialyl linkages in several oligosaccharides and glycoproteins [12,39,40,42]. The enzyme does not hydrolyze this linkage in gangliosides; hence storage substances that have so far been identified consist of sialic acid-containing oligosaccharides and glycoproteins. Other lysosomal acid hydrolases, including β-galactosidase, are within the normal range of activity.

Studies with human-mouse somatic cell hybrids show that two genes are necessary for the expression of α-neuraminidase; they are located on chromosomes 10 and 20 [29]. Fusion of cell hybrids lacking chromosome 10 or 20 with neuraminidase-deficient fibroblasts confirmed by complementation analysis that the sialidosis disorder results from a mutation on chromosome 10 that encodes the structural gene for neuraminidase. Mutation of the second gene required for neuraminidase expression on chromosome 20 causes another closely related disorder, galactosialidosis, discussed here.

Sialidosis Type II

This severe disorder has its onset in early infancy, although congenital as well as juvenile forms have also been described. Similar to sialidosis type I, cherry-red macular spots and myoclonus are the presenting symptoms. In addition, however, this form of sialidosis is accompanied by abnormal somatic features, including coarse facies and other features of dysostosis multiplex [15,16,26]. Joint stiffness, visceromegaly, and mental retardation are frequently seen, although the severity in individual cases is highly variable [9]. Tortuosity and saccular aneurysms of conjunctival and retinal vessels have also been described [16,37]. Death usually occurs during the first or second decade; however, living patients 25 years of age have been reported [16]. A high proportion of reported cases are of Japanese origin. The juvenile form of type II sialidosis was initially called Goldberg's syndrome [17], but this disorder is now classified as galactosialidosis (see Sec. III.C).

Despite the coarse facies and other skeletal changes resembling those found in some of the MPS, there is no mucopolysacchariduria, nor is there any evidence for storage of glycosaminoglycans (GAG). The biochemical defect, a deficiency of α-neuraminidase, is similar to that found in sialidosis type I.

B. Mucolipidosis IV

Clinical Features. Mucolipidosis IV is a lysosomal storage disorder with autosomal recessive inheritance [3]. The most striking presenting sign in virtually all cases of mucolipidosis IV is moderate to severe corneal clouding at birth or in early infancy. The intraocular pressure in all cases is normal. This disorder was first reported in Israel [11], and although the early cases studied suggested a high frequency among Ashkenazi Jews, several non-Jewish patients have also been described [14,34,35]. The clinical spectrum and developmental features of children from 20 Israeli families have been reviewed in detail [3]; other cases with similar clinical findings have been reported in the United States [19,31,41]. The true extent of this disorder is difficult to estimate because the presenting signs, corneal clouding and delayed motor development, are not always recognized as a distinct clinical entity; however, in addition to the preceding 20 cases, there are probably at least 40 additional known or highly suspect cases.

Psychomotor retardation and visual disturbances during the first year of life are the major presenting signs. Language development during the next few years is severely reduced or nonexistent. However, the patients are not completely devoid of cognitive function. Organomegaly, skeletal abnormalities, and other signs of MPS are absent in ML-IV; however, growth decelerates markedly by 2–3 years even though food intake is adequate. Facial dysplasia, kyphoscoliosis, and other severe physical changes have been observed in older patients, ages 21 and 23 [31,35]. The disorder has a protracted course, and life expectancy may be into the third decade or beyond.

Ocular Manifestations.   The most striking presenting sign in virtually all cases of mucolipidosis IV is moderate to severe corneal clouding at birth or in early infancy. The intraocular pressure in all cases is normal. Bilateral corneal clouding is a characteristic feature of ML-IV, although the onset of opacities may vary from early infancy to 5 years of age [3]. The corneal clouding varies from slight to dense and involves mainly the epithelium; it remains static in some patients, but in others it may continue to deteriorate or even to improve. The opacity involves mainly the anterior stroma and consists of punctate dots extending from the center of the cornea to the periphery [28,31]. There is no corneal edema.

Although the retina appears normal in most infants, electroretinograms (ERG) may be severely diminished or extinct [2]. Retinal changes are often difficult to evaluate because of the corneal clouding; however, subnormal [27] or extinguished [31] ERG, involving both the photopic and scotopic components, have been observed in two patients aged 2 and 14, respectively. A 9-year-old patient had an extinct ERG, flat visual evoked potentials, and progressive rod-cone impairment [1]. Severe optic atrophy has been observed in several patients [31,35,41].

Apart from corneal and retinal changes, esotropia and photophobia are present in nearly all patients [3]. They appear early in the course of the disease.

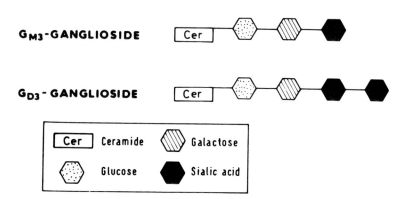

Figure 1 Structural forms of gangliosides accumulating in mucolipidosis type IV.

Electron microscopy of the cornea [14,19,28,35] reveals epithelial cells engorged with single-membrane–limited cytoplasmic vacuoles, some of which contain fibrillogranular material, whereas others are optically empty (Fig. 1). The corneal fibroblasts are somewhat distended and contain laminated structures in addition to the single-membrane–limited vacuoles. Bowman's layer is normal. The massive involvement of the corneal epithelium, with the stromal keratocytes relatively spared, is an important feature of ML-IV. Keratoplasty would be of little value because the replacement of donor epithelium by the host would be expected to bring about renewed clouding [19]. However, epithelial removal combined with transplantation of healthy conjunctiva in a 28-month-old patient resulted in improved corneal clarity that continued during the 1 year follow-up period [14].

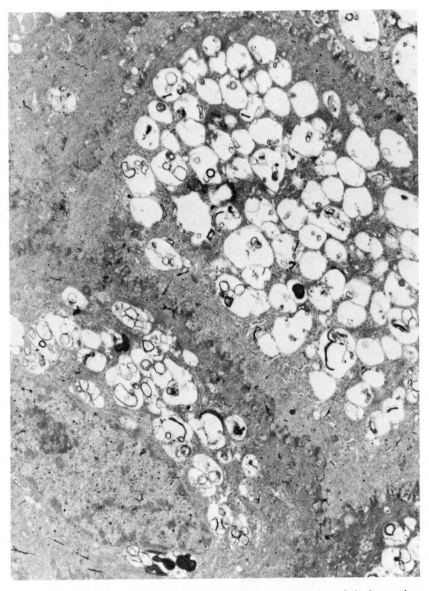

Figure 2 Corneal epithelium in mucolipidosis type IV showing accumulation of single-membrane–limited vacuoles, most of them optically empty but some of them containing lamellar deposits. (×6000) (Reproduced by courtesy of Dr. N. Livni.)

Striking changes have been noted in the conjunctiva [11,23,35], which provides one of the most reliable tissues for diagnosing this disorder. Epithelial cells as well as fibroblasts are filled with abnormal inclusion bodies similar to those found in the cornea (Fig. 2). The ultrastructural abnormalities are especially prominent in the conjunctival epithelium.

Postmortem examination of an eye from a 23-year-old patient revealed widespread changes, not only in the corneal epithelium and conjunctiva but also in other cells [35]. Light microscopy revealed a markedly disorganized and atrophic retina, with loss of photoreceptors together with intraretinal migration of pigment-laden macrophages. Electron microscopy revealed two types of storage bodies (membrane-limited vacuoles containing fibrillogranular material and lamellar whorls) in ciliary epithelial cells, Schwann cells, retinal ganglion cells, and vascular endothelial cells. The presence of these characteristic cytoplasmic inclusions is consistent with the storage of GAG and lipids.

Biochemistry.   The activities of lysosomal enzymes in leukocytes, plasma, and fibroblasts are within normal limits [11,31,35,41]. Those examined include α-fucosidase, β-glucuronidase, β-galactosidase, α-iduronidase, α-mannosidase, hexosaminidases A and B, and sulfatidase. Although the primary storage substances are not known with certainty, excess gangliosides have been detected in brain [41] and in cultured fibroblasts of several patients [5]. These have been identified as GM_3 and GD_3 gangliosides (Fig. 3), which differ from GM_1 and GM_2 gangliosides in that they lack N-acetylgalactosamine residues. They are classified as hematosides and are normally found mainly in extraneural tissues. In addition, despite normal GAG excretion, there is some evidence for abnormal intracellular metabolism of GAG in ML-IV.

A specific deficiency of a lysosomal ganglioside sialidase has been demonstrated in cultured fibro-

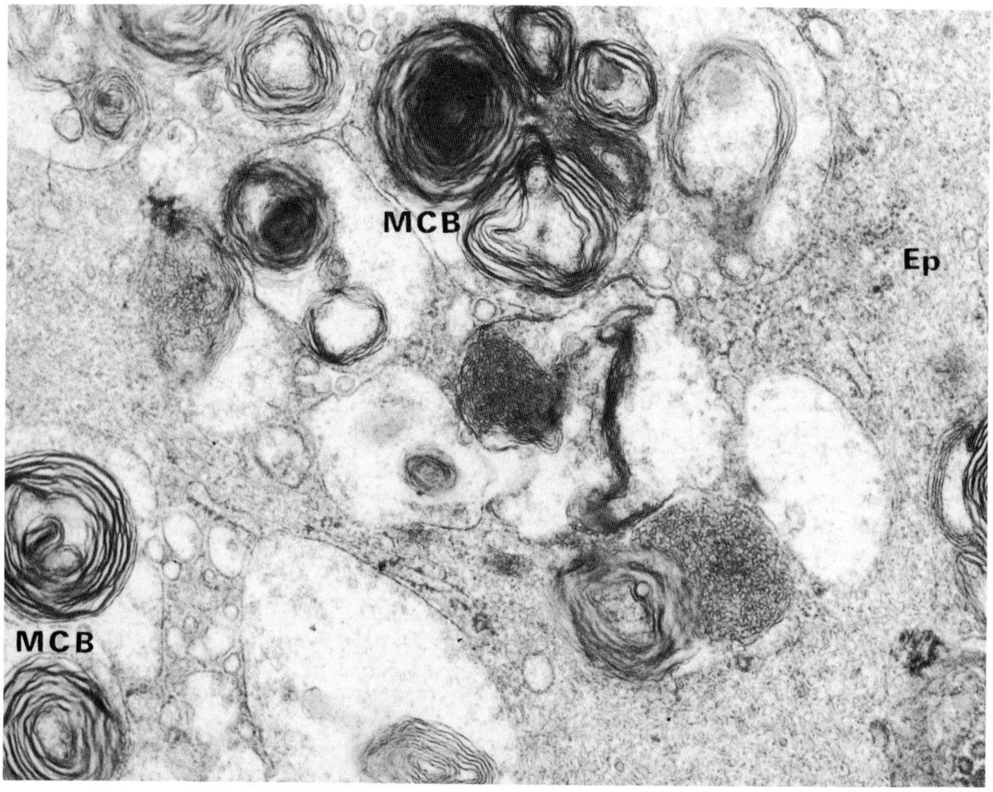

Figure 3   Conjunctival epithelial cell in mucolipidosis type IV filled with single-membrane–limited vacuoles and membranous lamellar bodies (MCB). Many of the lamellar deposits are contained within the vacuoles. Ep, epithelium. (×30,200) (Reproduced with permission from S. Merin, N. Livni, E.R. Berman, and S. Yatziv. Mucolipidosis IV: Ocular, systemic, and ultrastructural findings. *Invest. Ophthalmol. 14*:437–448, 1975.)

blasts of ML-IV patients [6]. Measurements of this enzyme activity often yield ambiguous results, however, leaving some doubt about whether this is the primary enzymatic defect [7]. Nevertheless, fibroblasts from ML-IV patients consistently accumulate larger amounts of exogenously supplied gangliosides than normal controls [47]. This finding provides a basis for accurate diagnosing of ML-IV patients.

Abnormalities in phospholipid metabolism have also been demonstrated in cultured fibroblasts from several patients [7,8]. These substances are identified as phosphatidylethanolamine, phosphatidylcholine, lysobisphosphatidic acid, and lysophosphatidylcholine. Pulse-chase experiments indicate a catabolic defect, yet all phospholipase enzymes measured showed normal activity. Phosphatidylcholine accumulates specifically in the lysosomal fraction of cultured fibroblasts, as well as in closely related endosomes. The defect leading to the accumulation of lysosomal phospholipids remains to be established, but as in several ganglioside storage disorders (see Chap. 29), the possibility of a defect in an activator protein cannot be excluded.

III. DISORDERS OF GLYCOPROTEIN DEGRADATION

A. Mannosidosis

Clinical and Ocular Manifestations.   At first thought to represent a variant of Hurler syndrome, mannosidosis is recognized clinically by coarse facies, psychomotor retardation, neural hearing loss, hepatosplenomegaly, gingival hyperplasia, and dysostosis multiplex [9,20,46].

Considerable heterogeneity is evident in this autosomal recessive disorder from reports of over 60 cases, who are now classified in two groups: type I is the severe infantile form with early death, and type II is the milder juvenile-adult phenotype with survival into adulthood [9]. Vacuolated lymphocytes are present in nearly all cases.

Ocular findings in mannosidosis are distinctive, especially lenticular lesions, which constitute the major ophthalmological manifestation in both forms of mannosidosis [4,22,30,46]. Moreover, the specific appearance of the lens opacity may provide an important tool for distinguishing between the two forms of the disease. A study of 42 cases of mannosidosis [22] showed that the type I (severe) form is almost always associated with confluent opacities forming a spokelike pattern in the posterior lens cortex [9,46]. This type of opacity is considered pathognomonic for type I mannosidosis by some investigators (Fig. 4). By contrast, only 4 of 17 patients with mannosidosis type II manifested lenticular changes, and these consisted of punctate opacities scattered randomly throughout the tissue rather than the wheellike patterns found in type I patients.

Other ocular findings are not consistent in all cases of mannosidosis [46]. Thus, corneal opacities are occasionally present, whereas fundus changes were noted in only 4 of the 42 patients examined by Letson and Desnick [22]. As in all the other mucolipidoses and MPS, the lysosomal nature of the disorder is expressed in the conjunctiva [23,46], where abnormal single-membrane–limited vacuoles containing fibrillogranular material are present in the fibroblasts (Fig. 5). They represent an intralysosomal accumulation of complex carbohydrates. Lipid storage is manifested either in the form of electron-dense globules or as lamellar bodies.

Biochemistry.   No mucopolysacchariduria is found in these patients. Instead, there is increased urinary excretion and tissue accumulation of mannose-rich asparagine-linked oligosaccharides, the principal one having the structure Man($\alpha1\rightarrow3$)-Man($\beta1\rightarrow4$)N-acetylglucosamine [2,9]. The failure to catabolize oligosaccharides of this type is due to a generalized deficiency of the heat-stable lysosomal acid form of α-mannosidase [9,20]. Another form of this enzyme, a heat-labile cytoplasmic glycosidase with optimum activity at about pH 6, is normal in mannosidosis patients. Most diagnoses have been made using either leukocytes or cultured fibroblasts, with the enzyme assayed at pH 4.0 or lower using substrate concentrations not exceeding 1 mM. Tears are an excellent source of α-mannosidase isoenzymes, in which normal levels are 10-fold higher than in serum or leukocytes (see Chap. 26). In five proven cases of α-mannosidosis, only about 7–20% of normal activity was present in tear fluid [45].

Immunological studies suggest that mannosidosis is caused by a defect of a structural gene, leading to the formation of an enzyme with lower, although not totally lacking, affinity for its substrate. Studies with human-mouse and human-Chinese hamster somatic cell hybrids have led to the assignment of the acid α-mannosidase structural gene to chromosome 19 in humans [13], and more recent investigations have mapped the gene locus to 19p13.2-q12 [9].

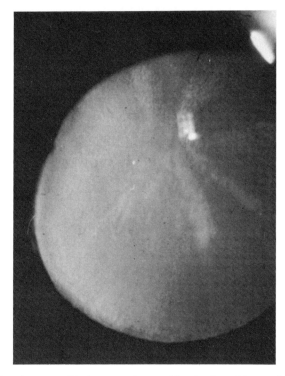

Figure 4 Cataractous lens in mannosidosis as seen by retroillumination with magnification. The opacities, in the form of spokes radiating from a central hub, are composed of small round vacuoles lying at different depths in the lens. (Reproduced courtesy of Dr. A. Linn Murphree.)

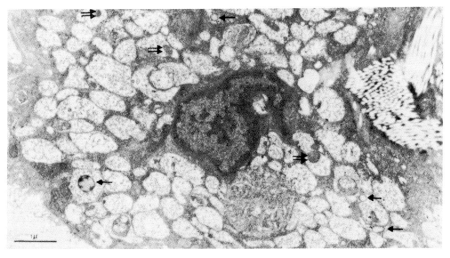

Figure 5 Conjunctival fibroblast in a 25-year-old patient with mannosidosis, mild type. The cytoplasm is engorged with single-membrane–limited vacuoles containing fibrillogranular material. Opaque lipid deposits (arrows) and dense round bodies (double arrows) are also found inside the vacuoles. (×10,400) (Reproduced with permission from J. Libert. Discussion. *Birth Defects* 12(3):329–330, 1976.)

Analyses of the storage products in mannosidosis have contributed to our understanding of both the normal pathway(s) of glycoprotein degradation and the aberrant pathways in mannosidosis patients [2]. The lysosomal catabolism of glycoproteins containing asparagine-linked oligosaccharides in normal cells proceeds in two steps. First, the polypeptide chain is degraded by the action of endopeptidases (cathepsins), peptidases, and carboxyexopeptidases, resulting in the release of amino acids and asparagine-linked oligosaccharides. The latter are then degraded at the reducing terminus by aspartyl N-acetylglucosaminidase and endohexosaminidase and at the nonreducing terminus by exoglycosidases. The lysosomal enzyme α-mannosidase is an exoglycosidase that cleaves α-mannosidic linkages present in complex, hybrid, and high-mannose N-linked oligosaccharides. In the lysosomal storage disease mannosidoses, oligosaccharides with α-linked mannose residues at the non-reducing terminus are not hydrolyzed. As a result, these oligosaccharides accumulate in the tissues and are also excreted in large quantities in the urine.

B. Fucosidosis

Clinical and Ocular Manifestations.   This rare autosomal recessive disorder is characterized by progressive psychomotor retardation, coarse facies, mild dysostosis multiplex, growth retardation, and often but not always mild hepatosplenomegaly and cardiomegaly. At least 40 cases of this disorder have been reported in the world literature [9]. As in other lysosomal disorders, genetic heterogeneity is also an important feature of fucosidosis. A fatal infantile form, referred to as type I, accounts for about 60% of the patients. The type II phenotype is characterized by psychomotor retardation beginning during the first or second year of life. The other clinical signs are similar to those found in type I, except that angiokeratomatous lesions resembling those in Fabry's disease are present in type II fucosidosis; moreover, there is longer survival, often to adulthood, and mental retardation appears later than in the type I phenotype [24,36].

The major ocular abnormality in fucosidosis is tortuosity of conjunctival vessels, always present in the severe form but not always seen in the adult phenotype [24]. The conjunctival vessels are dilated and tortuous and have local fusiform and saccular microaneurysms. Similarly, the retinal veins are dilated and tortuous. Corneal opacities are variable and may not be directly related to the disease.

Several specific ultrastructural changes that may be pathognomonic for fucosidosis are found in the conjunctiva by transmission electron microscopy [24]. The epithelial cells contain numerous single-membrane–bound inclusion bodies measuring 0.3–0.4 μm in diameter and filled with both fibrillogranular and concentric lamellar material (Fig. 6). Conjunctival fibroblasts are distended and contain two types of abnormal storage bodies (Fig. 7). The most abundant appear as clear vacuoles containing delicate reticular material. They are similar in structure to those found in both the epithelium and connective tissue cells of the conjunctiva in the MPS. The second type of inclusion body is unique to fucosidosis and consists of dark, dense granules with homogeneous matrices. The latter are not generally found in other mucolipidoses or in the sphingolipidoses. Two types of membrane-limited vacuoles also accumulate in the endothelial cells of the conjunctival capillaries. The most common of these consist of electron-lucent inclusion bodies often containing fine reticular material. The other less frequent type appears as round or oval electron-dense vacuoles. Lamellar material is occasionally present in both types. These changes are probably responsible for the vascular tortuosities in the mild phenotype of fucosidosis. The important and specific changes present in the conjunctiva provide an easily accessible tissue for biopsy and a tissue diagnosis of fucosidosis [24]. Cytoplasmic inclusion bodies are also found in conjunctival and corneal epithelium, conjunctival, corneal, and scleral fibroblasts, corneal endothelium, and other ocular tissues, but the lysosomal swelling is not as severe and hence causes no functional impairment.

Biochemistry and Molecular Genetics.   In both types of fucosidosis, there is a generalized deficiency of the lysosomal enzyme α-L-fucosidase, with concomitant accumulation of fucose-containing sphingolipids and oligosaccharides in body tissues. Ultrastructural studies of biopsy specimens from liver reveal foamy cytoplasm in hepatocytes and in Kupffer's cells; these cells contain vacuoles that are heterogeneous in appearance, as in conjunctiva described earlier.

The major glycolipid accumulating is the H antigen glycolipid: Fuc(α1→2)Gal(β1→4)N-acetyl-glucosamine-α-Gal-ceramide [9]. At least 22 other oligosaccharides and asparagine-linked oligosaccharides have also been isolated and identified in urine and tissues of fucosidosis patients. Blood group substances are determined by oligosaccharide chains linked to proteins or lipids. The H, Le[a], and Le[b] antigens are determined by the presence of fucosyltransferases. The genotype at these loci may determine

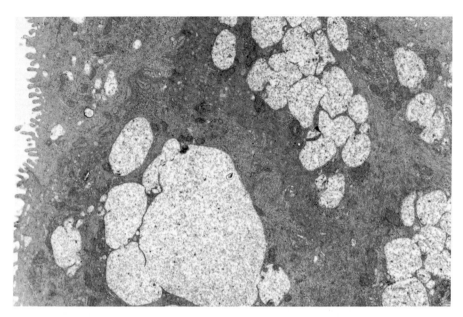

Figure 6 Superficial layer of the conjunctival epithelium in a child with the severe form of fucosidosis. The cytoplasm contains numerous single-membrane–limited vacuoles filled with fibrillogranular material. (×8700) (Reproduced with permission from J. Libert, F. van Hoof, and M. Tondeur. Fucosidosis: Ultrastructural study of conjunctiva and skin and enzyme analysis of tears. *Invest. Ophthalmol. 15*:626–639, 1976.)

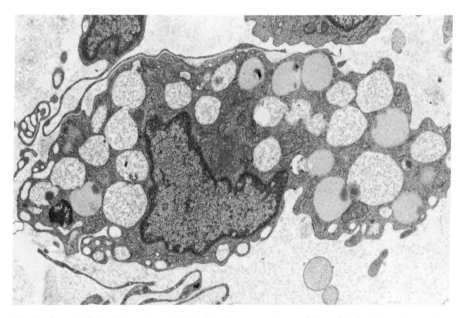

Figure 7 Conjunctival fibroblasts in a child with the severe form of fucosidosis. Two abnormal types of inclusion bodies are present: single-membrane–limited vacuoles filled with fibrillogranular material and dense inclusion bodies with homogeneous matrix often containing small dense aggregates within. (×9600) (Reproduced with permission from J. Libert, F. van Hoof, and M. Tondeur. Fucosidosis: Ultrastructural study of conjunctiva and skin and enzyme analysis of tears. *Invest. Ophthalmol. 15*:626–639, 1976.)

the exact nature of the stored material in fucosidosis patients and could in part explain the heterogeneous types of material stored in these patients.

Studies with cDNA clones have established that the lysosomal enzyme α-L-fucosidase is a tetramer composed of four identical 50 kD subunits [9]. Detailed kinetic analysis has revealed four active sites per tetrameric complex. The enzyme is located on chromosome 1 and has recently been mapped to band p34 [9]. Using molecular cloning techniques, a cDNA has been isolated that codes for at least 80% of the mature α-L-fucosidase protein. Molecular evidence for the presence of heterogeneity among fucosidosis patients is now available. The structural locus for the enzyme is designated FUCA1 [9] and is associated with an electrophoretic polymorphism with three alleles, one of which is the silent allele causing fucosidosis.

C. Galactosialidosis

Clinical Features. Galactosialidosis has been recognized as a distinct lysosomal storage disorder only during the past few years, although the phenotype was first described by Goldberg and coworkers more than two decades ago [17]. This disorder has often been misdiagnosed as either GM_1 gangliosidosis or juvenile-onset sialidosis type II [16,34]. It has also been termed the cherry-red spot with dementia syndrome. The finding that this specific phenotype is associated with a combined deficiency of β-galactosidase and α-neuraminidase, as discussed later, has greatly enhanced our understanding of this disorder, now known to be transmitted as an autosomal recessive trait.

Galactosialidosis, like virtually all other inherited lysosomal disorders, is heterogeneous in clinical signs, age of onset, and severity [34]. Myoclonus is found in all cases, but other clinical features are variable. The presenting signs in the early infantile form include edema, ascites, skeletal dysplasia, and macular cherry-red spots. A late infantile form that develops after 6 or 12 months of age is characterized by dysostosis multiplex, mild mental retardation, visceromegaly, and macular cherry-red spots. The largest number of patients observed to date have a late juvenile form with onset at any time between infancy and adulthood. These patients, mainly of Japanese origin, have somewhat different presenting signs from those found in the first two phenotypes. The major features of the late juvenile form are skeletal dysplasia, Hurler-like facies, dysmorphism, progressive neurological deterioration, angiokeratomatous rash, corneal clouding, and macular cherry-red spots. Survival is usually into adulthood.

Ocular Manifestations. Macular cherry-red spots are pathognomonic for all forms of galactosialidosis. Corneal clouding is observed only in the late infantile type. Detailed histochemical and electron microscopic studies in a 13-year-old patient with this form of galactosialidosis disclosed an extensive loss of ganglion cells and optic atrophy [44]. The ganglion cells that remained were swollen and had numerous cytoplasmic inclusion bodies and abnormal accumulations of lipids and proteins that were tentatively characterized as phospholipids and lipofuscinlike substances. Amacrine cells had similar storage substances. Rather unexpectedly, macular cherry-red spots were not observed in this patient before death. Usui and colleagues [44] reasoned that the cherry-red spots were probably present at an early age, while abnormal storage substances were accumulating. Afterward they may have faded owing to the extensive loss of ganglion cells. The optic atrophy was considered secondary to ganglion cell death.

Biochemistry and Molecular Genetics. All forms of galactosialidosis are characterized by deficiencies in two lysosomal enzymes, β-galactosidase and α-neuraminidase [16,34]. The disorder was distinguished from GM_1 gangliosidosis on the basis of complementation analyses using somatic cell hybridization, which showed that the two diseases resulted from different gene mutations [34]. Other studies using human-mouse somatic cell hybrids have in addition differentiated sialidosis from galactosialidosis; the former results from a mutation on chromosome 10 that encodes the neuraminidase structural gene and latter from a mutation in a second gene on chromosome 20 that is required for neuraminidase expression [29].

Combined deficiencies of two enzymes in an inherited lysosomal disorder are unusual and difficult to understand in terms of molecular genetics. However, one explanation has been forthcoming from the observation that galactosialidosis patients have a severe deficiency of a 32 kD protective protein that prevents intralysosomal proteolytic degradation of the two enzymes [34]. In normal cells this protective protein, which is coded by a locus on chromosome 22, is thought to form a multimolecular aggregate with β-galactosidase and α-neuraminidase that stabilizes the enzymes and prevents their proteolysis. In its absence, the two enzymes may be partially degraded and hence lose their catalytic activity. This interesting hypothesis requires further study [34].

IV. DISORDERS OF LYSOSOMAL ENZYME PHOSPHORYLATION AND LOCALIZATION

Two disorders, I-cell disease (ML-II) and pseudo-Hurler polydystrophy (ML-III) are now recognized as belonging to a distinct subgroup of mucolipidoses (Table 1). They are inherited as autosomal recessive traits, and although closely linked biochemically, with both phenotypes manifesting multiple lysosomal enzyme deficiencies, the clinical features of the two disorders are strikingly different.

A. I-Cell Disease (Mucolipidosis II)

Clinical Features. I-cell disease is a very severe neurodegenerative disorder having many features in common with Hurler syndrome (MPS I-H). A unique characteristic of ML-II, noted in its first description as a clinical entity, is the presence of inclusion bodies throughout the cytoplasm of fibroblasts from affected individuals [32]. The cells were termed inclusion cells (I cells), and the disorder was subsequently named I-cell disease. Evidence, albeit indirect, for storage of both lipids and complex carbohydrates led to its classification as a mucolipidosis [38]. This disorder is characterized by an early onset of psychomotor retardation, craniofacial abnormalities, course facial features, severe skeletal abnormalities, restricted joint movement, visceromegaly, and gingival hyperplasia. There is no mucopolysacchariduria. In the next few years, developmental delay and failure to thrive are prominent features; facial and skeletal changes become more pronounced. Cardiorespiratory complications usually lead to death during the fifth to seventh years, although cases of longer survival have been reported [32].

Ocular Manifestations. Corneal clouding is not always obvious in ML-II; for example, mild opacities consisting of diffuse stromal granularities were seen on slit-lamp examination in only 14 of 35 ML-II patients [25]. They generally appear as a late clinical development. This correlates well with ultrastructural changes, since the keratocytes are not extensively swollen and Bowman's layer is normal in infants under 8 months of age; moreover, extracellular deposits in the stroma are not observed and the collagen fibrils are regularly arranged. However, the keratocytes are grossly distended by the accumulation of membrane-limited inclusion bodies in older patients (Fig. 8) with ophthalmoscopically visible corneal clouding [25].

As in other MLS and in the MPS, the genetic defect is expressed in characteristic ultrastructural changes in the conjunctiva (Fig. 9). Connective tissue cells are ballooned and packed with two types of storage vacuole, single-membrane–limited inclusions with fibrillogranular material similar to those found in the MPS and membranous lamellar bodies resembling the inclusion bodies in the sphingolipidoses. The severity of the conjunctival abnormalities is not related to the corneal changes, since corneal clouding, even when present, is relatively mild in ML-II.

B. Pseudo-Hurler Polydystrophy (Mucolipidosis III)

Clinical Features. ML-III (pseudo-Hurler polydystrophy) is a relatively mild condition, without obvious neurological signs, and compatible with a reasonably long life span [32]. Onset is usually between 2 and 4 years of age. Stiffness of hands and restriction of shoulder movements are among the earliest signs. About 50% of ML-III patients have learning disabilities, and mild mental retardation is thought to be present in all patients. The disease is slowly progressive, and by about 6 years of age, claw-hand deformities, scoliosis, and short stature are obvious. Progressive destruction of the hip joints develops early, and skeletal dysplasia is also apparent in hands, elbows, and shoulders. Severe pelvic and vertebral changes develop during the second decade of life and are considered characteristic of ML-III; they are more severe in males than in females, for unknown reasons [32]. Survival is into the fourth or fifth decade.

Ocular Manifestations. Fine discrete stromal opacities, observable by slit-lamp and best seen by biomicroscopy with scleral scatter illumination, are found in virtually all ML-III patients [15,43]. The opacities involve both the central and peripheral regions of the cornea but do not interfere with vision. No ultrastructural studies of the cornea are available, but conjunctival biopsies have revealed changes similar, although not completely identical, to those found in ML-II [43]. The conjunctival fibroblasts are filled to varying degrees with single-membrane–limited inclusion bodies containing fibrillogranular material. Lamellar inclusions are seen only rarely in the fibroblasts but are abundant in the capillary endothelial cells. The conjunctival epithelium is normal.

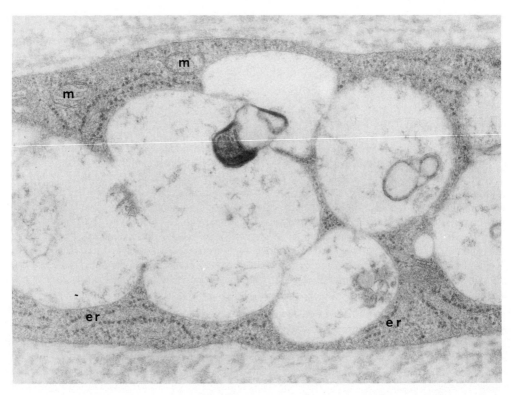

Figure 8   Corneal fibroblasts in mucolipidosis type II are distended by clear single-membrane–limited vacuoles containing fine fibrillogranular material nonhomogeneously dispersed and occasional lamellar whorls. Both the mitochondria (m) and the endoplasmic reticulum (er) are normal in appearance. (×40,000) (Reproduced with permission from J. Libert, F. van Hoof, J.P. Farriaux, and D. Toussaint. Ocular findings in I-cell disease (mucolipidosis type II). *Am. J. Ophthalmol. 83*:617–628, 1977.)

There appears to be no obvious relationship between the severity of the ultrastructural changes in the conjunctiva and the degree of corneal clouding in ML-II and ML-III. Conjunctival abnormalities are considered more severe in ML-II than in ML-III, yet corneal clouding, which is a constant feature of ML-III, is either mild or totally absent in ML-II [25]. It is curious that despite the similar biochemical defect in these two MLS, the clinical signs in the cornea and the pathological changes in the conjunctiva are distinctly different.

Hyperopic astigmatism, optic disk edema, and surface wrinkling maculopathy have been described in several ML-III patients [43]. Visual field defects were found in three of four patients examined; visual acuity is relatively stable despite mild retinopathy.

Biochemistry and Molecular Genetics.   Early studies using cultured fibroblasts from ML-II [18] and ML-III [10] patients showed a striking intracellular deficiency of eight or more lysosomal acid hydrolases and a concomitant excess, extracellularly, in the culture medium. Similarly, in patients with these disorders cells of mesenchymal origin show the same pattern of intracellular enzyme deficiency combined with greatly elevated levels of acid hydrolases in serum, body fluids, and urine [21]. This is one of the most striking biochemical features of ML-II and ML-III and provides the basis for diagnosis of affected individuals [32]. Serum levels in these patients are 10–20 times higher than in normal controls; cultured fibroblasts can also be used, and in this case the ratios of extracellular to intracellular enzyme activities are a reliable parameter in the diagnosis.

A key observation by Hickman and Neufeld [18] led to the hypothesis that the major defect in ML-II fibroblasts is the inability to internalize lysosomal enzymes secreted into the medium. These experiments suggested that lysosomal enzymes contain a recognition marker for uptake and transport from the

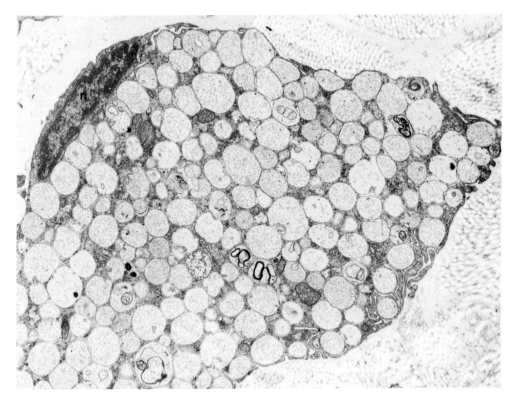

Figure 9 Distended conjunctival fibroblast from a patient with mucolipidosis II. The cell is engorged with single-membrane–limited inclusion bodies containing fine granular material of various density. The nucleus (n) of the fibroblast is displaced to the periphery. (×12,000) (Reproduced with permission from J. Libert, F. van Hoof, J.P. Farriaux, and D. Toussaint. Ocular findings in I-cell disease (mucolipidosis type II). *Am. J. Ophthalmol. 83*:617–628, 1977.)

extracellular medium to the lysosomes and that the lysosomal hydrolases from ML-II fibroblasts lacked the required marker. This hypothesis proved to be correct, and a decade or more of investigations in many laboratories has elucidated not only the normal pathway(s) for lysosomal enzyme biogenesis, but also the specific defect in ML-II and ML-III patients.

The biogenesis of soluble lysosomal acid hydrolases was described in Chapter 26, and a detailed summary of this process has been presented by Nolan and Sly [32]. The major steps in the biosynthesis and transport of lysosomal enzymes are presented here. Lysosomal enzymes, together with many membrane proteins and proteins destined for secretion, are synthesized on endoplasmic reticulum-bound ribosomes. They contain a specific "signal sequence" that promotes the formation of a complex with a signal recognition particle (SRP). This complex then binds to an SRP and is transported into the lumen of the endoplasmic reticulum. The signal peptide is then cleaved, and the acid hydrolases are modified in the endoplasmic reticulum by the addition of high-mannose oligosaccharides. These enzymes are trimmed and modified and are then transferred to the Golgi apparatus for further processing. It is in the cis (or early) Golgi apparatus [13a] that many acid hydrolases are specifically modified by the addition of the mannose 6-phosphate (Man-6-P) marker. This addition occurs in two enzymatic steps. The first is the addition of an α-N-acetylglucosamine-1-phosphate residue to the 6 position of mannose, resulting in the formation of a phosphodiester intermediate. This step is catalyzed by a lysosomal N-acetylglucaminylphosphotransferase, the phosphotransferase. The second step involves removal of the N-acetylglucosamine residue to expose the Man-6-P marker.

Only acid hydrolases containing the Man-6-P marker can be recognized by specific membrane receptors that direct their transfer to lysosomes. One, which does not require divalent cations for binding activity, is called the cation-independent mannose phosphate receptor. The cDNA for this receptor has been cloned, and amino acid sequencing studies indicate a molecular mass of about 270 kD [13a]. The second receptor has a smaller mass, 46 kD, and requires divalent cations; it has also been cloned and sequenced. The relative role of these two receptors in the targeting of Man-6-P-containing lysosomal enzymes is not entirely clear, but both are active in binding acid hydrolases. These complexes are transferred to a prelysosomal compartment thought to be an endosomelike vesicle, in which the Man-6-P-containing lysosomal enzyme is dissociated from the receptors. The latter are recycled to the Golgi apparatus, and the acid hydrolases are transported to lysosomes to form primary lysosomes.

In certain cell types, such as fibroblasts, lysosomal enzymes may be internalized from the medium, a process mediated by cation-independent Man-6-P receptors [13a]. These plasma membrane-associated receptors account for only about 10–20% of the total cellular complement of receptors in fibroblasts and are negligible in most other cell types [13a]. However, it was the discovery of the plasma membrane receptors that led to the identification of a defect in this pathway in ML-II (and, later, in ML-III).

The primary enzymatic defect in all ML-II and ML-III patients is the phosphotransferase enzyme [32]. All other steps in the complex biogenesis of lysosomal enzymes in these patients are normal. The phosphotransferase enzyme can now be assayed in fibroblasts: there is little or no detectable activity in ML-II patients, whereas in ML-III patients, residual activity representing about 2–20% of that found in normal fibroblasts has been detected [32]. This is consistent with the clinical course of the two disorders, but further understanding of these disorders awaits cloning of the phosphotransferase enzyme and identification of mutant alleles.

REFERENCES

1. Abraham, F.A., Brand, N., and Blumenthal, M. Retinal function in mucolipidosis IV. *Ophthalmologica 191*:210–214, 1985.
2. Al Daher, S., de Gasperi, R., Daniel, P., Hall, N., Warren, C.D., and Winchester, B. The substrate-specificity of human lysosomal αD-mannosidase in relation to genetic α-mannosidosis. *Biochem. J. 277*:743–751, 1991.
3. Amir, N., Zlotogora, J., and Bach, G. Mucolipidosis type IV: Clinical spectrum and natural history. *Pediatrics 79*:953–959, 1987.
4. Arbisser, A.I., Murphree, A.L., Garcia, C.A., and Howell, R.R. Ocular findings in mannosidosis. *Am. J. Ophthalmol. 82*:465–471, 1976.
5. Bach, G., Cohen, M.M., and Kohn, G. Abnormal ganglioside accumulation in cultured fibroblasts from patients with mucolipidosis IV. *Biochem. Biophys. Res. Commun. 66*:1483–1490, 1975.
6. Bach, G., Zeigler, M., Schaap, T., and Kohn, G. Mucolipidosis type IV ganglioside sialidase deficiency. *Biochem. Biophys. Res. Commun. 90*:1341–1347, 1979.
7. Bargal, R., and Bach, G. Phospholipid accumulation in mucolipidosis IV cultured fibroblasts. *J. Inherited Metab. Dis. 11*:144–150, 1988.
8. Bargal, R., and Bach, G. Phosphatidylcholine storage in mucolipidosis IV. *Clin. Chim. Acta 181*:167–174, 1989.
9. Beaudet, A.L., and Thomas, G.T. Disorders of glycoprotein degradation: Mannosidosis, fucosidosis, sialidosis, and aspartylglycosaminuria. In *The Metabolic Basis of Inherited Disease*, 6th ed., C.R. Scriver, A.L. Beaudet, W.S. Sly, and D. Valle (Eds.), McGraw-Hill, New York, pp. 1603–1621, 1989.
10. Berman, E.R., Kohn, G., Yatziv, S., and Stein, H. Acid hydrolase deficiencies and abnormal glycoproteins in mucolipidosis III (pseudo-Hurler polydystrophy). *Clin. Chim. Acta 52*:115–124, 1974.
11. Berman, E.R., Livni, N., Shapira, E., Merin, S., and Levij, I.S. Congenital corneal clouding with abnormal systemic storage bodies: A new variant of mucolipidosis. *J. Pediatr. 84*:519–526, 1974.
12. Cantz, M., Gehler, J., and Spranger, J. Mucolipidosis I: Increased sialic acid content and deficiency of an α-N-acetylneuraminidase in cultured fibroblasts. *Biochem. Biophys. Res. Commun. 74*:732–738, 1977.
13. Champion, M.J., and Shows, T.B. Mannosidosis: Assignment of the lysosomal α-mannosidase B gene to chromosome 19 in man. *Proc. Natl. Acad. Sci. USA 74*:2968–2972, 1977.
13a. Dahms, N.M., Lobel, P., and Kornfeld, S. Mannose 6-phosphate receptors and lysosomal enzyme targeting. *J. Biol. Chem. 264*:12115–12118, 1989.
14. Dangel, M.E., Bremer, D.L., and Rogers, G.L. Treatment of corneal opacification in mucolipidosis IV with conjunctival transplantation. *Am. J. Ophthalmol. 99*:137–141, 1985.
15. Dangel, M.E., and Mauger, T. Mucolipidoses. In *The Eye in Systemic Disease*, D.H. Gold and T.A. Weingeist (Eds.), J. B. Lippincott, Philadelphia, pp. 369–372, 1990.
16. Deutsch, J.A., and Asbell, P.A. Sialidosis and galactosialidosis. In *The Eye in Systemic Disease*, D.H. Gold and T.A. Weingeist (Eds.), J. B. Lippincott, Philadelphia, pp. 376–377, 1990.
17. Goldberg, M.F., Cotlier, E., Fichensher, L.G., Kenyon, K., Enat, R., and Borowsky, S.A. Macular cherry-red

spot, corneal clouding, and β-galactosidase deficiency. Clinical, biochemical, and electron microscopic study of a new autosomal recessive storage disease. *Arch. Intern. Med. 128*:387–398, 1971.

18. Hickman, S., and Neufeld, E.F. A hypothesis for I-cell disease: Defective hydrolases that do not enter lysosomes. *Biochem. Biophys. Res. Commun. 49*:992–999, 1972.

19. Kenyon, K.R., Maumenee, I.H., Green, W.R., Libert, J., and Hiatt, R.L. Mucolipidosis IV-histopathology of conjunctiva, cornea and skin. *Arch. Ophthalmol. 97*:1106–1111, 1979.

20. Kistler, J.P., Lott, I.T., Kolodny, E.H., Friedman, R.B., Nersasian, R., Schnur, J., Mihm, M.C., Dvorak, A.M., and Dickersin, R. Mannosidosis. New clinical presentation, enzyme studies, and carbohydrate analysis. *Arch. Neurol. 34*:45–51, 1977.

21. Kress, B.C., and Miller, A.L. Urinary lysosomal hydrolases in mucolipidosis II and mucolipidosis III. *Biochem. J. 177*:409–415, 1979.

22. Letson, R.D., and Desnick, R.J. Punctate lenticular opacities in type II mannosidosis. *Am. J. Ophthalmol. 85*: 218–224, 1978.

23. Libert, J. Discussion. *Birth Defects 12*(3):329–330, 1976.

24. Libert, J. Fucosidosis. In *The Eye in Systemic Disease*, D.H. Gold and T.A. Weingeist (Eds.), J. B. Lippincott, Philadelphia, pp. 358–360, 1990.

25. Libert, J., van Hoof, F., Farriaux, J.P., and Toussaint, D. Ocular findings in I-cell disease (mucolipidosis type II). *Am. J. Ophthalmol. 83*:617–628, 1977.

26. Lowden, J.A., and O'Brien, J.S. Sialidosis: A review of human neuraminidase deficiency. *Am. J. Hum. Genet. 31*:1–18, 1979.

27. Merin, S., Livni, N., Berman, E.R., and Yatziv, S. Mucolipidosis IV: Ocular, systemic, and ultrastructural findings. *Invest. Ophthalmol. 14*:437–448, 1975.

28. Merin, S., Nemet, P., Livni, N., and Lazar, M. The cornea in mucolipidosis IV. *J. Pediatr. Ophthalmol. 13*:289–295, 1976.

29. Mueller, O.T., Henry, W.M., Haley, L.L., Byers, M.G., Eddy, R.L., and Shows, T.B. Sialidosis and galacto-sialidosis: Chromosomal assignment of two genes associated with neuraminidase-deficiency disorders. *Proc. Natl. Acad. Sci. USA 83*:1817–1821, 1986.

30. Murphree, A.L., Beaudet, A.L., Palmer, E.A., and Nichols, B.L., Jr. Cataract in mannosidosis. *Birth Defects 12*(3):319–325, 1976.

31. Newell, F.W., Matalon, R., and Meyer, S. A new mucolipidosis with psychomotor retardation, corneal clouding, and retinal degeneration. *Am. J. Ophthalmol. 80*:440–449, 1975.

32. Nolan, C.M., and Sly, W.S. I-Cell disease and pseudo-Hurler polydystrophy: Disorders of lysosomal enzyme phosphorylation and localization. In *The Metabolic Basis of Inherited Disease*, 6th ed., C.R. Scriver, A.L. Beaudet, W.S. Sly, and D. Valle (Eds.), McGraw-Hill, New York, pp. 1589–1601, 1989.

33. O'Brien, J.S. The cherry red spot-myoclonus syndrome: A newly recognized inherited lysosomal storage disease due to acid neuraminidase deficiency. *Clin. Genet. 14*:55–60, 1978.

34. O'Brien, J.S. β-Galactosidase deficiency (GM$_1$ gangliosidosis, galactosialidosis, and Morquio syndrome type B); ganglioside sialidase deficiency (mucolipidosis IV). In *The Metabolic Basis of Inherited Disease*, 6th ed., C.R. Scriver, A.L. Beaudet, W.S. Sly, and D. Valle (Eds.), McGraw-Hill, New York, pp. 1797–1806, 1989.

35. Riedel, K.G., Zwann, J., and Kenyon, K.R. Ocular abnormalities in mucolipidosis IV. *Am. J. Ophthalmol. 99*: 125–136, 1985.

36. Snyder, R.D., Carlow, T.J., Ledman, J., and Wenger, D.A. Ocular findings in fucosidosis. *Birth Defects 12*(3): 241–251, 1976.

37. Sogg, R.L., Steinman, L., Rathjen, B., Tharp, B.R., and O'Brien, J.S. Cherry-red spot-myoclonus syndrome. *Ophthalmology 86*:1861–1870, 1979.

38. Spranger, J.W., and Wiedemann, H.R. The genetic mucolipidoses: Diagnosis and differential diagnosis. *Humangenetik 9*:113–139, 1970.

39. Spranger, J., Gehler, J., and Cantz, M. Mucolipidosis I-a sialidosis. *Am. J. Med. Genet. 1*:21–29, 1977.

40. Swallow, D.M., Evans, L., Stewart, G., Thomas, P.K., and Abrams, J.D. Sialidosis type I: Cherry red spot–myoclonus syndrome with sialidase deficiency and altered electrophoretic mobility of some enzymes known to be glycoproteins. II. Enzyme studies. *Ann. Hum. Genet. 43*:27–35, 1979.

41. Tellez-Nagel, I., Rapin, I., Iwamoto, T., Johnson, A.B., Norton, W.T., and Nitowsky, H. Mucolipidosis IV. Clinical, ultrastructural, histochemical, and chemical studies of a case, including a brain biopsy. *Arch. Neurol. 33*:828–835, 1976.

42. Thomas, G.H., Tipton, R.E., Ch'ien, L.T., Reynolds, L.W., and Miller, C.S. Sialidase (α-N-acetyl neuraminidase) deficiency: The enzyme defect in an adult with macular cherry-red spots and myoclonus without dementia. *Clin. Genet. 13*:369–379, 1978.

43. Traboulsi, E.I., and Maumenee, I.G. Ophthalmologic findings in mucolipidosis III (pseudo-Hurler polydystrophy). *Am. J. Ophthalmol. 102*:592–597, 1986.

44. Usui, T., Sawaguchi, S., Abe, H., Iwata, K., and Oyanagi, K. Late-infantile type galactosialidosis. Histopathology of the retina and optic nerve. *Arch. Ophthalmol. 109*:542–546, 1991.

45. van Hoof, F., Libert, J., Aubert-Tulkens, G., and Serra, M.V. The assay of lacrimal enzymes and the ultrastructural analysis of conjunctival biopsies: New techniques for the study of inborn lysosomal diseases. *Metab. Ophthalmol. 1*:165–171, 1977.

46. Weiss, A.H. Mannosidosis. In *The Eye in Systemic Disease*, D.H. Gold and T.A. Weingeist (Eds.), J. B. Lippincott, Philadelphia, pp. 368–369, 1990.

47. Zeigler, M., and Bach, G. Internalization of exogenous gangliosides in cultured skin fibroblasts for the diagnosis of mucolipidosis IV. *Clin. Chim. Acta 157*:183–190, 1986.

31

Disorders of Amino Acid Metabolism and Melanin Pigmentation

Gordon K. Klintworth

Duke University Medical Center, Durham, North Carolina

I. DISORDERS OF PHENYLALANINE AND TYROSINE METABOLISM

Of the many genetic disorders that express themselves as specific defects of amino acid metabolism, some, including two of Garrod's four original "inborn errors of metabolism" (albinism and alkaptonuria), produce significant abnormalities in the ocular tissues (88). Several abnormalities in the metabolism of the essential amino acid phenylalanine and its oxidized derivative tyrosine are recognized. From the standpoint of the eye, albinism, alkaptonuria, and tyrosinemia are the most important.

A. Albinism

The appellation "albinism" (Latin *albus*, white) embraces a heterogeneous collection of genetically determined conditions typified by decreased melanin pigmentation in the eye and skin (157,218,272, 282,284,286). Albinism is common, and its various forms affect about 1 in 10,000 births in the United States. An additional 1–2% of the population has normal pigmentation but is heterozygous for a recessive allele for albinism (286). Albinism exemplifies an inherited deficiency of a metabolic product (a partial or total reduction in melanin deposition on melanosomes). Of the various forms of human albinism, some affect all melanins, others only eumelanin. The distribution of the abnormality also varies in different types of albinism, melanin being deficient in the eye (ocular albinism) or in the most severe forms the skin and hair of the entire body as well as the eyes (oculocutaneous albinism).

Melanin and Melanogenesis

Albinism has been recognized since antiquity, and an understanding of it requires an appreciation of melanogenesis. A review of melanin and its synthesis is beyond the scope of this book, so only a few salient points are stressed. Melanins range in color from brown to black, but not all pigments with these colors are melanin. Eumelanin is a black or brown polymer of high molecular weight with many quinone groups and as yet an incompletely resolved complicated molecular structure. It is insoluble in virtually all solvents but can be solubilized in 0.1 M sodium dodecyl sulfate and 8 M urea without degrading the proteinaceous components (114). In contrast to the yellow and red pheomelanins, eumelanin is insoluble in dilute alkali and resistant to degradation by other chemicals. Eumelanin and the pheomelanins are derived from the same precursors [tyrosine and 3,4-dihydroxyphenylalanine (dopa)], and their synthesis is interrelated, although they are end products of separate metabolic pathways controlled by different genetic loci.

Tyrosinase (EC 1.14.18.1), a copper-containing oxidase within melanosomes, is believed to mediate two of the metabolic steps between tyrosine and melanin: the oxidation of tyrosine to dopa and its conversion to dopaquinone (Fig. 1). Much is known about the biosynthetic pathway of melanin in nature, and many alleles at different loci on different chromosomes influence it. The regulation of pigmentation is governed at numerous disparate steps. For instance, more than 150 distinct mutations are known to affect

939

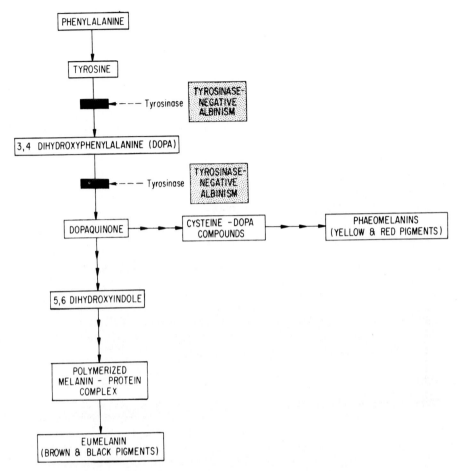

Figure 1   Site of metabolic defect in albinism. (Modified from G.K. Klintworth and M.B. Landers, III. *The Eye: Structure and Function in Disease*, Williams and Wilkins, Baltimore, 1976.)

pigmentation in the mouse, and these involve more than 50 separate genetic loci (115). Yet little is known about the extremely complex genetic control of human melanogenesis, the synthesis of tyrosinase and the regulation of its activity being only part of the complex chain of events (218).

Melanosomes form in two ways. Tyrosinase and the structural proteins of melanosomes are synthesized by the ribosomes of the rough endoplasmic reticulum (ER) and then transferred through its cisternae to the Golgi apparatus, where the proteins segregate within membrane-limited vesicles. An alternative method of melanosome development takes place in some cells, including the retinal pigment epithelium (RPE), where premelanosomes appear to form in the cisternae of a specialized hydrolase-rich region of the smooth ER (184,190). In such cases the tyrosinase is closely associated with acid phosphatase and other lysosomal enzymes, and although melanin granules in such situations are often designated "melanolysosomes," the melanin is probably not being degraded by the lysosomes.

The stages of melanosome formation have been numbered I–IV. Stage I consists of a spherical membrane-delineated vesicle with tyrosinase activity or filaments with the distinctive melanosomal periodicity, stage II is an oval organelle with numerous membranous filaments of distinctive periodicity, stage III is a further advancement in which the inner structure is partly obscured by electron-dense material, and stage IV is an electron-opaque oval organelle without discernible internal structure in routine preparations (Fig. 2) (218).

Melanin is synthesized predominantly by melanocytes derived from the neural crest. These cells migrate throughout the embryo and settle in many tissues, including the skin. In the ocular tissues, where

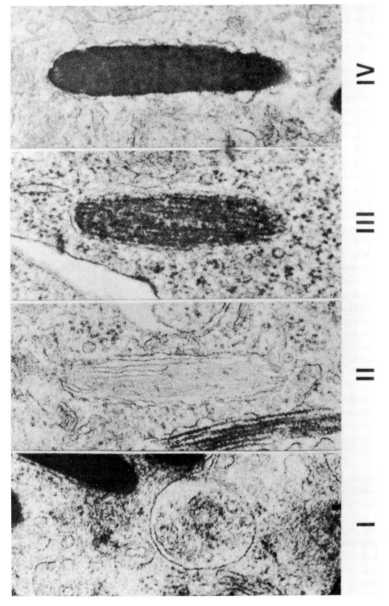

Figure 2 Types of melanosomes. (Reproduced with permission from W.C. Quevedo, Jr., T.B. Fitzpatrick, G. Szabó, and K. Jimbow. Biology of the melanin pigmentary system. In *Dermatology in General Medicine: Textbook and Atlas*, 3rd ed., T.B. Fitzpatrick, A.Z. Eisen, K. Wolff, I.M. Freedberg, and K.F. Austen (Eds.), McGraw-Hill, New York, pp. 224–251, 1987.

melanin is a significant constituent, this pigment is found especially in the eyelids, conjunctiva, and stroma of the iris, ciliary body, and choroid. Melanin is also produced within the eye by another cell population derived embryologically from neuroectoderm (the pigment epithelium of the retina, ciliary body, and iris). The normal melanosomes of the ocular pigmented epithelia range in shape from oval to spherical and tend to be larger than those within the uveal melanocytes.

Classification of Albinism

Albinism is traditionally divided into oculocutaneous albinism, in which the melanin deficiency is manifest in both the skin and eyes, and ocular albinism, in which the skin and hair are clinically of normal color.

However, the connotation of ocular albinism is a misnomer because melanogenesis is affected in the integument in "ocular" albinism despite the predominant ocular involvement and the apparent lack of participation of the hair and skin (192,193). Hypopigmented skin patches occur in ocular albinism, and macromelanosomes are present even in clinically unremarkable skin (192,193,295) (Figs. 3 and 4). Nevertheless, the terms "oculocutaneous" and "ocular albinism" are so entrenched in the literature that authorities on the subject retain the terms, and for this reason they are considered separately in this chapter.

An additional semantic difficulty stems from the traditional, but clearly oversimplified, restriction of the term "albinism" for congenital heritable hypomelanosis that is apparently limited to the eye or that involves the eye and integument and in which nystagmus, photophobia, and decreased visual acuity are present. Thus, some disorders with impaired pigmentation, such as the Cross-McKusick-Breen syndrome (9,68) and the black locks-albinism-deafness syndrome (283), do not fit this strict definition of albinism (186), even though some investigators include such entities under this umbrella.

The designation "albinoidism" pertains to hypomelanotic disorders that lack photophobia, nystagmus, and diminished visual acuity (286). Oculocutaneous forms of albinoidism or partial albinism may occur in Menkes' kinky hair disease (X-linked copper malabsorption syndrome; see Chap. 37) and Waardenburg's syndrome (interoculoiridic-dermatoauditive dysplasia; see Chap. 25). Albinoidism is also an inconstant finding in acrocephalosyndactyly (Apert syndrome; exophthalmos, exotropia, optic atrophy, partial ophthalmoplegia, and cataracts) (177). Other forms of albinoidism include piebaldism (leukism), which may be associated with heterochromia iridis (56).

Oculocutaneous Albinism. An absence or diminution of melanin in the skin, hair, and eyes in oculocutaneous albinism gives rise to a congenital pink-white skin, snow-white hair, photophobia, nystagmus, and decreased visual acuity.

A total of 14 varieties of oculocutaneous albinism can be differentiated on clinical, biochemical, genetic, and morphological features:

1. Type IA, tyrosinase negative
2. Type IB, yellow mutant albinism
3. Type IC, platinum albinism
4. Type II, tyrosinase-positive albinism
5. Type III, minimal pigment albinism
6. Type IV, brown albinism
7. Type V, red or rufous albinism
8. Type VIA, Hermansky-Pudlak syndrome
9. Type VIB, Chédiak-Higashi syndrome
10. Type VII, autosomal dominant albinism
11. Oculocerebral hypopigmentation, hypopigmentation-microphthalmos, Cross-McKusick-Breen syndrome*
12. Albinism with immune deficiency*
13. Black locks-albinism-deafness syndrome*
14. X-linked albinism-deafness syndrome*

---

*These varieties of "albinism" have not been designated a specific type, and some are regarded as albinoidism by some investigators.

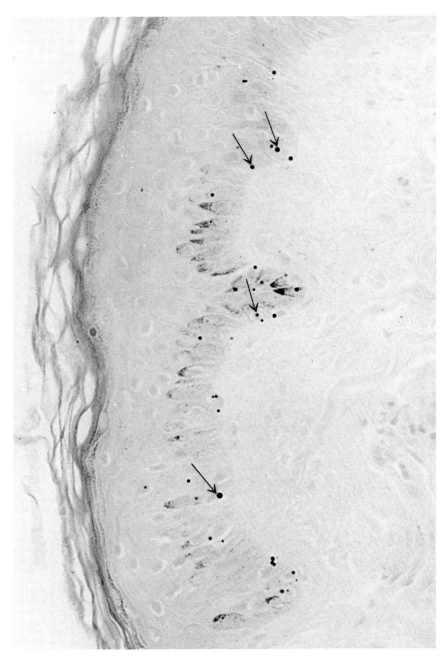

Figure 3 Giant melanin granules (arrows) in the basal epidermis of a patient with ocular albinism. (Fontana's stain, × 500) (Courtesy of Prof. A. Garner.)

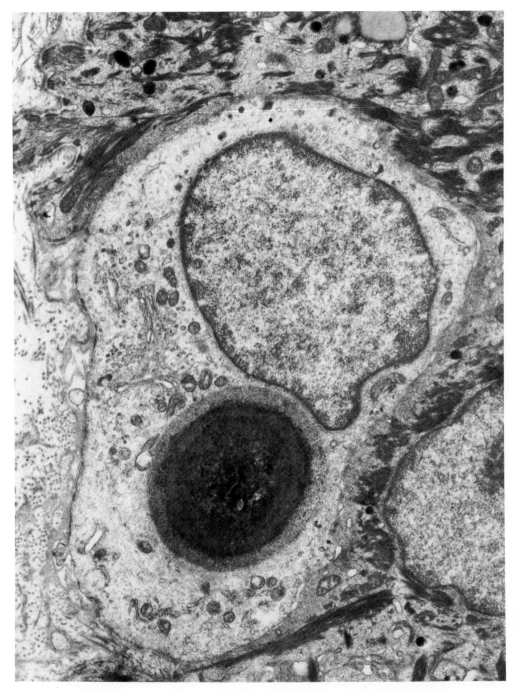

Figure 4   Electron micrograph of giant melanosome in skin of patient with ocular albinism. (× 135,000) (Courtesy of Prof. A. Garner.)

With the exception of autosomal dominant oculocutaneous albinism and the X-linked albinism-deafness syndrome, other varieties of oculocutaneous albinism are inherited as autosomal recessive traits. Three forms of oculocutaneous albinism (types IA–IC) appear to result from different mutations of the same genetic allele located on chromosome 11.

Most albinos express albinism only in the homozygous state, and it is not clear whether all types represent the homozygous state of two identical genes or whether some reflect compounds of two allelic but different genes. It remains uncertain whether type II and type III albinism portray disparate genetic entities (286).

The lack of skin pigment predisposes individuals with oculocutaneous albinism, especially in the tropics, to sun-induced neoplasms, such as lentigines, solar keratoses, and well-differentiated squamous cell carcinoma of the skin, but it is noteworthy that the prevalence of melanomas in albinos is low (286).

Type IA, Tyrosinase-Negative Oculocutaneous Albinism. In type IA oculocutaneous albinism the irides appear gray to blue-gray and the retinal fundus is readily seen through it. The macula is hypoplastic, and visual acuity is markedly diminished. Ultraviolet light causes the hair to become yellow, presumably because of its affect on keratin. According to most authorities the melanocytes contain only stage I and II premelanosomes (286), but type IV mature melanosomes have been observed by transmission electron microscopy (TEM) in the iris from a tyrosinase-negative human albino (180).

Type IB, Yellow Mutant Albinism. At birth, individuals affected with type IB oculocutaneous albinism, also termed yellow or xanthous albinism, lack pigment at birth, have fair skin, and are indistinguishable from other tyrosinase-negative albinos. The condition is common in Amish and some other communities. These albinos eventually develop yellow to yellow-red or yellow-brown hair and yellow-brown irises. Sunlight tans the skin slightly. Stage I, II, and III melanocytes are evident by transmission microscopy in affected persons, but the matrices of these organelles, which are unevenly pigmented, resemble pheomelanosomes (218) and are probably derived from the interaction between dopaquinone and cysteine. Incubation of melanosomes from yellow mutant albinos with L-tyrosine and cysteine intensifies the yellow or red pheomelanin. Nevocellular nevi in yellow mutant albinos are pigmented.

Type IC, Platinum Albinism. In contrast to the white hair of tyrosinase-negative albinos, the hair of some albinos has a color reminiscent of platinum. These so-called platinum albinos acquire small quantities of pigment in their eyes and hair during late childhood. The melanosomes in type IC albinism are predominantly of the early stage III variety, with faint linear pigmentation of the matrix (286).

Type II, Tyrosinase-Positive Albinism). Type II oculocutaneous albinism (formerly called complete perfect albinism) is the most common type of albinism in the United States and in several other countries (218). Because individuals with this variety of albinism form some melanin granules in their hair, skin, and eyes, they may appear darker than normal blond whites. In such individuals a red color follows illumination of the fundus ("red reflex"), but in albinos of heavily pigmented races this may be absent. The presence of some iris pigment imparts a blue, yellow, hazel, or brown color to the eye. Some pigment accumulates with age, and cutaneous melanocytes contain abundant stage I–III premelanosomes, but rarely stage IV melanosomes. However, the premelanosomes mature to stage IV on incubation with L-tyrosine.

Type III, Minimal Pigment Albinism. At birth persons suffering from type III oculocutaneous albinism lack pigment in the skin and eye, and their hair is white and their irises are blue. Minimal quantities of pigment accumulate in the iris during the first decade of life. The ultrastructure of the cutaneous melanocytes is unremarkable, and variations in premelanosomal pigmentation correlate with tyrosinase activity. In contrast to other forms of oculocutaneous albinism, the tyrosinase activity may be low in one parent but normal in the other parent (156).

Type IV, Brown Albinism. Albinos in pigmented races with the tyrosinase-positive type IV oculocutaneous albinism have a tan to olive skin, which contains all stages of melanosomes (155). A faint tan develops with sun exposure (154).

The irises are blue, hazel, or light brown with a punctate and radial translucency (154). The color in the peripheral and central portions may differ (154). Other ocular abnormalities include an impaired visual acuity, a moderate pendular nystagmus, exotropia, a muted foveal reflex, and reduced retinal pigment (154).

Type V, Red or Rufous Albinism. A mahogany-red-brown skin is associated with deep mahogany to sandy red hair in some African-American albinos in the United States and in some albinos in New Guinea. The iris in such persons with type V oculocutaneous albinism is red-brown in color.

Type VIA, Albinism–Hemorrhagic Diathesis, Hermansky-Pudlak Syndrome.   The Hermansky-Pudlak syndrome consists of the triad of tyrosinase-positive oculocutaneous albinism, a hemorrhagic diathesis, and a widespread accumulation of a ceroidlike substance. Although rare in most parts of the world, the gene and heterozygote frequencies for this syndrome are 1:12 and 1:6, respectively, in a small Valais village (164).

The epidermal melanocyte population is of normal density, and incubation of hair bulbs and epidermis in L-dopa reveals tyrosinase activity (81). Stage I–III melanosomes are found, but stage IV melanosomes are rare. A striking feature of the Hermansky-Pudlak syndrome is the presence of numerous atypical large, irregularly pigmented round melanosomes with spotted pigment that resemble pheomelanosomes and vacuolated melanocytes (81,164). The giant melanosomes resemble those reported in various hyperpigmented skin lesions (81).

The hemorrhagic diathesis is manifest by a susceptibility to bruises, epistaxis, gingival hemorrhage, hemoptysis, and excessive bleeding after tooth extraction and childbirth. The platelet count is normal, but the function of these cellular elements is defective as a consequence of an impaired storage of normal components of their dense granules (Ca^{2+}, nucleotides, and amines) (81,164). TEM and fluorescence microscopy have disclosed a lack of dense granules within platelets, as well as in the megakaryocytes (164).

A ceroidlike substance accumulates in macrophages, lymphocytes, and several other cell types in the oral and intestinal mucosa, lung, liver, kidney, and other organs that become discolored. The ceroidlike substance is also excreted in the urine. Interstitial pulmonary fibrosis is associated with the deposition of this material in alveolar macrophages (255). Pseudomelanosis coli and ulcerative colitis, as well as renal and cardiac failure, are frequent manifestations of the condition.

The basic defect in the Hermansky-Pudlak syndrome is poorly understood, and as in many other inherited syndromes, it remains to be determined whether the manifestations reflect different expressions of the same gene or the combined effects of closely linked genes. Because the ceroidlike pigment accumulates within lysosomes, the possibility of a deficient lysosomal enzyme has been raised (255).

Type VIB, Chédiak-Higashi Syndrome.   The Chédiak-Higashi syndrome is a rare autosomal recessive disease of childhood characterized by partial oculocutaneous albinism, the presence of giant granules in most, but not all, granule-containing cells, a marked susceptibility to recurrent pyogenic infection from an early age, and a hemorrhagic diathesis (16,28,161,251). Subjects with the Chédiak-Higashi syndrome exhibit a peripheral granulocytopenia, defective granulocyte regulation, and intramedullary granulocyte destruction (26). Affected individuals have an accelerated lymphomalike phase of the disease, and death almost invariably occurs during childhood or in the early teens from infection, hemorrhage, or malignant lymphomas (258).

This form of partial oculocutaneous albinism is of interest to ophthalmologists, because it causes irises that are blue-violet to brown in color, photophobia, nystagmus, decreased retinal pigmentation, and sometimes strabismus. Tissue examinations of the eye have disclosed a diminished amount of pigment within the pigmented epithelia and melanocytes and an inflammatory cell infiltrate in the choroid, optic nerve, and other ocular structures (32,130,249).

Histological observations of skin, hair, and eyes has disclosed the basis of the partial albinism to be a clumping of melanin granules and a pigmentary dilution. The abnormal granules appear to result from an abnormal fusion of preexisting granules of more normal size. The melanocytes are of normal size and number and contain fully melanized stage IV melanosomes. Such granules are also found in hair follicles (185), RPE, and the choroid plexus, as well as in the pia-arachnoid mater covering the central nervous system (CNS) (15,172,277). Some melanosomes are of normal size; others are abnormally large, probably as a result of fusion between melanosomes and are probably not created as giant melanosomes (186).

Despite its rarity the disease has attracted much attention, as reflected by the voluminous bibliography that has accumulated on the subject. Like many other inherited diseases, the Chédiak-Higashi syndrome provides the investigator with an opportunity to study basic mechanisms and functions of tissues, cells, and organelles. This feat is facilitated by the availability of suitable animal models of this disease (202,214,215).

Aside from humans, a variety of animal species, including mink (165,204), cattle (204,217), mice (173,202,216,270), cats (159), and even the killer whale (259), are known to develop the Chédiak-Higashi syndrome. Homology between the syndrome in some of these species has been established (72,203).

Most investigators have failed to demonstrate a reduced amount of lysosomal enzymes in granulocytes from subjects with the Chédiak-Higashi syndrome. Partly because of this, the lysosomal defect in this disease has been thought to involve the membrane of the various granules rather than their content (203,276).

The Chédiak-Higashi syndrome has provided insight into such varied phenomena as polymorphonuclear leukocyte migration (197,287), bactericidal activity, and the function of platelets (18,34,57). The polymorphonuclear leukocytes of affected individuals manifest impaired chemotaxis and defective lysosomal degranulation following phagocytosis (202). Although most granules in these cells are morphologically normal, some are extremely large (275) and apparently represent secondary lysosomes formed by the fusion of primary granules with ingested or autophagocytosed material rather than enlarged primary granules or multiple fused lysosomes (72). Experimental evidence supports the hypothesis that the abnormalities of neutrophils in Chédiak-Higashi syndrome reflect defective microtubules (197).

The giant cytoplasmic inclusions are maintained in culture (27,71) and can be exaggerated by growing fibroblasts from affected subjects for several days after they reach confluence (198).

The discovery of a severe reduction in the levels of elastase in azurophilic granules within neutrophils of both humans and mice with the Chédiak-Higashi syndrome suggests that this enzyme may contribute to the killing of certain microorganisms to which patients with the Chédiak-Higashi syndrome are susceptible.

The beige mouse, an animal model of the Chédiak-Higashi syndrome, offers opportunities to investigate the interrelationships between the RPE and the photoreceptors. Using this mutant of the C57 black mouse, Robinson and colleagues (228) concluded that the primary lysosomes fuse with the enlarged melanin granules. Many cell types, including the RPE, manifest a defective lysosomal degradation of substances ingested by endocytosis (203). By cross-breeding, Robinson and Kuwabara (227) obtained albino-beige mice with giant granules, which should be particularly useful for studying the possible roles of the RPE in the maintenance of photoreceptors and in their recovery from light damage and other injuries. The RPE also contains enlarged granules of variable size and shape (228). Aside from containing structural evidence of melanin, such granules also exhibit acid phosphatase activity, indicating lysosomal activity.

Type VII, Oculocutaneous Albinoidism, Autosomal Dominant Albinism. In the rare autosomal dominant inherited oculocutaneous albinoidism (76), the skin, hair, and eyes contain less melanin than normal. The skin is white to cream, and the hair bulbs form melanin from tyrosine. The hair ranges in color from white to yellow or red. The irises are gray to blue, nystagmus is mild or absent, and visual acuity is normal. A defect in melanosomal membranes has been proposed but not confirmed (286).

Oculocerebral Hypopigmentation (Hypopigmentation-Microphthalmos) Syndrome (Cross-McKusick-Breen Syndrome). A unique syndrome was detected in three members of an Amish family with multiple consanguineous marriages from the state of Ohio (68). The Cross-McKusick-Breen syndrome, named after its discoverers, has been found elsewhere in the United States, as well as in Italy (9) and Uruguay. The syndrome is characterized by retarded growth, tyrosinase-negative oculocutaneous albinism, impaired cerebral function (athetoid movements and mental retardation), dental defects, and ocular abnormalities (including bilateral microphthalmos with cloudy corneas, iris atrophy, cataracts, and a jerky nystagmus). The fundamental defect in this syndrome remains unknown, but melanosomes are scarce in the skin (58) and small clusters of them in all stages of development have been found in the few melanocytes that are present. Tyrosinemia has been detected in one case, but the significance of this observation, if any, remains to be determined (9).

Albinism with Immune Deficiency. Separate families have been documented with pigment dilution, frequent pyogenic infections, neutropenia, thrombocytopenia, hepatosplenomegaly, and impaired immunity (hypogammaglobulinemia, defective antibody synthesis, impaired delayed hypersensitivity, and deficient helper T lymphocytes) (101). Such individuals have pale skin, sometimes with a tinge of gray, and the hair is silvery gray. The melanocytes contain unremarkable melanosomes but lack the dendrites that normally transfer melanosomes into the epidermis. This, together with a relatively higher number than normal of melanosomes in melanocytes compared to keratinocytes, hints at defective melanosome transfer (218).

Black Locks, Albinism, Deafness Syndrome. At least two kindreds have been documented with a syndrome consisting of congenital sensory deafness, oculocutaneous albinism, and some pigmentation. Almost all of the skin and hair lacks melanin pigment, but affected individuals have locks of black hair and brown cutaneous macules. Ocular involvement includes marked nystagmus, poor visual acuity, gray irides, and hyperpigmented and hypopigmented zones on fundoscopy (283).

X-Linked Albinism-Deafness Syndrome.   The X-linked albinism-deafness syndrome, which may affect the migration of neural crest-derived precursors of the melanocytes, is characterized by congenital nerve deafness and piebaldness. A linkage analysis and hybridization studies suggest that the locus for the accountable gene is on the long arm of the X chromosome at the Xq26 locus (241).

Other Possible Types of Albinism.   The aforementioned clearly does not reflect the entire story of oculocutaneous albinism: other incompletely characterized varieties of albinism have been documented. Other cases of oculocutaneous albinism have been observed in association with microcephaly, hypoplasia of the distal phalanx of several fingers of both hands and agenesis of the distal end of the big toe (43), and infantile neuroaxonal dystrophy (281), but time will tell if these connections are more than fortuitous.

Ocular Albinism.   Six types of ocular albinism have been documented (131,192,193):

1. Nettleship-Falls or Vogt ocular albinism (type 1 ocular albinism)
2. Forsius-Eriksson ocular albinism (Åland Island eye disease, type 2 ocular albinism)
3. Ocular albinism cum pigmento (type 3 ocular albinism)
4. Punctate ocular albinism
5. Autosomal dominant ocular albinism
6. Ocular albinism with neural deafness

Four of these varieties of ocular albinism (Nettleship-Falls or Vogt type, Forsius-Eriksson type, ocular albinism cum pigmento, and ocular albinism with neural deafness) are inherited as X-linked disorders. The other types of ocular albinism have autosomal dominant modes of transmission.

Type 1 Ocular Albinism (Nettleship-Falls or Vogt Type).   The most common variety of ocular albinism (type 1) is typified by normal or minimally diminished ocular pigmentation, variable degrees of photophobia, horizontal nystagmus, strabismus, impaired visual acuity, and foveal hypoplasia (192,193), but these clinical manifestations vary considerably even within the same sibship (254). A moderately pigmented fundus and lack of iris translucency have been noted in affected Japanese with type 1 ocular albinism (111). Female carriers manifest a normal visual acuity but have an abnormal mosaic pattern of the retinal pigment (254).

Fewer melanosomes than normal and giant melanosomes (up to 12 μm in diameter) are present in the neuroepithelium-derived pigmented epithelia of the eye, as well as within melanocytes and keratinocytes of the skin (111,193,244). Melanocytes of the uvea are lightly pigmented, but macromelanosomes are present in them. Dopa oxidase-positive giant pigment granules are found within melanocytes in the epidermis and dermis, with slate-colored parts of skin having numerous macromelanosomes and hypopigmented areas containing very few granules (Fig. 3) (193). In black individuals with type 1 ocular albinism, hypomelanotic macules and vitiligo have been observed (218), but macromelanosomes have not been noted in the hypomelanotic macules, which contain only a few melanosomes (218).

The mutant gene for type 1 ocular albinism is located at the Xp22.3 locus on the short arm of the X chromosome close to the Xg blood group (181,209).

Type 2, Forsius-Eriksson Type, Aland Island Eye Disease.   The so-called X-linked type 2 ocular albinism (also known as Forsius-Eriksson albinism or Åland Island eye disease) was originally reported in 1964 in a family on the Aland Islands (77). This condition is typified by hypopigmentation of the fundus (less severe than in type 1 ocular albinism), diminished visual acuity, progressive axial myopia, astigmatism, nystagmus, foveal hypoplasia, defective dark adaptation, and protanomalous red-green color blindness.

At one time this disorder was regarded as a type of ocular albinism, but the skin melanocytes are normal. Also, in contrast to type 1 ocular albinism, female heterozygotes do not manifest mosaic retinal patterns but have a latent nystagmus and mild defects in color discrimination (267). Furthermore, in contradistinction to other forms of ocular and oculocutaneous albinism, there is no misrouting of the optic pathway (see ophthalmic manifestations of albinism) and the opticokinetic nystagmus does not resemble that of most albinos. The ocular abnormalities in this X-linked disorder are probably due to a high-grade axial myopia with stretching of the RPE.

Aland Island eye disease differs from congenital stationary night blindness with myopia (also an X-linked recessive disorder) in that the scotopic functions are only moderately affected and the peripheral photopic visual fields are not restricted (267). However, congenital stationary night blindness and Aland Island eye disease may be caused by mutations in the same gene (2).

Linkage studies indicate that the location of the responsible gene is probably in the pericentromeric region of the long arm of the X chromosome (Xq13-q21) (2). An individual with Åland Island eye disease has also expressed a contiguous gene syndrome with features of congenital adrenal hypoplasia, glycerol kinase deficiency, and Duchenne muscular dystrophy (212). Using molecular genetic techniques, this deletion has been mapped to the Xp21.3-21.2 portion of the X chromosome (2).

Type 3, Ocular Albinism cum Pigmento. Macromelanosomes occur in the skin in darkly pigmented individuals with an X-linked recessive type of ocular albinism in which the fundus is often moderately pigmented (192).

Type 4, Punctate Ocular Albinism. A diffuse, fine punctate depigmentation of the iris and RPE have been documented in a woman and two of her children with light-colored skin and hair (22). Other associated abnormalities in this autosomal dominant condition are reduced visual acuity and elevated central cone thresholds. The hair bulb test was positive for tyrosinase.

Autosomal Dominant Ocular Albinism. A predisposition to multiple sun-induced brownish cutaneous spots (lentigines) may be inherited in an autosomal dominant fashion with congenital sensory deafness and vestibular abnormalities (168). In this entity, macromelanosomes are detected in the lentigines but not in the normal skin.

Ocular Albinism with Neural Deafness. Winship and colleagues detected a large Afrikaner kindred in South Africa with an X-linked recessive type of ocular albinism and late-onset neural deafness (278).

Nature of Melanosomes in Albinism. In most forms of albinism melanocytes in the skin are present in normal numbers and contain morphologically normal premelanosomes but lack mature melanosomes. There are usually fewer melanin granules than normal, but Masson-Fontana and dopa-positive giant melanin granules (macromelanosomes or melanin macroglobules) are present in keratinocytes and melanocytes of the skin of most albinos (oculocutaneous albinism type VIA, Chédiak-Higashi syndrome, ocular albinism types 1 and 3, and X-linked ocular albinism with deafness) (111,192,193,254) and even in heterozygotes with some types of albinism (type 1 ocular albinism and X-linked ocular albinism with deafness) (254). Ultrastructurally macromelanosomes are composed of a dense core and a less profuse surrounding mantle (295). Although absent in the normal skin, such macromelanosomes are present in the lentigines of autosomal dominant albinism as well as in numerous other disorders, including von Recklinghausen's neurofibromatosis and xeroderma pigmentosa (186).

The number of giant melanocytic cells is increased in intradermal, compound, and junctional nevi of patients with both tyrosinase-negative and tyrosinase-positive oculocutaneous albinism (210), and presumably as a reflection of skin sensitivity to ultraviolet light, marked solar elastosis surrounds the nevi, even when the lesions are covered by clothing (210).

Pathobiology of Albinism. The basic pathobiology of almost all varieties of albinism is poorly understood. The defect in type IA oculocutaneous albinism, which is also termed imperfect albinism, is an inability to synthesize tyrosinase. Some forms of tyrosinase-positive albinism are conceivably due to one or more inhibitors of this enzyme. Tyrosinase uses tyrosine as a substrate, and almost any peptide or protein with an exposed tyrosine or phenylalanine residue can function as a competitive inhibitor (115). Indeed, several endogenous melanogenic inhibitors of this enzyme have been purified and partially characterized (115), but such substances have not yet been detected in albinos. Tyrosinase is synthesized in type II oculocutaneous albinism, but evidence for an inhibitor of this enzyme in type II oculocutaneous albinism is lacking (218). Some types of tyrosinase-positive albinism may result from an impaired transfer of melanin to cells that normally acquire it, such as keratinocytes in the skin. The latter mechanism may be involved in oculocutaneous albinism associated with immune deficiency (218). Defects in melanosome synthesis can also lead to albinism. Arrested melanosomal development with a partial block in the distal eumelanin pathway may occur in brown oculocutaneous albinism (154). Defective melanosomal membranes may lead to diminished pigmentation, as has been suggested but not shown in type VII oculocutaneous albinism (286). Pigment dilution due to the presence of fewer melanosomes than normal can account at least in part for the hypopigmentation of the Chédiak-Higashi syndrome. Other potential reasons for albinism include failure of melanocytes to migrate to target tissues or their failure to survive in hypopigmented regions. A partial block in the distal eumelanin pathway in brown oculocutaneous albinism has been proposed on the basis of ultrastructural findings in the skin (154).

Ophthalmic Features of Albinism. The eye is hypopigmented in both oculocutaneous and ocular forms of albinism. The melanin-containing cells of the eye (melanocytes in the conjunctiva, eyelid, iris, ciliary body, choroid, and orbit and pigment epithelia of retina, ciliary body, and iris) are hypopigmented. The iris is usually abnormally translucent and light gray to blue in color (but sometimes dark) and is often hypoplastic. Iris pigmentation increases with age in ocular albinism. Albinism is manifest clinically in the most severe cases by nystagmus, photophobia, and decreased visual acuity. The severity of these manifestations varies in the different types of albinism, and they are most marked in those forms having a marked deficiency of ocular pigment (oculocutaneous albinism types IA and II, the black locks-albinism-deafness syndrome, and type 1 ocular albinism). In the other varieties of albinism individual variations in the ocular abnormalities are conspicuous, and in some albinos these are often relatively mild (oculocutaneous type V and albinism with immune deficiency) or absent (oculocutaneous type VII). In several forms of oculocutaneous albinism (types IB and II), clinical examination of the translucent iris discloses radial opacities, but such "cartwheeling" is absent in some types of albinism, such as type IA oculocutaneous albinism.

In ocular albinism the melanin in the pigment epithelium of the retina, ciliary body, and iris is absent or severely reduced. In oculocutaneous albinism, melanin is usually present in the pigment epithelia of the retina, ciliary body, and iris, although it is diminished in quantity. The paucity of pigment in the RPE and choroid enables the choroidal blood vessels to be visualized with the ophthalmoscope, and illumination of the fundus commonly imparts a red color ("red reflex").

Heterozygous females with some types of X-linked ocular albinism (type 1 ocular albinism and X-linked ocular albinism with deafness) have a characteristic mosaic pattern of pigmentation in the fundi as a result of the random inactivation of one X chromosome in each cell during development (Lyon hypothesis) (231). This aids in the recognition of the carrier state and in the clinical diagnosis of X-linked albinism.

The presence of melanin within the eye influences several biological phenomena that separate albinos from individuals with normal melanin pigmentation. These events include a failure of the fovea centralis to develop, the projection of retinal axons from the temporal retina to the contralateral side of the brain, the retinal light-mediated suppression of the synthesis of the pineal gland hormone melatonin, and perhaps anterior chamber angle development.

The albinotic macula is abnormal, owing possibly to the failure of the fovea centralis to develop because of the inability of the RPE to absorb light.

The optic fibers decussate in the optic chiasm in all vertebrates with laterally placed eyes (213). With the appearance of both eyes in a frontal position and the evolution of stereoptic vision, some fibers from the temporal retina project to the brain on the same side as the eye from which they arose. The extent of the uncrossed fibers varies in different species. In humans almost half of the axons fail to decussate, and those arising in the ganglion cells of the temporal retina normally project to neurons in the CNS on the same side as the eye of origin. However, in virtually all types of human (6,7,29,30,41,42,55,57,60–66,106, 153,285) and animal albinism (59,75,90,91,102,103,105,107,108,167,171,234,235,236) evaluated, an abnormal decussation of the optic tracts has been detected, and nerve fibers from the temporal retina cross to the opposite side of the brain (lateral geniculate body in humans and that site or the optic tectum in animals). An apparent exception to this rule, based on neurophysiological observations on a patient, is type 2 ocular albinism, but as pointed out earlier this entity is no longer regarded as a type of albinism (267). The anomalous decussation of axons in the optic tract of albinos results in an inability to perceive binocular vision. This abnormal decussation has been shown with neurophysiological, morphological, and horseradish peroxidase tracer studies (75,286).

At one time the abnormal axonal projections were thought perhaps to be secondary to the loss of a nonmelanin neuronal function of tyrosinase or to a separate mutation in the region of the tyrosinase gene. However, anatomical studies of brains from both tyrosinase-negative and tyrosinase-positive human albinos have disclosed that the anomalous decussations are independent of the type of albinism (104,106). Several investigators have postulated that the anomalous chiasmatic decussation is a sequel to any defect that results in an absence of pigment in the developing optic cup during the critical stage of ontogeny when optic cup neurons normally become programmed to approach targets within the growing brain (286). The development of abnormal retinogeniculocortical pathways is apparently not specific for the albino state, however, because it has been observed in both homozygous albino cats and in normally pigmented cats carrying a recessive allele for albinism (167).

Stimulation of the retina by light normally suppresses melatonin synthesis by the pineal gland in rats. Eye pigmentation enhances this reaction but does not seem to be the critical factor in determining the sensitivity of the rat pineal gland to retinal photic stimulation (174). Light also suppresses melatonin production by the pineal gland in albino rats, but at higher levels of irradiance than needed for pigmented rats (174).

Anterior chamber angle imperfections of the Axenfeld type have been documented in too many cases of albinism to be considered a coincidence (3,20,31,109,111,170,222,266). This developmental anomaly is not related to the type of albinism or to the chromosomal location of the mutant gene. It has been associated with ocular albinism (3,111,222,266), as well as tyrosinase-negative (170) and tyrosinase-positive oculocutaneous albinism (286). Presumably, a deficiency of melanin in the developing eye significantly influences the formation of the anterior chamber.

Impaired Hearing in Albinism.   Although hearing is usually only mildly affected in albinism, sensory deafness is a prominent feature of some types of albinism (X-linked albinism-deafness syndrome, black locks-albinism-deafness syndrome, and ocular albinism with late-onset neural deafness) (278) and certain forms of albinoidism (286). The impairment of hearing in albinism is probably not a chance association, but the reason some forms of albinism are more prone to sensory deafness remains to be determined. Melanin is a normal constituent of the inner ear and is believed to protect it from the traumatic effect of noise. Also, as in the visual system, melanin normally influences the neuronal decussation of auditory neurons. In oculocutaneous albinism the decussation of nerve fibers from the cochlea is reduced or absent at the level of the superior olive (286). The otic abnormalities in albinism are reviewed by Witkop and colleagues (285).

Animal Models.   Many animal models of albinism and albinoidism exist that affect the eye, including the Waardenburg-Klein syndrome, and offer opportunities for detailed investigation (21). In quails with a sex-linked recessive form of albinism, several ocular abnormalities develop over time in the mutant quails (eye enlargement, hazy corneas, lens opacities, deep anterior chambers, retinal degeneration, optic disk degeneration and excavation, and cavernous optic atrophy) (256).

B. Alkaptonuria (Ochronosis)

Alkaptonuria inherited as an autosomal recessive trait, results from the absence of an enzyme that exists primarily in the kidney and liver and oxidizes homogentisic acid (homogentisic acid oxidase; EC 1.13.11.5) (163). Homogentisic acid is an intermediate compound in the metabolic conversion of tyrosine to maleylacetoacetic acid, the latter in turn being oxidized through the citric acid cycle to yield energy (Fig. 5). A deficiency of homogentisic acid oxidase results in an abnormal accumulation of homogentisic acid, which becomes oxidized to by-products that polymerize to a melaninlike pigment. Because it is rapidly excreted in the urine (163), the serum levels of homogentisic acid are usually not elevated. The urine is dark or turns dark on standing in affected individuals, and the presence of homogentisic aciduria is diagnostic, even in infancy. The condition is often detected later in life, when the progressive deposition of blackish pigment in connective tissue occurs, especially in the cartilage of the nose, ears, and joints.

The most striking ocular abnormalities involve the sclera and peripheral cornea (4,8,11,23, 35,69,79,87,110,140,200,229,230,232,240,245,246,279), and several reports document microscopic examinations of the ocular tissue in this disease (4,8,69,229,230,240). Triangular patches of brownish black scleral pigmentation develop in both eyes midway between the margin of the cornea and the insertions of the horizontal rectus muscles. These lesions usually become evident during the third decade of life. The sclera is pigmented and frequently needs to be bleached to evaluate the underlying tissue. Documented abnormalities include abnormal elastic fibers, loss of cellularity, and the presence of pigment-containing cells in the region of the lateral and medial rectus muscle insertions. Subepithelial pigmented globules that resemble oil drops have been noted near the corneoscleral limbus, and the episclera may contain lesions that resemble pigmented pingueculae. The scleral pigmentation, although asymptomatic, is of practical importance to the ophthalmologist, because it must be differentiated from a transscleral extension of a melanoma. Indeed, an only eye has been enucleated from a patient as a result of such a misdiagnosis (245). A similar scleral pigmentation can occur as an occupational hazard after prolonged ocular exposure to hydroquinones or quinones (5,183). Such exogenous ochronosis can also blacken the skin after the oral or intramuscular administration of quinine and other antimalarial drugs (33) or after the topical treatment of leg ulcers with phenol or the topical use of hydroquinone-containing bleaching creams by black people (122,211). It is noteworthy that these exogenously induced forms of ochronotic skin pigmentation manifest morphological similarities to those that accompany alkaptonuria (33,122,211).

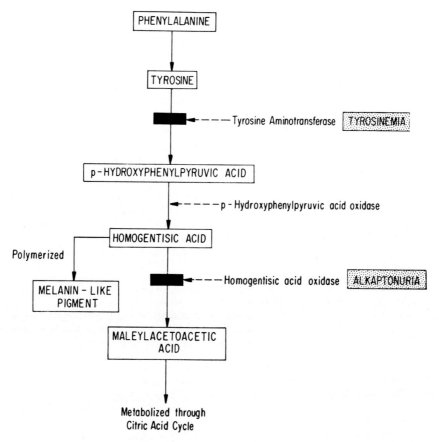

Figure 5 Site of metabolic defect in alkaptonuria and tyrosinemia. (Reproduced with permission from G.K. Klintworth and M.B. Landers, III. *The Eye: Structure and Function in Disease*, Williams and Wilkins, Baltimore, 1976.)

C. Tyrosinemia

Tyrosinemia and tyrosinuria are manifestations of several metabolic disorders, and the two main types of tyrosinemia have an autosomal recessive mode of inheritance (94,97). Type I tyrosinemia (tyrosinosis, congenital tyrosinosis, and fumarylacetoacetate hydrolase deficiency) occurs as a consequence of a defect in tyrosine catabolism caused by the inhibition of hepatic enzymes. In tyrosinemia type II (Richner-Hanhart syndrome or Oregon tyrosinosis), tyrosine accumulates as a result of an enzymatic defect in its metabolism.

The primary defect in type I tyrosinemia does not involve tyrosine metabolism and results from an inherited deficiency of fumarylacetoacetate hydrolase (EC 3.7.1.2), which presumably leads to elevated levels of fumarylacetoacetate and maleylacetoacetate and the formation of succinylacetoacetone and succinylacetone. These compounds have toxic effects, particularly on the kidney and liver, and the acute and chronic manifestations of tyrosinemia type I include features of disordered liver and renal function. Tyrosinemia is only one manifestion of this toxicity. In contrast to tyrosinemia type II, and for reasons that are not clear, the eye and skin are not specifically affected.

Tyrosinemia type II is one of the very few diseases with toxic effects due to the accumulation of an amino acid that is inadequately metabolized. It results from a deficiency of the liver enzyme tyrosine aminotransferase (EC 2.6.1.5; Fig. 5) (150). The gene encoding for this enzyme, which converts tyrosine to *p*-hydroxyphenylpyruvic acid, has been localized to the long arm of human chromosome 16 (16q22-

q24) (13). The deficiency of this catabolic enzyme of tyrosine results in elevated plasma tyrosine, and this is followed by a rise in tyrosine metabolites in the urine.

The high plasma tyrosine results in a distinct syndrome with prominent ocular and cutaneous manifestations (25,37,38,40,45,54,78,95,96,118,128,253). Tyrosine crystallizes in the cornea, producing photophobia with shallow dendritic corneal erosions that resemble herpetic keratitis and, sometimes, corneal epithelial proliferation. In the epidermis of the palms and soles, tyrosine leads to erosions, crusting, and then punctate hyperkeratotic lesions. Sometimes mental retardation is a prominent feature of this entity. It is important for clinicians to make an early diagnosis because the severity of tyrosinemia can be diminished by dietary restriction of phenylalanine and tyrosine and proteins containing them (97,176,188).

Corneal crystals are not specific for tyrosinemia type II: they have been observed as a temporary phenomenon in a neonate with tyrosinemia due to other causes. For example, transient neonatal tyrosinemia is relatively common in infants who are premature or ingest a high-protein diet, or both (73).

Tyrosinemia type II occurs in mink (46,47,54,98) and dogs (162), and a disorder with almost identical features can be produced in rats by feeding them a high-tyrosine low-protein diet (14,39,40,92,223,226). When tyrosinemia is reproduced in young rats by a high-tyrosine diet, pinpoint corneal epithelial opacities evolve into larger ones resembling snowflakes. The earliest morphological abnormality occurs in the epithelium, where birefringent crystals are evident in alcohol-fixed and fresh tissue (40). Tyrosine crystals dissolve during tissue processing, and in TEM micrographs needle-shaped lucent areas traverse the corneal epithelial cells at sites where crystals were presumably originally located. Epithelial lesions in the cornea are followed by a prominent infiltration of polymorphonuclear leukocytes and blood vessels. In the animal model, the cornea, which initially becomes opaque in the axial region, regains its transparency spontaneously with time. The tyrosine-induced keratopathy in rats can almost be prevented by the induction of tyrosine aminotransferase with adrenal corticosteroids (39) or by decreasing the leukocytic infiltrate with cyclophosphamide (226).

I. DISORDERS OF SULFUR-CONTAINING AMINO ACIDS

A. Homocystinuria

The activity of the enzyme cystathionine β-synthetase (EC 4.2.1.22) is markedly reduced in homocystinuria, an entity with numerous phenotypical similarities to Marfan syndrome. This enzyme catalyzes an important step in the metabolism of methionine to cysteine (Fig. 6). Pyridoxine-responsive and nonresponsive varieties of homocystinuria are recognized (152), and the mutant genes accountable for both types are localized in the same locus on the long arm of chromosome 21 (21q22.3) (187). Cystathionine β-synthetase requires pyridoxal-5'-phosphate as a cofactor, and in pyridoxine-responsive homocystinuric individuals the mutant synthetase has a markedly reduced affinity for both its coenzyme and cosubstrates (L-homocysteine and L-serine) and is much more thermolabile than the normal enzyme. The molecular abnormality in the pyridoxine-responsive mutant enzyme seems to be in the apoenzyme (catalytically inactive enzyme lacking its cofactor), which impairs coenzyme binding. This results in a reduced total enzyme activity by reducing its holoenzyme (catalytically active enzyme-coenzyme complex) formation and by accelerating apoenzyme degradation. Pharmacological amounts of pyridoxine presumably increase holoenzyme formation modestly, thereby enhancing catalytic activity and slowing apoenzyme turnover (152). In both forms of homocystinuria, methionine, homocystine, and homocysteine levels are elevated in the serum, excess sulfur-containing amino acids are excreted in the urine, and a cyanide-nitroprusside test of the urine is positive (112). Cystathionine synthetase activity in cultured skin fibroblasts is negligible, and this activity may increase only slightly with pyridoxine therapy (112).

The ocular manifestations of homocystinuria include subluxated lenses, spherophakia, and high myopia (36,67,166). Ectopia lentis is common and is frequently the presenting clinical manifestation of homocystinuria, the lens usually being dislocated downward, often into the anterior chamber, and its forward displacement may occlude the pupil and produce pupillary block glaucoma (67,112,139). Occasionally the spherophakic lens becomes cataractous. A single case report documents bilateral band keratopathy decades after bilateral intracapsular cataract extractions (252). Retinal detachment is common even in the absence of cataract surgery, and the globe is often elongated and myopic. Peripheral cystoid degeneration of the retina is marked and evident at an earlier age than usual.

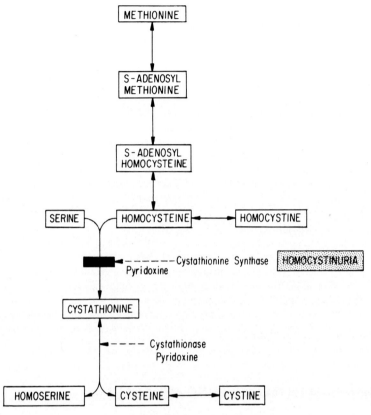

Figure 6   Site of metabolic defect in homocystinuria. (Reproduced with permission from G.K. Klintworth and M.B. Landers, III. *The Eye: Structure and Function in Disease*, Williams and Wilkins, Baltimore, 1976.)

Another important expression in homocystinuria of practical significance to ophthalmologists is the frequent tendency to thrombosis (about 50% of cases) (166). Thromboembolism is a potential postoperative complication of procedures to extract a displaced lens or to treat retinal detachment. Thrombi may develop at a young age in veins (such as the common iliac and deep leg veins), as well as in intermediate-sized arteries throughout the body, including those of the eye, such as the central retinal artery. The thrombotic tendency may lead to embolic complications. Thromboembolic occlusions of retinal vessels may even be the presenting manifestion of the disorder (265).

The thrombotic tendency in individuals with homocystinuria probably results from both platelet activation and abnormalities in blood coagulation. The plasma level of several proteins involved in blood coagulation (antithrombin III, factor VII, and protein C antigen) may be lower than normal in homocystinuria (19,205). Evidence of platelet activation (such as an elevated serum β-thromboglobulin) is evident in some cases. These abnormalities may return to normal during pyridoxine therapy, and although the essence of these changes remains unsure, their amelioration during treatment implies that the disordered transsulfuration of homocystinuria affects the production or activity of some liver-dependent coagulation factors (205). In the pyridoxine-responsive patient general anesthesia is not hazardous if platelet function can be controlled by the vitamin (112).

How homocystinuria with its autosomal recessive mode of inheritance causes its diverse manifestations remains unknown, but a morphological explanation for the tendency of the lens to dislocate exists in the region of the zonules and ciliary body. The ciliary body is often small and has been variably interpreted as underdeveloped or atrophic. Deficient zonules recoil onto a markedly thickened basal lamina of the nonpigmented ciliary epithelium (116,220). A thickening of this basal lamina is not specific for homocystinuria and also occurs in Marfan syndrome and Weill-Marchesani syndromes (Fig. 7). Because cystine

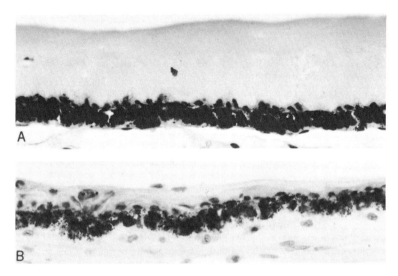

Figure 7 Thickened basement membrane of nonpigmented epithelium of ciliary body in Weill-Marchesani syndrome. (B) Appearance of normal ciliary body at same magnification. (Hematoxylin and eosin, × 325)

is a normal constituent of zonules (288), a defect in the metabolism of this amino acid may be significant in the genesis of the abnormal zonules. Decreased collagen cross-links have been detected in skin biopsies from three patients (141).

B. Cystinosis (Cystine Storage Disease)

Another rare autosomal recessive metabolic disorder of amino acid metabolism that affects most parts of the eye is cystinosis. Childhood (nephropathic), juvenile, and adult forms of this condition are recognized (83). Cystinosis leads to the widespread accumulation of cystine crystals in ocular tissues, as well as in bone marrow, liver, spleen, lymph nodes, and kidneys. Despite differences in clinical expression, all varieties of cystinosis are characterized by an intralysosomal storage of cystine, but plasma cystine and cysteine levels are not consistently elevated. Cystine is stored within leukocytes and other cell types within membrane-bound cytoplasmic vacuoles as fine granular noncrystalline material. The lysosomal identity of the intracytoplasmic inclusions is supported by the associated acid phosphatase activity (290). Available morphological observations suggest that the storage of cystine precedes its crystallization. The excessive accumulation of cystine within cells is a consequence of the impaired transport of cystine from lysosomes (see also Chap. 26) (82,83,86).

Childhood cystinosis, the most severe form, is associated with defective renal tubular reabsorption and the Fanconi syndrome (polyuria, generalized aminoaciduria, proteinuria, glycosuria, phosphaturia, and rickets). Renal failure is common, but dialysis and renal transplantation have prolonged the lives of individuals with nephropathic cystinosis, and by 1986 at least 80 affected individuals in the United States and Canada had survived until aged at least 10 years (84). At least 1 patient has reached 31 years of age (137). Death is usually from uremia secondary to renal failure, and the median survival time of cystinotic patients is 8.5 years (100). The survival of individuals with infantile and adolescent types of cystinosis is not significantly different (100).

The ocular manifestations of cystinosis are well established (80,83,133,237). The presence of multiple delicate scintillating crystals in the cornea (chiefly in the region of the corneoscleral limbus and in the anterior corneal stroma) and conjunctiva is characteristic of all forms of cystinosis (51,52,80,83, 89,149,160,296). Crystals may also be present in the iris and other parts of the uvea (83,273), retina, and sclera (83). Although the corneal crystals were once regarded as pathognomonic of cystinosis, other conditions, including hypergammaglobulinemia (discussed in Chap. 32), also produce corneal crystals and need to be differentiated clinically from cystinosis. The corneal crystals are absent at birth and during early infancy but are usually evident by 1 year of age (83). Early in life the corneal crystals involve the anterior central corneal stroma and the entire thickness of the peripheral cornea (50,83), but as the patient ages the crystals become located in the posterior cornea (182). Pupillary block glaucoma has been attributed to a cystine accumulation in the iris stroma (273).

From an ocular standpoint, individuals with cystinosis generally complain only of photophobia and glare, and the glare presumably results from the ocular cystine crystals (143). A markedly decreased corneal sensitivity has been detected in persons with cystinosis (145), and the cornea may thicken, perhaps as a sequel to subclinical corneal edema (147). The ocular symptoms may necessitate corneal transplantation (134,135,144,146,147,225). Following keratoplasty, the graft may remain free of cystinosis for as long as 2 years (134,135), but in some cases crystals reappear in the graft and may be evident within 6 weeks (144,146). A markedly decreased corneal sensitivity compared to age-matched controls has been detected in cystinosis, possibly resulting from an altered function of the basal epithelial neural plexus (145). Loss of contrast sensitivity (a psychophysical parameter of visual function) has been found in individuals with cystinosis, especially at higher spatial frequencies (142), and could result from the corneal, retinal, or CNS abnormalities, but most of the contrast sensitivity probably reflects the corneal lesions.

Long-term ocular complications of nephropathic cystinosis in patients who have survived into adulthood as a result of dialysis and renal transplantation include blepharospasm, photophobia, corneal erosions, posterior synechiae, the deposition of crystals on the anterior lens surface, and reduced visual acuity (83,85,133).

A mottled pigmentary retinopathy is common in cystinosis (224,237,291). The RPE degenerates, and this layer of cells may be lost, particularly in the peripheral retina. A patchy depigmentation of the RPE with pigment clumping intensifies from the macula toward the preequator area and gives the fundus a "salt and pepper" appearance (224). Focal depigmentation, atrophy, and hypertrophy of the RPE, without intraretinal pigment migration, have been noted, and the abnormalities of the RPE may precede the corneal crystals (291). When the RPE is extensively affected, the macula acquires a unique yellow mottling (237). Abnormalities in the RPE begin early in life, and vacuoles have been detected in these cells in an 18-week-old fetus with cystinosis (239). The pigmentary retinopathy is absent at birth but has been noted in a 5-week-old infant girl (44). Crystals have been documented in the retina of at least one case by photography (133).

Cystine crystals are insoluble in absolute ethanol and can easily be seen with polarized light in tissue sections prepared without aqueous solutions, which dissolve them. In cystinosis, needle-shaped, rectangular, or hexagonal crystals have been found in ocular tissues, the fusiform crystals being identified only in the cornea and sclera (Fig. 8) (50,237). By TEM intracytoplasmic electron lucencies indicate the sites of crystalline inclusions. They have been identified within membrane-bound vesicles in different cell types in the cornea (149,237), conjunctiva (149,237,250,273,290), and iris (273) and in the RPE (237). It is extremely doubtful that cystine crystallizes outside cells despite reports of extracellular conjunctival crystals by light microscopy (289). In adult cystinosis profiles of cystine crystals have been identified extracellularly adjacent to degenerated cells (250), but they have apparently not yet been reported in this site in childhood cystinosis. Whether this difference is real still needs to be determined. TEM has almost always disclosed profiles of crystalline outlines only within cells.

Cultured fibroblasts from patients with cystinosis accumulate cystine within secondary lysosomes, and cystine is depleted with cysteamine (mercaptoamine) (99). This cystine-depleting agent also appears to be beneficial after renal transplantation (85), and when applied topically to the eye, such medication may clear the corneal crystals in some (132,137) but not in all patients (175).

The eye is not affected in cystinuria, in contrast to cystinosis, with which it is sometimes confused. Cystine, lysine, arginine, and ornithine are excreted in excess in cystinuria, a disorder with a transport defect involving renal tubules and the intestinal tract.

C. Sulfocysteinuria

Sulfite oxidase (EC 1.8.3.1), a molybdenum-containing enzyme involved in the oxidation of sulfites to sulfates (53), is deficient in an extremely rare inherited disorder with severe neurological defects, which include mental deficiency and seizures (126,247). Bilateral dislocated lenses are a prominent clinical feature, and other ocular abnormalities (hypoplasia of ciliary body, diminished ganglion cells and thinning of the nerve fiber layer in the retina, and absence of myelin in the optic nerve) have also been noted (247).

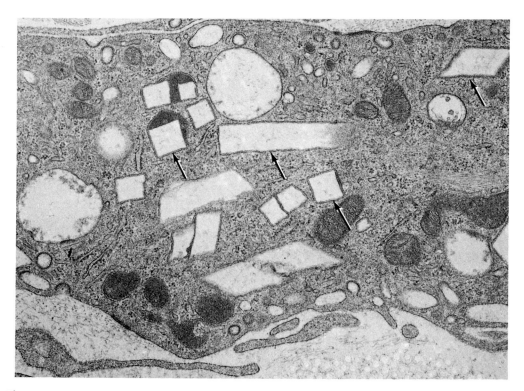

Figure 8 Profiles of crystalline inclusions within cytoplasm of a histiocyte in cystinosis. (Reproduced with permission from V.G. Wong, T. Kuwabara, P. Brubaker, W. Olson, J. Schulmar, and J.E. Seegmiller. Intralysosomal cystine crystals in cystinosis. *Invest. Ophthalmol.* 9: 83–88, 1970.)

There is an increased urinary excretion of sulfite ions (SO_3^{2-}), thiosulfate ions ($S_2O_3^{2-}$), and the amino acid S-sulfo-L-cysteine, but sulfate ions in the urine are markedly diminished or absent (126). S-sulfo-L-cysteine may also be elevated in the plasma.

III. DISORDERS OF MISCELLANEOUS AMINO ACIDS

A. Hyperornithinemia (Chorioretinal Gyrate Atrophy)

Gyrate atrophy of the retina and choroid is an inherited progressive degenerative retinopathy with an autosomal recessive mode of inheritance. The disorder, which is particularly prevalent in Finland and in individuals of Finnish ancestry, is associated with elevated ornithine (an amino acid not found in protein) in the blood and urine and a reduction or absence of the mitochondrial matrix enzyme ornithine aminotransferase (L-ornithine:2-oxoacid aminotransferase, OAT; EC 2.6.1.13), which converts ornithine to proline through the intermediates glutamic-γ-semialdehyde and Δ'-pyrroline 5-carboxylate (Fig. 9) (194,257). Vitamin B$_6$ is required as a coenzyme for ornithine aminotransferase (Fig. 9). The clinical picture of gyrate atrophy of the choroid and retina can occur in the absence of hyperornithinemia (129).

cDNA for human ornithine aminotransferase mRNA has been cloned and characterized (119, 124,125,219), and genes encoding for this enzyme have been localized by somatic cell hybrids and in situ hybridization to human chromosome 10 (10q26), as well as to the X chromosome (Xp11.2) (12). The mature protein consists of 407 residues, and the amino acid sequence of the enzyme is known (125). Lys292 is the residue that binds the coenzyme pyridoxal phosphate. The site of posttranslational proteolysis occurs at Ala25-Thr26 (243).

Developmental differences of specific ornithine ketoacid aminotransferase activities have been detected between ocular tissues and liver (242). The retina and choroid have a relatively low activity after

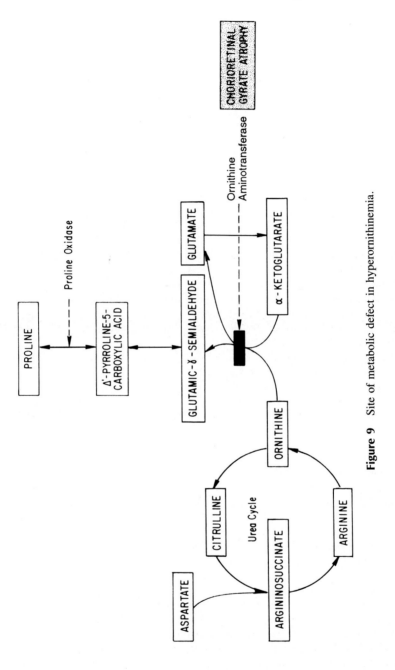

Figure 9   Site of metabolic defect in hyperornithinemia.

birth and an increased activity at 2.5 weeks, which remains high thereafter. The ciliary body and iris also manifest a relatively low activity at birth and a rapid increase at 1 week, which remains so for about 14 weeks before a gradual decrease occurs (242). Retinoblastoma cells express OAT at a high level (125).

In the early stages of gyrate atrophy, the margins of the atrophic retina appear by funduscopy as curved circular segments, and the term "gyrate atrophy" stems from this clinical appearance (Latin *gyratus*, turned around). The chorioretinal lesions are confined to the peripheral retina in older cases and are minimal in younger patients. However, a dystrophy of the macular may be a manifestation of gyrate atrophy (117). Electroretinographic evidence points to marked involvement of the cone and rod systems (138).

Despite a generalized deficiency of ornithine aminotransferase, clinical manifestations are limited to the eye (264). Individuals with gyrate atrophy of the choroid and retina are not weak, but type 2 muscles are atrophic and have tubular aggregates (See Chap. 54) (244). Bizarrely shaped mitochondria have been noted in the liver and in cultured skin fibroblasts of patients with gyrate atrophy (195). Because similar abnormalities can be induced in normal fibroblasts grown in culture media containing a high ornithine concentration (195), these are probably a sequel to hyperornithinemia.

TEM studies of the iris in patients with gyrate atrophy have disclosed atrophy, abnormal mitochondria, and tubular aggregates (structures similar to those found in skeletal muscle) in the dilator pupillae. Degenerative changes, such as extracted cellular matrix, dropout of cellular organelles, and dilated intercellular spaces, occur in the pigmented posterior epithelium and the anterior iris epithelium (269).

Some individuals with gyrate atrophy respond to high doses of vitamin B_6 by lowering their serum ornithine level and improving their electroretinogram (274). Also, with a partial deficiency of ornithine ketoacid transaminase activity, the residual activity may be stimulated in vitro by high concentrations of pyridoxal phosphate (17).

The level of ornithine aminotransferase activity in transformed lymphocytes in obligate heterozygous carriers is approximately 50% of the normal value (263).

A deficiency of the enzyme's product proline is unlikely to be important in the pathogenesis of the retinal degeneration, because this amino acid can be derived from other sources (194). Also, proline is an important constituent of collagen, but there is no clinical evidence of a systemic disorder of this ubiquitous protein. A candidate for possible toxicity to the retina in OAT deficiency is glyoxalate (221). Arginine glycine transmidinase activity was not detectable in human retina; thus a previously postulated creatine phosphate deprivation in OAT deficiency may not be applicable to the pathogenesis of the disease.

Clinical and biochemical heterogeneity has been detected in hyperornithinemia, and the response to vitamin B_6 also varies (274).

The molecular genetic flaw in gyrate atrophy has been demonstrated by finding a defect in the ornithine aminotransferase gene, mRNA, and protein (123). Very low levels of the enzyme have been identified in some affected individuals by immunoradioassay (196). Some ornithine aminotransferase activity has been detected in homogenates of liver biopsies of some cases of chorioretinal gyrate atrophy (268). However, in these individuals the kinetics of the residual ornithine aminotransferase differed from that of normal ornithine aminotransferase, suggesting that an abnormal enzyme rather than an absent one may occur in hyperornithinemia.

The ornithine aminotransferase activity in cultured skin fibroblasts from patients with gyrate atrophy is markedly decreased or not detected (194,260,263), not as a result of production of a structurally altered enzyme lacking catalytic activity but because of decreased production of enzyme protein (196).

The view that hyperornithinemia is toxic to the retina and choroid and causally related to chorioretinal gyrate atrophy finds support in several observations. The retina and choroid atrophy markedly in both monkeys and rats following an intravitreal injection of ornithine (127). The plasma ornithine level diminished fivefold in an affected individual who was maintained on an arginine-deficient diet for 20 months (136), and this was associated with a subjective improvement in visual function 15 months after institution of the diet.

In newly hatched chicks the subcutaneous injection of formoguanamine (2,4-diamino-*s*-triazine) induces a rapid decrease in the specific activity of ornithine aminotransferase (localized exclusively in the mitochondria of RPE) and of the content of vitamin B_6, degeneration of pigment epithelium and photoreceptors, acute retinal detachment, and a secondary gliosis in the outer nuclear layer (191). The retinal Δ^1-pyrroline-5-carboxylate reductase, an enzyme in the retinal cytosol, did not change (191).

Using human OAT cDNA to probe genomic DNA, evidence of gene deletion or rearrangement has not been found in patients with gyrate atrophy (219). The size and apparent amount of OAT mRNA in fibroblasts and/or lymphoblasts in some cases with gyrate atrophy who display a marked reduction in OAT activity is normal.

B. Familial Hyperlysinemia

The protein α-aminoadipic semialdehyde synthase has two enzyme activities, lysine-ketoglutarate reductase (EC 1.14.11.4) and saccharopine dehydrogenase (EC 1.5.1.10), that catabolize L-lysine. Lysine-ketoglutarate reductase is needed for the conversion of lysine to saccharopine, which saccharopine dehydrogenase converts to α-aminoadipic acid semialdehyde (70). In familial hyperlysinemia the activity of both of these enzymes is diminished, leading to hyperlysinemia and an excess excretion of lysine in the urine. An occasional individual with this rare autosomal recessive disorder has bilateral spherophakia or dislocated lenses (248). The question of whether the ocular changes are related to the metabolic defect remains unresolved.

C. Oculocerebrorenal (Lowe) Syndrome

In 1952, Lowe and colleagues (169) drew attention to the oculocerebrorenal syndrome, an X-linked recessive disorder with ocular and cerebral abnormalities and an aminoaciduria (1,169).

Congenital cataracts in both eyes are characteristic (262). The lens is small and spherical (spherophakia) and often has a conical posterior surface (posterior lenticonus). Total, nuclear, or posterior polar cataracts are evident at birth or during early infancy in most cases. Peculiar excrescences on the anterior and equatorial lens capsule (261) resemble those found in trisomy 21 (Down syndrome) and in Miller's syndrome (see Chap. 17).

About 50% of cases have congenital glaucoma, and many affected individuals have congenital anomalies of the retina and other ocular structures. Bilateral corneal keloids have been reported in a boy with Lowe syndrome without signs of perforating corneal trauma or iridocorneal incarceration in either eye (48). The cause of the keloids remains obscure, and the combination of corneal keloids with Lowe syndrome is probably coincidental in view of the rarity of the association.

The genetic defect in Lowe syndrome is manifest early in embryogenesis, as evidenced by the finding of both congenital cataract and iridocorneal angle dysgenesis in the eyes of a fetus obtained from a woman with a previous child having Lowe syndrome (74). All lens cells are presumably affected in males expressing the Lowe syndrome gene, and defective formation and subsequent degeneration of the primary posterior lens fibers account for the characteristic flattened, diskoid, or ring-shaped lens opacities. Some lens abnormalities, such as anterior polar cataract, subcapsular fibrous plaque, capsular excrescences, bladder cells, and posterior lenticonus, are not specific for Lowe syndrome (265).

Cerebral atrophy, which may be detectable clinically by computed tomography (280), causes mental retardation, hypotonia, and other neurological manifestations.

Involvement of the kidney accounts for many attributes of Lowe syndrome and many of the systemic effects, including proteinuria, excretion of undersulfated chondroitin sulfate A, sialic aciduria, generalized aminoaciduria, renal tubular acidosis, renal rickets, and a reduced ammonia production, reflect renal tubular dysfunction.

Other nonocular manifestations include physical retardation and frontal bossing. Studies of skin biopsy specimens in individuals with Lowe syndrome have disclosed cytoplasmic, membrane-bound, electron-lucent vacuoles and some electron-dense membranous inclusion bodies in fibroblasts and Schwann cells, as well as axonal degeneration and vascular changes (280).

As in other X-linked inherited disorders, one of the two X chromosomes is presumably randomly deactivated early in ontogeny in heterozygous female carriers (Lyon hypothesis), who develop punctate opacities occur in the lens with a relatively high frequency, and these opacities in the female lens probably reflect abnormal lens cells that express the mutant gene on the X chromosome. Carriers of Lowe syndrome develop variably shaped cortical dots, which become more numerous with age, as well (49,120,158). Rarely, Lowe syndrome occurs in girls without a positive family history (121,206,233). It may be accompanied by a balanced X/3 translocation, with a breakpoint at Xq25 (121), presumably as a result from a disruption of the X chromosome within the Lowe syndrome gene locus and a nonrandom inactivation of the normal X chromosome.

cDNAs for a Lowe syndrome gene have been isolated, and the predicted gene product resembles inositol polyphosphate-5-phosphatase, suggesting that Lowe syndrome may result from an inborn error of inositol phosphate metabolism (10). An earlier theory postulates that the basic defect in Lowe syndrome involves electron transport in mitochondria before the cytochromes (93). This view finds support in the observation of a marked diminution in the respiratory controls of mitochondria from muscle, with substrates reducing nicotinamide adenine dinucleotide (glutamate plus malate) and with a flavoprotein-linked substrate (succinate). Oxygen consumption with ascorbate and tetramethylphenylenediamine as substrates is normal with mitochondria from persons with Lowe syndrome (93), but the mitochondria manifest a decreased adenosine diphosphate phosphorylate-oxygen ratio, indicating partial uncoupling of the mitochondrial electron transport system. However, other disorders of mitochondria do not express the features of Lowe syndrome.

The possibility that manifestations of Lowe syndrome are attributable to the defective metabolism of glycosaminoglycans has been proposed (see Chap. 28) (151,280,293,294). Also, because cultured skin fibroblasts from patients with Lowe syndrome synthesize substantially less collagen than normal (207), the issue of whether other extracellular matrix abnormalities are present has also been raised.

D. Canavan's Disease

Canavan's disease (spongy degeneration of the brain) is a rare autosomal recessive lethal disorder of infancy characterized by a spongy state of the white matter in the brain and defective myelination. The salient clinical manifestations include an onset in early infancy of blindness, megalocephaly, severe mental retardation, atonia of the neck muscles, hyperextension of the legs, and flexion of the arms. Death ensues before the end of the second year of life. Congenital, infantile, and late-onset forms of the disorder are recognized (179). Most documented cases have been Jewish and can be traced to Eastern Europe (164). Many cases have been identified in Saudi Arabia (201). N-acetylaspartic acid is elevated in the plasma and urine (178,179), as well as in the cerebrospinal fluid (179), and a deficiency of aspartoacylase (EC 3.5.1.15) has been detected in some affected individuals (178,201). As in many other inherited disorders with the same type of inheritance, obligate carriers of the mutant gene express enzyme levels of less than 50% of control values (179).

E. Taurine Deficiency

Cholesterol is normally converted into trihydroxycoprostanoate and then into cholyl coenzyme A, an activated intermediate in the synthesis of bile salts. The amino group of the sulfur-containing amino acid taurine, which is not a constituent of any protein, reacts with cholyl coenzyme A to form the bile salt taurocholate. Although it remains uncertain whether taurine has other roles in the human, taurine is the most bountiful amino acid in the vertebrate retina (208,271), where it is synthesized. Taurine is particularly abundant in the RPE and the photoreceptors (148,189,199,271), and it is suspected of having antioxidant, osmoregulatory, and membrane-stabilizing functions in the retina (292). Taurine appears to be important in retinal function at least in the cat, in which a deficiency of this amino acid leads to retinal degeneration and blindness (113,238). Cats fed a taurine-free casein diet manifest a central photoreceptor (both rods and cones) degeneration after plasma and retinal taurine deficiency (24,113,238).

ACKNOWLEDGMENT

Supported in part by research grant EY0146 from the National Eye Institute.

REFERENCES

1. Abbassi, V., Lowe, C.U., and Calcagno, P.L. Oculo-cerebro-renal syndrome: A review. *Am. J. Dis. Child.* *115*:145–168, 1968.
2. Alitalo, T., Kruse, T.A., Forsius, H., Eriksson, A.W., and de la Chapelle, A. Localization of the Åland Island eye disease locus to the pericentromeric region of the X chromosome by linkage analysis. *Am. J. Hum. Genet.* *48*:31–38, 1991.
3. Alkemade, P. *Dysgenesis Mesodermalis of the Iris and the Cornea*, Van Gorcum, Assen, the Netherlands, 1969.

4. Allen, R.A., O'Malley, C., and Straatsma, B.R. Ocular findings in hereditary ochronosis. *Arch. Ophthalmol.* 65:656–668, 1961.
5. Anderson, B. Corneal and conjunctival pigmentation among workers engaged in manufacture of hydroquinone. *Arch. Ophthalmol.* 38:812–826, 1947.
6. Apkarian, P., Reits, D., and Spekreijse, H. Component specificity in albino VEP asymmetry: Maturation of the visual pathway anomaly. *Exp. Brain Res.* 53:285–294, 1984.
7. Apkarian, P., Reits, D., Spekreijse, H., and Van Doorp, D. A decisive electrophysiological test for human albinism. *Electroencephalogr. Clin. Neurophysiol.* 55:513–531, 1983.
8. Ashton, N., Kirker, J.G., and Lavery, F.S. Ocular findings in a case of hereditary ochronosis. *Br. J. Ophthalmol.* 48:405–415, 1964.
9. Assensio, A.M., Cascone, C., Fracassi, A., Parisi, S.G., Lubrano, R., and Giardini, O. Albinismo oculo-cutaneo e tirosinuria. Desrizione di un caso clinico. *Minerva Pediatr.* 35:99–103, 1983.
10. Attree, O., Olivos, I.M., Okabe, I., Bailey, L.C., Nelson, D.L., Lewis, R.A., McInnes, R.R., and Nussbaum, R.L. The Lowe's oculocerebrorenal syndrome gene encodes a protein highly homologous to inositol polyphosphate-5-phosphatase. *Nature* 358: 239–242, 1992.
11. Babel, J. Rheumatisme et oeil. *Arch. Ophtalmol. (Paris)* 33:341–354, 1973.
12. Barrett, D.J., Bateman, J.B., Sparkes, R.S., Mohandas, T., Klisak, I., and Inana, G. Chromosomal localization of human ornithine aminotransferase gene sequences to 10q26 and Xp11.2. *Invest. Ophthalmol. Vis. Sci.* 28:1037–1042, 1987.
13. Barton, D.E., Yang-Feng, T.L., and Francke, U. The human tyrosine aminotransferase gene mapped to the long arm of chromosome 16 (region 16q22-q24) by somatic cell hybrid analysis and in situ hybridization. *Hum. Genet.* 72:221–224, 1986.
14. Beard, M.E., Burns, R.P., Rich, L.F., and Squires, E. Histopathology of keratopathy in the tyrosine-fed rat. *Invest. Ophthalmol.* 13:1037–1041, 1974.
15. Bedoya, V. Pigmentary changes in Chédiak-Higashi syndrome. *Br. J. Dermatol.* 85:336–347, 1971.
16. Beguez-Cesar, A. Neutropenia crónica maligna familiar con granulaciones atípicas de los leucocitos. *Bol. Soc. Cubana Pediatr.* 15:900–922, 1943.
17. Behrens-Baumann, W., König, U., Schröder, K., Hansmann, I. and Langenbeck, U. Biochemical and therapeutical studies in a case of atrophia gyrata. *Graefes Arch. Clin. Exp. Ophthalmol.* 218:21–24, 1982.
18. Bell, T.G., Meyers, K.M., Prieur, D.J., Fauci, A.S., Wolff, S.M., and Padgett, G.A. Decreased nucleotide and serotonin storage associated with defective function in Chédiak-Higashi syndrome cattle and human platelets. *Blood* 48:175–184, 1976.
19. Ben Dridi, M.F., Karoui, S., Kastally, R., Gharbi, H.A., Zaimi, I., and Ben Osman, R. L'homocystinurie: Forme avec thrombose vasculaire et deficit en factor VIII. *Arch. Fr. Pediatr.* 43:41–44, 1986.
20. Benson, W. Oculocutaneous albinism with Axenfeld's anomaly (letter). *Am. J. Ophthalmol.* 92:133–134, 1981.
21. Bergsma, D.R., and Brown, K.S. Animal models of albinism. *Birth Defects* 12:409–426, 1976.
22. Bergsma, D.R., and Kaiser-Kupfer, M. A new form of albinism. *Am. J. Ophthalmol.* 77:837–844, 1974.
23. Berman, E.R. Biochemical diagnostic tests in genetic and metabolic eye disease. In *Genetic and Metabolic Eye Disease*, M.F. Goldberg (Ed.), Little, Brown, Boston, pp. 94–95, 1974.
24. Berson, E.L., Hayes, K.C., Rabin, A.R., Schmidt, S.Y., and Watson, G. Retinal degeneration in rats fed casein. II. Supplementation with methionine, cysteine or taurine. *Invest. Ophthalmol.* 15:52–58, 1975.
25. Bienfang, D.C., Kuwabara, T., and Pueschel, S.M. The Richter-Hanhart syndrome: Report of a case with associated tyrosinemia. *Arch. Ophthalmol.* 94:1133–1137, 1976.
26. Blume, R.S., Bennett, J.M., Yankee, R.A., and Wolff, S.M. Defective granulocyte regulation in the Chédiak-Higashi syndrome. *N. Engl. J. Med.* 279:1009–1015, 1968.
27. Blume, R.S., Glade, P.R., Gralnick, H.R., Chessin, L.N., Haase, A.T., and Wolff, S.M. The Chédiak-Higashi syndrome: Continuous suspension cultures derived from peripheral blood. *Blood* 33:821–832, 1969.
28. Blume, R.S., and Wolff, S.M. The Chédiak-Higashi syndrome: Studies in four patients and a review of the literature. *Medicine (Baltimore)* 51:247–280, 1972.
29. Boylan, C., Clement, R.A., and Harding, G.F.A. Lateralization of the flash visual evoked cortical potential in human albinos. *Invest. Ophthalmol. Vis. Sci.* 25:1448–1450, 1984.
30. Boylan, C., and Harding, G.F. Investigation of visual pathway abnormalities in human albinos. *Ophthalmic Physiol. Opt.* 3:273–285, 1983.
31. Bradley, W.F., Richardson, J., and Frew, I.J.C. The familial association of neurofibromatosis, peroneal muscular atrophy, congenital deafness, partial albinism and Axenfeld's defect. *Brain* 97:521–532, 1974.
32. Bregeat, P., and Dhermy, P., and Hamard, H. Manifestations oculaires du syndrome de Chédiak Higashi. *Arch. Ophtalmol. (Paris)* 26:661–676, 1966.
33. Bruce, S., Tschen, J.A., and Chow, D. Exogenous ochronosis resulting from quinine injections. *J. Am. Acad. Dermatol.* 15:357–361, 1986.
34. Buchanan, G.R., and Handin, R.L. Platelet function in the Chédiak-Higashi syndrome. *Blood* 47:941–948, 1976.
35. Bunim, J.J., McGuire, J.S., Jr., Hilbish, T.F., Laster, L., La Du, B.N., Jr., and Seegmiller, J.E. Alcaptonuria: Clinical staff conference at the National Institutes of Health. *Ann. Intern. Med.* 47:1210–1224, 1957.

36. Burke, J.P., O'Keefe, M., Bowell, R., and Naughten, E.R. Ocular complications in homocystinuria—early and late treated. *Br. J. Ophthalmol. 73*:427–431, 1989.
37. Burns, R.P. The tyrosine aminotransferase deficiency: An unusual cause of corneal ulcers. *Am. J. Ophthalmol. 73*:400–402, 1972.
38. Burns, R.P. Soluble tyrosine aminotransferase deficiency in an unusual cause of corneal ulcers. *Am. J. Ophthalmol. 73*:400–402, 1972.
39. Burns, R.P., Beard, M.E., Weimar, V.L., and Squires, E.L. Modification of L-tyrosine-induced keratopathy by adrenal corticosteroids. *Invest. Ophthalmol. 13*:39–45, 1974.
40. Burns, R.P., Gipson, I.K., and Murray, M.J. Keratopathy in tyrosinemia. *Birth Defects 12*:169–180, 1976.
41. Carroll, W.M., Jay, B.S., McDonald, W.I., and Halliday, A.M. Two distinct patterns of visual evoked response asymmetry in human albinism. *Nature 286*:604–606, 1980.
42. Carroll, W.M., Jay, B.S., McDonald, W.I., and Halliday, A.M. Pattern evoked potentials in human albinism. *J. Neurol. Sci. 48*:265–287, 1980.
43. Castro-Gago, M., Pombo, M., Novo, I., Tojo, R., and Peña, J. Sindrome familiar de microcefalia con albinismo oculoctáneo y anomalies digitales. *An. Esp. Pediatr. 19*:128–131, 1983.
44. Chan, A.M., Lynch, M.J.G., Bailey, J.D., Ezrin, C., and Fraser, D. Hypothyroidism in cystinosis. *Am. J. Med. 48*:678–692, 1970.
45. Charlton, K.H., Binder, P.S., Wolziak, L., and Digby, D.J. Pseudodendritic keratitis and systemic tyrosinosis. *Ophthalmology 88*:355–360, 1981.
46. Christensen, K., Fischer, P., Knudsen, K.E.B., Larsen, S., Sorensen, H., and Venge, O. A syndrome of hereditary tyrosinemia in mink (*Mustela vison* Schreb). *Can. J. Comp. Med. 43*:333–340, 1979.
47. Christensen, K., Henriksen, P., and Sorensen, H. New forms of hereditary tyrosinemia type II in mink: Hepatic tyrosine aminotransferase defect. *Hereditas 104*:215–222, 1986.
48. Cibis, G.W., Tripathi, R.C., Tripathi, B.J., and Harris, D.J. Corneal keloid in Lowe's syndrome. *Arch. Ophthalmol. 100*:1795–1799, 1982.
49. Cibis, G.W., Waeltermann, J.M., Whitcraft, C.T., Tripathi, R.C., and Harris, D.J. Lenticular opacities in carriers of Lowe's syndrome. *Ophthalmology 93*:1041–1045, 1986.
50. Cogan, D.G., and Kuwabara, T. Ocular pathology of cystinosis. *Arch. Ophthalmol. 63*:51–57, 1960.
51. Cogan, D.G., Kuwabara, T., Kinoshita, J., Sheehan, L., and Merola, L. Cystinosis in an adult. *JAMA 164*:394–396, 1957.
52. Cogan, D.G., Kuwabara, T., Kinoshita, J., Sudarsky, D., and Ring, H. Ocular manifestations of systemic cystinosis. *Arch. Ophthalmol. 55*:36–41, 1956.
53. Cohen, H.J., Betcher-Lange, S., Kessler, D.L., and Rajagopalan, K.V. Hepatic sulfite oxidase: Congruency in mitochondria of prosthetic group and activity. *J. Biol. Chem. 247*:7759–7766, 1972.
54. Colditz, P.B., Yu, J.S., Billson, F.A., Rogers, M., Molloy, H.F., O'Halloran, M., and Wilcken, B. Tyrosinaemia II. *Med. J. Aust. 141*:244–245, 1984.
55. Coleman, J., Sydnor, C.F., Wolbarsht, M.L., and Bessler, M. Abnormal visual pathways in human albinos studied with visually evoked potentials. *Exp. Neurol. 65*:667–679, 1979.
56. Comings, D.E., and Odland, G.F. Partial albinism. *JAMA 195*:519–523, 1966.
57. Costa, J.L., Fauci, A.S., and Wolff, S.M. A platelet abnormality in the Chédiak-Higashi syndrome of man. *Blood 48*:517–520, 1976.
58. Courtens, W., Broeckx, W., Ledoux, M., and Vamos, E. Oculocerebral hypopigmentation syndrome (Cross syndrome) in a Gipsy child. *Acta Paediatr. Scand. 78*:806–810, 1989.
59. Creel, D.J. Visual system anomaly associated with albinism in the cat. *Nature (Lond) 231*:465–466, 1971.
60. Creel, D. Problems of ocular miswiring in albinism, Duane's syndrome, and Marcus Gunn phenomenon. *Int. Ophthalmol. Clin. 24*:165–176, 1984.
61. Creel, D., Boxer, L.A., and Fauci, A.S. Visual and auditory anomalies in Chediak-Higashi syndrome. *Electroencephalogr. Clin. Neurophysiol. 55*:252–257, 1983.
62. Creel, D., King, R.A., Witkop, C.J., Jr., and Okoro, A.N. Visual system anomalies in human albinos. In *Pigment Cell, Pathophysiology of Melanocytes*, S.N. Klaus (Ed.), Karger, New Haven, CT, pp. 21–27, 1979.
63. Creel, D., O'Donnell, F.E., Jr., and Witkop, C.J., Jr. Visual system anomalies in human ocular albinos. *Science 201*:931–933, 1978.
64. Creel, D., Spekreijse, H., and Reits, D. Evoked potentials in albinos: Efficacy of pattern stimuli in detecting misrouted optic fibers. *Electroencephalogr. Clin. Neurophysiol. 52*:595–603, 1981.
65. Creel, D., Witkop, C.J., Jr., and King, R.A. Asymmetric visually evoked potentials in human albinos: Evidence for visual system anomalies. *Invest. Ophthalmol. 13*:430–440, 1974.
66. Creel, D.J., Bendel, C.M., Wiesner, G.L., Wirtschafter, J.D., Arthur, D.C., and King, R.A. Abnormalities of the central visual pathways in Prader-Willi syndrome associated with hypopigmentation. *N. Engl. J. Med. 314*:1606–1609, 1986.
67. Cross, H.E., and Jensen, A.D. Ocular manifestations in the Marfan syndrome and homocystinuria. *Am. J. Ophthalmol. 75*:405–520, 1973.
68. Cross, H.E., McKusick, V.A., and Breen, W. A new oculocerebral syndrome with hypopigmentation. *J. Pediatr. 70*:398–406, 1967.

69. Daicker, B., and Riede, U.N. Histologische und ultrastrukturelle Befunde bei alkaptonurischer Ochronosis oculi. *Ophthalmologica 169*:377–388, 1974.

70. Dancis, J., and Cox, R.P. Errors of lysine metabolism. In *The Metabolic Basis of Inherited Disease*, 6th ed., Vol. 1, C.R. Scriver, A.L. Beaudet, W.S. Sly, and D. Valle (Eds.), McGraw-Hill, New York, Chap. 21, pp. 665–670, 1989.

71. Danes, B.S., and Bearn, A.G. Cell culture and the Chédiak-Higashi syndrome. *Lancet 2*:65–67, 1967.

72. Davis, W.C., Spicer, S.S., Greene, W.B., and Padgett, D.V.M. Ultrastructure of bone marrow granulocytes in normal mink and mink with the homology of the Chédiak-Higashi trait of humans. I. Origin of the abnormal granules present in the neutrophils of mink with the C-HS trait. *Lab. Invest. 24*:303–317, 1971.

73. Driscoll, D.J., Jabs, E.W., Alcorn, D., Maumenee, I.H., Brusilow, S.W., and Valle, D. Corneal tyrosine crystals in transient neonatal tyrosinemia. *J. Pediatr. 113*:91–93, 1988.

74. Dufier, J.L., Dhermy, P., Farriaux, J.P., Amedee-Manesme, P., Broyer, M., and François, P. Contribution au diagnostic anténatal dun syndrome de Lowe par l'examen histologique des yeux du foetus. *J. Fr. Ophtalmol. 9*:361–366, 1986.

75. Dunn-Meynell, A.A., Prasada Rao, P.D., and Sharma, S.C. The ipsilateral retinotectal projection in normal and albino channel catfish. *Neurosci. Lett. 36*:25–31, 1983.

76. Fitzpatrick, T.B., Jimbow, K., and Donaldson, D.D. Dominant oculo-cutaneous albinism (summary). *Br. J. Dermatol. (Suppl.) 10*:23, 1974.

77. Forsius, H., and Eriksson, A.W. Ein neues Augensyndrom mit X-chromosomaler Transmission. Eine Sippe mit Fundusalbinismus, Foveahypoplasie, Nystagmus, Myopie, Astigmatismus und Dyschromatopsi. *Klin. Monatsbl. Augenheilkd. 144*:447–457, 1964.

78. Franceschetti, A.T., Schnyder, U.W., and Felgenhauer, W.R. Die Cornea beim Richter-Hanhart Syndrom. Bericht über die 71, Zusammenkunft der Deutchen Ophthalm. Gesellschaft in Heidelburg, 1979, p. 109.

79. Francois, J. Ocular manifestation in aminoacidopathies. *Monogr. Hum. Genet. 6*:99–113, 1972.

80. Francois, J., Hanssens, M., Coppieters, R., and Evens, L. Cystinosis: Clinical and histopathologic study. *Am. J. Ophthalmol. 73*:643–650, 1972.

81. Frenk, E., and Lattion, F. The melanin pigmentary disorder in a family with Hermansky-Pudlak syndrome. *J. Invest. Dermatol. 78*:141–143, 1982.

82. Gahl, W.A., Bashan, N., Tietze, F., Bernardini, I., and Schulman, J.D. Cystine transport is defective in isolated leukocyte lysosomes from patients with cystinosis. *Science 217*:1263–1265, 1982.

83. Gahl, W.A., Renhund, M., and Thoene, J.G. Lysosomal transport disorders: Cystinosis and sialic acid storage disorders. In *The Metabolic Basis of Inherited Disease*, 6th ed., Vol. 2, C.R. Scriver, A.L. Beaudet, W.S. Sly, and D. Valle (Eds.), McGraw-Hill, New York, Chap. 107, pp. 2619–2647, 1989.

84. Gahl, W.A., Schneider, J.A., Thoene, J.G., and Chesney, R. Course of nephropathic cystinosis after age 10 years. *J. Pediatr. 109*:605–608, 1986.

85. Gahl, W.A., Thoene, J.G., Schneider, J.A., O'Regan, S., Kaiser-Kupfer, M.I., and Kuwabara, T. NIH conference. Cystinosis: Progress in a prototypic disease. *Ann. Intern. Med. 109*:557–569, 1988.

86. Gahl, W.A., Tietze, F., Bashan, N., and Steinherz, J.D. Defective cystine exodus from isolated lysosome-rich fractions of cystinotic leukocytes. *J. Biol. Chem. 257*:9570–9575, 1982.

87. Garrett, E.E. Ocular ochronosis with alkaptonuria. *Am. J. Ophthalmol. 55*:617–620, 1963.

88. Garrod, A. *Inborn Errors of Metabolism*, Frowde, London, 1909.

89. Garron, L.K. Cystinosis. *Trans. Am. Acad. Ophthalmol. Otolaryngol. 63*:99–108, 1959.

90. Giolli, R.A., and Creel, D.J. The primary optic projections in pigmented and albino guinea pigs: An experimental degeneration study. *Brain Res. 55*:25–39, 1973.

91. Giolli, R.A., and Guthrie, M.D. The primary optic projections in the rabbit: An experimental degeneration study. *J. Comp. Neurol. 136*:99–125, 1969.

92. Gipson, I.K., Burns, R.P., and Wolfe-Lande, J.D. Crystals in corneal epithelial lesions of tyrosine-fed rats. *Invest. Ophthalmol. 14*:937–941, 1975.

93. Gobernado, J.M., Lousa, M., Gimeno, A., and Gonsalvez, M. Mitochondrial defects in Lowe's oculocerebrorenal syndrome. *Arch. Neurol. 41*:208–209, 1984.

94. Goldsmith, L.A. Tyrosinemia II: Lessons in molecular pathophysiology. *Pediatr. Dermatol. 1*:25–34, 1983.

95. Goldsmith, L.A. Tyrosinemia II. *Int. J. Dermatol. 24*:293–294, 1985.

96. Goldsmith, L.A., Kang, E., Beinfang, D.C., Jimbow, K., Gerald, P., and Baden, H.P. Tyrosinemia with plantar and palmar keratosis and keratitis. *J. Pediatr. 83*:798–805, 1973.

97. Goldsmith, L.A., and Laberge, C. Tyrosinemia and related disorders. In *The Metabolic Basis of Inherited Disease*, 6th ed., Vol. 1, C.R. Scriver, A.L. Beaudet, W.S. Sly, and D. Valle (Eds.), McGraw-Hill, New York, Chap. 16, pp. 547–562, 1989.

98. Goldsmith, L.A., Thorpe, J.M., and Marsh, R.F. Tyrosine aminotransferase deficiency in mink *Mustela vison*: A model for human tyrosinemia II. *Biochem. Genet. 19*:687–693, 1981.

99. Greene, A.A., Jonas, A.J., Harms, E., Smith, M.L., Pellett, O.L., Bump, E.A., Miller, A.L., and Schneider, J.A. Lysosomal cystine storage in cystinosis and mucolipidosis type II. *Pediatr. Res. 19*:1170–1174, 1985.

100. Gretz, N., Manz, F., Augustin, R., Barrat, T.M., Bender-Götze, C., Brandis, M., Bremer, H.J., Brodehl, J., Broyer, M., Bulla, M., Callis, L., Chantler, C., Diekmann, L., Dillon, M.J., Egli, F., Ehrich, J.H., Endres, W.,

Fanconi, A., Feldhoff, C., Geisert, J., Gekle, D., Geschöll-Bauer, B., Grote, K., Grüttner, R., Hagge, W., Haycock, C.B., Hennemann, H., Klare, B., Leupold, D., Löhr, H., Michalk, D., Oliveira, A., Ott, F., Pistor, K., Rau, J., Schärer, K., Schindera, F., Schmidt, H., Schulte-Wissermann, H., Verrier-Jones, K., Weber, H.P., Willenbockel, U., and Wolf, H. Survival time in cystinosis. A collaborative study. *Proc. Eur. Dial. Transplant Assoc.* 19:582–589, 1983.

101. Griscelli, C., Durandy, A., Guy-Rand, D., Daguillard, F., Herzog, C., and Prunieras, M. A syndrome associating partial albinism and immunodeficiency. *Am. J. Med.* 65:691–702, 1978.

102. Guillery, R.W. An abnormal retinogeniculate projection in Siamese cats. *Brain Res.* 14:739–741, 1969.

103. Guillery, R.W. An abnormal retinogeniculate projection in the albino ferret (*Mustela furo*). *Brain Res.* 33:482–485, 1971.

104. Guillery, R.W. Neuronal abnormalities in albinos. *Trends Neurosci.* 9:364–367, 1986.

105. Guillery, R.W., and Kaas, J.H. Genetic abnormality of the visual pathways in a "white" tiger. *Science* 180:1287–1289, 1973.

106. Guillery, R.W., Okoro, A.N., and Witkop, C.J., Jr. Abnormal visual pathways in the brain of a human albino. *Brain Res.* 96:373–377, 1975.

107. Guillery, R.W., Scott, G.L., Cattanach, B.M., and Deol, M.S. Genetic mechanisms determining the central visual pathways of mice. *Science* 179:1014–1016, 1973.

108. Guillery, R.W., Sitthi Amorn, C., and Eighmy, B.B. Mutants with abnormal visual pathways: An explanation of anomalous geniculate laminae. *Science* 174:831–832, 1971.

109. Hales, R.H. Albinism with Axenfeld's syndrome. *Rocky Mt. Med. J.* 65:51–52, 1968.

110. Hatch, J.L. Hereditary alkaptonuria with ochronosis. *Arch. Ophthalmol.* 62:575–578, 1959.

111. Hayakawa, M., Kato, K., Nakajima, A., Yoshiike, T., and Ogawa, H. Nettleship-Falls X-linked ocular albinism with Axenfeld's anomaly: A case report. *Ophthalmol. Paediatr. Genet.* 7:109–114, 1986.

112. Hayasaka, S., Asano, Y., Tateda, H., Hoshi, K., and Koga, Y. Lens subluxation in homocystinuria: A case report. *Acta Ophthalmol. (Copenh.)* 62: 425–431, 1984.

113. Hayes, K.C., Carey, R.E., and Schmidt, S.Y. Retinal degeneration associated with taurine deficiency in the cat. *Science* 188:949–951, 1975.

114. Hearing, V.J., and Lutzner, M.A. Mammalian melanosomal proteins: Characterization by polyacrylamide gel electrophoresis. *Yale J. Biol. Med.* 46:553–559, 1973.

115. Hearing, V.J., and Tsukamoto, K. Enzymatic control of pigmentation in mammals. *FASEB J.* 5:2902–2909, 1991.

116. Henkind, P., and Ashton, N. Ocular pathology in homocystinuria. *Trans. Ophthalmol. Soc. UK* 85:21–38, 1965.

117. Hennekes, R., and Gerding, H. Atrophia gyrata mit Makuladystrophie. *Klin. Monatsbl. Augenheilk.* 187:216–218, 1985.

118. Hill, A., and Zaleski, W.A. Tyrosinosis: Biochemical studies of an unusual case. *Clin. Biochem.* 4:263–271, 1971.

119. Himeno, M., Mueckler, M.M., Gonzalez, F.J., and Pitot, H.C. Cloning of DNA complementary to ornithine aminotransferase mRNA. *J. Biol. Chem.* 257:4669–4672, 1982.

120. Hittner, H.M., Carroll, A.J., and Prchal, J.T. Linkage studies in carriers of Lowe oculo-cerebro-renal syndrome. *Am. J. Hum. Genet.* 34:966–971, 1982.

121. Hodgson, S.V., Heckmatt, J.Z., Hughes, E., Crolla, J.A., Dubowitz, V., and Bobrow, M.S. A balanced de novo X/autosome translocation in a girl with manifestations of Lowe syndrome. *Am. J. Med. Genet.* 23:837–847, 1986.

122. Hoshaw, R.A., Zimmerman, K.G., and Menter, A. Ochronosislike pigmentation from hydroquinone bleaching creams in American blacks. *Arch. Dermatol.* 121:105–108, 1985.

123. Inana, G., Hotta, Y., Zintz, C., Takki, K., Weleber, R.G., Kennaway, N.G., Nakayasu, K., Nakajima, A., and Shiono, T. Expression defect of ornithine aminotransferase gene in gyrate atrophy. *Invest. Ophthalmol. Vis. Sci.* 29:1001–1005, 1988.

124. Inana, G., Totsuka, S., Redmond, M., Dougherty, T., Nagle, J., Shiono, T., Kominamini, E., and Katunuma, N. Molecular cloning of ornithine aminotransferase mRNA. *Proc. Natl. Acad. Sci. USA* 83:1203–1207, 1986.

125. Inana, G., Totsuka, S., Redmond, M., Dougherty, T., Nagle, J., Shiono, T., Ohura, T., Kominami, E., and Katunuma, N. Molecular cloning of human ornithine aminotransferase mRNA. *Proc. Natl. Acad. Sci. USA* 83:1203–1207, 1986.

126. Irreverre, F., Mudd, S.H., Heizer, W.D., and Laster, L. Sulfite oxidase deficiency: Studies of a patient with mental retardation, dislocated ocular lenses, and abnormal urinary excretion of S-sulfo-L-cysteine, sulfite, and thiosulfate. *Biochem. Med.* 1:187–217, 1967.

127. Ishikawa, Y., Kuwabara, T., and Kaiser-Kupfer, M.I. Toxic effects of ornithine to the pigment epithelium. *Invest. Ophthalmol. Vis. Sci. (Suppl.)* 20:120, 1981.

128. Jaeger, W., Gallasch, G., Schnyder, U.W., Lutz, P., and Schmidt, H. Tyrosinämie ais Urasche einer doppelseitigen herpetiformen Hornhaut-Spithel-Dystrophie (Richner-Hanhart-Syndrom). *Klin. Monatsobl. Augenheilkd.* 173:506–515, 1978.

129. Jaeger, W., von Kettler, J., Hilsdorf, C., and Lutz, P. Gibt es verschiedene Typen der Atrophia gyrata choroideae et retinae? (Atrophie gyrata chorioideae et retinae mit und ohne Ornithinämie). In *Kunststoffimplantate in der Ophthalmologie*, W. Jaeger (Ed.), J.F. Bermann, Munich, pp. 655–663, 1977.

130. Johnson, D.L., Jacobson, L.W., Toyama, R., and Monahan, R.H. Histopathology of eyes in Chédiak-Higashi syndrome. *Arch. Ophthalmol. 75*:84–88, 1966.

131. Johnson, G.J., Gillan, J.G., and Pearce, W.G. Ocular albinism in Newfoundland. *Can. J. Ophthalmol. 6*:237–248, 1971.

132. Jones, N.P., Postlethwaite, R.J., and Noble, J.L. Clearance of corneal crystals in nephropathic cystinosis by topical cysteamine 0.5%. *Br. J. Ophthalmol. 75*:311–312, 1991.

133. Kaiser-Kupfer, M.I., Caruso, R.C., Minckler, D.S., and Gahl, W.A. Long-term ocular manifestations in nephropathic cystinosis. *Arch. Ophthalmol. 104*:706–711, 1986.

134. Kaiser-Kupfer, M.I., Datiles, M.B., and Gahl, W.A. Corneal transplant in boy with nephropathic cystinosis (letter). *Lancet 1*:331, 1987.

135. Kaiser-Kupfer, M.I., Datiles, M.B., and Gahl, W.A. Clear graft two years after keratoplasty in nephropathic cystinosis (letter). *Am. J. Ophthalmol. 105*:318–319, 1988.

136. Kaiser-Kupfer, M.I., de Monasterio, F.M., Valle, D., Wasler, M., and Brusilow, S. Gyrate atrophy of the choroid and retina and improved visual function following reduction of plasma ornithine by diet. *Science 210*:1128–1131, 1980.

137. Kaiser-Kupfer, M.I., Gazzo, M.A., Datiles, M.B., Caruso, R.C., Kuehl, E.M., and Gahl, W.A. A randomized placebo-controlled trial of cysteamine eye drops in nephropathic cystinosis. *Arch. Ophthalmol. 108*:689–693, 1990.

138. Kaiser-Kupfer, M.I., Ludwig, I.H., de Monasterio, F.M., Valle, D., and Krieger, I. Gyrate atrophy of the choroid and retina. Early findings. *Ophthalmology 92*:394–401, 1985.

139. Kalra, B.R., Ghose, S., and Sood, N.N. Homocystinuria with bilateral absolute glaucoma. *Ind. J. Ophthalmol. 33*:195–197, 1985.

140. Kampik, A., Sani, J.N., and Green, W.R. Ocular ochronosis: Clinicopathological, histochemical, and ultrastructural studies. *Arch. Ophthalmol. 98*:1441–1447, 1980.

141. Kang, A.H., and Trelstad, R.L. A collagen defect in homocystinuria. *J. Clin. Invest. 52*:2571–2578, 1973.

142. Katz, B., Melles, R.B., and Schneider, J.A. Contrast sensitivity function in nephropathic cystinosis. *Arch. Ophthalmol. 105*:1667–1669, 1987.

143. Katz, B., Melles, R.B., and Schneider, J.A. Glare disability in nephropathic cystinosis. *Arch. Ophthalmol. 105*:1670–1671, 1987.

144. Katz, B., Melles, R.B., and Schneider, J.A. Recurrent crystal deposition after keratoplasty in nephropathic cystinosis. *Am. J. Ophthalmol. 104*:190–191, 1987.

145. Katz, B., Melles, R.B., and Schneider, J.A. Corneal sensitivity in nephropathic cystinosis. *Am. J. Ophthalmol. 104*:413–416, 1987.

146. Katz, B., Melles, R.B., and Schneider, J.A. Crystal deposition following keratoplasty in nephropathic cystinosis. *Arch. Ophthalmol. 107*:1727–1728, 1989.

147. Katz, B., Melles, R.B., Schneider, J.A., and Rao, N.A. Corneal thickness in nephropathic cystinosis. *Br. J. Ophthalmol. 73*:665–668, 1989.

148. Kennedy, A.J., and Voaden, M.J. Free amino acids in the photoreceptor cells of the frog retina. *J. Neurochem. 23*:1093–1095, 1974.

149. Kenyon, K.R., and Sensenbrenner, J.A. Electron microscopy of cornea and conjunctiva in childhood cystinosis. *Am. J. Ophthalmol. 78*:68–76, 1974.

150. Kida, K., Takahashi, M., Fujisawa, Y., Matsuda, H., Machino, H., and Miki, Y. Hepatic tyrosine aminotransferase in tyrosinaemia type II. *J. Inherited Metab. Dis. 5*:229–230, 1982.

151. Kieras, F.J., Houck, G.E., Jr., French, J.H., and Wisniewski, K. Low sulfated glycosaminoglycans are excreted in patients with the Lowe syndrome. *Biochem. Med. 31*:201–210, 1984.

152. Kim, Y.J., and Rosenberg, L.E. On the mechanism of pyridoxine responsive homocystinuria. II. Properties of normal and mutant cystathionine β-synthase from cultured fibroblasts. *Proc. Natl. Acad. Sci. USA 71*:4821–4825, 1974.

153. King, R.A., Creel, D., Cervenka, J., Okoro, A.N., and Witkop, C.J. Albinism in Nigeria with delineation of a new recessive oculocutaneous type. *Clin. Genet. 17*:259–270, 1980.

154. King, R.A., Lewis, R.A., Townsend, D., Zelickson, A., Olds, D.P., and Brumbaugh, J. Brown oculocutaneous albinism: Clinical, ophthalmological, and biochemical characterization. *Ophthalmology 92*:1496–1505, 1985.

155. King, R.A., and Rich, S.S. Segregation analysis of brown oculocutaneous albinism. *Clin. Genet. 29*:496–501, 1986.

156. King, R.A., Wirtschafter, J.D., Olds, D.P., and Brumbaugh, J. Minimal pigment: A new type of oculocutaneous albinism. *Clin. Genet. 29*:42–50, 1986.

157. Kinnear, P.E., Jay, B., and Witkop, C.J., Jr. Albinism. *Surv. Ophthalmol. 30*:75–101, 1985.

158. Koniszewski, G., and Rott, H.-D. Der Lyon-Effekt an der Linse: Konduktorinnen befunde bei X-chromosomal gebundender Katarakt und beim Lowe-Syndrom. *Klin. Monatsbl. Augenheilk. 187*:525–528, 1985.

159. Kramer, J.W., Davis, W.C., and Prieur, D.J. The Chédiak-Higashi syndrome of cats. *Lab. Invest. 36*:554–562, 1977.

160. Kraus, E., and Lutz, P. Ocular cystine deposits in an adult. *Arch. Ophthalmol. 85*:690–694, 1971.

161. Kritzler, R.A., Terner, J.Y., Lindenbaum, J., Magidson, J., Williams, R., Preisig, R., and Phillips, G.B. Chédiak-Higashi syndrome cytoplasmic and serum lipid observations in a case and family. *Am. J. Ophthalmol. 36*:583–594, 1964.

162. Kunkle, G.A., Jezyk, P.F., West, C.S., Goldschmidt, M.H., and O'Keefe, C.O. Tyrosinemia in a dog. *J. Am. Anim. Hosp. Assoc. 20*:615–620, 1984.

163. La Du, B.N. Alcaptonuria. In *The Metabolic Basis of Inherited Disease*, 6th ed., Vol. 1, C.R. Scriver, A.L. Beudet, W.S. Sly, and D. Valle (Eds.), McGraw-Hill, New York, Chap. 27, pp. 775–790, 1989.

164. Lattion, F., Schneider, P., Da Prada, M., Lorez, H.P., Richards, J.G., Picotti, G.B., and Frenck, E. Syndrome d'Hermansky-Pudlak dans un village valaisan. *Helv. Paediatr. Acta 38*:495–512, 1983.

165. Leader, R.W., Padgett, G.A., and Gorham, J.R. Studies of abnormal leukocyte bodies in the mink. *Blood 22*: 477–484, 1963.

166. Leuenberger, S., Faulborn, J., Sturrock, G., Gloor, B., Rehorek, R., and Baumgartner, R. Vasculäre und okuläre Komplikationen bei einem Kind mit Homocystinurie. *Schweiz. Med. Wochenschr. 114*:793–798, 1984.

167. Leventhal, A.G., Vitek, D.J., and Creel, D.J. Abnormal visual pathways in normally pigmented cats that are heterozygous for albinism. *Science 229*:1395–1397, 1985.

168. Lewis, R.A. Ocular albinism and deafness. Twenty-ninth Annual Meeting of Human Genetics. Vancouver, p. 57A, 1978.

169. Lowe, C.U., Terrey, M., and MacLachlan, E.A. Organic-aciduria, decreased renal ammonia production, hydrophthalmos and mental retardation: A clinical entity. *Am. J. Dis. Child. 83*:164–184, 1952.

170. Lubin, J.R. Oculocutaneous albinism associated with corneal mesodermal dysgenesis. *Am. J. Ophthalmol. 91*:347–350, 1981.

171. Lund, R.D. Uncrossed visual pathways of hooded and albino rats. *Science 149*:1506, 1965.

172. Luntzner, M. Ultrastructure of giant melanin granules in the beige mouse during ontogeny. *J. Invest. Dermatol. 54*:91, 1969.

173. Lutzner, M.A., Lowrie, C.T., and Jordan, H.W. Giant granules in leukocytes of the beige mouse. *J. Hered. 58*:299–300, 1967.

174. Lynch, H.J., Deng, M.H., and Wurtman, R.J. Light intensities required to suppress nocturnal melatonin secretion in albino and pigmented rats. *Life Sci. 35*:841–847, 1984.

175. MacDonald, I.M., Noel, L.P., Mintsioulis, G., and Clarke, W.N. The effect of topical cysteamine drops on reducing crystal formation within the cornea of patients affected by nephropathic cystinosis. *J. Pediatr. Ophthalmol. Strabismus 27*:272–274, 1990.

176. Machino, H., Miki, Y., Kawatsu, T., Kida, K., and Matsuda, H. Successful dietary control of tyrosinemia II. *J. Am. Acad. Dermatol. 9*:533–539, 1983.

177. Margolis, S., Siegel, I.M., Choy, A., and Bleinin, G.M. Oculocutaneous albinism associated with Apert's syndrome. *Am. J. Ophthalmol. 84*:830–839, 1977.

178. Matalon, R., Kaul, R., Casanova, J., Michals, K., Johnson, A., Rapin, I., Gaskoff, P., and Deanching, M. Aspartocylase deficiency: The enzyme defect in Canavan disease. *J. Inherited Metab. Dis. 12 (Suppl. 2)*:329–331, 1989.

179. Matalon, R., Michals, K., Sebesta, D., Deanching, M., Gaskoff, P., and Casanova J. Aspartocylase deficiency and N-acetylasparticaciduria in patients with Canavan disease. *Am. J. Med. Genet. 29*:463–471, 1988.

180. McCartney, A.C., Spalton, D.J., and Bull, T.B. Type IV melanosomes of the human albino iris. *Br. J. Ophthalmol. 69*:537–541, 1985.

181. McKusick, V.A. *Mendelian Inheritance in Man. Catalogs of Autosomal Dominant, Autosomal Recessive and X-linked Pheotypes*, 10th ed., Johns Hopkins University Press, Baltimore, 1992.

182. Melles, R.B., Schneider, J.A., Rao, N.A., and Katz, B. Spatial and temporal sequence of corneal crystal deposition in nephropathic cystinosis. *Am. J. Ophthalmol. 104*:598–604, 1987.

183. Miller, S.J.H. Ocular ochronosis. *Trans. Ophthalmol. Soc. UK 74*:349–366, 1954.

184. Mishima, H., Hasebe, H., and Fujita, H. Melanogenesis in the retinal pigment epithelial cell of the chick embryo. Dopa-reaction and electron microscopic autoradiography of ^{3}H-dopa. *Invest. Ophthalmol. Vis. Sci. 17*:403–411, 1978.

185. Moran, T.J., and Estevez, J.M. Chédiak-Higashi disease: Morphologic studies of a patient and her family. *Arch. Pathol. 88*:329–339, 1969.

186. Mosher, D.B., Fitzpatrick, T.B., Ortonne, J.-P., and Hori, Y. Disorders of pigmentation. In *Dermatology in General Medicine: Textbook and Atlas*, 3rd ed., T.B. Fitzpatrick, A.Z. Eisen, K. Wolff, I.M. Freedberg, and K.F. Austen (Eds.), McGraw-Hill, New York, pp. 794–876, Chap. 79, 1987.

187. Munke, M., Kraus, J., Watkins, P., Tanzi, R., Gusella, J., Millington Ward, A., Watson, M., and Francke, U. Homocystinuria gene on human chromosome 21 mapped with cloned cystathione beta-synthase probe and in situ hybridization of other chromosomal 21 probes (abstract). *Cytogenet. Cell Genet. 40*:706–707, 1985.

188. Ney, D., Bay, C., Schneider, J.A., Kelts, D., and Nyhan, W.W.L. Dietary management of oculocutaneous tyrosinemia in an 11-year old child. *Am. J. Dis. Child. 137*:995–1000, 1983.

189. Nishimura, C., Ida, S., and Kuriyama, K. Taurine biosynthesis in the frog retina: Effects of light and dark adaptions. *J. Neurosci. Res. 9*:59–67, 1983.

190. Novikoff, A.B., Leuenberger, P.M., Novikoff, P.M., and Quintana N. Retinal pigment epithelium: Interrelations of endoplasmic reticulum and melanolyosososmes in the black mouse and its beige mutant. *Lab. Invest. 40*:155–165, 1979.

191. Obara, Y., Matsuzawa, T., Kuba, N., and Fujita, K. Retinal damage in hatched chicks induced by formoguanamine: Decrease in ornithine aminotransferase activity and vitamin B_6 content. *Exp. Eye Res. 41*:519–526, 1985.

192. O'Donnell, F.E., Green, W.R., Fleischman, J.A., and Hambrick, G.W. X-linked ocular albinism in blacks: Ocular albinism cum pigmento. *Arch. Ophthalmol. 96*:1189–1192, 1978.

193. O'Donnell, F.E., Jr., Hambrick, G.W., Jr., Green, W.R., Iliff, W.J., and Stone, D.L. X-linked ocular albinism: An oculocutaneous macromelanosomal disorder. *Arch. Ophthalmol. 94*:1883–1892, 1976.

194. O'Donnell, J.J., Sandman, R.P., and Martin, S.R. Gyrate atrophy of the retina: Inborn error of L-ornithine: 2-oxoacid aminotransferase. *Science 200*:200–201, 1978.

195. O'Donnell, J.J., Wood, I., and Hopkins, S.R. Mitochondrial abnormalities in cultured fibroblasts from a gyrate atrophy patient. *Invest. Ophthalmol. Vis. Sci. (Suppl.) 20*:79, 1981.

196. Ohura, T., Kominami, E., Tada, K., and Katunuma, N. Gyrate atrophy of the choroid and retina: Decreased ornithine aminotransferase concentration in cultured skin fibroblasts from patients. *Clin. Chim. Acta 136*:29–37, 1984.

197. Oliver, J.M. Impaired microtubule function correctable by cyclic GMP and cholinergic agonists in the Chédiak-Higashi syndrome. *Am. J. Pathol. 85*:395–418, 1976.

198. Oliver, J.M. Cell biology of leukocyte abnormalities—membrane and cytoskeletal function in normal and defective cells: Leukocyte abnormalities. *Am. J. Pathol. 93*:221–270, 1978.

199. Orr, H.T., Cohen, A.I., and Lowry, O.H. The distribution of taurine in the vertebrate retina. *J. Neurochem. 26*:609–611, 1976.

200. Osler, W. Ochronosis: The pigmentation of cartilages, sclerotics, and skin in alkaptonuria. *Lancet 1*:10–11, 1904.

201. Ozand, P.T., Gascon, G.G., and Dhalla, M. Aspartoacylase deficiency and Canavan disease in Saudi Arabia. *Am. J. Hum. Gent. 35*:266–268, 1990.

202. Padgett, G.A. Neutrophilic function in animals with the Chédiak-Higashi syndrome. *Blood 29*:906–915, 1967.

203. Padgett, G.A., Holland, J.M., Prieur, D.J., Davis, W.C., and Gorham, J.R. The Chédiak-Higashi syndrome: A review of the disease in man, mink, cattle and mice. *Anim. Models Biomed. Res. 3*:1–12, 1970.

204. Padgett, G.A., Leader, R.W., Gorham, J.R., and O'Mary, C.C. The familial occurrence of the Chédiak-Higashi syndrome in mink and cattle. *Genetics 49*:505–512, 1964.

205. Palareti, G., Salardi, S., Piazzi, S., Legnani, C., Poggi, M., Grauso, F., Caniato, A., Coccheri, S., and Cacciari, E. Blood coagulation changes in homocystinuria: Effects of pyridoxine and other specific therapy. *J. Pediatr. 109*:1001–1006, 1986.

206. Pallisgaard, G., and Goldschmidt, E. Oculo-cerebro-renal syndrome of Lowe in four generations of one family. *Acta Paediatr. Scand. 60*:146–148, 1971.

207. Palmieri, M.J., O'Hara, J., States, B., and Segal, S. Decreased procollagen production in cultured fibroblasts from patients with Lowe's syndrome. *J. Inherited Metab. Dis. 8*:187–192, 1985.

208. Pasantes-Morales, H., Kleithi, J., Ledig, M., and Mandel, P. Free amino acids of chicken and rat retina. *Brain Res. 41*:494–497, 1972.

209. Pearce, W.G., Johnson, C.J., and Sanger, R. Ocular albinism and Xg. *Lancet 1*:1072, 1971.

210. Perez, M.I., and Sanchez, J.L. Histopathologic evaluation of melanocytic nevi in oculocutaneous albinism. *Am. J. Dermatopathol. (Suppl.) 7*:23–28, 1985.

211. Phillips, J.I., Isaacson, C., and Carman, H. Ochronosis in black South Africans who used skin lighteners. *Am. J. Dermatopathol. 8*:14–21, 1986.

212. Pillers, D.A., Towbin, J.A., Chamberlain, J.S., Wu, D., Ranier, J., Powell, B.R., and McCabe, E.R.B. Deletion mapping of Åland Island eye disease to Xp21 between DXS67 (B24) and Duchenne muscular dystrophy. *Am. J. Hum. Genet. 47*:795–801, 1990.

213. Polyak, S. In: *The Vertebrate Visual System*, H. Klüver (Ed.), University of Chicago Press, Chicago, 1957.

214. Prieur, D.J. *A Bibliography of the Chédiak-Higashi Syndrome of Man and Animals*, Washington State University, Pullman, WA, pp. 1–23, 1976.

215. Prieur, D.J., and Collier, L.L. Animal model of human disease: Chédiak-Higashi syndrome. *Am. J. Pathol. 90*:533–536, 1978.

216. Prieur, D.J., Davis, W.C., and Padgett, G.A. Defective function of renal lysosomes in mice with the Chédiak-Higashi syndrome. *Am. J. Pathol. 67*:227–240, 1972.

217. Prieur, D.J., Holland, J.M., Bell, T.G., and Young, D.M. Ultrastructural and morphometric studies of platelets from cattle with the Chédiak-Higashi syndrome. *Lab Invest. 35*:197–204, 1976.

218. Quevedo, W.C., Jr., Fitzpatrick, T.B., Szabó, G., and Jimbow, K. Biology of the melanin pigmentary system. In *Dermatology in General Medicine: Textbook and Atlas*, 3rd ed. T.B. Fitzpatrick, A.Z. Eisen, K. Wolff, I.M. Freedberg, and K.F. Austen (Eds.), McGraw-Hill, New York, pp. 224–251, 1987.

219. Ramesh, V., Shaffer, M.M., Allaire, J.M., Shih, V.E., and Gusella, J.F. Investigation of gyrate atrophy using a cDNA clone for human ornithine aminotransferase. *DNA 5*:493–501, 1986.

220. Ramsey, M.S., Yanoff, M., and Fine, B.S. The ocular histopathology of homocystinuria: A light and electron microscopic study. *Am. J. Ophthalmol. 74*:377–385, 1972.

221. Rao, G.N., and Cotlier, E. Ornithine delta-aminotransferase activity in retina and other tissues. *Neurochem. Res. 9*:555–562, 1984.

222. Ricci, B., Lacerra, F., and Lubins, J.R. Oculocutaneous albinism and corneal mesodermal dysgenesis (letter). *Am. J. Ophthalmol. 92*:587, 1987.

223. Rich, L.F., Beard, M.E., and Burns, R.P. Excess dietary tyrosine and corneal lesions. *Exp. Eye Res. 17*:87–97, 1973.

224. Richard, G., and Kroll, P. Netzhautveränderungen bei Zystinose. *Ophthalmologica 186*:211–218, 1983.

225. Richler, M., Milot, J., Quigley, M., and O'Regan, S. Ocular manifestations of nephropathic cystinosis: The French-Canadian experience in a genetically homogeneous population. *Arch. Ophthalmol. 109*:359–362, 1991.

226. Ripple, R.E., Lohr, K.M., Twining, S.S., Hyndiuk, R.A., and Cayag, J.G. Role of leukocytes in ocular inflammation of tyrosinemia II. *Invest. Ophthalmol. Vis. Sci. 27*:926–931, 1986.

227. Robinson, W.G., and Kuwabara, T. A new, albino-beige mouse: Giant granules in retinal pigment epithelium. *Invest. Ophthalmol. Vis. Sci. 17*:365–370, 1978.

228. Robinson, W.G., Kuwabara, T., and Cogan, D.G. Lysosomes and melanin granules of the retinal pigment epithelium in a mouse model of the Chédiak-Higashi syndrome. *Invest. Ophthalmol. 14*:312–317, 1975.

229. Rodenhauser, J.H. Über die Augenpigmentierung bei Alkaptonurie (Ochronosis oculi). *Klin. Monatsbl. Augenheidk. 131*:202–205, 1957.

230. Rones, B. Ochronosis oculi in alkaptonuria. *Am. J. Ophthalmol. 49*:440–446, 1960.

231. Rott, H.D., and Rix, R. Konduktorinnenstatus bei X-gebundenem, okurärem Albinismus: Ein Belegfür die Gültigkeit der Lyon-Hypothese beim Menchen. *Klin. Monatsbl. Augenheilk. 184*:128–129, 1984.

232. Royer, M.J., and Rollin. Les manifestations oculaires de l'ochronose. *Bull. Soc. Ophtalmol. Fr. 65*:500–502, 1965.

233. Sagel, I., Ores, R.O., and Yuceoglu, A.M. Renal function and morphology in a girl with oculocerebrorenal syndrome. *J. Pediatr. 77*:124–127, 1970.

234. Salceda, R., Carabex, A., Pacheco, P., and Pasantes-Morales, H. Taurine levels, uptake and synthesizing enzyme activities in degenerated rat retinas. *Exp. Eye Res. 28*:137–146, 1979.

235. Sanderson, K.J. Normal and abnormal retinogeniculate pathways in rabbits and mink. *Anat. Rec. 172*:398, 1972.

236. Sanderson, K.J., Guillery, R.W., and Shackelford, R.M. Congenitally abnormal visual pathways in mink (*Mustela vision*) with reduced retinal pigment. *Comp. Neurol. 154*:225–298, 1974.

237. Sanderson, P.O., Kuwabara, T., Stark, W.J., Wong, V.G., and Collins, E.M. Cystinosis: A clinical, histopathologic, and ultrastructural study. *Arch. Ophthalmol. 91*:270–274, 1974.

238. Schmidt, S.Y., Berson, E.L., and Hayes, K.C. Retinal degeneration in cats fed casein. 1. Taurine deficiency. *Invest. Ophthalmol. 15*:47–52, 1976.

239. Schneider, J.A., Verroust, F.M., Kroll, W.A., Garvin, A.J., Horger, E.O., III, Wong, V.G., Spear, G.S., Jacobson, C., Pellett, O.L., and Becker, F.L.A. Prenatal diagnosis of cystinosis. *N. Engl. J. Med. 290*:878–882, 1974.

240. Seitz, R. Über die ochronotischen Pigmentierungen am Auge. *Klin. Monatsbl. Augenheilk. 125*:432–440, 1954.

241. Shiloh, Y., Litvak, G., Ziv, Y., Lehner, T., Sandkuyl, L., Hildesheimer, M., Buchris, V., Cremers, F.P.M., Szabo, P., White, B.N., Holden, J.J.A., and Ott, J. Genetic mapping of X-linked albinism-deafness syndrome (ADFN) to Xq26.3-q27.1. *Am. J. Hum. Genet. 47*:20–27, 1990.

242. Shiono, T., Hayasaka, S., and Mizuno, K. Development of ornithine ketoacid aminotransferase in rabbit ocular tissues and liver. *Invest. Ophthalmol. Vis. Sci. 23*:419–424, 1982.

243. Simmaco, M., John, R.A., Barra, D., and Bossa, F. The primary structure of ornithine aminotransferase: Identification of active-site sequence and site of post-translational proteolysis. *FEBS Lett. 199*:39–42, 1986.

244. Sipila, I., Simell, O., Rapola, J., Sainio, K., and Tuuteri, L. Gyrate atrophy of the choroid and retina with hyperornithinemia: Tubular aggregates and type 2 fiber atrophy in muscle. *Neurology 29*:996–1005, 1979.

245. Skinsnes, O.K. Generalized ochronosis: Report of an instance where it was misdiagnosed as melanosarcoma, with resultant enucleation of an eye. *Arch. Pathol. 45*:552–558, 1948.

246. Smith, J.W. Ochronosis of the sclera and cornea complicating alkaptonuria: Review of the literature and report of four cases. *JAMA 120*:1282–1288, 1942.

247. Smith, R.S. Ocular pathology in sulfite oxidase deficiency. *Invest. Ophthalmol. Vis. Sci. (Suppl.) 17*:247, 1978.

248. Smith, T.H., Holland, M.E., and Woody, N.C. Ocular manifestations of familial hyperlysinemia. *Trans. Am. Acad. Ophthalmol. Otolaryngol. 75*:355–360, 1971.

249. Spencer, W.H., and Hogan, M.J. Ocular manifestations of Chédiak-Higashi syndrome. *Am. J. Ophthalmol. 50*:1197–1203, 1960.

250. Stefani, F.H., and Vogel, S. Adult cystinosis: Electron microscopy of the conjunctiva. *Graefes Arch. Clin. Exp. Ophthalmol. 219*:143–145, 1982.

251. Stigmaier, O.C., and Schneider, L.A. Chédiak-Higashi syndrome. *Arch. Dermatol. 91*:1–9, 1965.

252. Sudarshan, A., and Kopietz, L. Corneal changes in homocystinuria. *Ann. Ophthalmol. 18*:60, 1986.

253. Suveges, I. Kongenitale Hornhautdysplasie vergesellschaftet mit Richner-Hanhart-Syndrom. *Klin. Monatsbl. Augenheilkd.* 157:493–499, 1970.

254. Szymanski, K.A., Boughman, J.A., Nance, W.E., Olansky, D.C., and Weinberg, R.S. Genetic studies of ocular albinism in a large Virginia kindred. *Ann. Ophthalmol.* 16:183–185, 188–191, 1984.

255. Takahashi, A., and Yokoyama, T. Hermansky-Pudlak syndrome with special reference to lysosomal dysfunction. A case report and review of the literature. *Virchows Arch. [A] 402*:247–258, 1984.

256. Takatsuji, K., Ito, H., Watanabe, M., Ikushima, M., and Nakamura, A. Histopathological changes of the retina and optic nerve in the albino mutant quail (*Coturnix coturnix japonica*). *J. Comp. Pathol.* 94:387–404, 1984.

257. Takki, K. Gyrate atrophy of the choroid and retina associated with hyperornithinaemia. *Br. J. Ophthalmol.* 58:3–23, 1974.

258. Tan, C., Etcubanas, E., Lieberman, P., Isenberg, H., King, O., and Murphy, M.L. Chédiak-Higashi syndrome in a child with Hodgkin's disease. *Am. J. Dis. Child.* 121:135–139, 1971.

259. Taylor, R.F., and Farrell, R.F. Light and electron microscopy of peripheral blood neutrophils in a killer whale affected with Chédiak-Higashi syndrome. *Feb. Proc.* 32:822, 1973.

260. Trijbels, J.M.F., Sengers, R.C.A., Bakkeren, J.A.J.M., Dekort, A.F., and Deutman, A.F. L-ornithine-ketoacid-transaminase deficiency in cultured fibroblasts of a patient with hyperornithinaemia and gyrate atrophy of the choroid and retina. *Clin. Chim. Acta* 79:371–377, 1977.

261. Tripathi, R.C., Cibis, G.W., and Tripathi, B.J. Lowe's syndrome. *Trans. Ophthalmol. Soc. UK 100*:132–139, 1980.

262. Tripathi, R.C., Cibis, G.W., and Tripathi, B.J. Pathogenesis of cataracts in patients with Lowe's syndrome. *Ophthalmology 93*:1046–1051, 1986.

263. Valle, D., Kaiser-Kupfer, M.I., and Del Valle, L.A. Gyrate atrophy of the choroid and retina: Deficiency of ornithine aminotransferase in transformed lymphocytes. *Proc. Natl. Acad. Sci. USA* 74:5159–5161, 1977.

264. Valle, D., and Simell, O. The hyperornithinemias. In *Metabolic Basis of Inherited Disease*, 6th ed., Vol. 1, C.R. Scriver, A.L. Beudet, W.S. Sly, and D. Valle (Eds.), McGraw-Hill, New York, Chap. XX, pp. 599–627, 1989.

265. Van Der Berg, W., Verbraak, F.D., and Bos, P.J. Homocystinuria presenting as central retinal artery occlusion and longstanding thromboembolic disease. *Br. J. Ophthalmol.* 74:696–697, 1990.

266. Van Dorp, D.B., Delleman, J.W., and Loewer-Sieger, D.H. Oculocutaneous albinism and anterior chamber cleavage malformations: Not a coincidence. *Clin. Genet.* 26:440–444, 1984.

267. Van Dorp, D.B., Eriksson, A.W., Delleman, J.W., van Vliet, A.G., Collewijn, H., van Balen, A.T., and Forsius, H.R. Åland eye disease: No albino misrouting. *Clin. Genet.* 28:526–531, 1985.

268. Vannas-Sulonen, K., O'Donnell, J.J., and Sipila, I. Gyrate atrophy of the retina: Kinetic mutation of liver ornithine aminotransferase. *Invest. Ophthalmol. Vis. Sci. (Suppl.)* 20:210, 1981.

269. Vannas-Sulonen, K., Vannas, A., O'Donnell, J.J., Sipila, I., and Wood, I. Pathology of iridectomy specimens in gyrate atrophy of the retina and choroid. *Arch. Ophthalmol. (Copenh.)* 61:9–19, 1983.

270. Vassali, J.-D., Granelli-Piperno, A., Griscelli, C., and Reich, E. Specific protease activity in polymorphonuclear leukocytes of Chédiak-Higashi syndrome and beige mice. *J. Exp. Med.* 147:1285–1290, 1978.

271. Voaden, M.J., Lake, N., Marshall, J., and Morjaria, B. Studies on the distribution of taurine and other neuroactive amino acids in the retina. *Exp. Eye Res.* 25:249–257, 1977.

272. Waardenburg, P.J. *Remarkable Facts in Human Albinism and Leukism*, Van Gorcum, Assen, the Netherlands, pp. 1–103, 1970.

273. Wan, W.L., Minckler, D.S., and Rao, N.A. Pupillary-block glaucoma associated with childhood cystinosis. *Am. J. Ophthalmol.* 101:700–705, 1986.

274. Weleber, R.G., Wirtz, M.K., and Kennaway, N.G. Gyrate atrophy of the choroid and retina: Clinical and biochemical heterogeneity and response to vitamin B$_6$. *Birth Defects* 18:219–230, 1982.

275. White, J.G. The Chédiak-Higashi syndrome: A possible lysosomal disease. *Blood* 28:143–156, 1966.

276. Windhorst, D.B., Zelickson, A.S., and Good, R.A. Chédiak-Higashi syndrome: Heredity giantism of cytoplasmic organelles. *Science 151*:81–83, 1966.

277. Windhorst, D.B., Zelickson, A.S., and Good, R.A. A human pigmentary dilution based on a heritable subcellular structural defect—the Chédiak-Higashi syndrome. *J. Invest. Dermatol.* 50:9–18, 1968.

278. Winship, I., Gericke, G., and Beighton, P. X-linked inheritance of ocular albinism with late-onset sensorineural deafness. *Am. J. Med. Genet.* 19:797–803, 1984.

279. Wirtschafter, J.D. The eye in alkaptonuria. *Birth Defects 12*:279–289, 1976.

280. Wisniewski, K.E., Kieras, F.J., French, J.H., Houck, G.E., Jr., and Ramos, P.L. Ultrastructural, neurological, and glycosaminoglycan abnormalities in Lowe's syndrome. *Ann. Neurol.* 16:40–49, 1984.

281. Wisniewski, K.E., Laure-Kamionowska, M., Sher, J., and Pitter, J. Infantile neuroaxonal dystrophy in an albino girl: A cliniconeuropathologic study. *Acta Neuropathol. (Berl.)* 66:68–71, 1985.

282. Witkop, C.J., Jr. Albinism. In *Advances in Human Genetics*, Vol. 2, H. Harris and K. Hirschhorn (Eds.), Plenum, New York, pp. 61–142, 1971.

283. Witkop, C.J., Jr. Depigmentation of the general and oral tissues and their genetic foundations. *Ala. J. Med. Sci.* 16:330–343, 1979.

284. Witkop, C.J., Jr., Hill, C.W., Desnick, S., Thies, J.K., Thorn, H.L., Jenkins, M., and White, J.G. Ophthalmologic, biochemical, platelet and ultrastructural defects in the various types of oculocutaneous albinism. *J. Invest. Dermatol. 60*:443–456, 1973.

285. Witkop, C.J., Jr., Jay, B., Creel, D., and Guillery, R.W. Optic and otic neurologic abnormalities in oculocutaneous and ocular albinism. *Birth Defects 18*:299–318, 1982.

286. Witkop, C.J., Jr., Quevedo, W.C., Jr., Fitzpatrick, T.B., and King, R.A. Albinism. In *The Metabolic Basis of Inherited Disease*, 6th ed., Vol. 2, C.R. Scriver, A.L. Beaudet, W.S. Sly, and D. Valle (Eds.), McGraw-Hill, New York, Chap. 119, pp. 2905–2947, 1989.

287. Wolff, S.M., Dale, D.C., Clark, R.A., Root, R.K., and Kimball, H.R. The Chédiak-Higashi syndrome: Studies of host defenses. *Ann. Intern. Med. 76*:293–306, 1972.

288. Wollensak, J. Zonula Zinnii histologische und chemische Untersuchungen, insbesondere über Zonolysis enzymatica und Syndroma Marfan. *Fortschr. Augenheildk. 16*:240–335, 1965.

289. Wong, V.G. Ocular manifestations in cystinosis. *Birth Defects 12*:181–186, 1976.

290. Wong, V.G., Kuwabara, T., Brubaker, R., Olson, W., Schulman, J., and Seegmiller, J.E. Intralysosomal cystine crystals in cystinosis. *Invest. Ophthalmol. 9*:83–88, 1970.

291. Wong, V.G., Lietman, P.S., and Seegmiller, J.E. Alterations of pigment epithelium in cystinosis. *Arch. Ophthalmol. 77*:361–369, 1967.

292. Wright, C.E., Tallan, H.H., and Lin. Y.Y. Taurine: Biological update. *Annu. Rev. Biochem. 55*:427–453, 1986.

293. Yamashina, I., Yoshida, H., Fukui, S., and Funakoshi, I. Biochemical studies on Lowe's syndrome. *Mol. Cell. Biochem. 52*:107–124, 1983.

294. Yokoi, T., Taniguchi, N., and Ikawa, K. Impaired synthesis of intracellular heparan sulfate in skin fibroblasts of Lowe's syndrome. *J. Lab. Clin. Med. 100*:461–468, 1982.

295. Yoshiike, T., Manabe, M., Hayakawa, M., and Ogawa, H. Macromelanosomes in X-linked ocular albinism (XLOA). *Acta Derm. Venereol. (Stockh.) 65*:66–69, 1985.

296. Zimmerman, T.J., Hood, I., and Gasset, A.R. "Adolescent" cystinosis: A case presentation and review of the recent literature. *Arch. Ophthalmol. 92*:265–268, 1974.

32

Proteins in Ocular Disease

Gordon K. Klintworth
Duke University Medical Center, Durham, North Carolina

I. INTRODUCTION

Because proteins are the product of DNA transcription, all genetically determined disorders basically result from the synthesis of abnormal proteins or from the failure of certain essential proteins to be produced (see Chap. 24). In some inherited and acquired diseases, proteins accumulate within ocular tissues. An understanding of these disorders requires identification of the particular protein in question. This is particularly important in inherited diseases because it can lead to the identification of the basic genetic defect. Histochemical techniques play an important role in the recognition of proteins, but an unfortunate limitation in the characterization of unknown proteins in tissue sections stems from the fact that most histochemical techniques only demonstrate reactive groups in amino acids. Although different proteins vary in size, amino acid sequence, and tertiary structure, amino acid analyses of proteins have disclosed that the majority contain similar proportions of the amino acids (378). In view of this, most proteins have indistinguishable histochemical attributes, exceptions being proteins with atypical amino acid profiles, such as collagen and elastin, in which a particular amino acid may predominate. When specific proteins are suspected immunocytochemical methods are important, but they suffer from the inherent weakness that antibodies may react with portions of molecules that are basically dissimilar.

Advances in molecular biology have made it possible to insert parts or entire foreign genes into bacteria and to make them synthesize the protein product of the gene in question (141). These so-called recombinant bacteria can be grown easily at low cost, and the applications of this intricate methodology are enormous. Such molecular biological procedures have extended our knowledge about many diseases, including some that are discussed in other chapters, and about certain ocular proteins, such as those of the lens (31,33), retina (62,467), and cornea (65,66). The technology of contemporary molecular biology offers considerable promise in future research on certain pathological conditions of the eye, especially inherited disorders.

II. EXTRACELLULAR MATRIX PROTEINS

Owing largely to special staining characteristics, histologists have long recognized different types of extracellular fibrous components in tissues. A considerable amount of information related to the molecular biology of some of these components is known, and a discussion of them is beyond the scope of this text. The interested reader should look elsewhere for details (8,20,356,392).

A. Collagen and Related Proteins

Collagen is discussed in Chap. 33.

973

Reticulin

The designation *reticulin* was originally introduced for the argyrophilic fibrous structure that forms a delicate network (reticulum) around certain cells, such as those of the hepatic parenchyma. Reticulin, which adsorbs metallic silver when treated with alkaline solutions of reducible silver, is not present in all tissues, and its precise nature still needs to be established, but current evidence favors the concept that reticulin consists of collagen fibers of a finer diameter than usual. Reticular fibers are interwoven in delicate networks rather than in coarse bundles and stain much more intensely than typical collagenous fibers with silver impregnation techniques. In electron micrographs, reticulin possesses the periodic ultrastructure that typifies collagen, and fibers with the properties of reticulin precede typical collagenous fibers, which gradually replace them in the differentiation of mesenchyme into loose connective tissue. Reticular fibers persist around certain cells, however, such as adipose cells and the endothelium of capillaries. Past analyses of the protein portion of reticulin suggested collagen with more carbohydrate (4.25 against 0.55%) and 10% bound fatty acids (57).

The composition of reticulin remains uncertain, and it may vary in different tissues. Some reticulin fibers have been found to contain laminin and type III collagen (224,225); others seem to consist of type III collagen (23,134,473), which retains its aminopropeptide (224), type I and type III collagen (195, 244,286), or hybrids of type I and type III collagen (110).

From the standpoint of ocular disease, abundant reticulin often surrounds neoplastic melanoma cells in the choroid. Indeed, at one time its presence was thought to be of prognostic significance, a view that is no longer accepted. In neoplasms of capillaries, the location of the reticulin can aid in the differentiation between hemangioendotheliomas and hemangiopericytomas. Reticulin is also conspicuous around capillaries in diabetic retinopathy.

B. Elastic and Related Fibers

Mature elastic fibers possess two distinct components: elastin and elastic fiber microfibrillary protein. These constituents are discernible in different tissues by transmission electron microscopy (TEM) as a central homogeneous component (elastin) enveloped by tubular microfibrils. Elastic fibers occur in close proximity to collagen, proteoglycans, glycoproteins, and other constituents of the extracellular matrix in most tissues but vary considerably in amount. This structural component of connective tissue can be demonstrated with a variety of stains, including orcein, aldehyde fuchsin, Weigert's resorcin-fuchsin, Verhoeff's iron hematoxylin stain, and orcinol-new fuchsin (orcinol-new fuchsin has a high degree of specificity for elastic fibers, but some dyes, such as aldehyde fuchsin, also react with other substances) (123). Elastic microfibrils possess an affinity for cationic substances, such as lead or uranyl acetate; anionic stains like phosphotungstic acid have an affinity for the nonfilamentous component (389,390).

From the standpoint of the eye, elastic fibers are present in Bruch's membrane, the sclera, the conjunctiva, and the walls of some blood vessels but are curiously absent from the normal cornea.

Elastin and Tropoelastin

Elastin surrounds elastic tissue microfibrils. Pure elastin is rich in glycine, proline, alanine, and valine, and these uncharged hydrophobic residues render the molecule insoluble in water. Elastin contains multiple cross-links between the polypeptide chains of the molecule that impart rubberlike properties to elastic tissue. Lysine plays a significant role in the formation of these cross-linkages, and this is achieved in part by lysinonorleucine and the two amino acid isomers, desmosine and isodesmosine (Greek *desmos*, band). Elastin, the most insoluble of all connective tissue elements, can apparently be solubilized only after cleavage of peptide bonds by either chemical or enzymatic procedures.

The gene for elastin has been cloned and mapped to the long arm of chromosome 2 (2q31-2qter) (103) and to chromosome 7 (290). The initial translational product of the elastin gene is known as tropoelastin (molecular mass 72 kD). This soluble precursor of elastin is a linear polymer of about 800 amino acids (molecular mass about 67 kD) (398,399). It is highly hydrophobic and has an amino acid composition that is similar but not identical to that of mature elastin. Tropoelastin has a higher content of lysine than elastin but lacks the desmosine, isodesmosine, and lysinonorleucine components known to participate in cross-links or to be precursors of cross-links.

The enzyme elastase, which possesses general proteolytic as well as elastolytic activity, degrades the homogeneous elastin component of elastic fibers more than the microfibrils (390). The elastic fiber microfibrils, but not elastin, are digested by trypsin, chymotrypsin, and pepsin (390). All other mammalian proteinases either do not act on elastin or their activity is very slow. However, several nonmammalian proteinases (papain, pronase, ficin, bromelain, and nagarase) possess marked elastolytic activity.

Disorders of Elastin. Pseudoxanthoma elasticum and the Buschke-Ollendorff syndrome are suspected of being genetic defects of elastin (388). In Menkes' syndrome (see Chap. 37) the synthesis of elastin is defective as a consequence of deficient cross-linking of elastin secondary to a deficiency of the enzyme lysyl oxidase, which needs both copper and pyridoxal as cofactors (74).

Pseudoxanthoma elasticum. Pseudoxanthoma elasticum is a rare progressive inherited disorder of elastic tissue with prominent, clinically significant manifestations in the skin, eye, and cardiovascular system. The elastic tissue fibers become fragmented and calcify. The disorder derives its name from small yellow cutaneous macules, papules, and plaques that form especially in the flexural areas. Angioid streaks are common (see Chap. 20). Considerable heterogeneity exists in pseudoxanthoma elasticum, and several forms are recognized (364,477). These include autosomal dominant (363) and autosomal recessive types. Two types of autosomal dominant pseudoxanthoma elasticum are recognized: type I (associated with "severe choroiditis") and type II (with myopia and blue sclera).

Buschke-Ollendorff syndrome. Cataracts are common in Buschke-Ollendorff (osteopoikilosis) syndrome (379), a rare autosomal dominant disorder characterized by asymptomatic circumscribed areas of bony sclerosis and multiple skin lesions with abnormal elastic fibers (disseminated dermatofibrosis). In contrast to pseudoxanthoma elasticum, elastic fiber fragmentation and calcification are not features of this disorder.

Elastic Microfibrils

Each elastic fiber microfibril measures approximately 11 nm in diameter and a glycoprotein is associated with the microfibrillary protein in the elastic fibers (389). The microfibrillar protein in elastic tissue differs from both elastin and collagen in being rich in cystine, aspartic acid, glutamic acid, and glycine, relatively poor in neutral and basic amino acids, and containing no hydroxyproline, hydroxylysine, desmosine, or isodesmosine (390). A component of the elastin-associated microfibrils is a glycoprotein known as fibrillin. Two human genes encode for it. One has been mapped to the long arm of chromosome 15 (15q15-21.3) (84); the other involves a locus on human chromosome 5 (5q23-31) (267).

Disorders of Fibrillin. *Marfan syndrome.* Marfan syndrome, one of the most common connective tissue disorders, has an autosomal dominant mode of inheritance, but almost 15% of cases occur sporadically (289). Cardinal features of Marfan syndrome involve the eye as well as the cardiovascular and skeletal systems. Affected persons tend to be tall, with elongated scrawny limbs and long slender spidery fingers and toes (arachnodactyly). A shortened lifetime of persons with Marfan syndrome is attributed to the cardiovascular manifestations, which include (1) an enfeebling aortic media that occasionally culminates in a deathly dissecting aneurysm, most frequently in the ascending aorta; and (2) pulmonary artery and aortic ring dilatation and a stretching of the aortic cusps that may result in marked aortic regurgitation. Skeletal anomalies include kyphoscoliosis, a prominent sternum (pectus carinatum) and/or undue depression in the sternum (pectus excavatum). The joints are often hypermobile, with redundant ligaments and capsules.

A characteristic ocular abnormality in Marfan syndrome is ectopia lentis, which occurs in approximately 50–80% of affected persons (Fig. 1) (70,289,370). Slit lamp biomicroscopy discloses thin, redundant, and occasionally severed zonules. The crystalline lens tends to dislocate upward, perhaps because of particularly weak zonular attachments between the inferior portion of the lens and the ciliary body. Unlike homocystinuria (70), the lens rarely becomes displaced into the anterior chamber. The reason for this probably rests in the clinical observation that the pupil is nearly always miotic and generally unresponsive to mydriatics. As a consequence of the lens dislocation, the unsupported iris trembles with ocular movement (iridodonesis).

Individuals with Marfan syndrome often have a myopic refractive error for which two potential reasons exist: an enlarged globe and microphakia (479). The markedly elongated globe, which sometimes enlarges under normal intraocular pressure, perhaps reflects involvement of scleral elastic tissue. Surgical treatment may become necessary for a resultant staphyloma (147). The elongated myopic eye that forms in

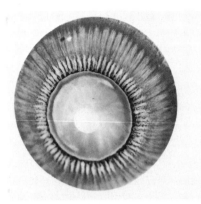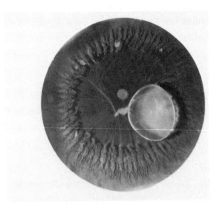

Figure 1 Crystalline lens, ciliary body, and iris viewed from behind. In contrast to the normal eye (left), the lens in Marfan syndrome is small, spherical, and displaced. The pupil of the abnormal eye is miotic. (Reproduced with permission from G.K. Klintworth and M.B. Landers, III. *The Eye: Structure and Function in Disease*, Williams and Wilkins, Baltimore, 1976.)

persons with Marfan syndrome probably predisposes these individuals to retinal detachment, especially after lens extraction (289). The sclera of persons with Marfan syndrome is thinner than normal, and this causes an apparent blue color of this tissue in some cases (35). The pathological state may also affect the cornea and cause keratoconus (18).

After immunohistochemical studies pointed to a defect in fibrillin in Marfan syndrome, a metabolic abnormality of fibrillin was identified in many patients with Marfan syndrome (267). The gene for Marfan syndrome has been mapped to the fibrillin gene on chromosome 15 (84,267). A missense mutation in this fibrillin gene has also been detected in patients with sporadic Marfan syndrome (84), and a condition with phenotypic similarities to Marfan syndrome has been linked to the fibrillin gene on chromosome 5 (267).

Investigators once suspected Marfan syndrome of being a disorder of collagen, and this view found minor support in observations on tissue or cells derived from some cases of Marfan syndrome. Such findings included a heightened solubility of skin collagen in certain solutions (417), an abnormal synthesis by fibroblasts of collagen (250,368), including less collagen α_2 chains (417), a higher soluble collagen content (368), or the production of less type I and more type III collagen by an aortic organ culture (250) than normal.

Abnormalities of glycosaminoglycan metabolism (261,300) have also been detected in fibroblasts secured from patients afflicted with Marfan syndrome (see Chap. 28).

Oxytalan

In 1958, Fullmer and Lillie (122) discovered by serendipity a connective tissue fiber with some attributes of elastic tissue. The fibers were more resistant to acid hydrolysis than collagen and were hence designated oxytalan (Greek *oxys*, acid and *talas*, enduring). Such structures become apparent in tissue with certain stains for elastic tissue (aldehyde fuchsin, orcein, and Weigert's resorcin-fuchsin) after an exposure of tissue to a strong oxidizing agent, such as peracetic acid, performic acid, or potassium peroxymonosulfate, but not otherwise (122). The grouping with which orcinol-new fuchsin and Verhoeff's stain reacts is absent in oxytalan both before and after oxidation with peracetic acid. That oxidation is required for fiber staining suggests that it may contain a reduced form of some component of elastic fibers. Elastase is only able to digest formalin-fixed oxytalan fibers after oxidation with peracetic acid or other appropriate oxidizing agents (122). Oxytalan is also susceptible to β-glucuronidase after oxidation (but not before it). The precise composition of oxytalan remains unknown, however, although the fibers do not contain cystine, arginine, tryptophan, tyrosine, or disulfide reactive sites in amounts detectable by histochemical procedures (122,123). Hence oxytalan fibers appear to have a protein portion and a stainable component digestible with β-glucuronidase after oxidation (123). TEM has disclosed that oxytalan fibers consist of fibrils (approximately 10–15 nm in diameter) (123) that resemble the fibrotubular component of elastic fibers, and like elastic fibers they are sometimes associated with variable amounts of a homogeneous material.

Oxytalan has been identified in several tissues (122) but has also been observed in the cornea, a tissue normally devoid of elastic tissue.

Oxytalan in Pathological States. Oxytalan has been identified beneath the epithelium of the cornea in keratoconus (10) and in postinflammatory or posttraumatic scarring, but not in normal corneas (Fig. 2) (9,10,130). Oxytalan has also been demonstrated in the excrescences on Descemet's membrane in Fuchs' corneal dystrophy (130).

Elaunin

Fibers that stain with orcein, Weigert's resorcin, and aldehyde fuchsin without previous oxidation, but not with Verhoeff's method, were designated elaunin (Greek *elauno*, I stretch) by Gawlik (135). Such fibers have been identified in tendons, fibrous cartilage, and elastic laminae of developing aortas but have not yet been identified in the eye.

Histochemical as well as light microscopic and TEM observations on tissues at different stages of development have permitted a tentative identification of the interrelationship between elastic fibers, oxytalan, and elaunin. In the embryo, elastic fibers consist mainly of microfibrils, and developing elastic tissue passes through a stage in which its histochemical attributes are indistinguishable from those of oxytalan (123). Current histochemical techniques cannot distinguish developing elastic fibers from oxytalan, but these fibers can be set apart by their appearance with TEM (123) and yet they are sufficiently alike to suggest that oxytalan is an incomplete or modified type of elastic fiber (123). Gawlik (135) found that in fetal and newborn arteries oxytalan fibers appear first and are followed by elaunin and finally elastic fibers. Light microscopic and TEM observations are also consistent with the concept that oxytalan fibers appear first and that elaunin is an intermediate between them and elastic fibers.

C. Other Extracellular Matrix Proteins

Fibronectin

Fibronectin is a sizable glycoprotein (220 kD) constituent of cell surfaces as well as of the extracellular matrix, many basal lamina, and media of cultured fibroblasts (393). Fibronectin, or an immunologically similar protein, is also found in the plasma (plasma fibronectin). A short amino acid sequence consisting of arginine-glycine-aspartate (Arg-Gly-Asp) is responsible for the attachment of cells to fibronectin (371).

Available evidence suggests that fibronectin plays a role in cell-to-cell and cell-to-connective tissue relationships, including cell adhesion. Although Descemet's membrane of the normal cornea alone contains immunologically detectable fibronectin, this glycoprotein accumulates, especially in the subepithelial zone, during corneal reepithelialization.

Vitronectin

Human serum and plasma contain another distinct cell adhesive protein known as vitronectin (serum spreading factor) (170). Although sharing some similarities and properties with fibronectin, including the presence of an Arg-Gly-Asp sequence, vitronectin is antigenically and structurally distinct from fibronectin. Immunohistochemical studies using monoclonal antibodies indicate that vitronectin (molecular mass 70 kd) exists in tissues and as an extracellular matrix protein (170). The cDNA of vitronectin has been cloned. Vitronectin has amino acid sequences which like the fibronectin receptor recognize Arg-Gly-Asp (371).

Laminin

Another noncollagenous glycoprotein known to be localized in the basal lamina of several tissues, including the eye, is laminin (111). Laminin is biochemically and immunologically distinct from both type IV collagen (see Chap. 33) and fibronectin. In contrast to fibronectin, laminin is not found in serum. By immunofluorescence microscopy laminin is located in Bruch's membrane and in the basal lamina of retinal and choroidal blood vessels (111).

The role of fibronectin and laminin in ocular diseases remains a fruitful field for future investigation, especially in view of the many basal laminae in the eye and the numerous pathological states that affect these structures.

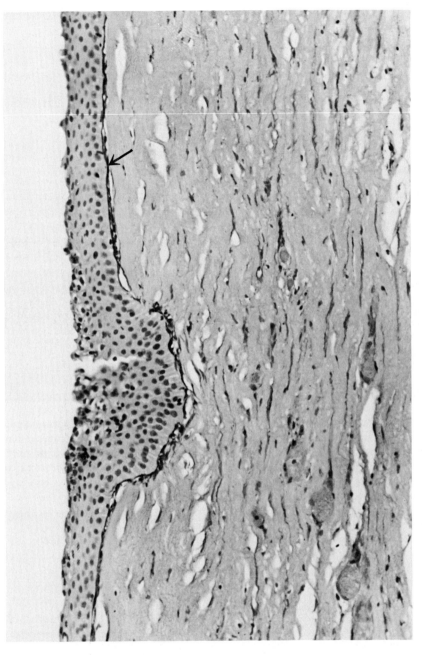

Figure 2 Oxytalan fibers in cornea. (peracetic acid–orcein, ×245) (Reproduced with permission from R.A. Alexander and A. Garner. Oxytalan fibre formation in the cornea: A light and electron microscopical study. *Histopathology I*:189–199, 1977.)

Tenascin

Tenascin (hexabrachion, cytotactin, or brachionectin) is an exceptionally large six-armed adhesion extracellular matrix protein (molecular mass > 1000 kD) consisting of a heximer of disulfide-linked subunits (55). The molecule contains several epidermal growth factor–like segments and portions related to part of fibronectin (fibronectin type III repeats). In contrast to fibronectin, with which it frequently colocalizes, tenascin is not found in the serum. Tenascin has a wide tissue distribution and is transiently found in wound healing. The function of tenascin remains uncertain, but like other components of the extracellular matrix it may modulate cell function. The chick vitreous contains abundant tenascin (498), but this molecule is rare in the mammalian vitreous (380).

III. CYTOSKELETAL PROTEINS

The cytoskeleton of eukaryotes contains three types of filaments (actin, microtubules, and intermediate filaments), which function in many important cellular events in normal and pathological processes (8). These filaments contribute to cell structure and motility. They are also involved in the attachment of cells to each other and to the extracellular matrix. Because of this they play a cardinal role in intercellular and extracellular matrix-cell communication. Specific proteins are major components of these filaments.

A. Tubulin

The globular polypeptide tubulin (molecular mass 50 kD) consists of a dimer composed of two closely related polypeptides (α and β tubulin). Polymers of tubulin molecules become assembled together to form microtubules, and within cilia these microtubules are precisely organized to form the typical 9 + 2 arrangement that characterizes the cross-sectional profile that electron microscopists established years ago (Fig. 14 in Chap. 1). Within cilia specific proteins (dynein and nexin) retain this configuration by forming links between adjacent doublets (nexin) and the side arms (dynein).

B. Actin

Actin filaments (F actin or microfilaments) consist of globular subunits (G actin) arranged into two helical fibrils. The globular molecules are stabilized by tightly bound calcium ions and are covalently bound to ATP. Hydrolysis of the terminal phosphate of the bound ATP causes G actin to polymerize into the actin filaments.

Actin is a constituent of virtually all cells, and in cells with the zonula adherens type of cell junctions they converge on this intermediate cell junction. Mammals express at least six actin genes, and some of them are restricted to specific cell types (two sarcomeric actins, α cardiac and α skeletal actins, two smooth muscle actins, α vascular smooth muscle actin and γ cytoplasmic actins) (8,410,411). The practical value of this information has already emerged. For example, analyses of the actin isoforms in leiomyosarcomas support the assumption that these smooth muscle tumors are heterogeneous in nature (410,411). Also, the immunohistochemical demonstration of sarcomeric α skeletal actin in tumor cells is useful in establishing the diagnosis of rhabdomyosarcoma (58).

Several proteins bind to actin, including α-actinin, filamin, fimbrin, gelsolin (see elsewhere in this chapter), myosin (muscle and nonmuscle), profilin, tropomyosin, and villin, as well as proteins that specifically bind to an end of the actin filaments (capping proteins). Organized bundles of actin filaments and associated proteins are referred to as stress fibers. Stress fibers terminate at specialized areas of the plasma membrane (adhesion plaques), where an anchoring protein (vinculin) links actin to the plasma membrane.

C. Intermediate Filaments

The intermediate filaments (10 nm in diameter and 21 nm axial periodicity) form a filamentous intracytoplasmic system in eukaryotic cells. These filaments, which are morphologically similar in all cell types, can be divided into six distinct classes by biochemical and immunological methods: cytokeratins (64,119,263,264,316,464), glial fibrillary acid protein (GFAP), vimentin, desmin (137), neurofilaments, and nestin (463). All have sequence similarities and form a complex multigene family (137).

Immunocytochemical studies with the immunoperoxidase technique using monoclonal antibodies that recognize specific intermediate filaments can help classify tumors derived from mesenchymal, muscle, epithelial, glial, or neural cells and are useful in confirming histopathological diagnoses and in differentiating among different diagnostic possibilities (58,339,410,452).

Cytokeratin is the major structural protein of all epithelial cells but is not specific for epithelial cells. Tonofilaments (cytokeratins), the most complex and highly developed of the various classes of intermediate filaments, anchor into desmosomes. The cytokeratins are a heterogeneous group of intermediate filaments, each of which is encoded by its own mRNA. In the human 19 different keratin species are recognized, and they are encoded by two distinct gene families (119). Keratins have been classified into the smaller acid keratins (10–19, keratin I, pH 4.5–5.3, 40–56.5 kD) and the larger basic keratins (1–8, keratin II; pH 5.5–7.5, 52–67 kD).

Most epithelia express several cytokeratins. The type of cytokeratin expressed varies with the species and tissue epithelium and the cell's state of differentiation and keratinization. The cornea contains some specific cytokeratins (cytokeratins 3 and 12) that can be detected with particular monoclonal antibodies (382).

Nestin is expressed abundantly in neuroepithelial stem cells early in embryogenesis (463).

D. Cytoskeletal and Other Proteins in Cell-Cell Adherens Junctions

In certain cells cytoskeletal components, such as actin and myosin, are linked in juxtaposed cells at adherens junctions that are composed of several proteins. Structural proteins at the cytoplasmic face of these sites of tight adhesion to the substrate, where actin filaments attach to the plasma membrane, include the following.

Vinculin

Vinculin, a major constitutive cytoskeletal protein (molecular mass 130 kD) of the adherens junctions (136), has some amino acid sequence similarity to E cadherin. Vinculin is associated with both cell-cell and cell-extracellular matrix adherens cell junctions. Vinculin is capable of interacting with α-actinin.

Talin

Talin, which binds to vinculin and to the cytoplasmic tail of integrin, is present with vinculin at the termini of cytoplasmic stress fiber bundles.

Other Proteins in Cell-Cell Adherens Junctions

As from vinculin and talin, cell-cell adherens junctions contain filamin, α-actinin (an actin cross-linking protein), dystrophin (only muscle), calpain II, protein kinase C, paxillin, tensin and zyxin, radixin, tenuin, and plaglobin (8,471,472).

IV. CELL ADHESION MOLECULES

Externally several proteins are involved in cell-cell and cell extracellular matrix adhesion. These proteins play an important role in mediating fundamental interactions between cells and between cells and the extracellular matrix. Such interactions are vital in normal and pathological processes, including the control of cellular growth and neoplasia, migration and differentiation, and cell-to-cell inflammatory and immunological reactions, as well as angiogenesis. Such mechanisms involve cell surface recognition mediated through a variety of independent sets of molecules. These processes involve several extracellular cell adhesion molecules, including fibronectin, vitronectin, laminin, collagens, and probably some proteoglycans. Several proteins have been identified in focal cell adhesions and presumably relate to linkages between actin filaments and the various cell adhesion molecules, such as integrins, and extracellular matrix receptors.

Focal contacts between the extracellular matrix and the plasma membrane of cells form a structural complex with the cytoskeleton, including its actin network. The discovery of numerous cell adhesion molecules by different investigators in disparate species and systems has led to a confusing and apparently illogical nomenclature that makes the subject particularly difficult for the noninitiated to follow. Several distinct families of trans–plasma membrane glycoproteins mediate cell-cell adhesion: cell adhesion molecules (CAM) (6,7), integrins (49,341,438), cadherins (17,298,453,458,483), and selectins (30,125,168, 438). Although the precise function of many of these molecules remains incompletely understood, the structure of most of these transmembrane glycoproteins has been determined and the cDNA encoding many of them have been cloned and sequenced (7,125,360).

Cell Adhesion Molecules

The CAM, which are products of the immunoglobulin gene superfamily, differ in function and tissue distribution. Some CAM become expressed during development (neural cell adhesion molecule, N-CAM), the inflammatory reaction (intercellular adhesion molecules 1 and 2, ICAM-1 and ICAM-2, vascular cell adhesion molecule 1, VCAM-1), and oncogenesis (carcinoembryonic antigen). The expression of ICAM-1 is amplified by certain cytokines [interferon-γ (IFN-γ), interleukin-1β (IL-1β), and tumor necrosis factor (TNF)] (94,361). Both ICAM-1 and ICAM-2 bind to the lymphocyte function-associated antigen 1 (LFA-1, now designated CD11a/CD18) on all leukocytes. ICAM-1 has been identified by immunohistochemistry in cultured human corneal endothelial cells, and its expression is increased after exposure to IL-1β, TNF-Mα, and IFN-γ (102).

Integrins

The integrin protein family comprises transmembrane receptors that mediate leukocyte-leukocyte and leukocyte-endothelial cell adhesion, as well as cellular interactions with specific components of the extracellular matrix (collagen, tenascin, laminin, fibrinogen and fibronectin, and vitronectin) (5,7,199, 246,393,462). Potential functions of integrins include the anchorage of cells to the extracellular matrix, cell migration, cytoskeletal organization, extracellular matrix and cell-cell interactions, and the transduction of differentiation signals (245). Some integrins are also referred to as VLA (very late activation) adhesion molecules because the first two members appeared unusually late after in vitro activation of T lymphocytes. Each integrin consists of two subunits (an α and a β subunit) noncovalently linked to each other. The different subclasses of the integrin family share the same β subunit but have variable distinct α subunits. The β_1-integrins share a β_1 subunit (molecular mass 130 kD). Many integrins bind to their respective extracellular receptor at sites containing the tripeptide sequence Arg-Gly-Asp (5).

The β_2 family of integrins embraces the leukocyte adhesion molecules (188). These include CD11a/CD18 (previously also known as LFA-1), which is expressed on all leukocytes, CD11b/DC18 (Mac-1, expressed on monocytes and polymorphonuclear leukocytes, PMN) (82), p150,95, and GP11b/11a. The ligand for this integrin is ICAM-1 (discussed later in this section). Some integrins are believed to mediate interactions between the extracellular matrix and the cytoskeleton (47). Members of the integrin family are summarized in Table 1.

Using monoclonal antibodies, integrin β (β_1, β_3, and β_4) and α subunits (α_2–α_6 and α_V) have been identified in the human corneal epithelium (266,462) and endothelium (266). Whether α_1 is present within normal corneal epithelium is debatable (266,462). Corneal fibroblasts (keratocytes) in the normal human cornea express the β_1 chain but not α chains. The expression of α_1, α_3, α_4, and α_5 chains is upregulated in young and older corneal scars, but α_2 chains have been noted only in older scars (266).

Selectins

The selectins, also known as LEC CAM (lectin–epithelial growth factor–complement binding adhesion molecules) bind leukocytes to vascular endothelial cells. They include endothelial leukocyte adhesion molecule 1 (ELAM-1), GMP-140 [granule membrane protein, molecular mass 140 kD (also known as CD62)], platelet activation-dependent granule external membrane protein (PADGEM), and the lymphocyte homing receptor (MEL-14 in mice and lectin–epidermal growth factor complement adhesion molecule, LECAM-1, in humans). The glycoprotein GMP-140 is present in the α granules of platelets as well as in the limiting membrane of the Weibel-Palade bodies of vascular endothelium (125) and becomes transiently displaced to the cell surface following certain stimuli, such as histamine (168). The selectin ELAM-1, despite not being present in resting vascular endothelium, mediates the adhesion of PMN to vascular endothelium activated by TNF or IL-1 (30). ELAM-1 has a structural similarity to the lymphocyte

Table 1   Classification of Integrins Based on Binding Characteristics

Integrin subunit	Ligand
I. Integrins functioning as cell-adhesion molecules	
β_1 family α_4/β_1 (VLA-4)	VCAM-1, lymphocyte homing receptor
β_2 family α_L/β_2 (LFA-1)	ICAM-1
α_M/β_2 (MAC-1)	ICAM-1, C3bi, endotoxin
α_X/β_2 (gp150, 95)	?
II. Integrins that bind primarily to basement membrane constituents	
β_1 family α_1/β_1 (VLA-1)	Collagen/laminin
α_2/β_1 (VLA-2)	Collagen/laminin
α_3/β_1 (VLA-3)	Fibronectin/laminin/collagen
α_6/β_1 (VLA-6)	Laminin
β_4 family α_6/β_4	Laminin
III. Integrins that bind primarily to matrix proteins in inflammation, wound healing, and development.	
β_1 family $\alpha_4/\beta1$	Fibronectin (CSII site)
α_5/β_1	Fibronectin (RGD site)
α_V/β_1	Fibronectin
α_5/β_1 (VLA-5)	Fibronectin (RGD site)
β_3 family α_V/β_3	Vitronectin, fibrinogen, thrombospondin, von Willebrand's factor
β_5 family α_V/β_5	Vitronectin

Source: Modified from Albelda (5).

homing receptor for peripheral lymph node high endothelial venules, which is present on both PMNs and lymphocytes (124,360).

Cadherins

The cadherins are a group of developmentally regulated structurally related glycoproteins that mediate calcium-dependent adhesion in a tissue-specific manner (5,230,327,458). Each cadherin consists of a transmembrane domain, a longer extracellular domain (N-terminal side), and a shorter cytoplasmic domain (C-terminal side) (453). The human genes for some of these molecules have been located to specific chromosomes.

The cadherin family contains many related members, each of which is known by several names (453). The cadherins include P cadherins (found in cells of placenta and epidermis) (453), N cadherins (A-CAM, adherens junction-specific CAM, found in nerve, heart, and crystalline lens cells) (17,453), R cadherin (202), M cadherin (found in mouse myoblasts) (176), XB cadherin (in early *Xenopus* development) (176), E cadherin (uvomorulin or liver cell adhesion molecule, found in many epithelial cells) (327,345,346,453), and U cadherin (457). Some cadherins have been identified in the retina [R cadherin (202) and N cadherin (89,301,453)] and lens (N cadherin) (17,298).

Pathological states due to abnormalities in cadherins have not been documented but might be anticipated in certain ocular developmental anomalies.

V. CYCLINS

A class of proteins called cyclins accumulate during the cell cycle before DNA replication. Some cyclins appear during the S phase (cyclin A), G_1 phase (C, D, and E cyclins), or G_2 phase (B$_1$ and B$_2$ cyclins). At least some cyclins activate kinases that phosphorylate one or more target proteins (93,500). One of the targets for cyclin-kinase complexes is the retinoblastoma protein (pRb; see Chap. 24) (184). Some cyclins are identical to previously recognized oncogenes. For example, cyclin D$_1$ has been identified as PRAD-1 (BCL-1), which is located on chromosome 13 (11q13) and rearranged with the gene for parathyroid hormone in a subset of parathyroid adenomas (326).

VI. PROTEINS OF THE BLOOD

The ocular tissues may be affected adversely by abnormalities in hemoglobin and in the circulating plasma proteins, such as the immunoglobulins.

A. Hemoglobin

The story of hemoglobin, the vital protein responsible for the transport of oxygen to all tissues, is unique. More information about its molecular structure, synthesis, function, genetic control, and clinical relevance in health and disease is known than about any other protein. This remarkable progress stems from several factors: large quantities of human hemoglobin are readily available, and amino acid sequences of both the α and β subunits of adult hemoglobin (HbA) have been known since 1963; mRNA for hemoglobin was one of the first to be purified, because hemoglobin is the only major protein synthesized by immature erythrocytes.

From the standpoint of ocular pathobiology, an understanding of hemoglobin is particularly important in sickle cell disease and because of the concepts that the hemoglobinopathies provide about other inherited disorders. Human hemoglobin consists of two pairs of dissimilar polypeptide chains (containing 574 amino acid residues), with a heme group (ferro protoporphyrin IX) linked covalently to a specific site in each globin polypeptide chain. Five structurally different globin polypeptide chains, designated α, β, γ, δ, ϵ are synthesized. The α chains contain 141 amino acids in linear sequence; the β, δ, and γ chains have 146 residues. In adult erythrocytes HbA ($\alpha_2\beta_2$) comprises over 90% of the total hemoglobin, and about 2.5% is A_2 ($\alpha_2\delta_2$). During fetal development fetal hemoglobin (HbF; $\alpha_2\gamma_2$) is produced, but the ϵ globin chains are only detected during the first 3 months of gestation.

At present more than 500 hemoglobins have been characterized, with new ones discovered at an unabated pace, but the potential number of hemoglobinopathies is enormous. The defect in most known abnormal hemoglobins is in the α or β chains. Many of them are rare and not of ophthalmological importance. The hemoglobinopathies represent the prototype of genetic abnormalities that can occur at a mutant site. The amino acid composition of the polypeptide chains of the globin fraction of hemoglobin is altered in the hemoglobinopathies, and in these genetically determined disorders there is usually substitution of a single amino acid.

One of the most widespread and best known genetic diseases is sickle cell anemia. In this disorder, a simple base chain in the nucleic acid alters the mRNA triplet coding for glutamic acid (GAG) in the sixth position from the N terminus of the β polypeptide chain to a triplet coding for valine (GUG; Fig. 3). This single amino acid change causes deoxygenated hemoglobin S (HbS) to associate into long fibers that distort the erythrocytes into a characteristic sickle shape. Up to 20% of the population in parts of Central and West Africa have the gene for sickle cell disease. Hypoxic states, such as respiratory infections or high-altitude flying, reduce HbS to relatively insoluble long rods. The eye is commonly affected in sickle cell disease because of occlusive vascular disease (see Chap. 52).

In hemoglobin C (HbC), the second hemoglobinopathy to be discovered, lysine is substituted for glutamic acid in the sixth position of the β polypeptide chain. HbC occurs most frequently in West Africa in the vicinity of North Ghana, where from 17 to 28% of the population possess this hemoglobin (98); 2–3% of the black population in the United States have hemoglobin C (409). Individuals who are heterozygous for both HbA and HbC (HbC trait) are asymptomatic, but a moderate chronic hemolytic anemia with splenomegaly occurs in individuals homozygous for HbC disease (HbCC disease) and HbSC disease. In hemoglobin SC disease there is a high incidence of vasoocclusive disorders and the retina is significantly affected (see Chap. 52).

B. Immunoglobulins

Immunoglobulins are synthesized by lymphocytes and plasma cells, and variable amounts of these constituents of the plasma exist in normal ocular tissues. For example, immunofluorescence microscopy has disclosed several immunoglobulins (IgA, IgD, IgE, and IgG) in the epithelium and stroma of the normal human cornea, but only occasionally trace amounts of IgM (12). (See also Chap. 4 for immunoglobulins in other ocular tissues.) Several abnormalities of the immunoglobulins affect the ocular tissues.

BETA CHAIN contains 146 of the amino acid links in the massive **hemoglobin molecule**

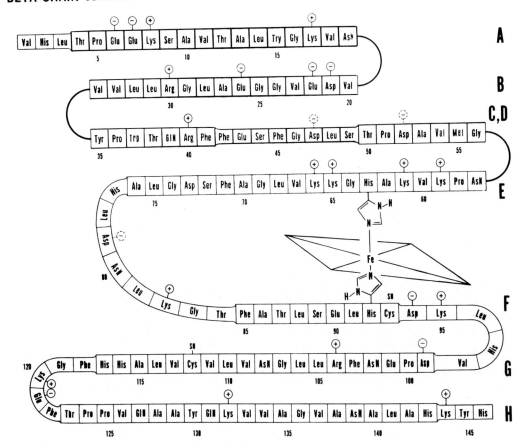

Figure 3 Amino acid sequence of hemoglobin. [Reproduced with permission from M. Murayama. Molecular mechanism of human red cell (with HbS) sickling. In *Molecular Aspects of Sickle Cell Hemoglobin, Clinical Application*, R.M. Nalbandian (Ed.), C.C. Thomas, Springfield, IL, 1971.]

Hypergammaglobulinemia

Plasma cell neoplasms, such as multiple myeloma, extramedullary plasmacytoma, solitary osseous plasmacytoma, Waldenström's macroglobulinemia, heavy-chain disease, plasma cell leukemia, and monoclonal gammopathy of undetermined significance, synthesize and secrete into the serum electrophoretically homogeneous immunoglobulins ("M components"). Various designations, including dysproteinemia, paraproteinemia, dysgammaglobulinemia, paraneoplastic gammopathies, and paraimmunoglobulinopathy, have been applied to conditions with an excessive proliferation of a single clone of immunoglobulin-producing cells. Some monoclonal gammopathies possess deletions in the variable portions of the light and heavy chains (80), but because most monoclonal immunoglobulins are normal, the aforementioned terms, which imply the existence of abnormal proteins, have met with disrepute. The more popular designation of plasma cell dyscrasias has much to commend it.

  Several manifestations of plasma cell dyscrasias (including a predisposition to infections, hemorrhages, cold sensitivity, and the hyperviscosity syndrome) result from the physicochemical properties of the excessive immunoglobulins that accumulate, such as an intrinsic high viscosity, the ability to form complexes with coagulation factors and other serum proteins, and cold insolubility (cryoglobulins).

  Macroglobulinemia. An excessive proliferation of plasma cells and lymphocytes that synthesize IgM results in the syndrome of macroglobulinemia, first recognized by Waldenström in 1944 (480).

Bleeding manifestations and anemia are accompanied by symptoms related to the presence of excessive quantities of monoclonal (M type) IGM globulins (macroglobulins) in the plasma.

Ocular Manifestations of Hypergammaglobulinemia. *Corneal deposits.* Hypergammaglobulinemia is relatively common and not usually associated with ocular disease. However, rarely, intra- and extracellular deposits accumulate in the cornea, conjunctiva, and other tissues in patients with multiple myeloma (14,21,24,36,46,109,115,116,189,239,445), rheumatoid arthritis (132,315,347), lymphoproliferative diseases (Hodgkin's and non-Hodgkin's lymphomas) (21,132,315), "reticulohistiocytosis" (337), or monoclonal gammopathies of undetermined significance (52,53,99,109,249,258,260,278,334, 340,359,383,437) and probable monoclonal gammopathy of undetermined significance (309) and indeed may be the first indication of the systemic disorder (239).

The corneal opacities are bilateral, and the clinical appearance varies considerably from case to case (437). The opacities may form a superficial thin gray crystalline ring concentric to the corneoscleral limbus, spongy fissures in the posterior corneal layers, or gray-brown homogeneous spots (115). Frequently, iridescent, polychromatic, or yellow-white punctate or linear delicate scintillating crystals appear within the cornea, bulbar conjunctiva, or lens, but corneal noncrystalline deposits with other appearances also occur. A diffuse corneal opacification due to deep hyalinelike corneal deposits has been reported in a patient with 38% plasma cells in the sternal marrow but who surprisingly did not manifest hypergammaglobulinemia or other confirmatory evidence of multiple myeloma (116). Corneal immunoglobulin deposits may account for the clinical entity designated "deep filiform corneal dystrophy" (503) and may simulate end-stage lattice dystrophy (except for the absence of a family history and a late onset) (437).

The location of the corneal immunoglobulin deposits varies considerably from case to case. They may involve the central (239,503), peripheral (99), or midperipheral (383) cornea or may be diffusely dispersed throughout the tissue. Some deposits occupy the epithelium (Figs. 4 and 5) (239,445), Bowman's layer and superficial stroma (52,99,347), the entire corneal stroma (21,315), posterior stroma (337), and the stroma immediately anterior to Descemet's membrane (189,383,503). They have also been observed within corneal fibroblasts (keratocytes) (21,52,340,445,503) as well as extracellularly (99,239,315,383,503). Small deposits of apparently similar material has been noted in the ciliary body (including the ciliary processes) and choroid (315).

Some investigators once thought that the crystals of plasma cell dyscrasias were composed of cholesterol (14) or cholesteryl stearate (89), but the nature of the crystals became apparent only after their recognition in tissue sections. That they could be identified in tissue that had passed through lipid solvents indicated that lipid was not a significant component (192,239,359,383). Like many other proteins, the crystals are eosinophilic but difficult to recognize in hematoxylin-eosin–stained preparations. They appear a brilliant red with the commonly used modified Masson's trichrome stain (containing the red dyes Ponceau 2R, acid fuchsin, and azophloxine) (239,315) and are also readily seen after staining with Movat's pentachrome technique (red), the Warthin-Starry method (black), and the Danielli reaction for tyrosine-rich proteins (red; Fig. 5a) (21).

TEM has disclosed elongated crystals of variable length (up to 32.5 mm) and width (up to 7.5 mm) within the corneal epithelium (Figs. 6 and 7). In nonocular tissue similar intracellular crystals have been identified within the cisternae of the rough endoplasmic reticulum (Fig. 8) as well as extracisternally (221). The crystals form in the renal tubular epithelium and extracellularly in multiple myeloma (206,221), as well as intracytoplasmically within neoplastic or reactive plasma cells. Such crystals are hexagonal in cross section and possess parallel sides when cut longitudinally (239). The crystals have an internal periodicity of approximately 10–11 nm (21,132,239,383).

Several lines of evidence indicate that the crystals are composed of immunoglobulin (239,383). They react positively with antisera against immunoglobulins (132,239,437,445) and closely resemble crystallized immunoglobulins (80). Crystals of isolated IgG are elongated and range in length (up to 180 mm) and in width (to about 10 mm) (80).

In multiple myeloma ($IgG_2\kappa$), spontaneously crystallizing cryoglobulin microtubules are hexagonal in cross section and possess internal and external diameters of about 10 and 20 nm, respectively. Such tubules have been observed within plasma cells and extracellularly in tissue (221), as well as in serum (38), and apparently aggregate into larger structures composed of tightly packed parallel nonbranching subunits. Crystals of this nature vary in length and appear hexagonal when cut perpendicular to the long axis. In cross-sectional profile the crystals have a fine honeycombed lattice pattern consisting of alternating

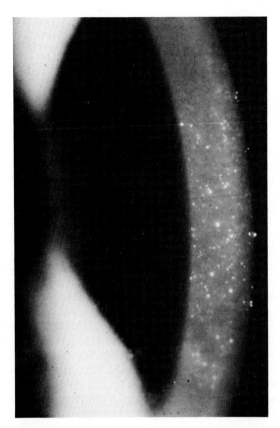

Figure 4　Slit lamp photograph of cornea in patient with multiple myeloma showing numerous crystals. (Reproduced with permission from G.K. Klintworth, S.J. Bredehoeff, and J.W. Reed. Analysis of corneal crystalline deposits in multiple myeloma. *Am. J. Ophthalmol. 86*:303–313, 1978.)

electron-dense and electron-lucent lines with a periodicity of about 6–9 nm (average 7.5 nm) (206). In multiple myeloma the periodicity of longitudinal sections of crystals in the serum is about 11 nm (277). The ultrastructural pattern of immunoglobulin crystals varies with the type of immunoglobulin. For example, the appearance of human cryoglobulins varies with the nature of the involved immunoglobulin. Monoclonal IgGκ 1 and 3 cryoglobulins with antibody activity form crystalline rods and annuli (22 nm diameter) (448). Polyclonal cryoglobulins, on the other hand, form filaments (6 nm wide), and cryoprecipitates of mixed IgG and IgM appear as cylindrical and annular bodies (12 nm internal diameter; 62 nm total diameter) (448). When IgM predominates over IgG, globular condensations result (30 nm diameter) (448). Fingerprintlike periodic condensations occur with mixtures in which IgG is more abundant than IgM (448).

The spontaneous crystallization of extracellular immunoglobulin in the absence of a tissue infiltration by cells with cytoplasmic crystals accounts for virtually all corneal immunoglobulin deposits (192,239, 383), but the corneal crystals have been associated with intracytoplasmic crystals or granular accumulations of conjunctival plasma cells (189,359).

Some hypergammaglobulinemic patients with corneal crystals have had crystalline inclusions within plasma cells of the bone marrow (14,260,359). Tears, aqueous, and the extravascular interstitial fluid contain immunoglobulins derived from plasma and neighboring plasma cells, and in hypergammaglobulinemia increased quantities of immunoglobulins presumably reach the cornea from these sites. Immunoglobulin may diffuse into the conjunctiva and corneal stroma after passing through the conjunctival microcirculation. Alternatively, plasma cells in the conjunctiva and other ocular tissues can produce immunoglobulins, and it is noteworthy that corneal crystals are sometimes preceded by episodes of conjunctivitis or anterior uveitis, which perhaps provide an increased number of crystalline-containing

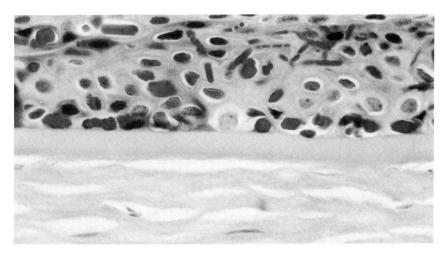

Figure 5 Crystalline deposits sectioned at variable depths in the corneal epithelium. (Masson's trichrome, ×680) (Reproduced with permission from G.K. Klintworth, S.J. Bredehoeff, and J.W. Reed. Analysis of corneal crystalline deposits in multiple myeloma. *Am. J. Ophthalmol. 86*:303–313, 1978.)

plasma cells. The possibility has been raised that immunoglobulin accumulation within the cornea may follow its local synthesis by corneal fibroblasts (503), but this view is contrary to the prevailing belief that immunoglobulins are products only of plasma cells and their precursor B lymphocytes. However, crystals that react immunochemically with antibodies to immunoglobulins and with a comparable structure to those in plasma cell dyscrasias have been observed in the absence of detectable serum immunoglobulin abnormalities using standard methods (503).

Crystals have not been identified in tissue sections of the lens in hypergammaglobulinemia but have been observed clinically within the lens in multiple myeloma (239). Because cells do not invade the intact lens capsule, immunoglobulins presumably can diffuse into the lens and crystallize there. In multiple myeloma the corneal (189) and lenticular crystals (239) may diminish in number while on chemotherapy, suggesting that crystallized immunoglobulins can resolubilize in the patient.

Why immunoglobulins should crystallize so rarely in individuals with hypergammaglobulinemia remains an enigma. The deposits do not appear to reflect a specific immunoglobulin because they have been associated with IgGκ (21,52,132,189,260,340,437,445), IgGλ (109,182,503), and IgAκ (334). In some instances nonocular crystals have been associated with spontaneously crystallizing cryoglobulin in the plasma (221). An understanding of the crystallization of immunoglobulin in the cornea clearly would have broad biological importance, as γ globulin crystallizes spontaneously so uncommonly (63) and the induction of crystals by purified immunoglobulin is difficult in the laboratory (77). Some patients with corneal crystals have had a relatively benign outcome even before the advent of therapy (239), but because of the extremely variable clinical course in patients with multiple myeloma, the question of whether corneal deposits are a favorable prognostic indicator remains unanswered.

The precipitation from serum of IgA, IgG, or IgM at temperatures below 37°C (cryoglobulins) is common in multiple myeloma, plasma cell dyscrasias, and a variety of systemic diseases (including rheumatoid arthritis). Seeing that cryoglobulins precipitate below the normal body temperature, one might anticipate that in affected patients this phenomenon would occur spontaneously in the cornea, where the temperature is normally about 35°C. Indeed, corneal opacities have accompanied cryoglobulinemia on rare occasions (249,309,337,347). If temperature is important, however, deposition should be maximal at the interpalpebral level, which is the coolest region in the cornea. Experience does not confirm that this is so.

Cysts of the ciliary body. Multiple cysts of the ciliary body develop in individuals with hypergammaglobulinemia due to multiple myeloma, plasma cell dyscrasias, systemic lupus erythematosus, a variety of liver diseases, and other conditions (15,19,215,216,400,401,427). The cysts are lined on the inner surface by the nonpigmented epithelium of the ciliary body and externally by this tissue's pigmented

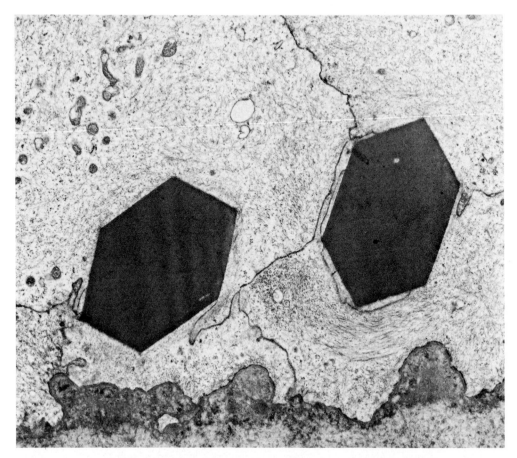

Figure 6   Hexagonal profiles of immunoglobulin crystals in basal portion of corneal epithelium of patient with multiple myeloma (×10,000) (Reproduced with permission from G.K. Klintworth, S.J. Bredehoeff, and J.W. Reed. Analysis of corneal crystalline deposits in multiple myeloma. *Am. J. Ophthalmol.* 86:303–313, 1978.)

epithelium. They most often involve the pars plicata but can also affect the corona ciliaris and orbiculus ciliaris of the ciliary body (19). In all likelihood an elevated serum gammaglobulin reaches the ciliary body by way of the circulation, passes through its pigmented epithelium, and becomes entrapped in the potential space separating the pigmented and nonpigmented epithelia of the ciliary body. The cysts vary considerably in size and may reach a sufficient dimension to sublux the lens partially and displace it and the iris anteriorly (19). In one reported patient multiple myeloma and unilateral angle-closure glaucoma were associated with such displacements and recurrent iridocyclitis (19). The cysts contain immunoglobulins and other proteins, and in multiple myeloma they have been shown by immunoelectrophoresis to contain the M protein, which is elevated in the serum (216). When observed clinically the ciliary cysts are translucent (19), and they remain so until the eye is placed in a fixative that precipitates the protein, making the cyst milky white (Fig. 9) (19,216). Similar cysts sometimes develop in the choroid plexus of the brain in individuals with hypergammaglobulinemia. Why ciliary body cysts do not occur in all individuals with hypergammaglobulinemia remains unknown, but the presence or absence of cysts and their size are not related to the serum gamma globulin level at the time of death (215).

Hyperviscosity manifestations.   The hyperviscosity of the plasma that occurs especially in primary macroglobulinemia (IgM globulins) and in certain cases of multiple myeloma and other plasma cell dyscrasias with monoclonal IgG results in a microcirculatory stasis. This accounts for a variety of retinal

Figure 7   Higher magnification of electron-dense immunoglobulin crystal in cornea showing a periodic inner structure. (×83,300) (Reproduced with permission from G.K. Klintworth, S.J. Bredehoeff, and J.W. Reed. Analysis of corneal crystalline deposits in multiple myeloma. *Am. J. Ophthalmol. 86*:303–313, 1978.)

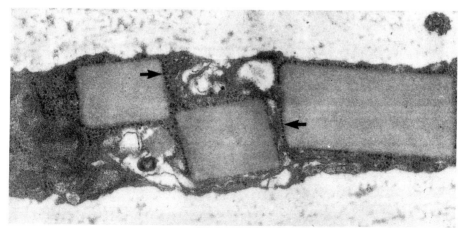

Figure 8   Monoclonal gammopathy. Crystals lined by ribosomes (arrows) are present within the cytoplasm of a keratocyte. (×23,000) (Reproduced with permission from C.C. Barr, H. Gelender, and R.L. Font. Corneal crystalline deposits associated with dysproteinemia: Report of two cases and review of the literature. *Arch. Ophthalmol. 98*:884–889, 1980.)

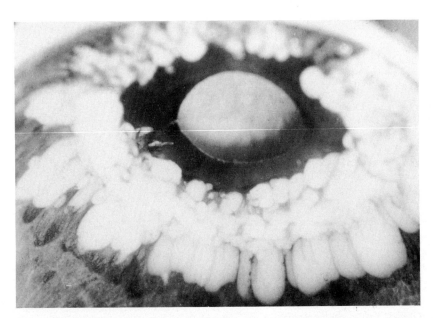

Figure 9 Milky white cysts of ciliary body in formalin-fixed eye from individual with multiple myeloma. (Reproduced with permission from T.R. Baker and W.H. Spencer. Ocular findings in multiple myeloma: A report of two cases. *Arch. Ophthalmol. 91*:110–113, 1974.)

vascular lesions (dilated veins, retinal hemorrhages, microaneurysms, and exudates) (2,16,50,59, 73,88,191).

Increased susceptibility to infection. In multiple myeloma, and to a lesser extent in macroglobulinemia, an increased susceptibility to infection results partly from an impaired capacity for antibody formation. This is reflected by a decreased serum concentration of normal IgA, IgG, and IgM (489). A metastatic bacterial endophthalmitis has been documented (19).

Hemorrhagic manifestations. Hemorrhages can follow thrombocytopenia or coagulation defects in patients with multiple myeloma. Some of the latter may be related to the formation of a complex between the specific M-type globulins and coagulation factors (including platelets, fibrinogen, factors V, VII, and VIII, and prothrombin) (489).

Amyloidosis. Amyloid may deposit in the ocular tissues in multiple myeloma (see section on amyloidosis).

Hypogammaglobulinemia

In a variety of conditions the serum level of one or more immunoglobulins is diminished or absent.

Light-Chain and Light- and Heavy-Chain Deposition Disease

On rare occasions monoclonal plasma cell populations, especially malignant plasma cell proliferations, produce abundant quantities only of immunoglobulin light chains. Under such circumstances the immunoglobulin light chains deposit in the kidney and various other tissues (126,288,376). A retinal vasculopathy has been documented in light chain disease, but without histopathological confirmation (104).

C. Amyloid-Related Blood Proteins

Aside from immunoglobulins, several other normal constituents of the blood (serum protein AA, β_2-microglobulin, transthyretin, and apolipoprotein A_1) are related to various forms of amyloid (discussed later in this chapter).

D. Fibrinogen and Fibrinoid Material

In several disorders including malignant hypertension, systemic lupus erythematosus, rheumatoid arthritis, rheumatic fever, periarteritis nodosa, and the endotoxin-induced Schwartzman phenomenon, an acellular, eosinophilic proteinaceous material, with the staining attributes of fibrin accumulates in the walls of the ocular blood vessels or in the connective tissue. The term "fibrinoid" stems from the resemblance of this material to precipitated fibrin. Its composition is variable, however, and depends on the circumstances in which it is deposited. Both immunofluorescent microscopy and TEM indicate that fibrin is usually if not always an important component. Fibrin has a characteristic ultrastructure with an axial periodicity of about 25 nm (less than half the periodicity of collagen). Fibrinoid material probably results from the insudation or exudation of several plasma proteins, including immunoglobulins, complement, and fibrinogen. Fibrin accumulation also occurs with excessive formation or defective fibrinolysis.

Ligneous conjunctivitis

In the chronic pseudomembranous variety of conjunctivitis known as ligneous conjunctivitis, the conjunctiva acquires a hard woody character due to the accumulation of an amorphous acellular eosinophilic hyaline material that has been shown by histochemical and immunohistochemical stains, as well as TEM, to contain fibrin (97,179,190,287), but immunofluorescence studies have also disclosed that immunoglobulins (especially IgG) are a prominent component of the hyaline material (179,190).

VII. SPECIFIC OCULAR PROTEINS

A. Retinal Proteins

Proteins of Rod Outer Segments

Rhodopsin.   Much is known about the biosynthesis and basic composition of rhodopsin, the light-sensitive pigment and predominant protein within membranes of retinal rod outer segments. Rhodopsin is synthesized within the inner segments of rods and is then inserted into the membranes of their outer segments (348) in such a manner that it is oriented across the membrane of the rod outer segments with its carboxyl-terminal region on the cytoplasmic surface of the disk bilayer (167). Autoradiographic and immunocytochemical studies of opsin indicate that after synthesis on ribosomes of the rough endoplasmic reticulum the apoprotein of rhodopsin passes through the Golgi apparatus (351,352), probably on water-insoluble membranes of its inner segment (349). Oligosaccharides of known structure are attached to two asparagine sites (Asn2 and Asn15) on rhodopsin (120,275).

The gene encoding rhodopsin, the rod photoreceptor pigment, is closely linked to a locus on the long arm of chromosome 3 (330). Autosomal dominant retinitis pigmentosa (adRP; see Chap. 41) is an extremely heterogeneous disorder resulting from a range of defects in rhodopsin and can have a locus or loci elsewhere in the genome (200). One type of adRP has been linked to the same locus as the rhodopsin gene (296). A point mutation resulting in a proline-to-histidine substitution has been observed in exon 1 at codon 23 of the rhodopsin gene in about 12% of U.S. patients with adRP, but this mutation was not been found in 91 European pedigrees with adRP (107), stressing the heterogeneity in adRP. A different mutation that deletes one of the two isoleucine monomers at codons 255 and 256 (200) in the fourth exon of the rhodopsin gene has been identified in another adRP family.

Peripherin and Other Proteins.   The term "peripherin" has unfortunately been coined to designate two separate and unrelated proteins. One is a type II intermediate filament with its gene on murine chromosome 15 and on human chromosome 12 (15q12-13) (323); the other peripherin (molecular mass 39 kD) is a glycoprotein localized to the rim of the photoreceptor cell disk membrane. Retinal peripherin has marked amino acid sequence similarity to the mouse protein encoded by the normal *rds* gene (62). Isolated rod outer segments also contain a larger protein, which varies in size in different species, having molecular masses of about 290 kD in the frog and about 230 kD in cattle (350,352). The latter protein, which comprises about 1–3% of the rod outer segment mass, is localized to the incisures that divide the disks into lobes and to the disk margin (352).

Mice homozygous for the mutant *rds* (retinal degeneration slow) gene fail to develop the outer segment of photoreceptors. The *rds* mutation is caused by a 10 kb insertion of exogenous sequence into the protein-coding exon of the gene (467). Some human cases of adRP have a mutated retinal peripherin gene (see Chap. 41).

Recoverin

Recoverin is a calcium-sensitive protein that is apparently unique to the human and bovine retina (also known as p26) (86,262,466). Similar, and perhaps functionally equivalent, proteins have been isolated from the retina of chicken (visinin) and frogs (sensitivity-modulating protein, or S-modulin). This modulator protein stimulates guanylate cyclase to resynthesize cGMP when calcium concentrations are low, inducing reopening of the sodium-calcium ion channels in the retinal photoreceptors. This allows the rods and cones to react to further photons of light that traverse the retina, even in the absence of calcium. The serum of a certain subset of patients with malignant neoplasms that have not invaded the retina or nervous system but who develop a cancer-associated retinopathy (see Chap. 20) contains antibodies to this protein (362).

Arrestin (S-antigen)

Retinal S-antigen, a well-characterized soluble protein present in the photoreceptor layer of the retina and in the pineal gland, is highly immunogenic, and severe cell-mediated autoimmune uveitis and pinealitis develop in previously sensitized rats (see Chap. 5) (90,91). Immunization to several small synthetic peptides corresponding to certain amino acid sequences in bovine S-antigen induces the same reaction as the native S-antigen, suggesting that multiple uveitopathogenic sites may be present in the molecule (419,420). An analysis of purified S-antigen from the retina in several species, as well as from the pineal gland, has disclosed a considerable amount of sequence similarity among species and between S-antigen in the retina and pineal gland. Such studies have also revealed the presence of the same consensus phosphoryl binding site that characterizes many GTP/GDP binding proteins and a homologous sequence found in the C terminus of α-transducin. These sequences may play a role in the action of S-antigen in transmembrane signal transduction (1,470). S-antigen (also called 48K protein) is now designated arrestin and is implicated in the negative control of visual transduction. It binds to phosphorylated rhodopsin and interferes with the interaction of rhodopsin with transducin (247).

B.   Corneal Proteins

Aside from those cellular proteins that are common to all cells and the extracellular matrix, such as proteoglycans (see Chap. 28), collagen (see Chap. 33), laminin, and fibronectin (discussed elsewhere in this chapter), the cornea contains other proteins that are apparently tissue specific or highly expressed in the cornea. Major deficiency exists in our knowledge about most corneal proteins, but knowledge about some of them is gradually accumulating.

Aldehyde Dehydrogenase (Major Corneal Soluble Protein)

Aldehyde dehydrogenase (ADH, molecular mass about 54 kD), the major soluble protein of the mammalian cornea (65), accounts for 30% of the soluble corneal proteins (11,242,253,418,474). The precise cellular localization of ADH remains uncertain. One study found it concentrated just above the nuclei in the basal corneal epithelium in a pattern corresponding to the cell membranes (105); in isolated bovine and human corneal epithelial cells in another study ADH was almost exclusively on the inner surface of the plasma membrane by immunofluorescence microscopy using rabbit anti-ADH antibodies, but not on the cell surface (242). The finding that rabbit antibovine ADH reacts with the corneas of many species, including rabbit, suggests that the antigen is not only conserved in many species but normally sequestered within corneal cells.

Immunofluorescence microscopy has disclosed ADH in the rat corneal and conjunctival epithelium but also in the fibroblasts and extracellular matrix of the corneal stroma, the corneal endothelium, the lens epithelium, and ciliary body, but not in other parts of the eye (105).

Soluble corneal proteins, such as ADH, may be important antigens involved in immunologically mediated diseases. Using the indirect immunofluorescence assay on whole corneal sections and enzyme-linked immunosorbent assay for ADH antibodies, circulating antibodies to ADH and other corneal proteins have been detected in a high percentage of patients with anterior uveitis without apparent corneal disease (including heterochromic cyclitis) and in almost one-quarter (26%) of patients with various corneal diseases but in only 4% of controls (172,251–253,259,474). Despite the presence of anticorneal antibodies in 88% of patients with Fuchs' heterochromic cyclitis using the immunofluorescence test, humoral immunity to ADH was detected in only about half the patients and in 17% of individuals with posterior uveitis (474), indicating that some anticorneal antibodies detected by the immunofluorescence test in these patients are directed at antigens other than ADH. Antibody production to corneal epithelium can be triggered after corneal damage (251). In the macrophage inhibition factor (MIF) assay the lymphocytes in patients with uveitis also have an increase in responsiveness to ADH (474), and the incidence of positive responses has been highest in patients with Fuchs' heterochromic cyclitis (20 of 28 patients) compared to individuals with posterior uveitis (2 of 14 patients). Only 1 healthy control (a person who had previous corneal injury) had a positive reaction in the study of van der Gaag and colleagues (474). The significance of the immune response to ADH in these conditions remains to be clarified. Perhaps because of its normally sequestered intracytoplasmic localization within the cornea, ADH functions as an autoantigen in the initiation and development of immunopathological processes in uveitis and some chronic keratopathies following its leakage from injured corneas. Also, the question of whether the anti-ADH immune response is of predictive value in the long-term outcome of these diseases remains to be determined. However, doubts exist concerning the role of the humoral autoantibody against the ADH in the pathogenesis of ocular disease. Although antibody production to corneal epithelial antigens is easily triggered, these antibodies do not bind to the corneal epithelium in rats following the intravenous injection of rabbit ADH antiserum (105). Instead, immunoglobulins deposit weakly in the corneal stroma and sclera but do not enter the corneal epithelium (105). Eype and colleagues (105) postulate that the corneal mucoprotein layer protects the corneal epithelial surface from the antibodies and that this barrier must be disrupted before immunoglobulins can penetrate the corneal surface cells. The antigenic sites on the molecule remain unknown, and all immunological studies on it have used polyclonal antibodies with undetermined specificity.

Tamm-Horsfall–Related Glycoprotein

An antigen in the human corneal endothelium is recognized by a monoclonal antibody (MoAb, 2B4.14.1) that also recognizes Tamm-Horsfall glycoprotein in the kidney (194), but the corneal antigen is presumably not Tamm-Horsfall glycoprotein because it is not recognized by a Tamm-Horsfall glycoprotein-specific MoAb. The nature and relevance of this antigen to corneal graft rejection remains unknown.

VIII. AMYLOID

Rokitansky (387) is usually credited with the first description of amyloid, which he included under the comprehensive term "lardaceous disease," but the designation "amyloid" was introduced by Virchow (271) because of its resemblance to starch (amylose) (60) in developing a violet hue after treatment with iodine and sulfuric acid. However, amyloid, is largely protein, not carbohydrate in composition (60). In tissue amyloid is eosinophilic, with characteristic tinctorial attributes. It stains metachromatically with certain triphenylmethane (crystal violet) and thiazine dyes (toluidine blue), most consistently when fresh unfixed tissue is examined. Elastic tissue and some other components of connective tissue may stain with Congo red, but amyloid has a unique green birefringence and dichroism when viewed in a polarizing microscope after staining with this dye. Amyloid is often naturally fluorescent (autofluorescent) and exhibits fluorescence after staining with thioflavin-T or S. In tissue, all types of amyloid appear by TEM as fine nonbranching fibrils (approximately 10 nm in diameter) organized in random array.

Virtually identical TEM and histochemical staining characteristics exist in all situations in which amyloid proteins accumulate. The diameter of isolated amyloid fibrils (7–7.5 nm) is thinner than those in tissue sections (about 10 nm), and a subunit of about 3.5 nm has also been identified.

Native amyloid fibrils are poorly immunogenic, but antigenic determinants are liberated when such material is treated with 0.1 M sodium hydroxide. Antiserum elaborated against such degraded amyloid is capable of reacting with native amyloid (118).

A. Causation and Types of Amyloidosis

Localized and systemic amyloid deposition occurs in numerous settings (29).

Systemic Amyloidoses

Primary Idiopathic Systemic Amyloidosis.   One variety of amyloidosis occurs in the absence of a positive family history without significant antecedent or coexistent disease (257).

   Myeloma and Plasma Cell-Associated Amyloidosis.   Amyloidosis occurs in approximately 15% of cases of multiple myeloma and may be associated with Waldenström's macroglobulinemia and other plasma cell dyscrasias.

   Reactive Systemic Amyloidosis (Secondary Systemic Amyloidosis).   Reactive amyloidosis, the most frequently observed variety of amyloidosis, may follow chronic infections (tuberculosis, tertiary syphilis, chronically infected burns, leprosy, infections with paraplegia, and Whipple's disease), chronic inflammatory diseases (regional enteritis, Reiter's syndrome, and ulcerative colitis), autoimmune conditions (rheumatic carditis, rheumatoid arthritis, scleroderma, systemic lupus erythematosus, and other "collagen vascular diseases"), and certain malignant neoplasms (renal cell carcinoma and Hodgkin's disease). Reactive systemic amyloidosis can be produced experimentally with powerful antigenic stimulants, such as casein and Freund's adjuvant.

   Primary Heredofamilial Amyloidoses.   The term "primary familial amyloidosis," widely used in the literature, lacks precision. Several distinct heredofamilial types of amyloidosis exist (13,297,310,391): amyloid nephropathy of Ostertag, familial Mediterranean fever (recurrent polyserositis), urticaria-deafness-amyloid nephropathy, cold hypersensitivity, cardiac amyloidosis, and the familial amyloid neuropathies (type I, Andrade or Portuguese type, type II, Rukavina or Indiana type, type IIA, Mahloudji, Maryland type, type III, Van Allen or Iowa type, and type IV, Meretoja or Finnish type or lattice corneal dystrophy type II; Table 1). FAP is now classifiable by the precise point mutations in transthryretin apolipoprotein A1 or gelsolin that result in single amino acid substitutions (Table 3) (27–29,68,143).

   With the exception of familial Mediterranean fever, which is transmitted by a recessive gene, all systemic primary heredofamilial varieties of amyloidoses have an autosomal dominant mode of inheritance.

   Amyloidosis of Aging.   Small deposits of amyloid are commonly seen postmortem in the central nervous system (CNS), aorta, pancreas, seminal vesicles, and several other organs in the elderly (499).

Localized Amyloidoses

Solitary or multiple small localized deposits of amyloid may occur in the skin, respiratory tract, bladder, urethra, and other tissues, sometimes simulating neoplasms clinically. The cornea, conjunctiva, orbit, and eyelid may be involved (discussed elsewhere in this chapter). In the brain of person's with Alzheimer's disease, the senile plaques, but not the neurofibrillary tangles, contain amyloid (see Chap. 53) (492).

   Localized forms of cutaneous amyloidosis may be associated with miscellaneous lesions of the skin (including basal cell carcinoma, calcifying epithelioma of Malherbe, and psoriasis). Several types of familial cutaneous amyloidosis have been documented: a bullous type with an onset at about 10–13 years of age (79), a hyperpigmented papular variety (396), a localized amyloidosis of the skin associated with psoriasis (203), and familial lichen amyloidosis (344).

   Cells that arise from the neural crest and secrete polypeptide hormones have been designated APUD (amine precursor uptake and decarboxylation) cells. Neoplasms derived from these cells (apudomas; pheochromocytomas, medullary carcinomas of the thyroid gland, gastrinomas, and insulinomas) produce a variety of localized forms of amyloid (apudamyloid) (355).

B. Nature of Amyloid

Because of variations in the staining attributes of amyloid in various situations, amyloid has long been suspected of being heterogeneous in nature. The chemical heterogeneity of amyloid has been established as a result of the isolation and analysis of purified amyloid fibrils from patients with a variety of amyloidoses (including primary systemic amyloidosis, familial Mediterranean fever, familial amyloid neuropathy types I, II, IIA, III, and IV, apudamyloidosis, Alzheimer's disease, hemodialysis amyloid, and secondary systemic amyloidosis), as well as from animals with experimentally produced secondary systemic amyloidosis (26,60,117,144,204,205,423,461).

   At least 15 distinct fibrillary amyloid proteins have been identified in deposits of amyloid in different situations. Most of these molecular species are modications of serum protein precursors. Thus immunoglobulin light chains (AL), amyloid protein AA, apolipoprotein A_1, transthyretin (prealbumin), β_2-microglobulin, and gelsolin (51,213) are major constituents of some forms of amyloid. Other types of amyloid involve cystatin c, procalcitonin, insulin, islet amyloid polypeptide, atrial natriuretic factor, β protein precursor (Alzheimer's disease and Down syndrome), amyloid precursor protein, and a cell membrane-related protein (prions; transmissible spongiform encephalopathy) (42).

Differences in the composition of amyloid in various locations result from the nature of the amyloid fibrils and in part from disparate associated macromolecules, including glycosaminoglycans, collagen, fibrinogen, lipoproteins, and complement components.

Terminology of Amyloid Proteins

Initially, the terminology of amyloid proteins was confusing because of the lack of a standardized nomenclature. A system for naming amyloid fibril proteins and related serum components recommended by an international committee has clarified the situation immensely (197). When possible the amyloid should be classified by the fibril protein that has been characterized by amino acid sequencing. The term "protein precursor" refers to the protein from which the amyloid fibril is believed to arise. Tissue-derived amyloid protein A is designated protein AA, and the tissue-derived P component protein is termed protein AP. For tissue-derived amyloid proteins of the immunoglobulin type, the established immunoglobulin chain nomenclature is used. For example, amyloid κI or λII chains are referred to as AκI and AλII, respectively. In situations in which new, inadequately characterized amyloid proteins are detected in tissue, the prefix A is followed by a provisional term to identify the particular protein, such as the first letters of the patient's name, for example A_{EH}. The prefix S is employed for serum protein components related to tissue-derived amyloid protein, whereas those serum proteins related to amyloid protein AA and AP are, for instance, designated SAA and SAP, respectively. For serum components corresponding to the immunoglobulin type of amyloid protein, the chain designation in the immunoglobulin system is given (for example, κ_1 and λII).

Proteins in Systemic Amyloidoses

Immunoamyloid (Amyloid Light-Chain Proteins). Almost four decades ago, Vazquez and Dixon (476) using immunofluorescence microscopy, identified gamma globulin in amyloid deposits in secondary amyloidosis. Subsequently, it became recognized that the major components of amyloid fibril in certain forms of amyloidosis (primary nonfamilial systemic amyloidosis or multiple myeloma and other plasma cell-related amyloidosis) are light-chain fragments of immunoglobulin (145,205,257,423,461). This amyloid, now designated AL (amyloid light-chain protein, previously designated protein B) (144,204), is considered to consist of polymerized fragments of entire light chains alone (461) or in combination with fragments of light chains (κ or λ), which probably consist of the variable portion and part of the constant-region portion of the light chain (145). These subunits consist of the first 30 residues of light chains. Data from detailed structural analyses on two amyloid-related Bence Jones proteins of different types (κ and λ) are known (343). Antisera to amyloid preparations cross-react with κ or λ light polypeptide chains (Bence Jones proteins) (204), but interestingly, antisera to κ and λ chains do not react with amyloid fibrils even when they are closely related to light chains (117), perhaps because of differences in tertiary structure. Human light-chain–related amyloidosis can be induced experimentally by injecting Bence Jones proteins obtained from patients with amyloidosis AL into mice (432). Under such circumstances amyloid deposits in the spleen, liver, and other organs. However, following their inoculation with non–amyloid-associated Bence Jones proteins, mice do not develop amyloidosis, indicating that only some light chains and Bence Jones proteins are amyloidogenic (432). Bone marrow cells from patients with AL amyloidosis, as well as from either light-chain or light- and heavy-chain deposition disease, have invariably synthesized monoclonal light chains corresponding to the class found in the tissue deposits (48).

Amyloid Protein AA. Amyloid fibrils in human and animal secondary amyloidosis and familial Mediterranean fever contain a unique fibrillar protein (amyloid protein AA) with an amino acid sequence different from that of immunoglobulin (26). The amino-terminal end of the individual polypeptide chains alternately face in opposite directions, and hence the protein is designated an antiparallel pleated sheet protein. Human protein AA (molecular mass 8–8.5 kD) has sequence similarities to comparable proteins in certain animals. A protein lacking the last 30 residues of AA may be the product of proteolytic digestion of a larger precursor.

Serum Protein AA

The serum of normal individuals contains minute quantities of a protein designated SAA (molecular mass about 80 kD). ApoSAA from plasma is found in the lipoprotein fraction (mainly with the high-density lipoproteins) (497). There are four different isotypes of SAA (SAA1, SAA2, SAA3, and SAA4), and different genes encode for these different proteins. High-density lipoprotein-associated apoSAA is the product of two genes (SAA1 and SAA2). In the mouse two of the genes are located on the same chromosome (SAA2 and SAA4) (497).

Although present in human serum from the time of birth, the serum SAA level usually becomes strikingly elevated after 70 years of age without relation to age-related disease. The serum SAA also rises in acute inflammatory diseases (an acute-phase protein), as well as in pregnancy (18,424). Antibodies to SAA cross-react with protein AA. The SAA levels are significantly increased in patients with primary, secondary, and multiple myeloma-associated amyloidosis (that is, even in forms of amyloidosis in which amyloid fibrils are devoid of AA protein), but from the standpoint of diagnosing and distinguishing different types of amyloidosis, the serum SAA level is of no practical value. SAA gene products are found in amyloid fibers of certain types of amyloidosis. SAA1 is a component of human reactive amyloidosis (associated with chronic inflammatory diseases) and murine amyloidosis, but both SAA1 and SAA2 are found in the amyloid deposits of familial Mediterranean fever (497).

Transthryretin Amyloidoses

Transthyretin (prealbumin, molecular mass about 56 kD) is a normal constituent of human plasma and cerebrospinal fluid. It is synthesized predominantly in the liver but is also produced in the choroid plexus of the brain (83), and in the eye by the retinal pigment epithelium (RPE) (78,174). This acid protein displays an affinity for thyroxine and retinol binding protein and partakes in their plasma transportation. On electrophoresis it migrates in front of albumin, hence the older term "prealbumin." It is made up of four identical subunits, each consisting of a known sequence of 127 amino acids. Approximately half of the amino acid chain forms a β-pleated sheet. The gene encoding for transthyretin has been mapped to the long arm of human chromosome 18 (18q11.2-q12.1) (436).

At least 46 distinct point mutations in the transthyretin gene have been identified, and most of them are associated with systemic deposits of amyloid (Table 3) (198). An amazing aspect of transthyretin-derived amyloid that still defies explanation is the varied tissue distribution of the amyloid deposition and the diverse clinical manifestations that occur with the different mutations. Mutations in positions 30 (Val-30-Met), 58 (Leu-58-His), 60 (Thr-60-Ala), or 84 (Ile-84-Ser) cause a familial polyneuropathy (FAP) (333,481). It is noteworthy that the substitution of alanine for threonine in position 60 results in FAP with major deposits in the heart (unlike the other mutations), and in contrast to many other transthyretin-related amyloidoses (including FAP types I and II), the eye is not involved (481). A methionine substitution for leucine at position 111 in transthyretin does not cause FAP but produces amyloid to deposit predominantly in the heart (198). Senile systemic amyloidosis occurs when isoleucine replaces valine in position 127 (151). Moreover, some mutations such as a valine substitution for tyrosine at position 116 of transthryrein have no pathological consequences (449).

A characteristic manifestation of transthyretin amyloidosis is a polyneuropathy, sometimes first becoming manifest with a carpal tunnel syndrome. A cardiomyopathy is often associated and may cause the death of the patient (67). Vitreous deposits of amyloid are features of some mutations in transthyretin (Table 3). All forms of transthyretin amyloid have autosomal dominant modes of transmission.

Familial Amyloid Polyneuropathy Type I (Andrade or Portuguese Type, Transthryretin Methionine Substitution for Valine at Position 30). FAP type I, first described by Andrade in 1952 (13) in patients from a small area in northwestern Portugal, starts in the lower extremities with thermal, superficial pain, touch, and position sense lost, in that order. In this disease early impotence in the male, perforating ulcers of the feet, diarrhea, sphincter disturbances, and weight loss are common. Amyloid deposits in blood vessels throughout the body and in almost all organs, but clinically significant renal disease is conspicuously absent. The pupils become irregular in contour, unequal in size, and dilated, with absent or sluggish reactions to light and accommodation. The pupil develops a characteristic scalloped appearance (13), which may also be a feature of other types of FAP (270). Ocular signs and symptoms may result from the neuropathy, vascular fragility, or vitreous opacification.

Table 2 Some Familial Amyloid Polyneuropathies

Characteristic	Type I (Andrade, Portuguese type)	Type II (Rukavina, Indiana, Swiss type), type IIB (Mahloudji Maryland type)	Type III (Van Allen, Iowa type)	Type IV (Meretoja, Finnish type)
Usual age at onset	Third decade	Fifth decade	Fourth decade	Third decade
Site of onset	Feet	Hands	Feet and hands	Cornea
Gastrointestinal complaints	Common	Rare	Common	Rare
Impotence and sphincter disturbances	Common	Rare	Common	Rare
Trophic ulcers	Common	Rare	Rare	Rare
Average duration of illness	4–12 years	14–40+ years	12 years	69 years
Nephropathy	Rare	Absent	Invariable	Common, usually mild
Eye	Abnormal pupils	Vitreal amyloid	Cataracts (sometimes)	Lattice corneal dystrophy
Type of amyloid	Transthyretin	Transthyretin	Apolipoprotein A_1	Gelsolin

Source: Modified from Mahloudji and colleagues (297).

The amyloid fibrils in FAP type I lack both AA and AL proteins, but a major component is a protein (molecular mass about 14 kD) with antigenic determinants and an electrophoretic mobility similar to that of transthyretin. Amino acid sequence analysis of the purified amyloid has disclosed it to consist of part of a variant transthyretin in which methionine is substituted for valine in position 30 (405). This mutation has been identified in persons of Portuguese, Japanese, Swedish, Greek, and other origins (290,459).

Familial Amyloid Polyneuropathy Type II (Rukavina, Indiana, or Swiss Type; Transthyretin 84 Isoleucine to Serine). FAP II starts later in life and progresses more slowly than FAP I, and the hands are affected, the carpal tunnel syndrome being a distinguishing feature (297). Ecchymoses of the eyelids, extraocular muscle weakness, internal ophthalmoplegia, and anisocoria may occur (106). In a postmortem study of an eye from a patient with this variety of amyloidosis, extensive deposits of amyloid have been found in blood vessels, ciliary nerves, and extraocular muscles, but not in the iris sphincter muscle or cornea (354). The amyloid in this condition is a variant of transthyretin with a serine substitution for isoleucine at position 84 (481).

Familial Amyloid Polyneuropathy Type IIA (Mahloudji, Maryland Type; Transthyretin 58 Histidine to Leucine). This type of amyloid polyneuropathy resembles FAP II clinically, but the mutation in the transthyretin gene encodes for a histidine substitution for leucine at position 58 (333).

Other Variants of Transthyretin Autosomal Dominant Amyloidosis. Another variant of transthyretin autosomal dominant amyloidosis, discovered in a patient of German descent with peripheral neuropathy and bowel dysfunction, involves the substitution of tyrosine for serine at position 77 (482). One variety of familial amyloidosis that has a predilection for the heart (cardiac amyloidosis, Denmark type) is characterized by a methionine substitution for leucine at position 111 in transthyretin (198). Some investigators have found the amyloid fibrils of senile systemic amyloidosis to be derived from normal transthyretin (487); others have found them to be related to mutated transthyretin in which isoleucine replaces valine in position 127 (151).

Apolipoprotein A_1-Derived Amyloid

The serum lipoproteins (see Chap. 35) include high-density lipoprotein, which has apolipoprotein A_1 as its major apoprotein. The gene for apolipoprotein A_1 has been assigned to human chromosome 11 (11q13-qter)

Table 3   Some Point Mutations in Transthyretin Causing Amyloidosis[a]

Position	Amino acid substitution	Synonyms	Clinical symptoms	References
30	Met for Val	FAP I	LLN, bowel, AN, vitreous	402, 403, 422, 459
30	Ala for Val		FAP	218
33	Ile for Phe	FAP (Jewish)	LLN, vitreous	29, 166, 329
33	Leu for Phe		FAP	
36	Pro for Ala		Vitreous with or without FAP	219, 397
49	Ala for Thr	FAP	FAP, cardiopathy, vitreous	397
49	Gly for Thr	FAP	FAP, cardiopathy	367
58	His for Leu	FAP IIA	FAP, not vitreous	333
60	Ala for Thr	FAP (Appalachian)	AN, CTS, heart	481
77	Tyr for Ser	FAP II (German)	LLN, kidney, bowel	482
84	Ser for Ile	FAP II	Heart, CTS, vitreous	96, 482
84	Asn for Ile		Vitreous, CTS, heart	426
90	Asn for His		FAP	421
111	Met for Leu	Cardiac amyloidosis (Danish)	Heart, no FAP	198, 335
116	Val for Tyr		No pathological effect	449
127	Ile for Val	Senile systemic amyloidosis	Heart, not FAP	151

[a]Abbreviations: FAP = familial amyloid polyneuropathy; CTS = carpal tunnel syndrome; AN = autonomic nervous system; LLN = lower limb neuropathy; Ala = alanine; Asn = asparagine; His = histidine; Leu = leucine; Met = methionine; Ser = serine; Thr = threonine; Tyr = tyrosine; Ile = isoleucine; Val = valine.

(54), and at least one mutation of this gene encodes for a variant of apolipoprotein A_1 that constitutes the main component of a certain type of amyloid, namely, FAP type III (Van Allen or Iowa type). Arginine is substituted for glycine in position 26 of apolipoprotein A_1 in the amyloid of this condition (332). Involvement of the nerves in all four extremities dominates the clinical picture at the onset in this disorder. Severe peptic ulcers may be present, and cataracts sometimes develop (290). A nephrotic syndrome commonly develops, and amyloid nephropathy is the usual cause of death.

Gelsolin-Derived Amyloid

Gelsolin, an actin binding protein, is a constituent of normal plasma (485). It is a calcium-dependent actin fragmenting protein that is present in virtually all cells. The amyloid protein in FAP type IV (Meretoja or Finnish type, lattice corneal dystrophy type II) has been identified as a 71 amino acid long fragment (7–12 kD) of gelsolin with an asparagine at codon 187 instead of aspartic acid (139,161,256,272,305–308) (see LCD type II). The same mutation has been found in an American family of Irish descent (149) and in a Japanese family (451a) with FAP type IV. A different mutation at the same codon that substitutes tyrosine for aspartic acid accounts for Danish and Czech families with FAP type IV. A gelsolin mutation probably causes FAP type IV, because clinical disease cosegregates with the mutant gelsolin in Finnish patients (183).

Cystatin C-Derived Amyloid

One variety of familial amyloidosis (cerebral amyloid angiopathy) has a predilection for cerebral arteries and arterioles, and affected individuals die from cerebral hemorrhage before they reach 40 years of age. The condition has an autosomal dominant mode of inheritance and was first described in Iceland (158). It has also been recognized among populations of fishermen along the Dutch North Sea Coast (284). Following purification and amino acid sequence analysis, the amyloid in this condition was identified as cystatin c, a potent inhibitor of several human cysteine proteinases (157,273). Interestingly, the amyloid found in the clinically similar Dutch form of cerebral amyloid angiopathy has an amino acid sequence similarity to the β protein of Alzheimer's disease and Down syndrome, not to cystatin c (475). This observation stresses that different proteins can be responsible for phenotypically similar forms of amyloidosis. Although the ocular vasculature could conceivably be affected in cerebral amyloid angiopathy, amyloid deposits have thus far not been documented within the eye or its adnexal tissues in cerebral amyloid angiopathy.

β_2-Microglobulin-Derived Amyloid

β_2-Microglobulin is a normal serum constituent with a β-pleated sheet structure. It has amino acid sequence similarities to the immunoglobulins and is coded by the HLA gene on human chromosome 15 (290). β_2-Microglobulin is present on the surface of all cells as the light chain of the human HLA complex (358). It is also a secretory product of plasma cells (22). After long-term hemodialysis for severe renal disease, β_2-microglobulin deposits particularly in the synovium and bone of patients, where it takes on the fibrillary pattern of amyloid, causing an osteoarthropathic syndrome (carpal tunnel syndrome, arthropathy, and lytic bone lesions that are prone to spontaneous fractures; hemodialysis-related amyloidosis) (138,285). β_2-Microglobulin-derived amyloid is coupled with a codeposition of calcium. This form of amyloid has not been identified within ocular tissues.

C.   Proteins of Localized Amyloidoses

The composition of amyloid in most localized and inherited varieties of amyloidosis has not yet been thoroughly investigated.

Alzheimer's Amyloid

The amyloid of Alzheimer's disease is highly conserved in evolution, and the gene encoding for it has been mapped to human chromosome 21 (148).

Immunoamyloid

An example of pulmonary nodular localized amyloidosis has been found to contain a λ light polypeptide chain (145).

Apudamyloid

Amyloid associated with neoplasms stemming from APUD cells may be derived from the nonhormone residue of the relevant prohormone or a polypeptide produced concomitantly with the hormone itself. Apudamyloid differs from immunoamyloid in not demonstrating yellow autofluorescence when examined under ultraviolet light and in lacking tryptophan and tyrosine.

Prion Amyloid

A sialoglycoprotein designated prion protein is believed to be the causative agent of Creutzfelt-Jakob disease and scrapie (see Chap. 53). The scrapie isoform of this protein (PrP^{sc}), as well as the component that is found in the CNS of normal individuals (PrP^c), polymerizes into amyloid rods (prion amyloid) (314).

D.   Other Associated Components

Aside from these major components, amyloid is associated with other proteins and glycosaminoglycans.

Amyloid Plasma Component (P Component)

A small constituent of amyloid is a plasma protein known as the pentagonal unit (P component) (425). Rod or doughnut-shaped particles (measuring up to 8–10 nm in diameter) are present in large amounts in partially purified tissue extracts of amyloid but have not been recognized in tissue sections of amyloid (425). These structures are composed of five small subunits, each 2–2.5 nm in diameter, clustered around a clear central zone, stacks of the pentagonal structures sometimes forming regularly beaded rods. These components, which constitute a small fraction of amyloid, correspond to the plasma component (P component, protein AP), which is immunologically identical with a globulin of normal human plasma but its amino acid sequence is distinct. The serum C-reactive protein possesses a similar pentagonal structure and some amino acid sequence similarities with the amyloid P component (AP). Protein AP exists in normal serum (SAP) as well as in association with amyloid fibrils, yet the SAP levels do not vary significantly with the presence of amyloidosis (424). Protein AP has been detected by indirect immuno-fluorescence techniques in normal cultured human skin fibroblasts, suggesting that it may be a product of such cells (435).

E. Topography of Amyloid Deposits

Amyloidosis of virtually any type can involve any organ, yet characteristically specific tissues tend to be affected, and even in the eye amyloid deposition occurs in different sites. Heller and colleagues (171) classified amyloidosis into perireticulin and pericollagen types depending upon the site of initial amyloid deposition. In primary and myeloma-associated amyloidosis, the heart, tongue, gastrointestinal tract, skin, and nerves are frequently affected, and the amyloid tends to deposit in mesenchymal tissue, where collagen fibrils prevail ("pericollagenous amyloid"; adventitia of arteries and veins, connective tissue, sarcolemma of muscle, and neurolemma of nerves, mesenchymal tissue distribution pattern I). In amyloidosis associated with an overt inflammatory disease or malignancy (secondary amyloidosis), on the other hand, the amyloid occurs especially in parenchymal locations rich in reticulin. With this so-called perireticulin pattern, the liver, spleen, kidneys, intestine, and adrenal glands are generally involved, but the heart and other organs may be affected, too. Why amyloid is regularly distributed in some organs but rarely in others is not clear; perhaps the initial binding is a ligand-adhering reaction.

F. Ocular Amyloidosis

Corneal Amyloidosis

Amyloid deposits in the cornea in numerous apparently unrelated chronic nonspecific disorders (61,81,100,127,169,180,181,274,291,292,374,439) and in five distinct inherited diseases.

Familial Corneal Amyloidoses.   At least five distinct inherited varieties of corneal amyloidosis are recognized. These include the lattice corneal dystrophies (LCD) (152,235,237,413,431,434)—type I (Biber-Haab-Dimmer), type II (Meretoja), type III (Hida), and type IIIA (Stock)—as well as primary familial subepithelial amyloidosis (gelatinous droplike dystrophy of the cornea).

Lattice corneal dystrophy type I.   LCD type I was first described by Biber in three unrelated females (34) and later by Haab (159) and Dimmer (85), who drew attention to its hereditary nature. This disorder is manifest clinically by opacities that particularly affect the central cornea. Typically, a network of delicate interdigitating filamentous structures appears within the corneal stroma, but opacities of other shapes may also develop (375,502). The lattice pattern of the corneal deposits, which resemble nerves on cursory examination and from which the disease derives its name, coupled with a frequent diminution of corneal sensation, suggested a primary disorder of corneal nerves. This view was strengthened by the argyrophilia of lesions in silver impregnation preparations of affected tissue, but TEM has failed to disclose nerves in the involved areas. Recurrent epithelial erosions may complicate the superficial corneal deposits and even antecede them, and in some families with LCD type I recurrent epithelial erosions may appear in individuals who lack clinically recognizable stromal disease (75). LCD type I usually begins clinically in both eyes toward the end of the first decade of life, sometimes not until middle life, and rarely it may be apparent at 2 years of age (440). A considerable individual variation in the clinical course exists even within affected families, but the disease is slowly progressive, and marked visual impairment eventually ensues before the fifth or sixth decades. Most patients do not require keratoplasty until after the fourth decade, but some need one by 20 years of age (265). The disease is almost always bilateral and symmetrical, but from a clinical standpoint it may be asymmetrical or unilateral (265,372).

Available evidence indicates that the amyloid deposits in LCD type I are restricted to the cornea (Figs. 10 and 11) and that clinical systemic disease is usually not associated. However, in one family three sisters with LCD also had amyotrophic lateral sclerosis and cutis hyperelastica (232), and other probably incidental relationships have been reported between LCD and adult polycystic kidney disease (489) and Paget's disease of bone (37). Amyloid has not been observed in surgically excised tissue from several sites (skin, lymph nodes, cartilage, nerve, muscle, and the wall of Baker's cyst) in subjects with LCD type I (235,311). Nevertheless, all tissues have not yet been examined in any patient with this disease. Following keratoplasty amyloid may deposit in the grafted donor tissue some 2–14 years later in patients with LCD type I (175,240,265,282). Bowen and colleagues (39) described specific apple green fluorescence in the areas of the amyloid deposits in human LCD type I stained with fluorescein-labeled antiserum to human

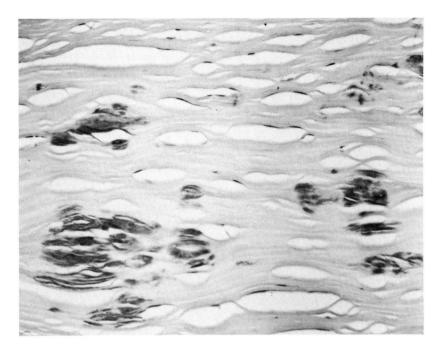

Figure 10   Histological section of cornea with lattice corneal dystrophy type 1 showing deposits of amyloid. (Congo red, ×200)

amyloid derived from amyloidotic (type not specified) human spleen and liver. The presence of proteins AA and AP has been reported in a case of LCD type I by immunofluorescent (325) and immunoperoxidase (488) techniques, but this has not been confirmed by others (152,240). Neither immunoglobulins nor their light chains have been detected in the amyloid deposits of LCD type I (240,325,488). A possible relationship of the amyloid in LCD type I (as well the amyloid in atypical LCD, polymorphic amyloid degeneration, primary familial subepithelial amyloidosis, and secondary corneal amyloidosis) to gelsolin has been raised because of positive immunohistoreactivity with a commercially available antigelsolin monoclonal antibody (281), but others have found the amyloid in LCD type I not to react with antibodies to mutant gelsolin (149). Also, the gene for LCD type I is not linked to the gelsolin gene on chromosome 9 (9q32–34) (489a).

Lattice corneal dystrophy type II.   Meretoja (310) drew attention to another variety of LCD with systemic amyloidosis in Finland (310–313), 2 years after the deposits in LCD were unequivocally shown to be amyloid (235). This entity was subsequently detected in the Netherlands (490), Denmark (40), and the United States (76,369,394,442). This condition, designated LCD type II (or FAP type IV, Finnish or Meretoja type), is associated with progressive facial and other cranial and peripheral nerve palsies, a dry and itchy skin with cutis laxa, protruding lips, blepharochalasis, and a "masklike" facial expression due to systemic amyloidosis. The disorder becomes apparent after the age of 20, and visual acuity usually remains good until after the age of 65 years; keratoplasty is rarely indicated. Aside from clinically detectable corneal lines due to amyloid deposition, asymptomatic amyloid deposits have been noted in scleral, choroidal, and adnexal blood vessels in the perineurium of ciliary nerves and in the lacrimal gland (311).

LCD type II differs in several respects from LCD type I. The corneal lines are located particularly in the peripheral cornea and are less numerous and more delicate than those in LCD type I. In heterozygotes the onset of the disease is later than in LCD type I, but the disease may begin earlier than usual in homozygotes. In contrast to LCD type I, amyloid deposits have been observed between the epithelium and Bowman's layer only rarely. As in LCD type I, the possibility that the corneal lesions involve nerves has been raised in view of the pronounced amyloid neuropathy elsewhere in this disease and the tendency for the opacities also to be located in the peripheral cornea. Light microscopic observations with silver impregnations have also supported this possibility (311), but unfortunately the techniques that have thus

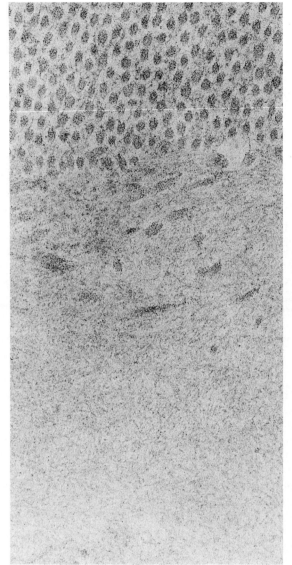

Figure 11 Transmission electron micrograph of amyloid deposit in corneal stroma of lattice corneal dystrophy type 1. The amyloid fibrils are adjacent to wider collagen fibers (right side). (×75,000)

far been utilized to demonstrate corneal nerve involvement in LCD type II are nonspecific and the question remains open, especially in view of experience with LCD type I. In eyes examined at necropsy amyloid has been identified predominantly in the corneal stroma in the heterozygous condition (311,313). Surgically excised corneal tissue has occasionally been examined following a superficial keratectomy or penetrating keratoplasty (369,442). In one case penetrating keratoplasty was complicated by a neurotrophic persistent epithelial defect (442). The corneal amyloid in LCD type II reacts with antibodies against amyloid P component (442) and the gelsolin mutant protein (150), but not with amyloid A protein or transthyretin antibodies (442). Postmortem examination of patients with LCD type II has disclosed amyloid in arterial walls of almost all organs, as well as in the heart, kidney (glomeruli), nerves, skin, and other tissues in addition to the ocular involvement.

Lattice corneal dystrophy type III.   An additional variety of LCD (type III) appears to have an autosomal recessive mode of inheritance (177,178). It does not become apparent until late in life and is characterized by lattice lines that are much thicker than normal and the absence of recurrent epithelial erosions. Proteins AA and AP, but not immunoglobulin light chains, have been detected in formalin-fixed paraffin-embedded corneal tissue from patients with LCD type III by the immunoperoxidase technique (177). Another variety of LCD (type IIIA) closely resembles type III in having thick ropy lattice lines, but it has associated corneal erosions and an autosomal dominant mode of inheritance (446).

Primary familial subepithelial corneal amyloidosis (gelatinous droplike dystrophy of the cornea). Aside from the LCD, at least one other type of inherited corneal amyloidosis is recognized. This is primary familial subepithelial amyloidosis, a bilateral corneal disorder first described in Japan (4,301,328, 338,456) but that has also been recognized in the United States (231,447), Tunis (101,486), the United Kingdom (133), and other countries (Fig. 12) (133). Most documented cases have been from Japan, where the disease has received the unfortunate designation of "gelatinous droplike dystrophy of the cornea," a term that is synonymous with chronic actinic keratopathy (see Chap. 23 and elsewhere in this chapter). The mode of inheritance is considered to be autosomal recessive. Primary familial subepithelial amyloidosis usually begins in the first or second decade of life with severe photophobia, tearing, and a corneal foreign body sensation. Multiple prominent nodular deposits of amyloid accumulate beneath the epithelium, producing a mulberry-shaped mass. There are no known associated systemic abnormalities, but the disease typically recurs in the graft following keratoplasty. One study claims that the amyloid in familial subepithelial amyloidosis reacts with a monoclonal antibody to gelsolin (281), but another investigation found no reactivity with antibodies to mutant gelsolin (149). In an immunofluorescent study of this form of corneal amyloidosis (324), the amyloid deposits have been noted to react with antibodies to protein AP but not with antibodies to protein AA, immunoglobulins, light chains, or transthyretin (prealbumin). Apparent sporadic cases of what may be the same condition have also been documented (274,374).

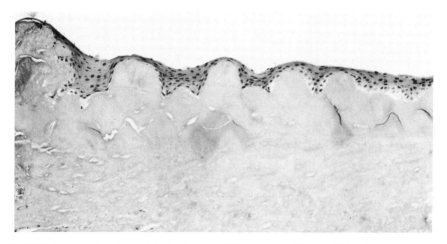

Figure 12   Nodular deposits of amyloid in the superficial cornea of in familial subepithelial corneal amyloidosis. (Hematoxylin and eosin, ×100)

Other forms of primary corneal amyloidosis.   Spontaneous nonfamilial deposits of amyloid have also been described under the designation "polymorphic amyloid degeneration" of the cornea (248,299). Loeffner and colleagues (281) reported a positive reactive of monoclonal antibodies to gelsolin with the amyloid of polymorphic amyloid degeneration, but others have reported no reactivity with antibodies to mutant gelsolin (149). Partington and colleagues (353) reported a family in which two males and seven females had brown pigmentation of the skin, the pigmentation mimicking incontinentia pigmenti in the females. In both sexes the skin was slightly hyperkeratotic with melanin in its basal layer. Amyloid was present in the papillary dermis. Neither male survived infancy, and one was almost blind, with amyloid deposits in the cornea.

Secondary Corneal Amyloidosis.   Amyloid deposits in the cornea without conjunctival involvement in a wide variety of long-standing and nonspecific conditions, such as the retinopathy of prematurity (retrolental fibroplasia) (292,439), trauma (61,127,292), keratoconus (291,292,444), phlyctenular keratoconjunctivitis (292), congenital glaucoma (81,233), glaucoma secondary to uveitis (292), endothelial decompensation secondary to glaucoma (233), sympathetic ophthalmia (292), trachoma (81,180), trichiasis (169), syphilitic interstitial keratitis (95,181), Schnyder's crystalline corneal dystrophy (100), lipid keratopathy (292), and chronic actinic keratopathy (304). In such instances the amyloid often occurs most conspicuously immediately beneath the corneal epithelium, but it may be scattered among the collagen fibers in the substantia propria. The literature contains an interesting, but single, example of bilateral corneal amyloidosis coupled with hypergammaglobulinemia (243).

Surprisingly, despite the deposition of amyloid within the cornea in the aforementioned conditions, this tissue is spared from amyloid deposition in other varieties of amyloidosis, including FAP type II (354), and in secondary systemic amyloidosis. This supports the notion that amyloid deposition depends on interaction with local tissue factors.

Vitreal Amyloidosis

Opaque vitreal deposits were first reported in 1953 by Kantarjian and de Jong (223). This complication of some forms of amyloidosis can impair vision and is often the first clinical manifestation of the systemic disease. Clinically the amyloid appears as bilateral vitreous opacities or floaters. Vitreal amyloidosis occurs in several types of FAP related to amino acid substitutions in transthyretin (106,186,223,227,228, 354, see also Chap. 22) yet not in FAP IIA (transthyretin Leu-58-His), or with some other point mutations of transthyretin (Table 2).

In FAP type II, vitreal involvement is most conspicuous. Rarely amyloid has been observed in the vitreous in the absence of a positive family history or overt systemic manifestations (108,186,403,412, 426). In one such case who was thoroughly studied, a transthyretin mutation was detected (426). In another family with a point mutation in transthyretin (Ala-36-Pro), vitreous amyloidosis was isolated and not accompanied by amyloid polyneuropathy (397).

Clinical and histopathological observations suggest that the amyloid reaches the vitreous from the retinal blood vessels. In the retina perivascular sheathing is often a prominent early clinical manifestation of vitreal amyloidosis. Tissue sections of eyes with FAP (163,268,496) have disclosed an extension of amyloid from the walls of retinal blood vessels into the vitreous, and when amyloid does not deposit in the walls of retinal blood vessels vitreal amyloidosis does not seem to occur.

The type of amyloid found in the vitreous has thus far only been of the mutated transthyretin type (153,403,404,426). Although transthyretin reaches the eye from the circulation, another potential source is the RPE, which has been shown to synthesize transthyretin (78).

Amyloid fibrils composed of immunoglobulin light chains have not been detected in the vitreous. It is also noteworthy that amyloid deposition has not been documented in either the retinal vessels or vitreous in FAP types III (van Allen or Iowa type) or IV (Meretoja or Finnish type) and that amyloid may be absent from the vitreous and retinal blood vessels despite other extensive ocular deposits in both multiple myeloma and primary idiopathic systemic amyloidosis (69,469).

Vitreous amyloid is frequently mistaken clinically for old hemorrhage, and its presence is often not appreciated until cytological evaluation of a vitrectomy specimen (156). Pars plana vitrectomy offers not only an opportunity for diagnosing the nature of the vitreal opacities, but is currently the sole method for removing them. Vitrectomy can improve vision markedly (226,228), but the amyloid gradually reaccumulates over weeks to years (87,186,226,406).

Orbital Amyloidosis

Orbital amyloidosis is uncommon and generally not preceded by overt local disease (164,193,241,407). It may cause proptosis, but diplopia and loss of visual acuity are not prominent clinical manifestations. Ptosis may be a presenting feature of localized amyloidosis of the eyelid and orbit, and several cases have simulated myasthenia gravis (407). Exophthalmos may occur in FAP I (223) or FAP II (106), suggesting that amyloid deposits in the orbit in these varieties of amyloidosis, but this has not been confirmed by tissue examination at either biopsy or autopsy. Ophthalmoplegia is sometimes associated with amyloid infiltrations of the extraocular muscles in multiple myeloma (373). The types of amyloid found in the orbit include AL (multiple myeloma) (373), AA (chronic inflammation) (149), and transthyretin amyloid polyneuropathy, cardiopathy, or both (149).

Amyloidosis of Conjunctiva and Eyelid

The first documented example of ocular amyloidosis appears to involve the conjunctiva (173). Conjunctival amyloidosis usually affects both eyes in individuals between 20 and 30 years of age. As a rule it begins at the fornix and eventually extends into the bulbar and palpebral conjunctiva. Chronic conjunctivitis (especially trachoma), repeated pyogenic conjunctivitis, and chronic idiopathic conjunctivitis may lead to localized deposits of amyloid in the eyelid and conjunctiva, but sometimes amyloid accumulates in the absence of a known antecedent disorder as a painless swelling of the eyelid (25,193,430,441).

Other Forms of Ocular Amyloidosis

The fibers that accumulate in the pseudoexfoliation syndrome (see Chap. 19) manifest some ultrastructural and histochemical features of amyloid, including an affinity for thioflavines (381). Unlike most forms of amyloid, however, the fibers rarely exhibit dichroism after staining with Congo red.

Ocular Involvement in the Systemic Amyloidoses

Clinically significant corneal amyloidosis has usually indicated localized disease, whereas amyloid of the vitreous or eyelid is usually a hallmark of a systemic disorder. Although orbital amyloidosis is usually a localized disorder, it may be a manifestation of multiple myeloma (373). Deposits of amyloid apparently localized to the palpebral conjunctiva may also be a component of systemic amyloidosis (441), including multiple myeloma-associated amyloid (373). Amyloidosis of the eyelids is virtually pathognomonic of systemic amyloidosis (43,373). The incidence of ocular involvement in systemic amyloidosis is not known, but in a retrospective clinical review of a heterogeneous group of 154 published patients with primary systemic amyloidoses (391), an overall incidence of ocular involvement was found in 8.4% of the cases. This sample was biased, however, because of the inclusion of many cases of FAP, some types of which have a high incidence of vitreal amyloidosis.

Secondary Systemic Amyloidoses. Histopathological studies of ocular tissues in patients with the systemic amyloidoses have disclosed variable amounts of amyloid in ocular and adnexal tissues, particularly in the choroidal blood vessels. The vascular deposition of amyloid does not appear to interfere with the transport of nutrients across blood vessels: marked choroidal amyloidosis with occlusion of the choriocapillaris in a fatal case of multiple myeloma still had a morphologically normal overlying retina (469).

The vascular walls in the conjunctiva, retina, choroid, and extraocular muscles may contain amyloid in idiopathic primary systemic amyloidosis, as well as in some inherited varieties of amyloidosis mentioned earlier. In several histopathological studies of primary systemic amyloidosis, the uveal blood vessels, particularly those of the choroid, have contained variable amounts of amyloid.

Rarely small, clinically insignificant deposits of amyloid have been documented in the eyelid, sclera, conjunctiva, uvea, optic nerve, extraocular muscles, and other orbital tissues in systemic secondary amyloidosis (140,377,386). In lepromatous leprosy with secondary amyloidosis, amyloid has been noted in the vascular walls of the choriocapillaris and in larger choroidal blood vessels, as well as in Bruch's membrane (386), in the iris of a patient with leprosy (377). Amyloid deposits have not been documented in the retina or vitreous in secondary amyloidosis.

Vision may be severely affected as a result of vitreal involvement in FAP types I and II (see section on vitreal amyloidosis). Glaucoma can accompany vitreal amyloidosis (279,354), and amyloid has been noted in the trabecular meshwork of an eye with secondary open-angle glaucoma (354) but has not been documented in this part of the eye in patients with normal intraocular pressure. A hemorrhagic diathesis is common in systemic forms of amyloidosis, apparently due to a deficiency of clotting factor X, which seems to bind nonspecifically to amyloid fibrils. Ecchymoses of the eyelids and retinal hemorrhages can develop in such cases.

G. Pathogenesis of Amyloidosis

The disparate conditions included under the connotation "amyloidosis" do not represent a single disease. They share an extracellular deposition of proteinaceous material with common morphological, structural, and staining attributes. In each instance the major protein component shares a β-pleated configuration, and its deposition is an end product of a complex chain of reactions in which genetic and antigenic determinants are important.

Although not expressed overtly by all varieties of amyloidosis, an excessive antigenic stimulation characterizes chronic infections, autoimmune disorders, neoplasms, and many other conditions that may lead to amyloid production. The immune response in these situations may manifest itself in a production of normal or abnormal immunoglobulins or immunoglobulin light chains. Amyloid formation may depend on the characteristics of the immunoglobulin light chain: some of them form amyloid fibrils more easily than others, and not all individuals with Bence Jones proteins (light-chain polypeptides of immunoglobulin) develop amyloidosis. Also, fibrils obtained from the cleavage of some but not all Bence Jones proteins by peptic digestion manifest typical attributes of amyloid fibrils: characteristic green birefringence in the polarizing microscope after Congo red staining, a distinctive ultrastructure, and a typical x-ray diffraction pattern (142). Primary nonfamilial systemic amyloidosis is associated with a high incidence of serum and/ or urine immunoglobulin abnormalities, and a high percentage of such patients (92% of 50 patients) have Bence Jones proteinuria and characteristic M proteins (205). Nonspecific immunoglobulin abnormalities frequently occur in patients with secondary amyloidosis, but rarely if ever is a myeloma or Bence Jones protein detected in such individuals. Of 17 patients with secondary generalized amyloidosis, 53% had characteristic M proteins (144).

In many tissues investigators have alluded to a cellular origin of amyloid. Plasma cells, which synthesize and secrete immunoglobulins, undoubtedly play a cardinal role in the genesis of amyloid light-chain proteins in primary nonfamilial systemic amyloidosis and in amyloidosis associated with multiple myeloma and other plasma cell dyscrasias. Plasma cells presumably produce light chains, which are both excreted in the urine as Bence Jones proteins and subjected to proteolytic breakdown or polymerization with the formation of amyloid.

Macrophages and other phagocytic cells also seem to participate in the formation of amyloid. The fibroblast is suspected of playing a role in amyloidogenesis as well, and two normal serum proteins associated with amyloid (AP and AA) have been identified in fibroblasts, which may be the source of them (435).

Amyloid proteins that accumulate in certain tissues are constituents of serum and presumably reach tissues from the blood. Protein SAA is a probable precursor of the smaller but antigenically similar amyloid protein AA, the major component of secondary amyloidosis. Other serum proteins that contribute to various forms of amyloid include transthyretin, immunoglobulin light chains, apolipoprotein A_1, β_2-microglobulin, and gelsolin or variants of them.

At least some localized forms of amyloidosis, such as the apudamyloidoses and Alzheimer's amyloid, are produced by constituents of the affected tissue. It remains to be determined whether other types of localized amyloidosis are also locally produced or are derived from serum or cells that invade the affected tissue. Some localized deposits of amyloid in the conjunctiva and orbit are preceded by chronic inflammation and associated with a prominent infiltrate of lymphocytes and plasma cells (164,241), but in most instances this is not the case. The deposition of at least some types of amyloid (AA amyloid, AL amyloid, β-amyloid of Alzheimer's disease, and the transthyretin amyloid of senescence) requires the presence of a specific amyloid enhancing factor (AEF). AEF has yet to be characterized, and its cell of origin is unknown.

That amyloid can clearly deposit in the center of the avascular cornea in the absence of overt systemic disease suggests that amyloid can be produced locally within the cornea. From the standpoint of localized corneal amyloidoses, especially LCD types I, III, and IIIA, synthesis by tissue cells is a distinct possibility. The aforementioned evidence that fibroblasts play a role in amyloid production elsewhere, together with the intimate association of some corneal fibroblasts with amyloid and the prominent rough endoplasmic reticulum disclosed by TEM within such cells (187,235,365,502), supports the possibility that the amyloid may be a product of corneal fibroblasts. On the other hand, the amyloid could reach the cornea from elsewhere, for example by way of the aqueous or pericorneal vasculature. Whether this takes place or not remains an open question.

The possibility that corneal amyloid results from collagen disintegration or from precursors of collagen has been raised on ultrastructural grounds (295). This has been considered unlikely because isolated amyloid fibrils from other tissues are resistent to collagenase digestion, differ ultrastructurally from collagen, and have been shown conclusively to differ from collagen in amino acid composition. Until the deposits in all varieties of corneal amyloidosis are characterized at a molecular level, however, a relationship to collagen cannot be completely excluded.

Possibly relevant to the pathogenesis of corneal amyloidosis is the yet unconfirmed observation from Finland, where LCD II (FAP type IV) is common, that the corneal changes in cases of LCD with histological evidence of systemic amyloidosis are preceded by acute episodes reminiscent of iritis or scleritis, during which crystals are evident in the cornea, bulbar conjunctiva, and aqueous (229). The crystals stained positively with the performic acid alcian blue method and hence were thought to contain cystine or cysteine.

H.   Secondary Effects of Amyloid

In the past amyloid deposits were regarded as inert and dysfunctions in affected tissue were considered a result of the displacement of adjacent cells and extracellular constituents. Most clinical manifestations, including those in the eye, occur by virtue of the space that amyloid occupies. However, certain substances in the serum, such as the blood-clotting factors IX and X, bind to the polyanionic amyloid fibrils, possibly resulting in other secondary effects, such as a bleeding diathesis. Foreign body giant cells commonly surround amyloid in the ocular adnexa, as in primary orbital amyloidosis (164,193), but because amyloid in most situations does not elicit an inflammatory response, the giant cells may be an independent reaction to an underlying disease process.

IX.   UNIDENTIFIED PROTEINS

A.   Hyalinlike Proteins

On purely morphological grounds the designation "hyalin" has been applied to homogeneous, structure-less eosinophilic material occurring in the epithelium or connective tissue, but hyalin is not an entity and the term embraces several different substances. From the standpoint of ocular tissues this pigeonhole is applicable to the excrescences that occur on the periphery of Descemet's membrane in the cornea with aging (Hassall-Henle bodies) and to the almost identical nodules (cornea guttata) that extend across the entire cornea in Fuchs' corneal dystrophy (see Chap. 40), macular corneal dystrophy (see Chap. 28), and interstitial keratitis (484). In the latter situations, collagen is a major constituent of the hyalin, but other substances, such as glycoproteins, are probably involved as well. Thick bands of amorphous eosinophilic material occur in the walls of arterioles and medium-sized arteries in diabetes mellitus and hypertension of long standing. It, like the hyalin material in the walls of arterioles with arteriolosclerosis, is believed to be derived from an insudation of plasma proteins, as well as by local production. The hyalin present in connective tissue in certain diseases appears to consist of excessive amounts of glycoprotein deposited between the collagen fibrils and other constituents of the extracellular matrix. Hyalin is commonly observed in connective tissue with aging and in the conjunctiva in chronic conjunctivitis, notably trachoma, but the exact mechanism of its production in these situations is not clear.

Granular Corneal Dystrophy

Eosinophilic lesions possessing the characteristics of nonspecific hyalin deposit in the cornea in granular corneal dystrophy (GCD). This relatively benign inherited disorder is clinically confined to the cornea

(320). Multiple, discrete irregularly shaped white opacities accumulate within the corneal stroma, especially in the central and more superficial portions. The tissue between the opacities remains crystal clear, as does the extreme periphery of the cornea, usually. The deposits usually appear during the first decade of life and gradually enlarge and become more numerous with time. Visual acuity is more or less normal in children, who develop small, superficial corneal opacities, often arranged in lines and for the most part with a smooth exterior surface (320). In adult patients the external corneal surface is uneven and corneal opacities are larger and distributed superficially as well as more deeply in the corneal stroma (320). As in many genetic disorders interfamilial differences and intrafamilial similarities occur (317), and although some patients have only a few granules in the cornea, the cornea becomes markedly opaque in other patients. Probable examples of persons homozygous for the GCD gene have been detected in the offspring of marriages between two individuals with GCD (322). One probable homozygote had a more severe form of GCD than his or her parents, as well as an earlier onset and a severe course, with two grafts in each eye before the age of 17 (322). In contrast to this case, the offspring of two different affected individuals in another pedigree suggested that individuals heterozygous and homozygous for the GCD gene are identical (71).

GCD usually has an autosomal dominant mode of inheritance, but it apparently occurs sporadically on rare occasions (160). In some families the GCD gene has a 100% penetrance (321), but in others the penetrance is incomplete (71). The mutation rate has been estimated as about 0.3 in 1,000,000 (319).

Blood and saliva from 124 members of one family of GCD have been investigated with 35 genetic markers with the aim of localizing the mutant gene to a particular chromosome (321). The test of linkage between a marker and a gene of interest is based on the ratio L of the probability of noting their association under the hypothesis of linkage to the probability of finding no linkage. The highest decimal logarithm of L (the lod score) in this study was 1.04 in females at θ 0.00 to the locus C1R on the short arm of chromosome 12. This lod score, which indicates a probability of linkage to chromosome 12 of 1 in 10, is interesting and warrants further investigation. To be considered significant a lod score of greater than 3 (odds ratio of 1000:1) and preferably of more than 4 is desirable. Further work is clearly indicated before GCD can be assigned to a particular chromosome.

In most cases of GCD, visual acuity remains good until late in the course of the disease, so that many individuals never require corneal grafting. Vision is usually not sufficiently impaired to justify corneal grafting, but in one pedigree 14 patients were treated with corneal grafting and all grafts remained free of recurrence for at least 30 months (320). However, in persons undergoing keratoplasty the deposits may recur in the grafts within a year (196), usually being superficial to the donor tissue, even with lamellar grafts, or at the host/graft interface. Most histopathologically confirmed recurrences have been superficial to Bowman's layer in subepithelial nonvascularized collagenous tissue, with fibroblasts almost certainly of host origin (44,222,269,384a,414,450,468). The rare occurrence of characteristic deposits within the periphery (450) or stroma of the donor cornea (44,384a) probably result from an invasion of the graft by corneal fibroblasts of the recipient.

The light microscopic and TEM appearance and staining attributes of the corneal deposits in GCD are diagnostic (Fig. 13) (128,220). They appear brilliant red with Masson's trichrome stain, and with Wilder's reticulin stain the stromal lesions of GCD contain tangles of argyrophilic fibers (220).

By TEM characteristic electron-dense, discrete, rod-shaped or trapezoidal bodies are evident (Fig. 14) (3,44,212,238,254,255,303,336,450,455). Cross-sectional profiles of the corneal deposits are usually irregularly shaped but sometimes hexagonal, measuring 100–500 nm in diameter (3,212,222). By TEM, clusters of elongated bodies of varying shapes with discrete borders occur, particularly in the superficial corneal stroma. They may be present in the epithelial intercellular space (455) or within degenerated basal epithelial cells (222). Some rod-shaped structures appear homogeneous and an inner structure is not discernible; others, however, appear to be composed of an orderly array of closely packed filaments (70–100 nm in width) that are oriented parallel to the long axis; yet others appear moth-eaten, with variably shaped cavities containing fine filaments (Fig. 15) (44). Some superficial and most deep stromal deposits do not all possess the rod-shaped configuration (44).

The corneal endothelium and Descemet's membrane are normal in GCD.

The differentiation between GCD and Reis-Bücklers' dystrophy (discussed in Chap. 40) may not be possible without a tissue diagnosis in an affected member of the pedigree. Most individuals with "Reis Bücklers' dystrophy" (318) have nonspecific abnormalities or the morphological attributes of GCD. Most investigators believe that GCD can be differentiated from Reis-Bücklers' corneal dystrophy by ultrastructural features. However, because of comparable clinical qualities and the presence of the characteristic

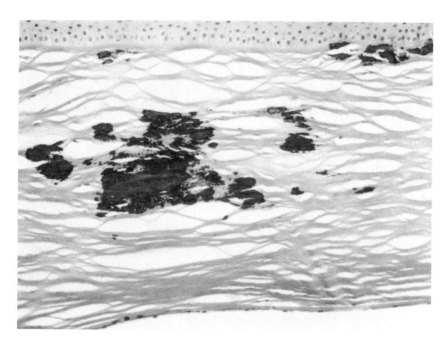

Figure 13 Corneal stromal deposits in granular corneal dystrophy. Note the tendency for the superficial stroma to be more extensively involved than the deeper stroma. (Masson's trichrome, ×170)

"rod-shaped" bodies of GCD in the superficial corneal stroma in some individuals with Reis-Bücklers' dystrophy (318), including some with the bona fide Reis-Bücklers' dystrophy (494), Møller postulates that they are the same condition (318).

Typical deposits of amyloid are uncommon in GCD, but fine filamentous structures that resemble amyloid have been observed in the corneal stroma in GCD (460). Some investigators have been impressed by an apparent increase in delicate filaments (about 5 nm in diameter) in corneas with GCD (44,212,303,460), and indeed, some studies have noted all granules within masses of delicate filaments (44). Such fibrils tend to be especially situated in the deepest stroma (Fig. 16), and their existence has led some authors to doubt the diagnosis of GCD, even to suspect LCD (3).

The distinction between GCD and LCD is customarily straightforward, but a possible relationship between these dystrophies has been raised (44,128,212) because the typical stromal lesions in GCD can be associated with amyloid (128,165,303,450). In three cases of GCD studied by Garner (128), some typical stromal deposits possessed the staining attributes of amyloid, and in one of these patients coexistent lesions in the deep stroma were indistinguishable from those in LCD by light microscopy. Although Akiya and Brown (3) did not find the stromal deposit to stain with Congo red, they observed an increased bi-refringence in the deep stroma, which they interpreted as a possible change similar to LCD. The occasional occurrence of amyloid in corneas with GCD cannot be taken as evidence that GCD and LCD are related. Because, as mentioned, amyloid precipitates in the cornea in many conditions, some corneas with GCD may conceivably contain independent secondary deposits of amyloid. The characteristic extracellular deposits of GCD are usually not observed in corneas of individuals with LCD, but in several families whose ancestry has been traced from the Avelline region of Italy, atypical GCD is accompanied by latticelike deposits of amyloid within the cornea (112). However, until the genes responsible for GCD and LCD have been isolated and sequenced, the concept that GCD and LCD are expressions of the same gene or that the association of the two dystrophies in the same family represents a distinct entity (Avellino corneal dystrophy) (112) remains speculative.

The basic nature and origin of the extracellular protein accumulates of GCD remain unknown. Insight into their identity has been provided by histochemical procedures (128,154,414,415), which indicate that they contain tryptophan, tyrosine, arginine, and sulfur-containing amino acids (128), like almost all known proteins. The granules stain positively with luxol fast blue (a stain that is not specific for phospholipid), and

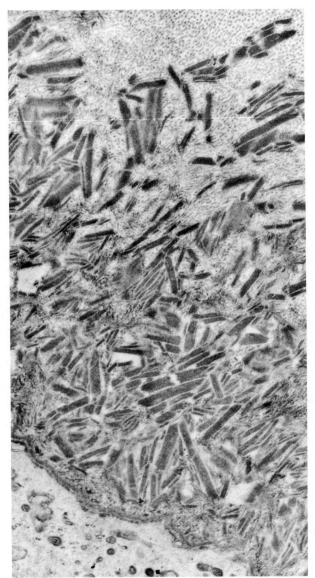

Figure 14 Rod-shaped crystalloid bodies in superficial corneal stroma in granular corneal dystrophy. (×19,500)

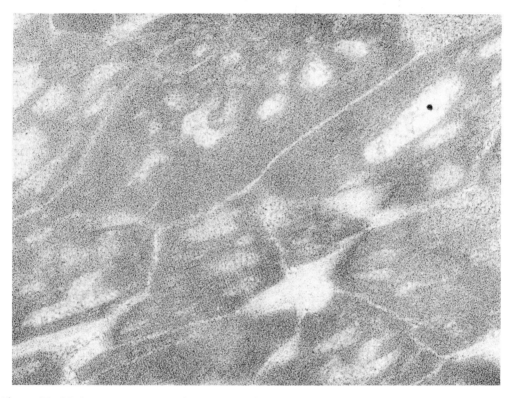

Figure 15 Moth-eaten appearance of corneal deposits in deep corneal stroma from patient with granular corneal dystrophy. (×126,000)

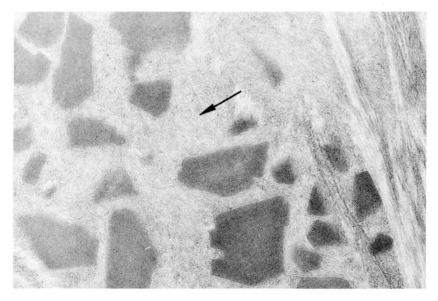

Figure 16 Delicate filaments (arrow) in cornea stroma with granular corneal dystrophy. Such filaments are frequently associated with larger, variably shaped electron densities. (×49,500)

fresh-frozen tissue from corneas with GCD stain positively with antibodies to microfibrillar protein (385). A primary abnormality in lipid metabolism seems most unlikely in GCD, but Rodrigues and colleagues (385) reported an increased lipid content in every phospholipid class in two corneas with GCD, although their cholesterol content was unchanged (385). They also observed alterations in the fatty acid profile of phospholipids in corneas with GCD. Specimens have been examined by analytical EM (222), but this technique has not disclosed any significant information about the identity of the deposits.

A limiting factor in the analysis of the composition of the corneal deposits in GCD is the scarcity of material available for refined analytical procedures. The eosinophilic lesions have been designated historically as a "hyaline degeneration" of the corneal stroma (113,220). In theory, the deposits could result from an alteration in preexisting extracellular components of the corneal stroma, be produced locally by corneal cells, or have an extracorneal origin. Observations derived from the mode of inheritance, morphological and cytochemical characteristics of the lesions, and the fate of the corneal grafts in patients with the disease may shed some light on the problem. Clinical observations indicate that convectional currents within the corneal stroma presumably do not move the stromal deposits. Because comparable deposits have not been found elsewhere in the body, it is possible that the protein is formed within the cornea, but until detailed postmortem studies are performed on all tissues the question of whether the dystrophy is restricted to the cornea will remain unanswered. Also, if the deposits reach the cornea by diffusion from a noncorneal origin, one might expect a high recurrence rate after corneal grafting and an inconstant relationship of recurrences to host tissue, but as mentioned this is not the case.

Relatively few investigators have attempted to interpret the basic events that give rise to the characteristic lesions of GCD (128,460). The corneal fibroblasts (keratocytes) have been implicated as the source of the extracellular material (3) because of the proximity of the latter to the characteristic abnormal accumulations. Circumstantial evidence suggests the most likely origin of the deposits to be stromal cells inherently present in the cornea. However, convincing morphological testimony to support this view is lacking. Corneal stromal cells lack specific ultrastructural alterations, and material with the same morphology as the extracellular deposits has not been observed within them. A variety of nonspecific and inconsistent degenerative cellular abnormalities have been observed by TEM (3,254,293,294,303, 433,450,460,468), yet some authors have interpreted such ultrastructural cellular findings, which could all represent secondary alterations, as cardinal to the disorder (433,460). An epithelial source warrants consideration despite the lack of morphological evidence of the abnormal protein emanating from diseased epithelial cells (128), yet if the proteinaceous material is derived from the epithelium recurrences in grafts should be the rule rather than the exception, because host epithelium soon replaces that of the donor.

Collagen-synthesizing cells secrete procollagen, which polymerizes into filaments of about 5 nm width outside the cell. Could the filamentous component of the lesions in GCD be an abnormal variety of collagen? Teng (460) interpreted cellular abnormalities as fundamental to the disease and proposed that the lesions in GCD resulted from a failure of newly formed precollagenous filaments to aggregate into mature collagen. If this is true, the deposits are expected to have the same chemical composition as collagen, but this is not the case. As Garner (128) pointed out, tyrosine, tryptophan, and sulfur-containing amino acids, which are conspicuous components of the lesions in GCD, are not significant constituents of collagen.

The nuclear DNA molecule presumably contains the fundamental defect in GCD. Taking into account the autosomal dominant mode of inheritance of the disease, the cytochemical attributes of the corneal deposits, ultrastructural morphological observations in the disease, experience with corneal grafts in the condition, and the known properties of the corneal grafts in the condition, the following hypothesis is proposed. A defective codon in the DNA presumably results in the synthesis and secretion by the corneal fibroblasts of an abnormal filamentous protein that is rich in trytophan, tyrosine, and sulfur-containing amino acids and hence structurally different from normal procollagen. It seems that these fibrils crystallize under specific but yet to be defined conditions, particularly in the superficial central corneal stroma. In the deeper corneal stroma, where the extracellular milieu is different, the fibrils aggregate into deposits of a different configuration, and in some areas abundant delicate fibrils remain unincorporated in a haphazard array. When this occurs, they appear by light microscopy, as with Wilder's reticulin stain, as argyophilic fibrils. The filamentous material that coexists with granular deposits in GCD is of approximately the same diameter (about 15 nm) as the fibrils in LCD, but the spatial arrangement of the fibrils usually differs (44). Depending upon the configuration of these fibrils some lesions may manifest different properties, such as an increased birefringence. The uneven distribution within the corneal stroma remains unexplained. Observations on corneal cells isolated from patients with GCD will, it is hoped, extend our knowledge about this disease, resolve unanswered questions about the nature of the deposits, and help to test the aforementioned hypothesis.

In 1961, Waardenburg and Jonkers (478) documented an autosomal dominant corneal dystrophy characterized by a superficial corneal granularity with clinical features of GCD but with several differences, including an earlier age of onset as well as an absence of radial lines and dots in the initial stage. Some authors considered it to be a specific corneal dystrophy (the corneal dystrophy of Waardenburg and Jonkers), but most authorities regarded it as a variant of GCD. The nature of this dystrophy was recently resolved. In a detailed follow-up study of the original pedigree, Wittebol-Post and colleagues (495) found that affected corneas have the characteristic "curly" fibers of Reis-Bücklers' dystrophy (see Chap. 40), not the deposits that typify GCD.

Especially in early childhood, deposits indistinguishable from those of typical GCD sometimes accumulate beneath or within the corneal epithelium (128,154,160,414,415) and produce snowflakelike opacities and a diffuse superficial corneal haze followed by epithelial erosions. Some authors (41,114) once regarded this probable variant of GCD as "progressive corneal dystrophy of Waardenburg and Jonkers," but as mentioned the corneal dystrophy of Waardenburg and Jonkers is now known to be Reis-Bücklers' dystrophy.

B. Miscellaneous Proteins

Chronic Actinic Keratopathy (Chronic Climatic Keratopathy)

Numerous extracellular granules and concretions of variable size accumulate in the cornea in a condition that is notorious for its numerous designations (chronic actinic keratopathy, spheroidal degeneration, chronic climatic keratopathy, climatic droplet keratopathy, noncalcific band keratopathy, and other terms; see also Chap. 23 (155). They are easily identified in unstained tissue secretions viewed by fluorescence microscopy because of their intense yellow autofluorescence. The concretions possess an affinity for certain histochemical and empirical stains, and these properties permit one to deduce that they are predominantly proteinaceous in nature, with phenyl, indole, guanidyl, and sulfhydryl reactive groups, and composed in part of sulfur-containing amino acids, as well as tyrosine, tryptophan, and arginine. Proteins with the latter components are not detectable in the normal cornea by histochemical methods. Yellow globules within the cornea in this keratopathy have been likened to oil droplets, but lipid is not a significant constituent (45,236). Despite the basophilia of some granules, calcification is rarely present by standard histochemical procedures. Although most concretions stain positively with some methods for elastic tissue (such as the Verhoeff-van Gieson technique) (45,56,217,236,384), others lack this affinity (131,217,236). Moreover, unlike normal elastic fibers (discussed elsewhere in this chapter), the accumulations do not stain with orcein or aldehyde fuchsin (131,217). Identical granules are commonly found in pingueculae (236), in actinic (solar) elastosis of the skin (236), and at the corneoscleral limbus of eyes with presumed sun-induced lesions, such as actinic keratosis, intraepithelial and invasive squamous carcinoma, and variable degrees of elastotic degeneration (45). In one investigation the deposits were resistant to elastase digestion (45), but this observation indicates nothing about the nature of the material because the cornea had been embedded in paraffin, making it an inappropriate substrate to evaluate by enzymatic digestion.

The claim that the material is of collagenous origin (72) is refuted by histochemical data. Since trypophan, tyrosine, and sulfur-containing amino acids are absent from collagen or are present in insignificant quantities, the denaturation of collagen should not release these reactive moieties. A different source for the concretions must be sought. It is conceivable that they are products of injured corneal and/or conjunctival cells or that they enter the damaged tissue from the conjunctival blood vessels or elsewhere. Impressed by histochemical similarities to keratin, Garner (129) originally suggested that the epithelium might be a potential source of the material, but this possibility is not supported by TEM observations.

That the concretions appear to be a protein rich in amino acids that are not normally detected in the cornea, combined with the absence of morphological evidence of their synthesis by corneal cells, suggests that the concretions are neither synthesized in the cornea nor formed there by the degradation of normal constituents. A possible site for their origin can be inferred from observations on eyes with the mild forms of the condition. In such instances, which presumably represent early stages in the genesis of the keratopathy, the concretions occur only in the superficial interpalpebral portion of the peripheral cornea. This finding, together with the coexistence of the keratopathy with pingueculae containing identical proteinaceous granules, suggests that the concretions may form in the conjunctiva. This hypothesis is underscored by the occasional presence of identical concretions in pingueculae of eyes that lack them in the cornea (236). One is led to suspect that a noncorneal protein progressively diffuses into the superficial cornea and accumulates there with time, resulting in larger globules that form by the coalescence of the smaller ones. Clinical findings in individuals with variable degrees of the keratopathy are consistent with this concept. From a clinical standpoint the first detectable droplets are restricted to the medial and lateral parts of the cornea in the interpalpebral fissure, and subsequent progression ensues by centripetal extension across the cornea. The observations that some concretions stain with histochemical procedures that demonstrate elastic fibers and that the corneal concretions coexist with pingueculae raise the possibility of the concretions being derived from constituents of conjunctival elastotic debris. Johnson and Overall (217) suggested that ultraviolet light may act upon plasma proteins in the subconjunctival tissue and as they diffuse through the cornea. An attempt has been made to identify the protein by analyzing specimens by sodium dodecyl sulfate–polyacrylamide gel electrophoresis, but because of the extreme insolubility of the protein it remains uncertain whether extracted high-molecular-weight proteins (molecular mass 20–300 kD) (454) are indeed identical to those that are evident histologically.

To learn more about the nature of the abnormal deposits that accumulate within the cornea in the corneal amyloidoses, GCD, and other corneal disorders characterized by the deposition of protein, investigators are trying to isolate the abnormal corneal proteins and to determine their amino acid sequence. This should, it is hoped, enable responsible genes to be isolated and characterized.

X. HEAT-SHOCK PROTEINS

As part of their response to unfavorable environmental alterations, such as heat stress and exposure to adverse chemical agents, eukaryotes synthesize specific proteins known as heat-shock proteins (280,408, 451). The α-crystallins are among the most abundant proteins in the crystalline lens of all vertebrates (491) and consist of two α-crystallin subunits (αA and αB), both of which are related to small heat-shock proteins (201,493). The αB subunit of the α-crystallins, which resides in many nonlenticular tissues (32,92,207, 209,210), has considerable amino acid sequence similarity to small heat-shock proteins (201), and its gene is regulated by stress (234).

Heat-shock protein has been identified by immunohistochemistry in the atrophic corneal epithelium of rats with an inherited retinal degeneration (Royal College of Surgeons dystrophic rats), perhaps as a response to products of degenerating rod outer segments (501).

In several disorders eosinophilic fibers (Rosenthal fibers) accumulate, especially in the white matter of the CNS, including Alexander's disease (see Chap. 53) and astrocytomas of the optic nerve (see Chap. 50). By TEM these structures are composed of condensations of microfilaments (146,162), and immunohistochemical methods have disclosed that they stain positively for the heat-shock protein ubiquitin (283). Examination of purified Rosenthal fibers has indicated that they consist of aggregates of αB-crystallin with glial fibrillary acid protein and ubiquitin (465).

A diffuse reactivity with antibodies to αB-crystallin has been detected in several characteristic lesions of tuberous sclerosis: dysgenetic giant cells in both the cerebral white and gray matter, subependymal nodules and neoplastic giant cells within subependymal giant cell astrocytomas, rhabdomyomas, renal and hepatic angiomyolipomas, a fetal cell adenoma of the thyroid gland, and hyperplastic renal tubule cells, as well as in smooth muscle proliferations surrounding lymphatics (lymphangioleiomyomatosis) in the lung and lymph nodes (208,211). This observation is particularly noteworthy because the gene responsible for one genetic form of tuberous sclerosis (discussed in Chap. 45) has been mapped to chromosome 11 (11q22-23) (214,366,428,429), which is the second locus for the αB-crystallin gene (331). Although a primary gene abnormality seems more likely in view of the close proximity of the tuberous sclerosis and αB-crystallin genes (211), because small heat-shock proteins are developmentally regulated it is also conceivable that the αB-crystallin is induced as a consequence of the hamartomas.

REFERENCES

1. Abe, T., Yamaki, K., Tsuda, M., Singh, V.K., Suzuki, S., McKinnon, R., Klein, D.C., Donoso, L.A., and Shinohara, T. Rat pineal S-antigen: Sequence analysis reveals presence of alpha-transducin homologous sequence. *FEBS Lett.* 247:307–311, 1989.
2. Ackerman, A.L. The ocular manifestations of Waldenström's macroglobulinemia and its treatment. *Arch. Ophthalmol.* 67:701–707, 1962.

3. Akiya, S., and Brown, S.I. Granular dystrophy of the cornea: Characteristic electron microscopic lesion. *Arch. Ophthalmol. 84*:179–192, 1970.
4. Akiya, S., Ho, K., and Matsui, M. Gelatinous drop-like dystrophy of the cornea: Light and electron microscopy study of superficial stromal lesion. *Jpn. J. Clin. Ophthalmol. 26*:815–826, 1972.
5. Albelda, S.M. Biology of disease: Role of integrins and other cell adhesion molecules in tumor progression and metastasis. *Lab. Invest. 68*:4–17, 1993.
6. Albelda, S.M., and Buck, C.A. Integrins and other cell adhesion molecules. *Fed. Am. Soc. Exp. Biol. J. 4*:2868–2880, 1990.
7. Albelda, S.M., Muller, W.A., Buck, C.A., and Newman, P.J. Molecular and cellular properties of PECAM-1(endoCAM/CD31): A novel vascular cell-cell adhesion molecule. *J. Cell Biol. 114*:1059–1068, 1991.
8. Alberts, B., Bray, D., Lewis, J., Raff, M., Roberts, K., and Watson, J.D. *Molecular Biology of the Cell*, 2nd ed., Gartland Publishing, New York, 1989.
9. Alexander, R.A., Clayton, D.C., Howes, R.C., and Garner, A. Effect of oxidation upon demonstration of oxytalan fibres: A light and electron microscopical study. *Med. Lab. Sci. 38*:91–101, 1981.
10. Alexander, R.A., and Garner, A. Oxytalan fibre formation in the cornea: A light and electron microscopical study. *Histopathology 1*:189–199, 1977.
11. Alexander, R.J., Silverman, G., and Henley, W.L. Isolation and characterization of BCP54, the major soluble protein of bovine cornea. *Exp. Eye Res. 32*:205–216, 1981.
12. Allansmith, M.R., Whitney, C.R., McClellan, B.H., and Newsome, L.P. Immunoglobulins in the human eye. *Arch. Ophthalmol. 89*:36–45, 1973.
13. Andrade, C. A peculiar form of peripheral neuropathy: Familiar atypical generalized amyloidosis with special involvement of the peripheral nerves. *Brain 75*:408–427, 1952.
14. Aronson, S.B., II, and Shaw, R. Corneal crystals in multiple myeloma. *Arch. Ophthalmol. 61*:541–546, 1959.
15. Ashton, N. Ocular changes in multiple myelomatosis. *Arch. Ophthalmol. 73*:487–494, 1965.
16. Ashton, N., Kok, D.A., and Foulds, W.S. Ocular pathology in macroglobulinaemia. *J. Pathol. Bacteriol. 86*:453–461, 1963.
17. Atreya, P.L., Barnes, J., Katar, M., Alacala, J., and Maisel, H. N-cadhedrin of the human lens. *Curr. Eye Res. 8*:947–956, 1989.
18. Austin, M.G., and Schaefer, R.F. Marfan's syndrome with unusual blood vessel manifestations: Primary medionecrosis dissection of right innominate, right carotid, and left carotid arteries. *Arch. Pathol. 64*:205–209, 1957.
19. Baker, T.R., and Spencer, W.H. Ocular findings in multiple myeloma: A report of two cases. *Arch. Ophthalmol. 91*:110–113, 1974.
20. Balazs, E.A. (Ed.) *Chemistry and Molecular Biology of the Intercellular Matrix*, Academic Press, New York, 1970.
21. Barr, C.C., Gelender, H., and Font, R.L. Corneal crystalline deposits associated with dysproteinemia: Report of two cases and review of the literature. *Arch. Ophthalmol. 98*:884–889, 1980.
22. Bataille, R., Greiner, J., and Commes, T. In vitro production of beta$_2$ microglobulin by human myeloma cells. *Cancer Invest. 6*:271–277, 1988.
23. Becker, U., Nowack, H., Gay, S., and Timpl, R. Production and specificity of antibodies against the aminoterminal region in type III collagen. *Immunology 31*:57–65, 1976.
24. Beebe, W.E., Webster, R.G., Jr., and Spencer, W.B. Atypical corneal manifestations of multiple myeloma: A clinical and immunohistochemical report. *Cornea 8*:274–280, 1989.
25. Behal, M.L. Secondary amyloid infiltration around the limbus. *Br. J. Ophthalmol. 48*:622–623, 1964.
26. Benditt, E.P., and Eriksen, N. Chemical classes of amyloid substance. *Am. J. Pathol. 65*:231–249, 1971.
27. Benson, M.D. Hereditary amyloidosis: Disease entity and clinical model. *Hosp. Pract.* March 15:165–181, 1988.
28. Benson, M.D., and Dwulet, F.E. Prealbumin and retinol binding protein serum concentrations in the Indiana type hereditary amyloidosis. *Arthritis Rheum. 26*:1493–1498, 1983.
29. Benson, M.D., and Wallace, M.R. Amyloidosis. In *The Metabolic Basis of Inherited Disease*, 6th ed., Vol. 2, C.R. Scriver, A.L. Beaudet, W.S. Sly, and D. Valle (Eds.), McGraw-Hill, New York, Chap. 97, pp. 2439–2460, 1989.
30. Bevilacqua, M.P., Pober, J.S., Mendrick, D.L., Cotran, R.S., and Gimbrone, M.A. Identification of an inducible endothelial-leukocyte adhesion molecule. *Proc. Natl. Acad. Sci. USA 84*:9238–9242, 1987.
31. Bhat, S.P., Jones, R.E., Sullivan, M.A., and Piatigorsky, P. Chicken lens crystallin DNA sequences show at least two α-crystallin genes. *Nature 284*:234–238, 1980.
32. Bhat, S.P., and Nagineni, C.N. αB subunit of lens-specific protein α-crystallin is present in other ocular and nonocular tissues. *Biochem. Biophys. Res. Commun. 158*:319–325, 1989.
33. Bhat, S.P., and Piatigorsky, J. Molecular cloning and partial characterization of δ-crystallin cDNA sequences in a bacterial plasmid. *Proc. Natl. Acad. Sci. USA 76*:3299–3303, 1979.
34. Biber, H. Ueber einige seltenere Hornhauterkrankungen: Die oberflachliche gittrige Keratitis. Inaugural Dissertation. A. Digglemann, Zurich, pp. 35–42, 1890.
35. Black, H.H., and Landay, L.H. Marfan's syndrome: Report of five cases in one family. *Am. J. Dis. Child. 89*:414–420, 1955.

36. Blobner, F. Kristallinsche degeneration der Bindehaut und Hornhaut. *Klin. Monatsbl. Augenheilkd. 100*:588–593, 1938.

37. Boehme, J.D., and Litwak, A.B. Juxtapapillary choroidal neovascular membrane in a patient with Paget's disease and lattice corneal dystrophy. *J. Am. Optom. Assoc. 80*:612–616, 1989.

38. Bogaars, H.A., Kaldenon, A.E., Cummings, F.J., Kaplan, S., Melnicoff, I., Park, C., Diamond, I., and Calabresi, P. Human IgG cryoglobulin with tubular crystal structure. *Nature New Biol. 245*:117–118, 1973.

39. Bowen, R.A., Hassard, D.T.R., Wong, V.G., DeLellis, R.A., and Glenner, G.G. Lattice dystrophy of the cornea as a variety of amyloidosis. *Am. J. Ophthalmol. 70*:822–825, 1970.

40. Boysen, G., Galassi, G., Kamieniecka, Z., Schlaeger, J., and Trojaborg, W. Familial amyloidosis with cranial neuropathy and corneal lattice dystrophy. *J. Neurol. Neurosurg. Psychiatr. 42*:1020–1030, 1979.

41. Bron, A.J., and Tripathi, R.C. Corneal disorders. In *Genetic and Metabolic Eye Disease*, M.F. Goldberg (Ed.), Little, Brown, Boston, pp. 281–323, 1974.

42. Brown, P., Goldfarb, L.G., and Gajdusek, D.C. The new biology of spongiform encephalopathy: Infectious amyloidosis with genetic twist. *Lancet 337*:1019–1022, 1991.

43. Brownstein, M.H., Elliot, R., and Helwig, E.B. Ophthalmologic aspects of amyloidosis. *Am. J. Ophthalmol. 69*:423–430, 1970.

44. Brownstein, S., Fine, B.S., Sherman, M.E., and Zimmerman, L.E. Granular dystrophy of the cornea: Light and electron microscopic confirmation of recurrence in a graft. *Am. J. Ophthalmol. 77*:701–710, 1974.

45. Brownstein, S., Rodrigues, M., Fine, B.S., and Albert, E.N. The elastotic nature of hyaline corneal deposits: A histochemical, fluorescent, and electron microscopic examination. *Am. J. Ophthalmol. 75*:799–809, 1973.

46. Burk, E.V. Über Hornhautveränderungen bei einem Fall von multiplem Myeloma (Plasmocytom). *Ophthalmologica 135*:565–572, 1958.

47. Burridge, K., Fath, K., Kelly, T., Nuckolls, G., and Turner, C. Focal adhesions: Transmembrane junctions between the extracellular matrix and the cytoskeleton. *Annu. Rev. Biol. 4*:487–525, 1988.

48. Buxbaum, J., Caron, D., and Gallo, G. AL amyloid, L-chain and L and H-chain deposition diseases: Comparison of Ig synthesis and tissue deposition. In *Amyloid and Amyloidosis*, J.B. Natvig, O. Forre, G. Husby, A. Husebekk, B. Skogen, K. Sletten, and P. Westermark (Eds.), Kluwer Academic, Dordrecht, pp. 197–200, 1991.

49. Carlos, T.M., and Harlan, J.M. Membrane proteins involved in phagocyte adherence to endothelium. *Immunol. Rev. 114*:5–28, 1990.

50. Carr, R., and Henkind, P. Retinal findings associated with serum hyperviscosity. *Am. J. Ophthalmol. 56*:23–31, 1963.

51. Castano, E.M., and Frangione, B. Human amyloidosis, Alzheimer's disease and related disorders. *Lab. Invest. 58*:122–132, 1988.

52. Cherry, P.M.H., Kraft, S., McGowan, H., Ghosh, M., and Shenken, E. Corneal and conjunctival deposits in monoclonal gammopathy. *Can. J. Ophthalmol. 18*:142–149, 1983.

53. Cherry, P.M.H., and Scott, J.G. Corneal and conjunctival deposits in monoclonal gammopathy: Addendum and correction (letter). *Can. J. Ophthalmol. 18*:256, 1983.

54. Cheung, P., Kao, F.-T., Law, M.L., Jones, C., Puck, T.T., and Chan, L. Localization of the structural gene for human apolipoprotein A-1 on the long arm of human chromosome 11. *Proc. Natl. Acad. Sci. USA 81*:508–511, 1984.

55. Chiquet-Ehrismann, R. What distinguishes tenascin from fibronectin? *FASEB J. 4*:2598–2604, 1990.

56. Christensen, G.R. Proteinaceous corneal degeneration: A histochemical study. *Arch. Ophthalmol. 89*:30–32, 1973.

57. Chvapil, M.L. *Physiology of Connective Tissue*, Butterworth, London, pp. 229–233, 1967.

58. Cintorino, M., Vindigni, C., Del Vecchio, M.T., Tosi, P., Frezzotti, R., Hadjistilianou, T., Leoncini, P., Silvestri, S., Skalli, O., and Gabbiani, G. Expression of actin isoforms and intermediate filament proteins in childhood orbital rhabdomyosarcomas. *J. Submicrosc. Cytol. Pathol. 21*:409–419, 1989.

59. Clarke, E. Ophthalmological complications of multiple myelomatosis. *Br. J. Ophthalmol. 39*:233–236, 1955.

60. Cohen, A.S., Cathcart, E.S., and Skinner, M. Amyloidosis: Current trends in its investigation. *Arthritis Rheum. 21*:153–160, 1978.

61. Collyer, R.T. Amyloidosis of the cornea. *Can. J. Ophthalmol. 3*:35–38, 1968.

62. Connell, G., Bascom, R., Molday, L., Reid, D., McInnes, R.R., and Molday, R.S. Photoreceptor peripherin is the normal product of the gene responsible for retinal degeneration in the *rds* mouse. *Proc. Natl. Acad. Sci. USA 88*:723–726, 1991.

63. Connell, G.E., Freedman, M.H., Nyburg, S.C., Painter, R.H., Parr, D.M., Pinteric, L., and Pruzanski, W. A human IgG myeloma protein crystallizing with rhombohedral symmetry. *Can. J. Biochem. 51*:1137–1141, 1973.

64. Cooper, D., Schermer, A., and Sun, T-T. Biology of disease. Classification of human epithelia and their neoplasms using antibodies to keratins: Strategies, applications, and limitations. *Lab. Invest. 52*:243–256, 1985.

65. Cooper, D.L., Baptist, E.W., Enghild, J.J., Isola, N., and Klintworth, G.K. Mixed oligonucleotide primed amplification cDNA cloning (MOPAC) of bovine corneal protein 54K (BCP 54) reveals it is a homologue of the tumor inducible (class 3) rat aldehydrogenase gene. *Gene 98*:201–207, 1991.

66. Cooper, D.L., Baptist, E.W., Enghild, J., Lee, H., Isola, N., and Klintworth, G.K. Partial amino acid sequence determination of bovine corneal protein 54K (BCP54). *Curr. Eye Res. 9*:781–786, 1990.

67. Cornwell, G.G., Westermark, O., Natvig, J.B., and Murdock, W. Senile cardiac amyloid evidence that fibrils contain a protein immunologically related to prealbumin. *Immunology 44*:447–452, 1981.

68. Costa, P.P., Figueira, A.S., and Bravo, F.R. Amyloid fibril protein related to prealbumin in familial amyloidotic polyneuropathy. *Proc. Natl. Acad. Sci. USA 75*:4499–4503, 1978.

69. Crawford, J.B. Cotton wool exudates in systemic amyloidosis. *Arch. Ophthalmol. 78*:214–216, 1967.

70. Cross, H.E., and Jensen, A.D. Ocular manifestations in the Marfan syndrome and homocystinuria. *Am. J. Ophthalmol. 75*:405–420, 1973.

71. Cuendet, J.F., Beuret-Niedzielsky, A., and Zografos, L. Hérédité de la dystrophie granuleuse de la cornée (Groenouw I). *Ophtalmologie 3*:265–266, 1989.

72. Cursino, J.W., and Fine, B.S. A histologic study of calcific and noncalcific band keratopathies. *Am. J. Ophthalmol. 82*:395–404, 1976.

73. Danis, P., Brauman, S., and Coppez, P. Lesions of the fundus of the eye found in certain hyperproteinemias, particularly those of myelomatous origin. *Acta Ophthalmol. (Copenh.) 33*:33–52, 1955.

74. Danks, D.M. Disorders of copper transport. In *The Metabolic Basis of Inherited Disease*, 6th ed., Vol. 1, C.R. Scriver, A.L. Beaudet, W.S. Sly, and D. Valle (Eds.), McGraw-Hill, New York, Chap. 54, pp. 1411–1431, 1989.

75. Dark, A.J., and Thompson, D.S. Lattice dystrophy of the cornea: A clinical and microscopic study. *Br. J. Ophthalmol. 44*:257–279, 1960.

76. Darras, B.T., Adelman, L.S., Mora, J.S., Bodziner, R.A., and Munsat, T.L. Familial amyloidosis with cranial neuropathy and corneal lattice dystrophy. *Neurology 36*:432–435, 1986.

77. Davies, D.R., Padlan, E.A., and Segal, D.M. Three-dimensional structure of immunoglobulins. *Annu. Rev. Biochem. 44*:639–667, 1975.

78. Defoe, D.M., Martone, R.L., Caldwell, R.B., Chang, C.-W., and Herbert, J. Transthyretin secretion by cultured rat retinal pigment epithelium. *Invest. Ophthalmol. Vis. Sci. (Suppl.) 33*:911, 1992.

79. De Souza, A.R. Amiloidose cutanea bulhosa familial observacao de 4 casos. *Rev. Hosp. Clin. Fac. Med. S. Paulo 18*:413–417, 1963.

80. Deutsch, H.F., and Suzuki, T. A crystallin γ-G human monoclonal protein with an excessive H chain deletion. *Ann. N.Y. Acad. Sci. 190*:472–486, 1971.

81. Dhermy, P., Pouliquen, Y., and Salvodelli, M. Amylose secondaire localisée de la cornée. *Arch. Ophtalmol. (Paris) 33*:501–523, 1973.

82. Diamond, M.S., Staunton, D.E., de Fougerolles, A.R., Stacker, S.A., Garcia-Aguilar, J., Hibbs, M.L., and Springer, T.A. ICAM-1(CD54): A counter-receptor for Mac-1(CD11b/CD18). *J. Cell Biol. 111*:3129–3139, 1990.

83. Dickson, P.W., and Schreiber, G. High levels of messenger RNA for transthyretin (prealbumin) in human choroid plexus. *Neurosci. Lett. 66*:311–315, 1986.

84. Dietz, H.C., Cutting, G.R., Pyeritz, R.E., Maslen, C.L., Sakai, L.Y., Corson, G.M., Puffenberger, E.G., Hamosh, A., Nathakumar, E.J., Curristin, S.M., Stetten, G., Meyers, D.A., and Francomano, C.A. Marfan's syndrome caused by a recurrent de novo missense mutation in the fibrillin gene (see comments). *Nature 352*:337–339, 1991.

85. Dimmer, F. Ueber oberflächliche gittrige Hornhauttrübung. *Z. Augenheilkd. 2*:354–361, 1899.

86. Dizhoor, A.M., Ray, S., Kumar, S., Niemi, G., Spencer, M., Brolley, D., Walsh, K.A., Philipov, P.P., Hurley, J.B., and Stryer, L. Recoverin: A calcium sensitive activator of retinal rod guanylate cyclase. *Science 251*:915–918, 1991.

87. Doft, D.H., Machemer, R., Skinner, M., Buettner, H., Clarkson, J., Crock, J., McLeod, D., Michels, R., Scott, J., and Wilson, D. Pars plana vitrectomy for vitreous amyloidosis. *Ophthalmology 94*:607–611, 1987.

88. Donnelly, E.J. Ocular complications of multiple myelomatosis. *Am. J. Ophthalmol. 47*:211–214, 1959.

89. Drazba, J., and Lemmon, V. The role of cell adhesion molecules in neurite outgrowth on Müller cells. *Dev. Biol. 138*:82–93, 1990.

90. Dua, H.S., Liversidge, J., and Forrester, J.V. Immunomodulation of experimental autoimmune uveitis using a rat antiretinal S-antigen specific monoclonal antibody: Evidence for a species difference. *Eye 3*:69–78, 1989.

91. Dua, H.S., Sewell, H.F., and Forrester, J.V. The effect of retinal S-antigen-specific monoclonal antibody therapy on experimental autoimmune uveoretinitis (EAU) and experimental autoimmune pinealitis (EAP). *Clin. Exp. Immunol. 75*:100–105, 1989.

92. Dubin, R.A., Wawrousek, E.F., and Piatigorsky, J. Expression of the murine αβ-crystallin gene is not restricted to the lens. *Mol. Cell. Biol. 9*:1083–1091, 1989.

93. Dulic, V., Lees, E., and Reed, S.I. Association of human cyclin E with a periodic G_1-S phase protein kinase. *Science 257*:1958–1961, 1992.

94. Dustin, M.L., Rothlein, R., Bhan, A.K., Dinarello, C.A., and Springer, T.A. Induction by IL 1 and interferon-gamma: Tissue distribution, biochemistry, and function of a natural adherence molecule (ICAM-1). *J. Immunol.* *137*:245–254, 1986.

95. Dutts, S., Elner, V.M., Soong, H.K., Meyer, R.F., and Sugar, A. Secondary localized amyloidosis in intersitial keratitis: Clinicopathologic findings. *Ophthalmology* 99:817–823, 1992.

96. Dwulet, F.E., and Benson, M.D. Characterization of a transthyretin (prealbumin) variant associated with familial amyloidotic polyneuropathy type II (Indiana/Swiss). *J. Clin. Invest.* 78:880–886, 1986.

97. Eagle, R.C., Jr., Brooks, J.S.J., Katowitz, J.A., Weiberg, J.C., and Perry, H.D. Fibrin as a major constituent of ligneous conjunctivitis. *Am. J. Ophthalmol.* *101*:493–494, 1986.

98. Eddington, G.N., and Lehmann, H. A case of sickle cell-hemoglobin C disease in a survey of hemoglobin incidence in West Africa. *Trans. World Soc. Trop. Med. Hyg.* 48:332–336, 1954.

99. Eiferman, R.A., and Rodrigues, M.M. Unusual superficial stromal corneal deposits in IgGk monoclonal gammopathy. *Arch. Ophthalmol.* 98:78–81, 1980.

100. Eiferman, R.A., Rodrigues, M.M., Laibson, P.R., and Arentsen, J.J. Schnyder's crystalline dystrophy associated with amyloid deposition. *Metab. Pediatr. Ophthalmol.* 3:15–20, 1979.

101. El Matri, L., Bachtobji, A., Ghorbal, M., Maamri, J., Kamoun, M., Ouertani, A., Bardi, R., and Triki, M.F. Forme familiale de dystrophie gélatineuse en gouttes de la cornée. *J. Fr. Ophtalmol.* *14*:125–129, 1991.

102. Elner, V.M., Elner, S.G., Pavilack, M.A., Todd, R.F., III, Yue, B.Y.J.T., and Huber, A.R. Intercellular adhesion molecule-1 in human corneal endothelium: Modulation and function. *Am. J. Pathol.* *138*:525–536, 1991.

103. Emanuel, B.S., Cannizzarol, L., Ornstein-Goldstein, N., Indik, Z.K., Yoon, K., May, M., Oliver, L., Boyd, C., and Rosenbloom, J. Chromosomal localization of the human elastin gene. *Am. J. Hum. Genet.* 37:873–882, 1985.

104. Enzenauer, R.J., Stock, J.G., Enzenauer, R.W., Pope, J., and West, S.G. Retinal vasculopathy associated with systemic light chain deposition disease. *Retina* *10*:115–118, 1990.

105. Eype, A.A., Kruit, P.J., van der Gaag, R., Neuteboom, G.H., Broersma, L., and Kijlstra, A. Autoimmunity against corneal antigens. II. Accessibility of the 54kD corneal antigen for circulating antibodies. *Curr. Eye Res.* 6:467–475, 1987.

106. Falls, H.F., Jackson, J., Carey, J.H., Rukavina, J.G., and Block, W.D. Ocular manifestations of hereditary primary systemic amyloidosis. *Arch. Ophthalmol.* 54:660–664, 1955.

107. Farrar, G.J., Kenna, P., Redmond, R., McWilliam, P., Bradley, D.G., Humphries, M.M., Sharp, E.M., Inglehearn, C.F., Bashir, R., Jay, M., Watty, A., Ludwig, M., Schinzel, A., Samanns, C., Gal, A., Bhattacharya, S., and Humphries, P. Autosomal dominant retinitis pigmentosa: Absence of the rhodopsin proline-histidine substitution (codon 23) in pedigrees from Europe. *Am. J. Hum. Genet.* 47:941–945, 1990.

108. Ferry, A.P., and Leiberman, T.W. Bilateral amyloidosis of the vitreous body: Report of a case without systemic and familial involvement. *Arch. Ophthalmol.* 94:982–991, 1976.

109. Firkin, F.C., Lee, N., Ramsay, R., and Robertson, I. Visual loss caused by corneal crystals in myeloma: Rapid improvement with plasma exchange and chemotherapy. *Med. J. Aust.* 2:677–678, 1979.

110. Fleischmajer, R., Jacobs, L., II, Perlish, J.S., Katchen, B., Schwartz, E., and Timpl, R. Immunochemical analysis of human kidney reticulin. *Am. J. Pathol.* *140*:1225–1235, 1992.

111. Foidart, J.M., Bere, E.W., Jr., Yaar, M., Rennard, S.I., Gullino, M., Martin, G.R., and Katz, S.I. Distribution and immunoelectron microscopic localization of laminin, a non-collagenous basement membrane glycoprotein. *Lab. Invest.* 42:336–342, 1980.

112. Folberg, R., Alfonso, E., Croxatto, J.O., Driezen, N.G., Panjawani, N., Laibson, P.R., Boruchoff, S.A., Baum, J., Malbran, E.S., Fernandez-Meijide, R., Morrison, J.A., Jr., Bernardino, V.B., Jr., Arbizo, V.V., and Albert, D.M. Clinically atypical granular corneal dystrophy with pathologic features of lattice-like amyloid deposits: A study of three families. *Ophthalmology* 95:46–51, 1988.

113. Franceschetti, A., and Babel, J., II. *The Heredo-Familial Degenerations of the Cornea. B. Pathological Anatomy.* XVI Concilium Ophthalmologicum, 1950, Britannia Acta, Vol. 1, British Medical Association, London, pp. 245–283, 1951.

114. Francois, J. Heredo-familial corneal dystrophies. *Trans. Ophthalmol. Soc. UK* 86:367–416, 1966.

115. Francois, J. Paraproteinaemic thesaurismosis of the cornea in Kahler's multiple myelomatosis. *Eye Ear Nose Throat Mon.* 46:857–860, 1967.

116. Francois, J., and Rabaey, M. Dystrophie cornéene et paraproteinemie. *Bull. Soc. Belge Ophtalmol.* *125*:1007–1017, 1960.

117. Franklin, E.C., and Pras, M. Immunologic studies of water-soluble human amyloid fibrils: Comparative studies of eight amyloid preparations. *J. Exp. Med.* *130*:797–808, 1969.

118. Franklin, E.C., Rosenthal, C.J., Pras, M., and Levin, M. Recent progress in amyloid. In *The Role of Immunological Factors in Infectious, Allergic, and Autoimmune Processes*, R.F. Beers and E.G. Basset (Eds.), Raven Press, New York, pp. 163–174, 1976.

119. Fuchs, E.V., Coppock, S.M., Green, H., and Cleveland, D.W. Two distinct classes of keratin genes and their evolutionary significance. *Cell* 27:75–84, 1981.

120. Fukuda, M.N., Papermaster, D.S., and Hargrave, P.A. Rhodopsin carbohydrate: Structure of small oligosaccharides attached at two sites near the NH_2 terminus. *J. Biol. Chem.* *254*:8201–8207, 1979.

121. Fullard, R.J., and Kissner, D.M. Purification of the isoforms of tear specific prealbumin. *Curr. Eye Res. 10*:613–628, 1991.
122. Fullmer, H.M., and Lillie, R.D. The oxytalan fiber: A previously undescribed connective tissue fiber. *J. Histochem. Cytochem. 6*:425–430, 1958.
123. Fullmer, H.M., Sheetz, J.H., and Narkates, A.J. Oxytalan connective tissue fibers: A review. *J. Oral Pathol. 3*:291–316, 1974.
124. Gallatin, W.M., Weissman, I.L., and Butcher, E.C. A cell-surface molecule involved in organ-specific homing of lymphocytes. *Nature 304*:30–34, 1983.
125. Gamble, J.R., Skinner, M.P., Berndt, M.C., and Vadas, M.A. Prevention of activated neutrophil adhesion to endothelium by soluble adhesion protein GMP140. *Science 249*:414–417, 1990.
126. Ganeval, D., Noel, L.H., Preud'homme, J.L., Droz, D., and Grünfeld, J.P. Light-chain deposition disease: Its relation with A1-type amyloidosis (editorial review). *Kidney Int. 26*:1–9, 1984.
127. Garner, A. Amyloidosis of the cornea. *Br. J. Ophthalmol. 53*:73–81, 1969.
128. Garner, A. Histochemistry of corneal granular dystrophy. *Br. J. Ophthalmol. 53*:799–807, 1969.
129. Garner, A. Keratinoid corneal degeneration. *Br. J. Ophthalmol. 54*:769–780, 1970.
130. Garner, A., and Alexander, R.A. Pre-elastic (oxytalan) fibres in corneal pathology. Proc. VIth Congress Eur. Soc. Ophthalmol., Academic Press and Royal Society of Medicine, London, pp. 213– 216, 1980.
131. Garner, A., Fraunfelder, F.T., Barras, T.C., and Hinzpeter, E.N. Spheroidal degeneration of cornea and conjunctiva. *Br. J. Opthalmol. 60*:437–478, 1976.
132. Garner, A., and Kirkness, G.M. Corneal gammopathy. *Cornea 7*:44–49, 1988.
133. Gartry, D.S., Falcon, M.G., and Cox, R.W. Primary gelatinous drop-like keratopathy. *Br. J. Ophthalmol. 73*:661–664, 1989.
134. Gay, S., Fletzek, P.P., Remberger, K., Eder, M., and Kuhn, K. Liver cirrhosis: Immunofluorescence and biochemical studies demonstrate two types of collagen. *Klin. Wochenschr. 53*:205–208, 1975.
135. Gawlik, Z. Morphological and morphochemical properties of the elastic system in the motor organ of man. *Folia Histochem. Cytochem. 3*:233–251, 1965.
136. Geiger, B., Tokuyasu, K.T., Dutton, A.H., and Singer, S.J. Vinculin, an intracellular protein localized at specialized sites where microfilament bundles terminate at cell membranes. *Proc. Natl. Acad. Sci. USA 77*:4127–4131, 1980.
137. Geisler, N., and Weber, K. The amino acid sequence of chicken muscle desmin provides a common structural model for intermediate filament proteins. *EMBO J. 1*:1649–1656, 1982.
138. Gejyo, F., Maruyama, S., Maruyama, N., Homma, N., Aoyayagi, R., Suzuki, Y., Hoque, E., and Arakawa, M. β_2-Microglobulin-derived amyloid and calcium in long-term dialysis patients. In *Amyloid and Amyloidosis*, J.B. Natvig, O. Forre, G. Husby, A. Husebekk, B. Skogen, K. Sletten, and P. Westermark (Eds.), Kluwer Academic, Dordrecht, pp. 377–380, 1991.
139. Ghiso, J., Haltia, A., Prelli, F., Novello, J., and Frangione, B. Gelsolin variant (ASN-187) in familial amyloidosis, Finnish type. *Biochem. J. 272*:827–830, 1990.
140. Giarelli, L., Bonito, L. Di., and Melato, M. Dans quelle mesure les tissue orbitaires (intra- et extra-oculaires) sont concernés dans l'amyloidose-Lignes de comportement déduites sur la base de 10 observations. *Arch. Ophtalmol. (Paris) 33*:757–762, 1973.
141. Gilbert, W., and Villa-Komaroff, L. Useful proteins from recombinant bacteria. *Sci. Am. 242*:74–94, 1980.
142. Glenner, G.G., Ein, D., Eanes, E.D., Bladen, H.A., Terry, W., and Page, D.L. Creation of amyloid fibrils from Bence-Jones proteins in vitro. *Science 174*:712–714, 1971.
143. Glenner, G.G., and Murphy, M.A. Amyloidosis of the nervous system. *J. Neurol. Sci. 94*:1–28, 1989.
144. Glenner, G.G., Terry, W., Harada, M., Isersky, C., and Page, D. Amyloid fibril proteins: Proof of homology with immunoglobulin light chains by sequence analysis. *Science 172*:1150–1151, 1971.
145. Glenner, G.G., Terry, W.D., and Isersky, C. Amyloidosis: Its nature and pathogenesis. *Semin. Hematol. 10*:65–86, 1973.
146. Gluszcz, A., Giernat, L., Habryka, K., Alwasiak, J., Lach, B., and Papierz, W. Rosenthal fibers, birefringent gliofibrillary changes and intracellular homogenous conglomerates in tissue cultures of gliomas. *Acta Neuropathol. (Berl.) 17*:54–67, 1971.
147. Goldberg, M.F., and Ryan, S.J. Intercalary staphyloma in Marfan's syndrome. *Am. J. Ophthalmol. 67*:329–335, 1969.
148. Goldgaber, D., Lerman, M.I., McBride, O.W., Saffiotti, U., and Gajdusek, D.C. Characterization and chromosomal localization of a cDNA encoding brain amyloid of Alzheimer's disease. *Science 235*:877–880, 1987.
149. Gorevic, P.D., Munoz, P.C., Gorgone, G., Purcell, J.J., Jr., Rodriques, M., Ghiso, J., Levy, E., Haltia, M., and Frangione, B. Amyloidosis due to a mutation of the gelsolin gene in an American family with lattice corneal dystrophy type II. *N. Engl. J. Med. 325*:1780–1785, 1991.
150. Gorevic, P.D., Munoz, P.C., Rodrigues, M., Haltia, M., Ghiso, J., and Frangione, B. Shared gelsolin antigenicity between familial amyloidosis Finnish type (FAF) and one form of familial lattice corneal dystrophy (LCD) with polyneuropathy from the United States. In *Amyloid and Amyloidosis*, J.B. Natvig, O. Forre, G. Husby, A. Husebekk, B. Skogen, K. Sletten, and P. Westermark (Eds.), Kluwer Academic, Dordrecht, pp. 423–435, 1991.

151. Gorevic, P.D., Prelli, F.C., Wright, J., Pras, M., and Frangione, B. Systemic senile amyloidosis. Identification of a new prealbumin (transthyretin) variant in cardiac tissue: Immunologic and biochemical similarity to one form of familial amyloidotic polyneuropathy. *J. Clin. Invest.* *83*:836–843, 1989.

152. Gorevic, P.D., Rodrigues, M.M., Krachmer, J.H., Green, C., Fujihara, S., and Glenner, G.G. Lack of evidence for protein AA reactivity in amyloid deposits of lattice corneal dystrophy and amyloid corneal degeneration. *Am. J. Ophthalmol.* *98*:216–224, 1984.

153. Gorevic, P.D., Rodrigues, M.M., Spencer, W.H., Munoz, P.C., Allen, A.W., Jr., and Verne, A.Z. Prealbumin is a major constituent of vitreous amyloid. *Ophthalmology 94*:792–798, 1987.

154. Goslar, H.G., and Seitz, R. Das histochemische Bild von Hornhautdegenerationen und -dystrophien in Beziehung zum ophthalmoskopischen Befund. *Acta Histochem. (Jena) 12*:289–304, 1961.

155. Gray, R.H., Johnson, G.J., and Freedman, A. Climatic droplet keratopathy. *Surv. Ophthalmol. 36*:241–253, 1992.

156. Green, W.R. Diagnostic cytopathology of ocular fluid specimens. *Ophthalmology 91*:726–749, 1984.

157. Grubb, A., Jensson, O., Gudmundsson, G., Arnason, A., Lofberg, H., and Malm, J. Abnormal metabolism of gamma-trace alkaline microprotein: The basic defect in hereditary cerebral hemorrhage with amyloidosis. *N. Engl. J. Med. 311*:1547–1549, 1984.

158. Gundmundsson, G., Hallgrimsson, J., Jonasson, T.A., and Bjarnason, O. Hereditary cerebral haemorrhage with amyloidosis. *Brain 95*:387–404, 1972.

159. Haab. Die gittrige Keratitis. *Z. Augenheilkd. 2*:235–246, 1899.

160. Haddad, R., Font, R.L., and Fine, B.S. Unusual superficial variant of granular dystrophy of the cornea. *Am. J. Ophthalmol. 83*:213–218, 1977.

161. Haltia, M., Prelli, F., Ghiso, J., Kiuru, S., Somer, H., Palo, J., and Frangione, B. Amyloid protein in familial amyloidosis (Finnish type) is homologous to gelsolin, an actin-binding protein. *Biochem. Biophys. Res. Commun. 167*:927–932, 1990.

162. Hamilton, A.M., Garner, A., Tripathi, R.C., and Sanders, M.D. Malignant optic nerve glioma: Report of a case with electron microscope study. *Br. J. Ophthalmol. 57*:253–264, 1973.

163. Hamburg, A. Unusual cause of vitreous opacities: Primary familial amyloidosis. *Ophthalmologica 162*:173–177, 1971.

164. Handousa, A. Localized intra-orbital amyloid disease. *Br. J. Ophthalmol. 38*:510–511, 1954.

165. Harada, T., Kojima, K., Hoshino, M., and Murakami, M. A light and electron microscopic study of heredo-familial corneal dystrophy (Groenouw I). *Acta Soc. Ophthalmol. Jpn. 81*:48–61, 1977.

166. Harding, J., Skare, J., and Skinner, M. A second transthyretin mutation at position 33 leu/phe associated with familial amyloidotic polyneuropathy. *Biochim. Biophys. Acta 1097*:183–186, 1991.

167. Hargrave, P.A., and Fong, S.L. The amino- and carboxyl-terminal sequence of bovine rhodopsin. *J. Supramol. Struct. 6*:559–570, 1977.

168. Hattori, R., Hamilton, K.K., Fugate, R.D., McEver, R.D., and Sims, P.J. Stimulated secretion of endothelial von Willebrand factor is accompanied by rapid redistribution to the cell surface of the intracellular granule membrane protein GMP-140. *J. Biol. Chem. 264*:7768–7771, 1989.

169. Hayasaka, S., Setogawa, T., and Ohmura, M. Secondary localized amyloidosis of the cornea caused by trichiasis. *Ophthalmologica 194*:77–81, 1987.

170. Hayman, E.G., Pierschbacher, M.D., Öhgren, Y., and Ruoslahti, E. Serum spreading factor (vitronectin) is present at the cell surface and in tissues. *Proc. Natl. Acad. Sci. USA 80*:4003–4007, 1983.

171. Heller, H., Missmahl, H.-P., Sohar, E., and Gafni, J. Amyloidosis: Its differentiation into peri-reticulin and peri-collagen types. *J. Pathol. Bacteriol. 88*:15–34, 1964.

172. Henley, W.L., and Kong, S. Antibody to corneal proteins in uveitis. *Pediatr. Res. (Suppl.) 20*:294A, 1986.

173. Herbert, H. Colloid degeneration of the conjunctiva. *Trans. Ophthalmol. Soc. UK 22*:261–266, 1902.

174. Herbert, J., Mizuno, R., and Cavallaro, T. Transthyretin gene expression in the developing rat retinal pigment epithelium (RPE). *Invest. Ophthalmol. Vis. Sci. (Suppl.) 32*:1011, 1991.

175. Herman, S.J., and Hughes, W.F. Recurrence of hereditary corneal dystrophy following keratoplasty. *Am. J. Ophthalmol. 75*:689–693, 1973.

176. Herrenknecht, K., Ozawa, M., Eckerskorn, C., Lottspeich, F., Lenter, M., and Kemler, R. The uvomorulin-anchorage protein α catenin is a vinculin homologue. *Proc. Natl. Acad. Sci. USA 88*:9156–9160, 1991.

177. Hida, T., Proia, A.D., Kigasawa, K., Sanfilippo, F.P., Burchette, J.L., Jr., Akiya, S., and Klintworth, G.K. Histopathologic and immunochemical features of lattice corneal dystrophy type III. *Am. J. Ophthalmol. 104*:249–254, 1987.

178. Hida, T., Tsubota, K., Kigasawa, K., Murata, H., Ogata, T., and Akiya, S. Clinical features of a newly recognized lattice corneal dystrophy. *Am. J. Ophthalmol. 104*:241–248, 1987.

179. Hidayat, A.A., and Riddle, P.J. Ligneous conjunctivitis: A clinicopathologic study of 17 cases. *Ophthalmology 94*:949–959, 1987.

180. Hidayat, A.A., and Risco, J.M. Amyloidosis of the corneal stroma in patients with trachoma: A clinico-pathologic study of 62 cases. *Ophthalmology 8*:1203–1211, 1989.

181. Hill, J.C., Maske, R., and Bowen, R.M. Secondary localized amyloidosis of the cornea associated with tertiary syphilis. *Cornea 9*:98–101, 1990.

182. Hill, J.C., and Mulligan, G.P. Subepithelial corneal deposits in IgG lambda myeloma. *Br. J. Ophthalmol.* 73: 552–554, 1989.

183. Hiltunen, T., Kiuru, S., Hongell, T., Helio, T., Palo, J., and Peltonen, L. Finnish type of familial amyloidosis: Cosegregation of ASP_{187} → ASN mutation of gelsolin with the disease in three large families. *Am. J. Hum. Genet.* 49:522–528, 1991.

184. Hinds, P.W., Mittnacht, S., Dulic, V., Arnold, A., Reed, S.I., and Weinberg, R.A. Regulation of retinoblastoma protein functions by ectopic expression of human cyclins. *Cell* 70:993–1006, 1992.

185. Hinzpeter, E.N., and Naumann, G. Zur sekundären Amyloidose der Hornhaut. *Graefes Arch. Clin. Exp. Ophthalmol.* 192:19–25, 1974.

186. Hitchings, R.A., and Tripathi, R.C. Vitreous opacities in primary amyloid disease: A clinical, histochemical, and ultrastructural report. *Br. J. Ophthalmol.* 60:41–54, 1976.

187. Hogan, M.J., and Alvarado, J. Ultrastructure of lattice dystrophy of the cornea: A case report. *Am. J. Ophthalmol.* 64:656–660, 1967.

188. Hogg, N. The leucocyte integrins. *Immunol. Today* 10:111–114, 1989.

189. Hoisen, H., Ringvold, A., and Kildahl-Anderson, O. Corneal crystalline deposits in multiple myeloma: A case report. *Arch. Ophthalmol. (Copenh.)* 61:493–500, 1983.

190. Holland, E.J., Chan, C.-C., Kuwabara, T., Palestine, A.G., Rowsey, J.J., and Nussenblatt, R.B. Immunologic findings and results of treatment with cyclosporine in ligneous conjunctivitis. *Am. J. Ophthalmol.* 107:160–166, 1989.

191. Holt, J.M., and Gordon-Smith, E.C. Retinal abnormalities in diseases of the blood. *Br. J. Ophthalmol.* 53:145–160, 1969.

192. Horácĕk, J. Kristallinische Augendegeneration als erstes Anzeichen der plasmozytären Myeloms. *Zentralbl. Allg. Pathol. Anat.* 104:264–267, 1963.

193. Howard, G.M. Amyloid tumours of the orbit. *Br. J. Ophthalmol.* 50:421–425, 1966.

194. Howell, D.N., Burchette, J.L., Jr., Paolini, J.F., Geier, S.S., Fuller, J.A., and Sanfillipo, F. Characterization of a novel human corneal endothelial antigen. *Invest. Ophthalmol. Vis. Sci.* 32:2473–2482, 1991.

195. Huang, T.W. Chemical and histochemical studies of human alveolar collagen fibers. *Am. J. Pathol.* 86:81–97, 1977.

196. Hughes, W.F. Discussion of Rodrigues, M.M., and McGavic, J.S. [384a].

197. Husby, G., Araki, S., Benditt, E.P., Benson, M.D., Cohen, A.S., Frangione, B., Glenner, G.G., Nativig, J.B., and Westermark, P. The 1990 guidelines for nomenclature and classification of amyloid and amyloidosis. In *Amyloid and Amyloidosis*, J.B. Natvig, O. Forre, G. Husby, A. Husebekk, B. Skogen, K. Sletten, and P. Westermark (Eds.), Kluwer Academic, Dordrecht, pp. 7–11, 1991.

198. Husby, G., Ranlov, P.J., Sletten, K., and Marhaug, G. Prealbumin nature of the amyloid in familial amyloid cardiomyopathy of Danish origin. In *Amyloidosis*, G.G. Glenner, E.F. Osserman, E.P. Benditt, E. Calkins, A.S. Cohen, and D. Zucker-Franklin (Eds.), Plenum, New York, pp. 391–399, 1986.

199. Hynes, R.O. Integrins: A family of cell surface receptors. *Cell* 48:549–554, 1987.

200. Inglehearn, C.F., Bashir, R., Lester, D.H., Jay, M., Bird, A.C., and Bhattacharya, S.S. A 3-bp deletion in the rhodopsin gene in a family with autosomal dominant retinitis pigmentosa. *Am. J. Hum. Genet.* 48:26–30, 1991.

201. Ingolia, T.D., and Craig, E.A. Four small *Drosophila* heat shock proteins are related to each other and to mammalian α-crystallin. *Proc. Natl. Acad. Sci. USA* 79:2360–2364, 1982.

202. Inuzuka, H., Miyatani, S., and Takeichi, M. R-cadherin: A novel Ca^{2+}-dependent cell-cell adhesion molecule expressed in the retina. *Neuron* 7:69–79, 1991.

203. Isaak, L. Localized amyloidosis cutis associated with psoriasis in siblings. *Arch. Dermatol. Syph.* 61:859–862, 1950.

204. Isersky, C., Ein, D., Page, E.L., Harada, M., and Glenner, G.G. Immunochemical cross-reactions of human amyloid proteins with human immunoglobulin light polypeptide chains. *J. Immunol.* 108:486–493, 1972.

205. Isobe, T., and Osserman, E.F. Patterns of amyloidosis and their association with plasma cell dyscrasia, monoclonal immunoglobulins and Bence-Jones protein. *N. Engl. J. Med.* 290:473–477, 1974.

206. Ito, S., Goshima, K., Niiomi, M., Horikoshi, N., Nomura, S., Sugiura, K., and Yamazaki, K. Electron microscopic studies of the crystalline inclusions in the myeloma cells and kidney of κ-Bence-Jones protein type myeloma. *Acta Haematol. Jpn.* 33:598–617, 1970.

207. Iwaki, A., Iwaki, T., Goldman, J.E., and Liem, R.K.H. Multiple mRNAs of rat brain α-crystallin B chain result from alternative transcriptional initiation. *J. Biol. Chem.* 265:22197–22203, 1990.

208. Iwaki, T., Iwaki, A., Miyazono, M., and Goldman, J.E. Preferential expression of αB-crystallin in astrocytic elements of neuroectodermal tumors. *Cancer* 68:2230–2240, 1991.

209. Iwaki, T., Kume-Iwaki, A., and Goldman, J.E. Cellular distribution of αB-crystallin in non-lenticular tissues. *J. Histochem. Cytochem.* 38:31–39, 1990.

210. Iwaki, T., Kume-Iwaki, A., Liem, R.K.H., and Goldman, J.E. αB-crystallin is expressed in non-lenticular tissues and accumulates in Alexander's disease brain. *Cell* 57:71–78, 1989.

211. Iwaki, T., and Takeishi, J. Immunohistochemical demonstration of αB-crystallin in hamartomas of tuberous sclerosis. *Am. J. Pathol.* 139:1303–1308, 1991.

212. Iwamoto, T., Stuart, J.C., Srinivasan, B.D., Mund, M.L., Farris, R.L., Donn, A., and DeVoe, A.G. Ultrastructural variation in granular dystrophy of the cornea. *Graefes Arch. Clin. Exp. Ophthalmol.* 194:1–9, 1975.

213. Jacobson, D.R., and Buxbaum, J.N. Genetic aspects of amyloidosis. *Adv. Hum. Genet. 20*:69–123, 1991.
214. Janssen, L.A.J., Povey, S., Attwood, J., Sandkuyl, L.A., Lindout, D., Flodman, P., Smith, M., Sampson, J.R., Haines, J.L., Merkens, E.C., Flery, P., Short, P., Amos, J., and Halley, D.J.J. A comparative study on genetic heterogeneity in tuberous sclerosis: Evidence for one gene on 9q34 and a second on 11q22-23: Tuberous sclerosis an allied diseases. *Ann. N.Y. Acad. Sci. 615*:306–315, 1991.
215. Johnson, B.L. Proteinaceous cysts of the ciliary epithelium. II. Their occurrence in non-myelomatous hyper-gammaglobulinemic conditions. *Arch. Ophthalmol. 84*:171–175, 1970.
216. Johnson, B.L., and Storey, J.D. Proteinaceous cysts of the ciliary body. I. Their clear nature and immuno-electrophoretic analysis in a case of multiple myeloma. *Arch. Ophthalmol. 84*:166–170, 1970.
217. Johnson, G.J., and Overall, M. Histology of spheroidal degeneration of the cornea in Labrador. *Br. J. Ophthalmol. 62*:53–61, 1978.
218. Jones, L.A., Skare, J.C., Cohen, A.S., Harding, J.A., Milunsky, A., and Skinner, M. Familial amyloidotic polyneuropathy: A new transthyretin position 30 mutation (alanine for valine) in a family of German descent. *Clin. Genet. 41*:70–73, 1992.
219. Jones, L.A., Skare, J.C., Harding, J.A., Cohen, A.S., Milunsky, A., and Skinner, M. Proline at position 36: A new transthyretin mutation associated with familial amyloidotic polyneuropathy. *Am. J. Hum. Genet. 48*:979–982, 1991.
220. Jones, S.T., and Zimmerman, L.E. Histopathologic differentiation of granular, macular and lattice dystrophies of the cornea. *Am. J. Ophthalmol. 51*:394–410, 1961.
221. Kalderon, A.E., Bogaars, H.A., Diamond, I., Cummings, F.J., Kaplan, S.R., and Calabresi, P. Ultrastructure of myeloma cells in a case with crystal cryoglobulinemia. *Cancer 39*:1475–1481, 1977.
222. Kanai, A., Yamaguchi, T., and Nakajima, A. The histochemical and analytical electron microscopic studies of the corneal granular dystrophy. *Acta Soc. Ophthalmol. Jpn. 81*:145–154, 1977.
223. Kantarjian, A.D., and de Jong, R.N. Familial primary amyloidosis with nervous system involvement. *Neurology 3*:399–409, 1953.
224. Karttunen, T., Alavaikko, M., Apaja-Sarkkinen, M., and Autio-Harmainen, H. An immunohistochemical study of laminin, type IV collagen and type III pN-collagen with relation to reticular fibres in Hodgkin's disease. *Int. J. Cancer 41*:52–58, 1988.
225. Karttunen, T., Sormunen, R., Risteli, L., Risteli, J., and Autio-Harmainen, H. Immunoelectron microscopic localization of laminin, type IV collagen and type III pN-collagen in reticular fibres of human lymph nodes. *J. Histochem. Cytochem. 37*:279–286, 1988.
226. Kasner, D., Miller, G., Taylor, W.H., Sever, R.J., and Norton, W. Surgical treatment of amyloidosis of the vitreous. *Trans. Am. Acad. Ophthalmol. Otolaryngol. 72*:410–421, 1968.
227. Kaufman, H.E. Primary familial amyloidosis. *Arch. Ophthalmol. 60*:1036–1043, 1958.
228. Kaufman, H.E., and Thomas, L.B. Vitreous opacities diagnostic of familial primary amyloidosis. *N. Engl. J. Med. 261*:1267–1271, 1959.
229. Kaunisto, N. Lattice dystrophy of the cornea: Its connection with preceding episodes of crystals and with subsequent amyloidosis. *Acta. Ophthalmol. (Copenh.) 51*:335–352, 1973.
230. Kemler, R., Ozawa, M., and Ringwald, M. Calcium-dependent cell adhesion molecules. *Curr. Opin. Cell Biol. 1*:892–897, 1989.
231. Kirk, H.G., Rabb, M., Hattenhauer, J., and Smith, R. Primary familial amyloidosis of the cornea. *Trans. Am. Acad. Ophthalmol. Otolaryngol. 77*:411–417, 1973.
232. Klaus, E., Freyberger, E., Kavka, G., and Vokcka, F. Familiäres Vorkommen von bulbärparalytischer Form der amyotrophischen Lateralskerose mit gittriger Hornhautdystrophie und Cutis hyperelastica bei drei Schwestern. *Psychiatr. Neurol. Basel 138*:79–97, 1959.
233. Klemen, U.M., Kulnig, W., and Radda, T.M. Secondary corneal amyloidosis: Clinical and pathological examinations. *Graefes Arch. Clin. Exp. Ophthalmol. 220*:130–138, 1983.
234. Klemenz, R., Fröhli, E., Steiger, R.H., Schafer, R., and Aoyama, A. αB-crystallin is a small heat shock protein. *Proc. Natl. Acad. Sci. USA 88*:3652–3656, 1991.
235. Klintworth, G.K. Lattice corneal dystrophy: An inherited variety of amyloidosis restricted to the cornea. *Am. J. Pathol. 50*:371–399, 1967.
236. Klintworth, G.K. Chronic actinic keratopathy: A condition associated with conjunctival elastosis (pingueculae) and typified by characteristic extracellular concretions. *Am. J. Pathol. 67*:327–348, 1972.
237. Klintworth, G.K. The cornea: Structure and macromolecules in health and disease. A review. *Am. J. Pathol. 89*:718–808, 1977.
238. Klintworth, G.K. Corneal dystrophies. In *Ocular Pathology Update*, D.H. Nicholson (Ed.), Masson, New York, pp. 23–54, 1980.
239. Klintworth, G.K., Bredehoeft, S.J., and Reed, J.W. Analysis of corneal crystals in multiple myeloma. *Am. J. Ophthalmol. 86*:303–313, 1978.
240. Klintworth, G.K., Ferry, A.P., Sugar, A., and Reed, J. Recurrence of lattice corneal dystrophy type 1 in the corneal grafts of two siblings. *Am. J. Ophthalmol. 94*:540–546, 1982.
241. Knowles, D.M., Jakobiec, F.A., Rosen, M., and Howard, G. Amyloidosis of the orbit and adnexae. *Surv. Ophthalmol. 19*:367–384, 1975.

242. Kong, S.A., Henley, W.L., and Luntz, M.H. Immunochemical localization of corneal protein BCP 54 in epithelial cells. *Invest. Ophthalmol. Vis. Sci. (Suppl.)* 30:519, 1989.

243. König, B., and Pur, S. Amyloidoza rohovky. *Cesk. Oftal.* 22:187–191, 1966.

244. Konomi, H., Sano, J., and Nagai, Y. Immunohistochemical localization of type I-III and IV (basement membrane) collagens in the lymph node: Codistribution of types I and III collagens in the reticular fibers. *Biomed. Res.* 2:536–545, 1981.

245. Korhonen, M., Ylänne, J., Laitinen, L., Cooper, H.M., Quaranta, V., and Virtanen, I. Distribution of the α1-α6 integrin subunits in human developing and term placenta. *Lab. Invest.* 65:347–356, 1991.

246. Korhonen, M., Ylänne, J., Laitinen, L., and Virtanen, I. Distribution of β_1 and β_2 integrins in human fetal and adult kidney. *Lab. Invest.* 62:616–625, 1990.

247. Kotake, S., Hey, P., Mirmira, R.G., and Copeland, R.A. Physicochemical characterization of bovine retinal arrestin. *Arch. Biochem. Biophys.* 285:126–133, 1991.

248. Krachmer, J.H., Dubord, P.J., Rodrigues, M.M., and Mannis, M.J. Corneal posterior crocodile shagreen and polymorphic amyloid degeneration. *Arch. Ophthalmol.* 101:54–59, 1983.

249. Kremer, I., Wright, P., Merin, S., Weiss, J., Pick, A.I., and Kaufman, H. Corneal subepithelial monoclonal kappa IgG deposits in essential cryoglobulinemia. *Br. J. Ophthalmol.* 73:669–673, 1989.

250. Krieg, T., and Müller, P.K. The Marfan syndrome: In vitro study of collagen metabolism in tissue specimens of the aorta. *Exp. Cell Biol.* 45:207–221, 1977.

251. Kruit, P.J., Broersma, L., van der Gaag, R., and Kijlstra, A. Clinical and experimental studies concerning circulating antibodies to corneal epithelium antigens. *Doc. Ophthalmol.* 64:43–51, 1986.

252. Kruit, P.J., van der Gaag, R., Broersma, L., and Kijlstra, A. Circulating antibodies to corneal epithelium in patients with uveitis. *Br. J. Ophthalmol.* 69:446–448, 1985.

253. Kruit, P.J., van der Gaag, R., Broersma, L., and Kijlstra, A. Autoimmunity against corneal antigens. I. Isolation of a soluble 54/Kd corneal epithelium antigen. *Curr. Eye Res.* 5:313–320, 1986.

254. Kuwahara, Y., Akiya, S., and Obazawa, H. Electron microscopic study of granular dystrophy, macular dystrophy and gelatinous drop-like dystrophy of the cornea. *Folia Ophthalmol. Jpn.* 18:434–435, 1967.

255. Kuwahara, Y., Akiya, S., and Obazawa, H. Electron microscopic study on the stromal lesion in granular dystrophy of the cornea. *Acta Soc. Ophthalmol. Jpn.* 74:1468–1478, 1970.

256. Kwiatkowski, D.J., Stossel, T.P., Orkin, S.H., Mole, J.E., Colten, H.R., and Yin, H.L. Plasma and cytoplasmic gelsolins are encoded by a single gene and contain a duplicated actin-binding domain. *Nature* 323:455–458, 1986.

257. Kyle, R.A. Primary systemic amyloidosis (AL) in 1990. In *Amyloid and Amyloidosis*, J.B. Natvig, O. Forre, G. Husby, A. Husebekk, B. Skogen, K. Sletten, and P. Westermark (Eds.), Kluwer Academic, Dordrecht, pp. 147–152, 1991.

258. Kyle, R.A., and Greipp, P.R. Monoclonal gammopathies of undetermined significance. In *Neoplastic Diseases of the Blood*, Vol. 2, P. H. Wiernik, G.P. Canellos, R.A. Kyle, and C.A. Schiffer (Eds.), Churchill Livingstone, New York, pp. 653–676, 1985.

259. La Hey, E., Baarsma, G.S., Rothova, A., Broersma, L., van der Gaag, R., and Kijlstra, A. High incidence of corneal epithelium antibodies in Fuch's heterochromic cyclitis. *Br. J. Ophthalmol.* 72:921–925, 1988.

260. Laibson, P.R., and Damiano, V.V. X-ray and electron diffraction of ocular and bone marrow crystals in paraproteinemia. *Science* 163:581–583, 1969.

261. Lamberg, S.I., and Dorfman, A. Synthesis and degradation of hyaluronic acid in the cultured fibroblasts of Marfan's disease. *J. Clin. Invest.* 52:2428–2433, 1973.

262. Lambrecht, H.-G., and Koch, K-W. A 26 kd calcium binding protein from bovine rod outer segments as modulator of photoreceptor guanylate cyclase. *EMBO J.* 10:793–798, 1991.

263. Lane, E.B. Monoclonal antibodies provide specific intramolecular markers for the study of epithelial tonofilament organization. *J. Cell Biol.* 92:665–673, 1982.

264. Lane, E.B., Bartek, J., Purkis, P.E., and Leigh, I.M. Keratin antigens in differentiating skin. *Ann. N.Y. Acad. Sci.* 455:241–258, 1985.

265. Lanier, J.D., Fine, M., and Togni, B. Lattice corneal dystrophy. *Arch. Ophthalmol.* 94:921–924, 1976.

266. Lauweryns, B., van den Oord, J.J., Volpes, R., Foets, B., and Missotten, L. Distribution of very late activation integrins in the human cornea. *Invest. Ophthalmol. Vis. Sci.* 32:2079–2085, 1991.

267. Lee, B., Godfrey, M., Vitale, E., Hori, H., Mattei, M.G., Sarfarazi, M., Tsipouras, P., Ramirez, F., and Hollister, D.W. Linkage of Marfan syndrome and a phenotypically related disorder to two different fibrillin genes (see comments). *Nature* 353:330–334, 1991.

268. Legrand, J., Guenel, J., and Dubigeon, P. Glaucome et opacification du vitré par amylose. *Bull. Soc. Ophtalmol. Fr.* 68:13–20, 1968.

269. Lempert, S.L., Jenkins, M.S., Johnson, B.L., and Brown, S.I. A simple technique for removal of recurring granular dystrophy in corneal grafts. *Am. J. Ophthalmol.* 86:89–91, 1978.

270. Lessell, S., Wolf, P.A., Benson, M.D., and Cohen, A.S. Scalloped pupils in familial amyloidosis. *N. Engl. J. Med.* 293:914–915, 1975.

271. Letterer, E. History and development of amyloid research. In *Amyloidosis*, Proceedings of the Symposium on Amyloidosis, University of Groningen, the Netherlands, September 24–28, 1967, E. Mandema, L. Ruinen, J.H. Scholten, and A.S. Cohen (Eds.), Excerpta Medica, Amsterdam, pp. 3–9, 1968.

272. Levy, E., Haltia, M., Fernandz-Madrid, I., Koivunen, O., Ghiso, J., Prelli, F., and Frangione, B. Mutation in gelsolin gene in Finnish hereditary amyloidosis. *J. Exp. Med. 172*:1865–1867, 1990.

273. Levy, E., Lopez-Otin, C., Ghiso, J., Geltner, D., and Frangione, B. Stroke in Icelandic patients with hereditary amyloid angiopathy is related to a mutation in the cystatin C gene, an inhibitor of cysteine proteases. *J. Exp. Med. 169*:1771–1778, 1989.

274. Lewkojewa, E.F. Ueber einen Fall primärer Degenerationamyloidose der Kornea. *Klin. Monatsbl. Augenheilk. 85*:117–137, 1930.

275. Liang, C.J., Yamashita, K., Muellenberg, C.G., Shichi, H., and Kobata, A. Structure of the carbohydrate moieties of bovine rhodopsin. *J. Biol. Chem. 254*:6414–6418, 1979.

276. Liaricos, S., and Streeten, B.W. Ophthalmological findings in primary systemic amyloidosis. *Bull. Greek Ophthalmol. Soc. 42*:152–162, 1974.

277. Lièvre, J.A., Camus, J.P., Lèvy, R., Badin, J., Bessis, M., and Tessier, F. Myéloma a globulin cristallisable: étude physiocochemique et microscopie electronique. *Nouv. Rev. Fr. Hematol. 1*:23–35, 1961.

278. Lightman, M.A. Essential and secondary monoclonal gammopathies. In *Hematology*, 4th. ed., W.J. Williams, E. Beutler, A.J. Erslev, and M.A. Lichtman (Eds.) McGraw-Hill, New York, pp. 1109–1114, 1990.

279. Limon, S., Rousselie, F., and Joseph, E. A propos d'une observation familiale d'amylose vitrénne héréditaire associée à un glaucome. *Arch. Ophtalmol. (Paris) 33*:525–528, 1973.

280. Linquist, S. The heat-shock response. *Annu. Rev. Biochem. 55*:1151–1191, 1986.

281. Loeffler, K.U., Edward, D.P., and Tso, M.O.M. An immunohistochemical study of gelsolin immunoreactivity in corneal amyloidosis. *Am. J. Ophthalmol. 113*:546–554, 1992.

282. Lorenzetti, D.W.C., and Kaufman, H.E. Macular and lattice dystrophies and their recurrence after keratoplasty. *Trans. Am. Acad. Ophthalmol. Otolaryngol. 71*:112–118, 1967.

283. Lowe, J., and Mayer, R.J. Ubiquitin, cell stress and diseases of the nervous system. *Neuropathol. Appl. Neurobiol. 16*:281–291, 1990.

284. Luyendiijk, W., and Bots, G.T.A.M. Hereditary cerebral haemorrhage (letter). *Scand. J. Clin. Lab. Invest. 46*:391, 1986.

285. McClure, J., Bartley, C.J., and Ackrill, P. Carpal tunnel syndrome caused by amyloid containing beta-2-micro-globulin: A new amyloid and a complication of long term haemodialysis. *Ann. Rheum. Dis. 45*:1007–1011, 1986.

286. McCurley, T.L., Gay, R.E., Gay, S., Glick, A.D., Haralson, M.A., and Collins, R.D. The extracellular protein in "sclerosing" follicular center cell lymphomas. *Hum. Pathol. 17*:930–938, 1986.

287. McGrand, J.C., Rees, D.M., and Harry, J. Ligneous conjunctivitis. *Br. J. Ophthalmol. 53*:373–381, 1969.

288. McKay, K., Striker, L., D'Amico, G., and Striker, G. Dysproteinemias and paraproteinemias. In *Renal Pathology*, C.C. Tisher and B.M. Brenner (Eds.), J.B. Lippincott, Philadelphia, pp. 1363–1416, 1989.

289. McKusick, V.A. *Heritable Disorders of Connective Tissue*, 4th ed., C.V. Mosby, St. Louis, MO, 1972.

290. McKusick, V.A. *Mendelian Inheritance in Man. Catalogs of Autosomal Dominant, Autosomal Recessive and X-linked Phenotypes*, 10th ed., Johns Hopkins University Press, Baltimore, 1992.

291. McPherson, S.D., Jr., and Kiffney, G.T., Jr. Some histologic findings in keratoconus. *Arch. Ophthalmol. 79*:669–673, 1968.

292. McPherson, S.D., Jr., Kiffney, G.T., Jr., and Freed, C.C. Corneal amyloidosis. *Trans. Am. Ophthalmol. Soc. 64*:148–162, 1966. Also in *Am. J. Ophthalmol. 62*:1024–1033, 1966.

293. McTigue, J.W. The electron microscope in corneal dystrophy. In *The Cornea, World Congress*, J.H. King and J.W. McTigue (Eds.), Butterworth, Washington, pp. 49–60, 1965.

294. McTigue, J.W. The human cornea: A light and electron microscopic study of the normal cornea and its alterations in various dystrophies. *Trans. Am. Ophthalmol. Soc. 65*:591–660, 1967.

295. McTigue, J.W., and Fine, B.S. The stromal lesion in lattice dystrophy of the cornea. *Invest. Ophthalmol. 3*:355–365, 1964.

296. McWilliam, P., Farrar, G.J., Kenna, P., Bradley, D.G., Humphries, M.M., Sharp, E.M., McDonnell, D.J., Lawler, M., Sheils, D., Ryan, C., Stevens, K., Daiger, S.P., and Humphries, P. Autosomal dominant retinitis pigmentosa (ADRP): Localization of an ADRP gene to the long arm of chromosome 3. *Genomics 5*:619–622, 1989.

297. Mahloudji, M., Teasdall, R.D., Adamkiewicz, J.J., Hartmann, W.H., Lambird, P.A., and McKusick, V.A. The genetic amyloidoses with particular reference to hereditary neuropathic amyloidosis, type II (Indiana or Rukavina type). *Medicine (Baltimore) 48*:1–37, 1969.

298. Maisel, H., and Atreya, P. N-cadherin detected in the membrane fraction of lens fiber cells. *Experientia 46*:222–223, 1990.

299. Mannis, M.J., Krachmer, J.H., Rodrigues, M.M., and Pardos, G.J. Polymorphic amyloid degeneration of the cornea. *Arch. Ophthalmol. 99*:1217–1223, 1981.

300. Matalon, R., and Dorfman, A. The accumulation of hyaluronic acid in cultured fibroblasts of the Marfan syndrome. *Biochem. Biophys. Res. Commun. 32*:150–154, 1968.

301. Matsui, M., Ito, K., and Akiya, S. Histochemical and electron microscopic examinations and so-called "gelatinous drop-like dystrophy of the cornea." *Folia Ophthalmol. Jpn. 23*:466–473, 1973.

302. Matsunaga, M., Hatta, K., and Takeichi, M. Role of N-cadherin cell adhesion molecules in the histogenesis of neural retina. *Neuron 1*:289–295, 1988.

303. Matsuo, N., Fujiwara, H., and Ofuchi, Y. Electron and light microscopic observations of a case of Groenouw's nodular corneal dystrophy. *Folia Ophthalmol. Jpn.* 18:436–447, 1967.
304. Matta, C.S., Tabbara, K.F., Cameron, J.A., Hidayat, A.A., and Al-Rajhi, A.A. Climatic droplet keratopathy with corneal amyloidosis. *Ophthalmology* 98:192–195, 1991.
305. Maury, C.P.J. Isolation and characterization of cardiac amyloid in familial amyloid polyneuropathy type IV (Finnish): Relation of amyloid protein to variant gelsolin. *Biochim. Biophys. Acta* 1096:84–86, 1990.
306. Maury, C.P.J., Alli, K., and Baumann, M. Finnish hereditary amyloidosis: Amino acid sequence homology between the amyloid fibril protein and human plasma gelsoline. *FEBS Lett.* 260:85–87, 1990.
307. Maury, C.P.J., Alli, K., and Baumann, M. Complete primary structure of amyloid protein in Finnish hereditary amyloidosis. Identification of a new type of amyloid protein derived from variant (Asn-187) gelsolin. In *Amyloid and Amyloidosis*, J.B. Natvig, O. Forre, G. Husby, A. Husebekk, B. Skogen, K. Sletten, and P. Westermark (Eds.), Kluwer Academic, Dordrecht, pp. 405–408, 1991.
308. Maury, C.P.J., Kere, J., Tolvanen, R., and de la Chapelle, A. Finnish hereditary amyloidosis is caused by a single nucleotide substitution in the gelsolin gene. *FEBS Lett.* 276:75–77, 1990.
309. Meesmann, A. Über eine eigenartige Hornhaut degeneration. (Ablagerung der Bence-Jonesschen Einweiss-korper in der Hornhaut). *Ber. Dtsch. Ophthalmol.* 50:311–315, 1934.
310. Meretoja, J. Familial systemic paramyloidosis with lattice dystrophy of the cornea, progressive cranial neuropathy, skin changes and various internal symptoms. I. A previously unrecognized heritable syndrome. *Ann. Clin. Res.* 1:314–324, 1969.
311. Meretoja, J. Comparative histopathological and clinical findings in eyes with lattice corneal dystrophy of two different types. *Ophthalmologica* 165:15–37, 1972.
312. Meretoja, J. Genetic aspects of familial amyloidosis with corneal lattice dystrophy and cranial neuropathy. *Clin. Genet.* 4:173–185, 1973.
313. Meretoja, J., and Teppo, L. Histopathological findings of familial amyloidosis with cranial neuropathy as principal manifestation. *Acta Pathol. Microbiol. Scand. (A)* 79:432–440, 1971.
314. Meyer, R.K., McKinley, M.P., Bowman, K.A., Braunfeld, M.B., Barry, R.A., and Prusiner, S.B. Separation and properties of cellular and scrapie proteins. *Proc. Natl. Acad. Sci. USA* 83:2310–2314, 1986.
315. Miller, K.H., Green, W.R., Stark, W.J., Wells, H.A., Mendelsohn, G., and Kanhofer, H. Immunoprotein deposition in the cornea. *Ophthalmology* 87:944–950, 1980.
316. Moll, R., Franke, W.W., Schiller, D.L., Greiger, B., Krepler, R. The catalog of human cytokeratins: Patterns of expression in normal epithelia, tumors and cultured cells. *Cell* 31:11–24, 1982.
317. Møller, H.U. Inter-familial variability and intrafamilial similarities of granular corneal dystrophy Groenouw type I with respect to biomicroscopical appearance and symptomatology. *Acta Ophthalmol. (Copenh.)* 67:669–677, 1989.
318. Møller, H.U. Granular corneal dystrophy Groenouw type I (GrI) and Reis-Bücklers' corneal dystrophy (R-B): One entity? *Acta Ophthalmol. (Copenh.)* 67:678–684, 1989.
319. Møller, H.U. Granular corneal dystrophy Groenouw type I. 115 Danish patients: An epidemiological and genetic population study. *Acta Ophthalmol. (Copenh.)* 68:297–303, 1990.
320. Møller, H.U. Granular corneal dystrophy Groenouw type I: Clinical aspects and treatment. *Acta Ophthalmol. (Copenh.)* 68:384–389, 1990.
321. Møller, H.U., Eiberg, H., and Kruse, T.A. Linkage relations of the locus for granular corneal dystrophy Groenouw type I with 35 polymorphic systems. *Acta Ophthalmol. (Copenh.)* 67:721–723, 1989.
322. Møller, H.U., and Ridgway, A.E. Granular corneal dystrophy Groenouw type I: A report of a probable homozygous patient. *Acta Ophthalmol. (Copenh.)* 68:97–101, 1990.
323. Moncla, A., Landon, F., Mattei, M.G., and Portier, M.M. Chromosomal localisation of the mouse and human peripherin genes. *Genet. Res.* 59:125–129, 1992.
324. Mondino, B.J., Rabb, M.F., Sugar, J., Sundar Raj, C.V., and Brown, S.I. Primary familial amyloidosis of the cornea. *Am. J. Ophthalmol.* 92:732–736, 1981.
325. Mondino, B.J., Sundar Raj, C.V., Skinner, M., Cohen, A.S., and Brown, S.I. Protein AA and lattice corneal dystrophy. *Am. J. Ophthalmol.* 89:377–380, 1980.
326. Motokura, T., Bloom, T., Kim, H.G., Juppner, H., Ruderman, J.V., Kronenberg, H.M., and Arnold, A. A novel cyclin encided by a bcl1-linked candidate oncogene (see comments). *Nature* 350:512–515, 1991.
327. Nagafuchi, A., Takeichi, M., and Tsukita, S. The 102 kd cadherin-associated protein: Similarity to vinculin and posttranscriptional regulation of expression. *Cell* 65:849–857, 1991.
328. Nagataki, S., Tanishima, T., and Sakimoto, T. A case of primary gelatinous drop-like corneal dystrophy. *Jpn. J. Ophthalmol.* 16:107–116, 1972.
329. Nakazato, M., Kangawa, K., Minamino, N., Tawara, S., Matsuo, H., and Araki, S. Revised analysis of amino acid replacement in a prealbumin variant (SKO-III) associated with familial amyloidotic polyneuropathy of Jewish origin. *Biochem. Biophys. Res. Commun.* 123:921–928, 1984.
330. Nathans, J., Piantanida, T.P., Eddy, R.L., Shows, T.B., and Hogness, D.S. Molecular genetics of inherited variation in human color vision. *Science* 232:203–210, 1986.
331. Ngo, J.T., Klisak, I., Dubin, R.A., Piatigorsky, J., Mohandas, T., Sparkes, R.S., and Bateman, J.B. Assignment of the αB-crystallin gene to human chromosome 11. *Genomics* 5:665–669, 1989.

332. Nichols, W.C., Dwulet, F.E., Liepnieks, J., and Benson, M.D. Variant apolipoprotein A1 as a major constituent of a human hereditary amyloid. *Biochem. Biophys. Res. Commun. 156*:762–768, 1988.

333. Nichols, W.C., Liepnieks, J.J., McKusick, V.A., and Benson, M.D. Direct sequencing of the gene for Maryland/German familial amyloidotic polyneuropathy type II and genotyping by allele-specific enzymatic amplification. *Genomics 5*:535–540, 1989.

334. Nik, N.A., Martin, W.F., and Berler, D.K. Corneal crystalline deposits and drusenosis associated with IgA-kappa chain monoclonal gammopathy. *Ann. Ophthalmol. 17*:303–307, 1985.

335. Nordlie, M., Sletten, K., Husby, G., and Ranløv, P.J. A new prealbumin variant in familial amyloid cardio-myopathy of Danish origin. *Scand. J. Immunol. 27*:119–122, 1988.

336. Offret, G., Pouliquen, Y., and Coscas, G. Une dystrophie cornéenne familiale: Étude clinique, histologique et ultrastructurale. *Arch. Ophtalmol. (Paris) 29*:537–550, 1969.

337. Oglesby, R.B. Corneal opacities in a patient with cryoglobulinemia and reticulohistiocytosis. *Arch. Ophthalmol. 65*:63–66, 1961.

338. Ohnishi, Y., Shinoda, Y., Ishibashi, T., and Taniguchi, Y. The origin of amyloid in gelatinous drop-like corneal dystrophy. *Curr. Eye Res. 2*:225–231, 1982.

339. Orcutt, J.C., Reeh, M.J., Gown, A.M., and Lindquist, T.D. Diagnosis of orbital and periorbital tumors: Use of monoclonal antibodies to cytoplasmic antigens (intermediate filaments). *Ophthal. Plast. Reconstruct. Surg. 3*:159–178, 1987.

340. Ormerod, L.D., Collin, H.B., Dohlman, C.H., Craft, J.L., Desforges, J.F., and Albert, D.M. Paraproteinemic crystalline keratopathy. *Ophthalmology 95*:202–212, 1988.

341. Osborn, L. Leucocyte adhesion to endothelium in inflammation. *Cell 62*:3–6, 1990.

342. Osborn, M., Altmannsberger, M., Debus, E., and Weber, K. Differentiation of the major human tumor groups using conventional and monoclonal antibodies specific for individual intermediate filament proteins. *Ann. N.Y. Acad. Sci. 455*:649–668, 1985.

343. Osserman, E.F. Analysis of amyloid-related Bence-Jones proteins (TEW BJκ and MCG BJλ) and the "non-immunoglobulin" amyloid protein AA: Hypervariable region homologies and their possible significance. In *Amyloidosis*, Proceedings of the Fifth Sigrid Jusélius Foundation Symposium, O. Wegelius and A. Pasternack (Eds.), Academic Press, New York, pp. 223–231, 1976.

344. Ozaki, M. Familial lichen amyloidosis. *Int. J. Dermatol. 23*:190–193, 1984.

345. Ozawa, M., Baribault, H., and Kemler, R. The cytoplasmic domain of the cell adhesion molecule in uvomorulin associates with three independent proteins structurally related to different species. *EMBO J. 8*:1711–1717, 1989.

346. Ozawa, M., Ringwald, M., and Kemler, R. Uvomorulin-catenin complex formation is regulated by a specific domain in the cytoplasmic region of the cell adhesion molecule. *Proc. Natl. Acad. Sci. USA 87*:4246–4250, 1990.

347. Palm, E. A case of crystal deposits in the cornea: Precipitation of a spontaneously crystallizing plasma globulin. *Acta Ophthalmol. (Copenh.) 25*:165–174, 1947.

348. Papermaster, D.S., Brustein, Y., and Schecter, I. Opsin mRNA isolation from bovine retina and partial sequence of the in vitro translation product. *Ann. N.Y. Acad. Sci. 343*:347–355, 1980.

349. Papermaster, D.S., Converse, C.A., and Siu, J. Membrane biosynthesis in the frog retina: Opsin transport in the photoreceptor cell. *Biochemistry 14*:1343–1352, 1975.

350. Papermaster, D.S., Converse, C.A., and Zorn, M. Biosynthetic and immunochemical characterization of a large protein in frog and cattle rod outer segment membranes. *Exp. Eye Res. 23*:105–115, 1976.

351. Papermaster, D.S., Schneider, B.G., Zorn, M.A., and Kraehenbuhl, J.P. Immunocytochemical localization of opsin in outer segments and Golgi zones of frog photoreceptor cells: An electron microscope analysis of cross-linked albumin-embedded retinas. *J. Cell Biol. 77*:196–210, 1978.

352. Papermaster, D.S., Schneider, B.G., Zorn, M.A., and Kraeherbuhl, J.P. Immunocytochemical localization of a large intrinsic membrane protein to the incisures and margins of frog rod outer segment disks. *J. Cell Biol. 78*:415–425, 1978.

353. Partington, M.W., Marriott, P.J., Prentice, R.S.A., Cavaglia, A., and Simpson, N.E. Familial cutaneous amyloidosis with systemic manifestations in males. *Am. J. Med. Genet. 10*:65–75, 1981.

354. Paton, D., and Duke, J.R. Primary familial amyloidosis: Ocular manifestations with histopathologic observations. *Am. J. Ophthalmol. 61*:736–747, 1966.

355. Pearse, A.G.E., Ewen, S.W.B., and Polak, J.M. The genesis of apudamyloid in endocrine polypeptide tumours: Histochemical distinction from immunoamyloid. *Virchows Arch. [B] 10*:93–107, 1972.

356. Pérez-Tamayo, R., and Rojkind, M. (Eds.). *Molecular Pathology of Connective Tissues*, Marcel Dekker, New York, 1973.

357. Perry, H.D., Fine, B.S., and Caldwell, D.R. Reis-Bücklers dystrophy: A study of eight cases. *Arch. Ophthalmol. 97*:664–670, 1979.

358. Peterson, P.A., Cunningham, B.A., Berggård, I., and Edelman, G.M. β$_2$-Microglobulin-a free immunoglobulin domain. *Proc. Natl. Acad. Sci. USA 69*:1697–1701, 1972.

359. Pinkerton, R.M.H., and Robertson, D.M. Corneal and conjunctival changes in dysproteinemia. *Invest. Ophthalmol. 8*:357–364, 1969.

360. Pober, J.S., and Cotran, R.S. What can be learned from the expression of endothelial adhesion molecules in tissues (editorial)? *Lab. Invest. 64*:301–305, 1991.

361. Pober, J.S., Gimbrone, M.A., Lapierre, L.A., Mendrick, D.L., Fiers, W., Rothlein, R., and Springer, T.A. Overlapping patterns of activation of human endothelial cells by interleukin-1, tumor necrosis factor and immune interferon. *J. Immunol. 137*:1893–1896, 1986.

362. Polans, A.S., Buczylko, J., Crabb, J., and Palczewski, K. A photoreceptor calcium binding protein is recognized by autoantibodies obtained from patients with cancer-associated retinopathy. *J. Cell Biol. 112*:981–989, 1991.

363. Pope, F.M. Autosomal dominant pseudoxanthoma elasticum. *J. Med. Genet. 11*:152–157, 1974.

364. Pope, F.M. Historical evidence for the genetic heterogeneity of pseudoxanthoma elasticum. *Br. J. Dermatol. 92*:493–509, 1975.

365. Pouliquen, Y., Dhermy, P., and Taillebourg, O. Étude au microscope électronique d'une dystrophie grillagée Haab-Dimmer. *Arch. Ophtalmol. (Paris) 33*:485–500, 1973.

366. Povey, S., Attwood, J., Janssen, L.A.J., Burley, M., Smith, M., Flodman, P., Morton, N.E., Edwards, J.H., Sampson, J.R., Yates, J.R.W., Haines, J.L., Amos, J., Short, M.P., Sandkuyl, L.A., Halley, D.J.J., Fryer, A.E., Bech-Hansen, T., Mueller, R., Al-Ghazali, L., Super, M., and Osborne, J. An attempt to map two genes for tuberous sclerosis using novel two-point methods: Tuberous sclerosis and allied diseases. *Ann. N.Y. Acad. Sci. 615*:298–305, 1991.

367. Pras, M., Prelli, F., Franklin, E.C., and Frangione, B. Primary structure of an amyloid prealbumin variant in familial polyneuropathy of Jewish origin. *Proc. Natl. Acad. Sci. USA 80*:539–542, 1983.

368. Priest, R.E., Moinuddin, J.F., and Priest, J.H. Collagen of Marfan syndrome is abnormally soluble. *Nature 245*:264–266, 1973.

369. Purcell, J.J., Jr., Rodrigues, M.M., Chishti, M.I., Riner, A.N., and Dooley, J.M. Lattice corneal dystrophy associated with familial systemic amyloidosis (Meretoja's syndrome). *Ophthalmology 90*:1512–1517, 1983.

370. Pyreritz, R.E., and McKusick, V.A. The Marfan syndrome: Diagnosis and management. *N. Engl. J. Med. 300*:772–777, 1979.

371. Pytela, R., Pierschbacher, M.D., and Ruoslahti, E. A 125/115-kDa cell surface receptor specific for vitronectin interacts with the arginine-glycine-aspartic acid adhesion sequence derived from fibronectin. *Proc. Natl. Acad. Sci. USA 82*:5766–5770, 1985.

372. Rabb, M.F., Blodi, F., and Bonuik, M. Unilateral lattice dystrophy of the cornea. *Trans. Am. Acad. Ophthalmol. Otolaryngol. 78*:440–444, 1974.

373. Raflo, G.T., Farrell, T.A., and Siossat, R.S. Complete ophthalmoplegia secondary to amyloidosis associated with multiple myeloma. *Am. J. Ophthalmol. 92*:221–224, 1981.

374. Ramsey, M.S., Fine, B.S., and Cohen, S.W. Localized corneal amyloidosis: Case report with electron microscopic observations. *Am. J. Ophthalmol. 73*:560–565, 1972.

375. Ramsey, R.M. Familial corneal dystrophy-lattice type. *Trans. Am. Ophthalmol. Soc. 65*:701–739, 1957.

376. Randall, R.E., Williamson, W.C., Mullinax, F., Tung, M.Y., and Still, W.J. Manifestations of systemic light chain deposition. *Am. J. Med. 60*:293–299, 1976.

377. Ratnaker, K.S., and Mohan, M. Amyloidosis of the iris. *Can. J. Ophthalmol. 11*:256–257, 1976.

378. Reeck, G.R., and Fisher, L. A statistical analysis of the amino acid compositions of proteins. *Int. J. Peptide Protein Res. 5*:109–117, 1973.

379. Reinhart, L.A., Rountree, C.B., and Wilkin, J.K. Buschke-Ollendorff syndrome. *Cutis 31*:94–96, 1983.

380. Ren, Z.X., Brewton, R.G., and Mayne, R. An analysis by rotary shadowing of the structure of the mammalian vitreous and zonular apparatus. *J. Ultrastruct. Biol. 106*:57–63, 1991.

381. Ringvold, A., and Husby, G. Pseudoexfoliation material: An amyloid-like substance. *Exp. Eye Res. 17*:289–299, 1973.

382. Rodrigues, M., Ben-Zvi, A., Krachmer, J., Schermer, A., and Sun, T.T. Suprabasal expression of a 64-kilodalton keratin (no. 3) in developing human corneal epithelium. *Differentiation 34*:60–67, 1987.

383. Rodrigues, M.M., Krachmer, J.H., Miller, S.D., and Newsome, D.A. Posterior corneal crystalline deposits in benign monoclonal gammopathy: A clinicopathologic case report. *Arch. Ophthalmol. 97*:124–128, 1979.

384. Rodrigues, M.M., Laibson, P.R., and Weinreb, S. Corneal elastosis: Appearance of band-like keratopathy and spheroidal degeneration. *Arch. Ophthalmol. 93*:111–114, 1975.

384a. Rodrigues, M.M., and McGavic, J.S. Recurrent corneal granular dystrophy: A clincopathologic study. *Trans. Am. Ophthalmol. Soc. 73*:306–316, 1975.

385. Rodrigues, M.M., Streeten, B.W., Krachmer, J.H., Laibson, P.R., Salem, N., Jr., Passonneau, J., and Chock, S. Microfibrillar protein and phospholipid in granular corneal dystrophy. *Arch. Ophthalmol. 101*:802–810, 1983.

386. Rodrigues, M., and Zimmerman, L.E. Secondary amyloidosis in ocular leprosy. *Arch. Ophthalmol. 85*:277–279, 1971.

387. Rokitansky, K. *Handbuch der Pathologischen Anatomie*, Vol. 3, Bramüller und Seidel, Vienna, pp. 311–312, 1842–1846.

388. Rosenbloom, J. Elastin: Relation of protein and gene structure to disease. *Lab. Invest. 51*:605–623, 1984.

389. Ross, R., and Bornstein, P. The elastic fiber. I. The separation and partial characterization of its macromolecular components. *J. Cell Biol. 40*:366–381, 1969.

390. Ross, R., and Bornstein, P. Studies of the components of the elastic fiber. In *Chemistry and Molecular Biology of Intercellular Matrix*, Vol. 1, E.A. Balazs (Ed.), Academic Press, New York, pp. 641–655, 1970.

391. Rukavina, J.G., Block, W.D., Jackson, C.E., Falls, H.F., Carey, J.H., and Curtis, A.C. Primary systemic amyloidosis: A review and an experimental, genetic and clinical study of 29 cases with particular emphasis on the familial form. *Medicine (Baltimore) 35*:239–334, 1956.

392. Ruoslahti, E. Structure and biology of proteoglycans. *Annu. Rev. Cell Biol. 4*:229–255, 1988.

393. Ruoslahti, E., and Pierschbacher, M.D. New perspectives in cell adhesion: RGD and integrins. *Science 238*:491–497, 1987.

394. Sack, G.H., Jr., Dumars, K.W., Gummerson, K.S., Law, A., and McKusick, V.A. Three forms of dominant amyloid neuropathy. *Johns Hopkins Med. J. 149*:239–247, 1981.

395. Sack, R.A., Tan, K.O., and Tan, A. Diurnal tear cycle: Evidence for a nocturnal inflammatory constitutive tear fluid. *Invest. Ophthalmol. Vis. Sci. 33*:626–640, 1992.

396. Sagher, F., and Shanon, J. Amyloidosis cutis: Familial occurrence in three generations. *Arch. Dermatol. 87*:171–175, 1963.

397. Salvi, G., Salvi, F., Volpe, R., Mencucci, R., Plasmati, R., Michelucci, R., Gobbi, P., Santangelo, M., Ferlini, A., Forabosco, A., and Tassinari, C.A. Transthyretin-related (TTR) hereditary amyloidosis of the vitreous body. Clinical and molecular characterization in two Italian families. *Ophthalmic Paediatrics and Genetics 14*:9–16, 1993.

398. Sandberg, L.B., Hackett, T.N., Jr., and Carnes, W.H. The solubilization of an elastin-like protein from copper deficient procine aorta. *Biochim. Biophys. Acta 181*:201–207, 1969.

399. Sanberg, L.B., Weissman, N., and Smith, D.W. The purification and partial characterization of a soluble elastin-like protein from copper deficient porcine aorta. *Biochemistry 8*:2940–2945, 1969.

400. Sanders, T.E., and Podos, S. Pars plana cysts in multiple myeloma. *Trans. Am. Acad. Ophthalmol. Otolaryngol. 70*:951–958, 1966.

401. Sanders, T.E., Podos, S.M., and Rosenbaum, L.J. Intraocular manifestations of multiple myeloma. *Arch. Ophthalmol. 77*:789–794, 1967.

402. Sandgren, O., Holmgren, G., and Lundgren, E. Vitreous amyloidosis associated with homozygosity for the transthyretin methionine-30 gene. *Arch. Ophthalmol. 108*:1584–1586, 1990.

403. Sandgren, O., Holmgren, G., Lundgren, E., and Steen, L. Restriction fragment length polymorphism analysis of mutated transthyretin in vitreous amyloidosis. *Arch. Ophthalmol. 106*:790–792, 1988.

404. Sandgren, O., Westermark, P., and Stenkula, S. Relation of vitreous amyloidosis to prealbumin. *Ophthalmic Res. 18*:98–103, 1986.

405. Saraiva, M.J.M., Costa, P.P., and Goodman, D.S. Biochemical marker in familial amyloidotic polyneuropathy, Portuguese type: Family studies on the transthyretin (prealbumin)-methionine-30 variant. *J. Clin. Invest. 76*:2171–2177, 1985.

406. Savage, D.J., Mango, C.A., and Streeten, B.W. Amyloidosis of the vitreous: Fluorescein angiographic findings and association with neovascularization. *Arch. Ophthalmol. 100*:1776–1779, 1982.

407. Savino, P.J., Schatz, N.J., and Rodrigues, M.M. Orbital amyloidosis. *Can. J. Ophthalmol. 11*:252–255, 1976.

408. Schesinger, M.J. Heat shock proteins: The search for function. *J. Cell Biol. 103*:321–325, 1986.

409. Schneider, R.G. Incidence of hemoglobin C trait in 505 normal negroes: A family with homozygous hemoglobin C and sickle-cell trait union. *J. Lab. Clin. Med. 44*:133–144, 1954.

410. Schürch, W., Skalli, O., Lagace, R., Seemayer, T.A., and Gabbiani, G. Intermediate filament proteins and actin isoforms as markers for soft tissue tumor differentiation and origin. III. Hemangiopericytomas and glomus tumors. *Am. J. Pathol. 136*:771–786, 1990.

411. Schürch, W., Skalli, O., Seemayer, T.A., and Gabbiani, G. Intermediate filament proteins and actin isoforms as markers for soft tissue tumor differentiation and origin. I. Smooth muscle tumors. *Am. J. Pathol. 128*:91–103, 1987.

412. Schwartz, M.F., Green, W.R., Michels, R.G., Kincaid, M.C., and Fogel, J. An unusual case of ocular involvement in primary systemic nonfamilial amyloidosis. *Ophthalmology 89*:394–401, 1982.

413. Seitelberger, F., and Nemetz, U.R. Beitrag zur Frage der gittrigen Hornhaut-dystrophie. *Graefes Arch. Ophthalmol. 164*:102–111, 1961.

414. Seitz, R., and Goslar, H.G. Über das Verhalten von transplantiertem Hornhautgewebe im Empfängerauge: Ein klinischer, morphologischer und histochemischer Beitrag. *Klin. Monatsbl. Augenheilk. 142*:943–969, 1963.

415. Seitz, R., and Goslar, H.G. Beitrag zur Kinik, Morphologie und Histochemie der verschiedenen Formen von Hornhautdystrophie. *Klin. Monatsbl. Augenheilk. 147*:673–691, 1965.

416. Selsted, M.E., and Martinez, R.J. Isolation and purification of bactericides from human tears. *Exp. Eye Res. 34*:305–318, 1982.

417. Siegal, R.C., and Chang, T.H. Defective α_2 chain synthesis in patients with sporadic Marfan syndrome. *Clin. Res. 26*:501A, 1978.

418. Silverman, B., Alexander, R.J., and Henley, W.L. Tissue and species specity of BCP 54, the major soluble protein of the bovine cornea. *Exp. Eye Res. 33*:19–29, 1981.

419. Singh, V.K., Nussenblatt, R.B., Donoso, L.A., Yamaki, K., Chan, C.C., and Shinohara, T. Identification of a uveitopathogenic and lymphocyte proliferation site in bovine S-antigen. *Cell. Immunol. 115*:413–419, 1988.

420. Singh, V.K., Yamaki, K., Donoso, L.A., and Shinohara, T. S-antigen: Experimental autoimmune uveitis induced in guinea pigs with two synthetic peptides. *Curr. Eye Res.* 7:87–92, 1988.

421. Skare, J.C., Milunsky, J.M., Milunsky, A., Skare, I.B., Cohen, A.S., and Skinner, M. A new transthyretin variant from a patient with familial amyloidotic polyneuropathy has asparagine substituted for histidine at position 90. *Clin. Genet.* 39:6–12, 1991.

422. Skare, J.C., Yazici, H., Erken, E., Dede, H., Cohen, A., Milunsky, A., and Skinner, M. Homozygosity for the met30 transthyretin gene in a Turkish kindred with familial amyloidotic polyneuropathy. *Hum. Genet.* 86:89–90, 1990.

423. Skinner, M., Benson, M.D., and Cohen, A.S. Amyloid fibril protein related to immunoglobulin λ-chains. *J. Immunol.* 114:1433–1435, 1975.

424. Skinner, M., Cohen, A.S., and Benson, M.D. Serum amyloid p-component (SAP) levels in normals, amyloidotic patients and in malignancy. *Fed. Proc.* 37:753, 1978.

425. Skinner, M., Cohen, A.S., Shirahama, T., and Cathcart, E.S. P-component (pentagonal unit) of amyloid: Isolation, characterization and sequence analysis. *J. Lab. Clin. Med.* 84:604–614, 1974.

426. Skinner, M., Harding, J., Skare, J., Jones, L.A., Cohen, A.S., Milunsky, A., and Skare, J. A new transthyretin mutation associated with amyloidotic vitreous opacities: Asparagine for isoleucine at position 84. *Ophthalmology* 99:503–508, 1992.

427. Slansky, H.H., Brownstein, M., and Gartner, S. Ciliary body cysts in multiple myeloma: Their relation to urethane, hyperproteinemia, and duration of the disease. *Arch. Ophthalmol.* 76:686–689, 1966.

428. Smith, M., Smalley, S., Cantor, R., Pandolfo, M., Gomez, M.I., Baumann, R., Yoshiyama, K., Nakamura, Y., Julier, C., Dumars, K., Haines, J., Trofatter, M., Spence, A., Weeks, D., and Conneally, M. Mapping of a gene determining tuberous sclerosis to human chromosome 11q14-q23. *Genomics* 6:105–114, 1990.

429. Smith, M., Yoshiyama, K., Wagner, C., Flodman, P., and Smith, B. Genetic heterogeneity in tuberous sclerosis. Map position of the TSC2 locus on chromosome 11q and future prospects. Tuberous sclerosis and allied diseases. *Ann. N.Y. Acad. Sci.* 615:274–283, 1991.

430. Smith, M.E., and Zimmerman, L.E. Amyloidosis of the eyelid and conjunctiva. *Arch. Ophthalmol.* 75:42–50, 1966.

431. Smith, M.E., and Zimmerman, L.E. Amyloid in corneal dystrophies: Differentiation of lattice from granular and macular dystrophies. *Arch. Ophthalmol.* 79:407–412, 1968.

432. Solomon, A., and Weiss, D.T. Experimental production of human amyloidosis AL. In *Amyloid and Amyloidosis*, J.B. Natvig, O. Forre, G. Husby, A. Husebekk, B. Skogen, K. Sletten, and P. Westermark (Eds.), Kluwer Academic, Dordrecht, pp. 193–196, 1991.

433. Sornson, E.T. Granular dystrophy of the cornea: An electron microscopic study. *Am. J. Ophthalmol.* 59:1001–1007, 1965.

434. de Souza Queiroz, L., and Brick, M. Degeneração reticular familial da cornea apresentaçãe de 10 casos e etudo histopathologico. *Arg. Inst. Penido Burnier, Sao Paulo* 18:94–106, 1961.

435. Spark, E.C., Shirahama, T., Skinner, M., and Cohen, A.S. Identification of amyloid p-component (protein AP) in normal cultured human fibroblasts. *Lab. Invest.* 38:556–559, 1978.

436. Sparkes, R.S., Sasaki, H., Mohandas, T., Yoshioka, K., Klisak, I., Sakaki, Y., Heinzmann, C., and Simon, M.I. Assignment of the prealbumin (PALB) gene (familial amyloidotic polyneuropathy) to human chromosome region 18q11.2-q12.1. *Hum. Genet.* 75:151–154, 1987.

437. Spiegel, P., Grossniklaus, H.E., Reinhart, W.J., and Thomas, R.H. Unusual presentation of paraproteinemic corneal infiltrates. *Cornea* 9:81–85, 1990.

438. Springer, T.A. Adhesion receptors of the immune system. *Nature* 346:425–433, 1990.

439. Stafford, W.R., and Fine, B.S. Amyloidosis of the cornea: Report of a case without conjunctival involvement. *Arch. Ophthalmol.* 75:53–56, 1966.

440. Stansbury, F.C. Lattice type of hereditary corneal degeneration: Report of five cases, including one of a child of two years. *Arch. Ophthalmol.* 40:189–217, 1948.

441. Stansbury, J.R. Conjunctival amyloidosis in association with systemic amyloid disease. *Am. J. Ophthalmol.* 59:24–29, 1965.

442. Starck, T., Kenyon, K.R., Hanninen, L.A., Beyer-Machule, C., Fabian, R., Gorn, R.A., McMullan, F.D., Baum, J., and McAdam, K.P.W.J. Clinical and histopathologic studies of two families with lattice corneal dystrophy and familial systemic amyloidosis (Meretoja syndrome). *Ophthalmology* 98:1197–1206, 1991.

443. Stephenson, W.V. Anterior megalophthalmos and arachnodactyly. *Am. J. Ophthalmol.* 28:315–317, 1945.

444. Stern, G.A., Knapp, A., and Hood, C.I. Corneal amyloidosis associated with keratoconus. *Ophthalmology* 95:52–55, 1988.

445. Steuhl, K.-P., Knorr, M., Rohrbach, J.M., Lisch, W., Kaiserling, E., and Thiel, H.-J. Paraproteinemic corneal deposits in plasma cell myeloma. *Am. J. Ophthalmol.* 111:312–318, 1991.

446. Stock, E.L., Feder, R.S., O'Grady, R.B., Sugar, J., and Roth, S.A. Lattice corneal dystrophy type IIIA: Clinical and histopathologic correlations. *Arch. Ophthalmol.* 109:354–358, 1991.

447. Stock, E.L., and Keilar, R.A. Primary familial amyloidosis of the cornea. *Am. J. Ophthalmol.* 82:266–271, 1976.

448. Stoeber, P., Renversez, J.C., Groulade, J., Vialtel, P., and Cordonnier, D. Ultrastructural study of human IgG and IgG-IgM crystalcryoglobulins. *Am. J. Clin. Pathol.* 71:404–410, 1979.

449. Strahler, J.R., Rosenblum, B.B., and Hanash, S.M. Identification and characterization of a human transthyretin variant. *Biochem. Res. Commun. 148*:471–477, 1987.

450. Stuart, J.C., Mund, M.L., Iwamoto, T., Troutman, R.C., White, H., and DeVoe, A.G. Recurrent granular corneal dystrophy. *Am. J. Ophthalmol. 79*:18–24, 1975.

451. Subjeck, J.R., and Shyy, T.-T. Stress protein systems of mammalian cells. *Am. J. Physiol. 250*:C1–17, 1986.

451a. Sunada, Y., Shimizu, T., Nakase, H., Ohta, S., Asaoka, T., Amano, S., Sawa, M., Kagawa, Y., Kanazawa, I., and Mannen, T. Inherited amyloid polyneuropathy type IV (gelsolin variant) in a Japanese family. *Ann. Neurol. 33*:57–62, 1993.

452. Sun, X.L., Zheng, B.H., Li, B., Li, L.Q., Soejima, K., and Kanda, M. Orbital rhabdomyosarcoma: Immuno-histochemical studies of seven cases. *Chin. Med. J. [Engl.] 103*:485–488, 1990.

453. Suzuki, S., Sano, K., and Tanihara, H. Diversity of the cadherin family: Evidence for eight new cadherins in nervous tissue. *Cell Regulation 2*:261–270, 1991.

454. Tabbara, K.F. Climatic droplet keratopathy. *Int. Ophthalmol. Clin. 26*:63–68, 1986.

455. Takagi, M., Ishizu, M., and Suzuki, H. An electron microscopic and histochemical study on a corneal granular dystrophy (Groenoew type I). *Folia Ophthalmol. Jpn. 22*:479–484, 1971.

456. Takahashi, M., Yokota, T., Yamashita, Y., Isihara, T., Uchino, F., Imada, N., and Matsumoto, N. Unusual inclusions in stromal macrophages in a case of gelatinous drop-like corneal dystrophy. *Am. J. Ophthalmol. 99*: 312–316, 1985.

457. Takeichi, M. Cadherins: Cell-cell adhesion molecules controlling animal morphogenesis. *Development 102*: 639–655, 1988.

458. Takeichi, M. The cadherins: A molecular family important in selective cell-cell adhesion. *Annu. Rev. Biochem. 59*:237–252, 1990.

459. Tawara, S., Nakazato, M., Kangawa, K., Matsuo, H., and Araki, S. Identification of amyloid prealbumin variant in familial amyloidotic polyneuropathy (Japanese type). *Biochem. Biophys. Res. Commun. 116*:880–888, 1983.

460. Teng, C.C. Granular dystrophy of the cornea: A histochemical and electron microscopic study. *Am. J. Ophthalmol. 63*:772–791, 1967.

461. Terry, W.D., Page, D.L., Kimura, S., Isobe, T., Osserman, E.F., and Glenner, G.G. Structural identity of Bence-Jones and amyloid fibril proteins in a patient with plasma cell dyscrasia and amyloidosis. *J. Clin. Invest. 52*:1276–1281, 1973.

462. Tervo, K., Tervo, T., van Setten, G.-B., and Virtanen, I. Integrins in human corneal epithelium. *Cornea 10*:461–465, 1991.

463. Tohyama, T., Lee, V. M.-Y., Rorke, L.B., Marvin, M., McKay, R.D.G., and Trojanowski, J.Q. Nestin expression in embryonic human neuroepithelium and in human neuroepithelial tumor cells. *Lab. Invest. 66*: 303–313, 1992.

464. Tölle, H.-G., Weber, K., and Osborn, M. Microinjection of monoclonal antibodies specific for one intermediate filament protein in cells containing multiple keratins allow insight into the composition of particular 10 nm filaments. *Eur. J. Cell Biol. 38*:234–244, 1985.

465. Tomokane, K., Iwaki, T., Tateishi, J., Iwaki, A., and Goldman, J.E. Rosenthal fibers share epitopes with αB crystallin, glial fibrillary acidic protein, and ubiquitin, but not vimentin: Immunoelectron microscopy with colloidal gold. *Am. J. Pathol. 138*:875–885, 1991.

466. Touchette, N. Recoverin illuminates mechanisms of visual adaptation. *J. NIH Res. 3*:58–64, 1991.

467. Travis, G.H., Sutcliffe, J.G., and Bok, D. The retinal degeneration slow (rds) gene product is a photoreceptor disc membrane-associated glycoprotein. *Neuron 6*:61–70, 1991.

468. Tripathi, R.C., and Garner, A. Corneal granular dystrophy: A light and electron microscopic study of its recurrence in a graft. *Br. J. Ophthalmol. 54*:361–372, 1970.

469. Ts'o, M.O.M., and Bettman, J.W. Occlusion of choriocapillaris in primary nonfamilial amyloidosis. *Arch. Ophthalmol. 86*:281–286, 1971.

470. Tsuda, M., Syed, K., Bugra, K., Whelan, J.P., McGinnis, J.F., and Shinohara, T. Structural analysis of mouse S-antigen. *Gene 73*:11–20, 1988.

471. Tsukita, S., Tsukita, S., and Nagafuchi, A. The undercoat of adherens junction: A key specialized structure in organogenesis and carcinogenesis. *Cell Struct. Funct. 15*:7–12, 1990.

472. Turner, C.E., and Burridge, K. Transmembrane molecular assemblies in cell-extracellular matrix interactions. *Curr. Opin. Cell Biol. 3*:849–853, 1991.

473. Unsworth, D.J., Scott, D.L., Almond, T.J., Beard, H.K., Hoborow, E.J., and Walton, K.W. Studies on reticulin I: Serological and immunohistological investigation of the occurrence of collagen type III, fibronectin and the noncollagenous glycoprotein of PRAS and GLYNN in reticulin. *Br. J. Exp. Pathol. 63*:154–166, 1982.

474. Van der Gaag, R., Broersma, L., Rothova, A., Baarsma, S., and Kijstra, A. Immunity to a corneal antigen in Fuchs' heterochromic cyclitis patients. *Invest. Ophthalmol. Vis. Sci. 30*:443–448, 1989.

475. Van Duinen, S.G., Castano, E.M., Prelli, F., Bots, G.T.A.M., Luyendijk, W., and Frangione, B. Hereditary cerebral hemorrhage with amyloidosis in patients of Dutch origin is related to Alzheimer's disease. *Proc. Natl. Acad. Sci. USA 84*:5991–5994, 1987.

476. Vazquez, J.J., and Dixon, F.J. Immunohistochemical analysis of amyloid by the fluorescence technique. *J. Exp. Med. 104*:727–736, 1956.

477. Viljoen, D.L., Pope, F.M., and Beighton, P. Heterogeneity of pseudoxanthoma elasticum: Delineation of a new form? *Clin. Genet. 32*:100–105, 1987.

478. Waardenburg, P.J., and Jonkers, G.H. A specific type of dominant progressive dystrophy of the cornea, developing after birth. *Acta Ophthalmol. (Copenh.) 39*:919–923, 1961.

479. Wachtel, J.G. The ocular pathology of Marfan's syndrome: Including a clinico-pathological correlation and an explanation of ectopia lentis. *Arch. Ophthalmol. 76*:512–522, 1966.

480. Waldenström, J. Incipient myelomatosis or "essential" hyperglobulinemia with fibrinogenopenia—a new syndrome? *Acta Med. Scand. 117*:216–247, 1944.

481. Wallace, M.R., Dwulet, F.E., Conneally, P.M., and Benson, M.D. Biochemical and molecular genetic characterization of a new variant prealbumin associated with hereditary amyloidosis. *J. Clin. Invest. 78*:6–12, 1986.

482. Wallace, M.R., Dwulet, F.E., Williams, E.C., Conneally, P.M., and Benson, M.D. Identification of a new prealbumin variant, Tyr-77 and detection of the gene by DNA analysis. *J. Clin. Invest. 81*:189–193, 1988.

483. Walsh, F.S., Barton, C.H., Putt, W., Moore, S.E., Kelsell, D., Spurr, N., and Goodfellow, P.N. N-cadherin gene maps to human chromosome 18 and is not linked to the E-cadherin gene. *J. Neurochem. 55*:805–812, 1990.

484. Waring, G.O., Font, R.L., Rodrigues, M.M., and Mulberger, R.D. Alterations of Descemet's membrane in interstitial keratitis. *Am. J. Ophthalmol. 81*:773–785, 1976.

485. Way, M., and Weeds, A. Nucleotide sequence of pig plasma gelsolin: Comparison of protein sequence with human gelsolin and other actin-severing proteins shows strong homologies and evidence for large internal repeats. *J. Mol. Biol. 203*:1127–1133, 1988.

486. Weber, F.L., and Babel, J. Gelatinous drop-like dystrophy: A form of primary corneal amyloidosis. *Arch. Ophthalmol. 98*:144–148, 1980.

487. Westermark, P., Sletten, K., Johansson, B., and Cornwell, G.G., III. Fibril in senile systemic amyloidosis is derived from normal transthyretin. *Proc. Natl. Acad. Sci. USA 87*:2843–2845, 1990.

488. Wheeler, G.E., and Eiferman, R.A. Immunohistochemical identification of the AA protein in lattice dystrophy. *Invest. Ophthalmol. Vis. Sci. (Suppl.) 20*:115, 1981.

489. Whitt, J.W., Wood, B.C., Sharma, J.N., and Crouch, T.T. Adult polycystic kidney disease and lattice corneal dystrophy: Occurrence in a single family. *Arch. Intern. Med. 138*:1167–1168, 1978.

489a. Wiens, A., Marles, S., Safneck, J., Kwiatkowski, D.J., Maury, C.P., Zelinski, T., Phillips, S., Ekins, M.B., and Greenberg, C.R. Exclusion of the gelsolin gene on 9q32–34 at the cause of familial lattice dystrophy type I. *Am. J. Hum. Genet. 51*:156–160, 1992.

490. Winkelman, J.E., Delleman, J.W., and Ansink, B.J.J. Ein hereditäres Syndrom, bestehend aus peripherer Polyneuropathie, Hautveränderungen und gittriger Dystrophie der Hornhaut. *Klin. Monatsbl. Augenheilkd. 159*:618–623, 1971.

491. Winstow, G.J., and Piatigorsky, J. Lens crystallins: The evolution and expression of proteins for a highly specialized tissue. *Annu. Rev. Biochem. 57*:479–504, 1988.

492. Wisniewski, H.M., and Terry, R.D. Reexamination of the pathogenesis of the senile plaque. In *Progress in Neuropathology*, Vol. 2, H.M. Zimmerman (Ed.), Grune and Stratton, New York, pp. 1–26, 1973.

493. Wistow, G. Evolution of a protein superfamily: Relationships between vertebrate lens crystallins and microorganism dormancy proteins. *J. Mol. Evol. 30*:140–145, 1990.

494. Wittebol-Post, D., and Pels, E. The dystrophy described by Reis and Bücklers: Separate entity or variant of granular dystrophy? *Ophthalmologica 199*:1–9, 1989.

495. Wittebol-Post, D., Van Schooneveld, M.J., and Pels, E. The corneal dystrophy of Waardenburg and Jonkers. *Ophthalmol. Paediatr. Genet. 10*:249–255, 1989.

496. Wong, V.G., and McFarlin, D.E. Primary familial amyloidosis. *Arch. Ophthalmol. 78*:208–213, 1967.

497. Woo, P., Betts, J., and Edbrooke, M. The human serum amyloid A genes and their regulation by inflammatory cytokines. In *Amyloid and Amyloidosis*, J.B. Natvig, O. Forre, G. Husby, A. Husebekk, B. Skogen, K. Sletten, and P. Westermark (Eds.), Kluwer Academic, Dordrecht, pp. 13–19, 1991.

498. Wright, D., and Mayne, R. Vitreous humor of chicken contains two fibrillar systems: An analysis of their structure. *J. Ultrastruct. Mol. Struct. Res. 100*:224–234, 1988.

499. Wright, J.R., Calkins, E., Breen, W.J., Stolte, G., and Schultz, R.T. Relationship of amyloid to aging: Review of the literature and systematic study of 83 patients derived from a general hospital population. *Medicine (Baltimore) 48*:39–60, 1969.

500. Xiong, Y., Zhang, H., and Beach, D. D type cyclins associate with multiple protein kinases and the DNA replication and repair factor PCNA. *Cell 71*:505–514, 1992.

501. Yamaguchi, K., Yamaguchi, K., Sheedlo, H.J., and Turner, J.E. Expression of heat shock protein in the atrophic corneal epithelium of the royal college of surgeon dystrophic rat. *Cornea 10*:161–165, 1991.

502. Yanoff, M., Fine, B.S., Colosi, N.J., and Katowitz, J.A. Lattice corneal dystrophy: Report of an unusual case. *Arch. Ophthalmol. 95*:651–655, 1977.

503. Yassa, N.H., Font, R.L., Fine, B.S., and Koffler, B.H. Corneal immunoglobulin deposition in the posterior stroma: A case report including immunohistochemical and ultrastructural observations. *Arch. Ophthalmol. 105*:99–103, 1987.

504. Zirm, M. Proteins in aqueous humor. *Adv. Ophthalmol. 40*:100–172, 1980.

33
Collagen and Its Disorders

J. Godfrey Heathcote
St. Joseph's Health Centre and The University of Western Ontario, London, Ontario, Canada

I. INTRODUCTION

In the 1970s research into collagen was focused primarily on the characterization of a few distinct types of collagen (42), the primary structures of their α chains (150), and the posttranslational modification of their respective procollagens (186,268). At the time of the first edition of *Pathobiology of Ocular Disease* in 1982, 5 different types of collagen had been identified. In the subsequent decade the number of genetically distinct collagens recognized has increased to 13, with more in the process of being characterized, and the genes for some of these types have been assigned to specific chromosomes. Immunohistochemical studies, notably those of Linsenmayer and his colleagues (see later), have dramatically increased our appreciation of the roles of the different collagens in the development of tissue structure, particularly in the eye. Advances in molecular genetics have answered many questions about generalized connective tissue disorders, such as osteogenesis imperfecta, and Marfan syndrome has now been shown to be primarily a disorder of fibrillin (550), not collagen, as once seemed likely (see Chap. 32).

This review of collagen and its disorders touches only briefly on the structure and biosynthesis of the different types of collagen, more emphasis being placed on the collagen fiber and its modification by cross-linking, interaction with other connective tissue macromolecules, and nonenzymatic glycosylation. The major part of the chapter deals with collagen as it contributes to the different structures within the eye and as it is altered by diseases involving these structures. Finally, some of the recent advances in understanding the major heritable connective tissue diseases that affect the eye are briefly reviewed.

Reviews specifically devoted to collagen within the eye have been published by Freeman (142) and Bailey (13).

II. COLLAGEN

A. Molecular Structure and Biosynthesis

A collagen may be defined as "an extracellular structural protein whose functional properties depend significantly upon a triple-helical domain" (52). The nomenclature of collagen biochemistry is complicated and a helpful glossary is provided by Weiss and Ayad (540); a shorter glossary, more relevant to the contents of this chapter, is provided in Table 1. At least 13 types of collagen, designated I–XIII, are now recognized, and for many of the constituent polypeptide chains the gene has been characterized and localized to a specific chromosome (Table 2) (529).

Collagens may be divided into two classes: those that form banded fibers with a 67 nm periodicity (types I, II, III, V, IX, XI, and XII) and those that do not. Some of the others, such as types VI and VII, form banded structures but without the classic 67 nm periodicity. In this section the fundamental features of collagen structure and biosynthesis, as exemplified by the classic collagens of interstitial connective tissues (types I–III), are briefly reviewed.

Table 1   Nomenclature of Collagen Biochemistry

α Chain   one polypeptide of the triple helical molecule, e.g., α_1(I)

β Subunit   two cross-linked polypeptides of triple helical molecules, e.g., $\beta_{12} = \alpha_1$(I)α_2(I)

γ Subunit   three cross-linked polypeptides of triple helical molecules, e.g., $[\alpha_1$(I)$]_2\alpha_2$(I)

FLS   fibrous long-spacing collagen, a fibrillar precipitate of collagen molecules with periodicity > 67 nm; similar aggregates may be seen within tissues

Gelatin   denatured form of collagen

NC domain   noncollagenous (i.e., non–triple-helical) domain within a collagen molecule

pC-collagen   procollagen lacking the amino propeptide

Pepsin-extracted collagen   collagen obtained from tissue digested with pepsin; it lacks telopeptides

pN-collagen   procollagen lacking the carboxy propeptide

Procollagen   secreted precursor form of some collagen types; globular extension peptides are present at N and C termini

Propeptides   extension peptide at each end of the procollagen molecule (amino propeptide and carboxy propeptide)

Protocollagen   newly synthesized intracellular collagen with proline residues not yet hydroxylated

Reconstituted collagen   collagen fibrils formed *in vitro* under certain conditions of temperature, pH, and ionic strength

SLS crystallite   segment long-spacing collagen, a precipitate of collagen in which the molecules are arranged with like features in an accurate transverse register

Telopeptide   short nonhelical peptide at the terminus of the α chain

Tropocollagen   intact triple-helical molecule (collagen fibril monomer) containing telopeptides

Tropocollagen is a rodlike molecule that consists of three chains, each a left-handed helix, coiled in a righthanded triple helix. Each α chain contains approximately 1050 amino acids, and every third residue is glycine: the primary structure is thus a polymer of (-Gly-*X*-*Y*-). A high proportion of the *X* and *Y* positions are occupied by proline and hydroxyproline, respectively. At each end of the α chain is a nonhelical telopeptide, 15–20 amino acids long, in which lysine and hydroxylysine residues involved in cross-linking may be found. In some collagen types, such as type IV, short nonhelical sequences are found within the triple helix and confer flexibility upon the molecules.

The transcription of the collagen genes is discussed elsewhere (529). The initially synthesized precursor of tropocollagen, procollagen, is composed of three chains, each with a large, globular noncollagenous polypeptide at the amino (N) and carboxyl (C) termini. During passage from the ribosome to the extracellular space, the polypeptides undergo a series of posttranslational modifications (165,268). These modifications include (1) hydroxylation of some proline residues in the *Y* position of the (-Gly-*X*-*Y*-) triplet; (2) hydroxylation of some lysine residues (there are no codons for the amino acids hydroxyproline and hydroxylysine); (3) glycosylation of hydroxylysine residues; and (4) sulfation of tyrosine residues. This last modification appears to be a widespread feature of secreted proteins and has been described in both type III procollagen (235) and type V procollagen (122); its significance remains uncertain (213). Hydroxyproline residues contribute to the stability of the triple helix through hydrogen bond formation. The folding of the polypeptides into the triple helix is facilitated by the presence of disulfide bridges between the extension peptides of the pro-α chains (268).

Once in the extracellular matrix, procollagen is converted to tropocollagen by proteolytic removal of the propeptides (Fig. 1), the order of removal differing between tissues and collagen types. The tropocollagen molecules spontaneously assemble to form fibrils. This process occurs in collagen solutions in vitro if conditions are favorable; in electron micrographs the resulting fibers are indistinguishable from those of intact tissues. Collagen fibers stained with phosphotungstic acid display a substructure of dark and light bands that repeat at intervals of 67 nm (designated *D*). The assembly of tropocollagen molecules 300 nm long into a banded fibril is governed by the primary structure. Regions rich in charged amino acids are distributed at intervals along the monomer (124), and adjacent monomers are aligned so that negative and positive charges on the surface are neutralized (283). Maximal interaction between amino acids of opposite charge and between hydrophobic residues occurs when parallel molecules overlap by *D* (234 residues) or an integral multiple of *D* (211). This arrangement leaves a gap between the ends of molecules in line because

300 nm is not an exact multiple of the D period. In each D repeat along the fibril, a "gap" zone and an "overlap" zone occur, and these correlate with the banding pattern seen in electron micrographs. The gap zone is believed to be the site of mineralization.

Although biosynthetic experiments with cell cultures suggest that procollagen is secreted as a monomer, it has been proposed that in vivo, where the local concentration would be high, the molecules may be released from the cell as segment long-spacing crystallites with a zero D stagger (210). Subsequent lateral aggregation and processing within the fibril would give rise to the D-staggered arrangement and characteristic axial periodicity. Indeed, the rate of removal of the N-terminal propeptide might regulate the diameter of collagen fibers in vivo (135, 209). Stabilization of the fiber is dependent upon the formation of intermolecular lysine-derived cross-links (see Sec. II.C).

B. Fibril Formation

As discussed in the previous section, the natural process of fibrillogenesis can be reproduced in vitro by warming a neutral salt solution of tropocollagen to 37°C, when the molecules spontaneously aggregate to form fibrils (220). The process, which can be measured turbidimetrically, involves a temperature-dependent conformational change in the telopeptides (394) followed by a nucleation phase in which two monomers form an end-to-end dimer overlapping by $4D$ (533). Finally there is a sigmoidal growth phase with lateral accretion of molecules.

The lateral aggregation of fibril monomers is subject to a number of controlling influences that are slowly being elucidated. Their importance is emphasized by a comparison of collagen fiber diameter in cornea, where it is very uniform, and sclera, where the variation in fiber diameter is considerable (Table 3) (388). In at least some soft tissues collagen fibers of large diameter have a slower rate of turnover than thinner ones, although it is not entirely clear which is the cause and which the effect (489). In a study antedating the identification of the numerous types of collagen, Grant and colleagues (166) suggested that the extent of glycosylation of polypeptidylhydroxylysine might have some effect on fiber diameter. Thus, in bovine cornea, in which the mean fiber diameter is 30 nm, polymeric collagen was found to contain 30 residues of hexose per 3000 amino acid residues; the corresponding figures in bovine sclera (mean fiber diameter 90 nm) and tendon (mean fiber diameter 100 nm) were 8 and 6 hexose residues, respectively. This idea could explain the absence of banded fibers from basement membranes, the collagen of which is highly glycosylated. A more recent study on collagen type I from bovine cornea, skin, and tendon confirmed that a high percentage of glycosylated hydroxylysine correlates with a low mean diameter of fibrils in vivo (520).

It is now accepted that different collagen types are to be found in the same fiber. When fibrils are precipitated in vitro from a mixture of purified type I and type V collagens, the mean fibril diameter increases as the proportion of type I collagen in the mixture increases (1). Type III collagen has been identified on the surface of 67 nm banded fibrils in a wide variety of tissues, including some, such as tendon, where it is only a minor component (251).

One important influence controlling fibrillogenesis appears to be the removal of the propeptides by procollagen proteinases (30). This is likely to be complicated if more than one collagen type is present in a given fiber. In dermatosparaxis, where the N-terminal proteinase is deficient, the dermal collagen fibers are twisted and lack uniformity and contain the aberrant pN form of type I collagen (545). Type III pN-collagen, however, appears to be a normal constituent of banded fibrils within the dermis (134).

Although glycoproteins have been shown to influence collagen fibrillogenesis in vitro (5,477), evidence for a close relationship between fiber architecture and glycosaminoglycan (GAG) content is stronger. A high total content of GAG in a tissue is associated with a low mean fibril diameter (347), but there is disagreement about whether the proportion of individual GAG is of comparable significance (347,389). There seems no doubt that a high concentration of chondroitin sulfate in a tissue has an inhibitory effect on fiber growth (347), a factor that may be of particular relevance to cornea (41).

Fetal tissues generally contain fibrils of narrow diameter with a unimodal distribution of diameters. With maturation the diameters increase and the distribution becomes broader and multimodal (93). The diameters of small collagen fibrils are multiples of about 8 nm, and it appears that growth occurs by accretion of units with a dimension of either 8 nm (if lateral deposition) or 4 nm (if circumferential deposition).

In healing wounds tensile strength is directly related to the diameter of the newly formed collagen

Table 2 The Collagen Family of Proteins

Type	Site	Chains	Gene	Chromosome	Trimer	Banded fibrils	Special features
I	Cornea Sclera Tendon	$\alpha1(I)$ $\alpha2(I)$	COL1A1 COL1A2	17q21.3–q22 7q21.3–q22	$[\alpha1(I)]_2\alpha2(I)$ $[\alpha1(I)]_3$	+	
II	Cartilage Vitreous	$\alpha1(II)$	COL2A1	12q13–q14	$[\alpha1(II)]_3$	+	
III	Skin Smooth muscle	$\alpha1(III)$	COL3A1	2q24.3–q31	$[\alpha1(III)]_3$	+	
IV	Basement membranes	$\alpha1(IV)$ $\alpha2(IV)$ $\alpha3(IV)$ $\alpha4(IV)$ $\alpha5(IV)$	COL4A1 COL4A2 COL4A3 COL4A4 COL4A5	13q34 13q34 xq22	$[\alpha1(IV)]_2\alpha2(IV)$	−	
V	Cartilage Liver Bone Cornea Placenta	$\alpha1(V)$ $\alpha2(V)$ $\alpha3(V)$	COL5A1 COL5A2 COL5A3	2q24.3–q31	$[\alpha1(V)]_3$ $[\alpha1(V)]_2\alpha2(V)$ $\alpha1(V)\alpha2(V)\alpha3(V)$	+	Mixed fibrils: I,V
VI	Cornea Cartilage Aorta	$\alpha1(VI)$ $\alpha2(VI)$ $\alpha3(VI)$	COL6A1 COL6A2 COL6A3	21q22.3 21q22.3 2q37	$\alpha1(VI)\alpha2(VI)\alpha3(VI)$	+	Microfibrils of 100 nm periodicity

Type	Tissue	Chain	Gene	Chromosome	Molecular composition	Present	Comments
VII	Subepithelial connective tissue, Skin, Cornea, Amnion	α1(VII)	COL7A1		$[\alpha1(VII)]_3$	+	Tissue form is anchoring fibril
VIII	Vascular subendothelium, Cartilage, Descemet's membrane, Sclera, Bruch's membrane	α1(VIII), α2(VIII)	COL8A1, COL8A2	3q11.1–q13.2, 1p32.3–p34.3	?	–	May occur in a highly insoluble form in Decemet's membrane as part of hexagonal lattice
IX	Cartilage, Cornea, Vitreous	α1(IX), α2(IX), α3(IX)	COL9A1, COL9A2, COL9A3	6q12–q14	$\alpha1(IX)\alpha2(IX)\alpha3(IX)$	–	Lateral association to type II Covalently bonded GAG
X	Cartilage (Hypertrophic chondrocytes)	α1(X)	COL10A1		$[\alpha1(X)]_3$	–	May be involved in calcification of cartilage
XI	Cartilage	α1(XI), 1α, α2(XI), 2α, α3(XI), 3α	COL11A1, COL11A2, COL2A1	1p21, 6q21.2, 12q13–q14	$1\alpha2\alpha3\alpha = \alpha1(XI)\alpha2(XI)\alpha3(XI)$	+	Mixed fibrils: II, IX, XI
XII	Tendon, Ligament	α1(XII)	COL12A1		$[\alpha1(XII)]_3$	+	Partially homologous to type IX. May be one of a family of molecules, associated with banded fibrils.
XIII	Epidermis, Intestinal mucosa	α1(XIII)	COL13A1	10q11–qter	?	?	α1 chains of different lengths

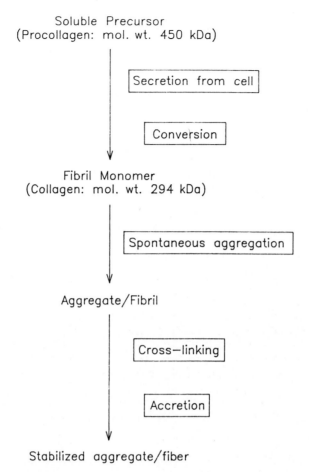

Figure 1   General outline of the assembly of the collagen fiber. [Reproduced with permission from J.G. Heathcote and M.E. Grant. Extracellular modification of connective tissue proteins. In *The Enzymology of Post-translational Modification of Proteins*, Vol. 1, R.B. Freedman and H.C. Hawkins (Eds.), Academic Press, London, pp. 457–506, 1980.]

fibers (108). Although fibrosis is a fundamental part of tissue repair, it is not always beneficial. Scarring within the vitreous, for example, has a detrimental effect on the retina, which may become detached. Although a number of drugs may interfere with collagen biosynthesis and cross-linking, none has yet been proved effective in the therapeutic control of fibrosis (298). Immunotherapy may ultimately prove of greater value since activated T lymphocytes may be seen in hypertrophic scars (227) and cytokines modulate the mobilization and proliferation of fibroblasts as well as fibrogenesis (530,531).

C. Cross-linking

Much of the structural strength of collagen depends on its relative insolubility and resistance to proteolytic digestion, properties in part attributable to intermolecular covalent cross-links derived from residues of lysine and hydroxylysine within the polypeptide chains. Two types of lysine-derived cross-link are recognized. The first, reducible cross-links, may be recovered from hydrolysates of collagen following mild reduction with tritiated borohydride ($NaBH_4$), which labels the cross-links and renders them stable to acid hydrolysis. The second type, mature cross-links, forms as the number of reducible cross-links declines during maturation (423) and may be derived from them, although apparently not by natural reduction (116).

Table 3 Collagen Fiber Diameter During Fetal Development in
Macaca mulatta

Gestational age (days)	Corneal stroma (nm)	Sclera (nm)	Fiber periodicity (nm)
43	29–33	26	—
60	33–37	30–58	70
95	35–37	112–118	73–80
125	31–35	55–130	75–80
2 postnatal	33–35	42–292	75–80

Source: Data from Ozanics and colleagues (388).

The first step in the formation of these cross-links, and the only one under enzymatic control, is oxidative deamination of specific lysine and hydroxylysine residues in the telopeptides. The reactive aldehydes generated, allysine and hydroxyallysine, respectively, react with ε-amino groups of hydroxy-lysine residues in the helical region of adjacent molecules to form aldimine cross-links. The specific residues involved are conserved in collagen types I, II, and III (116). The oxidative deamination is regulated by lysyl oxidase, a copper metalloenzyme that requires vitamin B_6 for optimal activity (33,366) and is most active on insoluble, fibrillar collagen (471). The enzyme is irreversibly inhibited by the lathyrogen, β-aminopropionitrile (BAPN).* The process of cross-linking may also be disturbed by D-penicillamine, which both inhibits lysyl oxidase and blocks the aldehyde groups (374).

The reactive aldehydes form the basis of two pathways of reducible cross-link formation.

(1) The allysine pathway involves the reaction of allysine with hydroxylysine to form dehydro-hydroxylysinonorleucine. This is the predominant pathway in both type I and type III collagen of adult skin (16) and cornea (301). Other possible cross-links include aldol-histidine, produced from two allysine residues and histidine, and its derivatives (116,301). The mature cross-link of this pathway has not yet been identified.

(2) The hydroxyallysine pathway involves the interaction of hydroxyallysine and hydroxylysine to form dehydrohydroxylysinohydroxynorleucine, which undergoes a spontaneous Amadori rearrangement to form the ketoamine hydroxylysino-5-ketonorleucine. There is now strong evidence that a mature cross-link of this pathway is pyridinoline (472). This may be formed by the reaction of two ketoamine cross-links with the elimination of a hydroxylysine residue. It has not been found in cornea or skin (116): its susceptibility to degradation by ultraviolet light (434) may make it unsuitable for these tissues. More of the pyridinoline is found in type II than type I collagen (116), and it has been identified in vitreous (476). Light and Bailey (304) localized the pyridinoline cross-link in type I collagen to a peptide at the carboxyl terminus of the α$_2$ chain. The major cross-linked material from the collagen, however, consisted of a polymer of a different peptide (303) that could be identified in a variety of mature tissues, including cornea, and did not contain pyridinoline (302,304). From their studies Light and Bailey (304) concluded that there was insufficient pyridinoline in type I collagen for this compound to be the mature cross-link.

The reducible cross-links have largely disappeared by the age of maturity, that is, at about 20 years in the human and 5 years in the ox (15,423). Their replacement by stable nonreducible cross-links is also complete by this age, at least in bovine tendon (100,226). Nevertheless, studies of human collagen derived from dura mater (275) and tendon (146) clearly demonstrate a progressive reduction in solubility with advancing age, and this may be the result of the formation of advanced Maillard products (see Sec. IV.C) (146). Certainly the progressive diminution in solubility is accelerated in diabetics (275).

Recently there has been renewed interest in the possibility of other types of cross-links, such as pyrroles. Scott and colleagues (256,456) have presented evidence for a cross-linking compound that reacts

---

*Lathyrism is a condition in animals in which connective tissues have a markedly reduced tensile strength and their collagen has increased solubility (21,299). Ingestion of BAPN, a toxic constituent of the sweet pea *Lathyrus odoratus*, is the usual cause. Topical BAPN has been shown to diminish symblepharon formation following an alkali burn of the conjunctiva (356). The lathyrogen, β,β′-iminodipropionitrile, causes cataracts and buphthalmos in rats (447).

with Ehrlich's reagent to give a pink color in a variety of connective tissues, including bone, skin, and cartilage. The chromogen is only found in polymeric collagen and has been identified in a three-chain peptide derived from type III collagen and the 7S cross-linking region of human placental type IV collagen (458).

In addition, type III collagen is distinguished by the presence of both intramolecular (80) and intermolecular (76) disulfide bridges. A cross-linked peptide containing the N-terminal regions of α_1(I) and α_1(III) has been isolated (197), supporting the existence of mixed fibrils of these collagen types.

Disulfide bridges play an important role in the stabilization of type IV collagen, but there is also strong evidence for lysine-derived cross-links. Heathcote and colleagues (184) were able to demonstrate the biosynthesis of hydroxylysino-5-ketonorleucine by intact rat lenses in tissue culture. Since the turnover of lens capsule collagen is low, the proportion of reducible cross-links in the capsules of mature animals is small (184), but the identity of the stable cross-link is unknown. It does not appear to be pyridinoline (190). Hydroxylysino-5-ketonorleucine was the only reducible cross-link identified in type IV collagen from human placenta, and again pyridinoline could not be identified (17).

Desmosine and isodesmosine were found unexpectedly in a study of the cross-links of bovine Descemet's membrane (190). These lysine-derived tetrafunctional compounds constitute the principal cross-links of elastic fibers and join two elastin polypeptides in alanine-rich regions (186). In Descemet's membrane they were identified in a relatively insoluble component that was also enriched in alanine. There is no evidence for the presence of elastin in Descemet's membrane, however, and the molecular site of these cross-links has yet to be established.

A further type of covalent cross-link, not derived from lysine, has been described in collagen from the cuticle of *Ascaris* (147). This is isotrityrosine, composed of three tyrosine residues joined by one biphenyl and one ether link. McNamara and Augusteyn (342) have isolated 3,3'-dityrosine from the capsule of both normal and cataractous human lenses, and such tyrosine derivatives may prove to be significant cross-links in basement membranes.

D. Degradation of Collagen

The early experimental work on the biological degradation of collagen and the conceptual framework in which that research was carried out have been reviewed by Gross (174). In recent years it has been recognized that classic vertebrate collagenase is simply one of a number of metalloproteinases involved in the degradation of extracellular matrix (330). The metalloproteinases are a group of proteolytic enzymes that can digest synergistically all the major matrix macromolecules (Table 4) (420). They are secreted in an inactive form and activated by proteolytic cleavage and/or a change in configuration (77,181); zinc is a cofactor, and calcium is required for stability. Since they are active at neutral pH they are ideally suited for operation within the extracellular space.

Most experimental work has been carried out on the collagenases. Their synthesis and release are largely controlled by cytokines in both normal tissues and tumors. Epithelial cells produce stimulators (molecular weight 19 and 54 kD) that increase the output of collagenase by mesenchymal cells through an increase in the amount of collagenase mRNA available for translation (229,230). Goslen and colleagues (161) isolated from basal cell carcinomas a similar 19 kD polypeptide that stimulated collagenase production by human skin fibroblasts. The idea that a tumor's invasive potential is linked to its capacity to produce collagenase (175) or hyaluronidase (508) or to its ability to induce the synthesis of these enzymes by host tissues is attractive, yet evidence suggests that the relative secretion of enzyme inhibitors may be equally

Table 4　Matrix Metalloproteinases

Enzyme	Substrate
Collagenases	Native collagen types I, II, and III
Stromelysins	Laminin, fibronectin, proteoglycans
Gelatinases	Denatured collagen types I, II, and III
	Native collagen types IV, V, and VII

important. TIMP (tissue inhibitor of metalloproteinase) is a 28 kD protein of widespread distribution that complexes with collagenase and stromelysin (420). More than one type has been identified (330). Hicks and colleagues (202) cultured fibrosarcoma cell lines of low and high invasive potential. Neither cell line produced collagenase, but the highly invasive line secreted 10- to 20-fold less TIMP. In actively remodeling scar tissue fibroblasts synthesize both collagenase and TIMP (195). In dermis the same cells appear to be responsible for the phagocytosis and intracellular degradation of collagen fibril fragments (176,490).

Gelatinases may be particularly important in tumor metastasis because of their ability to degrade type IV (basement membrane) collagen (311). At least two gelatinases have been identified: a high-molecular-weight (>90 kD) form produced by leukocytes and an enzyme of lower molecular weight (72 kD) synthesized by connective tissue cells (365). In normal human cornea the high-molecular-weight enzyme is a major product of the epithelium and the other a major product of the stromal keratocytes (127). In experimental thermal burns, the 92 kD gelatinase is produced by epithelial cells and/or neutrophils about 3 days after injury and may be responsible for dissolution of the corneal epithelial basement membrane. The low-molecular-weight form appears about 7 days after injury when remodeling of the stroma is beginning (331). The capacity to degrade type VII collagen (467) in addition to types IV and V collagen also supports a significant role for these enzymes in the pathogenesis of corneal ulcers.

III. THE COLLAGEN FAMILY OF PROTEINS

A. Types I, II, and III Collagen

The early understanding of collagen biochemistry was obtained from studies of these three classic collagens of interstitial connective tissue. Much of this was reviewed in the previous section, and further details can be obtained from a number of excellent reviews (42,349) and books (334,541).

B. Type IV Collagen

Many of the details of our current understanding of type IV collagen are discussed in the sections on basement membrane and the lens capsule. It is synthesized as a high-molecular-weight heterotrimer (540 kD) and is incorporated as such into the fabric of the basement membrane (184,192). Since there is no proteolytic conversion, the constituent polypeptides with N- and C-terminal extension peptides have been called pro-α chains by some. Studies of the matrix of the Engelbreth-Holm-Swarm tumor, which is a basement membrane–like material (386), have led to a network model for the structure of type IV collagen (506). In this model there is end-to-end association of two type IV collagen molecules at the C termini and an antiparallel association of the N termini of four such dimers. The association is stabilized by disulfide and lysine-derived cross-links at both the N terminus [the 7S domain (284)] and the C terminus (NC1; Table 1) (539). Although this arrangement may apply within the tumor matrix, the situation in true basement membranes is likely to be more complex with increased lateral association of the collagen molecules (20).

In a variety of basement membranes NC1 is composed of three major subunits, M1, M2*, and M3, all of which represent transitional zones between a small collagenous region and a predominant noncollagenous region. Two polypeptides are present in M1, and judged by their amino acid sequences, these are derived from the α_1(IV) and α_2(IV) collagen chains. The amino acid sequences of M2* and M3 are distinct and have been attributed to two additional polypeptide chains of type IV collagen, α_3(IV) and α_4(IV), respectively (59). Antisera from patients with Goodpasture's syndrome react with the M2* subunit, indicating the presence of the Goodpasture antigen within this basement membrane component (59). Comparative studies of bovine anterior lens capsule, glomerular basement membrane, and placental basement membrane have shown differences in the size, shape, and subunit composition of NC1 between the three basement membranes (289).

Type IV collagen is closely associated with other macromolecules in basement membranes. Heparin binds to type IV collagen by an electrostatic interaction at three sites, one in NC1 and two in the triple helix. The interaction inhibits the aggregation of type IV collagen (515), an effect that could influence the properties of a basement membrane in circumstances in which the concentration of heparan sulfate proteoglycan (perlecan) is reduced, for example in the diabetic glomerular basement membrane (470).

C. Type V Collagen

Type V collagen was initially prepared from human fetal membranes (53) but has now been identified in a variety of tissues, including bone, cartilage, muscle (striated and non-striated), cornea, and the desmoplastic stroma of invasive carcinomas (22). The three α chains may combine to form a homotrimer $[\alpha_1(V)]_3$ or heterotrimers $[\alpha_1(V)]_2\alpha_2$ (V) and $\alpha_1(V)\alpha_2$ (V)α_3(V) (123,379). Although it is synthesized as a procollagen and undergoes proteolytic conversion, the N-terminal propeptide is not completely removed. The presence of an additional globular domain at the N terminus may explain the thin (22 nm diameter) fibrils without an axial banding pattern produced in reconstitution experiments in vitro (47). In vivo, type V collagen has been identified by immunogold labeling in 9–16 nm unbanded fibrils (352). In the embryonic chick cornea type V collagen is masked by type I, except in Bowman's layer, where thin fibrils predominate (132,306).

D. Type VI Collagen

Type VI collagen is a heterotrimer, $\alpha_1(VI)\alpha_2(VI)\alpha_3(VI)$, that appears to have a widespread distribution in connective tissues. The constituent polypeptides have molecular weights of 140 kD $[\alpha_1(VI)$ and $\alpha_2(VI)]$ and 250 kD $[\alpha_3(VI)]$, and there are at least three variants of the α_2 chain generated by alternative splicing of mRNA (79). Rotary shadowing indicates that the molecule has large globular domains at either end of a 105 nm triple helix and is deposited in the tissues without proteolytic conversion. The collagen aggregates into tetramers that are stabilized by disulfide bridges and forms microfibrils with a 100 nm periodicity (50,51). No lysine-derived cross-links have been demonstrated within the aggregates (548), and the molecule can be quantitatively extracted from cartilage with 4 M guanidine hydrochloride (117). Earlier preparation methods utilizing pepsin digestion gave the misleading impression that type VI collagen was only a minor tissue component (512).

Despite its presence in elastic tissues, such as aorta and ligamentum nuchae (11), there is no apparent relation to the microfibrils of elastic fibers (10). A study of the effects of chronic hypertension on the cerebral vasculature has indicated increased type VI collagen in the walls of both intracerebral arterioles and meningeal arteries (425). In two cases with cerebral infarcts type VI collagen could be detected in the walls of vessels as small as capillaries.

E. Type VII Collagen

Type VII collagen was first isolated from pepsin digests of human amnion (27). It occurs in tissues as a 780 nm antiparallel dimer formed from two molecules 424 nm long with an overlap of 60 nm. This overlap includes a noncollagenous globular domain at the N terminus (NC2) and is the site of interchain disulfide bridges (359); before integration into the tissues this globular domain is excised (312). Immunofluorescence studies indicate a precise correlation between the presence of type VII collagen and anchoring fibrils in tissues (433). Both are present in cornea (Bowman's layer), skin, oral mucosa, and cervix, and the presence of immunoreactive collagen type VII within cultured epithelial cells supports an origin from this cell type, with perhaps a small contribution from a subpopulation of fibroblastic cells (54,433). Sakai and colleagues (433) suggested that anchoring fibrils are composed of an unstaggered parallel array of dimers. The fibrils are closely related to basement membranes (111), and the globular extensions (NC1) at the C termini of the type VII molecules are inserted into the lamina densa, often both ends of the dimer in skin, but more commonly only one in cornea (156). Usually the anchoring fibrils are inserted at one end into amorphous "anchoring plaques" composed in part of collagen type IV (252). The NC1 domain of collagen type VII has been shown to bind to the corresponding domain of type IV collagen (54). It is believed that the "sling" produced by the anchoring fibril serves to bind the lamina densa to the underlying stroma by trapping the banded collagenous fibers.

F. Type VIII Collagen

Type VIII collagen was first identified in biosynthetic studies of cultured corneal (28) and aortic (432) endothelial cells and designated EC. Three newly synthesized collagenous polypeptides with molecular weights of 180, 120, and 60 kD were thought to be derived from a triple-helical molecule (molecular weight 560 kD) with interruptions one-third and two-thirds of the way along its length (28). Subsequent studies, including sedimentation analysis, have indicated a trimer composed of short 61 kD chains of which a 10 kD segment can be removed by pepsin treatment (29). At each end of the triple helix there is a small noncollagenous domain: NC1 (molecular weight 14–15 kD), the site of strong covalent acid-labile inter-chain cross-links, and NC2 (molecular weight 4–5 kD). There is no evidence for proteolytic conversion in vivo (29). Type VIII collagen has been identified biochemically in bovine Descemet's membrane (287), and pepsin digestion released two polypeptides (molecular weight approximately 50 kD) with distinct amino acid compositions and N-terminal amino acid sequences (240). The primary structure of the α_1(VIII) chain has now been determined from the DNA sequence, and the gene has been localized to human chromosome 3; a gene on chromosome 1 encodes a distinct α_2(VIII) collagen chain (375). A variety of normal endothelial cells (aorta, vena cava, cornea, and retinal capillary) are capable of synthesizing type VIII collagen, as are some neoplastic cells (astrocytoma and Ewing's sarcoma) in culture (431). Interestingly, in the earliest biosynthetic study on corneal endothelium (255), a 55 kD collagenous polypeptide secreted by the endothelium was detected but not further characterized.

Immunohistochemical studies have confirmed the localization of type VIII collagen in the suben-dothelial zone of large blood vessels, arterioles, and venules (266,267) and, somewhat unexpectedly, in cartilage and perichondrium (241). Within the eye, type VIII collagen has a wide distribution, being present in the anterior one-third of human Descemet's membrane (the anterior banded zone), sclera, trabecular meshwork, lamina cribrosa (adult), and the dura of the optic nerve (241,494). Despite the results of biosynthetic studies (431), human retinal capillaries do not appear to contain type VIII collagen, although the molecule is present in the wall of the central retinal artery (494).

G. Type IX Collagen

Type IX collagen was originally described as a minor collagen of cartilage released by pepsin digestion (418), but it has now been identified in both cornea and vitreous (133). It is a 190 nm long heterotrimer α_1(IX)α_2(IX)α_3(IX) with a glycosaminoglycan side chain. Three triple-helical collagenous regions (COL1–3) separate four noncollagenous domains (NC1–4) with an oblique angle in the molecule in the NC3 domain. The GAG, predominantly chondroitin-4-sulfate in cartilage and chondroitin-6-sulfate in vitreous (549), is attached to a serine residue in the NC3 domain (208).

Morphological studies with rotary shadowing indicate that the long arm (NC1-COL1-NC2-COL2-NC3) of the molecule lies alongside the fibril of type II collagen to form a discontinuous sheath with a D-periodic distribution (524). A covalent cross-link, pyridinoline, has been identified between the N-terminal telopeptides of two α_1(II) chains and the N terminus of one α_2(IX) COL2 segment (521). In the vitreous of the developing avian eye, deposition of collagen types II and IX appears to be spatially and temporally coordinated (309), but this is not true of cornea (133). The NC4 domain is a basic protein that may interact with negatively charged GAG. Compared with avian cartilage, a major portion of this domain is missing in the cornea and vitreous (491,549), and a similar difference has been noted between mammalian cartilage and vitreous (463). The functional implications of this have yet to be determined, but in the vitreous at least the shorter form is more characteristic of later stages of development, when hyalocytes have taken over the formation of the vitreous from the neural retina.

H. Type X Collagen

The biosynthesis of a low-molecular-weight collagen by chick embryo sternal chondrocytes grown in a three-dimensional gel of type I collagen was first reported by Gibson and colleagues (155). Subsequently it became apparent that this collagenous species was expressed by chondrocytes as they became hypertrophic (154,286) and that it might be a prerequisite for calcification of the matrix (219,444). The presence of two sites in the molecule that are susceptible to vertebrate collagenase may allow rapid cleavage by the enzyme and fit the protein for a remodeling function (444). Immunoelectron microscopy indicates that the collagen is concentrated in a filamentous mat close to the chondrocyte surface; farther from the cell it is found on the surface of fibrils of type II collagen (444). The newly synthesized collagenous polypeptide has a molecular weight of 59 kD, but there is disagreement about whether this undergoes proteolytic conversion to an α chain of molecular weight 49 kD (168,487). The bulk of the tissue collagen appears to be a homotrimer of 59 kD chains (444).

I. Type XI Collagen

Type XI collagen is another minor collagen of cartilage, comprising 2–3% of the collagen in adult bovine articular cartilage (117). It is a heterotrimer composed of three distinct chains, α_1, α_2, and α_3 (358). The α_1 and α_2 polypeptides resemble $\alpha_1(V)$ and $\alpha_2(V)$, respectively, but α_3 is virtually identical to $\alpha_1(II)$ and may indeed be a product of the same gene (52,527). The close relationship of collagen types V and XI is emphasized by the presence of the $\alpha_1(XI)$ chain within type V collagen in bovine bone, possibly in the form of the heterotrimer $\alpha_1(V)\alpha_2(V)\alpha_1(XI)$ (378). Similarly, $\alpha_1(V)$ has been identified within type XI collagen prepared from bovine articular cartilage (117). In vitro chondrocytes switch from the biosynthesis of predominantly type II collagen to type I collagen as they become senescent; simultaneously, biosynthesis of type V collagen is substituted for type XI (335). In cartilage, collagen types II and XI have similar distributions, and in culture, some chondrocytes contain both collagen types (493). Close biosynthetic coordination may be necessary for type XI to form the core of mixed fibrils with types II and IX (346).

J. Type XII Collagen

Type XII collagen has a partial amino acid sequence similarity to type IX collagen and is a homotrimer of three α_1 chains with a molecular weight of 220 kD. A short triple-helical segment 75 nm long is joined to a three-legged subunit with a central globular domain at the N terminus (160). It is generally found in tissues rich in type I collagen, such as tendon or ligament; although present in periosteum and perichondrium, it has not been identified in either bone matrix or cartilage (160,486). Recently, two molecules of similar structure, TL-A and TL-B, were identified in fetal calf skin, bone, and articular cartilage. TL-A, but not TL-B, has been found in cornea. In skin, TL-A is found within the papillary dermis and TL-B in the reticular dermis; immunoelectron microscopy suggests that the molecules are located along the surface of banded fibers, rather in the way that type IX collagen is associated with type II (250,313).

K. Type XIII Collagen

Type XIII collagen has not been isolated, and characterization of the collagen has depended upon sequencing of cDNA and genomic DNA. The deduced polypeptide is composed of four noncollagenous domains separated by three collagenous segments (400). The gene is unusual in that alternative splicing of the primary transcript may give rise to a number of mRNA and collagenous domains of different lengths (503). The complete α_1 chain may thus vary in length from 566 to 654 residues. Northern blotting studies have confirmed the presence of mRNA in a variety of fetal tissues, and the cellular distribution of the collagen has been determined by in situ hybridization. Epidermis, both fetal and adult, intestinal mucosa, skeletal muscle, bone (including periosteum), and cartilage all seem to be major sites of synthesis, but it is not clear whether the different gene products have specific distributions (435).

IV. MACROMOLECULAR INTERACTIONS

A.   Collagen-Proteoglycan Interactions

The diversity of proteoglycan structure (see Chap. 28) permits numerous potential interactions with the different collagen types, and these interactions may profoundly affect the form and stability of the collagen (474). Much of the early work, reviewed by Scott (452), concentrated on the electrostatic interaction of polyanionic GAG with soluble collagen and the influence of GAG and proteoglycans on the precipitation of collagen and fibrillogenesis in vitro. On the basis of these studies, Scott (452) drew the following general conclusions:

1. GAG, such as dermatan sulfate, that interact strongly with collagen accelerate fibrillogenesis.
2. GAG are not incorporated into fibrils of collagen types I and II.
3. Chondroitin sulfate proteoglycan and dermatan sulfate proteoglycan interact strongly with type I collagen and become incorporated into the growing fibril even though they actually inhibit the overall process of fibrillogenesis.

It appears that the interaction of proteoglycan with collagen occurs primarily through the core protein (459,507).

Proof of the significance of any such interaction requires its demonstration within tissue. Routine preparation of tissues for transmission electron microscopy dehydrates the proteoglycans, which collapse and precipitate randomly in the specimen. Scott and his colleagues (179,452) have developed methods for staining the proteoglycans and fixing them with their molecular arrangement with respect to the fibrillar components of connective tissue essentially undisturbed. These methods employ cationic phthalocyanin dyes (cuprolinic blue and cupromeronic blue) at controlled electrolyte concentrations. Identification of individual GAG components within the preserved proteoglycan structures can then be achieved by the use of specific GAG-degrading enzymes.

In this way D-periodic arrays of a dermatan sulfate-rich proteoglycan were demonstrated in tendon, with the molecules organized at right angles to the fibers of type I collagen (457). These proteoglycan molecules appeared to be located in the gap zone of the quarter-staggered fibril. A similar arrangement of proteoglycan molecules has been identified in this zone of collagen fibrils (type II?) in articular cartilage (385) and type I fibrils in human and rabbit sclera (551). Additional proteoglycan molecules are arranged parallel to the fibril and transversely between fibrils (452,551), and these appear to be rich in chondroitin sulfate (455). The gap zone is thought to be the nucleation site for calcium deposition in mineralized connective tissues, and the dermatan sulfate-rich proteoglycan is absent from bone collagen: Scott and Haigh (453) suggested that this proteoglycan may prevent the calcification of soft tissues.

The presence of dermatan sulfate proteoglycan on the surface of collagen may explain its ability to restrict the lateral aggregation of newly formed fibrils (455,526), and a small dermatan sulfate proteoglycan has been located at the gap zone of corneal collagen fibers (454). In addition, in rat and rabbit cornea keratan sulfate proteoglycan (lumican) is present in the zone adjacent to the gap. Mouse cornea lacks keratan sulfate, and very little proteoglycan can be demonstrated morphologically in this region of the fiber. The absence of keratan sulfate from mouse cornea suggests that this GAG does not have a critical role in the maintenance of a constant interfibrillar distance. Nevertheless, in macular corneal dystrophy type I, in which no sulfated keratan sulfate can be demonstrated in the cornea, x-ray diffraction indicates a 20% reduction in interfibrillar spacing, sufficient to account for the observed central thinning of the cornea (413).

B. Basement Membranes

In the light of current knowledge, basement membranes represent the most highly developed macro-molecular interactions within connective tissues. The last 25 years has seen an explosion of interest in these structures as their importance in tissue development, function, and pathology has become appreciated. Several detailed reviews have discussed the biochemistry of the component macromolecules and their functional significance (167,187,325,326,505). The recognition of type IV collagen as the major component of apparently all basement membranes and its almost ubiquitous association with the glycoprotein laminin and perlecan (heparan sulfate) proteoglycan encouraged a unitary view of basement structure. However, by the early 1980s it had become obvious that there was considerable diversity in basement membrane morphology and function, probably reflecting different quantities and organizations of essentially the same molecular subunits (Table 5) (167,504).

Ashton (8) defined basement membranes as ". . . acellular hyaline sheets of gellike plasticity, which are eosinophilic, and intensely periodic acid Schiff positive, and lie extracellularly in intimate relation to epithelial cells, smooth muscle cells, endothelial cells, pericytes, and nerve sheaths, and other structures, characteristically occurring at the interface between cells and connective tissue, but often, as in the case of vascular walls, between the cellular components." This definition draws particular attention to the pericellular location of the basement membrane and to the fact that virtually all cells, with the exception of connective tissue cells, such as fibroblasts and blood cells, deposit a basement membrane (118). The periodic acid-Schiff–positive basement membrane seen under the light microscope can be resolved by transmission electron microscopy into three zones:

1. Lamina rara or lucida, an electron-lucent layer, approximately 10 nm wide, immediately adjacent to the plasmalemma
2. Lamina densa, an electron-dense layer of variable thickness (20–50 nm)
3. Lamina fibroreticularis, a product of connective tissue cells that forms a transitional zone between the basement membrane and the extracellular matrix proper

Table 5   Macromolecular Components of Basement Membranes

Collagen type IV	Molecular weight: 540 kDa (monomer). Capable of self-assembly into network by (i) end-to-end and (ii) lateral interactions (203). Highly cross-linked by: (i) intra-/inter-molecular disulfide bonds (ii) lysine-derived cross-links.
Laminin	Noncollagenous glycoprotein of molecular weight 900 kDa; 13% carbohydrate. Cross-shaped molecule composed of 3 disulfide-bonded polypeptides. Structural variants; discrete functional domains. Capable of polymerization. Binds to type IV collagen (intact helix). First matrix protein formed during embryogenesis.
Entactin (Nidogen)	Noncollagenous glycoprotein of molecular weight 150 kDa. 5% carbohydrate; sulfated tyrosine residue. Single polypeptide, highly sensitive to proteases. Binds to laminin (high affinity) and type IV collagen (weaker).
Heparan sulfate-proteoglycan (HSPG)	Molecular weight: 620–720 kDa. Protein core: (i) single polypeptide (500 kDa) and (ii) probable interaction site with laminin and type IV collagen. HS: 3 chains at one end of core protein. Possible storage site for growth factors (204).
BM-40	Ca-binding protein of molecular weight 40 kDa.
Others	Fibronectin (205), merosin (206), bullous pemphigoid antigen (207), amyloid P protein (208)

Zones (1) and (2) constitute the basal lamina, an ultrastructural term. In certain sites, most particularly the glomerular basement membrane, a second lamina rara is substituted for the lamina fibroreticularis since this basement membrane results from the fusion of two distinct cellular basement membranes (500).

The heterogeneity of basement membranes has been demonstrated in several ways. The susceptibility of laminin and type IV collagen to digestion by *Streptomyces griseus* proteinase differs between sites and also between normal basement membranes and those produced by malignant cells (296). Grant and Leblond (163) compared the distribution of type IV collagen, laminin, and heparan sulfate proteoglycan in a series of thick (such as Reichert's membrane) and thin (such as renal tubular) basement membranes and used the density of immunogold label to compare the concentrations of the macromolecules. They found the concentrations of collagen and laminin to be higher in thick basement membranes and that of proteoglycan to be higher in thin. Rat Descemet's membrane was the only ocular basement membrane studied, and the concentration of type IV collagen was relatively low, confirming the unusual nature of this structure (see Descemet's membrane Sec. V.A). In general, Grant and Leblond (163) were able to demonstrate all three components in both lamina densa and lamina rara. The early studies of glomerular basement membrane clearly localized the heparan sulfate proteoglycan to the laminae rarae (119), but subsequent reports have indicated considerable variation between basement membranes in the location of the glycan side chains (274).

There is general agreement that type IV collagen is principally located within the lamina densa. Although this has an amorphous, rather granular appearance, its fibrillar substructure may be revealed by treatment with proteolytic enzymes (71). The revealed fibrils have a diameter of 3–8 nm, most being about 4 nm. The concentration of macromolecules within the lamina densa, which in certain sites may include lipid (158), makes this the likely site of maximal interaction. Basement membrane macromolecules extracted in 2 M urea form a gel when dialyzed against 0.15 M NaCl at neutral pH and then warmed to 35°C for 1 h (269). The gel contains laminin (60%), collagen type IV (30%), heparan sulfate proteoglycan (3%), and noncollagenous glycoproteins (6%), linked by strong, but noncovalent, bonds. Ultrastructural examination of the gel reveals a network of electron-dense material resembling lamina densa and composed of 5 nm diameter fibrils. Most interestingly, the gel is able to support the adhesion, growth, and differentiation of a melanoma cell line, endothelial cells, and hepatocytes (269). Although there are a number of ways in which such macromolecular complexes could assemble into a basement membrane (560), they all depend on the flexibility of the triple helix of collagen type IV (504) and its ability to undergo end-to-end and lateral associations with other molecules of type IV collagen (559).

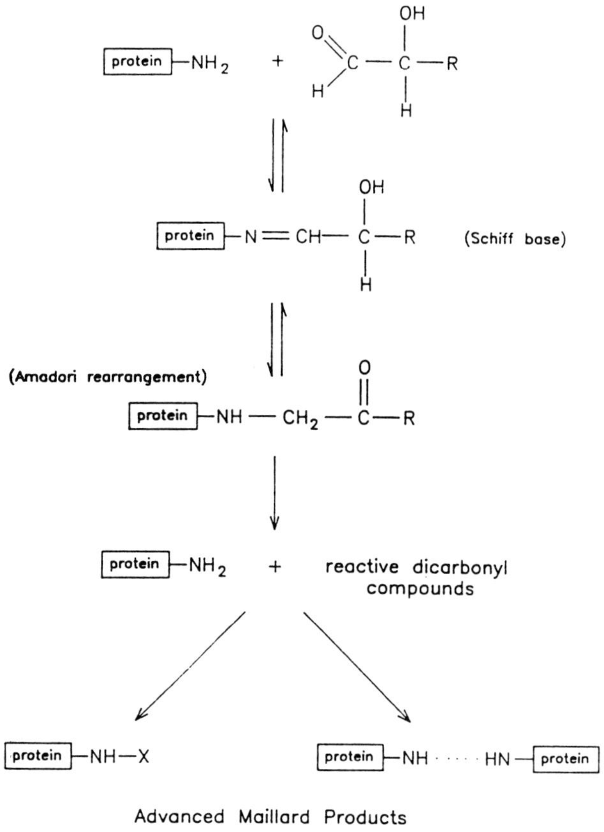

Advanced Maillard Products

Figure 2   The Maillard reaction.

C.   Nonenzymatic Glycosylation

It has been known for almost a century that nonenzymatic reactions between the carbonyl groups of sugar molecules and free amino groups of proteins result in the formation of insoluble brown products. Although initially of particular concern to the food industry, this nonenzymatic browning or Maillard reaction has become a focus of medical interest because of the value of glycosylated hemoglobin as an index of glycemic control in diabetes mellitus and the possible role of glycosylated proteins in the pathogenesis of the complications of this disorder (49,258). Also, since the changes of aging occur predominantly in tissues composed of proteins with a very low turnover rate, such as lens and arterial wall, accumulation of the end products of the Maillard reaction has been advanced as a mechanism for many of these changes (354).

The Maillard reaction (Fig. 2) commences with the nonenzymatic condensation of a reducing sugar with a free amino group on a protein molecule to form a Schiff base (380). An Amadori rearrangement results in the formation of a stable ketoamine, which may be transformed, however, into highly reactive compounds with α-dicarbonyl groups. These in turn may be degraded or react further with amino groups to form such compounds as pyrroles. Additional reactions generate brown, fluorescent compounds, such as 2-(2-furoyl)-4(5)-(2-furanyl)-1H-imidazole, that may serve to cross-link proteins (405).

Collagen in all its forms has numerous ϵ-amino groups of lysine and hydroxylysine along the polypeptide chain in addition to the α-amino group at the N terminus. The condensation of hexose residues with the ϵ-amino groups was demonstrated by the isolation of N-ϵ-hexosyllysine and N-ϵ-hexosyl-hydroxylysine from acid hydrolysates of borohydride-reduced collagen (422). The quantities of the hexosyl-amino acids were found to be increased in older tissues (423). Subsequent studies have indicated that these initial glycosylation products contribute to the formation of stable intermolecular bonds (14). Fibers of interstitial collagen, when incubated in vitro with glucose, display increased mechanical strength and shrinkage temperatures indicative of increased numbers of heat-stable covalent cross-links within the fibers. Cyanogen bromide digestion of the fibers reveals increased amounts of high-molecular-weight material. The chemical identity of these cross-links has not yet been clearly established, although 2-(2-furoyl)-4(5)-(2-furanyl)-1H-imidazole is one candidate (14).

In view of the slow turnover of collagen and its extracellular location, an increased level of glycosylation of the molecule in diabetics was not unexpected (448). This was associated with a decrease in the solubility of dermal collagen, particularly in juvenile-onset diabetics (448). It seems unlikely that the ketoamine cross-link is responsible for the decreased solubility of the collagen (317), but advanced Maillard products may be important. Following incubation of insoluble collagen with glucose, a covalently bound product is formed that fluoresces at 440 nm when excited at 370 nm. This fluorescence, probably associated with an advanced Maillard product, is increased twofold in dermal collagen from insulin-dependent diabetics, and the intensity of fluorescence (adjusted for age) increases with increased duration of diabetes and severity of retinopathy (355). The concentration of advanced Maillard products in the lens nucleus is correlated with the severity of retinopathic changes in diabetics (383). Diabetics are prone to a wide variety of connective tissue abnormalities, many characterized by an inappropriate deposition of collagen (95). Two of the more common abnormalities are Dupuytren's contracture (381) and limited joint mobility in the hand (428), and both of these are associated with the presence of diabetic retinopathy, particularly proliferative retinopathy (24,292,428). It is tempting to ascribe the fibrosis to the diminished solubility of glycosylated collagen. There is, however, no apparent difference in the level of nonenzymatic glycosylation of skin collagen between diabetics with limited joint mobility and those without (316). Nevertheless, levels of advanced Maillard products have not been determined, so differences in intermolecular cross-links cannot be excluded.

Nonenzymatic glycosylation of basement membrane collagen has been demonstrated both in vivo (87,398) and in vitro (14). Basement membrane collagen may indeed be more susceptible than interstitial collagen because of the thinner fibers and the higher content of lysine plus hydroxylysine. The studies of Bailey and Kent (14) on bovine lens capsule support the formation of additional intermolecular cross-links following glycosylation, and such modifications could alter the physical properties of the basement membrane.

Although much attention has been paid to the condensation of glucose with proteins, it should be remembered that all reducing sugars may participate in the Maillard reaction, together with other compounds, such as ascorbate (354). Indeed, pentoses, including fructose, are considerably more reactive than glucose. This may have relevance to diabetic retinopathy since fructose produces a similar retinopathy in rats fed a sucrose-rich diet (40). A pentose-derived cross-link, pentosidine, has been isolated from insoluble human skin collagen: levels increase with age and in type I diabetes mellitus with renal failure and retinopathy (465).

V. COLLAGEN IN THE EYE

A. Cornea

The anatomical simplicity of the cornea is deceptive. Within this tissue three types of cells, epithelial, endothelial, and fibroblastic, synthesize and interact with a variety of collagens and other matrix macromolecules to produce a strong, transparent tissue (182). The connective tissue elements are organized into four distinct layers: the corneal epithelial basement membrane, Bowman's layer, the stroma, and the corneal endothelial basement membrane (Descemet's membrane).

Epithelial Basement Membrane

The epithelial basement membrane of the cornea is synthesized by the epithelium and is composed of type IV collagen (92,277,371,488), the helical portion of which has been shown to promote both adhesion and migration of the epithelial cells (64). The collagen is less readily demonstrable by immunofluorescence in the corneal epithelial basement membrane than in the adjacent conjunctival basement membrane (84,145). In addition to type IV collagen, laminin, fibronectin, and bullous pemphigoid antigen have also been detected in the basement membrane (92,350).

In the central cornea the basal surface of the epithelium is flat and the basement membrane is composed of a lamina rara and a continuous lamina densa. At the periphery, where the basal surface undulates, the lamina densa is reduplicated, with apparent focal discontinuities (44). The unilaminar basement membrane of the central cornea is 105 ± 22.7 nm thick at birth and thickens with age at a rate of approximately 3 nm per annum (4). More importantly, after the second decade, foci of reduplication are seen, often within excavations of Bowman's layer. Eventually the central basement membrane becomes completely multilaminar and markedly thickened. In early life anchoring filaments penetrate deeply (as much as 2 μm) into Bowman's layer, contributing to epithelial adhesion (156). Later their length is insufficient to traverse the multilaminar basement membrane, and bullous separation becomes more frequent.

Corneal epithelial basement membrane thickening has been reported in diabetes mellitus (496) and as a secondary effect in epithelial dystrophies, such as Meesmann's (126,511) and map-dot-fingerprint "dystrophy" (see Chap. 23) (86,376,424).

Discontinuities in the basement membrane have been described in buphthalmos and may account for the diminished epithelial integrity in this condition (407,523).

Bowman's Layer

Although it is almost 150 years since Sir William Bowman recognized this distinct subepithelial layer in the human cornea, it remains something of an enigma. In histological sections it stands out as a 9–12 μm thick, acellular, homogeneous band separated from the epithelium by the basement membrane. Long considered to be a modified region of the anterior stroma (248), it is still uncertain whether it is synthesized by the corneal epithelium or the stromal keratocytes. Perhaps its most intriguing feature is its inability to regenerate following injury: defects are repaired by either a downgrowth of epithelium (an epithelial facet) or scar tissue.

Bowman's layer is essentially restricted to primate eyes and is composed of a random meshwork of collagen fibers, with a diameter approximately two-thirds that of the stromal fibers, 25 versus 33 nm (248) (Fig. 3). This random orientation is seen in both perpendicular and tangential sections. The posterior border merges with the lamellae of the stroma proper. The nature of the collagen has not been clearly established by immunofluorescence studies. Newsome and colleagues (371) reported the presence of both type I and type III collagen, whereas others have identified type IV (26) and type V (277). Immunogold localization of collagens within the human cornea indicates that types I, III, V, and VI are present in Bowman's layer, but not type IV (322,323). In the embryonic chick eye Bowman's layer is a 4 μm wide zone that represents the residue of the anterior primary stroma following formation of the secondary stroma. It is an epithelial product and is composed of types I, II, and V collagens (35,182). The collagen in this region of the avian stroma appears to be particularly stable (307).

Bowman's layer provides a barrier to corneal invasion by tumors and pathogenic organisms. It may be damaged in a number of diseases, including keratoconus, in which multiple breaks occur (see Chap. 23). Focal defects of Bowman's layer are a feature of Reis-Bücklers dystrophy (see Chap. 40). Bowman's layer dysgenesis has been described as a cause of congenital corneal opacification: it is characterized by uniform thickening with or without the presence of keratocytes and without apparent disturbance of the collagenous organization (6,194). The thickening is not always associated with corneal opacification, as in the Smith-Lemli-Opitz syndrome of microcephaly, ambiguous male genitalia, syndactyly, and failure to thrive (281). Absence of the central part of Bowman's layer occurs in various forms of anterior segment mesenchymal dysgenesis, including Peters' anomaly (368), sclerocornea (144), and posterior keratoconus (484), and complete agenesis, has been described (244).

Stroma

The stroma occupies about 90% of the thickness of the cornea and about 80% of its dry weight is collagen (332). The collagen fibers are arranged in lamellae that appear to extend from corneoscleral limbus to corneoscleral limbus. The posterior stromal lamellae are slightly thicker than those in the anterior one-third (0.2–2.5 versus 0.2–2.1 μm) and have a more definite orientation parallel to the corneal surface (276). This may explain the greater ease of dissection in the posterior stroma during lamellar keratoplasty. In the center of the cornea there is little or no interweaving of collagen fibers from adjacent lamellae, but this occurs peripherally and contributes to a greater interlamellar adhesive strength in this region (473). Between the lamellae there is a planar network of fibroblastic cells (keratocytes) that can be demonstrated by scanning electron microscopy following treatment of the cornea with trypsin and 8 M hydrochloric acid (377). Along the optic axis adjacent lamellae are arranged at an angle of slightly less than 90°; in humans

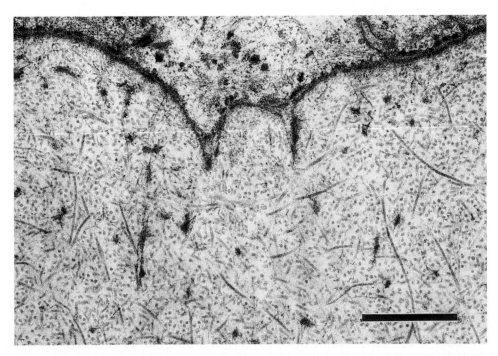

Figure 3   The anterior border of Bowman's layer in human cornea. The layer is composed of a random feltwork of fine collagen fibrils. (Uranyl acetate–lead citrate stain, scale bar 1.0 μm)

the collagen lamellae of the anterior stroma manifest little preferred orientation, but a more orthogonal pattern is seen in the posterior stroma (343).

The morphology of the individual collagen fibers has been the subject of many investigations. The most systematic study was undertaken by Craig and Parry (94), who measured fiber diameters in 28 species from all vertebrate groups. With the exception of adult bony fish, which had a mean fiber diameter of 16 nm, all species had the same mean fiber diameter of 24–25 nm, and contrary to many earlier reports, this was true at all levels of the cornea. There was a slight diminution in diameter to 17 nm in the region immediately anterior to Descemet's membrane in chick, rat, and magpie (94), and the collagen in this region is thought to have a greater stability (307). In rat and human cornea the mean fiber diameter in the fetus was 17 nm, the adult value being achieved shortly after birth (94). In addition to a smaller fiber diameter, bony fish also have a lower interfibrillar distance (<52 nm), calculated from the first-order equatorial diffraction ring, than birds and mammals (>59 nm) (288). Synchrotron x-ray diffraction has also revealed a unique feature of human cornea: there are preferred fiber orientations, inferior-superior and medial-lateral, that produce four distinct lobes of intensity in the diffraction ring (177).

The morphogenesis of the corneal stroma has been extensively studied in the embryonic chick (182). The corneal epithelium lays down a primary stroma of type I and type II (about 40%) collagen, which overlap in distribution (196,308). The epithelium also synthesizes and secretes type IX collagen, but this disappears relatively early in development (133,309), possibly triggering stromal swelling and subsequent infiltration by mesenchymal cells. The fibers of the primary stroma are arranged orthogonally, and the mesenchymal cells align themselves with a corresponding orthogonal orientation of the cell processes. The deposition of the collagen fibers of the secondary stroma occurs close to the cell surface, and the disposition of the cell processes ensures an orthogonal pattern of fibers as the lamellae of the secondary stroma form (34).

Some type II collagen is left in the subepithelial stroma (and Descemet's membrane), but this gradually decreases with time and is undetectable after hatching (196). The secondary stroma shows a uniform distribution of type I collagen together with types V and VI (36,310). Types I and V are closely associated, apparently within the same fiber (36). Based on the sensitivity of type V collagen to mammalian collagenase and the masking of its immunoreactivity unless fibrillar structure is disrupted, for example by acetic acid treatment, type V collagen appears to be buried within the fiber (131). Biosynthetic studies of stromal keratocytes obtained from late (>15 days) chick embryos indicate production of predominantly type I procollagen with 5–10% of type V collagen (239,406). The cells are also capable of synthesizing type III collagen, but this is probably repressed in vivo, perhaps by keratan sulfate proteoglycan (lumican) (89).

The morphogenesis of the mammalian stroma is simpler in that there is no primary stroma. The mesenchymal cells destined to be keratocytes migrate from the lip of the optic vesicle between the differentiating epithelia of lens and cornea. In the rabbit this occurs at about day 13–14 of gestation, and 1 day later 30 nm fibers may be seen between the stromal fibroblasts (82). The keratocytes deposit an orthogonal matrix of collagen, a property they retain in vitro (56). A number of different collagen types have been reported in the mammalian stroma, but there is general agreement that type I collagen is quantitatively the most important.

Type I constitutes 80–95% of the collagen in bovine (294,514), rabbit (83,293,542), and human (372) stroma. Cultures of human keratocytes synthesize predominantly type I together with type V collagen (37,554). As in the embryonic chick, type V collagen appears to be the second major component, comprising 6–15% of the collagen mass (83,101,293,294,372). Type III collagen has been reported in some (293,294,372,409,445,514) but not all (101,542) studies. Where it has been found the amount appears to diminish with aging (293,294,514): in the 2-day-old rabbit type III collagen accounts for 2.2% of the collagen solubilized by pepsin from the corneal stroma, whereas at 14 days and at 2 years the value has declined to 0.6 and 0.0% respectively (293). The proportion of type V collagen increased during this period from 4.8 to 8.1% (293). The mouse appears to be unusual in that not only is type I collagen demonstrable in the stroma but also type IV (408), in conjunction with laminin associated with an 8–11 nm diameter microfibril, and perhaps even type II collagen (180). The latter finding has yet to be confirmed. On the basis of chemical analysis (3,81,563) and immunohistochemical studies (78,362), type VI collagen has been added to the list of collagens found in mammalian as well as avian (310) stroma. Recent experiments suggest that fibroblastic cells bind more strongly to native type VI collagen than to type I collagen and type VI collagen provides a better environment for spreading of the cells (106). Immunoelectron microscopic studies of human cornea have confirmed the presence of collagen types I, III, V, and VI within the stroma (322,323).

Descemet's Membrane

Although similar to other basement membranes in that it stains intensely with the periodic acid-Schiff stain and contains type IV collagen, Descemet's membrane has many unusual features. It is appreciably thicker than most basement membranes, and in the human its thickness increases from 3 μm at birth to 12.5 μm or more in old age (231,363,537). Cogan (85) pointed out its affinity for elastic tissue stains and that its edges tended to curl when it was cut or broken. Furthermore, the basement membrane showed considerable, although not complete, resistance to penetration and destruction by either leukocytes or tumor cells (85). The provision of mechanical strength to the anterior segment of the eye appears to be a major function of Descemet's membrane. Thus exposure of the cornea to alkali (369) or to a fulminating bacterial infection (169) may cause extensive loss of the stroma until only Descemet's membrane persists, often in the form of a thinned bulging membrane (descemetocele), as the last barrier to perforation of the globe.

Early comparative studies on the ultrastructure of Descemet's membrane were carried out by Jakus (221), who observed in tangential sections a regular hexagonal array of electron-dense nodes connected by thick filaments, with an internodal distance of approximately 107 nm (Fig. 4). Transverse sections indicated that hexagonal arrays were stacked upon each other with the nodes aligned perpendicularly (Fig. 5). This arrangement was seen in bovine and chick Descemet's membrane (221). Human Descemet's membrane is particularly intriguing. As described by Jakus (221,222), the anterior 3 μm (the anterior banded zone), which is deposited during fetal life, is composed of 30–40 compacted lamellae, each a hexagonal array. Although the orientation of the lamellae is less precise than in bovine Descemet's membrane, they are held in alignment by fine interlamellar fibrils 170 nm long, 40 nm wide, and 110–120 nm apart (363). Postnatally the basement membrane thickens by the apposition of nonbanded material, such that by the age of 60 years it is 12.5 μm thick (363). In this posterior nonbanded zone occasional collagen fibers with characteristic 64 nm periodicity and fusiform bundles of long-spacing collagen (periodicity 120 nm) can be seen (363). Similar fusiform structures are present in the Hassall-Henle warts

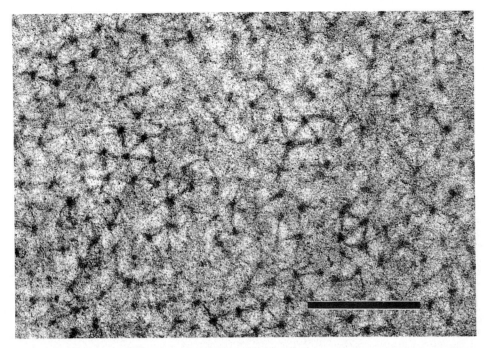

Figure 4   Tangential section of bovine Descemet's membrane. The hexagonal array of nodes and filaments is partially obscured by amorphous granular material. (Uranyl acetate–lead citrate stain, scale bar 0.5 μm)

Figure 5   Perpendicular section through bovine Descemet's membrane. The periodicity results from stacking of the nodes in vertical register. (Uranyl acetate–lead citrate stain, scale bar 0.5 μm)

that develop on peripheral Descemet's membrane with advancing years (121,222), but immunochemical identity has not been established and the relationship to the macromolecular components of the anterior banded zone is also unknown. Endothelial disturbances are reflected in an altered ultrastructure of Descemet's membrane, which thus provides a historical record of the fetal and postnatal function of the endothelium (12).

Following the demonstration by Pirie (403) that bovine lens capsule was collagenous in nature, Dohlman and Balazs (107) identified collagen as the major component of bovine Descemet's membrane and suggested that it was associated with a tyrosine-rich, noncollagenous protein. Kefalides and Denduchis (254) found considerable similarity between the amino acid compositions of anterior lens capsule and Descemet's membrane but noted the higher tyrosine content of the latter (21 versus 11 residues per 1000). Subsequently Kefalides (253) isolated type IV collagen from pepsin digests of both basement membranes. Further investigation with analytical, biosynthetic, and immunohistochemical studies has suggested a wide range of component macromolecules. Collagen types I, II, and V have been isolated from bovine Descemet's membrane in addition to type IV (294,514). This may simply be the result of stromal contamination, although bovine corneal endothelial cells in culture synthesize the same collagens with a predominance of type III collagen (436,513). Other studies of bovine Descemet's membrane have indicated the presence of collagen types IV and VIII as the major components (287,288), and this is supported by biosynthetic experiments in vitro with rabbit corneal endothelium (28,247,255,261). Immunohistochemical studies of human cornea have confirmed the presence of collagen types IV and VIII within Descemet's membrane (26,371,494).

Correlation of the morphology and function of Descemet's membrane with its biochemical composition is as yet fragmentary. The amino acid composition of the basement membrane changes with age, but the significance of this in terms of either subunit composition or function is unknown (143). Despite the elastic properties of the basement membrane, it is completely solubilized by treatment with 0.1 M sodium hydroxide at 100°C for 45 minutes and therefore cannot contain insoluble elastin (190). However, the lysine-derived cross-links of insoluble elastin, desmosine and isodesmosine, have been identified in bovine Descemet's membrane and are located within a relatively insoluble "core" enriched in tyrosine, alanine, and valine that is resistant to digestion with purified bacterial collagenase (190). Although the molecular site of these cross-links has yet to be established, ultrastructural examination of the core suggests that they are located within the nodes of the hexagonal arrays. Sawada (439) has confirmed that the nodes are relatively resistant to collagenase digestion. A report based on immunoelectron microscopy with horseradish peroxidase that the nodes in bovine Descemet's membrane were composed of types III and IV collagen (441) could not be substantiated when colloidal gold was substituted as label (440). Indeed, this report could find no evidence for collagen types I, II, III, IV, or VI in the hexagonal array (440). Marshall and colleagues (322,323), also using immunogold localization, were able to identify type IV collagen within the posterior nonbanded zone and, to a lesser extent, within the anterior banded zone.

Apart from providing mechanical strength to the anterior segment, perhaps by virtue of its desmosine cross-links and disulfide bonds (39), the Descemet's membrane–endothelial cell complex may contribute to stromal integrity (see Sect. VII.A).

B. Sclera

Despite its importance in protecting the delicate intraocular structures and in preventing distortion of the light-sensitive elements during movement of the globe, the sclera has received little attention. This in part reflects the limited involvement of the sclera in disease processes other than inflammation.

The differentiation of the periocular mesenchyme into sclera begins in the human fetus at about 6 weeks of gestation. Maturation proceeds in an anteroposterior direction and from the inner to the outer surface (388,466). Nonbanded, presumably collagenous fibers with a diameter of 27–29 nm are seen in the extracellular matrix at about 6 weeks, and as fiber diameter gradually increases, the fibers become organized into lamellae. By 13 weeks of gestation histological differences between the pre- and post-equatorial sclera have disappeared, and the adult organization is evident by 24 weeks (466). At this time the fiber diameter is the same in the inner and outer sclera; sometime thereafter this changes so that in the adult sclera the outer fibers are thicker than the inner (97,478,551). Published figures for fiber diameter in the adult human are somewhat variable, presumably reflecting differences in tissue fixation and, perhaps, age of the subjects (538), but those of Spitznas (478) are representative: average diameter of inner collagen fibers, 62 nm, and of outer collagen fibers, 125 nm. Changes in fiber diameter during scleral development have been well documented in *Macaca mulatta* (Table 3) (388). Of particular interest in this study was the relative constancy of corneal fiber diameter compared with sclera. This may result from differences in macromolecular interactions in the two tissues since it was also noted that cross-striations became apparent at a later stage of development in cornea and were never as clearly visible as in sclera (388).

Biochemical studies have shown that type I collagen is the major component in both bovine (445) and human (249) sclera. This type accounts for approximately 94% of the total collagen, the remainder being type III (142,249), although the proportion of the latter is higher in young animals (445). Type II collagen is found in the hyaline cartilage of the avian posterior sclera (509). These results have been confirmed in immunohistochemical studies using purified type-specific antibodies. Collagen types I and III are present in the fibrous sclera of the embryonic chick and type II in the cartilaginous sclera; the scleral perichondrium consists of type I collagen (528). Konomi and colleagues (278) were able to detect only type I collagen in the sclera of normal human eyes, type III being confined to the lamina cribrosa. In an eye from a 31-year-old patient with Marfan syndrome, the posterior scleral lamellae were in disarray and collagen type III was demonstrable in that area (278). Others have demonstrated type III as well as type I collagen in the scleral spur (364), possibly reflecting the need for this part of the eye wall to change configuration in response to accommodation and intraocular pressure.

Analytical studies indicate that scleral collagen is stabilized by divalent aldimine and ketoamine cross-links in the embryo; only the aldimine is detectable in young individuals, and mature sclera contains a complex cross-link but no pyridinoline (13).

In both human and rabbit sclera proteoglycans have been demonstrated by electron microscopic histochemistry on the surface of the collagen fibers and extending between adjacent fibers (551). The GAG of sclera (dermatan sulfate, chondroitin sulfate, and hyaluronic acid) are different from those in cornea (keratan sulfate and chondroitin), and this may be the basis of the larger diameter of scleral collagen fibers (41).

C. Trabecular Meshwork

The importance of the trabecular meshwork in aqueous outflow and its characteristic morphology have long drawn attention to this structure. An early idea that the accumulation of extracellular matrix material might provide a mechanical block to aqueous outflow and thus cause chronic simple glaucoma (125,426) focused attention on the matrix of the meshwork. The early ultrastructural studies documented the major components of the matrix but provided a somewhat confused picture, with descriptions of different kinds of plaques and fibers (314).

The major matrix structures are the focally discontinuous subendothelial basal lamina and loose granular connective tissue containing banded collagen fibrils and electron-dense cores surrounded by a sheath of wide-spacing collagen (341). In a morphometric study McMenamin and Lee (341) observed a decrease in the proportion of loose matrix with age and a corresponding increase in the proportion of the extracellular space occupied by the central dense core and the sheath of wide-spacing collagen. The proportion of basement membrane material did not change significantly, although above the age of 60 years there was a greater variation in the thickness of the basal lamina. It has not been conclusively proven that these changes are accentuated in glaucoma, and quantitative analysis of collagen within normal and glaucomatous meshwork by hydroxyproline estimation assay and sirius red dye binding has shown no significant difference (128). Such analyses are inherently crude and could easily miss small but important changes in the amounts of individual collagens.

Immunofluorescence studies with purified antibodies to connective tissue macromolecules have shed some light on the molecular complexity of the various matrix structures. Beneath the endothelial cells in the basement membrane zone, collagen types III and V, fibronectin, and basement membrane constituents (collagen type IV, laminin, and heparan sulfate proteoglycan) have been identified (364). Collagen type III, together with type I and elastin, is present within the central core. Collagen type I and elastin are not found in the juxtacanalicular region. The relative contributions of elastin and the collagens to the configurational response of the meshwork to intraocular pressure (233) remain unknown.

The sheath of wide-spacing collagen has been reported to increase in thickness with both age and chronic glaucoma (427). This wide-spacing collagen, which may also be found in the subendothelial basal lamina and beneath the inner wall of Schlemm's canal, has been identified as collagen type VI by means of immunoelectron microscopy using affinity-purified antibodies to human placental collagen type VI (315). It is not normally seen in mouse trabecular meshwork but can be induced in vitro by incubating segments of tissue with ATP at 37°C for 2 h under acid conditions (203), conditions in which type VI collagen forms 100 nm periodic fibrils (51). In a comprehensive immunoelectron microscopic study of the aged human outflow system, however, Marshall and colleagues (321) were unable to confirm that the material was type VI collagen and concluded from their review that at present "there is no justification for classifying this material as a collagen." These authors demonstrated type VI collagen, in association with type V, in a fine network around the striated fibrils of the cores of the trabecular beams. Somewhat surprisingly, the subendothelial basal lamina of the beams was found to contain collagen types I and III (321), in addition to the anticipated type IV (201,319). Type IV collagen was also present in the subendothelial material of the juxtacanalicular region (319).

Trabecular endothelial cells from a variety of species have been cultured and shown to synthesize collagenous proteins (types I, III, IV, V, and VI), noncollagenous glycoproteins (laminin and fibronectin), and proteoglycans (172,201,285,556,558). Grierson and colleagues (172) were unable to demonstrate the biosynthesis of type IV collagen by cultured bovine trabecular cells, consistent with the absence of a definite subendothelial basal lamina in the bovine trabecular beams, although type IV collagen has been recognized in the bovine endothelial cell matrix by immunohistochemical methods (285).

D. Lamina Cribrosa

Just as the trabecular meshwork may be considered a modification of the scleral coat, so may the lamina cribrosa. Tengroth and Ammitzboll (498) noted that in human eyes obtained postmortem the collagen content of both lamina and meshwork (estimated as nmol hydroxyproline per mg defatted, dried tissue) was considerably lower than in the sclera proper, 700 versus 350 (lamina cribrosa) and 440 (trabecular meshwork). In glaucoma the collagen contents of the optic disk and meshwork were increased, but this was not true of sclera. The increase achieved statistical significance only in the lamina. Since the increase was also found in eyes with raised intraocular pressure but no optic disk abnormality, the authors suggested that the change preceded the axonal degeneration and may represent the primary lesion in chronic open-angle glaucoma (498). Subsequent immunohistochemical studies from the same laboratory (419,499) indicated similarities in the collagen composition of the lamina cribrosa and trabecular meshwork (collagen types I, III, and IV), which was different from that of sclera (type I only). This finding is supported by the immunohistochemical report of Konomi and colleagues (278); the detection of small amounts of collagen type III in sclera by biochemical analysis (142,445) could have resulted from contamination of the sclera with lamina cribrosa, meshwork, or uvea. Although the idea of abnormal collagen metabolism underlying both the malfunction of the meshwork and the weakness of the lamina cribrosa is appealing, no firm evidence in its favor has yet been advanced.

A more detailed immunohistochemical analysis of the extracellular matrix of the lamina cribrosa in both normal and glaucomatous eyes is now available (198,199). The connective tissue plates contain a core of elastin, collagen types I, III, and VI, and a fine filamentous network of collagen type IV. At the edge of the plate collagen type VI can be found, and the plates are covered by a basement membrane, of presumed glial origin, composed of collagen type IV and laminin (198,200). The collagenous components of the laminar plates appear to increase with age, although the basement membrane covering the plates did not thicken (198). In cases of primary open-angle glaucoma the major changes were in respect to collagen types IV and VI, the amounts of which increased in the cores of the cribriform plates (199). Collagen type IV was also increased in the prelaminar region of the optic nerve head, where it is produced by glial cells (200). The change became more marked as the severity of the glaucoma increased. It has been reported that in glaucoma the distribution of collagen fiber diameter in the lamina cribrosa (normal mean 50 nm) is shifted toward that of sclera (normal mean 75 nm) (414), but the molecular basis of this change has not been established and the relationship to alterations in amounts of collagen types IV and VI is not readily apparent.

In experimental studies of glaucomatous optic atrophy in monkeys, Morrison and colleagues (361) noted a marked increase in the quantity of glial basal lamina and type IV collagen between the disorderly laminar plates. Similar changes were observed in optic atrophy secondary to transection of the optic nerve, although thickening of the basal lamina appeared to be specific for severe glaucomatous atrophy. Deposits of collagen types I and III were also seen between the laminar plates. These changes are presumably secondary since they were detected only in those monkeys with severe glaucomatous damage (361). Since the extracellular matrix of the optic nerve head may be altered by both aging and elevated intraocular pressure, it follows that the level of intraocular pressure an individual eye is able to tolerate may change with age. Although the significance of the molecular changes in the matrix is far from clear, the architectural features of the lamina (for review see Ref. 113) provide an explanation of the pattern of neural degeneration in glaucoma (see Chap. 16).

Observations on the connective tissue framework of the optic nerve, the retrolaminar pial septa, have, not surprisingly, shown considerable similarities in composition to the cribriform plates. The major macromolecular components appear to be collagen types I and III, with type IV in the basement membranes of the blood vessels and covering the septa (198,360,419). Collagen type VI has been identified at the edge of the septa (199). The elastin and collagen (types I and III) contents of the septa increase with age, but changes specific to glaucoma are not seen (198,199,361). In situ hybridization studies using radioactively labeled cDNA probes for mRNA of collagen types I and IV have confirmed that the collagen type IV on the surface of the septa is a product of glial cells located there (200). This material appears to be increased in amount in optic atrophy whatever the cause, presumably as a nonspecific response to axonal loss (361).

E. Uvea

All parts of the uvea show some degree of sclerosis with age, and this particularly affects the blood vessels (538). Atrophy of ciliary muscle in secondary glaucoma is accompanied by atrophy of the connective tissue stroma of the ciliary body and processes (518). Proliferation of nonpigmented ciliary epithelial cells in a coronal adenoma is accompanied by deposition of a periodic acid-Schiff–positive matrix containing predominantly collagen type IV with some type I (48).

The collagens of the uveal tract have not been well characterized. Following careful dissection of the uveal components from bovine eyes, Schmut (446) used pepsin to solubilize the collagen, which was subsequently purified by differential salt precipitation and analyzed by sodium dodecyl sulfate–polyacrylamide gel electrophoresis (SDS-PAGE) and cyanogen bromide (CNBr) digestion. The collagen constituted 49 ± 9, 41 ± 8, and $49\pm6\%$ of the dry weights of iris, ciliary body, and choroid, respectively. Within the iris the distribution of collagen was not uniform, accounting for 58% of the dry weight of the iris root but only 11% of the peripupillary iris (446). Collagen types I and III were identified (446) and appear to be the major components of the iris and choroidal stroma (278,279).

Immunoelectron microscopic studies have since confirmed the importance of these two collagen types in the iris blood vessels (279). Type I collagen occurred with type IV in the endothelial and pericyte basement membranes and with type III in the tunica adventitia. The signal intensity for type I was greater in the larger vessels, but this was not so for type IV. Within the blood vessels of the ciliary body there is a similar distribution of collagen types (324). Collagen type I was also identified in the basement membranes of the iris pigment epithelium and the dilator muscle (279). In the aged human eye the basement membranes of the nonpigmented and pigmented ciliary epithelia and the ciliary muscle contain not only collagen types I and IV but also type III, possibly reflecting the exposure to biomechanical forces of these structures (324).

F. Lens Capsule

The capsule is the only collagenous structure of the crystalline lens. It is the thickest basement membrane of the body, some 20–25 μm thick in the central anterior region (464), and turns over slowly (129,178). Because of its ease of isolation, it has been the subject of much intensive investigation since Pirie (403) first established its collagenous nature by chemical analysis and x-ray diffraction. Subsequent x-ray diffraction studies (429) indicated that the collagen had a poorly defined quarter-staggered structure consistent with the ultrastructural appearance of narrow (approximately 4 nm diameter), nonbanded filaments arranged in parallel (130). Morphological (384,449–451) and biosynthetic (184,186,192) studies clearly indicate that the filaments are composed of a molecule (type IV collagen) with globular, noncollagenous extensions at the amino and carboxyl termini, that is, one that is more akin to the procollagen form of type I. This molecule is synthesized by anterior subcapsular epithelial cells (193,553) that are also capable of incorporating a heparan sulfate proteoglycan into the basement membrane (185,189). The thinner posterior lens capsule has a chemical composition identical to that of the anterior capsule (148) but appears to be secreted by nucleated cortical fiber cells at a much slower rate (415,533). The identity of amino acid composition does not necessarily indicate an identical polypeptide substructure, and evidence of different collagenous polypeptides in the anterior and posterior capsules of embryonic chick lens has been presented (232).

As in other tissues, type IV collagen in lens capsule was initially thought to consist of a homotrimer of a single α_1(IV) polypeptide (102). Later it became apparent from both analytical and biosynthetic studies that there were at least two [α_1IV) and α_2(IV)], and perhaps more, distinct collagenous polypeptides (104,105,152,164,184,186,192,232,495). More recent studies of anterior lens capsule and glomerular basement membrane (GBM) have confirmed the existence of additional polypeptides within type IV collagen (see later). Much of the investigation in this area has been directed toward increased understanding of Goodpasture's syndrome and Alport's syndrome of hereditary nephritis. The noncollagenous domain of GBM type IV collagen (NC1) contains a number of polypeptides of molecular weight 24, 26, and 28 kD, together with their dimers. The origin of these polypeptides is not firmly established, but the 24 and 26 kD components are thought to be part of the α_1(IV) and α_2(IV) chains, respectively [i.e., M1 of Butkowski and colleagues (59)] and the 28 kD component, which includes the Goodpasture epitope, part of the α_3(IV) chain (437). In the GBM, at least, the Goodpasture antigen is composed of two polypeptides, designated M28$^+$ and M28^{3+} according to their charge. Monoclonal antibodies to these components react with normal human GBM and normal human anterior and posterior lens capsule (272). They do not react with GBM in Alport's syndrome (272), however. Patients with Alport's syndrome who have undergone renal transplantation occasionally develop anti-GBM nephritis in the allograft. Serum from such patients reacts with the distinct 26 kD polypeptide in the NC1 region of human GBM (243). In immunofluorescence studies the Alport antigen and Goodpasture antigen are located together in both GBM and lens capsule (270), and the antigenicity of both is lost from collagenase digests of GBM from Alport kidneys (438). The Alport antigen may thus be a prerequisite for integration of the 28 kD polypeptides within the GBM (271).

The 26 kD Alport antigen is unlikely to be derived from the α_1(IV) collagen polypeptide since the genes for both α(IV) and α_2(IV) collagen are located on chromosome 13 at the 13q34 locus (173) and Alport's syndrome is X linked. A distinct polypeptide present in GBM, α_5(IV) collagen, has been identified by isolating the appropriate cDNA clones with an oligonucleotide probe coding for a consensus sequence (Cys-Gln-Val-Cys-Met) in the NC1 domain of type IV collagen (206). This polypeptide appears to be a minor but specific component of GBM and is closely related in sequence and size to α_1(IV) collagen: its NC1 domain is 26 kD, and it has an 83% sequence identity with the α_1(IV) chain. The gene COL4A5 for this polypeptide has been localized to the long arm of the X chromosome (Xq22) (206,367), and mutations in the gene have been identified in Alport's syndrome (19).

The major clinical features of Alport's syndrome are familial progressive nephritis and neural deafness, although there is considerable phenotypic and genetic heterogeneity. The principal ocular manifestation is anterior lenticonus, which may occur in as many as 50% of patients (162,497). Spontaneous rupture of the cone may lead to anterior subcapsular cataract. In one study 11 of 17 patients (65%) from nine families had bilateral corneal endothelial changes of posterior polymorphous dystrophy (497). The marked thinning of the central anterior lens capsule (4 versus 16 μm in control lens) is accompanied by vertical dehiscences in the inner two-thirds (485). These dehiscences form a network of channels 0.09–2.00 μm wide and are less frequent and smaller in the peripheral capsule. The channels contain 3–6 nm filaments (slightly larger than normal lens capsule filaments) and membranous debris (485). The fragility of the capsule may reflect lack of the 26 kD component from the NC1 domain, which is an important cross-linking site (539).

Tangential splitting of the capsule may occur in "true exfoliation." This condition, also known as capsular delamination, was once mainly found in workers exposed to hot, open furnaces but may be seen in advanced age irrespective of occupation (74). Brodrick and Tate (46) observed fibrillar densities in the capsule at the plane of delamination, and these seem to be a feature of the capsule in later life (464). Although these have a periodic banded structure and resemble long-spacing collagen, their true nature remains unknown. Long-term cultures (8 months) of bovine lens epithelial cells deposit similar structures within a matrix of compacted 8–15 nm filaments (291). Compositional studies of aged human lens capsules suggest a relative diminution in collagen content (396).

Although age-related cataract is not accompanied by any specific capsular abnormalities, the thickness of the capsule at the anterior pole increases with advancing age, and lamination of the capsule becomes less prominent (129,464,482).

In anterior subcapsular cataracts the subcapsular epithelial cells assume a spindle shaped and become embedded in a fibrous matrix (138). The cells assume characteristics of modified (myo) fibroblasts, with basal lamina and subplasmalemmal bundles of fine (7 nm diameter) filaments containing electron-dense bodies: intercellular junctions can be seen, except where the cells are widely separated within the plaque (391). The transformation of lens epithelial cells into cells with mesenchymal characteristics has been accomplished in vitro by culturing them in gels of native type I collagen (170), and aging lens epithelial cells in culture synthesize less type IV collagen and more types I and III (290). The presence of a collagenous plaque containing contractile cells corrugates the overlying anterior capsule. The collagenous fibers are generally thin (average diameter 15–21 nm) and arranged in strata with alternating layers of basement membrane material (382). Broad fibrillar aggregates (>1000 nm in diameter) are also seen (382,392), and these resemble the amianthoid collagen (fused collagen fibrils) seen in degenerate cartilage (153).

G.   Vitreous

The collagenous nature of the insoluble residual protein of the vitreous was first inferred by Young in 1894 because of the reversible gel-liquid transformation of vitreous upon heating and cooling (460). Biochemical, biophysical (404), and ultrastructural (329) confirmation was only provided many years later. The structure, function, and pathology of the vitreous have been comprehensively reviewed (see Chap. 22) (460).

The characteristic property of vitreous is its gellike consistency, resulting from the trapping of water within a fibrillar network formed by the interaction of collagen fibers with the high-molecular-weight polyanion hyaluronic acid. In addition to hyaluronic acid, noncollagenous glycoproteins are associated with the collagen fibers, but their nature and function have yet to be fully established (460). The insoluble proteins of the rabbit vitreous, comprising approximately 30% of the dry weight, can be separated from the soluble components by centrifugation at 45,000 g for 50 minutes (205).

The collagenous fibers in normal vitreous from a variety of species are widely dispersed and of narrow diameter (7–23 nm), with a major axial period of 62 nm when positively stained with uranyl acetate (475). Rabbit fibrils have the smallest diameter (7 nm on average) and are associated with another extremely fine fibrillar structure that has not been identified. This may consist of pN-collagen type II, which has been detected together with type II collagen in the liquid phase of the rabbit vitreous (205). The fibril organization of rabbit vitreous collagen differs from that in other species since the fibrils have a lower thermal stability (judged by shrinkage temperature), although the melting temperatures of the pepsin-solubilized collagens are identical (475). pN-collagen II may be part of the rabbit vitreous fibril in the way that pN-collagen I occurs in the fine type I collagen fibrils of young human skin (135), the aminopropeptide in some manner preventing lateral growth of the fiber.

In the vitreous gel of adult chickens the collagen fibers, as viewed by rotary shadowing, have a diameter of 27.9 ± 2.4 nm (547). The fibrils are invested with a coat of chondroitin/dermatan sulfate proteoglycan in which tenascin molecules (see Chap. 32) are embedded. Others have identified a coat of GAG on the collagen fibers in bovine vitreous (7).

The detailed studies of Swann extending over many years have clearly shown that the major collagenous polypeptide of vitreous is the α_1(II) chain. This differs from the corresponding chain in cartilage in amino acid composition (reduced alanine content and higher degrees of hydroxylation of both lysine and proline) and carbohydrate content, which is increased (9,492). The thermal stability of vitreous collagen is less than that of articular cartilage collagen (476), probably because of the greater abundance of proteoglycans in the cartilage matrix (474). The major reducible cross-links of vitreous collagen, dihydroxylysinonorleucine and hydroxylysinonorleucine, are only half as numerous as in cartilage. Their numbers diminish with age as they mature into pyridinoline (476).

The presence of collagens other than type II has also been documented. Burke (55) suggested that the 3α chain was a significant component of rabbit vitreous, and type IX collagen, of which this polypeptide is an element, has been identified by others using both biochemical and morphological techniques (9, 133,547,549). As mentioned earlier, type IX collagen in avian vitreous differs in structure from that in avian cartilage, in size of the α_1(IX) chain and in size and composition of the GAG side chain (549). Rotary shadowing of vitreous gel from adult chicks indicates that the type IX collagen molecule lacks the NC4 globular domain on the short arm (547). The molecule can be visualized by immunoelectron microscopy in a D-periodic (66.9 nm) arrangement along the thin collagen type II fibrils (549). Biosynthetic studies of chick embryos indicate that vitreous collagen in the early embryo is synthesized by neural retina and later by hyalocytes (373). Immunofluorescence studies of the developing eyes indicate that the secretion of collagen types II and IX is stringently regulated. As the vitreous forms in the early embryo, only type II collagen can be detected. Type IX collagen appears as soon as the definitive vitreous is present (stage 20) and later becomes concentrated in the anterior hyaloid membrane (133).

Ayad and Weiss (9) identified additional cartilage collagens in bovine vitreous. These were initially named C-PS collagens (cartilage-phosphate soluble) but are now designated type XII. They were present in vitreous in an equimolar ratio, suggesting that they may occur in one larger molecule. They are cross-linked by disulfide bonds and may be bound to type II collagen by this mechanism, since Swann and Sotman (492) identified peptides that were released from type II collagen following reduction. A quantitative comparison of the collagenous species in bovine vitreous and nasal septal cartilage has been presented by Ayad and Weiss (9).

Penetrating ocular injuries may be complicated by fibrous tissue deposition within the vitreous. The collagen may be in the form of dense fibrous sheets continuous with the scleral perforation and is believed to be deposited by proliferating scleral fibroblasts (401). The contribution of vitreous hemorrhage to the fibrotic process is not really clear. In the rabbit vitreous Raymond and colleagues (416) found type I collagen only when a pars plana wound was accompanied by the introduction of autologous blood into the vitreous. The resorption of vitreous blood clots is slow and is accompanied by the formation of vitreous membranes, but these are composed of condensed vitreous collagen and are not associated with fibroblastic activity (140).

The highest density of collagen fibers is present normally in the vitreous base, with progressive diminution in the posterior vitreous cortex, anterior vitreous cortex, and central vitreous. Anterior to the ora serrata vitreous fibrils insert into spaces between the cells of the nonpigmented ciliary epithelium, and posterior to the ora they are attached to the inner limiting membrane to form a strong vitreoretinal junction. The strength of vitreoretinal adhesion is greater in young eyes (<21 years) and at the posterior pole, but the matrix components responsible have not been identified (461). The vitreous cortex is absent over the macula, and passage of vitreous fluid through this premacular "hole" into the retrohyaloid space disturbs the vitreolaminar adhesion (139). The major change in the vitreous with aging is a transformation from the gel to the liquid state, and this appears to result from changes in the vitreous collagen fibers. The clearest demonstration of this is seen in the South American owl monkey. The central vitreous gel of the baby monkey contains collagen fibers, but by the age of 2 years the vitreous is a viscous liquid containing hyaluronic acid and noncollagenous glycoproteins but devoid of collagen fibers (212).

The gradual but progressive liquefaction of the human vitreous (synchysis) begins in the central vitreous: as the liquid vitreous forms the collagen fibers aggregate into thick bundles of parallel fibers (460,462). The accumulation of pools of liquid vitreous results in clinically recognizable "lacunae" in the vitreous, and the escape of liquid vitreous through the premacular and peripapillary holes leads to vitreous collapse (syneresis) and posterior vitreous detachment (see Chap. 22).

H. Bruch's Membrane and Retinal Pigment Epithelium

Bruch's membrane is the connective tissue boundary between the retinal pigment epithelium (RPE) and the choriocapillaris. It is approximately 3 μm thick (2.3–4.2 μm) (351) and is composed of five layers: (1) the basal lamina of the RPE cells, 40–100 nm thick; (2) an inner collagenous zone composed of tightly woven fibers of uniform diameter (70 nm); (3) a fenestrated layer of mature elastin through which collagen fibers from the inner collagenous zone pass; (4) an outer collagenous zone of looser texture than the inner collagenous zone; and (5) the basal lamina of the endothelium of the choriocapillaris (157). This appearance, characteristic of young (<20 years) eyes, changes with age, particularly in the macular region (120). The major change is thickening as a result of the accumulation of membranous debris in the inner and outer collagenous zones (120). The debris is derived from the RPE cell cytoplasm and is thought to include remnants of phagocytosed photoreceptor outer segments (58,552). The presence of such lipid-rich material in Bruch's membrane may produce a hydrophobic barrier limiting water transport and predisposing to pigment epithelial detachment (393).

The most significant change that occurs with aging is the development of drusen on the inner aspect of Bruch's membrane (see Chap. 20). These deposits are formed from extension of the RPE cell cytoplasm into the membrane with subsequent degeneration. Evidence for penetration of a portion of the RPE cell cytoplasm through the basal lamina (58) has been contradicted by reports of the cytoplasmic extensions carrying the RPE basal lamina into the subepithelial space (216,217). However, it has been recognized that in advanced stages the basal lamina separating the RPE and the extracellular deposit may disappear completely (191,264). At least four types of drusen have been identified, and there is some understanding of their biological significance (516). Plasma membrane-derived macromolecules appear to form a significant element in developing drusen, but the contribution of connective tissue macromolecules is much less clear. Much of the basal linear deposit is composed of material resembling long-spacing collagen, with a periodicity of 115–140 nm interspersed with homogeneous material and electron-lucent spaces (522). Similar material may be found in papillary drusen and in the outer collagenous zone of Bruch's membrane in young people (522). The origin and chemical constitution of this collagen, if such is its nature, has not been determined. A recent immunoelectron microscopic study of drusen failed to identify any matrix macromolecules within them (99).

No definitive analyses of the macromolecular composition of Bruch's membrane have been published, although there are indications that it contains collagen types I, III, IV, and V and that the solubility of the collagen within the membrane diminishes substantially with aging (242). Immunoelectron microscopy has provided some information on the location within Bruch's membrane of both the collagenous and non-collagenous macromolecules (Table 6) (98).

The ability to grow RPE cells in culture has permitted some understanding of the formation of Bruch's membrane. Early studies of embryonic chick RPE cells revealed the biosynthesis of basement membrane and fibrillar collagen to be closely linked both spatially and temporally (370). Adult human RPE cells in culture deposit a matrix containing collagen types I–IV (but not V), together with laminin and fibronectin, all of which can be identified immunochemically within human Bruch's membrane (66,98). Other studies have also demonstrated the biosynthesis of collagen type IV (273,300,517), fibronectin (273), and laminin (517). (See Chap. 32.) The amount of matrix produced by RPE cells in culture is increased by the addition of macrophage-conditioned medium, which also promotes spindle cell metaplasia (328).

Similar effects are produced by the addition of vitreous and serum, with an increase in the proportion of type I collagen in the deposited matrix (327). In vitro, extracellular matrix derived from bovine RPE cells stimulates the growth of retinal glial cells (546). RPE cells, together with fibroblasts, contribute to the subretinal neovascular membrane in age-related macular degeneration that has been shown by immuno-electron microscopy to contain collagen types I, III, IV, V, and VI, as well as laminin and fibronectin (561).

I. Retina

The major collagenous structures in the retina are blood vessels and the inner limiting membrane, which is composed of the basement membranes of the Müller cell processes.

A variety of different collagens contribute to the retinal vessels (320), but attention has been concentrated on the basement membrane of the smallest vessels (capillaries), thickening of which has long been recognized to accompany both aging (297) and diabetes mellitus (8).

Segments of retinal capillaries can be isolated for study by forcing lightly homogenized retina through a nylon sieve with pores 86 μm in diameter (344). The segments that are retained by the sieve are essentially

Table 6 Topographical Distribution of Extracellular Matrix Macromolecules in Human Bruch's Membrane

RPE basement membrane	Collagens types IV and V, laminin, HSPG[a]
Inner collagenous zone	Collagens type I, III, and V, fibronectin, HSPG
Elastic layer	α-Elastin, collagen VI
Outer collagenous zone	Collagens I, III, and V, fibronectin, HSPG
Choriocapillaris basement membrane	Collagens types IV and V, laminin, HSPG

[a]Heparan sulfate proteoglycan (basement membrane type) (perlecan).
Source: Data from Das and colleagues (98).

devoid of nonvascular elements and are metabolically active. Morphological examination indicates that many are not true capillaries but rather arterioles and venules, being composed of endothelium with one or more layers of pericytes, as well as the investing basement membrane matrix (73). Isolation of the matrix from these segments by treatment with detergents reveals layers of basement membrane composed of fine filaments (3.0–3.5 nm diameter) and amorphous material (73). Incubation of the segments with radioactive precursors of collagen and glycoprotein results in deposition of radioactivity within the basement membrane (544).

The detergent extraction technique has been modified to allow preparation of the vascular bed of a single eye (345). Duhamel and colleagues (109) were able to solubilize 60% by weight of the entire retinal vascular bed and effect a separation of collagenous and noncollagenous polypeptides. The polypeptide composition of the vascular basement membrane proved to be unexpectedly complex (109), but digestion with pepsin and purification of the solubilized collagens by salt precipitation yielded both type I and type IV collagen (257).

The presence of type I and type IV collagen, together with type V collagen, in the basement membranes of retinal capillaries, arteries, and venules has been demonstrated by immunohistochemistry (223,257) and immunoelectron microscopy (114,320). In addition, Marshall and colleagues (320) found type VI collagen in larger blood vessels. Collagen type III was essentially confined to larger blood vessels (223,320). Hyalinization of large blood vessels was accompanied by increased deposition of collagen types I, VI, and also IV, the last reflecting duplication of basal lamina (320). The apparently close association of collagen type I with type IV in the capillary basement membrane may underlie the resistance to trypsin digestion that has proved so useful in experimental studies of the retinal vasculature.

Sophisticated ultrastructural analyses of isolated retinal capillaries have confirmed the contribution of three cell types to the matrix (70). The endothelium is separated by a discontinuous, subendothelial basal lamina (70 nm thick) from one or more layers of pericytes that are surrounded by their own basal laminae (each 80–110 nm thick). The presence of fenestrae in the subendothelial basal laminae reflects contact between endothelial and pericyte cell processes (69). An irregular layer of collagen fibers and pericyte matrix is surrounded by a continuous basal lamina (80–110 nm thick) laid down by perivascular Müller cells. Structural differences between the different basal laminae have been noted (70,72), and the biochemical basis for these is under investigation using independent cultures of endothelial cells and pericytes (60). Both cell types are capable of depositing extracellular matrix in vitro, and postconfluent cultures of endothelial cells form bilayers and also tubular structures (60). This corresponds to the "sprouting" phenotype shown by retinal endothelial cells cultured within a gel of collagen type I (67). Under these conditions of culture, Canfield and colleagues (67) noted a reduction in biosynthesis of type IV collagen and an increase in collagen types I and III. It appears that for both pericytes and endothelial cells collagen types I and IV are the major biosynthetic products, with type III collagen a minor product (67,257). These biosynthetic experiments were carried out in the presence of a lathyrogen, β-aminopropionitrile, and the related compound β,β'-iminodipropionitrile has been shown to produce retinal vascular abnormalities in rats (532).

The presence of collagen types IV and V has been demonstrated in the inner limiting membrane (114,443). Although under certain conditions regeneration of the inner limiting membrane may occur (91), breaks in the basement membrane are usually complicated by epiretinal membrane formation. Collagen fibers within epiretinal membranes generally have diameters in the range of 10–15 and 20–25 nm, although occasionally thicker fibers may be present (237). The finest fibers may represent incorporated vitreous collagen or type II collagen synthesized by RPE cells; there does not appear to be a significant diminution in the type II collagen content when vitrectomy has been previously performed (225). In one study neither RPE cells nor type II collagen was found in the epiretinal membranes of proliferative diabetic retinopathy (224), although Scheiffarth and colleagues (443) detected type II collagen in 12 of 13 proliferative diabetic retinopathy membranes. Immunohistochemical studies have demonstrated several collagen types within epiretinal membranes: types I and III appear to predominate, with lesser amounts of types IV and II (225,357). This distribution does not appear to change with increasing age of the epiretinal membranes (357). The presence of type IV collagen seems largely to depend on the presence of segments of inner limiting membrane and blood vessels within the epiretinal membranes (224,225). Type V collagen has been demonstrated by SDS-PAGE (443).

Studies of the development of the eye in avian embryos have implicated the neural retina in the formation of collagen types II and IX in the vitreous (305,309). Messenger RNA of collagen type II can be detected by in situ hybridization in the retinal cells over the entire optic cup in the early embryo but gradually becomes restricted to the developing ciliary region. Type IX collagen mRNA is confined to the ciliary region at all stages, perhaps related to the concentration of this collagen in the anterior hyaloid membrane (309). Type II collagen does not appear to be synthesized in vitro by the fibrous astrocytes of rabbit neural retina (57). Type I collagen comprises 90% of the collagen secreted by these cells into the culture medium; in addition, a small amount of type V collagen is produced.

VI. OCULAR MANIFESTATIONS OF GENERALIZED DISORDERS OF COLLAGEN

A. Keratoconus

Although keratoconus, and the rarer keratoglobus, are often acquired conditions associated with, for example, vernal keratoconjunctivitis (62), for many years the possibility of an association with a generalized connective tissue disturbance has been considered (see Chap. 23). Although there is a positive family history in a small percentage (6%) of cases of keratoconus (259) and there have been a number of reports of individuals with blue sclerae, hyperextensible joints and deafness (32,63,171), and perhaps Ehlers-Danlos syndrome (421), no definitive evidence of such an association has been found. A study of 95 keratoconus patients did not reveal a significant increase in joint hypermobility or mitral prolapse (483).

Immunohistochemical studies show no significant alteration in the distribution of collagen types within keratoconus corneas, apart from an increase in type III collagen in scarred areas (371). A similar conclusion was drawn from an analytical study, although no more than 35% of the corneal collagen could be solubilized (562). An early report of alterations in lysine-derived cross-links (68) has not been substantiated (96,387). The study of Yue and colleagues (557) favored biochemical heterogeneity, with some patients showing a diminished collagen content and rate of synthesis and others manifesting no abnormality of collagen. Recent interest has been focused on increased collagenolytic and gelatinolytic activity within the stroma (214,238,262), which might help to explain the disruption of Bowman's layer and loss of stromal substance, particularly if proteinase inhibitor levels are reduced (442).

B. Relapsing Polychondritis

Ocular inflammation is found in approximately 50% of cases of relapsing polychondritis (see Chap. 5) (215), with episcleritis and intractable scleritis the most frequent manifestations. Approximately one-third of patients with relapsing polychondritis have circulating antibodies to native type II collagen, the titer correlating with the severity of inflammation (136,348). Since there is no cartilage or type II collagen in human sclera, an indirect mechanism must be invoked for the scleritis, namely, an immune complex vasculitis (204).

C. Epidermolysis Bullosa

Epidermolysis bullosa comprises a large group of clinically distinct entities characterized by a tendency to blister formation after minor trauma. Three major subgroups are recognized, depending on the location of the bulla: (1) autosomal dominant "epidermolytic epidermolysis bullosa," in which the bulla forms within the epidermis; (2) autosomal recessive "junctional epidermolysis bullosa," in which separation occurs within the lamina rara of the subepidermal basal lamina; and (3) "dystrophic epidermolysis bullosa," which may be either dominant or recessive and in which the blister forms below the lamina densa (395). Ocular complications occur principally in the recessive dystrophic form and generally take the form of recurrent corneal erosions (151). As many as 82% of patients with this form display symblepharon, corneoscleral limbal broadening, and corneal opacity (338,339). Blistering of the cornea is accompanied by loss of Bowman's layer and anterior stromal scarring (103). Symblepharon does not appear to be a feature of junctional epidermolysis bullosa, in which recurrent corneal erosions are also common (340).

Because of its greater prevalence and severity, most investigations have concentrated on the recessive dystrophic variety, in which there is a complete absence of anchoring fibrils in both blistered and intact skin (502). Similar changes have been observed in conjunctiva by immunofluorescence with a monoclonal antibody to collagen type VII and by transmission electron microscopy (218,339). The cause of the deficiency, which is incomplete in the dominant dystrophic form (502), is not entirely clear since some epitopes of collagen type VII are detectable even in the absence of anchoring fibrils (54). The concentration of collagenase is increased in both blistered and intact skin, and cutaneous fibroblasts from epidermolysis bullosa patients have a greater biosynthetic capacity for collagenase than normal fibroblasts (23).

D. Osteogenesis Imperfecta

Over 70 mutations in the two genes for type I collagen have been defined in this condition. The mutations fall into two classes: those producing a reduction in the amount of type I collagen, generally characterized by milder manifestations, and those producing alterations in the structure of the molecule, with variable clinical severity (61,411). The most common mutations involve substitution of a single glycine residue at one of several positions along the pro-α(I) chains (61). Although there has been phenomenal progress in documenting the mutations and defining their effects on phenotype, it is not yet clear why a particular structural change in one part of the type I molecule may affect skin and the same change in another part of the molecule may produce major manifestations in bone (412). The ocular sign of blue sclera probably results from a reduction in collagen fiber diameter that increases the visibility of uveal pigment and blood through the sclera (75). Changes in fiber structure and size may also account for a diminution in ocular rigidity (236).

The homozygous Mov 13 transgenic mutant mouse model of osteogenesis imperfecta is unable to synthesize type I collagen because of an insertional mutation in the collagen type I gene. The corneal stroma in this mouse is reduced in amount and composed of collagen fibrils with an average diameter of 6 nm (18). The overall architecture of the cornea is surprisingly normal, suggesting a structural rather than organizational role for type I collagen and a failure to compensate for its absence with increased synthesis of other collagen types (18).

E. Ehlers-Danlos Syndrome

The Ehlers-Danlos syndrome (EDS) is characterized by hyperextensibilty and/or fragility of the skin with hypermobility of joints and a tendency to bruising. A least 10 types are recognized (519), and there is genetic and biochemical heterogeneity within some of the clinical types (88). Although a reduction in fiber diameter and imperfect alignment of fibers within bundles have been described in several types (38), for most the underlying abnormality is not known. The best characterized type is EDS IV, which results from a deficiency of type III collagen (112).

In EDS VI the cutaneous and joint problems are accompanied by prominent ocular abnormalities, including scleral fragility and retinal detachment (25,397). The cornea may also be abnormally small and thin (333). The biochemical defect in some cases of EDS VI is a deficiency of lysyl hydroxylase that results in fewer hydroxylysine residues in collagen (280,282), increases solubility of dermal collagen (402), and changes in reducible cross-links (115). Not all cases of apparent EDS VI, however, display diminished lysyl hydroxylase activity (234).

F. Miscellaneous Disorders

Brittle Cornea Syndrome

Blue sclerae, red hair, and corneal rupture following minor trauma have been linked in the autosomal recessive brittle cornea syndrome (501). Cultured skin fibroblasts from individuals with this syndrome display normal lysyl hydroxylase activity and synthesize procollagen types I and III in a normal ratio. The only tissue abnormalities recognized so far have been a slight reduction in collagen fiber diameter in the dermis and the presence of areas within the dermis that are completely devoid of collagen fibers (430).

Stickler Syndrome

The Stickler syndrome of premature osteoarthritis and vitreoretinal degeneration (see Chap. 22) has been linked in some, but not all, families to the gene for type II collagen on the long arm of chromosome 12 (141). In one family, a premature stop codon in the COL2A1 gene has been detected that would result in a truncated α_1(II) chain and diminished biosynthesis of type II procollagen (2).

VII. OCULAR DISORDERS INVOLVING COLLAGEN

A. Corneal Disorders

Corneal Stromal Degradation

The profound ocular morbidity associated with corneal infection and ulceration has maintained interest in the role of collagenase in stromal degradation. Although some organisms, such as *Acanthamoeba castellani* (183) and *Lasiodiplodia theobromae* (417), that cause severe corneal injury are able to produce collagenase, other organisms, such as *Pseudomonas aeruginosa* (265), do not, and the evidence points to either the injured keratocytes themselves or infiltrating neutrophils as the major sources of collagenase. An immunohistochemical examination of penetrating keratoplasty specimens (including a healed ulcer) revealed the presence of collagenase in the stroma, but not the epithelium, of all the ulcerated but none of the intact buttons (159). Although some of the ulcers were infective and contained a polymorphonuclear leukocytic infiltrate, in two cases (alkali burn and neuroparalytic keratitis) a cellular infiltrate was not present. The requirement for ulceration is not absolute: increased collagenolytic activity is present in the corneas of rabbits with herpetic interstitial keratitis (65). The ability of stromal cells to release a latent collagenase in vitro is modulated by epithelial cell products (229).

Collagenase has been shown to play a role in corneal ulceration following exposure to alkali. Although it was initially thought that the alkali itself did not significantly disturb the covalent structure of the collagen α chains (369), it now seems that both type I and type V stromal collagens can be degraded to polypeptides of molecular weight < 20 kD (31). Given time, even a low concentration of sodium hydroxide (0.25 M) can degrade the collagen; since alkali has a propensity to be retained within the eye (390), this may partially explain the difficulty in controlling alkali burns. The alkali-exposed collagen shows a greater susceptibility to proteinases, such as trypsin (369), and may stimulate the ingress and metabolic activation of neutrophils (399,543). Nevertheless, the best evidence supports an endogenous source for the collagenase (228,369).

Disorders of Descemet's Membrane

Focal interruptions of the Descemet's membrane–endothelial cell complex, as in anterior segment dysgenesis, may result in localized corneal scarring (194) and the production of abnormally thick (60 nm) stromal fibrils (536).

Although Descemet's membrane is unusual among basement membranes in that it does not thicken in diabetes mellitus (468), it frequently thickens in response to an endothelial disturbance. Because of the complicated developmental changes within the normal membrane, with formation of two zones of different structure and peripheral guttata, a variety of different patterns of thickening can be seen. Collagenous tissue posterior to the normal Descemet's membrane is termed a posterior collagenous layer and has been classified by Waring (535) into three ultrastructural categories: (1) banded, containing long-spacing material with a macroperiod of 55 or 110 nm; (2) fibrillar, containing nonbanded collagenous fibrils of diameter 20 nm; and (3) fibrocellular, containing fibroblastic cells in a compact mesh of banded collagen fibers 30–40 nm in diameter. Fuchs' endothelial dystrophy provides a good example of a banded posterior collagenous layer that may occur as simple guttate excrescences (see Chap. 40) (43,536). In this disease the posterior nonbanded zone is generally thin, suggesting that endothelial dysfunction has already commenced by the age of about 20 years. Biochemical studies of the posterior collagenous layer in Fuchs' dystrophy do not indicate any deviation from the expected composition of types IV and VIII collagen (263). In posterior polymorphous dystrophy, both the anterior banded zone and the posterior nonbanded zone may be abnormally thin (337,410), suggesting that an endothelial disturbance during intrauterine life resumes in early childhood. The generally normal overall thickness of Descemet's membrane may be attributed to a posterior collagenous layer, generally of the fibrillar category (337).

Rabbit corneal endothelial cells in vitro deposit an extracellular matrix with alternating layers of amorphous and fibrillar material (260). The factors that govern the type of posterior collagenous layer deposited have not been determined. Studies of normal endothelial cells suggest that the cells need an endothelial matrix to remain polygonal and on a fibroblastic matrix assume a spindle shape (207). It may be that an abnormal endothelial matrix also stimulates spindle cell metaplasia. Metaplastic rabbit endothelial cells switch from biosynthesis of type IV collagen to types I, III, and V, regulation taking place at the level of mRNA translation (245,246).

B. Disorders of Sclera

A major anatomical disorder of the sclera is the staphyloma, defined as local scleral ectasia lined by uveal tissue. It occurs frequently between the corneoscleral limbus and the equator as a result of prolonged raised intraocular pressure. Spontaneous scleral thinning may also occur in the paralimbal region (scleromalacia perforans) (318). No peculiarities of the collagen fibers in this region have been described, although the difference in average fiber diameter between inner and outer wall is less marked in this area (469).

Posterior scleral thinning with axial elongation of the eyeball is a feature of myopia. Unilateral eyelid fusion in monkeys results in high myopia, with axial elongation developing over many months (149). The scleral thickness is reduced by 35–45%, and the outer collagen fibers have a diameter more typical of inner fibers. The scleral thinning is greater than can be accounted for by stretching alone (149), suggesting that there may be an alteration in fibrillogenesis. This conclusion is supported by experiments on eyelid suture myopia in tree shrews, in which the axial elongation of the eyeball is exaggerated by the systemic administration of lathyrogens (336). Similar changes in thin fibers and abnormal star-shaped fibers in human myopia have also been taken to support the concept of defective fibrillogenesis (97). Myopia associated with scleral fragility and rupture has been described in a recessive form of Ehlers-Danlos syndrome (25).

Localized accumulation of alcianophilic material within the inner sclera has been described on a number of occasions. This was noted by Stefani and colleagues (480) in 11% of eyes enucleated because of a choroidal melanoma. He termed the condition spongiotic sclera and thought it might represent nothing more than localized edema induced by the tumor. A similar appearance, accompanied by changes in the scleral collagen, was found in an enucleated eye from a patient with bilateral retinal pigment epithelial mottling in the macular region (90). The inner two-thirds of the submacular sclera was lightly eosinophilic in histological sections and contained material that stained positively with alcian blue (at pH 1.0 and 2.5) and with the colloidal iron technique. The alcianophilia was resistant to digestion with testicular hyaluronidase and appeared to be a highly sulfated GAG, but not keratan sulfate. In the abnormal area the scleral collagen fibers had diameters up to twice normal (580 nm). Inner scleral collagen fibers with slightly increased diameters (160 versus 95 nm) have been described in a globe enlarged as a result of uveitic glaucoma (525). The enlargement occurred during adolescence, presumably because of an abnormality of the scleral collagen; no defects in collagen could be established in either skin or cornea.

The sclera is markedly thickened in nanophthalmos. In this syndrome the eye is also small, with a shallow anterior chamber and a tendency to uveal effusion, perhaps through compression of the vortex veins by the thick sclera (45). Partial-thickness sclerectomy has been used to treat the uveal effusion, and examination of the excised scleral specimen has indicated a disturbance of the lamellar arrangement of the collagen bundles (510,534,555). A careful analysis of 10 cases has shown increased variation in collagen fiber diameter (30–320 versus 50–250 nm in controls) and fraying of the ends of fibers into thin fibrils of 10–15 or 30–35 nm diameter (481). The severity of the collagen abnormality correlated with the reduction in ocular diameter. Two reports (510,534) have suggested increased deposition of glycosaminoglycan within the sclera that may result in disturbed collagen fibrillogenesis.

REFERENCES

1. Adachi, E., and Hayashi, T. In vitro formation of hybrid fibrils of type V collagen and type I collagen. Limited growth of type I collagen into thick fibrils by type V collagen. *Connect. Tissue Res.* 14:257–266, 1986.
2. Ahmad, N.N., Ala-Kokko, L., Knowlton, R.G., Jimenez, S.A., Weaver, E.J., Maguire, J.I., Tasman, W., and Prockop, D.J. Stop codon in the procollagen II gene (COL2A1) in a family with the Stickler syndrome (arthroophthalmology). *Proc. Natl. Acad. Sci. USA* 88:6624–6627, 1991.
3. Alper, R. The bovine corneal SGP-complex is related to the tissue form of type VI collagen. *Curr. Eye Res.* 7: 31–42, 1988.
4. Alvarado, J., Murphy, C. and Juster, R. Age-related changes in the basement membrane of the human corneal epithelium. *Invest. Ophthalmol. Vis. Sci.* 24:1015–1028.
5. Anderson, J.C., Labedz, R.I., and Kewley, M.A. The effect of bovine tendon glycoprotein on the formation of fibrils from collagen solutions. *Biochem. J.* 168:345–351, 1977.
6. Apple, D.J., Olson, R.J., Jones, G.R., Carey, J.C., Van Norman, D.K., Ohrloff, C., and Philippart, M. Congenital corneal opacification secondary to Bowman's layer dysgenesis. *Am. J. Ophthalmol.* 98:320–328, 1984.

7.   Asakura, A. Histochemistry of hyaluronic acid of the bovine vitreous body as studied by electron microscopy. *Acta Soc. Ophthalmol. Jpn.* 89:179–191, 1985.
8.   Ashton, N. Vascular basement membrane changes in diabetic retinopathy. Montgomery Lecture, 1973. *Br. J. Ophthalmol.* 58:344–366, 1974.
9.   Ayad, S., and Weiss, J.B. A new look at vitreous-humour collagen. *Biochem. J.* 218:835–840, 1984.
10. Ayad, S., Chambers, C.A., Berry, L., Shuttleworth, C.A., and Grant, M.E. Type VI collagen and glycoprotein MFP I are distinct components of the extracellular matrix. *Biochem. J.* 236:299–302, 1986.
11. Ayad, S., Chambers, C.A.C., Shuttleworth, C.A., and Grant, M.E. Isolation from bovine elastic tissues of collagen type VI and characterization of its form in vivo. *Biochem. J.* 230:465–474, 1985.
12. Bahn, C.F., Falls, H.F., Varley, G.A., and Meyer, R.F., Edelhauser, H.F., and Bourne, W.M. Classification of corneal endothelial disorders based on neural crest origin. *Ophthalmology* 9:558–563, 1984.
13. Bailey, A.J. Structure, function and aging of the collagens of the eye. *Eye* 1:175–183, 1987.
14. Bailey, A.J., and Kent, C.M.J. Non-enzymatic glycosylation of fibrous and basement membrane collagens. In *The Maillard Reaction in Aging, Diabetes and Nutrition*, J.W. Baynes and V.M. Monnier (Eds.), Alan R. Liss, New York, pp.109–122, 1989.
15. Bailey, A.J., and Shimokomaki, M.S. Age-related changes in the reducible cross-links of collagen. *FEBS Lett.* 16:86–88, 1971.
16. Bailey, A.J., and Sims, T.J. Chemistry of the collagen cross-links. Nature of the cross-links in the polymorphic forms of dermal collagen during development. *Biochem. J.* 153:211–215, 1976.
17. Bailey, A.J., Sims, T.J., and Light, N. Cross-linking in type IV collagen. *Biochem. J.* 218:713–723, 1984.
18. Bard, J.B.L., Bansal, M.K., and Ross, A.S.A. The extracellular matrix of the developing cornea: Diversity, deposition and function. *Development (Suppl.)* 103:195–205, 1988.
19. Barker, D.F., Hostikka, S.L., Zhou, J., Chow, L.T., Oliphant, A.R., Gerken, S.C., Gregory, M.C., Skolnick, M.H., Atkin, C.L., and Tryggvason, K. Identification of mutations in the COL 4A5 collagen gene in Alport syndrome. *Science* 248:1224–1227, 1990.
20. Barnard, K., Gathercole, L.J., and Bailey, A.J. Basement membrane collagen—evidence for a novel molecular packing. *FEBS Lett.* 212:49–52, 1987.
21. Barrow, M.V., Simpson, C.F., and Miller, E.J. Lathyrism: A review. *Q. Rev. Biol.* 49:101–128, 1974.
22. Barsky, S.H., Rao, C.N., Grotendorst, G.R., and Liotta, L.A. Increased content of type V collagen in desmoplasia of human breast carcinoma. *Am. J. Pathol.* 108:276–283, 1982.
23. Bauer, E.A., and Tabas, M. A perspective on the role of collagenase in recessive dystrophic epidermolysis bullosa. *Arch. Dermatol.* 124:734–736, 1988.
24. Beacom, R., Gillespie, E.L., Middleton, D., Sawhney, B., and Kennedy, L. Limited joint mobility in insulin-dependent diabetes: Relationship to retinopathy, peripheral nerve function and HLA status. *Q. J. Med.* 56:337–344, 1985.
25. Beighton, P. Serious ophthalmological complications in the Ehlers-Danlos syndrome. *Br. J. Ophthalmol.* 54:263–268, 1970.
26. Ben Ezra, D., and Foidart, J-M. Collagens and noncollagenous proteins in the human eye. I. Corneal stroma in vivo and keratocyte production in vitro. *Curr. Eye Res.* 1:101–110, 1982.
27. Bentz, H., Morris, N.P., Murray, L.W., Sakai, L.Y., Hollister, D.W., and Burgeson, R.E. Isolation and partial characterization of a new human collagen with an extended triple-helical doman. *Proc. Natl. Acad. Sci. USA* 80:3168–3172, 1983.
28. Benya, P.D. EC collagen: Biosynthesis by corneal endothelial cells and separation from type IV without pepsin treatment or denaturation. *Renal Physiol.* 3:30–35, 1980.
29. Benya, P.D., and Padilla, S.R. Isolation and characterization of type VIII collagen synthesized by cultured rabbit corneal endothelial cells. A conventional structure replaces the interrupted-helix model. *J. Biol. Chem.* 261:4160–4169, 1986.
30. Berg, R.A., Birk, D.E., and Silver, F.H. Physical characterization of type I procollagen in solution: Evidence that the propeptides limit self-assembly. *Int. J. Biol. Macromol.* 8:177–182, 1986.
31. Berry, S.M., Hong, B.-S., Lam, K.W., Haddox, J.L., and Pfister, R.R. Degradation of bovine corneal collagen by alkali. *Cornea* 8:150–154, 1989.
32. Biglan, A.W., Brown, S.I., and Johnson, B.L. Keratoglobus and blue sclera. *Am. J. Ophthalmol.* 83:225–233, 1977.
33. Bird, T.A., and Levene, C.I. Lysyl oxidase: Evidence that pyridoxal phosphate is a cofactor. *Biochem. Biophys. Res. Commun.* 108:1172–1180, 1982.
34. Birk, D.E., and Trelstad, R.L. Extracellular compartments in matrix morphogenesis: Collagen fibril, bundle and lamellar formation by corneal fibroblasts. *J. Cell Biol.* 99:2024–2033, 1984.
35. Birk, D.E., Fitch, J.M., and Linsenmayer, T.F. Organization of collagen types I and V in the embryonic chicken cornea. *Invest. Ophthalmol. Vis. Sci.* 27:1470–1477, 1986.
36. Birk, D.E., Fitch, J.M., Babiarz, J.P., and Linsenmayer, T.F. Collagen type I and type V are present in the same fibril in the avian corneal stoma. *J. Cell Biol.* 106:999–1008, 1988.
37. Birk, D.E., Lande, M.A., and Fernandez-Madrid, F.R. Collagen and glycosaminoglycan synthesis in aging human keratocyte cultures. *Exp. Eye Res.* 32:331–339, 1981.

38. Black, C.M., Gathercole, L.J., Bailey, A.J., and Beighton, P. The Ehlers-Danlos syndrome: An analysis of the structure of the collagen fibres of the skin. *Br. J. Dermatol. 102*:85–96, 1980.

39. Böck, P. The distribution of disulfide-groups in Descemet's membrane, lens capsule and zonular fibres. *Acta Histochem. (Jena) 63*:127–136, 1978.

40. Boot-Handford, R., and Heath, H. Identification of fructose as the retinopathic agent associated with the ingestion of sucrose-rich diets in the rat. *Metabolism 29*:1247–1252, 1980.

41. Borcherding, M.S., Blacik, L.J., Sittig, R.A., Bizzell, J.W., Breen, M., and Weinstein, H.G. Proteoglycans and collagen fibre organization in human corneoscleral tissue. *Exp. Eye Res. 21*:59–70, 1975.

42. Bornstein, P., and Sage, H. Structurally distinct collagen types. *Annu. Rev. Biochem. 49*:957–1003, 1980.

43. Bourne, W.M., Johnson, D.H., and Campbell, R.J. The ultrastructure of Descemet's membrane. III. Fuchs' dystrophy. *Arch. Ophthalmol. 100*:1952–1955, 1982.

44. Brewitt, H., and Reale, E. The basement membrane complex of the human corneal epithelium. *Graefes Arch. Clin. Exp. Ophthalmol. 215*:223–231, 1981.

45. Brockhurst, R.J. Nanophthalmos with uveal effusion. A new clinical entity. *Arch. Ophthalmol. 93*:1289–1299, 1975.

46. Brodrick, J.D., and Tate, G.W., Jr. Capsular delamination (true exfoliation) of the lens. Report of a case. *Arch. Ophthalmol. 97*:1693–1698, 1979.

47. Broek, D.L., Madri, J., Eikenberry, E.F., and Brodsky, B. Characterization of the tissue form of type V collagen from chick bone. *J. Biol. Chem. 260*:555–562, 1985.

48. Brown, H.H., Glasgow, B.J., and Foos, R.Y. Ultrastructural and immunohistochemical features of coronal adenomas. *Am. J. Ophthalmol. 112*:34–40, 1991.

49. Brownlee, M., Cerami, A., and Vlassara, H. Advanced glycosylation end products in tissue and the biochemical basis of diabetic complications. *N. Engl. J. Med. 318*:1315–1321, 1988.

50. Bruns, R.R. Beaded filaments and long-spacing fibrils: Relation to type VI collagen. *J. Ultrastruct. Res. 89*: 136–145, 1984.

51. Bruns, R.R., Press, W., Engvall, E., Timpl, R., and Gross, J. Type VI collagen in extracellular, 100-nm periodic filaments and fibrils: Identification by immunoelectron microscopy. *J. Cell Biol. 103*:393–404, 1986.

52. Burgeson, R.E. New collagens, new concepts. *Annu. Rev. Cell Biol. 4*:551–577, 1988.

53. Burgeson, R.E., El Adli, F.A., Kaitila, I.I., and Hollister, D.W. Fetal membrane collagens: Identification of two new collagen alpha chains. *Proc. Natl. Acad. Sci. USA 73*:2579–2583, 1976.

54. Burgeson, R.E., Lunstrum, G.P., Rokosova, B., Rimberg, C.S., Rosenbaum, L.M., and Keene, D.R. The structure and function of type VII collagen. *Ann. N.Y. Acad. Sci. 580*:32–43, 1990.

55. Burke, J.M. An analysis of rabbit vitreous collagen. *Connect. Tissue Res. 8*:49–52, 1980.

56. Burke, J.M., and Foster, S.J. Corneal stromal fibroblasts from adult rabbits retain the capacity to deposit an orthogonal matrix. *Dev. Biol. 108*:250–253, 1985.

57. Burke, J.M., and Kower, H.S. Collagen synthesis by rabbit neural retina in vitro and in vivo. *Exp. Eye Res. 31*:213–226, 1980.

58. Burns, R.P., and Feeney-Burns, L. Clinico-morphologic correlations of drusen of Bruch's membrane. *Trans. Am. Ophthalmol. Soc. 78*:206–225, 1980.

59. Butkowski, R.J., Langeveld, J.P.M., Wieslander, J., Hamilton, J., and Hudson, B.G. Localization of Good-pasture epitope to a novel chain of basement membrane collagen. *J. Biol. Chem. 262*:7874–7877, 1987.

60. Buzney, S.M., Massicotte, S.J., Hetu, N., and Zetter, B.R. Retinal vascular endothelial cells and pericytes. Differential growth characteristics in vitro. *Invest. Ophthalmol. Vis. Sci. 24*:470–480, 1983.

61. Byers, P.H., Wallis, G.A., and Willing, M.C. Osteogenesis imperfecta: Translation of mutation to phenotype. *J. Med. Genet. 28*:433–442, 1991.

62. Cameron, J.A., Al-Rajhi, A.A., and Badr, I.A. Corneal ectasia in vernal keratoconjunctivitis. *Ophthalmology 96*:1615–1623, 1989.

63. Cameron, J.A., Cotter, J.B., Risco, J.M., and Alvarez, H. Epikeratoplasty for keratoglobus associated with blue sclera. *Ophthalmology 98*:446–452, 1991.

64. Cameron, J.D., Skubitz, A.P.N., and Furcht, L.T. Type IV collagen and corneal epithelial adhesion and migration. Effects of type IV collagen fragments and synthetic peptides on rabbit corneal epithelial cell adhesion and migration in vitro. *Invest. Ophthalmol. Vis. Sci. 32*:2766–2773, 1991.

65. Campbell, R., Pavan-Langston, D., Lass, J., Berman, M., Gage, J., and Albert, D.M. Collagenase levels in a new model of experimental herpetic interstitial keratitis. *Arch. Ophthalmol. 98*:919–923, 1980.

66. Campochiaro, P.A., Jerdan, J.A., and Glaser, B.M. The extracellular matrix of human retinal pigment epithelial cells in vivo and its synthesis in vitro. *Invest. Ophthalmol. Vis. Sci. 27*:1615–1621, 1986.

67. Canfield, A.E., Schor, A.M., Schor, S.L., and Grant, M.E. The biosynthesis of extracellular-matrix components by bovine retinal endothelial cells displaying distinctive morphological phenotypes. *Biochem. J. 235*:375–383, 1986.

68. Cannon, D.J., and Foster, C.S. Collagen cross-linking in keratoconus. *Invest. Ophthalmol. Vis. Sci. 17*:63–65, 1978.

69. Carlson, E.C. Fenestrated subendothelial basement membranes in human retinal capillaries. *Invest. Ophthalmol. Vis. Sci. 30*:1923–1932, 1989.

70. Carlson, E.C. Human retinal capillary basement membrane leaflets are morphologically distinct: A correlated TEM and SEM analysis. *Exp. Eye Res. 49*:967–981, 1989.
71. Carlson, E.C., and Audette, J.L. Intrinsic fibrillar components of human glomerular basement membranes: A TEM analysis following proteolytic dissection. *J. Submicrosc. Cytol. Pathol. 21*:83–92, 1989.
72. Carlson, E.C., Audette, J.L., and Swinscoe, J.C. Ultrastructural evidence for morphological specificity in isolated bovine retinal capillary basement membranes. *J. Ultrastruct. Mol. Struct. Res. 98*:184–198, 1988.
73. Carlson, E.C., Brendel, K., Hjelle, J.T., and Meezan, E. Ultrastructural and biochemical analyses of isolated basement membranes from kidney glomeruli and tubules and brain and retinal microvessels. *J. Ultrastruct. Res. 62*:26–53, 1978.
74. Cashwell, L.F., Jr., Holleman, I.L., Weaver, R.G., and van Rens, G.H. Idiopathic true exfoliation of the lens capsule. *Ophthalmology 96*:348–351, 1989.
75. Chan, C.C., Green, W.R., de la Cruz, Z., and Hillis, A. Ocular findings in osteogenesis imperfecta congenita. *Arch. Ophthalmol. 100*:1459–1463, 1982.
76. Cheung, D.T., DiCesare, P., Benya, P.D., Libaw, E., and Nimni, M.E. The presence of intermolecular disulfide cross-links in type III collagen. *J. Biol. Chem. 258*:7774–7778, 1983.
77. Chin, J.R., Murphy, G., and Werb, Z. Stromelysin, a connective tissue-degrading metelloendopeptidase secreted by stimulated rabbit synovial fibroblasts in parallel with collagenase. Biosynthesis, isolation, characterization and substrates. *J. Biol. Chem. 260*:12367–12376, 1985.
78. Cho, H., Covington, H.I., and Cintron, C. Immunolocalization of type VI collagen in developing and healing rabbit cornea. *Invest. Ophthalmol. Vis. Sci. 31*:1096–1102, 1990.
79. Chu, M.L., Pan, T.-C., Conway, D., Saitta, B., Stokes, D., Kuo, H.-J., Glanville, R.W., Timpl, R., Mann, K., and Deutzmann, R. The structure of type VI collagen. *Ann. N.Y. Acad. Sci. 580*:55–63, 1990.
80. Chung, E., Keele, E.M., and Miller, E.J. Isolation and characterization of the cyanogen bromide peptides from the α1(III) chain of human collagen. *Biochemistry 13*:3459–3464, 1974.
81. Cintron, C., and Hong, B.-S. Heterogeneity of collagens in rabbit cornea: Type VI collagen. *Invest. Ophthalmol. Vis. Sci. 29*:760–766, 1988.
82. Cintron, C., Covington, H., and Kublin, C.L. Morphogenesis of rabbit corneal stroma. *Invest. Ophthalmol. Vis. Sci. 24*:543–556, 1983.
83. Cintron, C., Hong, B.-S., and Kublin, C.L. Quantitative analysis of collagen from normal developing corneas and corneal scars. *Curr. Eye Res. 1*:1–8, 1981.
84. Cleutjens, J.P.M., Havenith, M.G., Vallinga, M., Beek, C., and Bosman, F.T. Monoclonal antibodies to native basement membranes reveal heterogeneous immunoreactivity patterns. *Histochemistry 92*:407–412, 1989.
85. Cogan, D.G. Applied anatomy and physiology of the cornea. *Trans. Am. Acad. Ophthalmol. Otolaryngol. 55*:329–359, 1951.
86. Cogan, D.G., Kuwabara, T., Donaldson, D.D., and Collins, E. Microcystic dystrophy of the cornea. A partial explanation for its pathogenesis. *Arch. Ophthalmol. 92*:470–474, 1974.
87. Cohen, M.P., Urdanivia, E., Surma, M., and Wu, V.-Y. Increased glycosylation of glomerular basement membrane collagen in diabetes. *Biochem. Biophys. Res. Commun. 95*:765–769, 1980.
88. Cole, W.G., Evans, R., and Sillence, D.O. The clinical features of Ehlers-Danlos syndrome type VII due to a deletion of 24 amino acids from the pro-α1(I) chain of type I procollagen. *J. Med. Genet. 24*:698–701, 1987.
89. Conrad, G.W., Dessau, W., and von der Mark, K. Synthesis of type III collagen by fibroblasts from the embryonic chick cornea. *J. Cell Biol. 84*:501–512, 1980.
90. Conn, H., Green, W.R., de la Cruz, Z.C., and Hillis, A. Scleropachynsis maculopathy. *Arch. Ophthalmol. 100*:793–799, 1982.
91. Constable, I.J., Horne, R., Slatter, D.H., Chester, G.H., and Cooper, R.L. Regeneration of retinal limiting membranes after chorioretinal biopsy in dogs. *Invest. Ophthalmol. Vis. Sci. 20*:246–251, 1981.
92. Cowen, S.J., Anhalt, G.J., Wicha, M.S., Sugar, A., Labib, R.S., and Diaz, L.A. Distribution of pemphigus and pemphigoid antigens, laminin and type IV collagen in corneal epithelium. *Invest. Ophthalmol. Vis. Sci. 21*:879–882, 1981.
93. Craig, A.S., and Parry, D.A.D. Growth and development of collagen fibrils in immature tissues from rat and sheep. *Proc. R. Soc. Lond. [B] 212*:85–92, 1981.
94. Craig, A.S., and Parry, D.A.D. Collagen fibrils of the vertebrate corneal stroma. *J. Ultrastruct. Res. 74*:232–239, 1981.
95. Crisp, A.J., and Heathcote, J.G. Connective tissue abnormalities in diabetes mellitus. *J. R. Coll. Physicans Lond. 18*:132–141, 1984.
96. Critchfield, J.W., Calandra, A.J., Nesburn, A.B., and Kenney, M.C. Keratoconus. I. Biochemical studies. *Exp. Eye Res. 46*:953–963, 1988.
97. Curtin, B.J., Iwamoto, T., and Renaldo, D.P. Normal and staphylomatous sclera of high myopia. An electron microscopic study. *Arch. Ophthalmol. 97*:912–915, 1979.
98. Das, A., Frank, R.N., Zhang, N.L., and Turczyn, T.J. Ultrastructural localization of extracellular matrix components in human retinal vessels and Bruch's membrane. *Arch. Ophthalmol. 108*:421–429, 1990.
99. Das, A., Zhang, N.L., and Frank, R.N. Topographical variation in components of human Bruch's membrane: An ultrastructural immunocytochemical study. *Invest. Ophthalmol. Vis. Sci. (Suppl.) 32*:687, 1991.

100. Davison, P.F. Bovine tendons. Aging and collagen cross-linking. *J. Biol. Chem. 253*:5635–5641, 1978.

101. Davison, P.F., Hong, B.-S., and Cannon, D.J. Quantitative analysis of the collagens in bovine cornea. *Exp. Eye Res. 29*:97–107, 1979.

102. Dehm, P., and Kefalides, N.A. The collagenous component of lens basement membrane. The isolation and characterization of an α-chain size collagenous peptide and its relationship to newly synthesized lens components. *J. Biol. Chem. 253*:6680–6686, 1978.

103. Destro, M., Wallow, I.H.L., and Brightbill, F.S. Recessive dystrophic epidermolysis bullosa. *Arch. Ophthalmol. 105*:1248–1252, 1987.

104. Dixit, R., Harrison, W.M., and Dixit, S.N. Isolation and partial characterization of a novel basement membrane collagen. *Biochem. Biophys. Res. Commun. 130*:1–8, 1985.

105. Dixit, S.N., and Kang, A.H. Anterior lens capsule collagens: Cyanogen bromide peptides of the C chain. *Biochemistry 18*:5686–5692, 1979.

106. Doane, K.J., Yang, G., and Birk, D.E. Corneal type VI collagen may function in cell-matrix interactions during stromal development. *Invest. Ophthalmol. Vis. Sci. (Suppl.) 32*:874, 1991.

107. Dohlman, C.H., and Balazs, E.A. Chemical studies on Descemet's membrane of the bovine cornea. *Arch. Biochem. 57*:445–457, 1955.

108. Doillon, C.J., Dunn, M.G., Bender, E., and Silver, F.H. Collagen fibre formation in repair tissue: Development of strength and toughness. *Collagen 5*:481–492, 1985.

109. Duhamel, R.C., Meezan, E., and Brendel, K. Selective solubilisation of two polypeptides form bovine retinal basement membranes. *Exp. Eye Res. 36*:257–267, 1983.

110. Dyck, R.F., Kershaw, M., McHugh, N., Lockwood, C.M., Duance, V., Baltz, M.L., and Pepys, M.B. Amyloid P-component is a constituent of normal human glomerular basement membrane. *J. Exp. Med. 152*:1162–1174, 1980.

111. Eady, R.A.J. The basement membrane. Interface between the epithelium and the dermis: Structural features. *Arch. Dermatol. 124*:709–712, 1988.

112. Editorial. Type III collagen deficiency. *Lancet 1*:197–198, 1989.

113. Elkington, A.R., Inman, C.B.E., Steart, P.V., and Weller, R.O. The structure of the lamina cribrosa of the human eye: An immunocytochemical and electron microscopical study. *Eye 4*:42–57, 1990.

114. Essner, E., and Lin, W.-L. Immunocytochemical localization of laminin, type IV collagen and fibronectin in rat retinal vessels. *Exp. Eye Res. 47*:317–327, 1988.

115. Eyre, D.R., and Glimcher, M.J. Reducible cross-links in hydroxylysine-deficient collagens of a heritable disorder of connective tissue. *Proc. Natl. Acad. Sci. USA 69*:2594–2598, 1972.

116. Eyre, D.R., Paz, M., and Gallop, P.M. Cross-linking in collagen and elastin. *Annu. Rev. Biochem. 53*:717–748, 1984.

117. Eyre, D.R., Wu, J.J., and Apone, S. A growing family of collagens in articular cartilage: Identification of 5 genetically distinct types. *J. Rheumatol. (Suppl.) 14*:25–27, 1987.

118. Farquhar, M.G. Structure and function in glomerular capillaries. Role of the basement membrane in glomerular filtration. In *Biology and Chemistry of Basement Membranes*, N.A. Kefalides (Ed.), Academic Press, New York, pp. 43–80, 1978.

119. Farquhar, M.G. The glomerular basement membrane. A selective macromolecular filter. In *Cell Biology of Extracellular Matrix*, E.D. Hay (Ed.), Plenum Press, New York, pp. 335–378, 1981.

120. Feeney-Burns, L., and Ellersieck, M.R. Age-related changes in the ultrastructure of Bruch's membrane. *Am. J. Ophthalmol. 100*:686–697, 1985.

121. Feeney, M.L., and Garron, L.K. Descemet's membrane in the human peripheral cornea. A study by light and electron microscopy. In *The Structure of the Eye*, G.K. Smelser (Ed.), Academic Press, New York, pp. 367–377, 1961.

122. Fessler, L.I., Chapin, S., Brosh, S., and Fessler, J.H. Intracellular transport and tyrosine sulfation of procollagen V. *Eur. J. Biochem. 158*:511–518, 1986.

123. Fessler, L.I., Robinson, W.J., and Fessler, J.H. Biosynthesis of procollagen [proαV)2 (proαV)] by chick tendon fibroblasts and procollagen (proαV)3 by hamster lung cell cultures. *J. Biol. Chem. 256*:9646–9651, 1981.

124. Fietzek, P.P., and Kühn, K. The primary structure of collagen. *Int. Rev. Connect. Tissue Res. 7*:1–60, 1976.

125. Fine, B.S., Yanoff, M., and Stone, R.A. A clinico-pathologic study of four cases of primary open-angle glaucoma compared to normal eyes. *Am. J. Ophthalmol. 91*:88–105, 1981.

126. Fine, B.S., Yanoff, M., Pitts, E., and Slaughter, F.D. Meesmann's epithelial dystrophy of the cornea. *Am. J. Ophthalmol. 83*:633–642, 1977.

127. Fini, M.E., and Girard, M.T. Expression of collagenolytic/gelatinolytic metalloproteinases by normal cornea. *Invest. Ophthalmol. Vis. Sci. 31*:1779–1788, 1990.

128. Finkelstein, I., Trope, G.E., Basu, P.K., Hasany, S.M., and Hunter, W.S. Quantitative analysis of collagen content and amino acids in trabecular meshwork. *Br. J. Ophthalmol. 74*:280–282, 1990.

129. Fisher, R.F., and Pettet, B.E. The postnatal growth of the capsule of the human lens. *J. Anat. (Lond.) 112*:207–214, 1972.

130. Fisher, R.F., and Wakely, J. The elastic constants and ultrastructural organization of a basement membrane (lens capsule). *Proc. R. Soc. Lond. [B] 193*:335–358, 1976.

131. Fitch, J.M., Birk, D.E., Mentzer, A., Hasty, K.A., Mainardi, C., and Linsenmayer, T.F. Corneal collagen fibrils: Dissection with specific collagenases and monoclonal antibodies. *Invest. Ophthalmol. Vis. Sci. 29*:1125–1136, 1988.

132. Fitch, J.M., Gross, J., Mayne, R., Johnson-Wint, B., and Linsenmayer, T.F. Organization of collagen types I and V in the embryonic chicken cornea: Monoclonal antibody studies. *Proc. Natl. Acad. Sci. USA 81*:2791–2795, 1984.

133. Fitch, J.M., Mentzer, A., Mayne, R., and Linsenmayer, T.F. Acquisition of type IX collagen by the developing avian primary corneal stroma and vitreous. *Dev. Biol. 128*:396–405, 1988.

134. Fleischmajer, R., Perlish, J.S., Burgeson, R.E., Shaikh-Bahai, F., and Timpl, R. Type I and type III collagen interactions during fibrillogenesis. *Ann. N.Y. Acad. Sci. 580*:161–175, 1990.

135. Fleischmajer, R., Timpl, R., Tuderman, L., Raisher, L., Wiestner, M., Perlish, J.S., and Graves, P.N. Ultrastructural identification of extension amino propeptides of type I and III collagens in human skin. *Proc. Natl. Acad. Sci. USA 78*:7360–7364, 1981.

136. Foidart, J.-M., Abe, S., Martin, G.R., Zizic, T.M., Barnett, E.V., Lawley, T.J., and Katz, S.I. Antibodies to type II collagen in relapsing polychondritis. *N. Engl. J. Med. 299*:1203–1207, 1978.

137. Folkman, J., Klagsbrun, M., Sasse, J., Wadzinski, M., Ingber, D., and Vlodavsky, I. A heparin-binding angiogenic protein—basic fibroblast growth factor—is stored within basement membrane. *Am. J. Pathol. 130*:393–400, 1988.

138. Font, R.L., and Brownstein, S. A light and electron microscopic study of anterior subcapsular cataracts. *Am. J. Ophthalmol. 78*:972–984, 1974.

139. Foos, R.Y. Vitreoretinal juncture; epiretinal membranes and vitreous. *Invest. Ophthalmol. Vis. Sci. 16*:416–422, 1977.

140. Forrester, J.V., Grierson, I., and Lee, W.R. The pathology of vitreous hemorrhage. II. Ultrastructure. *Arch. Ophthalmol. 97*:2368–2374, 1979.

141. Francomano, C.A., Liberfarb, R.M., Hirose, T., Maumenee, I.H., Streeten, E.A., Meyers, D.A., and Pyeritz, R.E. The Stickler syndrome: Evidence for close linkage to the structural gene for type II collagen. *Genomics 1*:293–296, 1987.

142. Freeman, I.L. Special tissue collagen: The eye. In *Collagen in Health and Disease*, J.B. Weiss and M.I.V. Jayson (Eds.), Churchill Livingstone, Edinburgh, pp. 388–403, 1982.

143. Freeman, I.L., Vergnes, J.P., and Brown, S.I. Age-related biochemical changes in human Descemet's membrane. *Gerontology 26*:217–220, 1980.

144. Friedman, A.H., Weingeist, S., Brackup, A., and Marinoff, G. Sclero-cornea and defective mesodermal migration. *Br. J. Ophthalmol. 59*:683–687, 1975.

145. Fujikawa, L.S., Foster, C.S., Gipson, I.K., and Colvin, R.B. Basement membrane components in healing rabbit corneal epithelial wounds: Immunofluorescence and ultrastructural studies. *J. Cell Biol. 98*:128–138, 1984.

146. Fujimoto, D. Human tendon collagen: Aging and cross-linking. *Biomed. Res. 5*:279–282, 1984.

147. Fujimoto, D., Horiuchi, K., and Hirama, M. Isotrityrosine, a new cross-linking amino acid isolated from *Ascaris* cuticle collagen. *Biochem. Biophys. Res. Commun. 99*:637–643, 1981.

148. Fukushi, S., and Spiro, R.G. The lens capsule: Sugar and amino acid composition. *J. Biol. Chem. 244*:2041–2048, 1969.

149. Funata, M., and Tokoro, T. Scleral change in experimentally myopic monkeys. *Graefes Arch. Clin. Exp. Ophthalmol. 228*:174–179, 1990.

150. Galloway, D. The primary structure. In *Collagen in Health and Disease*, J.B. Weiss and M.I.V. Jayson (Eds.), Churchill Livingstone, Edinburgh, pp. 528–557, 1982.

151. Gans, L.A. Eye lesions of epidermolysis bullosa. Clinical features, management and prognosis. *Arch. Dermatol. 124*:762–764, 1988.

152. Gay, S., and Miller, E.J. Characterization of lens capsule collagen: Evidence for the presence of two unique chains in molecules derived from major basement membrane structures. *Arch. Biochem. Biophys. 198*:370–378, 1979.

153. Ghadially, F.N. Giant collagen fibrils and amianthoid fibres. In *Ultrastructural Pathology of the Cell and Matrix*, 2nd ed., Butterworths, London, pp. 898–903, 1982.

154. Gibson, G.J., and Flint, M.H. Type X collagen synthesis by chick sternal cartilage and its relationship to endochondral development. *J. Cell Biol. 101*:277–284, 1985.

155. Gibson, G.J., Schor, S.L., and Grant, M.E. Effects of matrix macromolecules on chondrocyte gene expression: Synthesis of a low molecular weight collagen species by cells cultured within collagen gels. *J. Cell Biol. 93*:767–774, 1982.

156. Gipson, I.K., Spurr-Michaud, S.T., and Tisdale, A.S. Anchoring fibrils form a complex network in human and rabbit cornea. *Invest. Ophthalmol. Vis. Sci. 28*:212–220, 1987.

157. Goldbaum, M.H., and Madden, K. A new perspective on Bruch's membrane and the retinal pigment epithelium. *Br. J. Ophthalmol. 66*:17–25, 1982.

158. Goldberg, M., Lecolle, S., Ruch, J.V., Staubli, A., and Septier, D. Lipid detection by malachite green-aldehyde in the dental basement membrane in the rat incisor. *Cell Tissue Res. 253*:685–687, 1988.

159. Gordon, J.M., Bauer, E.A., and Eisen, A.Z. Collagenase in human cornea. Immunologic localization. *Arch. Ophthalmol.* 98:341–345, 1980.
160. Gordon, M.K., Gerecke, D.R., Dublet, B., van der Rest, M., Sugrue, S.P., and Olsen, B.R. The structure of type XII collagen. *Ann. N.Y. Acad. Sci.* 580:8–16, 1990.
161. Golsen, J.B., Eisen, A.Z., and Bauer, E.A. Stimulation of skin fibroblast collagenase production by a cytokine derived from basal cell carcinomas. *J. Invest. Dermatol.* 85:161–164, 1985.
162. Govan, J.A.A. Ocular manifestations of Alport's syndrome: A hereditary disorder of basement membranes? *Br. J. Ophthalmol.* 67:493–503, 1983.
163. Grant, D.S., and Leblond, C.P. Immunogold quantitation of laminin, type IV collagen and heparan sulfate proteoglycan in a variety of basement membranes. *J. Histochem. Cytochem.* 36:271–283, 1988.
164. Grant, M.E., and Heathcote, J.G. A comparative study of lens capsule assembly. In *New Trends in Basement Membrane Research*, K. Kühn, H. Schoene, and R. Timpl (Eds.), Raven Press, New York, pp. 195–202, 1982.
165. Grant, M.E., and Jackson, D.S. The biosynthesis of procollagen. *Essays Biochem.* 12:77–113, 1976.
166. Grant, M.E., Freeman, I.L., Schofield, J.D., and Jackson, D.S. Variations in the carbohydrate content of human and bovine polymeric collagens from various tissues. *Biochim. Biophys. Acta 177*:682–685, 1969.
167. Grant, M.E., Heathcote, J.G., and Orkin, R.W. Current concepts of basement-membrane structure and function. *Biosci. Rep. 1*:819–842, 1981.
168. Grant, M.E., Kielty, C.M., Kwan, A.P.L., Holmes, D.F., and Schor, S.L. Partial characterization of collagen types IX and X synthesized by embryonic chick chondrocytes. *Ann. N.Y. Acad. Sci.* 460:443–444, 1986.
169. Gray, L.D., and Kreger, A.S. Rabbit corneal damage produced by *Pseudomonas aeruginosa* infection. *Infect. Immun.* 12:419–432, 1975.
170. Greenburg, G., and Hay, E.D. Epithelia suspended in collagen gels can lose polarity and express characteristics of migrating mesenchymal cells. *J. Cell Biol.* 95:333–339, 1982.
171. Greenfield, G., Romano, A., Stein, R., and Goodman, R.M. Blue sclerae and keratoconus: Key features of a distinct heritable disorder of connective tissue. *Clin. Genet.* 4:8–16, 1973.
172. Grierson, I., Kissun, R., Ayad, S., Phylactos, A., Ahmed, S., Unger, W.G., and Day, J.E. The morphological features of bovine meshwork cells in vitro and their synthetic activities. *Graefes Arch. Clin. Exp. Ophthalmol.* 223:225–236, 1985.
173. Griffin, C.A., Emanuel, B.S., Hansen, J.R., Cavenee, W.K., and Myers, J.C. Human collagen genes encoding basement membrane α1(IV) and α2(IV) chains map to the distal long arm of chromosome 13. *Proc. Natl. Acad. Sci. USA 84*:512–516, 1987.
174. Gross, J. An essay on biological degradation of collagen. In *Cell Biology of Extracellular Matrix*, E.D. Hay (Ed.), Plenum Press, New York, pp. 217–258, 1981.
175. Gross, J., Azizkhan, R.G., Biswas, C., Bruns, R.R., Hsieh, D.S.-T., and Folkman, J. Inhibition of tumor growth, vascularization and collagenolysis in the rabbit cornea by medroxyprogesterone. *Proc. Natl. Acad. Sci. USA 78*:1176–1180, 1981.
176. Gunson, D.E., Halliwell, R.E.W., and Minor, R.R. Dermal collagen degradation and phagocytosis. Occurrence in a horse with hyperextensible fragile skin. *Arch. Dermatol.* 120:599–604, 1984.
177. Gyi, T.J., Meek, K.M., and Elliott, G.F. Collagen interfibrillar distances in corneal stroma using synchrotron X-ray diffraction: A species study. *Int. J. Biol. Macromol.* 10:265–269, 1988.
178. Haddad, A., and Bennett, G. Synthesis of lens capsule and plasma membrane glycoproteins by lens epithelial cells and fibers in the rat. *Am. J. Anat.* 183:212–225, 1988.
179. Haigh, M., and Scott, J.E. A method of processing tissue sections for staining with cupromeronic blue and other dyes, using CEC techniques, for light and electron microscopy. *Basic Appl. Histochem.* 30:479–486, 1986.
180. Harnisch, J.P., Buchen, R., Sinha, P.K., and Barrach, H.J. Ultrastructural identification of type I and type II collagen in the cornea of the mouse by means of enzyme-labelled antibodies. *Graefes Arch. Clin. Exp. Ophthalmol.* 208:9–13, 1978.
181. Harris, E.D., Jr., Welgus, H.G., and Krane, S.M. Regulation of the mammalian collagenases. *Collagen 4*: 493–512, 1984.
182. Hay, E.D. Development of the vertebrate cornea. *Int. Rev. Cytol.* 63:263–322, 1980.
183. He, Y., Niederkorn, J.Y., McCulley, J.P., Stewart, G.L., Meyer, D.R., Silvany, R., and Dougherty, J. In vivo and in vitro collagenolytic activity of *Acanthamoeba castellani*. *Invest. Ophthalmol. Vis. Sci.* 31:2235–2240, 1990.
184. Heathcote, J.G., Bailey, A.J., and Grant, M.E. Studies on the assembly of the rat lens capsule. Biosynthesis of a cross-linked collagenous component of high molecular weight. *Biochem. J.* 190:229–237, 1980.
185. Heathcote, J.G., Bruns, R.R., and Orkin, R.W. Biosynthesis of sulphated macromolecules by rabbit lens epithelium. II. Relationship to basement membrane formation. *J. Cell Biol.* 99:861–869, 1984.
186. Heathcote, J.G., and Grant, M.E. Extracellular modification of connective tissue proteins. In *The Enzymology of Posttranslational Modification of Proteins*, Vol. 1, R.B. Freedman and H.C. Hawkins (Eds.), Academic Press, London, pp. 457–506, 1980.
187. Heathcote, J.G., and Grant, M.E. The molecular organization of basement membranes. *Int. Rev. Connect. Tissue Res.* 9:191–264, 1981.
188. Heathcote, J.G., and Grant, M.E. The macromolecular composition of the embryonic chick lens capsule.

Preliminary biosynthetic studies on the collagenous and noncollagenous glycoproteins. *Exp. Eye Res. 34*:985–1000, 1982.

189. Heathcote, J.G., and Orkin, R.W. Biosynthesis of sulphated macromolecules by rabbit lens epithelium. I. Identification of major macromolecules synthesized by lens epithelial cells in vitro. *J. Cell Biol. 99*:852–860, 1984.

190. Heathcote, J.G., Eyre, D.R., and Gross, J. Mature bovine Descemet's membrane contains desmosine and isodesmosine. *Biochem. Biophys. Res. Commun. 108*:1588–1594, 1982.

191. Heathcote, J.G., Schoales, B.A., and Willis, N.R. Incontinentia pigmenti (Bloch-Sulzberger syndrome): A case report and review of the ocular pathological features. *Can. J. Ophthalmol. 26*:229–237, 1991.

192. Heathcote, J.G., Sear, C.H.J., and Grant, M.E. Studies on the assembly of the rat lens capsule. Biosynthesis and partial characterization of the collagenous components. *Biochem. J. 176*:283–294, 1978.

193. Heathcote, J.G., Sear, C.H.J., and Grant, M.E. Biosynthesis of rat lens capsule collagen. In *Biology and Chemistry of Basement Membranes*, N.A. Kefalides (Ed.), Academic Press, New York, pp. 335–342, 1978.

194. Heathcote, J.G., Sholdice, J., Walton, J.C., Willis, N.R., and Sergovich, F.R. Anterior segment mesenchymal dysgenesis associated with partial duplication of the short arm of chromosome 2. *Can. J. Ophthalmol. 26*:35–43, 1991.

195. Hembry, R.M., and Ehrlich, H.P. Immunolocalization of collagenase and tissue inhibitor of metalloproteinases (TIMP) in hypertrophic scar tissue. *Br. J. Dermatol. 115*:409–420, 1986.

196. Hendrix, M.J.C., Hay, E.D., von der Mark, K., and Linsenmayer, T.F. Immunohistochemical localization of collagen type I and II in the developing chick cornea and tibia by electron microscopy. *Invest. Ophthalmol. Vis. Sci. 22*:359–375, 1986.

197. Henkel, W., and Glanville, R.W. Covalent cross-linking between molecules of type I and type III collagen. The involvement of the N-terminal, nonhelical regions of the α1(I) and α1(III) chains in the formation of inter-molecular cross-links. *Eur. J. Biochem. 122*:205–213, 1982.

198. Hernandez, M.R., Andrzejewska, W.M., and Neufeld, A.H. Changes in the extracellular matrix of the human optic nerve head in primary open-angle glaucoma. *Am. J. Ophthalmol. 109*:180–188, 1990.

199. Hernandez, M.R., Luo, X.X., Andrzejewska, W., and Neufeld, A.H. Age-related changes in the extracellular matrix of the human optic nerve head. *Am. J. Ophthalmol. 107*:476–484, 1989.

200. Hernandez, M.R., Wang, N., Hanley, N.M., and Neufeld, A.H. Localization of collagen types I and IV mRNAs in human optic nerve head by in situ hybridization. *Invest. Ophthalmol. Vis. Sci. 32*:2169–2177, 1991.

201. Hernandez, M.R., Weinstein, B.I., Schwartz, J., Ritch, R., Gordon, G.G., and Southren, A.L. Human trabecular meshwork cells in culture: Morphology and extracellular matrix constituents. *Invest. Ophthalmol. Vis. Sci. 28*:1655–1660, 1987.

202. Hicks, N.J., Ward, R.V., and Reynolds, J.J. A fibrosarcoma model derived from mouse embryo cells: Growth properties and secretion of collagenase and metalloproteinase inhibitor (TIMP) by tumour cell lines. *Int. J. Cancer 33*:835–844, 1984.

203. Hirano, K., Kobayashi, M., Kobayashi, K., Hoshino, T., and Awaya, S. Experimental formation of 100 nm periodic fibrils in the mouse corneal stroma and trabecular meshwork. *Invest. Ophthalmol. Vis. Sci. 30*:869–874, 1989.

204. Hoang-Xuan, T., Foster, C.S., and Rice, B.A. Scleritis in relapsing polychondritis. Response to therapy. *Ophthalmology 97*:892–898, 1990.

205. Hong, B.-S., and Davison, P.F. Identification of type II procollagen in rabbit vitreous. *Ophthalmic Res. 17*:162–167, 1985.

206. Hostikka, S.L., Eddy, R.L., Byers, M.G., Hoyhtya, M., Shows, T.B., and Tryggvason, K. Identification of a distinct type IV collagen chain with restricted kidney distribution and assignment of its gene to the locus of X chromosome-linked Alport syndrome. *Proc. Natl. Acad. Sci. USA 87*:1606–1610, 1990.

207. Hsieh, P., and Baum, J. Effects of fibroblastic and endothelial extracellular matrices on corneal endothelial cells. *Invest. Ophthalmol. Vis. Sci. 26*:457–463, 1985.

208. Huber, S., Winterhalter, K.H., and Vaughan, L. Isolation and sequence analysis of the glycosaminoglycan attachment site of type IX collagen. *J. Biol. Chem. 263*:752–756, 1988.

209. Hulmes, D.J.S. A possible mechanism for the regulation of collagen fibril diameter in vivo. *Collagen 3*:317–321, 1983.

210. Hulmes, D.J.S., Bruns, R.R., and Gross, J. On the state of aggregation of newly secreted procollagen. *Proc. Natl. Acad. Sci. USA 80*:388–392, 1983.

211. Hulmes, D.J.S., Miller, A., Parry, D.A.D., Piez, K.A, and Woodhead-Galloway, J. Analysis of the primary structure of collagen for the origins of molecular packing. *J. Mol. Biol. 79*:137–148, 1973.

212. Hültsch, E. The vitreous of the baby owl monkey. A model for rapid and complete gel-liquefaction. *Dev. Ophthalmol. 2*:1–7, 1981.

213. Huttner, W.B. Determination and occurrence of tyrosine O-sulfate in proteins. *Methods Enzymol. 107*:200–223, 1984.

214. Ihalainen, A., Salo, T., Forsius, H., and Peltonen, L. Increase in type I and type IV collagenolytic activity in primary cultures of keratoconus corneas. *Eur. J. Clin. Invest. 16*:78–84, 1986.

215. Isaak, B.L., Liesegang, T.J., and Michet, C.J., Jr. Ocular and systemic findings in relapsing polychondritis. *Ophthalmology 93*:681–689, 1986.

216. Ishibashi, T., Patterson, R., Ohnishi, Y., Inomata, H., and Ryan, S.J. Formation of drusen in the human eye. *Am. J. Ophthalmol. 101*:342–353, 1986.

217. Ishibashi, T., Sorgente, N., Patterson, R., and Ryan, S.J. Pathogenesis of drusen in the primate. *Invest. Ophthalmol. Vis. Sci. 27*:184–193, 1986.

218. Iwamoto, M., Haik, B.G., Iwamoto, T., Harrison, W., and Carter, D.M. The ultrastructural defect in conjunctiva from a case of recessive dystrophic epidermolysis bullosa. *Arch. Ophthalmol. 109*:1382–1386, 1991.

219. Iyama, K., Ninomiya, Y., Olsen, B.R., Linsenmayer, T.F., Trelstad, R.L., and Hayashi, M. Shift in spatial pattern of type X collagen expression in embryonic sterna undergoing endochondral ossification demonstrated by in situ hybridization and immunohistochemistry. *Ann. N.Y. Acad. Sci. 580*:529–531, 1990.

220. Jackson, D.S., and Fessler, J.H. Isolation and properties of a collagen soluble in salt solution at neutral pH. *Nature (Lond.) 176*:69–70, 1955.

221. Jakus, M.A. Studies on the cornea. II. The fine structure of Descemet's membrane. *J. Biophys. Biochem. Cytol. (Suppl.) 2*:243–255, 1956.

222. Jakus, M.A. The fine structure of the human cornea. In *The Structure of the Eye*, G.K. Smelser (Ed.), Academic Press, New York, 1961, pp. 343–366.

223. Jerdan, J.A., and Glaser, B.M. Retinal microvessel extracellular matrix: An immunofluorescent study. *Invest. Ophthalmol. Vis. Sci. 27*:194–203, 1986.

224. Jerdan, J.A., Michels, R.G., and Glaser, B.M. Diabetic preretinal membranes: An immunohistochemical study. *Arch. Ophthalmol. 104*:286–290, 1986.

225. Jerdan, J.A., Pepose, J.S., Michels, R.G., Hayashi, H., De Bustros, S., Sebag, M., and Glaser, B.M. Proliferative vitreoretinopathy membranes: An immunohistochemical study. *Ophthalmology 96*:801–810, 1989.

226. Jha, M. Age-related changes in pyridinoline content of rabbit collagen. *Exp. Gerontol. 17*:7–9, 1982.

227. Jimbow, K., Kobayashi, H., Ishii, M., Oyanagi, A., and Ooshimi, A. Scar and keloid lesions in progeria. *Arch. Dermatol. 124*:1261–1266, 1988.

228. Johnson-Wint, B. In vivo endogenous regulation of interstitial collagenase production in a mild alkali burn model in rabbit. *Invest. Ophthalmol. Vis. Sci. (Suppl.) 32*:1070, 1991.

229. Johnson-Wint, B., and Bauer, E.A. Stimulation of collagenase synthesis by a 20,000-Dalton epithelial cytokine. Evidence for pre-translational regulation. *J. Biol. Chem. 260*:2080–2085, 1985.

230. Johnson-Wint, B., and Gross, J. Regulation of connective tissue collagenase production: stimulators from adult and fetal epidermal cells. *J. Cell Biol. 98*:90–96, 1984.

231. Johnson, D.H., Bourne, W.M., and Campbell, R.J. The ultrastructure of Descemet's membrane. I. Changes with age in normal corneas. *Arch. Ophthalmol. 100*:1942–1947, 1982.

232. Johnson, M.C., and Beebe, D.C. Growth, synthesis and regional specialization of the embryonic chicken lens capsule. *Exp. Eye Res. 38*:579–592, 1984.

233. Johnstone, M.A., and Grant, W.M. Pressure-dependent changes in structures of the aqueous outflow system of human and monkey eyes. *Am. J. Ophthalmol. 75*:365–383, 1973.

234. Judisch, G.F., Waziri, M., and Krachmer, J.H. Ocular Ehlers-Danlos syndrome with normal lysyl hydroxylase activity. *Arch. Ophthalmol. 94*:1489–1491, 1976.

235. Jukkula, A., Risteli, J., Niemela, O., and Risteli, L. Incorporation of sulphate into type III procollagen by cultured human fibroblasts. Identification of tyrosine O-sulphate. *Eur. J. Biochem. 154*:219–224, 1984.

236. Kaiser-Kupfer, M.I., McCain, L., Shapiro, J.R., Polgon, M.J., Kupfer, C., and Rowe, D. Low ocular rigidity in patients with osteogenesis imperfecta. *Invest. Ophthalmol. Vis. Sci. 24*:432–436, 1983.

237. Kampik, A., Kenyon, K.R., Michels, R.G., Green, W.R., and de la Cruz, Z. Epiretinal and vitreous membranes. Comparative study of 56 cases. *Arch. Ophthalmol. 99*:1445–1454, 1981.

238. Kao, W.W.-Y., Vergnes, J.-P., Ebert, J., Sundar-Raj, C.V., and Brown, S.I. Increased collagenase and gelatinase activities in keratoconus. *Biochem. Biophys. Res. Commun. 107*:929–936, 1982.

239. Kao, W.W., Mai, S.H., and Chou, K.L. Biosynthesis of procollagens and collagens by tissue explants and matrix-free cells from embryonic chick cornea. *Invest. Ophthalmol. Vis. Sci. 23*:787–795, 1982.

240. Kapoor, R., Bornstein, P., and Sage, E.H. Type VIII collagen from bovine Descemet's membrane: Structural characterization of a triple-helical domain. *Biochemistry 25*:3930–3937, 1986.

241. Kapoor, R., Sakai, L.Y., Funk, S., Roux, E., Bornstein, P., and Sage, E.H. Type VIII collagen has a restricted distribution in specialized extracellular matrices. *J. Cell Biol. 107*:721–730, 1988.

242. Karwatowski, W.S.S., Jeffries, T.E., Duance, V.C., Albon, J., and Easty, D.L. Collagen and aging in Bruch's membrane. *Invest. Ophthalmol. Vis. Sci. (Suppl.) 32*:687, 1991.

243. Kashtan, C., Fish, A.J., Kleppel, M., Yoshioka, K., and Michael, A.F. Nephritogenic antigen determinants in epidermal and renal basement membranes of kindreds with Alport-type familial nephritis. *J. Clin. Invest. 78*:1035–1044, 1986.

244. Kasner, L., Mietz, H., and Green, W.R. Agenesis of Bowman's layer: A histopathological study of four cases. *Cornea 12*:163–170, 1993.

245. Kay, E.P. Expression of types I and IV collagen genes in normal and in modulated corneal endothelial cells. *Invest. Ophthalmol. Vis. Sci. 30*:260–268, 1989.

246. Kay, E.P., Cheung, C.C., Jester, J.V., Nimni, M.E., and Smith, R.E. Type I collagen and fibronectin synthesis by retrocorneal fibrous membrane. *Invest. Ophthalmol. Vis. Sci. 22*:200–212, 1982.

247. Kay, E.P., Smith, R.E., and Nimni, M.E. Basement membrane collagen synthesis by rabbit corneal endothelial cells in culture. Evidence for an α chain derived from a larger biosynthetic precursor. *J. Biol. Chem. 257*:7116–7121, 1982.

248. Kayes, J., and Holmberg, A. The fine structure of Bowman's layer and the basement membrane of the corneal epithelium. *Am. J. Ophthalmol. 50*:1013–1021, 1960.

249. Keeley, F.W., Morin, J.D., and Vesely, S. Characterization of collagen from normal human sclera. *Exp. Eye Res. 39*:533–542, 1984.

250. Keene, D.R., Lunstrum, G.P., Morris, N.P., Stoddard, D.W., and Burgeson, R.E. Two type XII-like collagens localize to the surface of banded collagen fibers. *J. Cell Biol. 113*:971–978, 1991.

251. Keene, D.R., Sakai, L.Y., Bächinger, H.P., and Burgeson, R.E. Type III collagen can be present on banded collagen fibrils regardless of fibril diameter. *J. Cell Biol. 105*:2393–2402, 1987.

252. Keene, D.R., Sakai, L.Y., Lunstrum, G.P., Morris, N.P., and Burgeson, R.E. Type VII collagen forms an extended network of anchoring fibrils. *J. Cell Biol. 104*:611–621, 1987.

253. Kefalides, N.A. Isolation of a collagen from basement membranes containing three identical α-chains. *Biochem. Biophys. Res. Commun. 45*:226–234, 1971.

254. Kefalides, N.A., and Denduchis, B. Structural components of epithelial and endothelial basement membranes. *Biochemistry 8*:4613–4621, 1969.

255. Kefalides, N.A., Cameron, J.D., Tomichek, E.A., and Yanoff, M. Biosynthesis of basement membrane collagen by rabbit corneal endothelium in vitro. *J. Biol. Chem. 254*:730–733, 1976.

256. Kemp, P.D., and Scott, J.E. Ehrlich chromogens, probably cross-links in elastin and collagen. *Biochem. Soc. Trans. 15*:711, 1987.

257. Kennedy, A., Frank, R.N., Mancini, M.A., and Lande, M. Collagens of the retinal microvascular basement membrane and of retinal microvascular cells in vitro. *Exp. Eye Res. 42*:177–199, 1986.

258. Kennedy, L., and Baynes, J.W. Non-enzymatic glycosylation and the chronic complications of diabetes: An overview. *Diabetologia 26*:93–98, 1984.

259. Kennedy, R.H., Bourne, W.M., and Dyer, J.A. A 48-year clinical and epidemiologic study of keratoconus. *Am. J. Ophthalmol. 101*:267–273, 1986.

260. Kenney, M.C., Benya, P.D., Nimni, M.E., and Smith, R.E. An ultrastructural study of retrocorneal fibrous membrane-like corneal endothelial metaplasia in vitro. *Ophthalmic Res. 12*:257–269, 1980.

261. Kenney, M.C., Benya, P.D., Nimni, M.E., and Smith, R.E. Stability of the collagen phenotype and decreased collagen production in serial subcultures of rabbit corneal endothelial cells. *Exp. Eye Res. 33*:131–140, 1981.

262. Kenney, M.C., Chwa, M., Escobar, M., and Brown, D. Altered gelatinolytic activity by keratoconus corneal cells. *Biochem. Biophys. Res. Commun. 161*:353–357, 1989.

263. Kenney, M.C., Labermeier, U., Hinds, D., and Waring, G.O. Characterization of the Descemet's membrane/posterior collagenous layer isolated from Fuchs' endothelial dystrophy corneas. *Exp. Eye Res. 39*:267–277, 1984.

264. Kenyon, K.R., Maumenee, A.E., Ryan, S.J., Whitmore, P.V., and Green, W.R. Diffuse drusen and associated complications. *Am. J. Ophthalmol. 100*:119–128, 1985.

265. Kessler, E., Kennah, H.E., and Brown, S.I. *Pseudomonas* protease. Purification, partial characterization, and its effect on collagen, proteoglycan and rabbit corneas. *Invest. Ophthalmol. Vis. Sci. 16*:488–497, 1977.

266. Kittelberger, R., Davis, P.F., and Greenhill, N.S. Immunolocalization of type VIII collagen in vascular tissue. *Biochem. Biophys. Res. Commun. 159*:414–419, 1989.

267. Kittelberger, R., Davis, P.F., Flynn, D.W., and Greenhill, N.S. Distribution of type VIII collagen in tissues. An immunohistochemical study. *Connect. Tissue Res. 24*:303–318, 1990.

268. Kivirikko, K.I., and Myllyla, R. Post-translational modifications. In *Collagen in Health and Disease*, J.B. Weiss and M.I.V. Jayson (Eds.), Churchill Livingston, Edinburgh, pp. 101–120, 1982.

269. Kleinman, H.K., McGarvey, M.L., Hassell, J.R., Star, V.L., Cannon, F.B., Laurie, G.W., and Martin, G.R. Basement membrane complexes with biological activity. *Biochemistry 25*:312–318, 1986.

270. Kleppel, M.M., and Michael, A.F. Expression of novel basement membrane components in the developing human eye. *Am. J. Anat. 187*:165–174, 1990.

271. Kleppel, M.M., Kashtan, C., Santi, P.A., Wieslander, J., and Michael, A.F. Distribution of familial nephritis antigen in normal tissue and renal basement membranes of patients with homozygous and heterozygous Alport familial nephritis. Relationship of familial nephritis and Goodpasture antigens to novel collagen chains and type IV collagen. *Lab. Invest. 61*:278–289, 1989.

272. Kleppel, M.M., Santi, P.A., Cameron, J.D., Wieslander, J., and Michael, A.F. Human tissue distribution of novel basement membrane collagen. *Am. J. Pathol. 134*:813–825, 1989.

273. Ko, M.K., and Choe, J.K. Extracellular matrix of the human retinal pigment epithelial cells in vitro. *Korean J. Ophthalmol. 2*:66–68, 1988.

274. Kogaya, Y., Kim, S., Haruna, S., and Akisaka, T. Heterogeneity of distribution at the electron microscopic level of heparan sulfate in various basement membranes. *J. Histochem. Cytochem. 38*:1459–1467, 1990.
275. Kohn, R.R. Effects of age and diabetes mellitus on cyanogen bromide digestion of human dura mater collagen. *Connect. Tissue Res. 11*:169–173, 1983.
276. Komai, Y., and Ushiki, T. The three-dimensional organization of collagen fibrils in the human cornea and sclera. *Invest. Ophthalmol. Vis. Sci. 32*:2244–2258, 1991.
277. Konomi, H., Hayashi,T., Nakayasu, K., and Arima, M. Localization of type V and type IV collagen in human cornea, lung and skin. Immunohistochemical evidence by anti-collagen antibodies characterized by immuno-electro-blotting. *Am. J. Pathol. 116*:417–426, 1983.
278. Konomi, H., Hayashi, T., Sano, J., Terato, K., Nagai, Y., Arima, M., Nakayasu, K., Tanaka, M., and Nakajima, A. Immunohistochemical localization of type I, III and IV collagens in the sclera and choroid of bovine, rat and normal and pathological human eyes. *Biomed. Res. 4*:451–458, 1984.
279. Konstas, A.G., Marshall, G.E., and Lee, W.R. Immunocytochemical localization of collagens (I–V) in the human iris. *Graefes Arch. Clin. Exp. Ophthalmol. 228*:180–186, 1990.
280. Krane, S.M., Pinnell, S.R., and Erbe, R.W. Lysyl-protocollagen hydroxylase deficiency in fibroblasts from siblings with hydroxylysine-deficient collagen. *Proc. Natl. Acad. Sci. USA 69*:2899–2903, 1972.
281. Kretzer, F.L., Hittner, H.M., and Mehta, R.S. Ocular manifestations of the Smith-Lemli-Opitz syndrome. *Arch. Ophthalmol. 99*:2000–2006, 1981.
282. Krieg, T., Feldmann, U., Kessler, W., and Müller, P.K. Biochemical characteristics of Ehlers-Danlos syndrome type VI in a family with one affected infant. *Hum. Genet. 46*:41–49, 1979.
283. Kühn, K. The structure of collagen. *Essays Biochem. 5*:59–87, 1969.
284. Kühn, K., Wiedemann, H., Timpl, R., Risteli, J., Dieringer, H., Voss, T., and Glanville, R.W. Macromolecular structure of basement membrane collagens. Identification of 7S collagen as a cross-linking domain of type IV collagen. *FEBS Lett. 125*:123–128, 1981.
285. Kurosawa, A., Elner, V.M., Yue, B.Y.J.T., Elvart, J.L., and Tso, M.O.M. Cultured trabecular-meshwork cells: Immunohistochemical and lectin-binding characteristics. *Exp. Eye Res. 45*:239–251, 1987.
286. Kwan, A.P.L., Freemont, A.J., and Grant, M.E. Immunoperoxidase localization of type X collagen in chick tibiae. *Biosci. Rep. 6*:155–162, 1986.
287. Labermeier, U., and Kenney, M.C. The presence of EC collagen and type IV collagen in bovine Descemet's membranes. *Biochem. Biophys. Res. Commun. 116*:619–625, 1983.
288. Labermeier, U., Demlow, T.A., and Kenney, M.C. Identification of collagens isolated from bovine Descemet's membrane. *Exp. Eye Res. 37*:225–237, 1983.
289. Langeveld, J.P.M., Wieslander, J,. Timoneda, J., McKinney, P., Butkowski, R.J., Wisdom, B.J., Jr., and Hudson, B.G. Structural heterogeneity of the non-collagenous domain of basement membrane collagen. *J. Biol. Chem. 263*:10481–10488, 1988.
290. Laurent, M., Kern, P., Courtois, Y., and Regnault, F. Synthesis of types I, III, and IV collagen by bovine lens epithelial cells in long-term culture. *Exp. Cell Res. 134*:23–31, 1981.
291. Laurent, M., Lonchampt, M., Regnault, F., Tassin, J., and Courtois, Y. Biochemical, ultrastructural and immunological study of in vitro production of collagen by bovine lens epithelial cells in culture. *Exp. Cell Res. 115*:127–142, 1978.
292. Lawson, P.M., Maneschi, F., and Kohner, E.M. The relationship of hand abnormalities to diabetes and diabetic retinopathy. *Diabetes Care 6*:140–143, 1983.
293. Lee, R.E., and Davison, P.F. Collagen composition and turnover in ocular tissues of the rabbit. *Exp. Eye Res. 32*:737–745, 1981.
294. Lee, R.E., and Davison, P.F. The collagens of the developing bovine cornea. *Exp. Eye Res. 39*:639–652, 1984.
295. Leivo, I., and Engvall, E. Merosin, a protein specific for basement membranes of Schwann cells, striated muscle and trophoblast, is expressed late in nerve and muscle development. *Proc. Natl. Acad. Sci. USA 85*:1544–1548, 1988.
296. Leu, F.-J., and Damjanov, I. Protease treatment combined with immunohistochemistry reveals heterogeneity of normal and neoplastic basement membranes. *J. Histochem. Cytochem. 36*:213–220, 1988.
297. Leuenberger, P. Ultrastructure of the ageing retinal vascular system, with special reference to quantitative and qualitative changes of capillary basement membranes. *Gerontologica 19*:1–15, 1973.
298. Levene, C.I. Possibilities for the therapeutic control of fibrosis. *Br. J. Dermatol. 112*:363–371, 1985.
299. Levene, C.I., and Gross, J. Alterations in state of molecular aggregation of collagen induced in chick embryos by β-aminopropionitrile (lathyrus factor). *J. Exp. Med. 110*:771–791, 1959.
300. Li, W., Stramm, L.E., Aguirre, G.D., and Rockey, J.H. Extracellular matrix production by cat retinal pigment epithelium in vitro: Characterization of type IV collagen synthesis. *Exp. Eye Res. 38*:291–304, 1984.
301. Lian, J.B., Morris, S., Faris, B., Albright, J., and Franzblau, C. The effects of acetic acid and pepsin on the cross-linkages and ultrastructure of corneal collagen. *Biochim. Biophys. Acta 328*:193–204, 1973.
302. Light, N., and Bailey, A.J. Collagen cross-links: Location of pyridinoline in type I collagen. *FEBS Lett. 182*:503–508, 1985.

303. Light, N.D. Bovine type I collagen. A study of cross-linking in various mature tissues. *Biochim. Biophys. Acta* *581*:96–105, 1979.
304. Light, N.D., and Bailey, A.J. The chemistry of the collagen cross-links. Purification and characterization of cross-linked peptide material from mature collagen containing unknown amino acids. *Biochem. J. 185*:373–381, 1980.
305. Linsenmayer, T.F., and Little, C.D. Embryonic neural retina collagen: In vitro synthesis of high molecular weight forms of type II plus a new genetic type. *Proc. Natl. Acad. Sci. USA 75*:3235–3239, 1978.
306. Linsenmayer, T.F., Fitch, J.M., Schmid, T.M., Zak, N.B., Gibney, E., Sanderson, R.D., and Mayne, R. Monoclonal antibodies against chicken type V collagen: Production, specificity and use for immunocytochemical localization in embryonic cornea and other organs. *J. Cell Biol. 96*:124–132, 1983.
307. Linsenmayer, T.F., Gibney, E., and Fitch, J.M. Embryonic avian cornea contains layers of collagen with greater than average stability. *J. Cell Biol. 103*:1587–1593, 1986.
308. Linsenmayer, T.F., Gibney, E., and Little, C.D. Type II collagen in the early embryonic chick cornea and vitreous: Immunoradiochemical evidence. *Exp. Eye Res. 34*:371–379, 1982.
309. Linsenmayer, T.F., Gibney, E., Gordon, M.K., Marchant, J.K., Hayashi, M., and Fitch, J.M. Extracellular matrices of the developing chick retina and cornea. Localization of mRNAs for collagen types II and IX by in situ hybridization. *Invest. Ophthalmol. Vis. Sci. 31*:1271–1276, 1990.
310. Linsenmayer, T.F., Mentzer, A., Irwin, M.H., Waldrep, N.K., and Mayne, R. Avian type VI collagen. Monoclonal antibody production and immunohistochemical identification as a major connective tissue component of cornea and skeletal muscle. *Exp. Cell Res. 165*:518–529, 1986.
311. Liotta, L.A. Tumour invasion and metastasis—role of the extracellular matrix: Rhoads Memorial Award Lecture. *Cancer Res. 46*:1–7, 1986.
312. Lunstrum, G.P., Kuo, H.J., Rosenbaum, L.M., Keene, D.R., Glanville, R.W., Sakai, L.Y., and Burgeson, R.E. Anchoring fibrils contain the carboxy-terminal globular domain of type VII procollagen but lack the amino-terminal globular domain. *J. Biol. Chem. 262*:13706–13712, 1987.
313. Lunstrum, G.P., Morris, N.P., McDonough, A.M., Keene, D.R., and Burgeson, R.E. Identification and partial characterization of two type XII-like collagen molecules. *J. Cell Biol. 113*:963–969, 1991.
314. Lütjen-Drecoll, E., Futa, R., and Rohen, J.W. Ultrahistochemical studies on tangential sections of the trabecular meshwork in normal and glaucomatous eyes. *Invest. Ophthalmol. Vis. Sci. 21*:563–573, 1981.
315. Lütjen-Drecoll, E., Rittig, M., Rauterberg, J., Jander, R., and Mollenauer, J. Immunomicroscopical study of type VI collagen in the trabecular meshwork of normal and glaucomatous eyes. *Exp. Eye Res. 48*:139–147, 1989.
316. Lyons, T.J., and Kennedy, L. Non-enzymatic glycosylation of skin collagen in patients with type 1 (insulin-dependent) diabetes mellitus and limited joint mobility. *Diabetologia 28*:2–5, 1985.
317. Lyons, T.J., and Kennedy, L. Effect of in vitro nonenzymatic glycosylation of human skin collagen on susceptibility to collagenase digestion. *Eur. J. Clin. Invest. 15*:128–131, 1985.
318. Mader, T.H., Stulting, R.D., and Crosswell, H.H., Jr. Bilateral paralimbal scleromalacia perforans. *Am. J. Ophthalmol. 109*:233–234, 1990.
319. Marshall, G.E., Konstas, A.G., and Lee, W.R. Immunogold localization of type IV collagen and laminin in the aging human outflow system. *Exp. Eye Res. 51*:691–699, 1990.
320. Marshall, G.E., Konstas, A.G., and Lee, W.R. Ultrastructural distribution of collagen types I-VI in aging human retinal vessels. *Br. J. Ophthalmol. 74*:228–232, 1990.
321. Marshall, G.E., Konstas, A.G.P., and Lee, W.R. Immunogold ultrastructural localization of collagens in the aged human outflow system. *Ophthalmology 98*:692–700, 1991.
322. Marshall, G.E., Konstas, A.G., and Lee, W.R. Immunogold fine structural localization of extracellular matrix components in aged human cornea. I. Types I-IV collagen and laminin. *Graefes Arch. Clin. Exp. Ophthalmol. 229*:157–163, 1991.
323. Marshall, G.E., Konstas, A.G., and Lee, W.R. Immunogold fine structural localization of extracellular matrix components in aged human cornea. II. Collagen types V and VI. *Graefes Arch. Clin. Exp. Ophthalmol. 229*:164–171, 1991.
324. Marshall, G.E., Konstas, A.G.P., Abraham, S., and Lee, W.R. Extracellular matrix in the aged human ciliary body: An immunoelectron microscopic study. *Invest. Ophthalmol. Vis. Sci. 33*:2546–2560, 1992.
325. Martin, G.R., and Timpl, R. Laminin and other basement membrane components. *Annu. Rev. Cell Biol. 3*:57–85, 1987.
326. Martinez-Hernandez, A., and Amenta, P.S. The basement membrane in pathology. *Lab. Invest. 48*:656–677, 1983.
327. Martini, B., Pandey, R., Ogden, T.E., and Ryan, S.J. Cultures of human retinal pigment epithelium. Modulation of extracellular matrix. *Invest. Ophthalmol. Vis. Sci. 33*:516–521, 1992.
328. Martini, B., Wang, H-M., Lee, M.B., Ogden, T.E., Ryan, S.J., and Sorgente, N. Synthesis of extracellular matrix by macrophage-modulated retinal pigment epithelium. *Arch. Ophthalmol. 109*:576–580, 1991.
329. Matoltsy, A.G., Gross, J., and Grignolo, A. A study of the fibrous components of the vitreous body of the electron microscope. *Proc. Soc. Exp. Biol. Med. 76*:857–860, 1951.
330. Matrisian, L.M. Metalloproteinases and their inhibitors in matrix remodeling. *Trends Genet. 6*:121–125, 1990.

331. Matsubara, M., Zieske, J.D., and Fini, M.E. Mechanism of basement membrane dissolution preceding corneal ulceration. *Invest. Ophthalmol. Vis. Sci. 32*:3221–3237, 1991.

332. Maurice, D.M. The structure and transparency of the cornea. *J. Physiol. 136*:263–286, 1957.

333. May, M.A., and Beauchamp, G.R. Collagen maturation defects in Ehlers-Danlos keratopathy. *J. Pediatr. Ophthalmol. Strabismus 24*:78–82, 1987.

334. Mayne, R., and Burgeson, R. (Eds.) *Structure and Function of Collagen Types*, Academic Press, New York, 1987.

335. Mayne, R., Elrod, B.W., Mayne, P.M., Sanderson, R.D., and Linsenmayer, T.F. Changes in the synthesis of minor cartilage collagens after growth of chick chondrocytes in 5-bromo-2'-deoxyuridine or to senescence. *Exp. Cell Res. 151*:171–182, 1984.

336. McBrien, N.A., and Norton, T.T. Experimental myopia in tree shrew is increased by treatment with lathyritic agents. *Invest. Ophthalmol. Vis. Sci. (Suppl.) 29*:33, 1988.

337. McCartney, A.C.E., and Kirkness, C.M. Comparison between posterior polymorphous dystrophy and congenital hereditary endothelial dystrophy of the cornea. *Eye 2*:63–70, 1988.

338. McDonnell, P.J., and Spalton, D.J. The ocular signs and complications of epidermolysis bullosa. *J. R. Soc. Med. 81*:576–578, 1988.

339. McDonnell, P.J., Schofield, O.M., Spalton, D.J., Mayou, B.J., and Eady, R.A.J. The eye in dystrophic epidermolysis bullosa: Clinical and immunopathological findings. *Eye 3*:79–83, 1989.

340. McDonnell, P.J., Schofield, O.M.V., Spalton, D.J., and Eady, R.A.J. Eye involvement in junctional epidermolysis bullosa. *Arch. Ophthalmol. 107*:1635–1637, 1989.

341. McMenamin, P.G., and Lee, W.R. Age-related changes in extracellular materials in the inner wall of Schlemm's canal. *Graefes Arch. Clin. Exp. Ophthalmol. 212*:159–172, 1980.

342. McNamara, M.K., and Augusteyn, R.C. 3,3'-Dityrosine in the proteins of senile nuclear cataracts. *Exp. Eye Res. 30*:319–321, 1980.

343. Meek, K.M., Blamires, T., Elliott, G.F., Gyi, T.J., and Nave, C. The organization of collagen fibrils in the human corneal stroma: A synchrotron-ray diffraction study. *Curr. Eye Res. 6*:841–846, 1987.

344. Meezan, E., Brendel, K., and Carlson, E.C. Isolation of a purified preparation of metabolically active retinal blood vessels. *Nature (Lond.) 251*:65–67, 1974.

345. Meezan, E., Nagle, R.B., Johnson, P., Wagner, C., White, R., and Brendel, K. Structural and functional properties of acellular histoarchitecturally intact basement membranes. *Front. Matrix Biol. 7*:101–119, 1979.

346. Mendler, M., Eich-Bender, S., Vaughan, L., Winterhalter, K.H., and Bruckner, P. Cartilage contains mixed fibrils of collagen types II, IX and XI. *J. Cell Biol. 108*:191–197, 1989.

347. Merrilees, M.J., Tiang, K.M., and Scott, L. Changes in collagen fibril diameters across artery walls including a correlation with glycosaminoglycan content. *Connect. Tissue Res. 16*:237–257, 1987.

348. Meyer, O., Cyna, J., Drill, A., Cywiner-Golenzer, C., Wassef, M., and Ryckewaert, A. Relapsing polychondritis—pathogenic role of anti-native collagen type II antibodies. A case report with immunological and pathological studies. *J. Rheumatol. 8*:821–824, 1981.

349. Miller, E.J. Biochemical characteristics and biological significance of the genetically distinct collagens. *Mol. Cell Biochem. 13*:165–192, 1976.

350. Millin, J.A., Golub, B.M., and Foster, C.S. Human basement membrane components of keratoconus and normal corneas. *Invest. Ophthalmol. Vis. Sci. 27*:604–607, 1986.

351. Mishima, H., Hasebe, H., and Kondo, K. Age changes in the fine structure of the human retinal pigment epithelium. *Jpn. J. Ophthalmol. 22*:476–485, 1978.

352. Modesti, A., Kalebic, T., Scarpa, S., Togo, S., Grotendorst, G., Liotta, L.A., and Triche, T.J. Type V collagen in human amnion is a 12 nm fibrillar component of the pericellular interstitium. *Eur. J. Cell Biol. 35*:246–255, 1984.

353. Mohan, P.S., and Spiro, R.G. Macromolecular organization of basement membranes. Characterization and comparison of glomerular basement membrane and lens capsule components by immunochemical and lectin affinity procedures. *J. Biol. Chem. 261*:4328–4336, 1986.

354. Monnier, V.M. Toward a Maillard reaction theory of aging. In *The Maillard Reaction in Aging, Diabetes and Nutrition*, J.W. Baynes and V.M. Monnier (Eds.), Alan R. Liss, New York, pp. 1–22, 1989.

355. Monnier, V.M., Vishwanath, V., Frank, K.E., Elmets, C.A., Dauchot, P., and Kohn, R.R. Relation between complications of type I diabetes mellitus and collagen-linked fluorescence. *N. Engl. J. Med. 314*:403–408, 1986.

356. Moorhead, L.C. Inhibition of collagen cross-linking: A new approach to ocular scarring. *Curr. Eye Res. 1*:77–83, 1981.

357. Morino, I., Hiscott, P., McKechnie, N.M., and Grierson, I. Variation in epiretinal membrane components with clinical duration of the proliferative tissue. *Br. J. Ophthalmol. 74*:393–399, 1990.

358. Morris, N.P., and Bachinger, H.P. Type XI collagen is a heterotrimer with the composition $(1\alpha, 2\alpha, 3\alpha)$ retaining non–triple-helical domains. *J. Biol. Chem. 262*:11345–11350, 1987.

359. Morris, N.P., Keene, D.R., Glanville, R.W., Bentz, H., and Burgeson, R.E. The tissue form of type VII collagen in an antiparallel dimer. *J. Biol. Chem. 261*:5638–5644, 1986.

360. Morrison, J.C., Jerdan, J.A., L'Hernault, N.L., and Quigley, H.A. The extracellular matrix composition of the monkey optic nerve head. *Invest. Ophthalmol. Vis. Sci. 29*:1141–1150, 1988.

361. Morrison, J.E., Dorman-Pease, M.E., Dunkelberger, G.R., and Quigley, H.A. Optic nerve head extracellular matrix in primary optic atrophy and experimental glaucoma. *Arch. Ophthalmol. 108*:1020–1024, 1990.

362. Murata, Y., Yoshioka, H., Iyama, K., and Usuku, G. Distribution of type VI collagen in the bovine cornea. *Ophthalmic Res. 21*:67–72, 1989.

363. Murphy, C., Alvarado, J., and Juster, R. Prenatal and postnatal growth of the human Descemet's membrane. *Invest. Ophthalmol. Vis. Sci. 25*:1402–1415, 1984.

364. Murphy, C.G., Yun, A.J., Newsome, D.A., and Alvarado, J.A. Localization of extracellular proteins of the human trabecular meshwork by indirect immunofluorescence. *Am. J. Ophthalmol. 104*:33–43, 1987.

365. Murphy, G., Hembry, R.M., McGarrity, A.M., Reynolds, J.J., and Henderson, B. Gelatinase (type IV collagenase) immunolocalization in cells and tissues: Use of an antiserum to rabbit bone gelatinase that identifies high and low Mr forms. *J. Cell Sci. 92*:487–495, 1989.

366. Murray, J.C., Fraser, D.R., and Levene, C.I., The effect of pyridoxine deficiency on lysyl oxidase activity in the chick. *Exp. Mol. Pathol. 28*:301–308, 1978.

367. Myers, J.C., Jones, T.A., Pohjolainen, E-R., Kadri, A.S., Goddard, A.D., Sheer, D., Solomon, E., and Pihlajaniemi, T. Molecular cloning of α5(IV) collagen and assignment of the gene to the region of the X chromosome containing the Alport syndrome locus. *Am. J. Hum. Genet. 46*:1024–1033, 1990.

368. Nakanishi, I., and Brown, S.I. The histopathology and ultrastructure of congenital central corneal opacity (Peters' anomaly). *Am. J. Ophthalmol. 72*:801–812, 1971.

369. Newsome, D.A., and Gross, J. Prevention by medroxyprogesterone of perforation in the alkali-burned rabbit cornea: Inhibition of collagenolytic activity. *Invest. Ophthalmol. Vis. Sci. 16*:21–31, 1977.

370. Newsome, D.A., and Kenyon, K.R. Collagen production in vitro by the retinal pigmented epithelium of the chick embryo. *Dev. Biol. 32*:387–400, 1973.

371. Newsome, D.A., Foidart, J-M., Hassell, J.R., Krachmer, J.H., Rodrigues, M.M., and Katz, S.I. Detection of specific collagen types in normal and keratoconus corneas. *Invest. Ophthalmol. Vis. Sci. 20*:738–750, 1981.

372. Newsome, D.A., Gross, J., and Hassell, J.R. Human corneal stroma contains three distinct collagens. *Invest. Ophthalmol. Vis. Sci. 22*:376–381, 1981.

373. Newsome, D.A., Linsenmayer, T.F., and Trelstad, R.L. Vitreous body collagen. Evidence for a dual origin from the neural retina and hyalocytes. *J. Cell Biol. 71*:59–67, 1976.

374. Nimni, M.E. Mechanism of inhibition of collagen cross-linking by penicillamine. *Proc. R. Soc. Med. (Suppl.) 70*(3):65–72, 1977.

375. Ninomiya, Y., Mattei, M-G., Muragaki, Y., Apte, S., Jacenko, O., Yamaguchi, N., and Olsen, B.R. α1(VIII) and α2(VIII) collagen chains, major constituents of Descemet's membrane, are encoded by genes located on the human chromosomes 3 and 1. *Invest. Ophthalmol. Vis. Sci. (Suppl.) 32*:1140, 1991.

376. Nirankari, V.S., Rodrigues, M.M., Jarmarwala, M.G., and Rajagopalan, S. An unusual case of epithelial basement membrane dystrophy. *Am. J. Ophthalmol. 107*:552–554, 1989.

377. Nishida, T., Yasumoto, K., Otori, T., and Desaki, J. The network structure of corneal fibroblasts in the rat as revealed by scanning electron microscopy. *Invest. Ophthalmol. Vis. Sci. 29*:1887–1890, 1988.

378. Niyibizi, C., and Eyre, D.R. Identification of the cartilage α1(XI) chain in type V collagen from bovine bone. *FEBS Lett. 242*:314–318, 1989.

379. Niyibizi, C., Fietzek, P.P., and van der Rest, M. Human placenta type V collagens. Evidence for the existence of an 1(V) 2(V) 3(V) collagen molecule. *J. Biol. Chem. 259*:14170–14174, 1984.

380. Njoroge, F.G., and Monnier, V.M. The chemistry of the Maillard reaction under physiological conditions: A review. In *The Maillard Reaction in Aging, Diabetes and Nutrition*, J.W. Baynes and V.M. Monnier (Eds.), Alan R. Liss, New York, pp. 85–107, 1989.

381. Noble, J., Heathcote, J.G., and Cohen, H. Diabetes mellitus in the aetiology of Dupuytren's disease. *J. Bone Joint Surg. [Br.] 66*:322–325, 1984.

382. Novotny, G.E.K., Pau, H., and Arnold, G. Organization of collagen and other extracellular material in anterior capsular cataract. *Anat. Anz. 168*:127–133, 1989.

383. Oimimi, M., Maeda, Y., Baba, S., Iga, T., and Yamamoto, M. Relation between levels of advanced-stage products of the Maillard reaction and the development of diabetic retinopathy. *Exp. Eye Res. 49*:317–320, 1989.

384. Olsen, B.R., Alper, R., and Kefalides, N.A. Structural characterization of a soluble fraction from lens capsule–basement membrane. *Eur. J. Biochem. 38*:220–228, 1973.

385. Orford, C.R., and Gardner, D.L. Proteoglycan association with collagen d band in hyaline articular cartilage. *Connect. Tissue Res. 12*:345–348, 1984.

386. Orkin, R.W., Gehron, P., McGoodwin, E.B., Martin, G.R., Valentine, T., and Swarm, R. A murine tumor producing a matrix of basement membrane. *J. Exp. Med. 145*:204–220, 1977.

387. Oxlund, H., and Simonsen, A.H. Biochemical studies of normal and keratoconus corneas. *Acta Ophthalmol. (Copenh.) 63*:666–669, 1985.

388. Ozanics, V., Rayborn, M., and Sagun, D. Some aspects of corneal and scleral differentiation in the primate. *Exp. Eye Res. 22*:305–327, 1976.

389. Parry, D.A.D., Flint, M.H., Gillard, G.C., and Craig, A.S. A role for glycosaminoglycans in the development of collagen fibrils. *FEBS Lett.* *149*:1–7, 1982.
390. Paterson, C.A., Pfister, R.R., and Levinson, R.A. Aqueous humour pH changes after experimental alkali burns. *Am. J. Ophthalmol.* *79*:414–419, 1975.
391. Pau, H., and Novotny, G.E.K. Ultrastructural investigations on anterior capsular cataract. Cellular elements and their relationship to basement membrane and collagen synthesis. *Graefes Arch. Clin. Exp. Ophthalmol.* *223*:41–46, 1985.
392. Pau, H., Novotny, G.E.K., and Arnold, G. Ultrastructural investigation of extracellular structures in subcapsular white corrugated cataract (anterior capsular cataract). *Graefes Arch. Clin. Exp. Ophthalmol.* *223*:96–100, 1985.
393. Pauleikhoff, D., Harper, C.A., Marshall, J., and Bird, A.C. Aging changes in Bruch's membrane. A histochemical and morphologic study. *Ophthalmology* *97*:171–178, 1990.
394. Payne, K.J., King, T.A., and Holmes, D.F. Collagen fibrillogenesis in vitro: An investigation of the thermal memory effect and of the early events occurring during fibril assembly using dynamic light scattering. *Biopolymers* *25*:1185–1207, 1986.
395. Pearson, R.W. Clinicopathologic types of epidermolysis bullosa and their non-dermatological complications. *Arch. Dermatol.* *124*:718–725, 1988.
396. Peczon, B.D., Peczon, J.D., Cintron, C., and Hudson, B.G. Changes in chemical composition of anterior lens capsules of cataractous human eyes as a function of age. *Exp. Eye Res.* *30*:155–165, 1980.
397. Pemberton, J.W., Freeman, H.M., and Schepens, C.L. Familial retinal detachment and the Ehlers-Danlos syndrome. *Arch. Ophthalmol.* *76*:817–824, 1966.
398. Perejda, A.J., and Uitto, J. Non-enzymatic glycosylation of collagen and other proteins: Relationship to development of diabetic complications. *Collagen* *2*:81–88, 1982.
399. Pfister, R.R., Haddox, J.L., Dodson, R.W., and Harkins, L.E. Alkali-burned collagen produces a locomotory and metabolic stimulant to neutrophils. *Invest. Ophthalmol. Vis. Sci.* *28*:295–304, 1987.
400. Pihlajaniemi, T., Tamminen, M., Sandberg, M., Hirvonen, H., and Vuorio, E. The $\alpha 1$ chain of type XIII collagen. Polypeptide structure, alternative splicing and tissue distribution. *Ann. N.Y. Acad. Sci.* *580*:440–443, 1990.
401. Pilkerton, A.R., Rao, N.A., Marak, G.E., and Woodward, S.C. Experimental vitreous fibroplasia following perforating ocular injuries. *Arch. Ophthalmol.* *97*:1707–1709, 1979.
402. Pinnell, S.R., Krane, S.M., Kenzora, J.E., and Glimcher, M.J. A heritable disorder of connective tissue. Hydroxylysine-deficient collagen disease. *N. Engl. J. Med.* *286*:1013–1020, 1972.
403. Pirie, A. Composition of ox lens capsule. *Biochem. J.* *48*:368–371, 1951.
404. Pirie, A., Schmidt, G., and Waters, J.W. Ox vitreous humour. 1. The residual protein. *Br. J. Ophthalmol.* *32*:321–339, 1948.
405. Pongor, S., Ulrich, P.C., Bencsath, F.A., and Cerami, A. Aging of proteins: Isolation and identification of a fluorescent chromophore from the reaction of polypeptides with glucose. *Proc. Natl. Acad. Sci. USA* *81*:2684–2688, 1984.
406. Pöschl, A., and von der Mark. Synthesis of type V collagen by chick corneal fibroblasts in vivo and in vitro. *FEBS Lett.* *115*:100–104, 1980.
407. Pouliquen, Y., and Saraux, H. Ultrastructure de la cornée d'un bupthalme. *Arch. Ophthalmol.* *27*:263–272, 1967.
408. Pratt, B.M., and Madri, J.A. Immunolocalization of type IV collagen and laminin in non-basement membrane structures of murine corneal stroma. *Lab. Invest.* *52*:650–656, 1985.
409. Praus, R., Brettschneider, I., and Adam, M. Heterogeneity of the bovine corneal collagen. *Exp. Eye Res.* *29*:469–477, 1979.
410. Presberg, S.E., Quigley, H.A., Forster, R.K., and Green, W.R. Posterior polymorphous corneal dystrophy. *Cornea* *4*:239–248, 1986.
411. Prockop, D.J. Mutations in collagen genes as a cause of connective-tissue diseases. *N. Engl. J. Med.* *326*:540–546, 1992.
412. Prockop, D.J., and Kivirikko, K.I. Heritable diseases of collagen. *N. Engl. J. Med.* *344*:376–386, 1984.
413. Quantock, A.J., Meek, K.M., Ridgway, A.E.A., Bron, A.J., and Thonar, E.J.-M.A. Macular corneal dystrophy—reduction in both corneal thickness and collagen interfibrillar spacing. *Curr. Eye Res.* *9*:393–398, 1990.
414. Quigley, H.A., Dorman-Pease, M.E., Dunkelberger, G., and Brown, A. Changes in collagen and elastin in the optic nerve head in chronic human and experimental monkey glaucoma. *Invest. Ophthalmol. Vis. Sci. (Suppl.)* *31*:564, 1990.
415. Rafferty, N.S., and Goossens, W. Growth and aging of the lens capsule. *Growth* *42*:375–389, 1978.
416. Raymond, L.A., Choromokos, E., Bibler, L.W., Spaulding, A.G., Alexander, D.W., and Kao, W.W.-Y. Change in vitreous collagen after penetrating injury. *Ophthalmic Res.* *17*:102–105, 1985.
417. Rebell, G., and Forster, R.K. Lasiodiplodia theobromae as a cause of keratomycosis. *Sabouraudia 14*:155–170, 1976.

418. Reese, C.A., and Mayne, R. Minor collagens of chicken hyaline cartilage. *Biochemistry* 20:5443–5448, 1981.
419. Rehnberg, M., Ammitzboll, T., and Tengroth, B. Collagen distribution in the lamina cribrosa and the trabecular meshwork of the human eye. *Br. J. Ophthalmol.* 71:886–892, 1987.
420. Reynolds, J.J. The molecular and cellular interactions involved in connective tissue destruction. *Br. J. Dermatol.* 112:715–723, 1985.
421. Robertson, I. Keratoconus and the Ehlers-Danlos syndrome: A new aspect of keratoconus. *Med. J. Aust.* 1:571–573, 1975.
422. Robins, S.P., and Bailey, A.J. Age-related changes in collagen: The identification of reducible lysine-carbohydrate condensation products. *Biochem. Biophys. Res. Commun.* 48:76–84, 1972.
423. Robins, S.P., Shimokomaki, M., and Bailey, A.J. The chemistry of the collagen cross-links. Age-related changes in the reducible components of intact bovine collagen fibres. *Biochem. J.* 131:771–780, 1973.
424. Rodrigues, M.M., Fine, B.S., Laibson, P.R., and Zimmerman, L.E. Disorders of the corneal epithelium. A clinicopathological study of dot, geographic and fingerprint patterns. *Arch. Ophthalmol.* 92:475–482, 1974.
425. Roggendorf, W., Opitz, H., and Schuppan, D. Altered expression of collagen type VI in brain vessels of patients with chronic hypertension. A comparison with the distribution of collagen IV and procollagen III. *Acta Neuropathol. (Berl.)* 77:55–60, 1988.
426. Rohen, J.W. Why is intraocular pressure elevated in chronic simple glaucoma? Anatomical considerations. *Ophthalmology* 90:758–765, 1983.
427. Rohen, J.W., Futa, R., and Lütjen-Drecoll, E. The fine structure of the cribriform meshwork in normal and glaucomatous eyes as seen in tangential sections. *Invest. Ophthalmol. Vis. Sci.* 21:574–585, 1981.
428. Rosenbloom, A.L., Silverstein, J.H., Lezotte, D.C., Richardson, K., and McCallum, M. Limited joint mobility in childhood diabetes mellitus indicates increased risk for microvascular disease. *N. Engl. J. Med.* 305:191–194, 1981.
429. Roveri, N., Ripamonti, A., Bigi, A., Volpin, D., and Giro, M.G. X-ray diffraction study of bovine lens capsule collagen. *Biochem. Biophys. Acta* 576:404–408, 1979.
430. Royce, P.M., Steinmann, B., Vogel, A., Steinhorst, U., and Kohlschuetter, A. Brittle cornea syndrome: An heritable connective tissue disorder distinct from Ehlers-Danlos syndrome type VI and fragilitas oculi, with spontaneous perforations of the eye, blue sclerae, red hair and normal collagen lysyl hydroxylation. *Eur. J. Pediatr.* 149:465–469, 1990.
431. Sage, H., Balian, G., Vogel, A.M., and Bornstein, P. Type VIII collagen. Synthesis by normal and malignant cells in culture. *Lab. Invest.* 50;219–231, 1984.
432. Sage, H., Pritzl, P., and Bornstein, P. A unique pepsin-sensitive collagen synthesized by aortic endothelial cells in culture. *Biochemistry* 19:5747–5755, 1980.
433. Sakai, L.Y., Keene, D.R., Morris, N.P., and Burgeson, R.E. Type VII collagen is a major structural component of anchoring fibrils. *J. Cell Biol.* 103:1577–1586, 1986.
434. Sakura, S., Fujimoto, D., Sakamoto, K., Mizuno, A., and Motegi, K. Photolysis of pyridinoline, a cross-linking amino acid of collagen, by ultraviolet light. *Can. J. Biochem.* 60:525–529, 1982.
435. Sandberg, M., Tamminen, M., Hirvonen, H., Vuorio, E., and Pihlajaniemi, T. Expression of mRNAs coding for the α1 chain of type XIII collagen in human fetal tissues: Comparison with expression of mRNA's for collagen types I, II and III. *J. Cell Biol.* 109:1371–1379, 1989.
436. Sankey, E.A., Bown, F.E., Morton, L.F., Scott, D.M., and Barnes, M.J. Analysis of the collagen types synthesized by bovine corneal endothelial cells in culture. *Biochem. J.* 198:707–710, 1981.
437. Saus, J., Wieslander, J., Langeveld, J.P.M., Quinones, S., and Hudson, B.G. Identification of the Goodpasture antigen as the α3(IV) chain of collagen IV. *J. Biol. Chem.* 263:13374–13380, 1988.
438. Savage, C.O.S., Noel, L.-H.., Crutcher, E., Price, S.R.G., Grunfeld, J.P., and Lockwood, C.M. Hereditary nephritis: Immunoblotting studies of the glomerular basement membrane. *Lab. Invest.* 60:613–618, 1989.
439. Sawada, H. The fine structure of the bovine Descemet's membrane with special reference to biochemical nature. *Cell Tissue Res.* 226:241–255, 1982.
440. Sawada, H., Furthmayr, H., Konomi, H., and Nagai, Y. Immunoelectron microscopic localization of extracellular matrix components produced by bovine corneal endothelial cells in vitro. *Exp. Cell Res.* 171:94–109, 1987.
441. Sawada, H., Konomi, H., and Nagai, Y. The basement membrane of bovine corneal endothelial cells in culture with β-aminopropionitrile: Biosynthesis of hexagonal lattices composed of a 160 nm dumbbell-shaped structure. *Eur. J. Cell Biol.* 35:226–234, 1984.
442. Sawaguchi, S., Twining, S.S., Yue, B.Y.J.T., Wilson, P.M., Sugar, J., and Chan, S.-K. Alpha-1 proteinase inhibitor levels in keratoconus. *Exp. Eye Res.* 50:549–554, 1990.
443. Scheiffarth, O.F., Kampik, A., Günther, H., and von der Mark, K. Proteins of the extracellular matrix in vitreoretinal membranes. *Graefes Arch. Clin. Exp. Ophthalmol.* 226:357–361, 1988.
444. Schmid, T.M., Popp, R.G., and Linsenmayer, T.F. Hypertrophic cartilage matrix. Type X collagen, supramolecular assembly and calcification. *Ann. N.Y. Acad. Sci.* 580:64–73, 1990.
445. Schmut, O. The identification of type III collagen in calf and bovine cornea and sclera. *Exp. Eye Res.* 25:505–509, 1977.
446. Schmut, O. The organization of tissues of the eye by different collagen types. *Graefes Arch. Clin. Exp. Ophthalmol.* 207:189–199, 1978.

447. Schneider, G., Oepen, H., and Klapproth, A. The effect of the neurolathyrogenic substance β,β'-iminodipropionitrile (IDPN) on some biological parameters in rats and mice. *Gen. Pharmacol.* 12:109–114, 1981.

448. Schnider, S.L., and Kohn, R.R. Effects of age and diabetes mellitus on the solubility and non-enzymatic glucosylation of human skin collagen. *J. Clin. Invest.* 67:1630–1635, 1981.

449. Schwartz, D., and Veis, A. Characterization of basement membrane collagen of bovine anterior lens capsule via segment-long-spacing crystallites and the specific cleavage of the collagen by pepsin. *FEBS. Lett.* 85:326–332, 1978.

450. Schwartz, D., and Veis, A. Structure of bovine anterior lens capsule collagen molecules from electron microscopy. *Biopolymers* 18:2363–2367, 1979.

451. Schwartz, D., and Veis, A. Characterization of bovine anterior lens capsule basement membrane collagen. 2. Segment-long-spacing precipitates: Further evidence for large N-terminal and C-terminal extensions. *Eur. J. Biochem.* 103:29–37, 1980.

452. Scott, J.E. Proteoglycan-fibrillar collagen interactions. *Biochem. J.* 252:313–323, 1988.

453. Scott, J.E., and Haigh, M. Proteoglycan-type I collagen fibril interactions in bone and non-calcifying connective tissues. *Biosci. Rep.* 5:71–81, 1985.

454. Scott, J.E., and Haigh, M. Keratan sulphate and the ultrastructure of cornea and cartilage: A "stand-in" for chondroitin sulphate in conditions of oxygen lack? *J. Anat.* 158:95–108, 1988.

455. Scott, J.E., and Hughes, E.W. Proteoglycan-collagen relationship in developing chick and bovine tendons. Influence of the physiological environment. *Connect. Tissue Res.* 14:267–278, 1986.

456. Scott, J.E., Hughes, E.W., and Shuttleworth, C.A. A collagen-associated Ehrlich chromogen: A pyrrolic cross-link? *Biosci. Rep.* 1:611–618, 1981.

457. Scott, J.E., and Orford, C.R. Dermatan sulphate-rich proteoglycan associates with rat tail-tendon collagen at the d band in the gap region. *Biochem. J.* 197:213–216, 1981.

458. Scott, J.E., Quian, R., Henkel, W., and Glanville, R.W. An Ehrlich chromogen in collagen cross-links. *Biochem. J.* 209:263–264, 1983.

459. Scott, P.G., Winterbottom, N., Dodd, C.M., Edwards, E., and Pearson, C.H. A role for disulphide bridges in the protein core in the interaction of proteodermatan sulphate and collagen. *Biochem. Biophys. Res. Commun.* 138:1348–1354, 1986.

460. Sebag, J. *The Vitreous. Structure, Function and Pathobiology*, Springer-Verlag, New York, 1989.

461. Sebag, J. Age-related differences in the human vitreo-retinal interface. *Arch. Ophthalmol.* 109:966–971, 1991.

462. Sebag, J., and Balazs, E.A. Morphology and ultrastructure of human vitreous fibers. *Invest. Ophthalmol. Vis. Sci.* 30:1867–1871, 1989.

463. Seery, C.M., Warman, M., Olsen, B., and Davison, P.F. Type IX collagen of the mammalian vitreous: The α1(IX) chain. *Invest. Ophthalmol. Vis. Sci. (Suppl.)* 32:1010, 1991.

464. Seland, J.H. Ultrastructural changes in the normal human lens capsule from birth to old age. *Acta Ophthalmol (Copenh.)* 52:688–706, 1974.

465. Sell, D.R., and Monnier, V.M. End-stage renal disease and diabetes catalyze the formation of a pentose-derived cross-link from aging human collagen. *J. Clin. Invest.* 85:380–384, 1990.

466. Sellheyer, K., and Spitznas, M. Development of the human sclera. A morphological study. *Graefes Arch. Clin. Exp. Ophthalmol.* 226:89–100, 1988.

467. Seltzer, J.L., Eisen, A.Z., Bauer, E.A., Morris, N.P., Glanville, R.W., and Burgeson, R.E. Cleavage of type VII collagen by interstitial collagenase and type IV collagenase (gelatinase) derived from human skin. *J. Biol. Chem.* 264:3822–3826, 1989.

468. Shetlar, D.J., Bourne, W.M., and Campbell, R.J. Morphological evaluation of Descemet's membrane and corneal endothelium in diabetes mellitus. *Ophthalmology* 96:247–250, 1989.

469. Shields, M.B., Shelburne, J.D., and Bell, S.W. The ultrastructure of human limbal collagen. *Invest. Ophthalmol. Vis. Sci.* 16:864–866, 1977.

470. Shimomura, H., and Spiro, R.G. Studies on macromolecular components of human glomerular basement membrane and alterations in diabetes. Decreased levels of heparan sulfate proteoglycan and laminin. *Diabetes* 36:374–381, 1987.

471. Siegel, R.C. Lysyl oxidase. *Int. Rev. Connect. Tissue Res.* 8:73–118, 1979.

472. Siegel, R.C., Fu, J.C.C., Uto, N., Horiuchi, K., and Fujimoto, D. Collagen cross-linking: Lysyl oxidase dependent synthesis of pyridinoline in vitro: Confirmation that pyridinoline is derived from collagen. *Biochem. Biophys. Res. Commun.* 108:1546–1550, 1982.

473. Smolek, M.K., and McCarey, B. Interlamellar adhesive strength in human eyebank corneas. *Invest. Ophthalmol. Vis. Sci.* 31:1087–1095, 1990.

474. Snowden, J.M. The stabilization of in vivo assembled collagen fibrils by proteoglycans/glycosaminoglycans. *Biochim. Biophys. Acta* 703:21–25, 1982.

475. Snowden, J.M., and Swann, D.A. Vitreous structure. V. The morphology and thermal stability of vitreous collagen fibres and comparison to articular cartilage (type II) collagen. *Invest. Ophthalmol. Vis. Sci.* 19:610–618, 1980.

476. Snowden, J.M., Eyre, D.R., and Swann, D.A. Vitreous structure. VI. Age-related changes in the thermal

stability and cross-links of vitreous, articular cartilage and tendon collagens. *Biochim. Biophys. Acta* 706:153–157, 1982.

477. Speranza, M.L., Valentini, G., and Calligaro, A. Influence of fibronectin on the fibrillogenesis of type I and type III collagen. *Collagen* 7:115–123, 1987.

478. Spitznas, M. The fine structure of human scleral collagen. *Am. J. Ophthalmol.* 71:68, 1971.

479. Stanley, J.R., Hawley-Nelson, P., Yaar, M., Martin, G.R., and Katz, S.I. Laminin and bullous pemphigoid antigen are distinct basement membrane proteins synthesized by epidermal cells. *J. Invest. Dermatol.* 78:456–459, 1982.

480. Stefani, F.H., Ebner, K., and Alexandridis, A. New observations on two common diseases of the eye. In *Abstracts of the Second Meeting of the International Society of Ophthalmic Pathology*, New Orleans, 1989, p. 10.

481. Stewart, D.H., III, Streeten, B.W., Brockhurst, R.J., Anderson, D.R., Hirose, T., and Gass, J.D.M. Abnormal scleral collagen in nanophthalmos. An ultrastructural study. *Arch. Ophthalmol.* 109:1017–1025, 1991.

482. Straatsma, B.R., Lightfoot, D.O., Barke, R.M., and Horwitz, J. Lens capsule and epithelium in age-related cataract. *Am. J. Ophthalmol.* 112:283–296, 1991.

483. Street, D.A., Vinokur, E.T., Waring, G.O., III, Pollak, S.J., Clements, S.D., and Perkins, J.V. Lack of association between keratoconus, mitral valve prolapse and joint hypermobility. *Ophthalmology* 98:170–176, 1991.

484. Streeten, B.W., Karpik, A.G., and Spitzer, K.H. Posterior keratoconus associated with systemic abnormalities. *Arch. Ophthalmol.* 101:616–622, 1983.

485. Streeten, B.W., Robinson, M.R., Wallace, R., and Jones, D.B. Lens capsule abnormalities in Alport's syndrome. *Arch. Ophthalmol.* 105:1693–1697, 1987.

486. Sugrue, S.P., Gordon, M.K., Seyer, J., Dublet, B., van der Rest, M., and Olsen, B.R. Immunoidentification of type XII collagen in embryonic tissues. *J. Cell Biol.* 109:939–945, 1989.

487. Summers, T.A., Irwin, M.H., Mayne, R., and Balian, G. Monoclonal antibodies to type X collagen. Biosynthetic studies using an antibody to the amino-terminal domain. *J. Biol. Chem.* 263:581–587, 1988.

488. Sundar-Raj, C.V., Freeman, I.L., and Brown, S.I. Selective growth of rabbit corneal epithelial cells in culture and basement membrane collagen synthesis. *Invest. Ophthalmol. Vis. Sci.* 19:1222–1230, 1980.

489. Svoboda, E.L.A., Howley, T.P., and Deporter, D.A. Collagen fibril diameter and its relation to collagen turnover in three soft connective tissues in the rat. *Connect. Tissue Res.* 12:43–48, 1983.

490. Svoboda, E.L.A., Shiga, A., and Deporter, D.A. A stereologic analysis of collagen phagocytosis by fibroblasts in three soft connective tissues with differing rates of collagen turnover. *Anat. Rec.* 199:473–480, 1981.

491. Svoboda, K.K., Nishimura, I., Sugrue, S.P., Ninomiya, Y., and Olsen, B.R. Embryonic chicken cornea and cartilage synthesize type IX collagen molecules with different amino-terminal domains. *Proc. Natl. Acad. Sci. USA* 85:7496–7500, 1988.

492. Swann, D.A., and Sotman, S.S. The chemical composition of bovine vitreous-humour collagen fibres. *Biochem. J.* 185:545–554, 1980.

493. Swoboda, B., Holmdahl, R., Stoss, H., and von der Mark, K. Cellular heterogeneity in cultured human chondrocytes identified by antibodies specific for $\alpha 2(XI)$ collagen chains. *J. Cell Biol.* 109:1363–1369, 1989.

494. Tamura, Y., Konomi, H. Sawada, H., Takashima, S., and Nakajima, A. Tissue distribution of type VIII collagen in human adult and fetal eyes. *Invest. Ophthalmol. Vis. Sci.* 32:2636–2644, 1991.

495. Taylor, C.M., and Grant, M.E. Assembly of chick and bovine lens-capsule collagen. *Biochem. J.* 226:527–536, 1985.

496. Taylor, H.R., and Kimsey, R.A. Corneal epithelial basement membrane changes in diabetes. *Invest. Ophthalmol. Vis. Sci.* 20:548–553, 1981.

497. Teekhasaenee, C., Nimmanit, S., Wutthiphan, S., Vareesangthip, K., Laohapand, T., Malasitr, P., and Ritch, R. Posterior polymorphous dystrophy and Alport syndrome. *Ophthalmology* 98:1207–1215, 1991.

498. Tengroth, B., and Ammitzboll, T. Changes in the content and composition of collagen in the glaucomatous eye—basis for a new hypothesis for the genesis of chronic open angle glaucoma. *Acta Ophthalmol. (Copenh.)* 62:999–1008, 1984.

499. Tengroth, R., Rehnberg, M., and Ammitzboll, T. A comparative analysis of the collagen type and distribution in the trabecular meshwork, sclera, lamina cribrosa and the optic nerve in the human eye. *Acta Ophthalmol. (Copenh.)* 63(Suppl. 173):91–93, 1985.

500. Thorning, D., and Vracko, R. Renal glomerular basal lamina scaffold. Embryologic development, anatomy and role in cellular reconstruction of rat glomeruli injured by freezing and thawing. *Lab. Invest.* 37:105–119, 1977.

501. Ticho, U., Ivry, M., and Merin, S. Brittle cornea, blue sclera and red hair syndrome (the brittle cornea syndrome). *Br. J. Ophthalmol.* 64:175–177, 1980.

502. Tidman, M.J., and Eady, R.A.J. Evaluation of anchoring fibrils and other components of the dermal-epidermal junction in dystrophic epidermolysis bullosa by a quantitative ultrastructural technique. *J. Invest. Dermatol.* 84:374–377, 1985.

503. Tikka, L., Pihlajaniemi, T., Henttu, P., Prockop, D.J., and Tryggvason, K. Gene structure for the $\alpha 1$ chain of a human short-chain collagen (type XIII) with alternatively spliced transcripts and translocation termination codon at the 5′ end of the last exon. *Proc. Natl. Acad. Sci. USA* 85:7491–7495, 1988.

504. Timpl, R. Structure and biological activity of basement membrane proteins. *Eur. J. Biochem.* 180:487–502, 1989.

505. Timpl, R., and Dziadek, M. Structure, development and molecular pathology of basement membranes. *Int. Rev. Exp. Pathol.* 29:1–112, 1986.

506. Timpl, R., Wiedemann, H., van Delden, V., Furthmayr, H., and Kühn, K. A network model for the organization of type IV collagen molecules in basement membranes. *Eur. J. Biochem.* 120:203–211, 1981.

507. Toole, B.P. Binding and precipitation of soluble collagens by chick embryo cartilage proteoglycan. *J. Biol. Chem.* 251:895–897, 1976.

508. Toole, B.P., Biswas, C., and Gross, J. Hyaluronate and invasiveness of the rabbit V2 carcinoma. *Proc. Natl. Acad. Sci. USA* 76:6299–6303, 1979.

509. Trelstad, R.L., and Kang, A.H. Collagen heterogeneity in the avian eye: Lens, vitreous body, cornea and sclera. *Exp. Eye Res.* 18:395–406, 1974.

510. Trelstad, R.L., Silbermann, N.N., and Brockhurst, R.J. Nanophthalmic sclera. Ultrastructural, histochemical and biochemical observations. *Arch. Ophthalmol.* 100:1935–1938, 1982.

511. Tremblay, M., and Dubé, I. Meesmann's corneal dystrophy: Ultrastructural features. *Can. J. Ophthalmol.* 17:24–28, 1982.

512. Trueb, B., Schreier, T., Brückner, P., and Winterhalter, K.H. Type VI collagen represents a major fraction of connective tissue collagens. *Eur. J. Biochem.* 166:699–703, 1987.

513. Tseng, S.C.G., Savion, N., Gospodarowicz, D., and Stern, R. Characterization of collagens synthesized by cultured bovine corneal endothelial cells. *J. Biol. Chem.* 256:3361–3365, 1981.

514. Tseng, S.C.G., Smuckler, D., and Stern, R. Comparison of collagen types in adult and fetal bovine corneas. *J. Biol. Chem.* 257:2627–2633, 1982.

515. Tsilibary, E.C., Koliakos, G.G., Charonis, A.S., Vogel, A.M., Reger, L.A., and Furcht, L.T. Heparin type IV collagen interactions: Equilibrium binding and inhibition of type IV collagen self-assembly. *J. Biol. Chem.* 263:19112–19118, 1988.

516. Tso, M.O.M. Pathogenetic factors of aging macular degeneration. *Ophthalmology* 92:628–635, 1985.

517. Turksen, K., Opas, M., and Kalnins, V.I. Cytoskeleton, adhesion and extracellular matrix of fetal human retinal pigmented epithelial cells in culture. *Ophthalmic Res.* 21:56–66, 1989.

518. Ueno, M., and Naumann, G.O.H. Uveal damage in secondary glaucoma. A morphometric study. *Graefes Arch. Clin. Exp. Ophthalmol.* 227:380–383, 1989.

519. Uitto, J., and Shamban, A. Heritable skin diseases with molecular defects in collagen or elastin. *Dermatol. Clin.* 5:63–84, 1987.

520. Valli, M., Leonardi, L., Strocchi, R., Tenni, R., Guizzardi, S., Ruggeri, A., and Balduini, C. "In vitro" fibril formation of type I collagen from different sources: biochemical and morphological aspects. *Connect. Tissue Res.* 15:235–244, 1986.

521. Van der Rest, M., and Mayne, R. Type IX collagen proteoglycan from cartilage is covalently cross-linked to type II collagen. *J. Biol. Chem.* 263:1615–1618, 1988.

522. Van der Schaft, T.L., de Bruijn, W.C., Mooy, C.M., Ketelaars, D.A.M., and de Jong, P.T.V.M. Is basal laminar deposit unique for age-related macular degeneration? *Arch. Ophthalmol.* 109:420–425, 1991.

523. Van Horn, D.L., Hyndiuk, R.A., Edelhauser, H.F., McDonald, T.O., and De Santis, L.M. Ultrastructural alterations associated with loss of transparency in the cornea of buphthalmic rabbits. *Exp. Eye Res.* 25:171–182, 1977.

524. Vaughan, L., Mendler, M., Huber, S., Brückner, P., Winterhalter, K.H., Irwin, M.I., and Mayne, R. D-periodic distribution of collagen type IX along cartilage fibrils. *J. Cell Biol.* 106:991–997, 1988.

525. Virgilio, L.A., Williams, R.J., and Klintworth, G.K. An unusually large human eye with abnormal scleral collagen. *Arch. Ophthalmol.* 94:101–105, 1976.

526. Vogel, K.G., and Trotter, J.A. The effect of proteoglycans on the morphology of collagen fibrils formed in vitro. *Collagen* 7:105–114, 1987.

527. Von der Mark, K., van Menxel, M., and Wiedemann, H. Isolation and characterization of new collagens from chick cartilage. *Eur. J. Biochem.* 124:57–62, 1982.

528. Von der Mark, K., von der Mark, H., Timpl, R., and Trelstad, R.L. Immunofluorescent localization of collagen types I, II and III in the embryonic chick eye. *Dev. Biol.* 59:75–85, 1977.

529. Vuorio, E., and De Crombrugghe, B. The family of collagen genes. *Annu. Rev. Biochem.* 59:837–872, 1990.

530. Wahl, S.M. Lymphocyte- and macrophage-derived growth factors. *Methods Enzymol.* 163:715–731, 1988.

531. Wahl, S.M. The role of lymphokines and monokines in fibrosis. *Ann. N.Y. Acad. Sci.* 460:224–231, 1985.

532. Wang, M.K., and Heath, H. Effect of β,β'-iminodipropionitrile and related compounds on the electroretinogram and the retinal vascular system of the rat. *Exp. Eye Res.* 7:56–61, 1968.

533. Ward, N.P., Hulmes, D.J.S., and Chapman, J.A. Collagen self-assembly in vitro: Electron microscopy of initial aggregates formed during the lag phase. *J. Mol. Biol.* 190:107–112, 1986.

534. Ward, R.C., Gragoudas, E.S., Pon, D.M., and Albert, D.M. Abnormal scleral findings in uveal effusion syndrome. *Am. J. Ophthalmol.* 106:139–146, 1988.

535. Waring, G.O. Posterior collagenous layer of the cornea. Ultrastructural classification of abnormal collagenous tissue posterior to Descemet's membrane in 30 cases. *Arch. Ophthalmol.* 100:122–134, 1982.

536. Waring, G.O., Bourne, W.M., Edelhauser, H.F., and Kenyon, K.R. The corneal endothelium. Normal and pathological structure and function. *Ophthalmology* 89:531–590, 1982.

537. Waring, G.O., Laibson, P.R., and Rodrigues, M.M. Clinical and pathological alterations of Descemet's membrane: With emphasis on endothelial metaplasia. *Surv. Ophthalmol. 18*:325–368, 1974.
538. Weale, R.A. *A Biography of the Eye: Development, Growth, Age*, H.K. Lewis and Co., London, 1982.
539. Weber, S., Engel, J., Wiedemann, H., Glanville, R.W., and Timpl, R. Subunit structure and assembly of the globular domain of basement membrane collagen type IV. *Eur. J. Biochem. 139*:401–410, 1984.
540. Weiss, J.B., and Ayad, S. An introduction to collagen. In *Collagen in Health and Disease*, J.B. Weiss and M.I.V. Jayson (Eds.), Churchill Livingstone, Edinburgh, pp. 1–17, 1982.
541. Weiss, J.B., and Jayson, M.I.V. *Collagen in Health and Disease*, Churchill Livingstone, Edinburgh, 1982.
542. Welsh, C., Gay, S., Rhodes, R.K., Pfister, R., and Miller, E.J. Collagen heterogeneity in normal rabbit cornea. I. Isolation and biochemical characterization of the genetically distinct collagens. *Biochim. Biophys. Acta 625*: 78–88, 1980.
543. Wentworth, J.S., Paterson, C.A., and Gray, R.D. Effect of a metalloproteinase inhibitor on established corneal ulcers after an alkali burn. *Invest. Ophthalmol. Vis. Sci. 33*:2174–2179, 1992.
544. White, R., Carlson, E.C., Brendel, K., and Meezan, E. Basement membrane biosynthesis by isolated bovine retinal vessels: Incorporation of precursors into extracellular matrix. *Microvasc. Res. 18*:185–208, 1979.
545. Wick, G., Olsen, B.R., and Timpl, R. Immunohistologic analysis of fetal and dermatosparactic calf and sheep skin with antisera to procollagen and collagen type I. *Lab. Invest. 39*:151–156, 1978.
546. Williams, D.F., and Burke, J.M. Modulation of growth in retina-derived cells by extracellular matrices. *Invest. Ophthalmol. Vis. Sci. 31*:1717–1723, 1990.
547. Wright, D.W., and Mayne, R. Vitreous humour of chicken contains two fibrillar systems: An analysis of their structure. *J. Ultrastruct. Mol. Struct. Res. 100*:224–234, 1988.
548. Wu, J.J., Eyre, D.R., and Slayter, H.S. Type VI collagen of the intervertebral disc. Biochemical and electron-microscopic characterization of the native protein. *Biochem. J. 248*:373–381, 1987.
549. Yada, T., Suzuki, S., Kobayashi, K., Kobayashi, M., Hoshino, T., Horie, K., and Kimata, K. Occurrence in chick embryo vitreous humor of a type IX collagen proteoglycan with an extraordinarily large chondroitin sulfate chain and short $\alpha 1$ polypeptide. *J. Biol. Chem. 265*:6992–6999, 1990.
550. Young, I. Understanding Marfan's syndrome. *Br. Med. J. 303*:1414–1415, 1991.
551. Young, R.D. The ultrastructural organization of proteoglycans and collagen in human and rabbit scleral matrix. *J. Cell Sci. 74*:95–104, 1985.
552. Young, R.W. Pathophysiology of age-related macular degeneration. *Surv. Ophthalmol. 31*:291–306, 1987.
553. Young, R.W., and Ocumpaugh, D.E. Autoradiographic studies on the growth and development of the lens capsule in the rat. *Invest. Ophthalmol. 5*:583–593, 1966.
554. Yue, B.Y.J.T., Baum, J.L., and Smith, B.D. Collagen synthesis by cultures of stromal cells from normal human and keratoconus corneas. *Biochem. Biophys. Res. Commun. 86*:465–472, 1979.
555. Yue, B.Y.J.T., Duvall, J., Goldberg, M.F., Puck, A., Tso, M.O.M., and Sugar, J. Nanophthalmic sclera. Morphologic and tissue culture studies. *Ophthalmology 93*:534–541, 1986.
556. Yue, B.Y.J.T., Kurosawa, A., Elvart, J.L., Elner, V.M., and Tso, M.O.M. Monkey trabecular meshwork cells in culture: Growth, morphological and biochemical characteristics. *Graefes Arch. Clin. Exp. Ophthalmol. 226*:262–268, 1988.
557. Yue, B.Y.J.T., Sugar, J., and Benveniste, K. Heterogeneity in keratoconus: Possible biochemical basis. *Proc. Soc. Exp. Biol. Med. 175*:336–341, 1984.
558. Yun, A.J., Murphy, C.G., Polansky, J.R., Newsome, D.A., and Alvarado, J.A. Proteins secreted by human trabecular cells. *Invest. Ophthalmol. Vis. Sci. 30*:2012–2022, 1989.
559. Yurchenko, P.D. Assembly of basement membranes. *Ann. N.Y. Acad. Sci. 580*:195–213, 1990.
560. Yurchenko, P.D., Tsilibary, E.C., Charonis, A.S., and Furthmayr, H. Models for the self-assembly of basement membrane. *J. Histochem. Cytochem. 34*:93–102, 1986.
561. Zhang, N.L., Puklin, J.E., Das, A., Stockfish, J., and Frank, R.N. Ultrastructural immunocytochemistry of a subretinal neovascular membrane due to age-related macular degeneration. *Invest. Ophthalmol. Vis. Sci. (Suppl.) 32*:686, 1991.
562. Zimmerman, D.R., Fischer, R.W., Winterhalter, K.H., Witmer, R., and Vaughan, L. Comparative studies of collagens in normal and keratoconus corneas. *Exp. Eye Res. 46*:431–442, 1988.
563. Zimmerman, D.R., Trueb, B., Winterhalter, K.H., Witmer, R., and Fischer, R.W. Type VI collagen is a major component of the human cornea. *FEBS Lett. 197*:55–58, 1986.

34
Disorders of Monosaccharide Metabolism

Anthony F. Winder

Royal Free Hospital and School of Medicine, University of London; and Institute of Ophthalmology and Moorfields Eye Hospital, London, England

I. SUGAR CATARACTS

The general process whereby excess of certain aldose sugars in the extracellular fluid can lead to cataracts has been well established for experimental animals, and there is good evidence that similar processes operate in humans, although not necessarily to the same extent [19,35,38–40,73]. Species differences can be considerable and important and may be underestimated in the extrapolation of animal data to human disease. The sugars are converted to the corresponding polyols by interaction with aldose reductase, an enzyme with broad specificity for aldoses and prominent in lens epithelium. The cofactor nicotinamide adenine dinucleotide in its reduced form (NADPH$^+$) is required, and this also functions as an allosteric activator for the enzyme, conversion to active forms being favored by an increase in NADP [19]. It is not known whether individual variation in the level of total lens aldose reductase activity or the degree of activation is significant in human cataractogenesis. As discussed later, the relationship between cataract and moderate deficiency of enzyme-dependent steps in the pathways of galactose metabolism suggests that additional secondary factors are involved.

Aldose reductase displays low affinity for galactose and glucose, particularly the latter, and the polyol pathway is dormant unless local concentrations of these sugars greatly increase through failure of other major pathways of utilization or the artificial presentation of an excessive load. Polyol production is then favored, the reaction being essentially irreversible. Polyols may be further metabolized in the lens by interaction with polyol dehydrogenase, although this stage is reversible. Thus, sorbitol from glucose may produce fructose, which may diffuse directly from the lens or form mannitol. Some polyols, such as arabitol and galactitol (dulcitol), are poor substrates for this enzyme. Polyols, and to a lesser extent ketose sugars, such as fructose, show a limited capacity to penetrate cell membranes: any osmotic consequences of fructose excess are therefore minor compared to those deriving from galactose. Intracellular accumulation in the lens of water-soluble solutes, such as polyols, leads to osmotic imbalance. Subsequent swelling and secondary damage affect fiber membranes and transport systems, with loss of the ability to maintain concentration gradients such that there is further entry of water, salts, and other solutes. Agglomeration of lens proteins to both, to each other, and to cell membranes occurs, with optical discontinuities and lens opacification [16,35,73]. At this stage the selective barrier to polyol escape is probably lost: dulcitol accumulation in the lens of the galactose-fed rat is not maintained when the cataract is fully developed. With experimentally induced galactose cataract, the lens swelling and failure of transport mechanisms correlates closely with the osmotic changes and the degree of polyol accumulation [35,40]. It is therefore evident that a simple osmotic mechanism can produce some cataracts, although it does not follow that cataracts in diabetics, for example, are produced in this way because the osmotic excess is minor, probably because fructose does not appear to accumulate to any great extent. There is strong evidence, however, that an osmotic mechanism is involved in the development of human cataracts associated with major derangements of the normal processes of galactose metabolism [35]. It is also noteworthy that lens has a very narrow range of biological responses and that any insult with direct or indirect nutritional consequences can lead to opacification.

II. INHERITED DISORDERS OF GALACTOSE METABOLISM

The major pathway for the utilization of dietary galactose in humans involves conversion to glucose-1-phosphate, and four enzyme-controlled steps are involved (Fig. 1). A range of genetically determined autosomal recessive defects, including variant enzyme forms with reduced activity, are now recognized at three of these steps [11,31,63]. Cataract formation is a major consequence of a severe deficiency affecting galactokinase and galactose-1-phosphate uridyl transferase and a systemically expressed deficiency of uridine diphosphate (UDP)-galactose-4-epimerase, with strong evidence that osmotic imbalance consequent to accumulation of galactose metabolites is involved.

A. Galactokinase Deficiency: Galactokinase Deficiency Galactosemia

The frequency of the homozygous form of this disorder may be 1 per 40,000 live births, and bilateral cataract formation within the first year of life is expected unless early diagnosis and restriction of galactose intake are achieved [17,63]. Regression or arrest of opacification has been reported after dietary treatment at an early stage, perhaps because early changes involve vacuolation rather than disorganization of lens proteins [35,39,43]. Symptoms suggestive of polyneuropathy have been reported for the occasional case, but cataract formation seems to be the sole characteristic clinical feature [11,63]. Laboratory findings in homozygous galactokinase deficiency include impaired galactose tolerance with an elevated fasting blood galactose and the presence of galactose and galactitol in the urine. Galactokinase is deficient in red cell lysates [6,71].

The frequency of the heterozygous form may approach 1%, and galactokinase activity is about 50% of normal. The heterozygous state is apparently associated with a moderate increase in the risk of cataract, almost invariably expressed in the first year of life [43,48,78]. This association has been shown by studies in families known to carry the abnormal gene and by screening for heterozygosity within unselected cataract populations, including mothers of children showing cataract in early life [7,8,43]. Some heterozygotes have an impaired galactose tolerance [40,65], and rather more have increased urinary output of galactitol after intravenous loading with galactose [66]. Allelic variation of galactokinase is not established, although this has been proposed as an explanation for differences in galactose tolerance among heterozygotes and for the skewed reduction in galactokinase activity found in black populations [46,68,72].

Generally similar metabolic pathways of galactose metabolism operate in the rat, and galactose feeding of pregnant rats induces cataract formation in utero [2]. In humans, mothers with a level of galactokinase activity at the low end of the normal distribution curve without evidence of genetic abnormality may carry an increased risk of producing a child with cataract, although the capacity of the child to metabolize galactose appears to be normal [27], and any real transmission of cataract may not operate through a galactose mechanism. Restriction of galactose intake by the mother in subsequent pregnancies may then be recommended [13]. This variable influence during pregnancy, also associated with the second enzyme galactose-1-phosphate uridyl transferase, together with the absence of cataract in most individuals heterozygous for galactokinase deficiency, suggests that other non-enzymatic factors influence the risk of cataract formation. Some possibilities are discussed here.

Galactokinase determination is most practically carried out on lysates of erythrocytes [6,71]. Since the enzyme is not stable, fresh cells are required and the lysate loses activity on storage at $-20°C$. The assay is also difficult and is not precise, and interpretation can also be difficult because the range of activity observed in apparently normal children may be about five times adult values in early life, falling to the adult range by about 5 years of age [51]. Homozygotes may be identified, but wider screening for heterozygotes is restricted by the lack of specificity of the present assay procedures, although it may be more useful in families known to carry the abnormal gene.

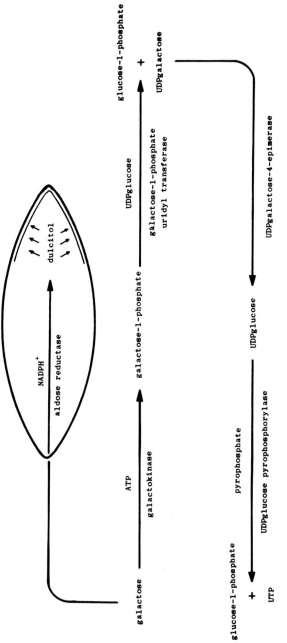

Figure 1 Galactose metabolism and the lens.

B. Galactose-1-Phosphate Uridyl Transferase Deficiency: Transferase Deficiency Galactosemia

The frequency of the homozygous form of this disorder is probably about 1 per 70,000 live births, with a carrier frequency approaching 1% [11,63]. The term "galactosemia" is usually reserved for a homozygous deficiency of the transferase enzyme. Presentation is in the form of widespread tissue damage, including hepatomegaly, mental deficiency, which may not be recognized until adulthood [18], ovarian atrophy but no testicular effects, septicemia, and bilateral cataracts [11,16,63]. This disorder, in contrast to galactokinase deficiency, involves the accumulation of galactose-1-phosphate as well as galactose and galactitol. Comparisons with galactokinase deficiency strongly suggest that accumulation of galactose-1-phosphate causes many of the adverse effects of galactosemia through as yet ill-defined mechanisms. Galactose-1-phosphate also causes product inhibition of galactokinase, with further promotion of the secondary pathway to galactitol [12]. A cataractous lens taken from a child with galactosemia contained an osmotically significant excess of galactitol and a lesser excess of galactose-1-phosphate [22]. Thus accumulation of the polyol appears to be responsible for the development of the cataract, as is presumed for galactokinase deficiency. The morphological changes in the late stages of the human galactosemic cataract are compatible with a pathogenesis similar to that of the more thoroughly studied experimental galactose cataract [35,39]. The observed changes include vacuolization of lens fibers, proceeding to fiber swelling and then rupture, with the later formation of interfibrillar clefts containing precipitated protein, as seen in human lenses [35,40]. In animal studies the initial changes are seen in the equatorial region, with subsequent progression to nuclear opacification as in human galactose-dependent cataract. The human galactosemic cataract is described as classically of oil drop appearance, an appearance that is probably more a function of the acute nature of the insult precipitating the lens changes than the general cause. Less acute galactose-related lesions can show a more varied appearance [78], as shown in Fig. 2.

Homozygotes manifest galactosemia, galactosuria, and an increase in galactose-1-phosphate in erythrocytes: this last has been used as an index of dietary compliance and response to treatment [13].

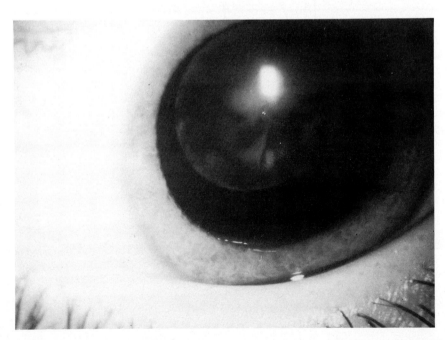

Figure 2 Cataract in a girl aged 10 years, with galactose intolerance and double partial deficiency of galactokinase and galactose-1-phosphate uridyl transferase deficiency. The opacities have lamellar and nuclear elements and were first noticed when she presented at age 7¾ years with an intermittent left divergent squint. (With permission from A.F. Winder, P. Fells, R.G. Jones, R.D. Kissun, I.S. Menzies, and J.N. Mount. Galactose intolerance and the risk of cataract. *Br. J. Ophthalmol.* 66:438–441, 1982.)

Galactosuria can be intermittent, perhaps as a function of intake, and diagnosis may in consequence be delayed [47]. The transferase enzyme may also be determined on erythrocyte lysates: activity is relatively stable and is not rapidly lost by storage at $-20°C$. The assay is technically less troublesome than for galactokinase, although interpretation must again consider some decline of mean normal activity in early life [4,5,53]. Enzyme activity in the simple blood spot test may be protected by the incorporation of dithiothreitol [3]. Antenatal diagnosis is also possible, by studies on cultured amniotic cells or by direct enzyme assay on fetal blood obtained at fetoscopy, amniotic fluid, or chorionic villi [11,14,59]. An automated procedure for analysis of neonatal blood spots from a screening program has also been described [25]. In affected families, restriction of maternal galactose intake during pregnancy has been associated with a reduced incidence of cataract [13], and the intelligence of the offspring may also possibly be protected by restriction of maternal galactose intake from early pregnancy [33]. Early and rigorous control of galactosemic children may also prevent cataract and other stigmata, although the protection against mental retardation and more subtle effects, such as shortened attention span, is less certain [63]. As with galactokinase deficiency, there is no good evidence that dietary control can be safely relaxed at maturity, although this may be difficult to avoid in consequence of adverse behavior, reduced understanding, and noncompliance.

Enzyme activity for heterozygotes is about 50% of normal values, and most show generally normal galactose tolerance and no excess excretion of galactitol [65,66]. From observations within known affected families, heterozygotes are generally believed to be clinically unaffected and without increased risk of cataract, although cataracts arose in two probable heterozygotes for whom further enzyme typing was not reported [56]. Lower than mean levels of activity in erythrocytes have also been recorded in some but not all studies of patients with infantile, presenile, and senile cataracts [27,67]. Galactosemic black subjects without detectable galactose-1-phosphate uridyl transferase activity in erythrocytes retain a limited capacity to metabolize galactose, apparently because of the residual activity of this enzyme in the tissues, as demonstrated for liver and intestine [63]. The gene encoding this enzyme was recently characterized, and missense mutations are reported for transferase-deficient galactosemia [58]; immunochemically reactive enzyme protein is also present in erythrocytes.

A range of probably allelic variant forms of the transferase enzyme has been detected by electrophoresis on various support media (Fig. 3) [50,61,62] and frequently named after the city or region of identification. The most common of these is the Duarte variant, and surveys in Europe, Australia, and North America suggest that Duarte/normal heterozygotes make up at least 10% of the general population [11,52,63,74]. Transferase activity is reduced to about 75% of normal in the Duarte/normal heterozygote and to 50% in the Duarte homozygote, without any known clinical effects in either case. Transferase activity in the Duarte/galactosemia heterozygote is reduced to about 25% of normal. Levy and colleagues [44] described 10 such heterozygotes without clinical stigmata or galactosemia on random blood sampling, for whom the response to milk feeding was in most cases also normal. However, Gitzelmann and colleagues [24] described a clinically normal case with evidence of galactose intolerance, and Wharton and colleagues [74] documented another asymptomatic case with impaired galactose tolerance and elevated erythrocyte galactose-1-phosphate for whom galactose restriction was considered prudent, an approach also taken with later cases [52]. The Indiana variant of the enzyme is less stable and consequently less active than the normal form [10]. Indiana/galactosemia heterozygotes express around 35% of normal transferase activity, with galactosemia and impaired galactose intolerance but no evident clinical stigmata. Heterozygotes for galactosemia and a further low-activity Rennes variant have about 10% of normal transferase activity, with galactose intolerance, cataract, and hepatomegaly [26]. Success in the prevention of cataract formation by dietary control consequent to early diagnosis in this condition has been reported. The Indiana and Rennes variants are probably rare, but their exact frequency has not been determined. An additional Los Angeles variant is more active than the normal form [49] and has a heterozygous frequency in southern California of about 5%: transferase activity is also increased in Down syndrome, owing to higher activity in leukocytes [32]. The discovery of further variant forms continues.

C. Deficiencies of Other Enzymes Involved in Galactose Metabolism

UDP-Galactose-4-Epimerase Deficiency: Epimerase Deficiency Galactosemia

An autosomal recessive deficiency of this enzyme but with expression limited to circulating blood cells can cause galactosemia and elevated erythrocyte galactose-1-phosphate. Galactose tolerance is not disturbed,

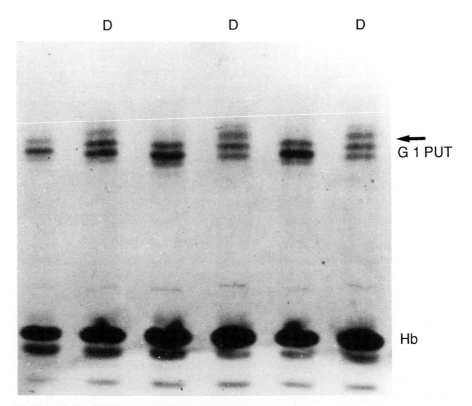

Figure 3 Isoelectrofocusing of erythrocyte hemolysates to show galactose-1-phosphate uridyl transferase activity (G1PUT) in the normal and variant, presumed Duarte (D) patterns for which there are reduced and additional (arrow) bands. Lower bands are hemoglobin (Hb) bands. (With permission from A.F. Winder, L.J. Claringbold, R.B. Jones, B. Jay, N.S.C. Rice, R.D. Kissun, I.S. Menzies, and J.N. Mount. Partial galactose disorders in families with premature cataracts. *Arch. Dis. Child.* 58:362–366, 1983.)

however, and there is normal mental and physical development with no other evident abnormal features [21]. A generalized deficiency of this enzyme is also described, again consistent with autosomal recessive inheritance, with major systemic effects similar to those of classic galactosemia but without cataracts in the very few cases described [11,31]. Levels of UDP-galactose are elevated, and cataract may not arise because the defect is distant from steps involving galactitol. Galactose restriction is recommended, but this cannot be complete because the defective enzyme step involves the production of UDP-galactose from UDP-glucose (Fig. 1). Some dietary galactose is required to produce UDP-galactose from galactose-1-phosphate and for the synthesis of galactolipids and other complex molecules.

UDP-Glucose Pyrophosphorylase

Defects in this fourth enzyme are described for *Escherichia coli* but have not been documented for humans.

III. GALACTOSE DISORDERS, GALACTOSE TOLERANCE, AND THE RISK OF CATARACT

There is strong evidence that cataracts associated with metabolic disorders involving galactose arise through a simple osmotic mechanism consequent to galactitol accumulation within the lens. Galactosylation of lens proteins is a possibility, but this process is not controlled by aldose reductase inhibitors, which in animal studies control the expression of experimental galactose cataract [35]. As discussed earlier, cataract may not have arisen in the rare major systemic epimerase deficiency galactosemia because the defect in the galactose metabolic pathway is distant from galactokinase. Associations between galactitol, galactose intolerance, and the risk of cataract are of particular interest because some quantitation of these associations could define the risk in a practically useful manner. They could similarly define any necessary prophylactic treatment protocols for patients with minor disorders affecting this pathway, including maternal deficiencies and their expression during pregnancy. Aspects of these associations are summarized in Table 1. Galactose intolerance may also arise through defects outside the main pathway of galactose metabolism as represented in Fig. 1 [1].

A major deficiency of galactokinase and of galactose-1-phosphate uridyl transferase, including low-activity variants, is associated with both galactose intolerance and a high risk of cataract in early life. The risk is reduced by early dietary intervention. Variant transferase forms and a range of compound deficiencies involving both the major enzymes can be associated with either galactose intolerance or cataract, or both, when the overall pathway activity falls below about 20% of normal reference values [52,54,77–79]. Heterozygous galactokinase deficiency shows a weak association with cataract, mainly seen in the first year of life: although enzyme activity is higher at that age [51], so is the dietary load of galactose in milk-based products. Occasional heterozygotes have expressed borderline galactose intolerance using an intravenous challenge, with increased urinary output of galactitol [66]. Heterozygous transferase deficiency galactosemia shows at most a weak cataract association, although heterozygous and other less severe partial deficiency has been reported on screening patients with presenile and senile cataract [27,56,67]. The real difficulties of establishing a causal association arise with such lesser deficiencies of both major enzymes, particularly in mothers identified after delivery of a child with cataract, since the children are usually then found to have a normal range of enzyme activity [27,77,79]. Three particular considerations arise: the nature of any galactose stress, secondary factors affecting expression of any such stress, and the reliability of the procedures used to establish enzymatic status. Galactose effects after birth involve responses to oral loads, and an oral test procedure incorporating intestinal and hepatic effects may be more relevant than intravenous loading. An oral procedure incorporating an inert internal standard to correct for variable absorption, however, did not define any simple relationship between intolerance (demonstrated in patients with partial single and compound defects) and expression of cataract for other direct or maternal effects [79]. It may be that such investigations in later life are not relevant to an earlier expression of cataract, including any influence during pregnancy. Any relationships between partial disorders of galactose metabolism and cataract may also be influenced by variable maturation and activity of fetal enzymes of galactose metabolism and of lens aldose reductase during pregnancy and in later life by diverse dietary habits of galactose intake and by relationships between galactose metabolism, liver function, and any compromising effects of ethanol intake. Activity of galactokinase and galactose-1-phosphate uridyl transferase is fully expressed early in development, from weeks 9 to 28 and increases further after birth: kinetic studies have not shown any differences between fetal and adult galactokinase [64]. The elimination of galactose may proceed at a slower rate in neonates than in adults, but responses vary and normal hepatic function is probably sufficient to prevent significant entry of galactose into the systemic circulation [28,29,34]. Any contribution from the endogenous production of galactose remains

Table 1 Galactose Disorders and Risk of Cataract

Galactoskinase deficiency
Homozygote	Strong assoication with cataract
Heterozygote	Weak association, mainly seen in first year of life
Low-normal	Occasional association of below mean level of maternal galactokinase activity and congenital cataracts in an enzymatically normal child

Galactose-1-phosphate uridyl transferase activity
Homozygote	Strong association with cataract
Heterozygote	At most a weak association with cataract
Variant forms	May be associated with cataract when multiple defects are present that cause overall pathway activity to fall below 25% of normal
Low-normal	Association occasionally reported between below mean activity in either mother or child and cataract in early life, but associations are weaker than for galactokinase

uncertain [23]. Variation in the extent of aldose reductase activity in the lens may also be important; animal studies on the relationship between cataract and hyperglycemia have shown a parallel relationship between activity and cataract. Activity in the human lens is at the lower end of the range recorded for various animal species and falls with age [36]. Fetal levels are not recorded, and individual variation may also affect polyol formation. Availability of free galactose can also be influenced by the gut bacterial flora, as is reported for kangaroos, a species apparently prone to dietary provocation of galactose-dependent cataract [69].

Cataract is common, and the possibility that expression is significantly related to minor deficiency of the enzymes of galactose metabolism, amenable to early dietary control of children or mothers at risk, is extremely attractive, but a causal connection is not well supported by present evidence. Dominant structural cataract may also affect some of the families reported; that is, any association with enzyme disorders may arise simply by chance, and the reported enzyme defects may also be erroneous because precision is hard to achieve, particularly for galactokinase as discussed earlier. The most important advance is likely to be improved techniques allowing reliable definition of the extent and nature of any monogenic or other enzyme deficiency, with clarification of any real relationship with cataract. Some molecular approaches to human disorders of galactose metabolism have now been developed, and further applications are awaited.

IV. DIABETES MELLITUS

The essential features of diabetes mellitus are inappropriate hyperglycemia, impaired glucose tolerance to an oral load, and a relative or absolute lack of insulin. Diabetes mellitus is a syndrome in which the insulin deficiency is central, but many other endocrine, genetic, and environmental influences may be involved. Different manifestations relate to the duration of the illness, the age of the patient, the degree of insulin deficiency and its consequent effects on intermediary metabolism, and other features of primary disorders of which diabetes may be a secondary feature. There is an extremely large literature on clinical, metabolic, and molecular features of diabetes mellitus, and extensive reviews are available [15,37,55].

The classification of diabetes mellitus and related disorders associated with impaired glucose tolerance has been reviewed by World Health Organization (WHO) expert committees and study groups [75,76]: it is helpful to emphasize that the distinctions are based overwhelmingly on clinical descriptive criteria and that individuals may be reclassified during progression of the disease. Classification based on the cause and primary defect is not yet secure: diabetes mellitus and related syndromes, particularly their clinical features, can be described in great detail, but the essential initiating events and some of the consequent cellular changes, at least for primary diabetes, remain speculative. Five main categories of diabetes mellitus are recognized [15,55,76].

A. Insulin-Dependent Diabetes

Insulin-dependent diabetes (IDDM) predominantly affects juveniles and young adults who are generally lean and who can present with sudden acute insulin deficiency, ketoacidosis, and dehydration. The resulting metabolic disturbance involves diminished glucose uptake by insulin-sensitive cells and stimulation of lipid catabolism in adipose tissue with release of fatty acids, mobilization of triglyceride by adipose tissue, β oxidation of fatty acids in liver as a major pathway for energy release, and consequent production of ketone bodies as 3-hydroxybutyrate, acetoacetate, and the decarboxylated product acetone. The switch away from glucose metabolism consequent to failure of insulin-dependent entry into cells also enhances gluconeogenesis, with protein catabolism, amino acid utilization, and further hyperglycemia. In long-standing IDDM, the pancreatic islets are essentially devoid of insulin-secreting islet beta cells. Immune factors appear to be important in the pathogenesis: circulating antibodies to islet cells and insulin are not only present but may precede clinical expression of diabetes. Partial or complete remission of insulin deficit may follow an initial acute presentation, although progression to IDDM is the general long-term result. Risk of IDDM is associated with expression of the HLA antigens, although the mechanisms of that association, including relationships with virally induced or autoimmune damage to islet beta cells, are obscure. Information on the genetic background of forms of diabetes mellitus has come from both animal and human studies, particularly those involving monozygotic twins, for whom the concordance rate for IDDM approaches 50%. Structural variation affecting HLA genes is reported, together with other probably indirect linkage associations at sites close to the insulin gene. There is thus significant genetic predisposition to IDDM, but the mechanisms of that expression are not yet well defined.

B. Non–Insulin-Dependent Diabetes Mellitus

Non–insulin-dependent diabetes mellitus (NIDDM) may occur in the young but is more common after middle age. The insulin lack is relative, and circulating levels of active insulin may even be elevated. Recent technical improvements in assay performance have suggested that inactive or partially inactive insulin may have also been measured and that NIDDM arises from a direct insufficiency of active insulin. It differs from IDDM in that the lipid mobilizing effect is not marked until the level of insulin has fallen well below that at which the effect on glucose entry into cells is lost. Insulin replacement is often unnecessary, at least until later life. There is a sluggish and diminished insulin response to a carbohydrate load, supporting the concept of insulin resistance; tolerance may improve after dietary change to reduce both obesity and the rate of postprandial glucose absorption. Most subjects are overweight, and the anatomical pattern of obesity may have a bearing on pathogenesis and prognosis. A genetic syndrome of insulin resistance with central obesity, hyperlipidemia, hypertension, and accelerated cardiovascular disease (Reaven's syndrome) has been proposed [57]. These associations may be fortuitous, however, in at least some cases, but that of IDDM with dyslipoproteinemia and large-vessel cardiovascular disease, including impaired renal function, is strong, and mortality and morbidity are both significantly increased. As with IDDM, genetic influences are evident without, however, any association with HLA patterns. Expression in the Pima Indians is both high at 50% and associated with a bimodal population distribution of glucose tolerance, compatible with a single gene effect for that group: concordance in monozygotic twins of IDDM, including lesser related abnormalities, approaches 100%. However, other data for most families is less clear-cut and is compatible with polygenic effects. Rare structural defects of the insulin molecule may cause IDDM, and some more common linkage associations with the insulin and insulin receptor genes are reported, but cause-effect relationships are not yet established.

C. Secondary Diabetes

Islet cell destruction, caused, for example, by pancreatitis or hemochromatosis, can progress to insulin-dependent diabetes with the long-term consequences characteristic of primary diabetes. Many other hormones than insulin affect the response to a glucose load, and responses may be impaired in the presence of disorders involving excess steroids, catecholamines, growth hormone, thyroid hormones, and glucagon. Hyperglycemia may also arise through medication, including thiazide diuretics in high dosage and, rarely, immune phenomena including antibodies to the insulin receptor. Rare genetic syndromes in which secondary IDDM may also arise include cystic fibrosis, type I glycogen storage disease, and other syndromes in which the metabolic connection with glucose intolerance is not as well defined, such as lipoatrophies and syndromes incorporating diabetes insipidus, diabetes mellitus, and optic atrophy (DIDMO syndromes).

D. Malnutrition-Related Diabetes

Malnutrition-related diabetes was introduced into the WHO classification in 1985 [76] to recognize different clinical associations arising in tropical developing countries. Associations involve pancreatic damage probably arising through malnutrition, particularly of protein, although the pathogenesis is not well defined.

E. Gestational Diabetes Mellitus

Gestational diabetes mellitus is also not well defined, but there is a moderate association between hyperglycemia identified during pregnancy and later clinical course and development of either IDDM or NIDDM, although such development is far from invariable and any latent period may be prolonged. There is some association with obesity and a family history of standard diabetes mellitus. Insulin therapy may be advised in the short term, together with long-term follow-up. Proposed influences include impaired expression of insulin receptors and of insulin secretion and postreceptor defects affecting glucose uptake and metabolism enhanced by other pregnancy-related endocrine changes [41,60]. The metabolic changes become apparent after midgestation, which may be why the associations with fetal maldevelopment seen in pregnancies involving known diabetic mothers are at most minor, although birth weight is generally increased. Unless formal diabetes mellitus develops, specific ophthalmological features are not described.

F. Impaired Glucose Tolerance

Delayed clearance of a standard oral glucose load, as defined by current WHO criteria for apparently normal individuals, is associated with a slightly increased risk of subsequent development of diabetes mellitus, and some of the metabolic associations even without formal conversion, including dyslipoproteinemia and vascular disease. Insulin resistance and obesity may be involved. Because of the cardiovascular associations, impaired glucose tolerance is commonly initially managed by dietary advice and attempted weight loss, but other specific objectives and benefits of intervention are not defined.

G. Metabolic Aspects of the Expression of Diabetes Mellitus

Defective metabolic control is displayed at some levels in all forms of diabetes. Some associated abnormalities are probably secondary to those metabolic derangements, whereas others follow tissue and vascular damage, as discussed in other chapters. Pathological changes may arise at least partly as a direct consequence of the hyperglycemia present in all forms of diabetes. Nonenzymic glycosylation of tissue proteins is a generalized phenomenon [9]. That of hemoglobin is of value in the monitoring of long-term glycemic control, although the changes in the oxygen dissociation curve are not of obvious functional significance, in contrast to proposed effects on other proteins. Incubation of rodent and bovine lenses and bovine lens extracts in solutions containing excess glucose induces glycosylation of lysine residues, particularly in γ-crystallins [70]. Glycosylation is associated with increased susceptibility of lens crystallins to sulfhydryl oxidation, with cross-linking, aggregation, and the development of turbidity in solution [70]. Glycosylation of crystallins in human lenses is also increased in diabetic patients, with some relationship to the degree of diabetic control achieved: changes in the organization of those proteins, with agglomeration, binding to fiber membranes, and resulting optical discontinuities as cataract, may then follow [20,45]. As outlined earlier, there is strong evidence that polyol production is involved in both experimental and human galactose cataract, but glycosylation is the more probable major influence in human diabetic cataract. Associations between levels of glucose and glycosylated hemoglobin in blood and the content of sorbitol within the human lens are expected and do not necessarily indicate a causal relationship with cataract [42]. The osmotically minor changes recorded for human lenses through accumulation of sorbitol and fructose may exert some further background influence, however, and this polyol pathway (and its potential modification by aldose reductase inhibitors) may contribute to damage at other sites, including nerves and blood vessels (see Chap. 52 for a discussion of the vascular changes) [19,30].

The most important advances in understanding the pathogenesis of diabetes mellitus will follow a clearer perception of the nature of the action of insulin at the cellular level. The structure and some aspects of the operation of the cell surface insulin receptor, including enhanced expression of transmembrane glucose transporter proteins facilitating glucose entry into cells, are now defined, but aspects of the presumed second messenger system amplifying the intracellular response to receptor activation remain obscure. Phosphorylation via a tyrosine kinase is one aspect of receptor activation, and wider phosphorylation via protein kinases with changes in the conformation and function of target proteins is also probably involved, but specific processes and any involvement of cyclic nucleotides have not yet been identified.

REFERENCES

1. Aperia, A., Bergqvist, G., Linne, T., and Zetterstrom, R. Familial Fanconi syndrome with malabsorption and galactose intolerance, normal kinase and transferase activity. *Acta Paediatr. Scand. 70*:527–533, 1981.
2. Bannon, S.L., Higginbottom, R.M., McConnell, J.M., and Kaan, H.W. Development of galactose cataract in the albino rat embryo. *Arch. Ophthalmol. 33*:224–228, 1945.
3. Berry, H.K., and Croft, C.C. Reagent that restores galactose-1-phosphate uridyl transferase in dry blood spots. *Clin. Chem. 33*:1471–1472, 1987.

4. Beutler, E., and Baluda, M.C. A simple spot screening test for galactosemia. *J. Lab. Clin. Med.* 68:137–141, 1966.
5. Beutler, E., and Baluda, M.C. Improved method for measuring galactose-1-phosphate uridyl transferase activity of erythrocytes. *Clin. Chim. Acta* 13:369–379, 1966.
6. Beutler, E., and Matsumoto, F. A rapid simplified assay for galactokinase activity in whole blood. *J. Lab. Clin. Med.* 82:818–821, 1973.
7. Beutler, E., Matsumoto, F. Galactokinase and cataracts. *Lancet* 1:1161,1978.
8. Beutler, E., Matsumoto, F., Kuhl, W., Krill, A., Levy, N., Sparkes, R., and Degnan, M. Galactokinase deficiency as a cause of cataracts. *N. Engl. J. Med.* 288:1203–1206, 1973.
9. Brownlee, M., Cerami, A., and Vlassara, H. Advanced glycosylation end-products in tissue and the biochemical basis of diabetic complications. *N. Engl. J. Med.* 318:1317–1320, 1988.
10. Chacko, C.M., Christian, J.C., and Nadler, H.L. Unstable galactose-1-phosphate uridyl transferase: a new variant of galactosemia. *J. Pediatr.* 78:454–460, 1971.
11. Cornblath, M., and Schwartz, R. Disorders of galactose metabolism. In *Disorders of Carbohydrate Metabolism in Infancy*, 3rd ed. Blackwell Scientific, Publications, Boston, pp. 295–324, 1991.
12. Cuatrecasas, P., and Segal, S. Mammalian galactokinase. *J. Biol. Chem.* 240:2382–2388, 1965.
13. Donnell, G.R., Koch, R., and Bergren, W.R. Observations on results of management of galactosemic patients. In *Galactosemia*, D.Y.Y. Hsia (Ed.), Charles C. Thomas, Springfield, IL, p. 247, 1969.
14. Fensom, A.H., Benson, P.F., Rodeck, C.K., Campbell, S., and Gould, J.D.H. Prenatal diagnosis of a galactosemia heterozygote by fetal blood enzyme assay. *BMJ* 291:22–29, 1979.
15. Foster, D.W. Diabetes Mellitus. In *The Metabolic Basis of Inherited Disease*, 6th ed., C.R. Scriver, A.L. Beaudet, W.S. Sly, and D. Valle (Eds.), McGraw-Hill, New York, pp. 375–398, 1989.
16. Francois, J. Ocular manifestations of inborn errors of carbohydrate and lipid metabolism. I. Classical galactosemia. *Bibl. Ophthalmol.* 84:2–10, 1975.
17. Francois, J. Ocular manifestations of carbohydrate and lipid metabolism. II. Galactokinase deficiency. *Bibl. Ophthalmol.* 84:11–12, 1975.
18. Friedman, J.H., Levy, H.L., and Bouslany, R.M. Late onset of distinct neurological syndromes in galactosemic siblings. *Neurology* 39:741–742, 1989.
19. Gabbay, K.H. The sorbitol pathway and the complications of diabetes. *N. Engl. J. Med.* 288:831–836, 1973.
20. Garlick, R.L., Mazer, J.S., Chylack, L.T., Jr., Tung, W.H., and Bunn, H.F. Non-enzymic glycation of human lens crystallin: Effects of aging and diabetes mellitus. *J. Clin. Invest.* 74:1742–1749, 1984.
21. Gitzelmann, R. Deficiency of UDPG-4-epimerase in blood cells of an apparently healthy infant. *Helv. Paediatr. Acta* 27:125–130, 1972.
22. Gitzelmann, R., Curtius, H.C., and Schneller, I. Galactitol and galactose-1-phosphate in the lens of a galactosaemic infant. *Exp. Eye Res.* 6:1–3, 1967.
23. Gitzelmann, R., Hauser, R.G., and Steinmann, B. Biogenesis of galactose, a possible mechanism of self-intoxication in galactosemia. In *Normal and Pathological Development of Energy Metabolism*, F.A. Hommes and C.J. van den Berg (Eds.), Academic Press, London, pp. 25–38, 1975.
24. Gitzelmann, R., Poley, J.R., and Prader, A. Partial galactose-1-phosphate uridyl transferase deficiency due to a variant enzyme. *Helv. Paediatr. Acta* 22:252–257, 1967.
25. Greenberg, C.R., Dilling, L.A., Thompson, R., Ford, J.D. Sergeant, L.E., and Haworth, J.C. Newborn screening for galactosemia: a new method used in Manitoba. *Pediatrics* 84:331–335, 1984.
26. Hammersen, G., Houghton, S., and Levy, H.L. Rennes-like variant of galactosemia: Clinical and biochemical studies. *J. Pediatr.* 87:50–57, 1975.
27. Harley, J.D., Irvine, S., Mutton, P., and Gupta, J.D. Maternal enzymes of galactose metabolism and the "inexplicable" infantile cataract. *Lancet* 2:259–261, 1974.
28. Haworth, J.C., and Ford, J.D. Variation of the oral galactose tolerance test with age. *J. Pediatr.* 66:276–282, 1963.
29. Haworth, J.C., Ford, J.D., and Robinson, T.J. Peripheral and portal vein blood sugar after lactose and galactose feedings. *Clin. Sci.* 29:83–92, 1965.
30. Hawthorne, G.C., Bartlett, K., Hetherington, C.S., and Alberti, K.G.M.M. The effect of high glucose on polyol pathway activity and myoinositol mechanism in cultured human endothelial cells. *Diabetologia* 32:63–166, 1989.
31. Holton, J.B., Gillett, M.G., MacFaul, R., and Young, R. Galactosemia: A new severe variant due to uridine diphosphate galactose-4-epimerase deficiency. *Arch. Dis. Child.* 56:885–887, 1981.
32. Hsia, D.Y.Y., Inouye, T., Wong, P., and South, A. Studies on galactose oxidation in Down's syndrome. *N. Engl. J. Med.* 270:1085–1088, 1964.
33. Hsia, D.Y., and Walker, F.A. Variability in the clinical manifestations of galactosemia. *J. Pediatr.* 59:872–883, 1961.
34. Hjelm, M., and Sjolin, S. Changes in the elimination rate from blood of intravenously injected galactose during the neonatal period. *Scand. J. Clin. Lab. Invest.* 92 (Suppl. 18):126–134, 1966.
35. Kador, P.F., Akagi, Y., and Kinoshita, J.H. The effect of aldose reductase and its inhibition on sugar cataract formation. *Metabolism* 35:15–19, 1986.

36. Kador, P.F., and Kinoshita, J.H. Diabetic and galactosaemic cataracts. *Human Cataract Formation*, CIBA Foundation Symposium 106, Pitman, London, pp. 110–131, 1978.
37. Keen, H., and Jarrett, J. (Eds.). *Complications of Diabetes*, 2nd ed., Edward Arnold, London, 1982.
38. Kinoshita, J.H., Cataracts in galactosemia. *Invest. Ophthalmol. 4*:786–799, 1965.
39. Kinoshita, J.H., Mechanisms initiating cataract formation. *Invest. Ophthalmol. 13*:713–724, 1974.
40. Kinoshita, J.H., Merola, K., and Dikmak, E. Osmotic changes in experimental galactose cataracts. *Exp. Eye Res. 1*:405–412, 1962.
41. Kuhl, C., Honnes, P.J., and Anderson, O. Etiology and pathophysiology of gestational diabetes mellitus. *Diabetes 34*(Suppl. 2):66–70, 1985.
42. Lerner, B.C., Varma, S.D., and Richards, R.D. Polyol pathway metabolites in human cataracts. Correlation of circulating glycosylated hemoglobin content and fasting blood glucose levels. *Arch. Ophthalmol. 102*:917–920, 1984.
43. Levy, N.S., Krill, A.E., and Beutler, E. Galactokinase deficiency and cataracts. *Am. J. Ophthalmol. 74*:41–48, 1972.
44. Levy, H.L., Sepe, S.J., Walton, D.S., Shih, V.E., Hammersen, G., Houghton, S., and Beutler, E. Galactose-1-phosphate uridyl transferase deficiency due to Duarte/galactosemia combined variation: Clinical and biochemical studies. *J. Pediatr. 92*:390–393, 1978.
45. Liang, J.N., Hershorin, L.L., and Chylack, L.T., Jr., Non-enzymatic glycosylation in human diabetic lens crystallins. *Diabetologia 29*:225–228, 1986.
46. Mellman, W.J., Rawnsley, B.E., Nichols, C.W., Needelman, B., Mennuti, M.T., Malone, J., and Tedesco, T. Galactose tolerance studies of individuals with reduced galactose pathway activity. *Am. J. Hum. Genet. 27*:748–754, 1975.
47. Monk, A.M., Mitchell, A.H., Milligan, J.W., and Holton, J.B. Diagnosis of classical galactosemia. *Arch. Dis. Child. 52*:943–946, 1977.
48. Monteleone, J.A., Beutler, E., Monteleone, P.L., Utz, C.L., and Casey, E.C. Cataracts, galactosuria and hypergalactosemia due to galactokinase deficiency in a child. *Am. J. Med. 50*:403–407, 1971.
49. Ng, W.G., Bergren, W.R., and Donnell, G.N. A new variant of galactose-1-phosphate uridyl transferase in man: The Los Angeles variant. *Ann. Hum. Genet. 37*:1–8, 1973.
50. Ng, W.G., Bergren, W.R., Fields, M., and Donnell, G.N. An improved electrophoretic procedure for galactose-1-phosphate uridyl transferase: Demonstration of multiple activity bands with the Duarte variant. *Biochem. Biophys. Res. Commun. 37*:354–362, 1969.
51. Ng, W.G., Donnell, G.N., and Bergren, W.R. Galactokinase activity in human erythrocytes of individuals at different ages. *J. Lab. Clin. Med. 66*:115–121, 1965.
52. Ng, W.G., Lee, J.S., and Donnell, G.N. Transferase-deficient galactosemia and the Duarte variant. *JAMA 257*:187–188, 1987.
53. Pesce, M.A., Bodourian, S.H., Harris, R.C., and Nicholson, J.F. Enzymatic micromethod for measuring galactose-1-phosphate uridyl transferase activity in human erythrocytes. *Clin. Chem. 23*:1711–1717, 1977.
54. Petterson, R., Dahlquist, A., Hattevig, G., and Kjellman, B. Borderline galactosemia. *Acta Pediatr. Scand. 69*:735–739, 1980.
55. Pickup, J., and Williams, G. (Eds.). *Textbook of Diabetes*, Blackwell Scientific, Oxford, 1991.
56. Prchal, J.T., Conrad, M.E., and Skalka, H.W. Association of presenile cataracts with heterozygosity for galactosemic states and with riboflavin deficiency. *Lancet 1*:12–13, 1978.
57. Reaven, G.M. Banting Lecture. Role of insulin resistance in human disease. *Diabetes 37*:1595–1607, 1988.
58. Reichardt, J.K.V., and Berg, P. Cloning and characterisation of a cDNA encoding human galactose-1-phosphate uridyl transferase. *Mol. Biol. Med. 5*:107–122, 1988.
59. Rolland, M.O., Mandou, G., Farriaux, J.P., and Dorche, E. Galactose-1-phosphate uridyl transferase activity in chorionic villi: A first trimester prenatal diagnosis of galactosemia. *J. Inherited Metab. Dis. 9*(Suppl. 2): 284–286, 1986.
60. Ryan, E.A., and Enns, L., Role of gestational hormones in the induction of insulin resistance. *J. Clin. Endocrinol. Metab. 67*:341–347, 1988.
61. Schapira, F., Gregori, C., and Banroques, J. Microheterogeneity of human galactose-1-phosphate uridyl transferase: Isoelectrofocussing results. *Biochem. Biophys. Res. Commun. 80*:291–297, 1978.
62. Schapira, F., Gregori, C., Banroques, J., Vidailhet, M., Despoisses, S., and Vigneron, C. Isoelectrofocussing of erythrocyte galactose-1-phospho-uridyl transferase in a family with both galactosemia and Duarte variants. *Hum. Genet. 46*:89–96, 1979.
63. Segal, S. Disorders of galactose metabolism. In *The Metabolic Basis of Inherited Disease* 6th ed., C.R. Scriver, A.L. Beaudet, W.S. Sly, and D. Valle (Eds.) McGraw-Hill, New York, pp. 453–480, 1989.
64. Shin-Buehring, Y.S., Beier, T., Tan, A., Osang, M., and Schaub, J. The activity of galactose-1-phosphate uridyl transferase and galactokinase in human fetal organs. *Pediatr. Res. 11*:1003–1009, 1977.
65. Sitzmann, F.C., and Kaloud, H. Biokinetics of galactose in the homozygotes and heterozygotes in both forms of galactosaemia. *Clin. Chim. Acta 72*:343–351, 1976.
66. Sitzman, F.C., Schmid, D., and Kaloud, H. Excretion of galactitol in the urine of heterozygotes of both forms of galactosaemia. *Clin. Chim. Acta 75*:313–319, 1977.

67. Skalka, H.W., and Prchal, J.T. Presenile cataract formation and decreased activity of galactosemic enzymes. *Arch. Ophthalmol. 98*:269–273, 1980.
68. Spielman, R.S., Harris, H., Mellman, W.J., and Gershowitz, H. Discussion of a continuous distribution: Red cell galactokinase activity in blacks. *Am. J. Hum. Genet. 30*:237–248, 1978.
69. Stephens, T.C., Crollini, C., Mutton, P., Gupta, J.D., and Harley, J.D. Galactose metabolism in relation to cataract formation in marsupials. *Aust. J. Exp. Biol. Med. Sci. 53*:233–239, 1975.
70. Stevens, V.J., Rouzer, C.A., Monniert, V.A., and Cerami, A. Diabetic cataract formation: Potential role of glycosylation of lens crystallins. *Proc. Natl. Acad. Sci. USA 75*:2918–2922, 1978.
71. Stocchi, V., Dacha, M., Bossu, M., and Fornaini, G. Modification of the radioactive method for erythrocyte galactokinase assay. *Clin. Chim. Acta 89*:371–374, 1978.
72. Tedesco, T.A., Miller, K.L., Rawnsley, B.E., Menniti, M.T., Spielman, R.S., and Mellman, W.J. Human erythrocyte galactokinase and galactose-1-phosphate uridyl transferase: A population survey. *Am. J. Hum. Genet. 27*:737–747, 1975.
73. Van Heyningen, R. The lens, metabolism and cataract. In *The Eye*, Vol. 1, H. Davson (Ed.), Academic Press, London, pp. 381–488, 1969.
74. Wharton, C.H., Berry, H.K., and Bofinger, M.K. Galactose-1-phosphate accumulation by a Duarte transferase deficiency double heterozygote. *Clin. Genet. 13*:171–175, 1978.
75. WHO Expert Committee on Diabetes Mellitus. Second Report, Geneva, Switzerland. *WHO Tech. Rep. Ser. 646*:1–80, 1980.
76. WHO Study Group, Geneva. Report on Diabetes Mellitus. *WHO Tech. Rep. Ser. 727*:1–113, 1985.
77. Winder, A.F., Claringbold, L.J., Jones, R.B., Jay, B., Rice, N.S.C., Kissun, R.D., Menzies, I.S., and Mount, J.N. Partial galactose disorders in families with premature cataracts. *Arch. Dis. Child. 58*:362–366, 1983.
78. Winder, A.F., Fells, P., Jones, R.B., Kissun, R.D., Menzies, I.S., and Mount, J.N. Galactose intolerance and the risk of cataract. *Br. J. Ophthalmol. 66*:438–441, 1982.
79. Winder, A.F., Fielder, A.R., Mount, J.N., and Menzies, I.S. Direct and maternal aspects of the risk of cataract with partial disorders of galactose metabolism. *Clin. Genet. 28*:199–206, 1985.

35

Disorders of Lipid and Lipoprotein Metabolism

Anthony F. Winder

Royal Free Hospital and School of Medicine, University of London; and Institute of Ophthalmology and Moorfields Eye Hospital, London, England

I. INTRODUCTION

Most plasma lipid is packaged in lipoproteins to facilitate transport in a water-soluble form [53,118]. Specific components can be identified in the plasma, most consistently in the fasting state, but essentially the system is in flux and after a fatty meal various transitional fractions can also be present. Increasing attention is being paid to rates of flow along lipoprotein metabolic pathways and between the various components involved, rather than to measurements recorded on a single sample, that merely give a static snapshot of this dynamic system.

II. THE PLASMA LIPOPROTEINS

Lipoproteins are conveniently classified on the properties through which they are most conveniently separated—size, the proportion of lipid to protein, which affects density, and which lipids and proteins are present—these differences also influencing the electrophoretic and immunochemical properties. A useful classification is based on electrophoretic mobility and uses the convention of prefixes applied to globulins, hence alpha-, prebeta-, and beta-lipoproteins. Alpha-lipoprotein contains several definable proteins, and those that are relatively specific for the alpha fraction are defined as the apolipoproteins A. Beta-lipoprotein contains essentially one protein only, apo B, and of the range of proteins in prebeta-lipoprotein the most specific is defined as apo C. This relatively neat arrangement has become blurred with the discovery of heterogeneity within the ABC system, hence apo A-I, A-II, A-IV, and so on, and of components not specific for any major fraction, such as the apo E series [20,53,118]. Various incomplete forms of apo B are defined by their size as a percentage of the major fraction, apo B-100, as apo B-48, for example.

The apoproteins are not merely inert carriers of lipid. Specific functions include activation of receptors for uptake into cells and of enzymes and intracellular transport: these are also under genetic control, and variation in their structure and turnover is extensive. The classification based on density into very low density lipoprotein (VLDL), with about 85% lipid by weight, intermediate- and low-density lipoproteins (IDL and LDL), with down to 70% lipid, and high-density lipoproteins (HDL), with down to about 44% lipid (equivalent to and formerly known as prebeta-, beta-, and alpha-lipoproteins) is now the convention, even though centrifugation and density are not commonly used in routine separation. However, the boundaries used to define these density-related fractions are applied to a continuous spectrum of components and may conceal true heterogeneity. Modified approaches to lipoprotein classification continue to arise in an attempt to make them more clinically useful.

The World Health Organization defined five broad types I–V of lipoprotein abnormalities in 1970 [10]. This classification was helpful but was based on the abnormality as expressed in plasma, rather than its primary cause, which is now preferred when possible. A convenient laboratory approach classifies disorders as mainly cholesterol excess, mainly triglyceride excess, or mixed excess of both.

III. OUTLINE OF LIPOPROTEIN METABOLISM

Essentially three major pathways are involved: from gut to liver, from liver to other peripheral sites, and prospects for reverse cholesterol transport from the tissues back to liver for excretion (Fig. 1).

A. Initial Processing of Dietary Lipid

Dietary lipid enters the circulation via the lymphatic ducts as chylomicrons, large particles containing about 99% lipid by weight. A small amount of low-molecular-weight lipid passes direct to liver via the hepatic portal vein. The main chylomicron protein is defined as apo B-48 because it represents 48% of the full apo B structure [20,53,118]. Lipid is removed from chylomicrons through the action of the endothelial enzyme lipoprotein lipase (LPL), which hydrolyses triglycerides into components then taken up mainly by adipose tissue and by transfer between other lipoproteins. Chylomicron clearance can be impaired by deficiency of LPL or apo C-II, which activates the enzyme, and by immunoglobulins and other circulating inhibitors [79]. The lipid-depleted chylomicron remnants are taken up by liver, almost certainly by a receptor-based mechanism interacting with apo E components on the remnant surface. Some genetic structural variants of apo E impair this uptake, and these mostly recessive disorders can express as *familial (type III) dysbetalipoproteinemia*. A second lipid disorder to overload the inadequate receptor pathway, usually diabetes, alcoholism, obesity, or hypothyroidism, is almost always necessary to cause major clinical expression, with accelerated arterial, particularly peripheral, obstructive disease [20,118]. Extra-vascular lipid deposits include xanthelasmata and corneal arcus, as well as the striking linear palmar xanthomata seen in about 50% of lipemic cases. Chylomicron-only excess with plasma forming a creamy upper layer over a clear infranatant is rare: more common is a mixed excess with chylomicrons, remnants, and other triglyceride lipoproteins with upper and lower turbidity (Fig. 2). Any pattern of severe large

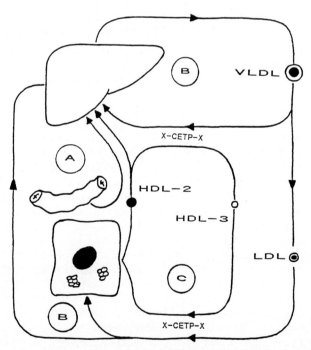

Figure 1   The three major pathways of lipoprotein metabolism. (A) Initial processing of dietary lipid: chylomicrons and remnants, from intestine to liver. (B) Endogenous lipoproteins and the lipoprotein cascade. Hepatic secretion of very low density lipoprotein (VLDL), with some reuptake and some conversion to low-density lipoprotein (LDL), which is then taken up by extrahepatic cells. (C) High-density lipoproteins (HDL) and reverse cholesterol transport, showing the major fractions HDL$_2$ and HDL$_3$ and the involvement of cholesterol ester transfer protein (CETP) in exchange X of lipid with VLDL/LDL components in the lipoprotein cascade.

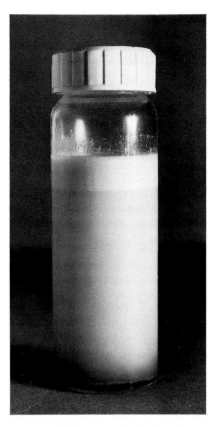

Figure 2 Plasma sample from a patient with lipemia retinalis showing major chylomicronemia as the upper creamy layer, plus an excess of smaller and somewhat denser very low density lipoprotein as the turbid infranatant.

triglyceride particle excess can lead to *lipemia retinalis*, sometimes with a history of eruptive xanthomata lasting a few days on the trunk and limbs and of abdominal pains suggestive of intermittent pancreatitis arising from the release of irritant fatty acids in the pancreas from hydrolysis of extravasated triglyceride particles by pancreatic lipase. Retinal angiography during a lipemic phase has not shown filling defects [40], but rates of perfusion are probably reduced.

B. Endogenous Lipoproteins and the Lipoprotein Cascade

The liver synthesizes triglyceride-rich VLDL. Intravascularly this undergoes similar transformations to the chylomicrons, with triglyceride hydrolysis and release, reduction in size, and transfer of lipid and protein between tissues and other lipoproteins. They are progressively modified to smaller, denser, and cholesterol-enriched lipoproteins, intermediate- and low-density lipoproteins (IDL and LDL), in a process termed the lipoprotein cascade. Disorders of VLDL excess are commonly secondary to other disorders, particularly overproduction, as in diabetes mellitus or alcoholism, but poorly understood genetic disorders also arise [53,118]. In the human, about 50% of VLDL of hepatic origin is partially metabolized as just mentioned but then taken up again by the liver. Excess of chylomicrons or their remnants is rare in fasting plasma and then involves defects, as discussed. Hypertriglyceridemia generally indicates excess of VLDL: similarly, except in the presence of uncommon high levels of HDL, LDL excess underlies hypercholesterolemia because it transports about 70% of plasma cholesterol. Mixed excess of triglycerides and cholesterol, and thus of VLDL and LDL, is also common.

All cells so far tested in the human have the capacity to synthesize cholesterol but normally do so to a very limited extent because needs are met by delivery in LDL via its uptake through specific high-affinity cell surface receptors binding to specific regions of LDL apo B. Because the receptors can also bind to apo E, they are defined as BE receptors. The internalized LDL is hydrolyzed, and while the lipid enters cellular pools, the apoprotein is degraded and receptors are recycled to the cell surface [26]. A complex system of cell signaling and sterol regulatory elements senses cholesterol availability within the cellular pools and controls expression of LDL receptors and of the endogenous cholesterol synthetic pathway to stabilize intracellular pool size [64].

In *Niemann-Pick type C disease* (see Chap. 29), cells become loaded with free cholesterol, but they appear to bind, endocytose, and hydrolyze LDL normally, without suppression of LDL receptor expression or intracellular cholesterol synthesis, implying defects in the pool system and the intracellular signaling processes [86].

Familial hypercholesterolemia (FH) results from a range of defects affecting the structure, expression, and efficacy of the high-affinity LDL cell surface receptor system or in the apo B-100 structure affecting binding to the BE receptors. Normal rates of clearance of LDL are maintained, but at approximately twice the normal levels of LDL in plasma [53,63]. In northern Europe and North America, about 1 in 500 of the general population are heterozygous for one of these defects, and perhaps 1 per million are the severely clinically affected homozygotes or double heterozygotes. The manifestations of FH are rather variable but are generally associated with accelerated coronary heart disease and extravascular lipid-rich deposits, such as tendon xanthomata, corneal arcus, and xanthelasmata, particularly if some hypertriglyceridemia is also present. Cardiovascular disease may be more severe if levels of the trace variant LDL lipoprotein Lp(a), incorporating a further apoprotein, apo(a), with amino acid sequence similarity to plasminogen, is also present in excess [72,135]. Diagnosis is still mainly clinical from the personal and family background of LDL excess, tendon xanthomata and other deposits, and heart disease, because about 180 different receptor gene sequence defects with the same general clinical result have now been defined, and many more are expected. Molecular approaches may help if specific information on the defect or linkage is available for an affected family or when, through founder effects, a population group has a preponderance of one or a few known FH defects, as in French Canadians or Afrikaners [63].

There is a general association between LDL excess in plasma and tissue accumulation of cholesterol and cholesterol esters. In recent deposits, at least, apo B-100 is present and the lipid acyl pattern resembles that of LDL. Accumulation may be facilitated by the established affinity of apo B-100 for glycosaminoglycans, as found in arterial walls and the peripheral cornea [17,76,128]. Some patients with accelerated atherosclerosis but relatively normal levels of total lipids in the plasma have LDL with less lipid per molecule of apo B than usual, resulting in hyperapobetalipoproteinemia [125]. Other receptor systems also facilitate uptake of lipoproteins into cells [130]: minor variation in composition, as perhaps occurs with VLDL in type II diabetics and with LDL modified by oxidative interaction with vascular endothelial cells [130], may also enhance accumulation of lipoprotein lipid within cells because receptor uptake for these modified lipoproteins may be avid and uncontrolled.

A report that *juvenile neuronal ceroid lipofuscinosis* (Batten disease; see Chap. 29) is associated with markedly low levels of circulating VLDL but no deficiency in its metabolic product LDL [11] is unexplained and has not been confirmed.

C. High-Density Lipoproteins and Reverse Cholesterol Transport

Precursor apoprotein and lipid material released from liver (with apo A-II), intestine (apo A-I and A-II), and spare surface coat shed during the breakdown of large triglyceride particles matures in plasma through transfer of lipid and protein from tissues and other lipoproteins. Two major fractions may then be defined: small, relatively dense HDL_3 and larger, more lipid-rich and thus less dense HDL_2. (HDL_1 is a larger, less dense, and apo E-enriched component found in trace amounts after lipid feeding: other trace HDL components can also be defined.) Metabolic transformations of HDL fractions are of particular ophthalmological interest (Figs. 1 and 3). There is strong but still partly indirect evidence that transfer of cholesterol from cells involves interaction of HDL_2 with surface receptors, expression of which is upregulated when cells are overloaded with cholesterol. Cholesterol mobilized by diffusion to the surface of the HDL_3 particle is then esterified by the enzyme lecithin-cholesterol acyltransferase (LCAT), associated in plasma with HDL and activated by apo A-I. Because it is nonpolar, the esterified cholesterol then sinks into the core of the progressively larger and less dense HDL_{2b} particle and the process continues

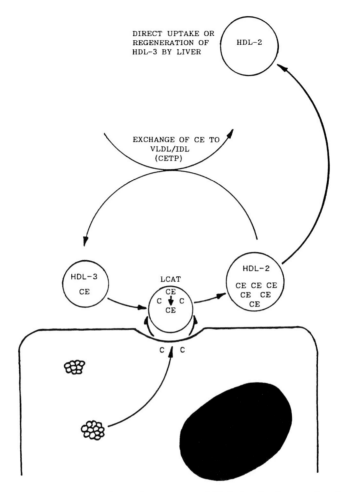

Figure 3 Cellular aspects of reverse cholesterol transport and high-density lipoproteins. Unesterified (free) cholesterol (C) is mobilized from intracellular sites, possibly through the action of apo A-I, diffuses from the cell surface across the extracellular space to the surface of the HDL_3 particle bound to the proposed receptor, and enlarges to HDL_2. The surface cholesterol (C) is esterified to cholesterol ester (CE) through the action of lecithin:cholesterol acyltransferase (LCAT), and this nonpolar CE product sinks into the hydrophobic core of the progressively enlarging HDL_2 particle. HDL_3 may be regenerated through lipid exchange from HDL_2 with VLDL/IDL components in plasma facilitated by cholesterol ester transfer protein or by interaction with hepatic triglyceride lipase; HDL_2 lipid may also be directly metabolized in liver. (HDL, VLDL, IDL, and LDL, high-density, very low density, intermediate-density, and low-density lipoproteins in plasma. CETP, cholesterol ester transfer protein.)

[97,107]. Further metabolism can involve transfer of cholesterol ester to triglyceride lipoproteins in the VLDL/LDL series in the lipoprotein cascade and some reverse exchange of triglyceride, a process requiring the plasma components known as cholesterol ester transfer protein (CETP) [108,153]. This process may be advantageous if the matured but potentially atherogenic VLDL/LDL are also rapidly cleared from the circulation, particularly if this proceeds through hepatic uptake. Finally, interaction with hepatic triglyceride lipase (HTGL) removes triglyceride from HDL_{2b}, regenerating HDL_3. Some direct uptake of HDL_2 by liver may also occur [107].

HDL can be subdivided by other criteria than density, such as particle size or apoprotein composition. Definition as HDL_3 and HDL_2 involves a particle mix similar but not identical to that produced on classification into large and small HDL or into apo A-1 with A-II and apo A-I-only particles [42,53]. These differences are important in defining the nature of any clinical advantage from elevated levels or increased turnover of HDL. Below average expression of coronary heart disease is associated with enhanced levels of HDL_2, particularly of HDL particles containing apo A-I but not apo A-II [105], these being the most effective species in promoting cholesterol efflux from cells in tissue culture. Further evidence now suggests that through as yet undefined mechanisms apo A-I may enhance the intracellular mobilization of cholesterol to the cell surface and thus promote transfer [97]. Although ethanol excess raises levels of HDL as defined by density, the excess is predominantly HDL_3, without increase in apo A-I-only material. Ophthalmological aspects of disorders involving HDL are discussed later. Corneal aspects of lipid disorders were reviewed recently [7].

IV. SPECIFIC LIPOPROTEIN DISORDERS AFFECTING THE EYE AND VISION

A. Abetalipoproteinemia and Related Disorders

These disorders involved impaired expression of forms of apo B in plasma, with effects on circulating lipoproteins and their functions notably transport of dietary fat and fat-soluble vitamins, particularly vitamin E [78]. Deficiency of these vitamins is likely to be the essential cause of any ophthalmological and particularly retinal features.

Abetalipoproteinemia is a rare autosomal recessive disorder in which apo B is not expressed in plasma. Thus the normal mechanisms of lipid transport from the intestine and liver are impaired, and chylomicrons, VLDL, and LDL are not formed. All plasma lipids are reduced, and plasma cholesterol rarely exceeds 1.0 mM (40 mg per 100 ml), almost all present as material in the HDL and particularly the HDL_2 density range at about half-normal levels, including apo E-enriched HDL. This fraction is probably the means of delivery of cholesterol to extrahepatic cells through interaction with the apolipoprotein BE receptors also internalizing LDL and thus preventing the major upregulation of endogenous local synthesis that would otherwise be predictable from the delivery defect [13,16]. Some vitamin E is transported in HDL: in normal plasma much greater amounts are transported in LDL. The presence of free apo(a) indicates that it can be secreted independently of LDL [72].

Recent molecular approaches, particularly linkage studies in consanguineous affected families, have shown that the apo B gene is discordant with the clinical disorder [132]. Transmission of the gene within affected families does not correlate with clinical affect, excluding a mutation in or near that gene is the seat of the disorder. The apo B gene in the intestine and liver appears normal, apo B and its mRNA are expressed within cells, and the disorder may arise through defects affecting synthesis, assembly, and/or secretion of apo B lipoproteins [41,84]. This conclusion applies to at least most patients studied, but the failure to identify apo B within intestinal epithelium using immunochemical methods in occasional patients leaves open the prospect of heterogeneity, some patients being unable to synthesize apo B at all or perhaps to produce immunochemically normal apo B [59,66].

Obligate heterozygotes are normolipemic and clinically normal, and the disorder usually presents in infancy with a reported mild male preponderance. Clinical features include steatorrhea, spinocerebellar ataxia and peripheral neuropathy, myopathy with ceroid deposits in the muscle fibers, retinal degeneration, and anemia with acanthocytosis [78]. Intellectual impairment, skeletal abnormalities, and cardiomyopathy with dysrhythmias may also be present. Without treatment the disorder carries a poor prognosis, with increasing visual and neuromuscular defects and death in early adult life. Ocular features include widespread destruction of rods and cones, with pigmentary changes initially sparing the macula, and electroretinographic (ERG) evidence of damage that may precede the morphological changes [30,78]. Ptosis, strabismus, nystagmus, and isolated oculomotor paresis may also occur [151]. Histological studies in a case with ophthalmoplegia suggested that the defects in that case were not myopathic in origin [151], although ceroid inclusions in muscle fibers have been reported [81]. Histological data on the retinal changes are available only for the late stages of the disease [114].

Cellular aspects of this disorder have been approached by studies of the composition and properties of the spiny erythrocytes (acanthocytes). The lipid composition of erythrocytes and their membranes is abnormal, with a relative increase in sphingomyelin, a reduction in phosphatidylcholine and other phospholipids, and very little linoleate [35,140]. The abnormalities of shape and composition are not changed by incubation in normal plasma, and normal erythrocytes are not modified by incubation in affected serum. Acanthocytosis is likely to be a response to abnormal membrane composition; the anemia is probably a less specific consequence of malabsorption and nutritional imbalance. Activities in the plasma of the enzymes LPL, HTGL, and LCAT are reduced to about half-normal, but this is probably secondary and unlikely to be of pathological significance because substantial activity remains. Plasma retinol binding protein is also reduced below normal, but this is also likely to be secondary, not significant, because levels tend to increase toward normal on vitamin A supplementation. Vitamin E tends to protect against lipid peroxidation, and the increased accumulation of lipofuscin in various tissues, including the heart, suggests that lipid peroxidation is a feature of abetalipoproteinemia. Vitamin E protects the erythrocytes of abetalipoproteinemic patients from hydrogen peroxide-induced hemolysis [39], but the decrease in red cell membrane fluidity is not affected by vitamin E and is therefore unlikely to result from fatty acid peroxidation [34]. Studies with mixed lipid monolayers using phospholipid with unsaturated acyl residues suggest that vitamin E may have both an antioxidant and a structural role, the latter influencing the density of membrane packing [89]. Although mainly erythrocyte membranes have been studied in this disorder because they are both accessible and abnormal, other cell membranes, such as those of retinal outer segments, may also be abnormal. Rod outer segments are enriched with vitamin E, polyunsaturated lipids, and superoxide dismutase, all with a potential for involvement in free radical inactivation. Phagocytosis of abnormal retinal components by the retinal pigment epithelium (RPE) could be impaired, although evidence of such membrane defects remains to be established.

Clinical features and their control relate to the defects in absorption and transport of fat. Some reduction in steatorrhea after infancy may indicate undefined adaptive changes, and thereafter bowel symptoms may be controlled by major restriction of dietary triglycerides. Hydrolysis of medium-chain triglycerides releases fatty acids that are then transported directly to the liver via the portal system, bound to plasma albumin. Supplementation with this source of energy is recommended in severely malnourished cases but not routinely because hepatic fibrosis has been associated with this approach [75]. Effects on polyunsaturated fatty acids and on vitamin A and K may contribute, but the clinically important effect is at least substantially impaired intake and distribution of vitamin E, overlapping responses probably arising because vitamin E may protect retinal vitamin A stores from oxidation [109]. Definite visual and other improvement arises in some but not all patients after massive supplementation with vitamin A [30,65]. Combined treatment with vitamins A and E, in some cases also with polyunsaturated lipids, has produced clear and objective evidence of stabilization or improvement in symptoms affecting nerve, muscle, and vision [92,113]. These included prevention of retinopathy in cases treated early and stabilization of, or improvement in, retinal electrophysiological responses and dark adaptation. However, some adult cases treated with vitamins A and E showed stable visual performance but progressive neuropathy, albeit at a reduced rate [88]. It seems important to start treatment early and adequately. Liver vitamin stores can be replenished by water-based vitamin preparations in a very high dosage of grams per day, although plasma levels remain low. Supplementation with vitamin K is recommended when evidence of deficiency, such as bleeding or bruising, is evident: a deficiency of vitamin D does not occur because different transport systems are involved [78].

The diagnosis of abetalipoproteinemia may be suspected on clinical grounds, supported by plasma lipoprotein studies demonstrating the absence of circulating immunochemically reactive apo B and confirmed by family studies and by jejunal biopsy, which reveals abnormal fat-laden cells, helpful when the diagnosis is not otherwise definitely confirmed. Clinical and lipoprotein studies should be performed on parents and close family members to confirm the lack of affect in heterozygotes and to exclude familial hypobetalipoproteinemia (see later), a related disorder with different manifestations in the heterozygote. Molecular techniques can be used for further definition of the defect in this second disorder but not as yet in abetalipoproteinemia, except to exclude other forms of apo B deficiency.

Familial hypobetalipoproteinemia is regarded as an autosomal dominant disorder in that heterozygotes are also affected to a limited and variable extent. Homozygotes are clinically and biochemically very similar to those with homozygous abetalipoproteinemia, but often with traces of immunochemically reactive apo B material in plasma, normal activity of lipoprotein lipase and hepatic triglyceride lipase on release into plasma, neuromuscular effects of variable but generally lesser severity, and retinal changes that may also be more benign and of later onset [78,152]. Heterozygous forms may be common, with an incidence of 1 per 3000 live births in one North American study [61], and they are probably largely unrecognized because a severe clinical affect is uncommon. Heterozygotes show moderate and variable lipoprotein changes, generally reduced levels of the apo B-containing lipoproteins LDL and VLDL, but at levels extending into the normal reference range. Plasma cholesterol does not respond to dietary loading.

They also show increased life expectancy and a remarkable freedom from atherosclerosis [60]. Most heterozygotes have no obvious neuromuscular problems, but posterior column and cerebellar lesions and peripheral neuropathy have been described, with clinical effects in early childhood. Some also contain a few acanthocytes, described as reverting to normal shape on exposure to normal plasma. Fundus changes in the form of a slight irregularity and clumping of the RPE may occur, but significant effects on acuity have not been reported [61,78,152].

All cases analyzed to date have contained mutations within the coding sequence of the apo B gene [32,74]. The disorder is heterogeneous: 11 truncated forms are now reported over the range 25–89% of the full sequence, hence apo B-25 to B-89. The apo B-25 and B-29 defects are sufficiently severe to prevent expression in plasma. Clinical expression of the apo B-25 variant is severe, but otherwise there is no obvious correlation between variant size and clinical affect for homozygotes or for heterozygotes in whom one apo B gene is normal. Most homozygotes are compound heterozygotes, and one or both variants may be sufficiently complete to allow expression of normal apo B-48 and thus chylomicrons and absorption of lipid from intestine.

Diagnosis and treatment are as for abetalipoproteinemia, with confirmation of a genetic effect by family studies, possible further analysis to identify truncated forms of apo B, and vitamin E supplements for heterozygotes because of the significant expression of neurological disease. Hypobetalipoproteinemia can also be secondary to a wide spectrum of other disorders [90], including fat malabsorption, hyperthyroidism, and hepatic necrosis.

Other structural variants of apo B are reported, but there are no specific ocular features.

B.   Disorders Affecting High-Density Lipoproteins

HDL components are involved in the flux of lipids between tissues and circulating lipoproteins, and anomalies in this system can have major systemic and ophthalmological effects, notably lipid accumulation in and clouding of the cornea [47,115]. Lipoproteins are also present in normal bovine and human aqueous, HDL and apo A-I being prominent, and a nutritional role in supplying lipid for lens is suggested [31]. At least 20 structural variants of apo A-I and further polymorphisms close to the A-I gene coding sequence compatible with reduced gene expression are associated with a substantial reduction of levels of HDL in plasma [4,20]. A gene cluster codes for the apoproteins A-I, C-III, and A-IV, and homozygotes for major rearrangements of this gene complex have no HDL in the plasma, premature cardiovascular disease, tissue lipid accumulation, and corneal clouding assumed to be lipid by analogy with confirmed deposits in other HDL syndromes [20].

Tangier Disease (Familial High-Density Lipoprotein Deficiency)

There are about 40 confirmed cases of the rare autosomal recessive disorder known as Tangier disease [5]. In plasma, HDL is present in traces only and is of abnormal composition, with levels of apo A-I and apo A-II measuring <1 and <10%, respectively, of reference levels. LDL and total cholesterol are low but with a normal proportion in the ester form, and triglyceride-rich chylomicrons and VLDL may be in moderate excess. The basic defect is not yet defined: all components of HDL are present, and apo A-I and A-II are of normal structure. Vitamin deficiencies are not known to be involved. From studies in tissue culture, defects of intracellular lipid and lipoprotein trafficking and rapid catabolism of HDL may be involved, with structural abnormalities of organelles, including lysosomes, and further effects on cellular phospholipid metabolism [108,116]. Any accelerated catabolism does not seem to involve adipose tissue [50]. Tissues accumulate phospholipid and cholesterol mainly in ester form (LCAT activity is not impaired) consequent to defective mobilization and transport through the virtually absent HDL system. The extent to which ingestion of modified lipoprotein or, alternatively, local synthesis contributes to the accumulation of lipid is not known, but abnormal circulating particles are more obvious after splenectomy and decrease in number after diet [71]. Uptake of such particles by phagocytosis into macrophages and impaired mobilization of tissue lipid is therefore likely: deposits in most tissues are intracellular and occur in cells with a vacuolated cytoplasm ("foam cells"). Sites of major tissue accumulation of lipid in homozygotes include the spleen, liver, lymphatic and reticuloendothelial systems, tonsils, and cornea. Peripheral neuropathy with various clinical manifestations is an important feature. Lipid deposits in Schwann cells and extracellularly within nerve bundles may explain occasional cardiac abnormalities, including conduction defects.

Corneal involvement with punctate panstromal extracellular deposits without an obvious clear zone at the periphery has been a feature of all reported cases, although this development may be delayed well into adult life. Vision is not significantly affected, although impairment can arise through ectropion of the eyelid, incomplete eyelid closure, exposure keratopathy, and corneal infiltration and ulceration [22, 50,104]. Refractory strabismus [49] and raised yellow linear conjunctival deposits, presumably lipid, may also occur. Tonsillar enlargement with yellow discoloration is a striking feature, possibly accentuated by the ambient coolness of the oropharynx, which could restrict melting and mobilization of the cholesterol esters present, since the transition temperatures of these liquid crystal deposits are close to body temperature [37,123]. Spaeth noted that the deposits in the peripheral cornea were more evident in the 3 o'clock position [126], although this distribution is not necessarily obvious with older patients, particularly when secondary corneal abnormalities have arisen [50]. This pattern differs from the 6 and 12 o'clock pattern seen with early corneal arcus and is consistent with a temperature-dependent accumulation. Thus arcus forms at sites of insudation promoted by temperature [44], Tangier deposits reflect a failure of mobilization accentuated at reduced temperature. Arcus is discussed later, but the proposed Tangier effect has now been directly supported by chemical and thermographic analysis of the corneas of a Canadian patient now deceased [50]. The presence of myelin figures with accumulation of phospholipid, and cholesterol with a normal proportion in ester form, confirmed that lipid was in excess as at other sites and that this excess formed the basis of the corneal opacification [148]. Tangier material also showed additional transition temperatures in the range 30–35°C in comparison with normal cornea [148], consistent with the idea that accumulation is influenced by the relationship between lipid transition temperatures and ambient corneal temperature, which like tonsil is below body core temperature in the affected corneal areas.

The disorder is relatively benign, with many patients surviving beyond 50 years, although the degree of disability may then be severe. Accelerated coronary heart disease is a minor feature of homozygotes only, perhaps because levels of LDL are low. Heterozygotes are clinically unaffected, although abnormal storage of lipid may be detected by rectal biopsy and plasma levels of HDL are often reduced, whereas apo A-I levels are always lower than normal. Diagnosis is made on the clinical presentation, lipoprotein profile, and tissue biopsy of tonsils or rectal mucosa to show foam cells: nerve conduction studies may also be performed. In contrast to LCAT deficiency (see later), the proportion of cholesterol present in plasma in ester form is normal at about 70%. In homozygotes, levels of triglyceride-rich lipoproteins may be controlled by diets [71], but no specific benefits have been confirmed and a treatment plan has not been defined.

Familial Lecithin: Cholesterol Acyltransferase Deficiency

The action of lecithin:cholesterol acyltransferase was outlined earlier in this chapter. Over 50 cases of absent or markedly reduced activity of this enzyme have been documented [95]. Immunoreactive protein is present in some cases [1], and the condition is compatible with an autosomal recessive inheritance [95]. The deficiency is associated with a marked reduction in the production of intravascular cholesterol esters (the presence of some ester is due to a different enzyme present in intestinal mucosa), initially on components of HDL but with secondary effects on the composition and organization of all other lipoprotein classes and on lipid exchange between the plasma and the tissues [95]. In most cases, immature and abnormal forms in the VLDL, LDL, and HDL density ranges are present in plasma, together with intra- and extracellular deposition of lipid in membranous and other forms (Fig. 4). Lipid also accumulates in macrophages, and the lipid composition of membranes of erythrocytes and other cells is altered. As in plasma, the proportion of cholesterol present in ester form is invariably reduced within cell membranes and in extracellular deposits like those found in the corneal stroma and atheromatous plaques [95,146,149].

Clinical features include accelerated atherosclerosis, renal impairment, and anemia, and lipid enriched with free cholesterol accumulates notably in the liver, spleen, cornea, conjunctiva, bone marrow, and arterial wall [95]. Some deposits are membranous, consistent with the presence of mixed phospholipid and cholesterol material. Arteriolar thickening in the kidney and foam cells in glomerular tufts are associated with proteinuria, uremia, and hypertension. The kidneys are pale, fatty, and enlarged, and similar lesions develop in renal transplants. Occasional patients retain good renal function well into adult life, and renal damage may be linked to the presence of high-molecular-weight components within the LDL density range [18,58]. Because expression of this abnormal LDL and of renal impairment varies among affected members of the same family, genetic heterogeneity is unlikely to apply [93]. The abnormal LDL is also less obvious in hypocholesterolemic patients and may be controlled by low-lipid diets, which have therefore been recommended in treatment although definite benefits to renal function are not confirmed [58,93]. Like membranes in other cells, those of erythrocytes possess an abnormal lipid composition. The

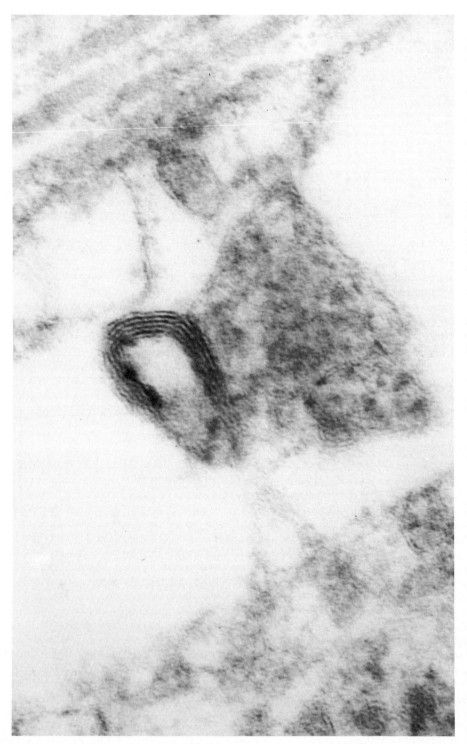

Figure 4   Electron micrograph of a portion of the central cornea of a patient with homozygous familial lecithin:cholesterol acyltransferase deficiency, showing a multilaminar myelinlike figure. (×100,000) The corneal inclusions are enriched with phospholipid and unesterified cholesterol.

altered erythrocytes are manifest by target cells and a decreased survival time [62] without obvious splenic hyperactivity. Moderate anemia is common, and the bone marrow contains foam cells.

Corneal opacification is a feature of all reported cases of LCAT deficiency, has been the cause of presentation, and may be evident in childhood [73,146]. A punctate stromal deposit is accentuated toward the periphery, where a circumferential clear zone may be present [23,73]. The presence of excess lipid, particularly of phospholipid and free cholesterol, has been demonstrated by microscopy and histochemistry of biopsy material and of corneas removed at transplantation, which were also subject to direct chemical analysis. The deposits are extracellular and some are membrane bound, and occasional multilayered myelinlike figures are also found (Fig. 4) [12,146,149]. The proportion and pattern of acyl residues in the cholesterol ester fraction differs from those in LCAT plasma (parallel differences are seen between normal plasma and associated corneal arcus; see later). The manner of entry or deposition of lipid in the cornea is unknown. The deposits do not appear to have an intracellular origin or location within the cornea, and the contribution of local synthesis or metabolism is also not known, but some such possibly general corneal effects seem to operate. Foam cells and fibroblasts with membrane-bound inclusions have been noted in the conjunctiva [146]. Retinal hemorrhages, angioid streaks, optic disk swelling, vascular occlusions, and total loss of vision may occur [73], but such changes are not characteristic and reported instances may have been secondary to associated renal or vascular disease.

Familial Partial LCAT Deficiency: Fish-eye Disease

Further patients have now been described with generally severe punctate corneal opacification as the only obvious clinical feature, associated with increased levels of triglyceride-rich lipoproteins and a marked deficiency of HDL in plasma but a normal or nearly normal proportion of plasma cholesterol in ester form [29]. The family background is consistent with autosomal recessive inheritance, and obligate heterozygotes may have reduced levels of HDL and LCAT activity in plasma. The description arose because corneal appearances resembled those of boiled fish, and visual impairment in the first cases was severe, leading to corneal transplantation. It was then found that an underlying cataractous lens not evident before corneal surgery was a substantial factor in the visual impairment and the ocular appearance: on analysis the corneal changes were very similar to those described for confirmed LCAT deficiency [100]. Further cases of probable fish-eye disease with minor corneal opacification have since been reported [3,51]. LCAT activity in association with apo A-I particles and HDL is markedly reduced, although as the proportion of cholesterol in ester form is adequate in other lipoproteins, some esterification, transfer, and exchange of cholesterol in plasma proceeds. Mutations have now been defined both in the LCAT sequence and in apo A-I [3,4], which seem to alter substrate specificity and impair interaction between LCAT and apo A-I HDL components, although transfer and esterification involving other lipoproteins can proceed. Fish-eye syndromes thus have at least some impairment of LCAT activity.

LCAT deficiency may be suspected from the clinical picture, notably corneal opacities, hypertension, and renal impairment, and from the lipid and lipoprotein abnormalities in plasma. Plasma LCAT activity may be assayed directly or indirectly by observing the (low) proportion of cholesterol present in ester form, which does not increase on prolonged incubation. The human LCAT gene has been sequenced, and direct diagnosis with oligonucleotide probes can be anticipated [3]. Fish-eye disease can also be defined from the clinical picture and plasma changes as discussed: specific molecular diagnostic approaches are also reported [4]. Sporadic cases of LCAT deficiency have been identified among various ethnic groups in several continents, but most cases may stem from a mutation in Norway some 300 years ago [95]. Presumed (obligate) heterozygotes are asymptomatic: LCAT activity in plasma is reduced in some cases, and minor increases in the proportion of phospholipid present in erythrocyte membranes are also found [52].

Other Disorders Affecting High-Density Lipoproteins

Corneal clouding may arise in other disorders affecting the levels, composition, and turnover of HDL in plasma [18,117,145]. Dyslipoproteinemia with marked deficiency of HDL was reported in a 48-year-old female presenting with diffuse planar xanthomata and moderate bilateral diffuse opacification of the cornea [67]. Minor lipoprotein abnormalities were found in other family members, but presentation in the index patient may have been modified by associated hypothyroidism and its treatment and by hepatic dysfunction implied by hepatomegaly. Levels of HDL are directly related to the activity of LPL and inversely to the activity of HTGL [83] and to levels of cholesterol ester transfer protein [127,153]. Although very high levels of HDL can be associated with longevity [60], the relationship is not simple and is expected to depend on the often poorly defined nature of the metabolic process involved. HDL excess as a consequence of reduced turnover may not be advantageous. Diffuse corneal clouding has been described in families with genetic hyperalphalipoproteinemia due to CETP deficiency [80,82]. The defect impairs transfer of cholesterol esters and exchange to triglyceride-rich lipoproteins in the lipoprotein cascade, leaving an excess of large and cholesterol ester-enriched HDL_2-like material. One major pathway of reverse cholesterol transport is therefore impaired, but circulating levels of lipid-enriched atherogenic LDL are also reduced, perhaps giving some balance of cardiovascular advantage: life expectancy can be above average. A defect in the CETP gene has been described in two siblings [25]. Because LCAT activity is adequate, the corneal clouding is assumed to result from delayed clearance of mainly esterified cholesterol, but direct analysis is not reported. Moderate alcohol intake also reduces CETP activity.

V. RELATED DISORDERS

A. Phytanic Acid α-Hydroxylase Deficiency (Refsum Disease)

Over 100 cases of this rare disorder are documented, in which activity of the mitochondrial enzyme catalyzing an early stage in the oxidation and degradation of phytanic acid either is absent or is present at less than 5% of normal activity [129]. The clinical and biochemical background is consistent with autosomal recessive inheritance. The branched-chain phytanic acid is a normal trace component of plasma, with an apparently entirely exogenous origin related to dietary intake of phytanate and phytol precursor, derived particularly from ruminants and thus dairy products. Endogenous production of phytanate is not absolutely excluded, but all dietary sources of phytanate may not yet have been defined. Phytol may also be released from cooked green vegetables, but little absorption occurs in the human. The defect gives a progressive but fluctuating disorder with a variable clinical presentation from childhood to late adulthood [102] and a latency associated with demyelination. Most cases present by age 20 years, with a range from childhood to late adulthood. The essential features are motor and sensory peripheral neuropathy, cerebellar ataxia, pigmentary retinopathy and other ocular defects, and an excess of protein in the cerebrospinal fluid. Characteristically, lipid accumulates in various organs, particularly in the liver, kidney, and parts of the brain [2,28,47,129]. An interstitial neuropathy develops, and cardiac deposition may form the basis of myocardial fibrosis and of electrocardiographic changes, disorders of rhythm, and occasionally sudden death [2].

Ophthalmological changes include atypical pigmentary retinopathy with variable early fundoscopic appearances. Night blindness may precede any pigmentary change, although this may not be obvious if impaired pupillary dilatation in the dark is taken into account [68]. Cone function may be unimpaired [68]. Cataract, generally posterior subcapsular and bilateral, occurs in about one-third of cases [106]. Cystic alterations were evident in the whole of the cystic epithelium in one case [13]. Diminished pupillary reactions, glaucoma and a keratopathy, nystagmus, and optic nerve degeneration may also occur. The retina and RPE are laden with lipid in which phytanate can be identified [36], and lipid deposits are also found in the sclera, the trabecular meshwork, and the pupillary muscles [133]. Xanthomata, when present, have also been shown to contain phytanate. The ocular morphological alterations during the early stages of classic Refsum disease have not been reported.

The manner in which restricted metabolism of and accumulation of phytanate produces these various effects is not well defined. Structural effects on lipids incorporating phytanate in place of other lipid, such as the linear-chain congener palmitate, may be involved—the antimetabolite hypothesis—although tissue levels of phytanate at post-mortem examination have in some cases been surprisingly low [129]. Phytanic acid bears some structural resemblance to the aminophenoxyalkanes, particularly diaminophenoxyalkane, the most potent of this group of agents associated with experimental pigmentary degeneration of the retina [19].

Diagnosis of the typical disorder may be suspected on clinical grounds, sometimes after a period of uncertainty, which may be prolonged. Awareness of the implications of neurological and ophthalmological features is important. Lipid analysis of extracts of blood or tissue samples by thin-layer chromatography readily demonstrates the major excess components, and phytanate can be specifically confirmed by gas-liquid chromatography and mass spectroscopy [129]. Antenatal diagnosis can be made on amniotic cells [129]. Heterozygotes are asymptomatic, and such status can be confirmed by enzyme analysis on cultured fibroblasts, activity being some 50% of normal values [129]. Treatment involves dietary control of the intake of phytanate and its available precursors. Because a minor capacity to degrade or excrete phytanate is retained, it should be possible to deplete body stores, and stabilization or clinical improvement in various respects, including effects on vision [68], is reported on dietary control. Responses may be limited by the extent of any demyelination. Diets are unpalatable, however, and compliance may be erratic [2,129]. Intermittent fasting to mobilize tissue stores of lipid incorporating phytanate, and then plasma exchange, can also improve balance [57], but mobilization associated with rapid weight loss, or intercurrent illness, can produce clinical relapse. Earlier untreated cases manifested variable but progressive clinical decline.

B. Inherited Defects in Peroxisomal Biogenesis

A spectrum of dysmorphic, neurological, hepatic, and ocular features arises in a group of disorders broadly characterized biochemically by defective oxidation of long-chain fatty acids, including phytanate [85,129]. The disorders are biochemically similar, but differ in the pattern and extent of organ involvement. Peroxisomal processes are involved, apparently normal in classical Refsum disease, thus properly called phytanic acid α-hydroxylase deficiency, and with a mitochondrial defect, as opposed to the peroxisomal disorder *infantile Refsum syndrome*. The group also includes the *Zellweger syndrome* (see Chap. 37), *cerebrohepatorenal syndrome*, forms of *adrenoleukodystrophy* (see Chap. 53), and *hyperpipecolic acidemia*. It follows that the further metabolism of phytanate involves peroxisomal processes that are not defective in classical Refsum syndrome. These other peroxisomal defects produce a very wide range of overlapping clinical effects, perhaps substantially because lipids enriched with long-chain acyl species accumulate in brain, nerve and elsewhere [120]. Prenatal diagnosis is possible [101,103].

C. Lipoid Proteinosis (Urbach-Wiethe Syndrome)

Over 200 cases of this rare disorder with autosomal recessive inheritance are now described. It is a multisystem disorder involving accumulation of hyaline material in the skin, mucous membranes, various organs, and at other sites, with hoarseness, stiffening and thickening of the lips and tongue, and blotchy cutaneous lesions, particularly of the elbows, knees, face, and scalp. Neurological involvement, particularly psychomotor epilepsy and rage attacks, may stem from calcified intracerebral lesions [94]. Although sometimes present in infancy or early childhood, this chronic disorder has a generally benign course with low direct mortality except when severe laryngeal obstruction is not controlled. The periocular tissues are characteristically involved, with numerous waxy nodules forming in the eyelid margins in more than 60% of cases, together with loss of eyelashes [48]. Infiltration less commonly involves the cornea, conjunctiva, and Bruch's membrane.

Histologically, the characteristic lesion is an extracellular accumulation of hyaline material, which produces indurated tissue, regarded as the physical basis for the clinical signs [91]. The basal lamina of small blood vessels in the dermis are multilaminated from a neighboring deposition of fibrillar material, giving an onionskin appearance [45]. The hyaline material is diastase resistant and reacts positively with the periodic acid–Schiff sequence and with lipophilic stains, such as Sudan red and oil red O [48,77]. There is no established local or systemic lipid disorder, however [124]. There is now extensive evidence of disordered production of collagen subunits and of excess production of normal associated noncollagenous proteins [45,69,70,91,96]. One study of fibroblasts in tissue culture demonstrated membrane-bound inclusions consistent with a lysosomal storage disease [7], and this report highlights the difficulty of drawing general conclusions from a series of detailed studies of mostly single cases, of what could also be a heterogeneous disorder. A unifying hypothesis has not yet arisen, but there is some consensus that the type I to type III collagen ratio is reduced, mainly because of reduced synthesis of type I material, and that mRNA levels for type IV procollagen and laminin are upregulated, at least in cultured fibroblasts [96]. One case was reported to show steady clinical improvement on administration of oral dimethylsulfoxide [150], an agent reported to scavenge hydroxyl radicals and to cause the dissolution of collagen and amyloid.

The diagnosis is made from clinical observations; histology can be supportive but otherwise there are no specific tests.

D.   Central Crystalline Dystrophy of the Cornea: Schnyder's Dystrophy

This uncommon disorder presents in early life, and the clinical features are predominantly and probably entirely limited to the cornea; the occasional association with genu valgum may be fortuitous [38,138]. Family studies showing vertical transmission over at least three generations are consistent with autosomal dominant inheritance [111], plus occasional further sporadic cases. The essential defect remains obscure. Associated hyperlipidemia, particularly hypercholesterolemia and familial (type III) dysbetalipoproteinemia, has been reported, but other members of affected families may manifest corneal changes or hyperlipidemia alone [24]. The stromal neutral fat deposits in the cornea reported by Garner and Tripathi [55] were probably secondary to associated hyperlipidemia. Sysi [131] reported that the corneal opacities in a patient who was also hypercholesterolemic were much reduced by a low-cholesterol diet and that the corneal deposits increased when plasma cholesterol again became elevated. The general experience, however, is that there is no clear association between the corneal features and plasma lipid levels [24], and the corneal changes found in this dystrophy are not characteristic of any inherited or other form of dyslipoproteinemia, which are unlikely therefore to be a primary component of the corneal disorder.

The bilateral corneal changes involve a stromal haze more evident centrally, often associated with corneal arcus, or independently with a white limbal girdle [138]. Deposition may also involve Bowman's layer, which may also be replaced with connective tissue. There is no accompanying corneal vascularization. Affected corneal material has been examined by light microscopy, histochemistry, including extraction with organic solvents and the use of fluorescent markers of free cholesterol, and transmission electron microscopy [56,110,111,138,141]. The fine particles present are mostly extracellular, and unesterified cholesterol predominates in extensive crystalline arrays [111]. Histochemical evidence of oxalate was also reported [120]. Radioactively labeled cholesterol was administered intravenously to a patient with Schnyder's dystrophy 2 weeks before performance of full-thickness keratoplasty [27]. The cholesterol accumulated within the cornea, and the residual radioactivity in the corneal button at the time of the operation was greater than that remaining in plasma, suggesting that the cornea was able to accumulate cholesterol. Comparable data for normal subjects are not available, however. After keratoplasty, grafts have remained clear for at least 15 months [110], but recrystallization can occur and may be more obvious after a lamellar transplant rather than penetrating keratoplasty [38]. There may therefore be active uptake, storage, and metabolism of cholesterol by the cornea, the potential for which is suggested by the differences between plasma and corneal lipid profiles in corneal arcus and familial LCAT deficiency, as discussed earlier. The posterior layers may be particularly involved. Such processes may be more significant in Schnyder's corneal dystrophy, local corneal systems for lipid processing may be defective, and coexisting but independent hyperlipidemia may accentuate or promote the disorder by producing further local overload. It remains the case, however, that the underlying defect is obscure. The diagnosis is made on clinical grounds, together with evidence of family involvement, and no specific laboratory tests are currently available. Because coexistent dyslipoproteinemia is sometimes present, affected patients and, if positive, their families should be screened in view of the association with accelerated cardiovascular disease.

VI.   DYSLIPOPROTEINEMIA, CORNEAL ARCUS, AND XANTHELASMA

Corneal arcus is a lipid-rich and predominantly extracellular deposit forming in the stroma of the peripheral cornea. Lipid can be demonstrated by light microscopy of suitably stained frozen sections (Fig. 5). Lipid is evident in the periphery of Bowman's layer and extracellularly in the adjacent stroma between and occasionally within the corneal fibroblasts, as well as extending into the deeper cornea to the periphery of Descemet's membrane. Lipid also accumulates in the adjacent sclera and often also in the ciliary processes and iris. The clear zone can also be shown to contain lipid, but the optical characteristics of this accumulation do not seem to favor opacification.

Corneal arcus characteristically appears first in the upper or lower segment. In time it may extend to a full circle; an outer clear zone is also characteristic. Corneal arcus can occur in young adults, but in Western Europe and North America it is common in old age. Several large studies have shown that accelerated development is a general feature of hyperlipoproteinemia, particularly excess of LDL, although it may arise in the absence of any overt disorder of lipoprotein metabolism [10,54,99,112,117]. Premature corneal arcus has also been associated with accelerated coronary heart disease, although this not a simple

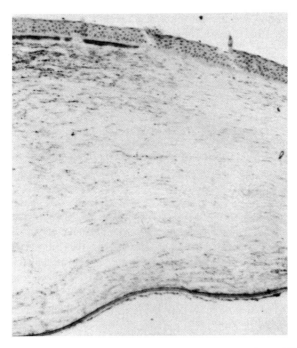

Figure 5 Corneal arcus is characterized histologically by extracellular subanophilic lipid deposits in the corneal stroma, particularly in Descemet's membrane and the periphery of Bowman's zone. (Oil red O, ×93) (Courtesy of Professor G. K. Klintworth.)

relationship [33,87]. Any contribution of additional variables, such as HDL or Lp(a), is not known. Further marked ethnic and individual variation, even within the severe genetic LDL excess syndromes, such as homozygous familial hypercholesterolemia [142], further confirms that factors other than the nature, extent, and duration of any associated dyslipoproteinemia are involved. The clear, general associations between corneal arcus, hyperlipidemia, and coronary heart disease are important in community policies for finding cases of lipemia but are less helpful in the management of the individual patient. Observer variation in the recognition and grading of corneal arcus is also considerable.

Studies within familial hypercholesterolemia have been informative in the context of the clinical associations of corneal arcus with LDL excess [10,54,117,142,143,144]. Homozygotes can develop arcus during early infancy, and arcus is common in heterozygotes by age 30 years, with an incidence in one large family of 100% [117]. In another study of over 200 unselected and predominantly unrelated heterozygotes, the mean age for both sexes at which arcus was detected in 50% of cases was 33 years [144]. The extent or rate of progression of arcus did not differentiate between those with and without clinical or electrocardiographic evidence of coronary heart disease in this high-risk group. The extent and progression of arcus was also strongly correlated with age rather than with the extent of LDL excess, which varied widely between the patients studied. This suggests that in markedly hyperbetalipoproteinemic individuals arcus formation is time dependent rather than dose dependent and that the relevant processes are saturated [143,144]. Unilateral arcus can arise in association with contralateral carotid artery stenosis, presumably as the reduced blood flow on the contralateral side restricts the processes leading to the accumulation of lipid within the cornea [44,124]. That insudation of lipoproteins at the corneoscleral limbus is a key element in these processes may be inferred from the altered pattern of arcus forming in the presence of anomalous vasculature at the corneoscleral limbus and by direct chemical analysis of the peripheral cornea. When intact human corneas with and without arcus obtained at postmortem are exposed to fluorescein-labeled antibody raised against human LDL (apo B), fluorescence is observed in the areas containing lipid deposits [136]. Apo B can be readily identified in peripheral corneas within 6 h of death, and the extent of reaction is unrelated to the presence or extent of corneal arcus [121]. The lipids present in human peripheral cornea with arcus involvement are of a more saturated pattern than those carried in plasma lipoprotein [21,134]; neither does the lipid-protein composition of saline extracts of peripheral cornea suggest a recent origin from plasma or a simple relationship with LDL [121]. The single major component extracted is of lower molecular weight and lipid-protein ratio than LDL and does not bind to glycosaminoglycans, and most preparations fail to react with antibody to apo B/LDL [121].

These clinical and laboratory studies on corneal arcus suggest that insudation of macromolecules at the corneoscleral limbus is a continuous process matched by clearance, some further process being required to build up a lipid-rich but not necessarily apo B- enriched arcus. Secondary processes are involved because the lipid present appears to originate from LDL, which has then been metabolized, with degradation of LDL apo B. Eyelid temperatures favor insudation at the upper and lower segments, and LDL-glycosaminoglycan interaction could trap LDL for modification as is proposed for other tissue deposits [76,128]. The peripheral cornea is enriched with dermatan sulfate [17], shown to interact with LDL in vitro, but specific corneal trapping effects are not described. Local lipid metabolism may also be involved, because although the deposits of corneal arcus are predominantly extracellular, their composition differs from that in plasma and LDL. A similar biochemical difference between plasma and cornea has also been detected with LCAT deficiency, compatible with as yet undefined metabolic activity in the cornea [149]. Resolution of corneal arcus on control of associated dyslipoproteinemia is described anecdotally in the human: the author has seen resolution in a heterozygote for familial hypercholesterolemia after 9 years of effective lipid-lowering therapy. Such regression may be impaired by the temperature gradient across the corneoscleral limbus as demonstrated by infrared thermography (Fig. 6). The accumulation of cholesterol esters becomes modified to include more long-chain saturated acyl residues, which are then trapped in an avascular area below their transition temperatures, as discussed for Tangier disease.

Xanthelasmata represent intracellular deposits of mixed lipids in which cholesterol esters predominate, forming superficially in the loose skin in and around the eyelids. They are a common feature of prolonged hyperlipoproteinemia, particularly when an element of hypertriglyceridemia and VLDL excess is also involved. In one series [43], 16 of 35 patients with xanthelasmata were hypercholesterolemic, with levels of cholesterol in plasma in excess of 7.8 mM (300 mg per 100 ml), and in a second series of heterozygotes for familial hypercholesterolemia, those with xanthelasmata had moderate but significant excess of plasma triglycerides and by implication of VLDL [142]. About 50% of subjects with xanthelasmata are broadly normolipemic, although detailed investigation may reveal some abnormalities of lipoproteins in the plasma, including reduced levels of HDL and some enrichment of LDL with triglycerides [139]. Modified triglyceride-rich lipoproteins may be particularly prone to cellular uptake by scavenger pathways of lipoprotein metabolism. Xanthelasmata can be regarded as one form of xanthomata, and as at other sites development may be accentuated by minor local trauma facilitating extravasation of lipoprotein [137], possibly here involving effects on periorbital skin vessels by frequent blinking and eye movements. Complete regression may be achieved by control of obese or lipemic subjects by diet or medication, particularly if the lesions have not been evident for more than a few months, after which partial regression with a darkening of color is more common. The rather variable relationship with patterns of lipoproteins in plasma suggests that local factors are important.

Previous studies on the lipid composition of various forms of xanthomata, including xanthelasmata, showed that in lesions present for a few months or less the lipid content closely resembles that in plasma, particularly that of any component in plasma present in excess [6,46,98]. With time, the composition of the accumulations progressively differs from that in plasma. Apoprotein is lost, much triglyceride and other lipid disappears, and the residue is enriched with cholesterol esters, also progressively modified to incorporate acyl residues, which are more saturated and of longer chain length than predominant components in plasma. Similar changes are involved in the natural history of corneal arcus, as discussed, and as with corneal arcus these changes and the relationship with local temperature may also contribute to the chronicity of established xanthelasmata. Studies of a mature xanthelasma by differential scanning calorimetry over the range 30–40°C are shown in Figure 7. This material, enriched with saturated cholesterol esters, manifests transition temperatures (lipid-phase transitions analogous to melting points) above local skin temperatures, suggesting that the physical form of this matured lipid is not compatible with remobilization [147].

Extensive animal studies on lipid accumulation in ocular tissues, including cornea, are not discussed in this chapter because lipoprotein systems differ markedly from those in the human and the results are difficult to interpret.

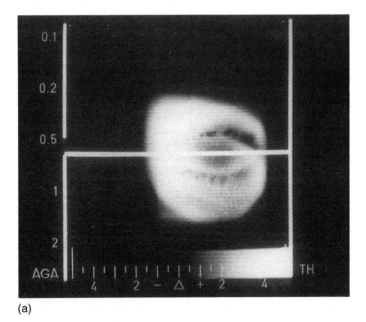

(a)

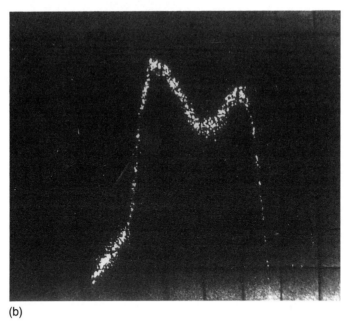

(b)

Figure 6   (a) Gray tone thermogram of the anterior surface of the eye. (b) Single-line temperature profile along the horizontal line shown in the upper part. The central trough corresponds to the relatively cool corneal center. (Reproduced with permission from A.R. Fielder, A.F. Winder, E.D. Cooke, and S.A. Bowcock. Arcus senilis and corneal temperature in man. In *The Cornea in Health and Disease*, VI Congress European Society for Ophthalmology, Royal Society of Medicine and Academic Press, London, pp. 1015–1020, 1981.

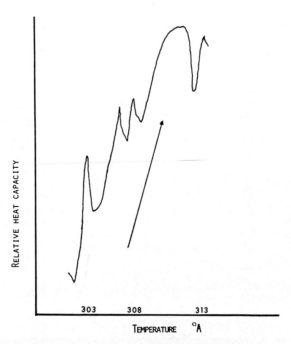

RELATIVE HEAT CAPACITY

303   308   313

TEMPERATURE   °A

Figure 7 Examination of xanthelasma material by differential scanning calorimetry, expressing change in enthalpy as a function of temperature in relative units. Measurements were in single-channel mode, and the baseline shift is shown. Peaks of deviation from this baseline trend indicate the midpoint temperature of phase changes occurring over the range 308–313K. (Reproduced with permission from A.F. Winder, K.R. Bruckdorfer, and A.R. Fielder. Thermal transition studies of a mature xanthelasma by differential scanning calorimetry. *Clin. Chim. Acta 151*:253–257, 1985.)

Corneal arcus and xanthelasma may also rarely present as minor features of two other rare human disorders of sterol metabolism associated with xanthomatosis, cerebrotendinous xanthomatosis and phytosterolemia [15]. Clinical and histological appearances can resemble those of familial hypercholesterolemia, but tissue deposits do not contain cholesterol and plasma levels are not in excess. Cerebrotendinous xanthomatosis can result in marked neurological features, and juvenile cataract formation is well recognized. Phytosterolemia has a more dermatological presentation.

REFERENCES

1. Albers, J.J., Chen, C.H., and Adolphson, J.L. Familial lecithin-cholesterol acyltransferase (LCAT) mass: Its relationship to LCAT activity and cholesterol esterification rate. *J. Lipid Res. 22*:1206–1213, 1981.
2. Allen, I.V., Swallow, M., Nevin, N.C., and McCormick, D. Clinico-pathological study of Refsum's disease with particular reference to fatal complications. *J. Neurol. Neurosurg. Psychiatr. 41*:323–332, 1978.
3. Assmann, G., von Eckardstein, A., and Funcke, H. Clinical, biochemical and genetic heterogeneity of lecithin:cholesterol acyltransferase syndromes. In *Disorders of HDL*, L.A. Carlson (Ed.), Smith-Gordon, London, pp. 169–175, 1990.
4. Assmann, G., von Eckardstein, A., and Funcke, H. Apoprotein A-I mutants and their significance for HDL metabolism. *J. Drug Dev. 3*(Suppl 1):57–62, 1990.
5. Assmann, G., Schmitz, G., and Brewer, H.B., Jr. Familial HDL deficiency: Tangier disease. In *The Metabolic Basis of Inherited Disease*, 6th ed., C.R. Scriver, A.L. Beaudet, W.S. Sly, and D. Valle (Eds.), McGraw-Hill, New York, pp. 1267–1282, 1989.
6. Baes, H., Van Gent, C.M., and Pries, C. Lipid composition of various types of xanthomata. *J. Invest. Dermatol. 51*:286–293, 1968.
7. Barchiesi, B.J., Eckel, R.H., and Ellis, P.P. The cornea and disorders of lipid metabolism. *Surv. Ophthalmol. 36*:1–22, 1991.

8. Bauer, E.A., Santa-Cruz, D.J., and Eisen, A.Z. Lipoid proteinosis: In vivo and in vitro evidence for a lysosomal storage defect. *J. Invest. Dermatol. 76*:119–125, 1981.

9. Beaumont, J.L., Carlson, L.A., Cooper, G.R., Fejfar, Z., Fredrickson, D.S., and Strasser, T. Classification of hyperlipidaemias and hyperlipoproteinaemias. *Bull. WHO 43*:891–915, 1970.

10. Beaumont, V., Jacotot, B., and Beaumont, J-L. Ischaemic disease in men and women with familial hypercholesterolaemia and xanthomatosis. *Atherosclerosis 24*:441–450, 1976.

11. Bennett, M.J., Gillis, W.S., Hosking, G.P., Galloway, J.H., and Cartwright, I.J. Lipid abnormalities in serum in Batten's disease. *Dev. Med. Child Neurol. 28*:814–823, 1986.

12. Bethell, W., McCulloch, C., and Ghosh, M. Lecithin:cholesterol acyltransferase deficiency: Light and electron microscopic findings from two corneas. *Can. J. Ophthalmol. 10*:494–501, 1975.

13. Bieri, J.G., Hoeg, J.M., Schaefer, E.J., Zech, L.A., and Brewer, H.B. Vitamin A and vitamin E replacement in abetalipoproteinaemia. *Ann. Inter. Med. 100*:238–239, 1984.

14. Billings, J.J., O'Callaghan, J., and O'Day, J. Refsum's syndrome: Heredopathia atactica polyneuritiformis. *Trans. Ophthalmol. Soc. Aust. 17*:131–136, 1957.

15. Bjorkem, I., and Skrede, S. Familial disorders of sterols other than cholesterol: Cerebrotendinous xanthomatosis and phytosterolemia. In *The Metabolic Basis of Inherited Disease*, 6th ed., C.R. Scriver, A.L. Beaudet, W.S. Sly, and D. Valle (Eds.), McGraw-Hill, New York, pp. 1283–1302, 1989.

16. Blum, C.B., Deckelbaum, R.J., Witte, L.D., Tall, A.R., and Cornicelli, J. Role of apolipoprotein E-containing lipoproteins in abetalipoproteinemia. *J. Clin. Invest. 70*:1157–1169, 1982.

17. Borcherding, M.S., Blacic, L.J., Sittig, R.A., Bizzell, J.W., Breen, M., and Weinstein, H.G. Proteoglycans and collagen fibre organisation in human corneoscleral tissue. *Exp. Eye Res. 21*:59–70, 1975.

18. Borysiewicz, L.K., Soutar, A.K., Evans, D.J., Thompson, G.R., and Rees, A.J. Renal failure in familial lecithin:cholesterol acyltransferase deficiency. *Q. J. Med. 204*:411–426, 1982.

19. Botermans, C.H. Primary pigmentary retinal degeneration and its association with neurological disease. In *Handbook of Clinical Neurology*, Vol. 13, *Neuroretinal Degenerations*, H.J. Vincken and G.W. Bruyn (Eds.), North Holland, Amsterdam, pp. 148–399, 1975.

20. Breslow, J.L. Apoprotein genetic variation in human disease. *Physiol. Rev. 68*:85–132, 1988.

21. Broeckhuyse, R.M. Lipids in tissues of the eye 14 (corneoscleral lipids during ageing and in arcus senilis). *Doc. Ophthalmol. 7*:313–322, 1976.

22. Bron, A.J. Dyslipoproteinaemias and their ocular manifestations. *Birth Defects 12*:257–270,1976.

23. Bron, A.J., Tripathi, R.C., Winder, A.F., Fosbrooke, A.S., and Lloyd, J.K. Familial LCAT deficiency disease. *XXII Concilium Ophthalmologicum*, Vol. 2, Masson, Paris, pp. 864–871, 1974.

24. Bron, A.J., Williams, H.P., and Carruthers, M.E. Hereditary crystalline stromal dystrophy of Schnyder I. Clinical features of a family with hyperlipoproteinaemia. *Br. J. Ophthalmol. 56*:383–399, 1972.

25. Brown, M.L., Inazu, A., Hesler, C.B., Agellon, L.B., Mann, C., Whitlock, M.E., Marcel, Y.L., Milne, R.W., Koizumi, J., Mabuchi, H., Takeda, R., and Tall, A.R. Molecular basis of lipid transfer protein deficiency in a family with increased high-density lipoproteins. *Nature 342*:448–451, 1989.

26. Brown, M.S., and Goldstein, J.L. A receptor-mediated pathway for cholesterol homoeostasis. *Science 232*:34–62, 1986.

27. Burns, R.P., Connor, W., and Gibson, I. Cholesterol turnover in hereditary crystalline corneal dystrophy of Schnyder. *Trans. Am. Ophthalmol. Soc. 76*:184–196, 1978.

28. Cammermeyer, J. Refsum's disease, neuropathological aspects. In *Handbook of Clinical Neurology*, Vol. 21, Part 1, *Systemic Disorders and Atrophies*, H.J. Vincken and G.W. Bruyn (Eds.), North Holland, Amsterdam, pp. 231–261, 1975.

29. Carlson, L.A. Fish-eye disease: A new familial condition with massive corneal opacities and dyslipoproteinaemia. *Eur. J. Clin. Lab. Invest. 12*:41–53, 1982.

30. Carr, R.E. Abetalipoproteinemia and the eye. *Birth Defects 12*:385–399, 1976.

31. Cenedella, R.J. Lipoproteins and lipids in cow and human aqueous humor. *Biochim. Biophys. Acta 793*:448–454, 1984.

32. Collins, D.R., Knott, T.J., Pease, R.J., Powell, L.M., Wallis, S.C., Robertson, S., Pullinger, C.R., Milne, R.W., Marcel, Y.L., Humphries, S., Talmud, P.J., Lloyd, J.K., Miller, N.E., Muller, D., and Scott, J. Truncated variants of apolipoprotein B cause hypobetalipoproteinaemia. *Nucleic Acids Res. 16*:8361–8375, 1988.

33. Cooke, N.T. Significance of arcus senilis in caucasians. *J. R. Soc. Med. 74*:1322–1324, 1981.

34. Cooper, R.A., Durocher, J.R., and Leslie, M.H. Decreased fluidity of red cell membrane lipids in abetalipoproteinaemia. *J. Clin. Invest. 60*:115–121, 1977.

35. Cooper, R.A., and Gulbrandsen, C.L. The relationship between serum lipoproteins and red cell membranes in abetalipoproteinaemia: Deficiency of lecithin:cholesterol acyltransferase. *J. Lab. Clin. Med. 78*:323–335, 1971.

36. Cumings, J.N. Inborn errors of metabolism in neurology (Wilson's disease, Refsum's disease and lipodoses). *Proc. R. Soc. Med. 64*:313–322, 1971.

37. Davis, G.J., Porter, R.S., Steiner, J.W., and Small, D.M. Thermal transitions of cholesterol esters of cholesterol esters of C18 aliphatic acids. *Mol. Crystals Liquid Crystals 10*:331–336, 1970.

38. Delleman, J.W., and Winkelman, J.E. Degeneratio corneae crystallinea hereditaria: A clinical, genetical and histological study. *Ophthalmologica 155*:409–426, 1968.
39. Dodge, J.T., Cohen, G., Kayden, H.J., and Phillips, G.P. Peroxidative haemolysis of red blood cells from patients with abetalipoproteinaemia (acanthocytosis). *J. Clin. Invest. 46*:357–368, 1967.
40. Dodson, P.M., Galton, D.J., and Winder, A.F. Retinal vascular abnormalities in the hyperlipidaemias. *Trans. Ophthalmol. Soc. UK 101*:17–21, 1981.
41. Dullart, A.P.F., Speelberg, B., Schuurman, H-J., Milne, R.W., Havekes, L.M., Marcel, Y.L., Geuze, H.J., Hulshof, M.M., and Erkelens, D.W. Epitopes of apolipoprotein B-100 and B-48 in both liver and intestine: Expression and evidence for local synthesis in recessive abetalipoproteinemia. *J. Clin. Invest. 78*:1397–1404, 1986.
42. Eisenberg, S. High density lipoprotein metabolism. *J. Lipid Res. 25*:1017–1058, 1984.
43. Epstein, M., Rosenmann, R.H., and Gofman, J.W. Serum lipids and cholesterol metabolism in xanthelasmata. *Arch. Dermatol. Syphilol. 65*:70–81, 1952.
44. Fielder, A.R., Winder, A.F., Cooke, E.D., and Bowcock, S.A. Arcus senilis and corneal temperature in man. In *The Cornea in Health and Disease*, VI Congress European Society for Ophthalmology, Royal Society of Medicine and Academic Press, London, pp. 1015–1020, 1981.
45. Fleischmajer, R., Krieg, T., Dziadek, M., Altchek, D., and Timpl, R. Ultrastructure and composition of connective tissue in hyalinosis cutis et mucosae skin. *J. Invest. Dermatol. 82*:252–258, 1984.
46. Fletcher, R.F. Lipid composition of xanthomas of different types. *Nutr. Metab. 15*:97–106, 1973.
47. Francois, J. Ocular manifestations of inborn errors of carbohydrate and lipid metabolism. V. Primary hyperlipoproteinaemias (hyperlipidaemias). *Bibl. Ophthalmol. 84*:150–159, 1975.
48. Francois, J., Bacskulin, J., and Follmann, P. Manifestations oculaires du syndrome d'Urbach-Wiethe. Hyalinosis cutis et mucosae. *Ophthalmologica 155*:433–448, 1968.
49. Fredrickson, D.S. Hereditary diseases of metabolism that affect the eye. In *The Eye and Systemic Disease*, F.A. Mausolt (Ed.), C.V. Mosby, St. Louis, pp. 8–33, 1975.
50. Frohlich, J., Fong, B., Julien, P., Despres, J-P., Angel, A., Hayden, M., McLeod, R., Chow, C., Davison, R.H., and Pritchard, H. Interaction of high-density lipoprotein with adipocytes in a new patient with Tangier disease. *Clin. Invest. Med. 10*:377–382, 1987.
51. Frohlich, J., Hoag, G., McLeod, R., Hayden, M., Godin, D.V., Wadsworth, L.D., Critchley, J.D., and Pritchard, P.H. Hypoalphalipoproteinaemia resembling fish-eye disease. *Acta Med. Scand. 221*:291–298, 1987.
52. Frohlich, J., McLeod, R., Pritchard, P.H., Fesmire, J., and McConathy, W. Plasma lipoprotein abnormalities in heterozygotes for familial lecithin:cholesterol acyltransferase deficiency. *Metabolism 37*:3–8, 1988.
53. Fruchart, J.-C., and Shepherd, J. (Eds.). *Human Plasma Lipoproteins*, de Gruyter, Berlin, pp. 1–398, 1989.
54. Gagne, C., Moorjani, S., Brun, D., Toussaint, M., and Lupien, P-J. Heterozygous familial hypercholesterolemia: Relationship between plasma lipids, lipoproteins, clinical manifestations and ischaemic heart disease in men and women. *Atherosclerosis 34*:13–24, 1979.
55. Garner, A., and Tripathi, R.C. Hereditary crystalline stromal dystrophy of Schnyder. II. Histopathology and ultrastructure. *Br. J. Ophthalmol. 56*:400–408, 1971.
56. Ghosh, M., and McCulloch, C. Crystalline dystrophy of the cornea: A light and electron microscopic study. *Can. J. Ophthalmol. 12*:321–329, 1977.
57. Gibberd, F.B., Page, N.G.R., Billimoria, J.D., and Retsas, S. Heredopathia atactica polyneuritiformis (Refsum's disease) treated by diet and plasma exchange. *Lancet 1*:575–578,1979.
58. Gjone, E., Blomhoff, J.P., and Skarbovic, A.J. Possible association between an abnormal low-density lipoprotein and nephropathy in lecithin:cholesterol acyltransferase deficiency. *Clin. Chim. Acta 54*:11–18, 1974.
59. Glickman, R.M., Green, P.H.R., Lees, R.S., Lux, S.E., and Kilgore, A. Immunofluorescence studies of apolipoprotein B in intestinal mucosa: Absence in abetalipoproteinemia. *Gastroenterology 76*:288–292, 1979.
60. Glueck, C.J., Gartside, P., Fallat, R.W., Sielski, J., and Steiner, P.M. Longevity syndromes: Familial hypobeta- and familial hyperalpha-lipoproteinemia. *J. Lab. Clin. Med. 88*:941–957, 1976.
61. Glueck, C.J., Mellies, M.J., Tsang, R.C., Steiner, P.M., and Stein, E.A. Neonatal hypobetalipoproteinemia. *Pediatr. Res. 12*:655–668, 1978.
62. Godin, D.V., Gray, G.R., and Frohlich, J. Erythrocyte membrane alterations in lecithin:cholesterol acyltransferase activity. *Scand. J. Clin. Lab. Invest. 38*(Suppl. 150):162–167, 1978.
63. Goldstein, J.L., and Brown, M.S. Familial hypercholesterolaemia. In *The Metabolic Basis of Inherited Disease*, 6th ed., C.R. Scriver, A.L. Beaudet, W.S. Sly, and D. Valle (Eds.), McGraw-Hill, New York, pp. 1215–1250, 1989.
64. Goldstein, J.L., and Brown, M.S. Regulation of the mevalonate pathway. *Nature 343*:425–433, 1990.
65. Gouras, P., Carr, R.E., and Gunkel, R.D. Retinitis pigmentosa in abetalipoproteinemia: Effects of vitamin A. *Invest. Ophthalmol. 10*:784–793, 1971.
66. Green, P.H.R., Lefkowitch, J.H., Glickman, R.M., Riley, J.W., Quinet, E., and Blum, C.B. Apolipoprotein localization and quantitation in the human intestine. *Gastroenterology 83*:1223–1230, 1982.
67. Gustafson, A., McConathy, W.J., Alaupovic, P., Curry, M.D., and Persson, B. Identification of lipoprotein families in a variant of human plasma apolipoprotein A deficiency. *Scand. J. Clin. Lab. Invest. 39*:377–387, 1979.

68. Hansen, E., Bachen, N.I., and Flage, T. Refsum's disease: Eye manifestations in a patient treated with a low phytol low phytanic acid diet. *Acta Ophthalmol. (Copenh.) 57*:899–913, 1979.

69. Harper, J.I., Duance, V.C., Sims, T.J., and Light, N.D. Lipoid proteinosis: An inherited disorder of collagen metabolism? *Br. J. Dermatol. 113*:145–151, 1985.

70. Hausser, I., Blitz, S., Rauterberg, E., Frosch, P.J., and Anton-Lamprecht, I. Hyalinosis cutis et mucosae (Morbus Urbach-Wiethe). Ultrastrukturelle und immunologische Merkmale. *Hautarzt 42*:28–33, 1991.

71. Herbert, P.N., Forte, T., Heinen, R.J., and Fredrickson, D.S. Tangier disease: One explanation of lipid storage. *N. Engl. J. Med. 299*:519–521, 1978.

72. Holmquist, L., Hamsten, A., and Dahlen, G.H. Free apolipoprotein (a) in abetalipoproteinaemia. *J. Intern. Med. 225*:285–286, 1989.

73. Horven, I., Gjone, E., and Egge, K. Ocular manifestations in familial LCAT deficiency. *Birth Defects 12*:271–278, 1976.

74. Huang, L.-S., Ripps, M.E., Korman, S.H., Deckelbaum, R.J., and Breslow, J.L. Hypobetalipoproteinemia due to an apolipoprotein B gene exon 21 deletion derived by Alu-Alu combination. *J. Biol. Chem. 264*:11394–11400, 1989.

75. Illingworth, D.R., Connor, W.E., and Miller, R.G. Abetalipoproteinemia: Report of two cases and review of therapy. *Arch. Neurol. 37*:659–662, 1980.

76. Iverius, P.H. The interaction between human plasma lipoproteins and connective tissue glycosaminoglycans. *J. Biol. Chem. 247*:2607–2613, 1972.

77. Jensen, A.D., Khodadoust, A.A., and Emery, J.M. Lipid proteinosis: Report of a case with electron microscopic findings. *Arch. Ophthalmol. 88*:273–277, 1972.

78. Kane, J.P., and Havel, R.J. Disorders of the biogenesis and secretion of lipoproteins containing the B apolipoproteins. In *The Metabolic Basis of Inherited Disease*, 6th ed., C.R. Scriver, A.L. Beaudet, W.S. Sly, and D. Valle (Eds.), McGraw-Hill, New York, pp. 1139–1164, 1989.

79. Kihara, S., Matsuzawa, Y., Kubo, M., Nozaki, S., Funahashi, T., Yamashita, S., Shuo, N., and Tarui, T. Autoimmune hyperchylomicronemia. *N. Engl. J. Med. 320*:1255–1259, 1989.

80. Koizumi, J., Mabuchi, H., Yoshimura, A., Michishita, I., Takeda, D.M., Itoh, H., Sakai, Y., Sakai, T., Ueda, K., and Takeda, R. Deficiency of serum cholesteryl-ester transfer activity in patients with familial hyperalpha-lipoproteinemia. *Atherosclerosis 58*:175–186, 1985.

81. Kott, E., Delpre, G., Kadish, U., Dziatelovsky, M., and Sandbank, U. Abetalipoproteinemia (Batten-Kornzweig syndrome). *Acta Neuropathol. (Berl.) 37*:255–258, 1977.

82. Kurasawa, T., Yokohama, S., Miyake, Y., Yamamura, T., and Yamamoto, A. Rate of cholesterol ester transfer between high and low density lipoproteins in human serum and a case with decreased transfer rate in association with hyperalphalipoproteinemia. *J. Biochem. 98*:1499–1508, 1985.

83. Kuusi, T., Ehnholm, C.E., Viikari, J., Harkonen, R., Vartiainen, E., Puska, P., and Taskinen, M-R. Postheparin plasma lipoprotein and hepatic lipase are determinants of hypo- and hyperalphalipoproteinemia. *J. Lipid. Res. 30*:1117–1126, 1989.

84. Lackner, K.J., Monge, J.C., Gregg, R.E., Hoeg, J.M., Triche, T.J., Law, S.W., and Brewer, H.B., Jr. Analysis of the apolipoprotein B gene and messenger ribonucleic acid in abetalipoproteinemia. *J. Clin. Invest. 78*:1707–1712, 1986.

85. Lazarow, P.W., and Moser, H.W. Disorders of peroxisosome biogenesis. In *The Metabolic Basis of Inherited Disease*, 6th ed., C.R. Scriver, A.L. Beaudet, W.S. Sly, and D. Valle (Eds.), McGraw-Hill, New York, pp. 1479–1509, 1989.

86. Liscum, L., Ruggiero, R.M., and Faust, J.R. The intracellular transport of low-density lipoprotein-derived cholesterol is defective in Niemann-Pick type C fibroblasts. *J. Cell. Biol. 108*:1625–1636, 1989.

87. Macaraeg, P.V.J., Lasagna, L., and Snyder, B. Arcus not so senilis. *Ann. Intern. Med. 68*:345–354, 1968.

88. MacGilchrist, A.J., Mills, P.R., Noble, M., Foulds, W.S., Simpson, J.A., and Watkinson, G. Abetalipoproteinaemia in adults: Role of vitamin therapy. *J. Inherited Metab. Dis. 11*:184–190, 1988.

89. Maggio, B., Diplock, A.T., and Lucy, J.A. Interaction of tocopherols and ubiquinone with monolayers of phospholipids. *Biochem. J. 161*:111–121, 1977.

90. Malloy, M.J., and Kane, J.P. Hypolipidemia. *Med. Clin. North Am. 66*:469–484, 1982.

91. Moy, L.S., Moy, R.L., Matsuoka, L.Y., Ohta, A., and Uitto, J. Lipoid proteinosis: Ultrastructural and biochemical studies. *J. Am. Acad. Dermatol. 16*:1193–1201, 1987.

92. Muller, D.P.R., Lloyd, J.K., and Bird, A.C. Long-term management of abetalipoproteinaemia: Possible role for vitamin E. *Arch. Dis. Child. 52*:209–214, 1977.

93. Naito, C., Teramoto, T., Kato, H., Watanabe, T., Yamanaka, T., and Iwamoto, A. Lipid composition of plasma major lipoproteins and lipoprotein lipase activity in hypolipidemic and hyperlipidemic siblings with familial LCAT deficiency. *Scand. J. Clin. Lab. Invest. 38*(Suppl. 150):168–176, 1978.

94. Newton, F.H., Rosenberg, R.N., Lampert, P.W., and O'Brien, J.S. Neurological involvement in Urbach-Wiethe's disease (lipoid proteinosis): A clinical, ultrastructural, and chemical study. *Neurology 21*:1205–1213, 1971.

95. Norum, K.R., Gjone, E., and Glomset, J.A. Familial lecithin:cholesterol acyltransferase deficiency, including

fish-eye disease. In *The Metabolic Basis of Inherited Disease*, 6th ed., C.R. Scriver, A.L. Beaudet, W.S. Sly, and D. Valle (Eds.), McGraw-Hill, New York, pp. 1181–1194, 1989.

96. Olsen, D.R., Chu, M.L., and Uitto, J. Expression of basement zone genes coding for type IV procollagen and laminin by human skin fibroblasts in vitro: Elevated alpha 1(IV) collagen mRNA levels in lipoid proteinosis. *J. Invest. Dermatol. 900*:734–738, 1988.

97. Oram, J.F. Cholesterol trafficking in cells. *Curr. Opin. Lipidol. 1*:416–421, 1990.

98. Parker, F., and Short, F.M. Xanthomatosis associated with hyperlipoproteinaemia. *J. Invest. Dermatol. 55*:71–88, 1970.

99. Parwaresch, M.R., Haacke, H., Mader, C.H., and Godt, C.H. Arcus lipoides corneae und hyperlipoproteinaemia. *Klin. Wochenschr. 54*:495–497, 1976.

100. Philipson, B.T. Fish-eye disease. *Birth Defects 18*:441–448, 1982.

101. Poll-The, B.T., Saudubray, J.M., Rocchiccioli, F., Scotto, J., Roels, F. Boue, J., Ogier, H., Dumez, Y., Wanders, R.J.A., Schutgens, R.B.H., Schram, A.W., and Tager, J.M. Prenatal diagnosis and confirmation of infantile Refsum's disease. *J. Inherited Metab. Dis. 10*(Suppl. 2):229–232, 1987.

102. Poulos, A., Pollard, A.C., Mitchell, J.D., Wise, G., and Mortimer, G. Patterns of Refsum's disease: Phytanic acid oxidase deficiency. *Arch. Dis. Child. 59*:222–229, 1984.

103. Poulos, A., Van Crugten, C., Sharp, P., Carey, W.F., Robertson, E., Becroft, D.M.O., Saudubray, J.M., Poll-The, B.T., Christensen, E., and Brandt, N. Prenatal diagnosis of Zellweger syndrome and related disorders: Impaired degradation of phytanic acid. *Eur. J. Paediatr. 145*:507–510, 1986.

104. Pressly, T.A., Scott, W.J., Ide, C.H., Winkler, A. and Reams, G.P. Ocular complications of Tangier disease. *Am. J. Med. 83*:991–994, 1978.

105. Puchois, P., Kandoussi, A., Fievet, P., Fourrier, J.L., Bertrand, M., Koren, E., and Fruchart, J.C. Apoprotein A-I-containing lipoproteins in coronary artery disease. *Atherosclerosis 68*:35–40, 1987.

106. Refsum, S. Heredopathia atactica polyneuritiformis: Phytanic acid storage disease (Refsum's disease). In *Handbook of Clinical Neurology*, Vol. 21, Part 1, *Systemic Disorders and Atrophies*, H.J. Vincken and G.W. Bruyn (Eds.), North Holland, Amsterdam, pp. 181–229, 1975.

107. Reichl, R., and Miller, N.E. Pathophysiology of reverse cholesterol transport: Insights from disorders of lipoprotein metabolism. *Arteriosclerosis 9*:785–797, 1989.

108. Robenek, H., and Schmitz, G. Abnormal processing of Golgi elements and lysosomes in Tangier disease. *Arteriosclerosis Thrombosis 11*:1007–1020, 1991.

109. Robison, W.G., Jr., Kuwabara, T., and Bieri, J.G. Deficiencies of vitamins E and A in the rat: Retinal damage and lipofuscin accumulation. *Invest. Ophthalmol. Vis. Sci. 19*:1030–1037, 1980.

110. Rodrigues, M.M., Kruth, H.S., Krachmer, J.H., and Willis, R.M. Unesterified cholesterol in Schnyder's corneal crystalline dystrophy. *Am. J. Ophthalmol. 104*:157–163, 1987.

111. Rodrigues, M.M., Kruth, H.S., Krachmer, J.H., Vrabek, M.P., and Blanchette-Mackie, J. Cholesterol localization in ultrathin frozen sections in Schnyder's corneal crystalline dystrophy. *Am. J. Ophthalmol. 110*:513–517, 1990.

112. Rosenman, R.H., Brand, R.J., Scholtz, M.S., and Jenkins, C.D. Relation of corneal arcus to cardiovascular risk factors and the incidence of coronary disease. *N. Engl. J. Med. 291*:1322–1324, 1974.

113. Runge, P., Muller, D.P.R., McAllister, J., Calver, D., Lloyd, J.K., and Taylor, D. Oral vitamin E supplements can prevent the retinopathy of abetalipoproteinaemia. *Br. J. Ophthalmol. 70*:166–173, 1986.

114. von Sallman, L., Gelderman, L.H., and Laster, L. Ocular histopathologic changes in a case of abetalipoproteinemia (Bassen-Kornzweig syndrome). *Doc. Ophthalmol. 26*:451–460, 1969.

115. Schaefer, E.J. Clinical, biochemical and genetic features in familial disorders of high density lipoprotein deficiency. *Arteriosclerosis 4*:303–312, 1984.

116. Schmitz, G., Fischer, H., Beuck, M., Hoecker, K-P., and Robenek, H. Dysregulation of lipid metabolism in Tangier monocyte-derived macrophages. *Arteriosclerosis 10*:1010–1019, 1990.

117. Schrott, A.G., Goldstein, J.L., Hazzard, W.R., McGoodwin, M.M., and Motulsky, A.G. Familial hypercholesterolemia in a large kindred: Evidence for a monogenic mechanism. *Ann. Intern. Med. 76*:711–720, 1972.

118. Scriver, C.R., Beaudet, A.L., Sly, W.S., and Valle, D. (Eds.). Lipoprotein and lipid metabolism disorders. In *The Metabolic Basis of Inherited Disease*, 6th ed., McGraw-Hill, New York, pp. 1129–1302, 1989.

119. Sedan, J., and Valles, A. Crystaux de cholesterol dans la cornee. *Bull. Soc. Fr. Ophtalmol. 59*:127–136, 1946.

120. Sharp, P., Johnson, D., and Poulos, A. Molecular species of phosphatidylcholine containing very long chain fatty acids in human brain: Enrichment in X-linked adrenoleukodystrophy brain and diseases of peroxisome biogenesis brain. *J. Neurochem. 56*:30–37, 1991.

121. Sheraidah, G.A., Winder, A.F., and Fielder, A.R. Lipid-protein constituents of human corneal arcus. *Atherosclerosis 40*:91–98, 1981.

122. Shore, R.N., Howard, B.V., Howard, W.J., and Shelley, W.B. Lipoid proteinosis. Demonstration of normal lipid metabolism in cultured cells. *Arch. Dermatol. 110*:591–594, 1974.

123. Small, D.M., Progression and regression of atherosclerotic lesions. Insights from lipid physical biochemistry. *Arteriosclerosis 8*:103–129, 1988.

124. Smith, J.L., and Susac, J.O. Unilateral corneal arcus senilis: Sign of occlusive disease of the carotid artery. *JAMA 226*:676–677, 1973.

125. Sniderman, A.D., Shapiro, S., Marpole, D., Skinner, B., Teng, B., and Kwiterovich, P.O. Association of coronary atherosclerosis with hyperapobetalipoprotienaemia (increased protein but normal cholesterol levels in human plasma low-density beta lipoprotein). *Proc. Natl. Acad. Sci. USA 77*:604–608, 1980.

126. Spaeth, G.L. Ocular manifestations of the lipodoses. In *Retinal Disease in Children*, W. Tasman (Ed.), Harper and Row, New York, pp. 127–206, 1971.

127. Sparks, D.L., Frohlich, J., Lacko, A.G., and Pritchard, P.H. Relationship between cholesteryl ester transfer activity and high density lipoprotein composition in hyperlipidemic patients. *Atherosclerosis 77*:183–191, 1989.

128. Srinivasan, S.R., Dolan, P., Radhakrishnamurthy, B., Pargaonkar, P.S., and Berenson, B.S. Lipoprotein-acid mucopolysaccharide complexes of human atherosclerotic lesions. *Biochim. Biophys. Acta 388*:58–70, 1975.

129. Steinberg, D., Refsum's disease. In *The Metabolic Basis of Inherited Disease*, 6th ed., C.R. Scriver, A.L. Beaudet, W.S. Sly, and D. Valle (Eds.), McGraw-Hill, New York, pp. 1533–1550, 1989.

130. Steinberg, D., Parthasarathy, S., Carew, T.E., Khoo, J.C., and Witztum, J.L. Beyond cholesterol: Modifications of low-density lipoproteins that increase its atherogenicity. *N. Engl. J. Med. 320*:915–924, 1989.

131. Sysi, R. Xanthoma corneae as hereditary dystrophy. *Br. J. Ophthalmol. 34*:369–374, 1950.

132. Talmud, P.J., Lloyd, J.K., Muller, D.P.R., Collins, D.R., Scott, J., and Humphries, S. Genetic evidence from two families that the apolipoprotein gene is not involved in abetalipoproteinaemia. *J. Clin. Invest. 82*:1803–1806, 1988.

133. Toussaint, D. and Davis, P. An ocular pathological study of Refsum's syndrome. *Am. J. Ophthalmol. 72*:342–347, 1971.

134. Tschetter, R.T. Lipid analysis of the human cornea with and without arcus senilis. *Arch. Ophthalmol. 76*:403–405, 1966.

135. Utermann, G. The mysteries of lipoprotein (a). *Science 246*:904–910, 1989.

136. Walton, K.W. Studies on the pathogenesis of corneal arcus formation. 1. The human corneal arcus and its relation to atherosclerosis as studied by immunofluorescence. *J. Pathol. 111*:263–273, 1973.

137. Walton, K.W., Thomas, C., and Dunkerley, E. The pathogenesis of xanthomata. *J. Pathol. 109*:271–289, 1973.

138. Waring, G.O., Rodrigues, M.M., and Laibson, P.R. Corneal dystrophies. 1. Dystrophies of the epithelium, Bowman's layer and stroma. *Surv. Ophthalmol. 23*:71–122, 1978.

139. Watanabe, A., Yoshimuna, A., Wakasugi, E., Ryozo, T., Ueda, K., Ueda, R., Haba, T., Kametani,T., Koizumi, J., Ito, S., Ohta, M., Miyamoto, S., Mabuchi, H., and Takeda, R. Serum lipids, lipoproteins and coronary heart disease in patients with xanthelasma palpebrarum. *Atherosclerosis 38*:283–290, 1980.

140. Ways, P., Reed, C.F., and Hanahan, D.J. Red cell and plasma lipids in acanthocytosis. *J. Clin. Invest. 42*:1248–1260, 1963.

141. Weller, R.O., and Rodger, F.C. Crystalline stromal dystrophy: Histochemistry and ultrastructure of the cornea. *Br. J. Ophthalmol. 64*:46–52, 1980.

142. Winder, A.F. Factors influencing the variable expression of xanthelasmata and corneal arcus in familial hypercholesterolaemia. *Birth Defects 18*:449–462, 1982.

143. Winder, A.F. Relationship between arcus and hyperlipidaemia is clarified by studies in familial hypercholesterolaemia. *Br. J. Ophthalmol. 67*:789–794, 1983.

144. Winder, A.F. Corneal arcus and prognosis in familial hypercholesterolaemia. *Atherosclerosis 68*:273, 1987.

145. Winder, A.F., and Borysiewicz, L.K. Corneal opacification and familial disorders affecting plasma high-density lipoprotein. *Birth Defects 18*:433–440, 1982.

146. Winder, A.F., and Bron, A.J. Lecithin-cholesterol acyltransferase presenting as visual impairment, with hypocholesterolaemia and normal renal function. *Scand. J. Clin. Lab. Invest. 38*(Suppl. 150):151–155, 1978.

147. Winder, A.F., Bruckdorfer, K.R., and Fielder, A.R. Thermal transition studies of a mature xanthelasma by differential scanning calorimetry. *Clin. Chim. Acta 151*:253–257, 1985.

148. Winder, A., Frohlich, J., Garner, A., Johnston, D., Vallance, D., and Alexander, R. The cornea in familial high density lipoprotein deficiency, Tangier disease. *Atherosclerosis 90*:222, 1991.

149. Winder, A.F., Garner, A., Sheraidah, G.A., and Barry, P. Familial lecithin:cholesterol acyltransferase deficiency. Biochemistry of the cornea. *J. Lipid Res. 26*:283–287, 1985.

150. Wong, C.K., and Lin, C.S. Remarkable response of lipoid proteinosis to oral dimethyl sulphoxide. *Br. J. Dermatol. 119*:541–544, 1988.

151. Yee, R.D., Cogan, D.B., and Zee, D.S. Ophthalmoplegia and dissociated nystagmus in abetalipoproteinemia. *Arch. Ophthalmol. 94*:571–575, 1976.

152. Yee, R.D., Herbert, P.N., Bergsma, D.R., and Breimer, J.J. Atypical retinitis pigmentosa in familial hypobetalipoproteinemia. *Am. J. Ophthalmol. 82*:64–71, 1976.

153. Zilversmit, D.B. Lipid transfer proteins. *J. Lipid Res. 25*:1563–1569, 1984.

36
Dysthyroid Eye Disease

Brian S. F. Shine
Stoke Mandeville Hospital, Aylesbury, England

I. INTRODUCTION

Dysthyroid eye disease (or endocrine or thyroid ophthalmopathy) is a chronic condition, characterized by inflammation and increased volume of the retrobulbar orbital contents, particularly the extraocular muscles, with consequent proptosis, limitation of eye movements, periorbital swelling, and the potential for optic nerve compression. A recent survey by Char [20] lists more than 25 names associated with dysthyroid eye disease, including those associated with early detailed clinical descriptions, such as Caleb Parry (1825), Robert Graves (1835), and Carl von Basedow (1840) [88]. Current evidence points to dysthyroid eye disease as part of the spectrum of autoimmune thyroid disease: nearly all patients with ophthalmopathy have demonstrable thyroid abnormalities, and most patients with autoimmune Graves' thyroid disease have orbital abnormalities. The responsible antigen(s) are elusive, but the most likely candidate is a 64 kD protein, which may be fibroblast rather than muscle related. The humoral immune responses so far identified may be secondary to damage mediated by other mechanisms.

II. INCIDENCE AND PREVALENCE

Several surveys of normal blood donors have reported a prevalence of antithyroid antibodies of more than 10%, with females outnumbering males about 2:1 [17,107]. One survey in the United Kingdom revealed a history of thyroid disease in 19 of 1000 women and 1.6 of 1000 men [113]; another found an annual incidence of 35.5 women and 9.2 men in 100,000 inhabitants [9]. It is estimated that up to 15% of females and 5% of males develop a dysthyroid condition in their lifetimes. Of these, only about 2–5% develop clinically significant ophthalmopathy [61]. Although it is received wisdom that the ratio of males to females is lower in dysthyroid eye disease than in thyroid disease alone, a recent study reported similar ratios both in Graves' hyperthyroidism with and without ophthalmopathy and in ophthalmopathy with and without overt thyroid disease [126].

III. PATHOLOGY

Dysthyroid eye disease affects many orbital components, the most prominent changes occurring in the extraocular muscles. The normal extraocular musculature has a rich arterial blood supply, which breaches the connective tissue compartments of the orbit, and the venous drainage respects the fascial planes. The nerve supply to the muscles is also particularly rich, with more motor end plates than other muscles and larger numbers of spindles [18,19]. The affected muscles have a firm, rubbery, and variably reddish appearance, and there may be a sevenfold increase in volume [19]. Histologically, the most striking pathological feature in early disease is infiltration of the muscles by lymphocytes (Fig. 1) and an increase in interstitial glycosaminoglycans (GAG). The infiltrate is focal, with groups of cells around the muscle cells, particularly perivascularly, and little involvement of the orbital fat. Immunohistochemistry reveals that

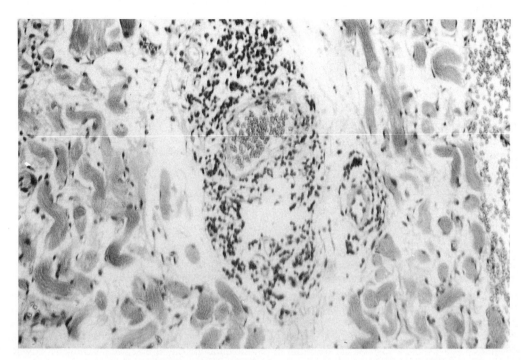

Figure 1   Section of extraocular muscle from a patient with dysthyroid eye disease, showing perivascular lymphocytic infiltration (Hematoxylin and eosin, × 100)

two-thirds of the infiltrating cells are T cells and one-third B cells, with scattered macrophages [108,119]. Some fibroblast proliferation occurs, with increased secretion of GAG into the intercellular matrix. GAG are hydrophilic and capable of 1000-fold increases in volume with increasing hydration [88,103]. HLA class II expression has been demonstrated by fibroblasts within the extraocular muscles and by endothelial cells [108,119]. Inflammation is followed by fibrosis, with destruction of the muscle structure.

IV.   CLINICAL FEATURES

A.   Ophthalmic Features

The most prominent ophthalmic features are exophthalmos, impairment of eye movements controlled by the extraocular muscles, eyelid retraction, surface irritation associated with lacrimation and photophobia, and optic nerve compression. The ophthalmopathy tends to run a waxing and waning course, typically becoming inactive after about 2 years, although active disease may persist for 5 years or more. Severe complications tend to occur within the first 6–9 months, and thus patients who do not have sight-threatening complications within this period are unlikely to experience permanent impairment of visual acuity, although residual strabismus and diplopia are common.

The most striking clinical feature is often proptosis, due to an increase in the volume of orbital contents, particularly the extraocular muscles, and the rigid nature of the orbit (Fig. 2). Although clinically significant proptosis is fairly rare (2–5% of patients with autoimmune thyroid disease), active autoimmune thyrotoxicosis is associated with a consistent increase in exophthalmometer readings [3] and abnormalities on ultrasonography [48], and computed tomographic scanning [57]. The proptosis is usually axial, with little deviation, and any lateral or medial displacement should lead to an intensive search for other causes. Proptosis is often associated with intermittent pain, which seems to be worse when the patient is anxious. An increase in orbital tension is usually demonstrable either by digital pressure or by mechanical measurement [39,58].

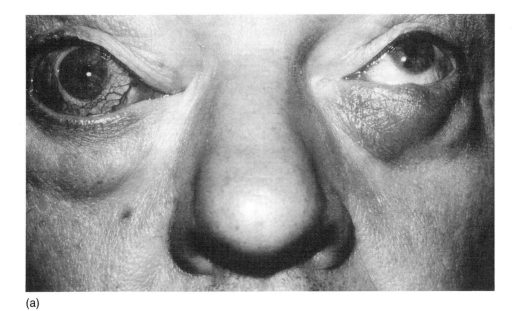

(a)

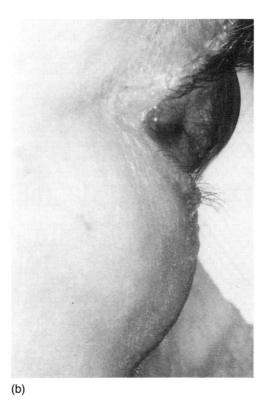

(b)

Figure 2 Ophthalmic features of dysthyroid eye disease, showing proptosis, almost complete absence of upward gaze on the right, hyperemia of the conjunctiva, dilated surface vessels laterally, and periorbital edema.

Bilateral proptosis is the rule, but may be unilateral in up to 15% of patients [126], with exophthalmometer readings differing by more than 2 mm [104]. This can cause diagnostic difficulties [87], although dysthyroid eye disease is the most common cause of unilateral proptosis [35,50,77]. Advances in radiological imaging techniques over the past decade have greatly improved diagnostic accuracy in proptosis [87].

The most commonly and earliest affected muscles are the inferior and medial recti [32,36,106], although any or all of the extraocular muscles may be affected. The inflammatory infiltration leads to an increase in the bulk of the muscles, demonstrable on computed tomography, ultrasonography, or magnetic resonance imaging (Fig. 3) [57,112]. Because of the initial increase in bulk and, later, fibrosis muscular control of eye movements is impaired. Tightness of the affected muscles leads to increased resistance to the action of opposing muscles, resulting in strabismus and diplopia (Fig. 2) [98,99].

Retraction of the upper and/or lower eyelids is another consistent feature [53,102]. Possible causes include sympathetic overactivity due to thyrotoxicosis (although retraction is often present in the absence of toxicosis), hypertrophy of the muscle fibers, inflammatory change with consequent fibrosis, and the mechanical effect of the proptosis [33,40,41]. Histological changes occur in the aponeurosis and in Müller's muscle [100,101]. Retraction may lead to reduced corneal and conjunctival cover, particularly when the patient is asleep. Corneal epithelial damage, demonstrable by stains, such as rose Bengal or fluorescein, may be followed by corneal ulceration and even endophthalmitis. Ptosis may also occur, leading to possible confusion over the diagnosis of dysthyroid eye disease.

Although poor cover may itself lead to increased lacrimation and damage to the front of the eye, the earliest symptoms are often surface irritation, photophobia, and lacrimation, especially on exposure to strong light, smoke, wind, or a dry atmosphere. The increased lacrimation may be a reaction to changes in the tear film secondary to decreased blink rate and widening of the palpebral fissure [47], and qualitative and quantitative changes in tear proteins have been detected [16,68,69]. Although obvious corneal damage is sometimes present, many patients lack obvious signs on examination. Superior limbic keratitis, seen as punctate staining with rose Bengal, is also common but by no means universal, and its presence does not correlate well with symptoms [35]. Other conjunctival signs include increased prominence of vessels and injection and inflammation of the insertion points of the rectus muscles (Fig. 2).

Periorbital changes include swelling of both upper and lower eyelids, with herniation of fat through the medial part of the aponeurosis of Müller's muscle and into the subcutaneous tissue (Fig. 2).

Optic neuropathy is the major vision-threatening complication. It may have a rapid onset [6] and is usually precipitated by increased pressure on the nerve from surrounding structures, especially at the orbital apex. Greatly increased extraocular muscle volume is usually seen on computer-assisted tomograms [10,31,32], and the orbital tension is greater than in noncompressive disease [38,39,58]. Optic neuropathy sometimes occurs without obvious involvement of the extraocular muscles [4,86]. The earliest sign is often reduction in color saturation, particularly for red targets, often with an increase in the physiological difference between the two eyes in color appreciation. This may be followed by a decrease in visual acuity, with a relative afferent pupillary reaction defect and reduced visual fields [46,129]. Less severe optic nerve compression may be relatively common, since computerized pattern reversal testing reveals a significant decrease in most patients with mild to moderate disease, even in the absence of clinical impairment [13,90]. This may mean that active treatment is indicated earlier and in a greater proportion of patients than has previously been appreciated. Occasionally optic neuropathy appears to be secondary to stretching of the optic nerve as a result of proptosis.

B. Thyroid Disease

Many patients have a history of autoimmune thyroid disease, and about 50% have clinically apparent thyroid disease at the time of diagnosis of dysthyroid eye disease. Thyrotoxicosis is very common, but approximately 5% have primary underactivity, probably due to Hashimoto's disease. Most patients with active autoimmune thyrotoxicosis have increased exophthalmometer readings, and ophthalmopathy commonly appears within 18 months of the thyroid condition [61,79,125], but they may be separated by many years. Dysthyroid eye disease may be precipitated by or worsen after radioactive iodine treatment of hyperthyroidism [11,65,114] but may regress following surgical thyroidectomy [80]. Gwinup's group was unable to show any difference between the progress of patients with different levels of thyroid function [51],

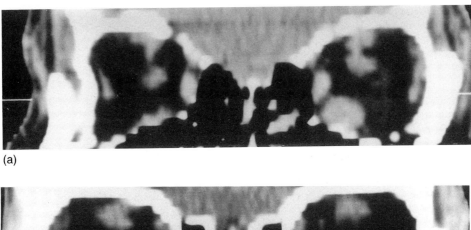

(a)

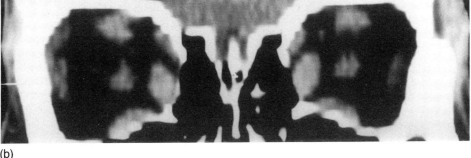

(b)

Figure 3   Orbital computed tomographic scans (coronal view) showing predominant increases in the bulk of (a) the left inferior rectus muscle and (b) both medial recti.

but DeGroot and colleagues [24] have reported that patients who required multiple doses of radioactive iodine had a greater tendency to develop eye disease.

V.   LABORATORY INVESTIGATIONS

The aims of investigation are to permit diagnosis, definition of the stage and prognosis of the disease, rational choice of therapy, and assessment of the likelihood of complications requiring intervention. To exclude an orbital tumor or pseudotumor, biopsy may be necessary in some patients in whom the diagnosis is not clear and in whom all other investigations are unhelpful. Unless the clinical differential diagnosis includes thyroid disease, the diagnosis may be missed even on biopsy because of the nonspecific nature of the infiltrate.

A.   Thyroid Function Tests

Tests of thyroid function are an essential part of the investigation, since approximately 50–60% of patients with dysthyroid eye disease have some abnormality of thyroid function. Thyrotropin is manufactured by the pituitary: its release is stimulated by the hypothalamic hormone, thyrotropin releasing hormone (TRH, or thyroliberin), and inhibited by triiodothyronine (T_3), which is produced by local conversion from tetraiodothyronine (T_4) in the pituitary cells. Thyrotropin causes both stimulation of the manufacture of T_4 and T_3 by the thyroid and release of the hormones into the peripheral circulation. In the circulation, both hormones are extensively (99.97% in the case of T_4 and 99.7% in the case of T_3) bound to binding proteins, principally thyroxine binding globulin (TBG). Although T_4 is present in much higher (about 30–50 times) concentrations than T_3, the latter is far more active metabolically, and the free T_4 levels are only 2–3 times those of T_3. Furthermore, most (approximately 80%) of the body's T_3 is produced by peripheral conversion from T_4 rather than in the thyroid.

Thyroid activity can be assessed by assaying total hormone levels (T_4 and T_3) or free hormone levels (free T_4 and free T_3) or by evaluating the control mechanisms through assay of thyrotropin. Total hormone levels are difficult to interpret in the presence of abnormal levels of the binding proteins, and there is a trend toward measurement of the free hormones, although technical problems have so far prevented these assays from being widely accepted as first-line tests. Thyrotropin levels are elevated in hypothyroidism of thyroid origin and suppressed in hyperthyroidism due to autonomous secretion (for example by an autonomous nodule) or autoimmune stimulation (classic Graves' disease). Because thyrotropin assays are efficient for diagnosing functional thyroid abnormalities, thyrotropin is often used as the first-line investigation for thyroid disease.

B. Thyroid Antibody Tests

Antibodies to several thyroid structures, including thyroglobulin, thyroid microsomes (thyroid perox-idase), and the thyrotropin receptor, have been detected in serum from most patients with dysthyroid eye disease. Thyroglobulin is the major protein of the thyroid, filling the thyroid colloid vesicles and acting as the reservoir for thyroid hormones previously manufactured inside the thyroid cells. Low levels of anti-thyroglobulin antibodies are present in most patients with thyroid disease. The active antigen in thyroid microsomes is thyroid peroxidase, the enzyme responsible for oxidation of iodide in the formation of iodothyronines [22,73,89]. Antimicrosomal antibodies are present in a higher proportion of patients with thyroid disease than are antithyroglobulin antibodies and seem to be a much more consistent marker for the disease. One or both of these antibodies is detectable in the serum of about 90% of patients with clinical dysthyroid eye disease [14,79,94]. The activity of the eye disease may be related to the levels of antithyroid antibodies [5].

Tests for antithyrotropin receptor antibodies can be classified [21,83] as either receptor binding assays, which measure thyrotropin binding inhibitory immunoglobulins (TBII; see, for instance, Refs. 42–44), or receptor stimulation assays, which measure thyroid stimulating immunoglobulins (TSI; see, for instance, Refs. 21 and 26), which show IgG subclass restriction [121]. Although some authors advocate the use of these assays in all patients with thyroid disease, they probably offer no advantage over clinical examination and thyroid function testing.

The interpretation of antibody tests requires caution, since antibodies are commonly detectable in apparently well subjects [17,107] and in up to 10% of pregnant women [127], even in the absence of other evidence of thyroid abnormalities.

VI. PATHOGENESIS: AUTOIMMUNITY

There is a strong consensus that dysthyroid eye disease is an autoimmune condition. Whether it is separate from autoimmune thyroid diseases or merely part of the spectrum of this group of conditions is not yet clear. The evidence for an autoimmune origin rests primarily upon its strong association with other autoimmune conditions, especially thyroid disease, diabetes mellitus, and myasthenia gravis. Approximately 5% of patients with myasthenia gravis develop Graves' disease, and about 0.2% of those with thyrotoxicosis develop myasthenia [45]. The conditions seem to have similar HLA and IgG heavy chain (Gm) associations and a strong familial tendency.

Any hypothesis proposing an autoimmune basis for thyroid eye disease must identify the antigens and explain the recognition of them and the mechanisms by which the immune response is mounted. The principles of autoimmune disease are reviewed elsewhere (see Chap. 3).

There are several candidates for the underlying antigen, including thyrotropin, thyroglobulin, and various cell surface proteins of the orbital muscles and/or fibroblasts. For nonorbital antigens, the possible mechanisms are preferential deposition of the antigen in the orbit (by mechanisms to be discussed) or cross-reaction with similar epitopes on different molecules.

The suggestion that thyrotropin or fragments of thyrotropin might be deposited in orbital tissue and lead to tissue changes [128] was stimulated by the largely anecdotal observation that hypothyroidism, which is associated with high circulating thyrotropin levels, may lead to a worsening of thyroid eye disease. Controlled clinical studies [51] do not support this impression, although as previously mentioned thyroid ophthalmopathy may be precipitated by or worsen following radioiodine treatment [11,65,114] and irradiation of the neck for Hodgkin's disease [60]. However, thyroid ophthalmopathy may improve after thyroidectomy [80], and it is thus possible that the worsening observed after radioiodine treatment is due to the immune response in which both B and T cell activation occur [2,111].

Another candidate antigen is thyroglobulin [75]. Antithyroglobulin antibodies are common in patients with thyroid disease, although levels tend to be higher in patients with Hashimoto's disease, which is not as strongly associated with thyroid ophthalmopathy as Graves' disease. The demonstration of amino acid sequence similarities between thyroglobulin and acetylcholinesterase makes a shared epitope a possibility [78] but does not explain the preferential involvement of the extraocular musculature. There are reports that monoclonal antibodies to thyroglobulin also cross-react with an orbital antigen [75]. Although the extraocular muscles have unique structural properties (reviewed in Refs. 61 and 88), no specific antigens have yet been demonstrated. The demonstration that thyroglobulin can travel by retrograde lymphatic spread from the neck to the orbit [74] has led to the proposal that this mechanism may underlie the pathogenesis of thyroid eye disease. Reports of thyroglobulin deposits in orbital tissue [72,84] have subsequently been denied [71]. Antithyroglobulin antibody levels do not correlate well with clinical signs [34], and levels of this antibody are usually much higher in Hashimoto's disease than in Graves' disease, although the latter is much more strongly associated with clinical eye disease.

Orbital muscle cell and fibroblast antigens have been extensively investigated. Three groups have reported finding specific antibodies to muscle and fibroblast cell membranes [29,66,70]. Kendall-Taylor's group has reported that antibodies to orbital antigens can be adsorbed by prior incubation with thyroid tissue [123], but these observations have not been confirmed by others [62,63,95]. The findings of Faryna and colleagues [29] have been both contradicted [97] and supported [8]. Some groups have used porcine muscle, and others have used human tissue, with consequent problems of cross-reaction with native immunoglobulins in the tissue, and this has led Wall's group to withdraw [82] its earlier claim [70]. Nevertheless, they have subsequently reported that positive antibodies on immunofluorescence correlate well with the clinical features of ophthalmopathy, although not with the titers of other antibodies [81]. An alternative to tissue immunofluorescence studies is to separate the proteins, as by sodium dodecyl sulfate–polyacrylamide gel electrophoresis, followed by immunoblotting to demonstrate antibodies to the antigens. Using this technique and human material, we have demonstrated serum antibodies to orbital antigens, but there was almost perfect correlation with antibody activity against skeletal muscle [120]. In immunoblotting studies, there was no apparent pattern in the antigens with which the antibodies reacted [120]. There have been claims of a specific 64 kD protein that reacts with antibodies in the serum of many patients with Graves' ophthalmopathy [110,130]. A 64 kD protein has been identified by other workers [1,123], but it was not considered the major autoantigen involved. It has been claimed [7] that the sera of Graves' disease patients contain antibodies to a 23 kD fibroblast protein with a much greater frequency than normal subjects. Wall et al. [115] propose that there is indeed a shared epitope between the thyroid and orbital tissue, with a molecular weight of 64 kD. This is an attractive hypothesis, which awaits confirmation by other groups. Recently, the presence of antibodies to a novel 64 kD protein serum from patients with Hashimoto's disease was reported. The protein was prepared from a cDNA library, and the mRNA coding for the protein has so far reportedly been identified only in thyroid and eye muscle cells, not in skeletal muscle [25].

Other antigens that have been considered possible triggers for the immune response include acetyl cholinesterase [109], α-galactosyl [27], and bacteria [14]. The possibility that antibodies are indeed responsible for the condition has been strengthened by the observation that plasmapheresis often causes a decrease in the activity of thyroid eye disease [15,23,49]. However, plasma exchange might remove some plasma factor other than antibodies, and there is at present no reliable report concerning the plasma fraction the removal of which is responsible for the improvement.

The mechanisms by which the immune response might be mounted have also been the subject of many studies. Although most of the reported studies of peripheral blood lymphocyte numbers and functions have been unilluminating, some interesting information has emerged from studies of the proportions of peripheral blood lymphocyte populations. One study [30] showed that patients with severe thyroid ophthalmopathy have an increase in the proportion of suppressor to cytotoxic CD8+ cells and that the proportion decreased following successful corticosteroid treatment. These patients also had an initial decrease in CD4/CD8 ratios. However, these results are difficult to interpret, since a preliminary statistical analysis was carried out and further tests were conducted only when a significant result was discovered. This may make the analysis faulty and calls into question the meaning of the results. In another recent study, increased activation of T cells was also reported [76]. Other cell-mediated immunity studies have included cell proliferation studies [120] and migration inhibition studies [85]. In our studies [120], we were unable to identify any unique reactivities.

An alternative mechanism proposed for cell damage is cell-mediated cytotoxicity. Wall's group has found evidence for this mechanism and has claimed that many antibodies identified by immunoblotting are capable of antibody-dependent cell-mediated cytotoxicity [54–56,130] rather than antibody-mediated complement-dependent cytotoxicity [116], with correlation between the degree of antibody-dependent cell-mediated cytotoxicity and clinical findings [54].

The principal suspected target of the immune response is the fibroblast. The evidence for this is based on examination of HLA class II (Ia) antigen expression, which is necessary for antigen recognition and presentation to the immune system (see Chap. 3). One mechanism by which autoimmunity may arise is the recognition of cell surface antigens by immune cells because of aberrant expression of Ia antigens, thus appearing to present antigen to T cells. Ia expression indeed occurs following viral infection and induction of interleukins and in thyroid eye disease [108,119]. In the last condition, expression seems to be confined to fibroblasts and some vascular endothelial cells [108,119]. If the fibroblast is the main target of the immune reaction, this may explain some of these findings: both monoclonal antibodies and sera of patients with Graves' ophthalmopathy are capable of stimulating proline uptake by fibroblasts [92,93], although these findings have not be reproduced by other investigators [109,124]; retrobulbar fibroblasts showed different responsiveness to thyroid and steroid hormones from dermal fibroblasts [103]; there is an increase in the urinary secretion of GAG in active thyroid ophthalmopathy, secretion decreasing with successful corticosteroid or radiotherapy treatment [64]. Interestingly, serum hyaluronic acid is not elevated [59]. Weetman [118] has proposed that the main actor is in fact the fibroblast and that stimulation to proliferation and production of collagen and other substances is mediated by cytokines derived from T cells and macrophages. An explanation of this type is attractive, although no antigenic differences between orbital and other fibroblasts have yet been discovered.

VII. GENETICS

Since there is an increased familial incidence of dysthyroid eye disease, with up to 50% concordance in monozygotic twins [28] and an association with other autoimmune diseases, it seems appropriate to pursue possible genetic markers. The well-characterized link between Graves' thyrotoxicosis and HLA-DR3 seems to hold for the thyroid ophthalmopathy. Frecker and colleagues have claimed a positive association between B8 and DR3 and thyroid eye disease in Hungarian patients and a protective effect of DR7 antigen and a further association with IgG heavy-chain (Gm) allotypes [37]. Cluster analysis of these data has revealed several groups of patients, with similar conclusions concerning the linkage with HLA antigens [91]. Some evidence of HLA-DR4 and HLA-DRw6 linkage has also been found in black patients in the United States, although the differences were not significant after correction for the number of comparisons [105]. These findings have not been confirmed in studies in the United Kingdom [67,117,122]. In our studies [122], DNA probes, rather than antibodies, were used to define the HLA genotypes of patients, and we were unable to show any association between HLA or Gm allotypes and dysthyroid eye disease. In the other study [67], only one of the many markers investigated, the P1 blood group, was significantly associated with dysthyroid eye disease. In this study, however, the quoted probability was not corrected for multiple comparisons, and our own unpublished P blood group data do not support the earlier conclusions. If the condition is really partly genetically determined, a more rewarding method of analysis may prove to be the investigation of markers within pedigrees, since this technique is far more powerful for detection of linkage than population studies. Unfortunately, the accumulation of enough data is likely to remain a problem for some time to come.

VIII. ENVIRONMENTAL INFLUENCES

If the evidence for genetic linkage is rather sketchy, a possible alternative is that the environment plays some part in the precipitation of the condition. Research on this aspect appears to have been neglected, and it is not possible to comment upon seasonality, activation by infection, or many other influences. Some study of antibodies to bacteria has been undertaken, but with inconclusive results [14].

Patients with thyroid ophthalmopathy commonly relate the onset or worsening of the condition to some traumatic event. It is tempting to ascribe some significance to this, but the same has been observed for many conditions, and there seems to be no reliable way of investigating this aspect. It is the author's personal observation, however, that the activity of the ophthalmopathy is influenced by the mood and general situation of the patient. However, an alternative explanation is that active disease is accompanied by an inability to cope normally with everyday stresses. This may be a fruitful area for research.

Several groups have shown a greater frequency of smoking in patients with active thyroid ophthalmopathy than in healthy controls or in patients with Graves' disease without ophthalmopathy [12,52,96]. However, this cannot be the only factor, since one-third of the patients in the severe ophthalmopathy group in one study had never smoked.

REFERENCES

1. Ahmann, A., Baker, J.R., Jr., Weetman, A.P., Wartofsky, L., Nutman, T.B., and Burman, K.D. Antibodies to porcine eye muscle in patients with Graves' ophthalmopathy: Identification of serum immunoglobulins directed against unique determinants by immunoblotting and enzyme-linked immunosorbent assay. *J. Clin. Endocrinol. Metab.* 64:454–460, 1987.
2. Althaus, B., Staub, J.J., Muller-Brand, J., Carmann, H., Viollier, M., Matter, L., and Berger, W. Profile of autoimmune antibodies in idiopathic hypothyroidism and hypothyroidism following radio-iodine treatment in Basedow's disease: Comparison with a group of normal subjects from the female population of Switzerland. *Schweiz. Med. Wochenschr.* 113:1319–1327, 1983.
3. Amino, N., Yuasa, T., Yabu, Y., Miyai, K., and Kumahara, Y. Exophthalmos in autoimmune thyroid diseases. *J. Clin. Endocrinol. Metab.* 51:1232–1234, 1980.
4. Anderson, R.L., Tweeten, J.P., Patrinely, J.R., Garland, P.E., and Thiese, S.M. Dysthyroid optic neuropathy without extraocular muscle involvement. *Ophthalmic Surg.* 20:568–574, 1989.
5. Atta, H.R., McCreath, G., McKillop, J.H., Forrester, J.V., Thomson, J.A., Wilson, R., and Gray, H.W. Ophthalmopathy in early thyrotoxicosis—relationship to thyroid receptor antibodies and effects of treatment. *Scott. Med. J.* 35:41–44, 1990.
6. Bahn, R.S., Bartley, G.B., and Gorman, C.A. Emergency treatment of Graves' ophthalmopathy. *Baillieres Clin. Endocrinol. Metab.* 6:95–105, 1992.
7. Bahn, R.S., Gorman, C.A., Johnson, C.M., and Smith, T.J. Presence of antibodies in the sera of patients with Graves' disease recognizing a 23 kilodalton fibroblast protein. *J. Clin. Endocrinol. Metab.* 69:622–628, 1989.
8. Balazs, C., Bokk, A., Molnar, I., Stenszky, V., and Farid, N.R. Graves' ophthalmopathy, eye muscle antibodies and HLA antigens. *Exp. Clin. Immunogenet.* 6:190–192, 1989.
9. Barker, D.J., and Phillips, D.I. Current incidence of thyrotoxicosis and past prevalence of goitre in 12 British towns. *Lancet* 2:567–570, 1984.
10. Barrett, L., Glatt, H.J., Burde, R.M., and Gado, M.H. Optic nerve dysfunction in thyroid eye disease: CT. *Radiology* 167:503–507, 1988.
11. Bartalena, L., Marcocci, C., Bogazzi, F., Panicucci, M., Lepri, A., and Pinchera, A. Use of corticosteroids to prevent progression of Graves' ophthalmopathy after radioiodine therapy for hyperthyroidism. *N. Engl. J. Med.* 321:1349–1352, 1989.
12. Bartalena, L., Martino, E., Marcocci, C., Bogazzi, F., Panicucci, M., Velluzzi, F., Loviselli, A., and Pinchera, A. More on smoking habits and Graves' ophthalmopathy. *J. Endocrinol. Invest.* 12:733–737, 1989.
13. Batch, J.A., and Lepre, F. Early diagnosis of Graves' optic neuropathy using visual evoked responses. *Postgrad. Med. J.* 66:664–666, 1990.
14. Bech, K. Thyroid antibodies in endocrine ophthalmopathy. A review. *Acta Endocrinol. (Copenh.)* 121(Suppl. 2):117–122, 1989.
15. Berlin, G., Hjelm, H., Lieden, G., and Tegler, L. Plasma exchange in endocrine ophthalmopathy. *J. Clin. Apheresis.* 5:192–196, 1990.
16. Berta, R., and Kalman, K. Tear protein tests in Graves' ophthalmopathy. *Radiobiol. Radiother.* 28:546–549, 1987.
17. Bjoro, T., Gaarder, P.I., Smeland, E.B., and Kornstad, L. Thyroid antibodies in blood donors: Prevalence and clinical significance. *Acta Endocrinol. (Copenh.)* 105:324–329, 1984.
18. Bleeker, G.M. Changes in the orbital tissues and muscles dysthyroid ophthalmopathy. *Eye* 2:193–197, 1988.
19. Campbell, J.R. Immunology of Graves' ophthalmopathy: Retrobulbar histology and histochemistry. *Acta Endocrinol. (Copenh.)* 121(Suppl. 2):9–16, 1989.
20. Char, D.H. The ophthalmopathy of Graves' disease. *Med. Clin. North Am.* 70:97–119, 1991.
21. Creagh, F., Teece, M., Williams, S., Didcote, S., Perkins, W., Hashim, F., and Rees-Smith, B. An analysis of thyrotrophin receptor binding and thyroid stimulating activities in a series of Graves' sera. *Clin. Endocrinol. (Oxf.)* 23:395–404, 1985.
22. Czarnocka, B., Ruf, J., Ferrand, M., Carayon, P., and Lissitzky, S. Purification of the human thyroid peroxidase

and its identification as the microsomal antigen involved in autoimmune thyroid diseases. *FEBS Lett. 190*: 147–152, 1985.

23. De Rosa, G., Menichella, G., Della, S., Rossi, P.L., Testa, A., Pierelli, L., Cecchini, L., Calla, C., and Mango, G. Plasma exchange in Graves' ophthalmopathy. *Prog. Clin. Biol. Res. 337*:321–325, 1990.

24. DeGroot, L.J., Mangklabruks, A., and McCormick, M. Comparison of RA 131I treatment protocols for Graves' disease. *J. Endocrinol. Invest. 13*:111–118, 1990.

25. Dong, Q., Ludgate, M., and Vassart, G. Cloning and sequencing of a novel 64-kDa autoantigen recognized by patients with autoimmune thyroid disease. *J. Clin. Endocrinol. Metab. 72*:1375–1381, 1990.

26. Ealey, P.A., Yateman, M.E., Holt, S.J., and Marshall, N.J. ESTA: A bioassay system for the determination of the potencies of hormones and antibodies which mimic their action. *J. Mol. Endocrinol. 1*:R1–R4, 1988.

27. Etienne-Decerf, J., Malaise, M., Mahieu, P., and Winand, R. Elevated anti-alpha-galactosyl antibody titres. A marker of progression in autoimmune thyroid disorders and in endocrine ophthalmopathy? *Acta Endocrinol. (Copenh.) 115*:67–74, 1987.

28. Farid, N.R. Immunogenetics of autoimmune thyroid disorders. *Endocrinol. Metab. Clin. North Am. 16*:229–245, 1987.

29. Faryna, M., Nauman, J., and Gardas, A. Measurement of autoantibodies against human eye muscle plasma membranes in Graves' ophthalmopathy. *Br. Med. J. 290*:191–192, 1985.

30. Felberg, N.T., Sergott, R.C., Savino, P.J., Blizzard, J.J., Schatz, N.J., and Amsel, J. Lymphocyte subpopulations in Graves' ophthalmopathy. *Arch. Ophthalmol. 103*:656–659, 1985.

31. Feldon, S.E., Muramatsu, S., and Weiner, J.M. Clinical classification of Graves' ophthalmopathy. Identification of risk factors for optic neuropathy. *Arch. Ophthalmol. 102*:1469–1472, 1984.

32. Feldon, S.E., Lee, C.P., Muramatsu, S.K., and Weiner, J.M. Quantitative computed tomography of Graves' ophthalmopathy. Extraocular muscle and orbital fat in development of optic neuropathy. *Arch. Ophthalmol. 103*:213–215, 1985.

33. Feldon, S.E., and Levin, L. Graves' ophthalmopathy, V. Aetiology of upper eyelid retraction in Graves' ophthalmopathy. *Br. J. Ophthalmol. 74*:484–485, 1990.

34. Feldt-Rasmussen, U., Kemp, A., Bech, K., Madsen, S.N., and Date, J. Serum thyroglobulin, its autoantibody and thyroid stimulating antibodies in the endocrine exophthalmos. *Acta Endocrinol. (Copenh.) 96*:192–198, 1981.

35. Fells, P. Thyroid-associated eye disease: Clinical management. *Lancet 338*:29–32, 1991.

36. Fells, P., and McCarry, B. Diplopia in thyroid eye disease. *Trans. Ophthalmol. Soc. UK 105*:413–423, 1986.

37. Frecker, M., Stenszky, V., Balazs, C., Kozma, L., Kraszits, E., and Farid, N.R. Genetic factors in Graves' ophthalmopathy. *Clin. Endocrinol. (Oxf.) 25*:479–485, 1986.

38. Frueh, B.R. Graves' eye disease: Orbital compliance and other physical measurements. *Trans. Am. Ophthalmol. Soc. 82*:492–598, 1984.

39. Frueh, B.R., Musch, D.C., Grill, R., Garber, F.W., and Hamby, S. Orbital compliance in Graves' eye disease. *Ophthalmology 92*:657–665, 1985.

40. Frueh, B.R., Garber, F.W., and Musch, D.C. The effects of Graves' eye disease on levator muscle function. *Ophthalmic Surg. 17*:142–145, 1986.

41. Frueh, B.R., Grill, R., and Musch, D.C. Lid protractor force generation in Graves' eye disease. *Ophthalmology 93*:8–13, 1986.

42. Gardas, A., Czarnocka, B., Faryna, M., Adler, G., Lewartowska, A., Krawcynski, K., and Nauman, J. Simple and sensitive method for estimation of antithyroid plasma membrane antibodies in serum of patients with autoimmune thyroid disorders: Comparison with other assays. *Acta Endocrinol. (Copenh.) 105*:492–499, 1984.

43. Gardas, A., Czarnocka, B., and Nauman, J. The presence of autoantibodies directed to thyroid plasma membrane antigens in sera of patients with thyroid disorders, estimated by the reaction with labelled protein A. *Acta Endocrinol. (Copenh.) 105*:500–504, 1984.

44. Gardas, A., and Rives, K.L. Enzyme-linked immunosorbent assay of autoantibodies reacting with thyroid plasma membrane antigens in sera of patients with autoimmune thyroid diseases. *Acta Endocrinol. (Copenh.) 113*:255–260, 1986.

45. Garlepp, M.J., and Dawkins, R.L. Graves' disease and myasthenia gravis. In *The Eye and Orbit in Thyroid Disease*, C.A. Gorman (Ed.), Raven Press, New York, pp. 121–127, 1984.

46. Gasser, P., and Flammer, J. Optic neuropathy of Graves' disease. A report of a perimetric follow-up. *Ophthalmologica 192*:22–27, 1986.

47. Gilbard, J.P., and Farris, R.L. Ocular surface drying and tear film osmolarity in thyroid eye disease. *Acta Ophthalmol. (Copenh.) 61*:108–116, 1983.

48. Given-Wilson, R., Pope, R.M., Michell, M.J., Cannon, R., and McGregor, A.M. The use of real-time orbital ultrasound in Graves' ophthalmopathy: A comparison with computed tomography. *Br. J. Radiol. 62*:705–709, 1989.

49. Glinoer, D., Etienne-Decerf, J., Schrooyen, M., Sand, G., Hoyoux, P., Mahieu, P., and Winand, R. Beneficial effects of intensive plasma exchange followed by immunosuppressive therapy in severe Graves' ophthalmopathy. *Acta Endocrinol. (Copenh.) 111*:30–38, 1986.

50. Grove, A.S., Jr. Evaluation of exophthalmos. *N. Engl. J. Med. 292*:1005–1013, 1975.

51. Gwinup, G., Elias, A.N., and Ascher, M.S. Effect on exophthalmos of various methods of treatment of Graves' disease. *JAMA* 247:2135–2138, 1982.
52. Hagg, E., and Asplund, K. Is endocrine ophthalmopathy related to smoking? *Br. Med. J.* 295:634–635, 1987.
53. Hedin, A. Eyelid surgery in dysthyroid ophthalmopathy. *Eye* 2:201–206, 1988.
54. Hiromatsu, Y., Fukazawa, H., and Wall, J.R. Cytotoxic mechanisms in autoimmune thyroid disorders and thyroid-associated ophthalmopathy. *Endocrinol. Metab. Clin. North Am.* 16:269–286, 1987.
55. Hiromatsu, Y., Fukazawa, H., How, J., and Wall, J.R. Antibody-dependent cell-mediated cytotoxicity against human eye muscle cells and orbital fibroblasts in Graves' ophthalmopathy—roles of class II MHC antigen expression and gamma-interferon action of effector and target cells. *Clin. Exp. Immunol.* 70:593–603, 1987.
56. Hiromatsu, Y., Fukazawa, H., Guinard, F., Salvi, M., How, J., and Wall, J.R. A thyroid cytotoxic antibody that cross-reacts with an eye muscle cell surface antigen may be the cause of thyroid-associated ophthalmopathy. *J. Clin. Endocrinol. Metab.* 67:565–570, 1988.
57. Holt, J.E., O'Connor, P.S., Douglas, J.P., and Byrne, B. Extraocular muscle size comparison using standardized A-scan echography and computerized tomography scan measurements. *Ophthalmology* 92:1351–1355, 1985.
58. Hurwitz, J.J., McGowan, H.D., Gentles, W., Weise, R.A., and Victor, W. Orbitotonography, the dynamic assessment of orbital tension. 2. Results in patients with orbital disease. *Can. J. Ophthalmol.* 23:308–310, 1988.
59. Imai, Y., Odajima, R., Shimizu, T., and Shishiba, Y. Serum hyaluronan concentration determined by radio-metric assay in patients with pretibial myxedema and Graves' ophthalmopathy. *Endocrinol. Jpn.* 37:749–752, 1990.
60. Jacobson, D.R., and Fleming, B.J. Graves' disease with ophthalmopathy following radiotherapy for Hodgkin's disease. *Am. J. Med. Sci.* 288:217–220, 1984.
61. Jacobson, D.H., and Gorman, C.A. Endocrine ophthalmopathy: Current ideas concerning etiology, pathogenesis, and treatment. *Endocr. Rev.* 5:200–220, 1984.
62. Kadlubowski, M., Irvine, W.J., and Rowland, A.C. The lack of specificity of ophthalmic immunoglobulins in Graves' disease. *J. Clin. Endocrinol. Metab.* 63:990–995, 1986.
63. Kadlubowski, M., Irvine, W.J., and Rowland, A.C. Anti-muscle antibodies in Graves' ophthalmopathy. *J. Clin. Lab. Immunol.* 24:105–111, 1987.
64. Kahaly, G., Schuler, M., Sewell, A.C., Bernhard, G., Beyer, J., and Krause, U. Urinary glycosaminoglycans in Graves' ophthalmopathy. *Clin. Endocrinol. (Oxf.)* 33:35–44, 1990.
65. Karlsson, F., Westermark, K., Dahlberg, P.A., Jansson, R., and Enoksson, P. Ophthalmopathy and thyroid stimulation (letter). *Lancet* 2:691, 1989.
66. Kendall-Taylor, P., Atkinson, S., and Holcombe, M. A specific IgG in Graves' ophthalmopathy and its relation to retro-orbital and thyroid autoimmunity. *Br. Med. J.* 288:1183–1186, 1984.
67. Kendall-Taylor, P., Stephenson, A., Stratton, A., Papiha, S.S., Perros, P., and Roberts, D.F. Differentiation of autoimmune ophthalmopathy from Graves' hyperthyroidism by analysis of genetic markers. *Clin. Endocrinol. (Oxf.)* 28:601–610, 1988.
68. Khalil, H.A., de Keizer, R.J., and Kijlstra, A. Analysis of tear proteins in Graves' ophthalmopathy by high performance liquid chromatography. *Am. J. Ophthalmol.* 106:186–190, 1988.
69. Khalil, H.A., de Keizer, R.J., Bodelier, V.M., and Kijlstra, A. Secretory IgA and lysozyme in tears of patients with Graves' ophthalmopathy. *Doc. Ophthalmol.* 72:329–334, 1989.
70. Kodama, K., Sikorska, H., Bandy-Dafoe, P., Bayly, R., and Wall, J.R. Demonstration of a circulating autoantibody against a soluble eye-muscle antigen in Graves' ophthalmopathy. *Lancet* 2:1353–1356, 1982.
71. Kodama, K., Sikorska, H., Bayly, R., Bandy-Dafoe, P., and Wall, J.R. Use of monoclonal antibodies to investigate a possible role of thyroglobulin in the pathogenesis of Graves' ophthalmopathy. *J. Clin. Endocrinol. Metab.* 59:67–73, 1984.
72. Konishi, J., Herman, M.M., and Kriss, J.P. Binding of thyroglobulin and thyroglobulin-antithyroglobulin immune complex to extraocular muscle membrane. *Endocrinology* 95:434–446, 1974.
73. Kotani, T., Umeki, K., Matsunaga, S., Kato, E., and Ohtaki, S. Detection of autoantibodies to thyroid peroxidase in autoimmune thyroid diseases by micro-ELISA and immunoblotting. *J. Clin. Endocrinol. Metab.* 62:928–933, 1986.
74. Kriss, J.P. Radioisotopic thyroidolymphography in patients with Graves' disease. *J. Clin. Endocrinol. Metab.* 31:315–324, 1970.
75. Kuroki, T., Ruf, J., Whelan, L., Miller, A., and Wall, J.R. Antithyroglobulin monoclonal and autoantibodies cross-react with an orbital connective tissue membrane antigen: A possible mechanism for the association of ophthalmopathy with autoimmune disorders. *Clin. Exp. Immunol.* 62:361–370, 1985.
76. Lai, K.N., Leung, J.C., Chow, C.C., and Cockram, C.S. T lymphocyte activation in euthyroid Graves' ophthalmopathy: Soluble interleukin 2 receptor release, cellular interleukin 2 receptor expression and inter-leukin 2 production. *Acta Endocrinol. (Copenh.)* 120:602–609, 1989.
77. Lawton, N.F. Exclusion of dysthyroid eye disease as a cause of unilateral proptosis. *Trans. Ophthalmol. Soc. UK* 99:226–228, 1979.
78. Ludgate, M., Swillens, S., Mercken, L., and Vassart, G. Homology between thyroglobulin and acetyl-cholinesterase: An explanation for pathogenesis of Graves' ophthalmopathy (letter)? *Lancet* 2:219–220, 1986.

79. Marcocci, C., Bartalena, L., Bogazzi, F., Panicucci, M., and Pinchera, A. Studies on the occurrence of ophthalmopathy in Graves' disease. *Acta Endocrinol. (Copenh.) 120*:473–478, 1989.

80. Marushak, D., Faurschou, S., and Blichert-Toft, M. Regression of ophthalmopathy in Graves' disease following thyroidectomy. A systematic study of changes of ocular signs. *Acta Ophthalmol. (Copenh.) 62*:767–779, 1984.

81. Mengistu, M., Laryea, E., Miller, A., and Wall, J.R. Clinical significance of a new autoantibody against a human eye muscle soluble antigen, detected by immunofluorescence. *Clin. Exp. Immunol. 65*:19–27, 1986.

82. Miller, A., Sikorska, H., Salvi, M., and Wall, J.R. Evaluation of an enzyme-linked immunosorbent assay for the measurement of autoantibodies against eye muscle membrane antigens in Graves' ophthalmopathy. *Acta Endocrinol. (Copenh.) 113*:514–522, 1986.

83. Morris, J.C., III, Hay, I.D., Nelson, R.E., and Jiang, N.S. Clinical utility of thyrotropin-receptor antibody assays: comparison of radioreceptor and bioassay methods. *Mayo Clin. Proc. 63*:707–717, 1988.

84. Mullin, B.R., Levinson, R.E., Friedman, A., Henson, D.E., Winand, R.J., and Kohn, L.D. Delayed hypersensitivity in Graves' disease and exophthalmos: Identification of thyroglobulin in normal human orbital muscle. *Endocrinology 100*:351–366, 1977.

85. Munro, R.E., Lamki, L., Row, V.V., and Volpé, R. Cell mediated immunity in the exophthalmos of Graves' disease as demonstrated by the migration inhibition factor (MIF) test. *J. Clin. Endocrinol. Metab. 37*:286–292, 1973.

86. Neigel, J.M., Rootman, J., Belkin, R.I., Nugent, R.A., Drance, S.M., Beattie, C.W., and Spinelli, J.A. Dysthyroid optic neuropathy. The crowded orbital apex syndrome. *Ophthalmology 95*:1515–1521, 1988.

87. Perrild, H., Feldt-Rasmussen, U., Bech, K., Ahlgren, P., and Hansen, J.M. The differential diagnostic problems in unilateral euthyroid Graves' ophthalmopathy. *Acta Endocrinol. (Copenh.) 106*:471–476, 1984.

88. Pope, R.M., Ludgate, M.E., and McGregor, A.M. Observations on Graves' ophthalmopathy; pathology and pathogenesis. In: *Immunology of Endocrine Diseases*, A.M. McGregor (Ed.); MTP, Lancaster, pp. 161–179, 1986.

89. Portmann, L., Hamada, N., Heinrich, G., and DeGroot, L.J. Anti-thyroid peroxidase antibody in patients with autoimmune thyroid disease: Possible identity with anti-microsomal antibody. *J. Clin. Endocrinol. Metab. 61*:1001–1003, 1985.

90. Potts, M. Falcao-Reis, F., Fells, P., Buceti, S., and Arden, G.B. Colour contrast sensitivity, pattern ERG's and cortical evoked potentials in dysthyroid optic neuropathy. *Invest. Ophthalmol. Vis. Sci. (Suppl.) 31*:189, 1990.

91. Preus, M., Frecker, M.F., Stenszky, V., Balazs, C., and Farid, N.R. A prognostic score for Graves' disease. *Clin. Endocrinol. (Oxf.) 23*:653–661, 1985.

92. Rotella, C.M., Zonefrati, R., Toccafondi, R., Valente, W.A., and Kohn, L.D. Ability of monoclonal antibodies to the thyrotropin receptor to increase collagen synthesis in human fibroblasts: An assay which appears to measure exophthalmogenic immunoglobulins in Graves' sera. *J. Clin. Endocrinol. Metab. 62*:357–367, 1986.

93. Rotella, C.M., Alvarez, F., Kohn, L.D., and Toccafondi, R. Graves' autoantibodies to extrathyroidal TSH receptor: Their role in ophthalmopathy and pretibial myxedema. *Acta Endocrinol. Suppl. (Copenh.) 281*:344–347, 1987.

94. Salvi, M., Zhang, Z.G., Haegert, D., Woo, M., Liberman, A., Cadarso, L., and Wall, J.R. Patients with endocrine ophthalmopathy not associated with overt thyroid disease have multiple thyroid immunological abnormalities. *J. Clin. Endocrinol. Metab. 70*:89–94, 1990.

95. Schifferdecker, E., Ketzler-Sasse, U., Boehm, B.O., Ronsheimer, H.B., Scherbaum, W.A., and Schoffling, K. Re-evaluation of eye muscle autoantibody determination in Graves' ophthalmopathy: Failure to detect a specific antigen by use of enzyme-linked immunosorbent assay, indirect immunofluorescence, and immunoblotting techniques. *Acta Endocrinol. (Copenh.) 121*:643–650, 1989.

96. Shine, B., Fells, P., Edwards, O.M., and Weetman, A.P. Association between Graves' ophthalmopathy and smoking. *Lancet 335*:1261–1263, 1990.

97. Sikorska, H., and Wall, J.R. Failure to detect eye muscle membrane specific autoantibodies in Graves' ophthalmopathy (letter). *Br. Med. J. 291*:604, 1985.

98. Simonsz, H.J., Kolling, G.H., Kaufman, H., and van Dijk, B. Intraoperative length and tension curves of human eye muscles, including stiffness in passive horizontal eye movement in awake volunteers. *Arch. Ophthalmol. 104*:1495–1500, 1986.

99. Simonsz, H.J., and Kommerell, G. Increased muscle tension and reduced elasticity of affected muscles in recent-onset Graves' disease caused primarily by active muscle contraction. *Doc. Ophthalmol. 72*:215–224, 1989.

100. Small, R.G. Enlargement of levator palpebrae superioris muscle fibers in Graves' ophthalmopathy. *Ophthalmology 96*:424–430, 1989.

101. Small, R.G. Upper eyelid retraction in Graves' ophthalmopathy: A new surgical technique and a study of the abnormal levator muscle. *Trans. Am. Ophthalmol. Soc. 86*:725–793, 1989.

102. Small, R.G., and Scott, M. The tight retracted lower eyelid. *Trans. Am. Ophthalmol. Soc. 87*:362–382, 1990.

103. Smith, T.J., Bahn, R.S., and Gorman, C.A. Hormonal regulation of hyaluronate synthesis in cultured human fibroblasts: Evidence for differences between retroocular and dermal fibroblasts. *J. Clin. Endocrinol. Metab. 69*:1019–1023, 1989.

104. Spiritus, M. Oculomotor disorders in orbital pathology. Thyroid ophthalmopathy. Involvement of the extraocular muscles. *J. Fr. Ophtalmol. 9*:679–683, 1986.

105. Sridama, V., Hara, Y., Fauchet, R., and DeGroot, L.J. HLA Immunogenetic heterogeneity in black American patients with Graves' disease. *Arch. Intern. Med. 147*:229–231, 1987.

106. Sterk, C.C., Bierlaagh, J.J., de Keizer, R.J. Motility disorders in endocrine ophthalmopathy. *Doc. Ophthalmol. 59*:71–75, 1985.

107. Tajiri, J., Higashi, K., Morita, M., Hamasaki, S., Yamasaki, H., Ohishi, S., Fujiyama, S., and Sato, T. Thyroid antibodies in healthy blood donors. *Endocrinol. Jpn. 31*:837–843, 1984.

108. Tallstedt, L., and Norberg, R. Immunohistochemical staining of normal and Graves' extraocular muscle. *Invest. Ophthalmol. Vis. Sci. 29*:175–184, 1988.

109. Tao, T.-W., Leu, S.-L., and Kriss, J.P. Glycosaminoglycans, DNA, and protein synthesis stimulating antibodies in pretibial myxedema. *Acta Endocrinol. (Copenh.) 121* (Suppl. 2):64–74, 1989.

110. Teboul, B., Triller, H., Chung, F., Bernard, N., Zhang, Z.G., Wall, J.R., and Salvi, M. Muscle and species reactivity of mouse monoclonal antibodies to human eye muscle membrane antigens. *Clin. Immunol. Immunopathol. 59*:104–116, 1991.

111. Teng, W.P., Stark, R., Munro, A.J., Young, S.M., Borysiewicz, L.K., and Weetman, A.P. Peripheral blood T cell activation after radioiodine treatment for Graves' disease. *Acta Endocrinol. (Copenh.) 122*:233–240, 1990.

112. Troelstra, A., Rijneveld, W.J., Kooijman, A.C., and Houtman, W.A. Correlation between NMR scans of extraocular muscles and clinical symptoms in Graves' ophthalmopathy. *Doc. Ophthalmol. 70*:243–249, 1989.

113. Tunbridge, W.M., Evered, D.C., Hall, R., Appleton, D., Brewis, M., Clark, F., Evans, J.G., Young, E., Bird, T., and Smith, P.A. The spectrum of thyroid disease in a community: The Whickham survey. *Clin. Endocrinol. (Oxf.) 7*:481–493, 1977.

114. Vestergaard, H., and Laurberg, P. Radioiodine and aggravation of Graves' ophthalmopathy (letter). *Lancet 2*:47, 1989.

115. Wall, J.R., Salvi, M., Bernard, N.F., Boucher, A., and Haegert, D. Thyroid-associated ophthalmopathy—a model for the association of organ-specific autoimmune disorders. *Immunol. Today 12*:150–153, 1991.

116. Wang, P.W., Hiromatsu, Y., Laryea, E., Wosu, L., How, J., and Wall, J.R. Immunologically mediated cytotoxicity against human eye muscle cells in Graves' ophthalmopathy. *J. Clin. Endocrinol. Metab. 63*:316–322, 1986.

117. Weetman, A.P., So, A.K., Warner, C.A., Foroni, L., Fells, P., and Shine, B. Immunogenetics of Graves' ophthalmopathy. *Clin. Endocrinol. (Oxf.) 28*:619–628, 1988.

118. Weetman, A.P. Thyroid-associated eye disease: Pathophysiology. *Lancet 338*:25–28, 1991.

119. Weetman, A.P., Cohen, S., Gatter, K.C., Fells, P., and Shine, B. Immunohistochemical analysis of the retrobulbar tissues in Graves' ophthalmopathy. *Clin. Exp. Immunol. 75*:222–227, 1989.

120. Weetman, A.P., Fells, P., and Shine, B. T and B cell reactivity to extraocular and skeletal muscle in Graves' ophthalmopathy. *Br. J. Ophthalmol. 73*:323–327, 1989.

121. Weetman, A.P., Yateman, M.E., Ealey, P.A., Black, C.M., Reimer, C.B., Williams, R.C., Jr., Shine, B., and Marshall, N.J. Thyroid-stimulating antibody activity between different immunoglobulin G subclasses. *J. Clin. Invest. 86*:723–727, 1990.

122. Weetman, A.P., Zhang, L., Webb, S., and Shine, B. Analysis of HLA-DQB and HLA-DPB alleles in Graves' disease by oligonucleotide probing of enzymatically amplified DNA. *Clin. Endocrinol. (Oxf.) 33*:65–71, 1990.

123. Weightman, D., and Kendall-Taylor, P. Cross-reaction of eye muscle antibodies with thyroid tissue in thyroid-associated ophthalmopathy. *J. Endocrinol. 122*:201–206, 1989.

124. Westermark, L.K., and Karlsson, F.A. Effects of sera and immunoglobulin preparations from patients with endocrine ophthalmopathy on the production of hyaluronate and the incorporation of tritiated thymidine in fibroblasts. *Acta Endocrinol. (Copenh.) 12* (Suppl. 2):85–89, 1989.

125. Wiersinga, W.M., Smit, T., van der Gaag, R., and Koornneef, L. Temporal relationship between onset of Graves' ophthalmopathy and onset of thyroidal Graves' disease. *J. Endocrinol. Invest. 11*:615–619, 1988.

126. Wiersinga, W.M., Smit, T., van der Gaag, R., Mourits, M., and Koornneef, L. Clinical presentation of Graves' ophthalmopathy. *Ophthalmic Res. 21*:73–82, 1989.

127. Wilson, R., McKillop, J.H., Walker, J.J., Gray, C.E., and Thomson, J.A. The incidence of clinical thyroid dysfunction in an unselected group of pregnant and post partum women. *Scott. Med. J. 35*:170–173, 1990.

128. Winand, R.J., and Kohn, L.D. Stimulation of adenylate cyclase activity in retro-orbital tissue membranes by thyrotropin and an exophthalmogenic factor derived from thyrotropin. *J. Biol. Chem. 250*:6522–6526, 1975.

129. Wirtschafter, J.D., Hard-Boberg, A.L., and Coffman, S.M. Evaluating the usefulness in neuro-ophthalmology of visual field examinations peripheral to 30 degrees. *Trans. Am. Ophthalmol. Soc. 82*:329–357, 1984.

130. Zhang, Z.-G., Medeiros-Neto, G., Iacona, A., Lima, N., Hiromatsu, Y., Salvi, M., Triller, H., Bernard, N., and Wall, J.R. Studies of cytotoxic antibodies against eye muscle antigens in patients with thyroid-associated ophthalmopathy. *Acta Endocrinol. (Copenh.) 121* (Suppl. 2):23–30, 1989.

37

Metabolic Disorders Involving Metals

Alec Garner

Institute of Ophthalmology, University of London, London, England

I. INTRODUCTION

The salts of many metals can act as external irritants if allowed to come into contact with the outer eye, giving rise to conjunctivitis and, in some instances, corneal ulceration. The ingestion of some metallic compounds, such as those containing gold, silver, or mercury, can cause a characteristic discoloration of the cornea or lens. Several metals are essential to tissue metabolism but if introduced in an abnormal form or manner can damage the tissues; in the ocular context foreign bodies composed of iron or copper produce marked degenerative changes in the eye (see Chap. 14), and excessive amounts of cobalt in the form of its chloride can result in cataractous lens changes in laboratory animals [1].

As opposed to allergic or direct toxic effects, a few metals essential to normal physiological processes can be associated with systemic disease because of an intrinsic defect in the metabolic sequences of which they are a part. This defect may be either inherited or acquired. Ocular disorders incurred in such a manner provide the subject of this chapter.

II. CALCIUM

Ocular lesions developing as part of a wider systemic involvement can be a result of either too much or too little calcium in the circulating blood.

A. Hypercalcemia

Hypercalcemia can be primary, in response to excessive parathormone secretion by a parathyroid tumor, or so-called primary hyperplasia, or secondary to hypervitaminosis D, sarcoidosis, multiple myeloma, certain carcinomas, and a number of other disorders. Parathormone acts primarily on the kidney and on bone, where it serves to promote increased calcium reabsorption by the renal tubules and release from the skeleton. Vitamin D also acts at a number of sites, but dietary excess chiefly affects the intestinal absorption of calcium. Sarcoidosis appears to incur an increased sensitivity to vitamin D [65]. The hypercalcemia associated with malignant neoplasia is often, but not always, attributable to osteolytic metastases.

Genetically determined disorders that incur hypercalcemia and ocular complications include hypophosphatasia and Alport's syndrome. Hypophosphatasia is an autosomal recessive disorder involving alkaline phosphatase activity. The associated hypercalcemia reflects reduced incorporation of calcium in bone because of inability to hydrolyze inorganic pyrophosphate, this serving as an inhibitor of hydroxyapatite crystal formation in the absence of adequate levels of alkaline phosphatase [27]. Corneal and conjunctival calcification are recognized complications [9,49]. Alport's syndrome shows a variable pattern of inheritance, although autosomal dominant transmission is most frequent [51] and is characterized by renal dysfunction, neural deafness, and a range of ocular problems, particularly with respect to the lens [32]. Deposition of calcium salts in the conjunctiva can occur as renal failure develops, when it may be

1137

associated with a foreign body response [10]. Clinical evidence of calcium deposits in the conjunctiva and peripheral cornea has been reported in patients with renal failure in general in association with either hypercalcemia [46] or, paradoxically, hypocalcemia (see later), but in both situations a raised serum calcium × phosphate product usually appertains [5,46].

The ocular complications of hypercalcemia in general relate principally to metastatic deposition of hydroxyapatite in the cornea [4], although calcification of the extrinsic muscles of the eye and their tendinous insertions has been described [38]. Calcification of the cornea commences at the nasal and temporal peripheries and gradually spreads to create a band-shaped opacity in the line of the interpalpebral fissure (see also Chap. 23) [16]. Initially, the deposits appear as fine basophilic amorphous particles in Bowman's zone of the substantia propria before spreading to the superficial stromal lamellae. The theory that seems to command most support for this anatomical distribution is that carbon dioxide loss, with consequent rise in pH and reduced calcium salt solubility, is likely to be greatest in the exposed interpalpebral region [14a,60].

B. Hypocalcemia

Low levels of serum calcium are a feature of the hypoparathyroidism that sometimes complicates thyroid surgery or that may occasionally arise spontaneously. Also recognized are individuals who are unresponsive to the renal effects of parathyroid hormone (pseudohypoparathyroidism). Hypocalcemia can also be a feature of chronic renal failure, the disturbance in calcium metabolism being due principally to inadequate conversion of 25-hydroxycholecalciferol to its more active form, 1,25-dihydrocholecalciferol, by the renal tubular epithelium [22].

Bilateral cataracts are the most frequent ocular complication of the hypocalcemia accompanying hypoparathyroidism, affecting over half the reported idiopathic cases [7,59] and developing after an average period of 11 years in cases in whom the lesion is secondary to thyroid surgery [35]. Typically, the cataracts present as numerous small discrete opacities in the anterior and posterior cortices of the lens, and although the precise pathogenesis is uncertain, osmotic changes resulting from ionic imbalance have been blamed [11]. That parathyroid hormone is able to regulate lens capsule permeability to calcium has been known for many years [14a].

Other reported ophthalmic effects of hypocalcemia include ptosis and impaired ocular motility [23], presumably on the basis of tetanic muscular contraction, pigmentary retinopathy [23], and edematous optic disk changes suggestive of ischemic optic neuritis [3].

Conjunctival calcification, which may impinge on the periphery of the cornea at the level of the interpalpebral fissure, is liable to develop in the hypocalcemia associated with chronic renal failure [5,6,36,60]. Although the serum calcium is low, the product obtained by multiplying the serum calcium and phosphorus levels may be increased as a result of impaired excretion of phosphate by the diseased kidneys. There is no adequate explanation for the conjunctival predilection for calcification or for the foreign body reaction and clinical irritation with which it is frequently linked [5].

III. COPPER

Trace amounts of copper are essential for the proper functioning of a number of intracellular enzyme systems. Diseases in humans referable to defective copper metabolism are genetically determined [18a].

A. Wilson's Disease

Wilson's disease, or hepatolenticular degeneration, is an autosomal recessively inherited disorder in which accumulation of copper in the liver is followed by its deposition in the renal tubules, brain, cornea, and other tissues. Although not established with certainty, it seems likely that the genetic abnormality exerts its primary effect in the liver to cause reduced incorporation of copper into ceruloplasmin and impaired excretion of copper into the bile [18a,64,72]. As a result, an increased proportion of the circulating plasma copper is loosely bound to albumin, in which state it is readily deposited in the tissues. Plasma levels of copper are usually low (less than 1.0 μmol/liter) and are associated with reduced levels of ceruloplasmin (below 20 mg per 100 ml).

The deposition of copper in the cornea to form the characteristic Kayser-Fleischer ring occurs early in the course of the disease and is contemporaneous with involvement of the basal ganglia [80]. The ring begins as an arc at the upper periphery of the cornea, followed by a similar arc in the lower cornea, before a complete circle, variably green to brown, is formed [80]. The copper is incorporated in Descemet's membrane, its presence having been confirmed by histochemical means [77] and by electron probe analysis [74]. The granular metallic deposits tend to be arranged in a linear fashion (Fig. 1), a pattern that has stimulated the suggestion that the copper enters the cornea by diffusion from the anterior chamber [37]. The precise nature of the copper in the membrane is not known, but it seems possible that it is in a chelated form [77] related to the proteoglycan component of Descemet's membrane. There is also evidence that the formation of discrete granules is preceded by combination with a sulfur-containing component [44]. The initial deposition in superior and inferior arcs has been attributed to a slower forward diffusion rate of corneal fluid in parts covered by the eyelids since surface evaporation is least in these areas: this would produce relative stagnation and an increased opportunity for copper deposition to occur [77]. Wilson's disease can be controlled and the corneal changes reversed by dosage with penicillamine, which has strong chelating properties. Note that Kayser-Fleischer rings can complicate other acquired disorders in which there is a high local concentration of copper [82].

The vast majority of patients develop Kayser-Fleischer rings, but a much smaller proportion, 17% in one series [80], also develop greenish cataracts. The cataracts are similar to those produced by copper-containing foreign bodies within the eye, the distribution of copper in the anterior capsule having been likened to a sunflower [12]. However, the finding that the metallic deposits in a case examined by electron microscopy [75] were most obvious close to the lenticular epithelium, rather than on the free surface of the capsule, has prompted the suggestion that deposition is related to cellular activity and cannot be accounted for solely by diffusion.

B.   Menkes' Disease (X-Linked Copper Malabsorption Syndrome)

Menkes' disease is an X-linked recessive disorder [53] attributable to a defect in the transport of copper across the intestinal mucosa that probably occurs at an intracellular level [19]. As a result the serum copper level is abnormally low, as is the ceruloplasmin, although the unconjugated apoceruloplasmin is present in normal amounts. Characteristically, affected male infants develop whitish, lusterless, short kinky hair within a few weeks of birth, together with skeletal abnormalities and progressive neuromuscular dysfunction. In untreated cases death ensues within 2–3 years.

The tissue effects are probably a result of copper deficiency, since the administration of copper within the first few weeks of life, before irreversible changes have taken place, has been claimed to arrest the disease [33].

Central to the metabolic disturbance is abnormal intracellular transport of copper and its excessive retention within fibroblasts and certain other cell types in association with increased amounts of metallothionein [18,47], the latter being a 10 kD sulfur-rich protein. In consequence there is reduced availability of copper for incorporation in copper-dependent enzyme systems, and it is to this that the tissue effects are attributable.

In the ophthalmic context the eyebrows are sparse with twisted and broken hairs, and the eyelashes are variably depigmented, scanty, and stubby. This defect, as with the pathognomonic kinky hair abnormality in general, is attributable to inadequate disulfide bonding because of reduced amine oxidase activity [41]. Deficient tyrosinase activity is linked with impaired melanin formation in the skin and retinal pigment epithelium (RPE) [41,84]. Abnormalities of Bruch's membrane [84] reminiscent of the fragmentation of the internal elastic lamina of arteries and considered due to inadequate cross-linkage of elastin can be linked to a deficiency of copper-dependent lysyl oxidase activity. Neuroretinal abnormalities are also common in the form of ganglion cell loss, and there is nerve fiber loss associated with myelin deficiency in the optic nerve [30,67,84]. Copper-deficient rats suffer a comparable demyelination affecting the post-laminar part of the optic nerve, together with neuronal swelling and vacuolation in the prelaminar region [17]. These changes are reflected in an abnormal electroretinogram (ERG) and diminished visually evoked response [50]. The neuronal disturbance is probably multifactorial since copper is needed for the cytochrome oxidase-dependent energy provision [50] and myelin formation [26].

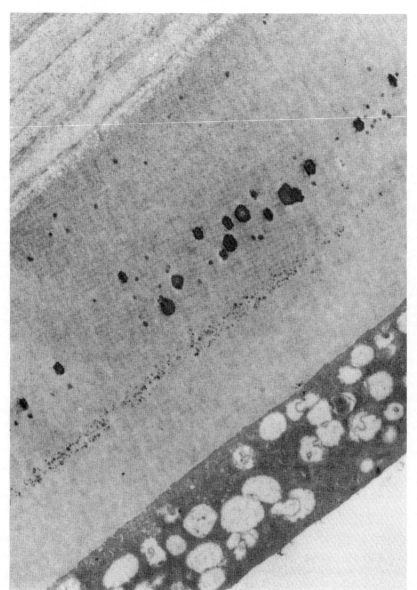

Figure 1 Kayser-Fleischer ring. Electron micrograph of posterior cornea showing granular deposits of copper in Descemet's membrane. The linear distribution of the metal with intervening uninvolved areas is suggestive of phasic deposition. (Uranyl acetate–lead citrate, ×10,000) (Reproduced with permission from J. Harry and R.C. Tripathi. Kayser-Fleischer ring: A pathological study. *Br. J. Ophthalmol. 54:794–800, 1970.*)

IV. IRON

Ocular disturbance caused by faulty metabolism of iron is extremely uncommon but has been described in hemochromatosis.

A. Hemochromatosis

Hemochromatosis is a clinical syndrome caused by the harmful effects of excessive quantities of iron, in the form of hemosiderin and ferritin, in the body tissues. Hemosiderin deposition in the skin, liver, and pancreas gives rise to a triad of skin pigmentation, hepatic cirrhosis, and diabetes mellitus. The primary form is inherited in an autosomal recessive manner and is attributable to a defective gene on chromosome 6 [25]. A distinct male preponderance is likely to be due to the female capacity to reduce her iron stores through menstruation. The nature of the basic defect is not known, although it clearly involves increased iron absorption by the tissues and intestinal absorption. Secondary hemochromatosis can result from a number of conditions characterized by iron overload, principal among which is multiple blood transfusions.

The ocular complications are usually attributable to secondary diabetic retinopathy, and a single case report of alleged corneal opacification [76] is open to doubt since the patient had none of the systemic manifestations of hemochromatosis; the histology of the deposits is suggestive of spheroidal droplet degeneration (see Chap. 23). Another report of three proven cases of primary hemochromatosis [62] described iron deposition in the ciliary epithelium and sclera, which was completely symptomless, but no corneal involvement. Iron has also been recognized in the RPE in both primary and secondary hemochromatosis [24], and conjunctival microaneurysms have been described [43]. Increased pigmentation of the conjunctiva and eyelid margins caused by melanin in the basal layers of epithelium is a feature in about 30% of cases [21].

B. Cerebrohepatorenal (Zellweger) Syndrome

Excessive amounts of iron in the tissues is a usual finding in the cerebrohepatorenal syndrome first described by Zellweger and his colleagues [8], and for a time it was considered that this was fundamental to the pathogenesis of the condition [56,70,78]. This conclusion now seems unfounded, and the inclusion of Zellweger syndrome in this chapter is justifiable only in terms of this earlier suspicion and editorial convenience. Conversely, there is now good evidence of a fundamental defect in peroxisomal function [31,66], and the cerebrohepatorenal syndrome is coming to be recognized as the prototype for a group of peroxisomal disorders that includes neonatal adrenoleukodystrophy, hyperpipecolic acidemia, infantile Refsum disease, and rhizomelic chondrodysplasia punctata [2,66]. In the context of Zellweger syndrome the evidence points to impaired synthesis of a peroxisomal membrane protein concerned with the orderly assembly of the constituent enzymes [63,68]. Not only has a point mutation in the peroxisome assembly factor-1 gene been described, but transfection of the intact gene into fibroblasts from a patient with Zellweger syndrome has been shown to restore normal function [68]. In line with the varied functions ascribed to peroxisomes, the metabolic expression of Zellweger syndrome is complex. Among the more characteristic abnormalities are high levels of circulating very long chain ($>$C22) fatty acids, 5-β-prostanoic acids, and pipecolic acid [45] and reduced amounts of the cell membrane constituent phosphatidylethanolamine [40,54]. The accumulation of pipecolic acid in the blood and urine stems from diversion of lysine through a normally minor catabolic pathway [20] and may be of particular relevance to the neurological manifestations of the syndrome.

The condition, which is probably an autosomal recessive disorder [56], is incompatible with life beyond a few months, and affected infants have a characteristic facial appearance caused by a high forehead with malformed external ears, flat supraorbital ridges, and epicanthal folds [8,29,56–58]. Central nervous system disturbance in the form of hypotonia and, less commonly, seizures and nystagmus is a constant feature [56–58]. Defective liver function, sometimes resulting in jaundice, and proteinuria are usual.

Ocular defects of one kind or another occur in most cases. Reported abnormalities include corneal opacification, glaucoma, cataract, Brushfield's spots, optic nerve atrophy, attenuated retinal vessels, and disturbances of the RPE [28,34,56–58,70,71]. Cataracts are common, and one report alludes to the presence of curvilinear bodies at the corticonuclear interface in an electron microscopic study of the lens of a heterozygote carrier of the syndrome [42]. Posterior segment changes, in the form of a rapidly progressive retinal dystrophy associated with extinction of the ERG, are a frequent and possibly constant feature. From the small number of eyes examined histologically, this appears to be due to loss of photoreceptor outer segments and degeneration of the RPE (Fig. 2) [15,29]. Deposits of an unidentified laminated material in the subretinal space have been described in ultrastructural studies [15,29].

The brain abnormalities are distinctive, consisting of coexistent abnormally small and broad gyri (pachymicrogyria), abnormal organization of cerebellar cortex neurons with myelin degeneration, and peculiar globoid cells with strongly sudanophilic cytoplasm in the gray matter [48,56]. The kidneys are usually small with numerous microcysts [8,69], whereas the liver tends to be enlarged, with cirrhotic changes attributed to intrahepatic biliary dysgenesis [69]. Unusually large amounts of iron have been reported in a number of tissues, especially the liver and kidneys [56,78], together with raised levels of iron in the serum [70]. As indicated earlier, such findings were initially taken to represent a congenital hemosiderosis caused possibly by defective genetic control of the placental transfer of iron in utero [56]. However, others [58] found that the total body iron in Zellweger syndrome (about 115 mg/kg) represents less than a 50% increase, which is negligible in comparison with the 25- to 50-fold elevation typical of hemochromatosis. Furthermore, Patton and coworkers [58] commented that of the five patients in whom serum iron levels were measured at the time of their review, two had normal levels. Consequently, these workers considered that the evidence in support of a congenital metabolic defect of iron metabolism was unconvincing and speculated that the increased amounts of this metal in the tissues might reflect deficient utilization secondary to growth retardation [58]. In two reported cases in whom appropriate stains were performed, iron was demonstrated in the corneal and nonpigmented ciliary body epithelium in one instance [79] but not in the other [34].

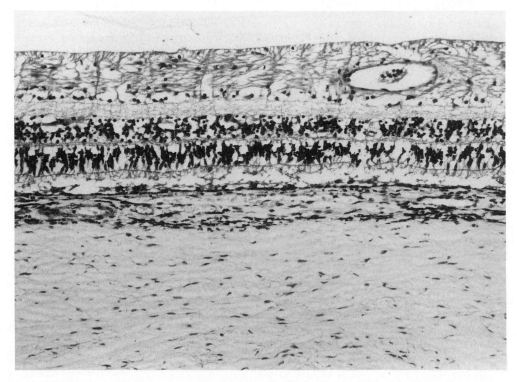

Figure 2   Zellweger syndrome. Section of retina from near the posterior pole showing atrophy of photoreceptor outer segments and pigment epithelium. (Hematoxylin and eosin, ×180)

V. ZINC

Traces of zinc are essential for the operation of several metalloenzymes, including some of ophthalmic importance, such as carbonic anhydrase and alcohol dehydrogenase. Zinc is also required for nucleic acid synthesis.

Intestinal malabsorption of zinc determined by an autosomal recessive gene defect [55] is the underlying cause of acrodermatitis enteropathica, a condition that presents in early infancy with a bullous pustular dermatitis and persistent diarrhea. The skin lesions develop in a symmetrical pattern around the body orifices and on the fingers and toes. Psychomotor and certain sensory dysfunctions, including disorders of smell [39], are also common, as are recurrent infections in the presence of impaired immune efficiency [73]. The latter is associated with thymic atrophy and relates primarily to T cell function [2]. In the absence of treatment in the form of zinc supplementation, the disease is usually fatal.

Photophobia, impaired dark adaptation, and reduced visual acuity are the principal ocular symptoms [14], and histological examination may reveal RPE degeneration at the posterior pole [13]. The eyelids share in the general skin disturbance, presenting with a vesicular eruption that later becomes psoriaform, and accompanying conjunctivitis is usual [14]. Less commonly, the corneal epithelium is affected and scarring of the immediately subjacent corneal stroma, with erosion of Bowman's zone can result [52,81,83]. An unexplained clinical finding described in each of these reports has been linear opacities radiating from the center of the cornea, which disappear following treatment of the basic condition. Cataract formation is also reported [14,61].

REFERENCES

1.   Alagna, G., and D'Aquino, S. Alterazioni oculari da cloruro di cobalto. *Arch. Ottalmol. 60*:5–29, 1956.
2.   Allen, J.I., Kay, N.E., and McClain, C.J. Severe zinc deficiency in humans: Association with a reversible T-lymphocyte dysfunction. *Ann. Intern. Med. 95*:154–157, 1981.
3.   Bajandas, F.J., and Smith, J.L. Optic neuritis in hypoparathyroidism. *Neurology 26*:451–454, 1976.
4.   Berkow, J.W., Fine, B.S., and Zimmerman, L.E. Unusual ocular calcification in hyperparathyroidism. *Am. J. Ophthalmol. 66*:812–824, 1968.
5.   Berlyne, G.M., and Shaw, A.B. Red eyes in renal failure. *Lancet 1*:4–7, 1967.
6.   Berlyne, G.M. Microcrystalline conjunctival calcification in renal failure. *Lancet 2*:366–370, 1968.
7.   Blake, J. Eye signs in idiopathic hypoparathyroidism. *Trans. Ophthalmol. Soc. UK 96*:448–451, 1976.
8.   Bowen, P., Lee, C.S.N., Zellweger, H., and Lindenberg, R. A familial syndrome of multiple congenital defects. *Bull. Johns Hopkins Hosp. 114*:402–414, 1964.
9.   Brenner, R.L., Smith, J.L., Cleveland, W.W., Bejar, R.L., and Lockhart, W.S., Jr. Eye signs in hypophosphatasia. *Arch. Ophthalmol. 81*:614–617, 1969.
10.   Buchbinder, M.C., Gindi, J.J., Schanzlin, D.J., and Rao, N. Conjunctival crystals in Alport's syndrome. *Ophthalmology (Suppl.) 91*:123, 1984.
11.   Bunce, G.E. Nutrition and cataract. *Nutr. Rev. 37*:337–343, 1979.
12.   Cairns, J.G., and Walshe, J.M. The Kayser-Fleischer ring. *Trans. Ophthalmol. Soc. UK 90*:187–190, 1970.
13.   Cameron, J.D., and McClain, C.J. Ocular histopathology of acrodermatitis enteropathica. *Br. J. Ophthalmol. 70*:662–667, 1986.
14.   Cameron, J.D., McClain, C.J., and Doughman, D.J. Acrodermatitis enteropathica. In *The Eye in Systemic Disease*, D.H. Gold and T.A. Weingeist (Eds.), J.B. Lippincott, Philadelphia, pp. 631–632, 1990.
14a.   Clark, J.H. The effect of parathyroid hormone on the permeability of the lens capsule to calcium. *Am. J. Physiol. 126*:136–141, 1939.
15.   Cohen, S.M., Brown, F.R., Martyn, L., Moser, H.W., Chen, W., Kistenmacher, M., Punnett, H., de la Cruz, Z.C., Chan, N.R., and Green, W.R. Ocular, histopathologic and biochemical studies of the cerebro-hepato-renal syndrome (Zellweger's syndrome) and its relationship to neonatal adrenoleukodystrophy. *Am. J. Ophthalmol. 96*:488–501, 1983.
16.   Cogan, D.G., Albright, F., and Barrter, F.C. Hypercalcemia and band keratopathy. *Arch. Ophthalmol. 40*:624–638, 1948.
17.   Dake, Y., and Amemiya, T. Electron microscopic study of the optic nerve in copper deficient rats. *Exp. Eye Res. 52*:277–281, 1991.
18.   Danks, D.M. Inborn errors of trace element metabolism. *Clin. Endocrinol. Metab. 14*:591–615, 1985.
18a.   Danks, D.M. Disorders of copper transport. In *The Metabolic Basis of Inherited Disease*, 6th ed. Vol. 1, C.R. Scriver, A.L. Beaudet, W.S. Sly, and D. Valle (Eds.), New York, McGraw-Hill, pp. 1411–1431, 1989.
19.   Danks, D.M., Campbell, P.E., Stevens, B.J., Mayne, V., and Cartwright, E. Menkes' kinky hair syndrome: An inherited defect in the intestinal absorption of copper with widespread effects. *Pediatrics 50*:188–201, 1972.

20. Danks, D.M., Tippett, P., Adams, C., and Campbell, P. Cerebro-hepato-renal syndrome of Zellweger: A report of eight cases with comments upon the incidence, the liver lesion, and a fault in pipecolic acid metabolism. *J. Pediatr.* 86:382–387, 1975.

21. Davies, G., Dymock, I., Harry, J., and Williams, R. Deposition of melanin and iron in ocular structures in haemochromatosis. *Br. J. Ophthalmol.* 56:338–342, 1972.

22. DeLuca, H.F. Recent advances in our understandings of the vitamin D endocrine system. *J. Lab. Clin. Med.* 87: 7–26, 1976.

23. Dralands, L., Evrard, P., Ponchon, P., Rommel, J., and Stanescu, B. Les complications oculaires de l'hypo-parathyroidie familiale chez l'enfant. *Bull. Soc. Belge. Ophthalmol.* 157:374–392, 1971.

24. Duke, J.R. Ocular effects of systemic siderosis in the human. *Am. J. Ophthalmol.* 44:158–172, 1957.

25. Edwards, C.Q., Carroll, M., Bray, P., and Cartwright, G.E. Hereditary hemochromatosis: Diagnosis in siblings and children. *N. Engl. J. Med.* 297:7–13, 1977.

26. Eversen, C.J., Schrader, R.E., and Wang, T.-I. Chemical and morphological changes in brains of copper deficient guinea pigs. *J. Nutr.* 96:115–125, 1968.

27. Fleisch, H., Russel, R.G.G., and Straumann, F. Effect of pyrophosphate on hydroxyapatite and its implication in calcium homeostasis. *Nature* 212:901–903, 1966.

28. Garner, A., and Fielder, A.R. Zellweger's syndrome: Cerebrohepatorenal syndrome. In *The Eye in Systemic Disease*, D.H. Gold and T.A. Weingeist (Eds.), J.B. Lippincott, Philadelphia, pp. 411–413, 1990.

29. Garner, A., Fielder, A.R., Primavesi, R., and Stevens, A. Tapetoretinal degeneration in the cerebro-hepato-renal (Zellweger's syndrome). *Br. J. Ophthalmol.* 66:422–431, 1982.

30. Geeraets, W.J. *Ocular Syndromes*, 3rd ed., Lea & Febiger, Philadelphia, p. 292, 1976.

31. Goldfischer, S., and Reddy, J.K. Peroxisomes (microbodies) in cell pathology. *Int. Rev. Exp. Pathol.* 26:45–84, 1984.

32. Gregg, J.B., and Becker, S.F. Concomitant progressive deafness, chronic nephritis, and ocular lens disease. *Ann. Ophthalmol.* 69:293–299, 1963.

33. Grover, W.E., and Scrutton, M.C. Copper infusion therapy in trichopoliodystrophy. *J. Pediatr.* 86:216–220, 1975.

34. Haddad, R., Font, R.L., and Friendly, D.S. Cerebro-hepato-renal syndrome of Zellweger. Ocular histopathologic findings. *Arch. Ophthalmol.* 94:1927–1930, 1976.

35. Hamilton, J.B. Hypoparathyroid cataract. *Trans. Asia-Pac. Acad. Ophthalmol.* 2:363–367, 1964.

36. Harris, L.S., Cohn, K., Toyofuku, H., Lonergan, E., and Galin, M.A. Conjunctival and corneal calcific deposits in uremic patients. *Am. J. Ophthalmol.* 72:130–133, 1971.

37. Harry, J., and Tripathi, R.C. Kayser-Fleischer ring: A pathological study. *Br. J. Ophthalmol.* 54:794–800, 1970.

38. Heath, P. Calcinosis oculi. *Am. J. Ophthalmol.* 54:771–781, 1962.

39. Henkin, R.I., Schechter, P.J., Hoye, R., and Mattern, C. Idiopathic hypogeusia with dysgeusia, hyposmia and dysosmia: A new syndrome. *JAMA* 217:434–440, 1971.

40. Heymans, H.S.A., Bosch, H.V.D., Schutgens, R.B.H., Tegelaers, W.H., Walther, J.U., Muller-Hocker, J., and Borst, P. Deficiency of plasmalogens in the cerebro-hepato-renal (Zellweger) syndrome. *Eur. J. Pediatr.* 142: 10–15, 1984.

41. Hiatt, R.L. Menkes' kinky hair syndrome. In *The Eye in Systemic Disease*, D.H. Gold and T.A. Weingeist (Eds.), J.B. Lippincott, Philadelphia, pp. 388–390, 1990.

42. Hittner, H.M., Kretzer, F.L., and Mehta, R.S. Zellweger syndrome: Lenticular opacities indicating carrier status and lens abnormalities characteristic of heterozygotes. *Arch. Ophthalmol.* 99:1977–1982, 1981.

43. Hudson, J.R. Ocular findings in haemochromatosis. *Br. J. Ophthalmol.* 37:242–246, 1953.

44. Johnson, R.E., and Campbell, R.J. Wilson's disease: Electron microscopic, x-ray energy spectroscopic, and atomic absorption spectroscopic studies of corneal copper deposition and distribution. *Lab. Invest.* 46:564–569, 1982.

45. Kelley, R.I. Review: The cerebro-hepato-renal syndrome of Zellweger, morphologic and metabolic aspects. *Am. J. Med. Genet.* 16:503–517, 1983.

46. Klaassen-Broeckema, N., and Bijsterveld, O.P. Red eyes in renal failure. *Br. J. Ophthalmol.* 76:268–271, 1992.

47. LaBadie, G.U., Hirschhorn, K., Katz, S., and Beratis, N.G. Increased copper metallothionein in Menkes' cultured skin fibroblasts. *Pediatr. Res.* 15:257–261, 1981.

48. De Léon, G.A., Grover, W.D., Huff, D.S., Morinigo-Mestre, G., Punnett, H.H., and Kistenmacher, M.L. Globoid cells, glial nodules, and peculiar fibrillary changes in the cerebro-hepato-renal syndrome of Zellweger. *Ann. Neurol.* 2:473–484, 1977.

49. Lessel, S., and Norton, E.W.D. Band keratopathy and conjunctival calcification in hypophosphatasia. *Arch. Ophthalmol.* 71:497–499, 1964.

50. Levy, N.S., Dawson, W.W., Rhodes, B.J., and Garnica, A. Ocular abnormalities in Menkes' kinky-hair syndrome. *Am. J. Ophthalmol.* 77:319–325, 1974.

51. McDonnell, P.J., Green, W.R., and Schanzlin, D.J. Alport's syndrome. In *The Eye in Systemic Disease*, D.H. Gold and T.A. Weingeist (Eds.), J.B. Lippincott, Philadelphia, pp. 499–502, 1990.

52. Matta, C.S., Felker, G.V., and Ide, C.H. Eye manifestations in acrodermatitis enteropathica. *Arch. Ophthalmol.* 93:140–142, 1975.

53. Menkes, J.H., Alter, M., Stiegleder, G.K., Weakley, D.R., and Sung, J.H. A sex-linked recessive disorder with retardation of growth, peculiar hair and focal cerebral and cerebellar degeneration. *Pediatrics* 29:764–779, 1962.

54. Monnens, L., Bakkeren, J., Parmentier, G., Janssen, G., van Haelst, U., Trijbels, F., and Eyssen, H. Disturbances in bile acid metabolism of infants with the Zellweger (cerebro-hepato-renal) syndrome. *Eur. J. Pediatr. 133*:31–35, 1980.
55. Moynahan, E.J., and Barnes, P.M. Zinc deficiency and a synthetic diet for lactose intolerance. *Lancet 1*:676–677, 1973.
56. Opitz, J.M., ZuRhein, G.M., Vitale, L., Shahidi, N.T., Howe, J.J., Chou, S.M., Shanklin, D.R., Sybers, H.D., Dood, A.R., and Gerritsen, T. The Zellweger syndrome (cerebro-hepato-renal syndrome). *Birth Defects 5*(2):144–158, 1969.
57. Passarge, E., and McAdams, A.J. Cerebro-hepato-renal syndrome. *J. Pediatr. 71*:691–702, 1967.
58. Patton, R.G., Christie, D.L., Smith, D.W., and Beckwith, J.B. Cerebro-hepato-renal syndrome of Zellweger: Two patients with islet cell hyperplasia, hypoglycemia, and thymic anomalies, and comments on iron metabolism. *Am. J. Dis. Child. 124*:840–844, 1972.
59. Pahjola, S. Ocular manifestations of idiopathic hypoparathyroidism: Case report and review of literature. *Acta Ophthalmol. (Copenh.) 40*:255–265, 1962.
60. Porter, R., and Crombie, A.L.I. Corneal and conjunctival calcification in chronic renal failure. *Br. J. Ophthalmol. 57*:339–343, 1975.
61. Racz, P., Kovacs, B., Varga, L., Vjlaki, E., Zombai, E., and Karbuckzy, S. Bilateral cataract in acrodermatitis enteropathica. *J. Pediatr. Ophthalmol. Strabismus 16*:180–182, 1979.
62. Roth, A.M., and Foos, R.Y. Ocular pathologic changes in primary hemochromatosis. *Arch. Ophthalmol. 87*:507–514, 1972.
63. Santos, M.J., Ojeda, J.M., Garrido, J., and Leighton, F. Peroxisomal organization in normal and cerebrohepatorenal (Zellweger) syndrome fibroblasts. *Proc. Natl. Acad. Sci. USA 82*:6556–6500, 1985.
64. Sass-Kortsak, A., and Bearn, A.G. Hereditary disorders of copper metabolism. In *The Metabolic Basis of Inherited Disease*, J.B. Stanbury, J.B. Wyngaarden, and D.S. Fredrickson (Eds.), McGraw-Hill, New York, pp. 1098–1126, 1978.
65. Scadding, J.F. *Sarcoidosis*, Eyre & Spottiswoode, London, 1967.
66. Schutgens, R.B.H., Heymans, H.S.A., Wanders, R.J.A., Bosch, H.V.D., and Tager, J.M. Peroxisomal disorders: A newly recognized group of genetic diseases. *Eur. J. Pediatr. 144*:430–440, 1986.
67. Seelenfreund, M.H., Gartner, S., and Vinger, F. The ocular pathology of Menkes' disease. *Arch. Ophthalmol. 80*:718–720, 1968.
68. Shimozawa, N., Tsukamoto, T., Suzuki, Y., Orii, T., Shirayoshi, T., Mori, T., and Fujuki, Y. A human gene responsible for Zellweger syndrome that affects peroxisome assembly. *Science 255*:1132–1134, 1992.
69. Smith, D.W., Opitz, J.M., and Inhorn, S.L. A syndrome of multiple developmental defects including polycystic kidneys and intrahepatic biliary dysgenesis in two siblings. *J. Pediatr. 67*:617–624, 1965.
70. Sommer, A., Bradel, E.J., and Hamondi, A.B. The cerebro-hepato-renal syndrome (Zellweger's syndrome). *Biol. Neonate 25*:219–229, 1974.
71. Stanescu, B., and Dralands, L. Cerebro-hepato-renal (Zellweger's) syndrome. *Arch. Ophthalmol. 87*:590–592, 1972.
72. Strickland, G.T., Beckner, W.M., Leu, M.L., and O'Reilly, S. Turnover studies of copper in homozygotes and heterozygotes for Wilson's disease and controls: Isotope tracer studies with ^{67}Cu. *Clin. Sci. 43*:605–615, 1972.
73. Sunderman, F.W. Current status of zinc deficiency in the pathogenesis of neurological, dermatological and musculoskeletal disorders. *Am. Clin. Lab. Sci. 5*:132–145, 1975.
74. Tripathi, R.C., and Ashton, N. Application of electron microscopy to the study of ocular inborn errors of metabolism. In *The Eye and Inborn Errors of Metabolism*, D. Bergsma, A.J. Bron, and E. Cotlier (Eds.), Alan R. Liss, New York, pp. 69–104, 1976.
75. Tso, M.O.M., Fine, B.S., and Thorpe, H.E. Kayser-Fleischer ring and associated cataract in a case of Wilson's disease. *Am. J. Ophthalmol. 79*:479–488, 1975.
76. Urrets-Zavalia, A., and Katz, C. Corneal hemochromatosis: A unique type of corneal dystrophy involving the anterior stroma and both limiting membranes. *Am. J. Ophthalmol. 72*:88–96, 1971.
77. Uzman, L.L., and Jakus, M.A. The Kayser-Fleischer ring: A histochemical and electron microscope study. *Neurology 7*:341–355, 1957.
78. Vitale, L., Opitz, J.M., and Shahidi, N.T. Congenital and familial iron overload. *N. Engl. J. Med. 280*:642–645, 1969.
79. Volpe, J.J., and Adams, R.D. Cerebro-hepato-renal syndrome of Zellweger: An inherited disorder of neuronal migration. *Acta Neuropathol. (Berl.) 20*:175–198, 1972.
80. Walshe, J.M. The eye in Wilson's disease. In *The Eye and Errors of Metabolism*, D. Bergsma, A.J. Bron, and E. Cotlier (Eds.), Alan R. Liss, New York, pp. 187–189, 1976.
81. Warshawsky, R.S., Hill, C.W., Doughman, D.J., and Harris, J.E. Acrodermatitis enteropathica: Corneal involvement with histochemical and electron microscopic studies. *Arch. Ophthalmol. 93*:194–197, 1975.
82. Wiebers, D.O., Hollenhorst, R.W., and Goldstein, P. The ophthalmologic manifestations of Wilson's disease. *Mayo Clin. Proc. 52*:409–416, 1977.
83. Wirsching, L. Eye symptoms in acrodermatitis enteropathica. *Acta Ophthalmol. (Copenh.) 40*:567–574, 1962.
84. Wray, S.H., Kuwabara, T., and Sanderson, P. Menkes' kinky hair disease: A light- and electron-microscopic study of the eye. *Invest. Ophthalmol. 15*:128–138, 1976.

38
Vitamin Deficiencies and Excesses

Gordon K. Klintworth
Duke University Medical Center, Durham, North Carolina

I. INTRODUCTION

Since the early years of this century it has been known that a diet containing purified fats, proteins, carbohydrates, and salts is insufficient to maintain experimental animals in healthy life, however liberally it is supplied. This observation eventually resulted in the discovery of the vitamins and the recognition that several ocular abnormalities result from vitamin deficiencies and excesses. Malnutrition and its consequences are a major global problem, particularly in the developing parts of the world, where the diet is inadequate for several reasons (climate, ignorance, primitive agricultural methods, poverty, lack of imported foods, and food taboos) [45]. Human vitamin deficiencies are usually associated with an inadequate intake of essential amino acids and protein, rarely limited to a single vitamin.

Vitamins play a crucial role in many metabolic reactions, and a deficiency of a specific vitamin at critical times during intrauterine development results in congenital anomalies in experimental animals. The timing, duration, and severity of the deficiency are related to the anomalies produced. Of the vitamins, only vitamin A and nicotinic acid have been found to be teratogenic in excess.

The biological effects of different vitamins are often interrelated. For example, subjects with elevated plasma levels of at least two of three antioxidant vitamins (vitamin E, vitamin C, and carotenoids) are at reduced risk of cataracts compared to individuals with low levels of one or more of these vitamins.

II. VITAMIN A

A. General Remarks

The designation "vitamin A" refers to the fat-soluble unsaturated 20-carbon cyclic colorless compounds that exhibit the biological activity of retinoids [11]. Vitamin A is mainly derived from preformed vitamin A in animal foods or from β-carotene in green plants. Vitamin A, which is produced only in animals, plays an important role in numerous biological processes, including vision, reproduction, and the maintenance of the epithelial and osseous tissues [54,130].

The small intestine absorbs both retinyl esters from animal tissues and provitamin A carotenoids from vegetables by diffusion at sites where lipid is taken up [55,161]. Retinyl esters are enzymatically converted to retinol in the lumen of the intestine and then absorbed by intestinal cells (enterocytes) [55,161]. Within the walls of the small intestine β-carotene and other carotenoids are cleaved by an oxygenase to form retinal (vitamin A aldehyde) [107], which becomes converted to the free alcohol (retinol, or vitamin A alcohol). By a different metabolic pathway retinal can also be irreversibly oxidized to retinoic acid (Fig. 1) [38]. Within the enterocytes retinyl esters are formed by a reaction of retinol with long-chain fatty acids, such as palmitic acid, and then become incorporated into chylomicrons. The esterification of retinol within the intestine involves acyl coenzyme A:retinol acyl transferase [68,69] and lecithin:retinol acyltransferase

1147

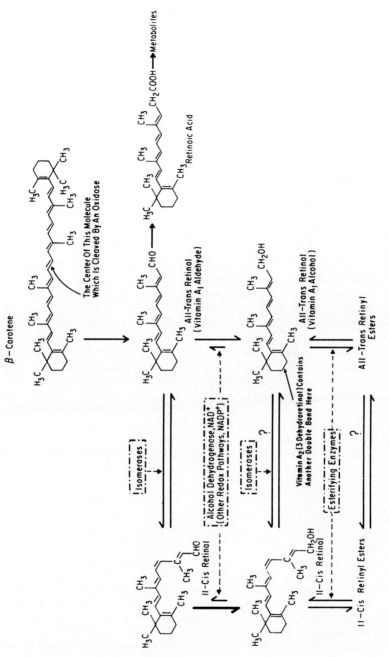

Figure 1 Metabolic pathways of vitamin A and related compounds.

[93,109]. Within the enterocytes retinol becomes bound to the intestinal intracytoplasmic retinol binding protein.

Vitamin A_1 (retinol), with its four unsaturated bonds, is transported in the plasma as chylomicrons mainly to the liver, where it is stored in relatively large quantities, mainly as retinyl palmitate, within lipid droplets of specialized stellate cells [70,85,146]. Of the total vitamin A content of the body, 70–95% is stored in the liver [158], which normally contains sufficient vitamin A to maintain an individual's nutritional needs for nearly a year. The level of retinol in cells may be controlled to some extent through membrane receptors or by excretion from the cell.

Retinol is transported in the plasma by a special retinol binding protein (molecular mass about 21 kD) associated with an acid protein (transthyretin; see Chap. 32) [111]. Normally the plasma retinol binding protein is almost saturated with retinol [102,144].

Retinoic acid, the most potent of the retinoids [138], modulates the expression of numerous proteins and gene transcription factors by interacting with specific receptors (retinoic acid receptors, RAR) inducing the transactivation of genes that possess retinoic acid response elements (RARE) [88]. The RAR include (1) RARα, which belongs to the family of steroid-thyroid hormone receptors and binds with high affinity to 13-*cis*-retinoic acid, all-*trans*-retinoic acid, and other differentiation effective retinoids; (2) RARβ; (3) RARγ, which is found almost exclusively in skin; and (4) RxARα, a nuclear retinoic acid receptor.

Numerous tissues, including the retina (amacrine neurons and, in some species, Müller cells) also contain intracytoplasmic receptor proteins that bind retinoids, retinol, and retinoic acids [40,106,108,152]. After cellular uptake retinol can be oxidized to retinoic acid, which diffuses into the nucleus and binds there to a nuclear RAR. All nuclear RAR appear to be ligand-dependent transcription factors that regulate gene expression by interacting with RARE in the vicinity of target genes.

B. Vitamin A and Vision

Vitamin A plays a crucial role in the vision of all species [18]. Under the influence of light, rhodopsin engages in a cycle of reactions with retinal (retinene, or vitamin A aldehyde) and retinol (vitamin A alcohol; Fig. 2) [128,147].

All visual pigments consist of vitamin A aldehyde (retinal) bound as a chromophore to opsin, a protein found in the outer segments of the photoreceptors. Opsins vary in rods and cones and are of two main types in the human: rod opsin and cone opsin, of which there are three kinds. Opsins trap retinal as quickly as it appears to form the visual pigments [147]. Retinol is oxidized to the corresponding retinal by alcohol dehydrogenases, which employ various coenzymes, such as nicotinamide adenine dinucleotide (NAD^+) or nicotinamide adenine dinucleotide phosphate ($NADP^+$). Because of the double bonds in the side chain of vitamin A, various geometrical confirmations of retinal and retinol are possible. The 11-cis isomer of retinal is found in rhodopsin, whereas the more stable configuration is all-trans retinal (Fig. 1). The only known action of light in vision is the isomerization of retinal from the 11-cis to the all-trans configuration [73,86]. 11-Cis-retinal is stable in the dark, but when visual pigment is bleached by light the retinal that

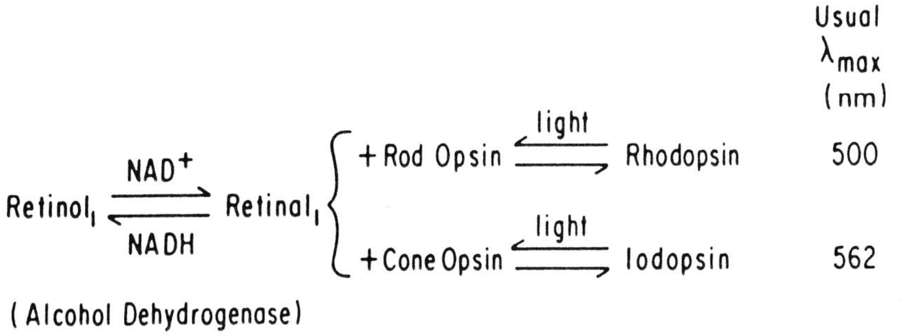

Figure 2 Light-induced reactions with visual pigments. (Modified from G. Wald. Molecular basis of visual excitation. *Science 162*:230–239, 1968.)

emerges within isolated retinal outer segments is all-trans and cannot combine with opsin to regenerate visual pigment [147].

The dark-adapted eye contains vitamin A in the rod outer segments [16], predominantly in the form of retinol, but stores most of the vitamin within the retinal pigment epithelium (RPE), where the vitamin is virtually all esterified and stored in microsomes or lipid droplets. Microsomes isolated from the RPE rapidly convert retinol into retinyl ester [9]. If contact with the RPE is maintained, most of retinol leaves the rod outer segments to become esterified and accumulate in the all-trans retinyl ester in the oil droplets of the RPE [16].

Lipid droplets in the RPE appear to be a physiological storage site of retinyl esters. Retinyl acetate is taken up into lipid droplets of the RPE, and these lipid droplets increase in number following injections of retinyl acetate or retinal palmitate (but not retinoic acid) [125]. Retinol has specific receptors in the RPE [153], where it becomes esterified, stored, and mobilized when needed [16,17,162]. Receptor sites for plasma retinol binding protein seem to be distributed along the basal and lateral surfaces of RPE cells [13]. Peroxisomes, cell organelles that contain catalase, often occur in close proximity to lipid droplets and may be involved in reactions that remove retinal from the plasma and esterify it [89,125].

C. Other Functions of Vitamin A

The role of vitamin A in epithelial cells is not clearly understood. Vitamin A causes a striking decrease in the production of fucose-containing glycopeptides, and it may have a direct action on the mannose-carrying lipid intermediary in glycoprotein synthesis [31]. This is supported by the finding of a diminution of specific glycoproteins in the corneal epithelium of vitamin A-deficient rats [84]. Mucous metaplasia can be induced with vitamin A [3,77]. Retinoic acid or some metabolite of vitamin A [24] may act as a regulatory molecule to transform undifferentiated epithelial cells into mucus-secreting cells. This possibility is supported by the finding that the addition of retinyl acetate to cell cultures of epidermis leads to an increase in cellular RNA [137] and that this effect is enhanced by the addition of insulin and glucocorticoids. It is plausible that these regulatory functions involve control of the transcription of the RNA and hence "turn on" or "turn off" genes specifying particular proteins.

Vitamin A lyses lysosomes in vitro [34], and rabbits are depleted of lysosomes by treatment with vitamin A [151]. Vitamin A and its analogs (retinoids) have a preventive and therapeutic effect on several experimental tumors in vivo [136]. Under some conditions, however, high doses of vitamin A may enhance tumor production by chemical carcinogens [90,122] and oncogenic viruses [116].

The possibility that carotenoids may protect against human cortical cataracts is raised by a study that found a reduced risk of cortical cataract in the presence of elevated serum carotenoids [78].

D. Vitamin A Deficiency

In most developed countries vitamin A requirements are satisfactorily met, but cases of deficiency sometimes occur, especially in newborns and pregnant and nursing women, whose nutritional needs are greatest.

In large areas of the world vitamin A deficiency remains endemic and continues to be a major cause of visual disability and mortality [119,134,142]. Estimates predict that more than 5 million children develop xerophthalmia annually and that a quarter million or more become blind from the effects of vitamin A deficiency. It is also a major pathway for measles-associated blindness, particularly in Africa [135].

Vitamin A deficiency can result from an inadequate intake, faulty absorption (as in sprue, celiac disease, cystic fibrosis, and other conditions causing steatorrhea) and less often from defective storage (as in liver disease). Healthy humans on a diet deficient in vitamin A and carotenoids develop evidence of the deficiency after time periods ranging from a few weeks to about a year.

Manifestations of vitamin A deficiency include cessation of growth, night blindness, and an increased susceptibility to infection. Epidemiological studies have shown an inverse relationship between cancer risk and vitamin A consumption, and much has been written about retinoids and neoplasms and about the ability of retinoids to modify cellular differentiation and proliferation [99,130].

The levels in the blood of retinol, retinol binding protein, and transthyretin are directly related. If malnourished children, who are deficient in vitamin A, are given vitamin A parenterally, the serum retinol binding protein does not increase for 24 h [133]. On the other hand, when protein and vitamin A are given to children with kwashiorkor or marasmus, the serum levels of retinol binding protein, transthyretin, and vitamin A all increase [132]. These observations point to an impaired hepatic release of vitamin A rather than to an actual vitamin A deficiency.

Rats deprived of vitamin A but fed retinoic acid become blind and sterile but otherwise appear healthy [132]. Evidently retinol or retinal functions in vision and reproduction whereas the maintenance of mucous secretions and some other functions of vitamin A requires only retinoic acid [24]. Giving retinoic acid to rats on a diet deficient in vitamin A and in carotenoids prevents all the signs of vitamin A deficiency, including the external ocular changes, except night blindness [38].

Retina

Ocular manifestations are an important clinical feature of vitamin A deficiency, and a rise in the visual threshold is the first sign of a deficiency of this vitamin [148], because the deficiency causes a failure of the formation of rhodopsin from retinal and the protein opsin. Initially the time required for dark adaptation increases, and eventually night blindness (nyctalopia) ensues as a result impaired function of the retinal rods. The cone function is also affected, but this is less apparent clinically.

Biochemical, morphological, and physiological changes occur in the retina of vitamin A-deficient animals. In rats on a vitamin A-deficient diet, the first sign of the deficiency is a rise in the threshold for eliciting the electroretinogram (ERG), and by 4–5 weeks [38,106] the level of rhodopsin within the retina is decreased. By 10 minutes no response can be elicited from the retinas of vitamin A-deficient rats [38]. Morphological alterations in the retina have been extensively studied in rats, and after 2 months of retinol deficiency the outer segments of the rods start to degenerate [37].

Structural degenerative alterations occur in the outer and inner segments of the retina [36,37,63] as well as in the photoreceptor nuclei [37,38,123]. These changes are accompanied by a loss of rhodopsin [23]. Some investigators have found opsin to decrease at a slower rate [23], but others maintain that the opsin density in the outer segments is unaffected [82]. The RPE remains more or less structurally normal, but the lipid droplets appear abnormal by transmission electron microscopy [23] and accumulate substantially fewer lipofuscin granules than non–vitamin A-deprived rats [83]. In vitamin A-deficient animals the lipid droplets appear homogeneous; in control animals the droplets are less homogeneous and often contain electron-lucent spots [23]. This appearance may relate to stored vitamin A or its metabolites, since similar lipid droplets form in mice receiving injections of vitamin A [125]. Rods degenerate earlier and with a strikingly greater susceptibility than cones, perhaps because of metabolic differences [23]. The first discernible morphological abnormality detectable at 7 weeks consists of a less intense staining of the distal two-thirds of the outer segments with toluidine blue [23]. After 16 weeks on a vitamin A-deficient diet some disks become distended, with small vesicles (0.19–0.35 μm in diameter), and the normal intimate contact between the RPE and the outer segments is destroyed.

Tadpoles born of vitamin A-deprived mothers and subsequently raised on a vitamin A-free diet sometimes manifest the vitamin deficiency, including impairment of the light-induced electrical response (b wave of the ERG). Morphological alterations in the rods of these animals are surprisingly subtle and consist of notching of the plasma membrane and, in some instances, invasion of the interdisk space by wedge-shaped clusters of vesicles [159]. In insects the biochemical events in vision are similar to those in vertebrates, and vitamin A deficiency causes a decreased visual sensitivity and morphological changes in the eyes [15].

Conjunctiva and Cornea

In vitamin A deficiency the epithelia of the skin and mucous membranes, including the ocular surface, thicken and keratinize. The designation "xerophthalmia" refers to the external ocular manifestations observed in vitamin A deficiency (xerosis of the conjunctiva and cornea, Bitot's spot, and keratomalacia). Xerophthalmia is prevalent in many parts of the world and progresses through several recognized stages: conjunctival xerosis (stage 1A), Bitot's spots with conjunctival xerosis (stage 1B), corneal xerosis (stage 2), corneal ulceration with xerosis (stage 3A), and keratomalacia (stage 3B) [114].

The conjunctiva becomes dry, opaque, thickened, wrinkled, and sometimes pigmented. This conjunctival xerosis is often followed by the appearance of small, variably shaped refractile plaques in the superficial bulbar conjunctiva (Bitot's spots). These lesions are usually bilateral, in the exposed interpalpebral fissure at the corneoscleral limbus and especially on the temporal side of the eye. Bitot's spots often have a silver-gray hue and foamy surface and usually occur in young children with night blindness. The foamy appearance is thought to be due to infection with *Corynebacterium xerosis*.

Xerosis of both corneas follows conjunctival xerosis and is characterized by corneal surfaces that lack the normal luster and have a fine, pebbly appearance. The dry corneas become keratinized and are prone to bacterial infection and ulceration. Such cloudy corneas often undergo a characteristic rapidly progressive, usually bilateral, corneal softening (keratomalacia), which results in partial or complete corneal perforation and the transformation of the cornea into a cloudy gelatinous mass. In developing countries this devastating keratomalacia is a major cause of blindness in young children and is usually associated with generalized malnutrition and infections, such as measles. Babies born of severely malnourished mothers sometimes have congenital keratomalacia. Since keratomalacia is not a feature of vitamin A deficiency in adults, vitamin A deficiency alone may not be responsible for the condition, but laboratory animals deficient from weaning solely in vitamin A and its precursor β-carotene develop all the manifestations of xerophthalmia, ending with perforation of the cornea and phthisis bulbi [114].

A collagenolytic system exists in xerophthalmic corneas [115]. Polymorphonuclear leukocytes (PMNs) infiltrate the ulcerating corneas extensively before the capillary invasion and perforation [114], suggesting that enzymes responsible for the melting could be contained in PMNs. This possibility is supported by the fact that PMNs contain several proteolytic enzymes.

In vitamin A-deficient animals the conjunctival goblet cells disappear [35,79,141,160] and the corneal and conjunctival epithelial cells lose the normal surface microprojections and become keratinized [7,160]. These changes and the desquamating superficial epithelial cells are dramatically illustrated by scanning electron microscopy [112]. Sometimes the corneal stroma becomes invaded by leukocytes [86] and vascularizes [160]. In some [7,79] but not other [112,160] experimental studies, corneal ulcers and keratomalacia have developed. Unlike the retinal abnormalities, the lesions in the conjunctiva and cornea of vitamin A-deficient animals are prevented by retinoic acid [37].

E. Vitamin A and Carotenoid Excess

Excessive ingestion of vegetables containing carotenoids over prolonged periods may result in the deposition of yellow pigment in the skin (carotenosis), beginning in the nasolabial folds and palms of the hands but, in contrast to jaundice, not in the conjunctiva. Excessive vitamin A intake results in benign intracranial hypertension (pseudotumor cerebri) and papilledema [42].

F. Vitamin A and Developmental Anomalies

Maternal vitamin A deficiency may cause fetal anophthalmia or xerophthalmia. Ocular and various systemic malformations develop in the offspring of vitamin A-deficient pigs [58], rats [76,157], hamsters [129], and rabbits [87]. The malformations include anophthalmia, microphthalmia, absence of the anterior chamber, iris, and ciliary body, colobomas and disorganization of the retina, failure or impairment of vitreous formation with the development in its place of fibrous retrolental membranes, and failure of the embryonic eyelids to fuse (the so-called congenital open eye). In calves blindness may follow constriction of the optic nerve caused by anomalous growth of the skeleton [100]. In the rat, the offspring born of vitamin A-deficient mothers may manifest abnormalities that resemble in some respects the retinopathy of prematurity. The abnormality varies considerably in degree in different lines [150], but approximately 75% of the offspring of female rats fed vitamin A-deficient diets before or during pregnancy develop ocular anomalies [149].

Hypervitaminosis A during pregnancy is teratogenic, some of its adverse effects reflecting an interference of crest cell migration [118]. Some of the defects of mandibulofacial dysostosis (Treacher Collins syndrome) develop in all offspring of pregnant rats given excess vitamin A at day 8.5 of gestation. Such treatment destroys neural crest cells of the facial and auditory primordia that normally migrate to the first and second branchial arches. The otomandibular defects thus produced are identical to those in humans with mandibulofacial dysostosis [117,118].

Embryos exposed to high levels of retinoids, such as vitamin A and retinoic acid, develop characteristic malformations of several structures, including the eye [4,52]. The pathogenesis of the ocular deformities, which include anophthalmos, microphthalmos, retinal defects, and cataract, remains unknown, but their incidence varies with the time of gestation at which the vitamin is administered [8,47,52,129].

An attempt has been made to mimic retinoid-induced teratogenesis in transgenic mice by linking a constitutively active retinoic acid receptor to the αA-crystallin promoter, which targets expression of the genes in the crystallin lens. The ocular lens in these transgenic mice express the active retinoic acid receptor but also manifest cataracts in association with microphthalmia [4].

III. VITAMIN B COMPLEX

A. General Remarks

The vitamin B complex comprises several independent water-soluble substances (thiamine, riboflavin, nicotinic acid, pantothenic acid, pyridoxine, choline, biotin, inositol, *para*-aminobenzoic acid, folic acid, and cyanocobalamin). Deficiencies of many of these vitamins produce ocular lesions in experimental animals, and deficiencies of some are suspected of causing ophthalmic manifestations in humans. It is noteworthy that the normal lens contains excessive amounts of inositol, but the significance of this is not known (see Chap. 18).

B. Vitamin B$_1$ (Thiamine)

A deficiency of thiamine (vitamin B$_1$), which in its phosphorylated form acts as a coenzyme (cocarboxylase) for the decarboxylation of pyruvate, leads to beriberi and Wernicke's syndrome (ophthalmoplegia, ataxia, and mental confusion). A peripheral neuropathy is a frequent complication of beriberi, especially of the chronic form. In beriberi, bilateral optic neuritis may occur and diffuse demyelination of the optic nerve has been observed postmortem [94]. Patchy demyelinization of the optic nerves and tracts has also been documented in thiamine-deficient rats [127]. The prominent nystagmus and ophthalmoplegia of Wernicke's encephalopathy result from lesions in the brain, and disturbances of vision are attributed to involvement of visual pathways. The optic chiasm may be severely gliosed [96], and the optic nerves may also be affected [20].

C. Vitamin B$_2$ (Riboflavin)

Riboflavin, a yellow pigment, is a precursor of flavin mononucleotide (FMN) and flavin adenine dinucleotide (FAD), coenzymes in several oxidation-reduction reactions involved in electron transfer [72,95,101]. Electrons are transferred from NADH to FMN during the chain of reactions in which these negatively charged particles are passed to oxygen.

The flavins are widely distributed throughout the body. Although present in various ocular structures, riboflavin, FMN, and FAD are abundant in several tissues of the eye and its adnexa [6,113]. In cattle they are most copious in the lacrimal and meibomian glands, and the corneal epithelium contains much more riboflavin than the corneal stroma or the aqueous [113]. In all rabbit ocular tissues the primary flavin is FAD, followed by FMN and riboflavin. The ratio of the flavins varies in different tissues. In the rabbit the FAD/FMN/riboflavin ratio has been found to be 6:2:1 in cornea, 42:3:1 in lens cortex, 68:3:1 in lens nucleus, and 49:13:1 in retina [6]. In the rabbit the cornea has the highest concentration of riboflavin, followed by retina, lens cortex, and lens nucleus [6], but FAD and FMN are present in highest concentration in the retina, followed by cornea and lens [6].

The flavins are light sensitive, and they rapidly degrade following exposure to visible or near ultraviolet light, producing inactive and toxic products [60,131]. Riboflavin-sensitized production of hydrogen peroxide has been demonstrated in the presence of light and oxygen, suggesting that the photooxidation is through a type I mechanism.

A deficiency of riboflavin becomes first manifest clinically in parts of the body exposed to ambient light, namely the skin and eye. Features of riboflavin deficiency include corneal vascularization, photophobia, angular stomatitis, seborrheic dermatitis, and growth retardation [53]. Studies in riboflavin-deficient rats have disclosed corneal vascularization [10,14], and cataracts have been a feature of some [28,67] but not all of such animals [10]. Cataracts and keratitis have also been produced in salmon [59] and rabbit [75] fed a riboflavin-deficient diet. Cataracts, but not corneal vascularization, have been documented in riboflavin-deficient mice [91], pigs [97], cats [48], monkeys [27,145], and chicks [29]. The possibility of riboflavin deficiency producing cataracts in humans has been raised on nebulous grounds [121]. Other lesions noted in experimental animals include angular blepharoconjunctivitis, "spectacle eye," keratitis, conjunctivitis, and optic atrophy.

The offspring of rodents on a riboflavin-deficient diet [57] or treated with the antimetabolite galacto-flavin [81,103] develop ocular anomalies, such as microphthalmos, anophthalmos, colobomas of the iris, and congenital "open eyes."

Excessively high doses of riboflavin are harmful. An increased fragility of the photoreceptor outer segments has been reported in normal Royal College of Surgeons rats maintained on a high dose [39]. Following the ingestion of a lethal dose, riboflavin crystallizes in the kidney and death ensues from renal failure [25,92].

D. Vitamin B$_{12}$ (Cyanocobalamin)

Addisonian pernicious anemia, in which the gastric mucosa is atrophic, is by far the most common cause of cyanocobalamin deficiency. Amblyopia may be an early indication of vitamin B$_{12}$ deficiency, and Heaton and colleagues [66] found the serum level of this vitamin to be lower than normal in 13 patients suffering from tobacco amblyopia. Freeman and Heaton [46] suggested that the optic atrophy and "retrobulbar neuritis" sometimes found in addisonian pernicious anemia may be tobacco amblyopia due to cyanide intoxication. This possibility is reinforced by evidence of a link between vitamin B$_{12}$ and the metabolism and detoxification of cyanide [155,156]. Some ocular manifestations of vitamin B$_{12}$ deficiency, such as retinal hemorrhages and cotton-wool spots, are probably a sequel to severe anemia.

Ocular developmental malformations (microphthalmos, anophthalmos, distortion of lens and retina, colobomas, decreased size of optic cup, and extension of everted retinal tissue into the optic nerve) have been reported in the offspring of vitamin B$_{12}$-deficient animals [57].

E. Folic Acid

Rats maintained on a folic acid-deficient diet give birth to pups with deformities of the eye (retinal colobomata, retinal folds, and lenticular abnormalities), face, and body or do not have viable embryos [50]. Deficiencies of folic acid and folate antagonists can also produce anophthalmos, microphthalmos, cataract, and coloboma [1].

F. Pantothenic Acid

Anophthalmia or microphthalmia occur in the offspring of pantothenic acid-deficient rats as well as of rats given an antimetabolite to pantothenic acid [12,49,51,104]. A deficiency of this vitamin, which is part of coenzyme A, appears to interfere with the normal inductive process because the telencephalon of the brain fails to divide into two hemispheres and give rise to optic cups [38].

G. Nutritional Amblyopia

A gradual impairment of central vision commonly develops along with other signs of malnutrition in malnourished individuals of all ages. This entity, designated nutritional amblyopia, was frequently observed among the World War II prisoners of war, especially in those maintained on deficient diets. Although the amblyopia is reversible in the early stages, it may become permanent. Impaired vision served by the papillomacular bundle results in central or paracentral scotomas, and fundoscopy discloses pallor of the temporal portions of the optic disks. In a postmortem study of 11 former prisoners of war with nutritional amblyopia, Fisher [44] observed degeneration of the papillomacular bundles in four cases.

The cause of nutritional amblyopia, which is generally associated with a deficiency of multiple essential nutrients, remains unknown, but a deficiency of one or more members of the vitamin B complex is believed to be particularly important. Some investigations consider thiamine to be important [147], but others disagree [32]. Many individuals with this ocular abnormality have a histamine-fast achlorhydria, but the extreme rarity of the condition in persons with true pernicious anemia mitigates against this association.

The so-called tobacco-alcohol amblyopia may be a variant of nutritional amblyopia (see Chap. 39) [22]. Folate deficiency is common in patients with tobacco-alcohol amblyopia, but the role of folic acid in this disorder has been underappreciated. The role of cyanide from tobacco smoke, folate, and other dietary deficiencies in tobacco-alcohol amblyopia is reviewed by Dang [26]. A new hypothesis of the pathogenesis of the amblyopia presumes an alteration of methionine and S-adenosyl-L-methionine metabolism.

IV. VITAMIN C (ASCORBIC ACID)

Only the human and the guinea pig are known to require ascorbic acid in the diet; other species are able to synthesize this compound. The amount of ascorbic acid in different tissues varies considerably among species. the lens has a high concentration, and its cortex has a higher level than the nucleus. Of the ocular constituents, however, the corneal epithelium contains the greatest concentration of vitamin C, and this almost reaches the high values normally found in the adrenal and pituitary glands [65].

Ascorbic acid, which is reversibly oxidized in the body to ascorbone (dehydroascorbic "acid"), plays an important role in maintaining connective tissues [56,124], being necessary for the hydroxylation of procollagen [5]. In addition to its well-established reducing properties, ascorbic acid is a weak acid with metal-complexing attributes: in the presence of ferric ions it promotes the generation of free radicals. High levels of ascorbic acid in guinea pigs lead to more rapid wound healing [62].

Hemorrhages caused by the increased capillary fragility is a prominent feature of scurvy, the disorder caused by a deficiency of ascorbic acid, and petechiae or larger hemorrhages can occur in the conjunctiva, eyelids, orbit, anterior chamber, vitreous, or other ocular structures [61]. It is noteworthy that despite the normal high concentration of ascorbic acid in the lens of many species, including the human, cataracts are not a feature of natural or experimentally produced scurvy.

In scorbutic guinea pigs intercellular edema of the corneal epithelium has been observed [140], and heat-induced corneal vascularization appears to be more easily produced in scorbutic than in healthy animals [21].

V. OTHER VITAMINS

A. Vitamin D (Calciferol)

The principal function of vitamin D is in the control of calcium metabolism, and this is accomplished through the mediation of polar hydroxylated metabolites, the most polar being 1,30,31-trihydroxy-cholecalciferol [30]. Both 1,25-dihydroxycholecalciferol and the trihydroxy derivative act on the intestinal mucosa to increase the uptake of calcium ions. A deficiency of vitamin D leads to rickets or osteomalacia, and although significant ocular manifestations are not produced, proptosis may be associated with deformities of the skull.

An excess ingestion of vitamin D causes hypercalcemia, and calcium often deposits in the conjunctiva and cornea to produce calcific band keratopathy (see Chap. 23). Corneal calcification can be induced experimentally in rabbits with vitamin D (see Chap. 23).

B. Vitamin E Family (Tocopherols)

Vitamin E (α-tocopherol), which was first recognized as a factor preventing sterility in rats, is a powerful antioxidant for unsaturated lipids and protects lipid membranes from attack by free radicals [98]. Small amounts of tocopherol inhibit the peroxidation of fats, presumably by trapping free radicals to form stable tocopherol radicals [105]. Since vitamin E is concentrated in the photoreceptor outer segments [34], a specific role in retinal function is expected and tocopherol may protect the outer segment of photoreceptor cells from excessive lipid peroxidation. Vitamins E and A may conceivably protect against age-related macular degeneration [41].

It is uncertain that a clinical deficiency of vitamin E exists in humans. However, monkeys [64] and rats [126] maintained on a vitamin E-deficient diet develop a retinal degeneration characterized by focal massive disruption of photoreceptor outer segments consistent with lipid peroxidation of these lipid-rich structures. When rats are maintained on a diet deficient in vitamin E but adequate in vitamin A, lipofuscin granules become much more numerous in the RPE, the cell that ingests photoreceptor outer segments [126]. In the monkey, cones may be more susceptible to vitamin E than vitamin A deficiency, and the macula is more extensively involved than the peripheral retina. Cataract formation has been induced by vitamin E deficiency in the rabbit [33] and turkey embryo [2,43]. The ceroid accumulation that occurs in chronic vitamin E deficiency resembles ceroid lipofuscinosis (see Chap. 29) [64].

Ocular developmental anomalies occur in the offspring of rabbits and rats on a vitamin E-deficient diet. These malformations include anophthalmos and microphthalmos and retinal abnormalities sugges- tive of the retinopathy of prematurity (ROP) [19].

Indeed, vitamin E was once considered effective in the prophylaxis of ROP [110]. Even today vitamin E is thought to pay a prophylactic role in the pathogenesis of ROP. Vitamin E partially retards the cytocidal effect of hyperoxia on rabbit vascular cells in vitro [143]. In a double-masked clinical trial of infants with a birth weight less than or equal to 2000 g or a gestational age less than or equal to 36 weeks, a decreased incidence of ROP was found in vitamin E-treated infants [80]. Treatment of moderate and severe ROP with vitamin E above physiological serum levels appears promising and warrants further investigation. Sepsis and late-onset necrotizing enterocolitis are potential complications, especially in infants weighing less than or equal to 1500 g at birth, if the vitamin E treatment continues for at least 8 days.

C. Vitamin K Family

Since the isolation of vitamin K (1,4-naphthoquinone), several related substances have been recognized to possess the activity of this vitamin: the phylloquinones (vitamin K_1), the menaquinones (vitamin K_2), and the synthetic menadione (vitamin K_3). Vitamin K, which is chemically related to vitamin E, plays an important role in blood coagulation. A deficiency results in the synthesis by the liver of an abnormal prothrombin, which lacks the ability to chelate calcium ions essential for the binding of prothrombin to phospholipids and for its activation to thrombin [139]. In vitamin K deficiency hemorrhages occur, and it has been claimed, on rather nebulous evidence, that retinal hemorrhages in the newborn are less frequent because of the prophylactic administration of vitamin K [120,154].

REFERENCES

1. Armstrong, R.C., and Monie, I.W. Congenital eye defects on rats following maternal folic-acid deficiency during pregnancy. *J. Embryol. Exp. Morphol. 16*:531–542, 1966.
2. Atkinson, R.L., Ferguson, T.M., Quisenberry, J.H., and Couch, J.R. Vitamin E and reproduction in turkeys. *J. Nutr. 55*:387–397, 1955.
3. Aydelotte, M.B. The effects of vitamin A and citral on epithelial differentiation in vitro. 2. The chick oesophageal and corneal epithelial and epidermis. *J. Embryol. Exp. Morphol. 11*:621–635, 1963.
4. Balkan, W., Klintworth, G.K., Bock, C.B., and Linney, E. Transgenic mice expressing a constitutively active retinoic acid receptor in the lens exhibit ocular defects. *Dev. Biol. 151*:622–625, 1992.
5. Barnes, M.J., and Kodicek, E. Biological hydroxylations and ascorbic acid with special regard to collagen metabolism. *Vitam. Horm. 30*;1–43, 1972.
6. Batey, D.W., and Eckhert, C.D. Analysis of flavins in ocular tissues of the rabbit. *Invest. Ophthalmol. Vis. Sci. 32*:1981–1985, 1991.
7. Beitch, I. The induction of keratinization in the corneal epithelium. *Invest. Ophthalmol. 9*:827–843, 1970.
8. Benke, P.J. The isoretinoin syndrome. *JAMA 251*:3267–3269, 1984.
9. Berman, E.R., Segal, N., and Horowitz, J. Distribution and metabolism of vitamin A in pigment epithelium. *Invest. Ophthalmol. Vis. Sci. (Suppl.) 18*:268, 1979.
10. Bessey, O.A., and Wolbach, S.B. Vascularization of the cornea of the rat in riboflavin deficiency, with a note on corneal vascularization in vitamin A deficiency. *J. Exp. Med. 69*:1–19, 1939.
11. Blomhoff, R., Green, M.H., Berg, T., and Norum, K.R. Transport and storage of vitamin A. *Science 250*:399–404, 1990.
12. Boisselot, J. Malformations foetales par insufficiance en acide pantothénique. *Arch. Fr. Pediatr. 6*:225–230, 1949.
13. Bok, D., and Heller, J. Transport of retinol from the blood of the retina: An autoradiographic study of the pigment epithelial cell surface receptor for plasma retinol-binding protein. *Exp. Eye Res. 22*:395–402, 1976.
14. Bowles, L.L., Allen, L., Sydenstricker, V.P., Hock, C.W., and Hall, W.K. The development and demonstration of corneal vascularization in rats deficient in vitamin A and in riboflavin. *J. Nutr. 32*:19–36, 1946.
15. Brammer, J.D., and White, R.H. Vitamin A deficiency: Effect on the mosquito eye ultrastructure. *Science 163*:821–823, 1969.
16. Bridges, C.D.B. Vitamin A and the role of the pigment epithelium during bleaching and regeneration of rhodopsin in the frog eye. *Exp. Eye Res. 22*:435–455, 1976.
17. Bridges, C.D.B., Hollyfield, J.G., Besharse, J.C., and Rayborn, M.E. Visual pigment loss after light-induced shedding of rod outer segments. *Exp. Eye Res. 23*:637–641, 1976.

18. Bridges, C.D.B., Hollyfield, J.G., Witkovsky, P., and Gallin, E. The visual pigment and vitamin A of *Xenopus laevis* embryos, larvae and adults. *Exp. Eye Res.* 24:7–13, 1977.

19. Callison, E.C., and Orent-Keiles, E. Anomalies of the eye occurring in young vitamin E-deficient rats. *Proc. Soc. Exp. Biol. Med.* 76:295–297, 1951.

20. Campbell, A.C.P., and Russell, W.R. Wernicke's encephalopathy: Clinical features and their probable relationship to vitamin B deficiency. *Q. J. Med.* 34:41–64, 1941.

21. Campbell, F.W., and Ferguson, I.D. The role of ascorbic acid in corneal vascularization. *Br. J. Ophthalmol.* 34:329–334, 1950.

22. Carroll, F.D. Toxic amblyopia. *Trans. Am. Acad. Ophthalmol. Otolaryngol.* 60:74–82, 1956.

23. Carter-Dawson, L., Kuwabara, T., O'Brien, P.J., and Bieri, J.G. Structural and biochemical changes in vitamin A-deficient rat retinas. *Invest. Ophthalmol. Vis. Sci.* 18:437–446, 1979.

24. Clamon, G.H., Sporn, M.B., Smith, J.M., and Saffiotti, U. α and β-retinyl acetate reverse metaplasias of vitamin A deficiency in hamster trachea in organ culture. *Nature* 250:64–66, 1974.

25. Cooperman, J.M., and Lopez, R. Riboflavin. In *Handbook of Vitamins*, L.J. Machlin (Ed.), Marcel Dekker, New York, pp. 283–310, 1991.

26. Dang, C.V. Tobacco-alcohol amblyopia: A proposed biochemical basis for pathogenesis. *Med. Hypotheses* 7:1317–1328, 1981.

27. Day, P.L. Vitamin G deficiency. *Am. J. Public Health* 24:603–608, 1934.

28. Day, P.L., Darby, W.J., and Cosgrove, K.W. The arrest of nutritional cataract by the use of riboflavin. *J. Nutr.* 15:83–90, 1938.

29. Day, P.L., and Langston, W.C. Further experiments with cataract in albino rats resulting from the withdrawal of vitamin G (B$_2$) from the diet. *J. Nutr.* 7:97–106, 1934.

30. DeLuca, H.F., and Schnoes, H.K. Metabolism and mechanism of action of Vitamin D. *Annu. Rev. Biochem.* 45:631–666, 1976.

31. DeLuca, L., Rosso, G., and Wolf, G. The biosynthesis of a mannolipid that contains a polar metabolite of 15-^{14}C-retinol. *Biochem. Biophys. Res. Commun.* 41:615–620, 1970.

32. Denny-Brown, D.E. Neurological conditions resulting from prolonged and severe dietary restriction (case reports in prisoners-of-war and general review). *Medicine (Baltimore)* 26:41–113, 1947.

33. Devi, A., Raina, P.L., and Singh, A. Abnormal protein and nucleic acid metabolism as a cause of cataract formation induced by nutritional deficiency in rabbits. *Br. J. Ophthalmol.* 49:271–275, 1965.

34. Dilley, R.A., and McConnell, D.G. Alpha-tocopherol in the retinal outer segment of bovine eyes. *J. Memr. Biol.* 2:317–323, 1970.

35. Dohlman, C.H., and Kalevar, V. Cornea in hypovitaminosis A and protein deficiency. *Isr. J. Med. Sci.* 8:1179–1183, 1972.

36. Dowling, J.E. The organization of vertebrate visual receptors. In *Molecular Organization and Biological Function*, J.M. Allen (Ed.), Harper and Row, New York, pp. 186–210, 1967.

37. Dowling, J.E., and Gibbons, I.R. The effect of vitamin A deficiency on the fine structure of the retina. In *The Structure of the Eye*, G. Smelser (Ed.), Academic Press, New York, pp. 85–99, 1961.

38. Dowling, J.E., and Wald, G. The biological function of vitamin A acid. *Proc. Natl. Acad. Sci. USA* 46:587–608, 1960.

39. Eckhert, C.D., Hsu, M.-H., and Batey, D.W. Effect of dietary riboflavin on retinal density and flavin concentrations. *Prog. Clin. Biol. Res.* 314:331–341, 1989.

40. Edwards, R.B., Adler, A.J., Dev, S., and Claycomb, R.C. Synthesis of retinoic acid from retinol by cultured rabbit Müller cells. *Exp. Eye Res.* 54:481–490, 1992.

41. Eldred, G.E. Vitamins A and E in RPE lipofuscin formation and implications for age-related macular degeneration. *Prog. Clin. Biol. Res.* 314:113–129, 1989.

42. Feldman, M.H., and Schlezinger, N.S. Benign intracranial hypertension associated with hypervitaminosis A. *Arch. Neurol.* 22:1–7, 1970.

43. Ferguson, T.M., Rigdon, R.H., and Couch, J.R. Cataracts in vitamin E deficiency: An experimental study in the turkey embryo. *Arch. Ophthalmol.* 55:346–355, 1956.

44. Fisher, M. Residual neuropathological changes in Canadians held prisoners of war by the Japanese. *Can. Serv. Med. J.* 11:157–203, 1955.

45. Follis, R.H., Jr. *Deficiency Diseases: Functional and Structural Changes in Mammalia, Which Result from Exogenous or Endogenous Lack of One or More Essential Nutrients*, Charles C. Thomas, Springfield, IL, 1958.

46. Freeman, A.G., and Heaton, J.M. The aetiology of retrobulbar neuritis in Addisonian pernicious anaemia. *Lancet* 1:908–911, 1961.

47. Geelen, J.A.G. Hypervitaminosis A induced teratogenesis. *CRC Crit. Rev. Toxicol.* 7:351–375, 1972.

48. Gershoff, S.N., Andrus, S.B., and Hegsted, D.M. The effect of the carbohydrate and fat content of the diet upon the riboflavin requirement of the cat. *J. Nutr.* 68:75–88, 1959.

49. Giroud, A., Delmas, A., Prost, H., and Lefebvres, J. Malformations encéphaliques par carence enacide pantothénique et leur interprétation. *Acta Anat. (Basel)* 29:209–227, 1957.

50. Giroud, A., Lefebvres, J., and Dupuis, R. Répercussions sur l'embryon de la carence en acide folique. *Int. Z. Vitaminforsch.* 24:420–429, 1952.

51. Giroud, A., Lefebvres, J., Prost, H., and Dupuis, R. Malformations des membres dues à des lésions vasculaires chez le foetus de rat déficient en acide pantothénique. *J. Embryol. Exp. Morphol. 3*:1–12, 1955.

52. Giroud, A., and Martinet, M. Tératogenèse par hautes doses de Vitamin A enfonction des stades du développement. *Arch. Anat. Microsc. 45*:77–98, 1956.

53. Goldsmith, G. Riboflavin deficiency. In *Riboflavin*, R.S. Rivlin (Ed.), Plenum Press, New York, pp. 221–238, 1975.

54. Goodman, D.S. Vitamin A and retinoids in health and disease. *N. Engl. J. Med. 310*:1023–1031, 1984.

55. Goodman, D.S., and Blaner, W.S. Biosynthesis, absorption, and hepatic metabolism of retinol. In *The Retinoids*, Vol. 2, M.B. Sporn, A.B. Roberts, and D.S. Goodman (Eds.), Academic Press, Orlando, FL, pp. 1–39, 1984.

56. Gould, B.S. Ascorbic acid and collagen fiber formation. *Vitam. Horm. 18*:89–120, 1960.

57. Grainger, R.B., O'Dell, B.L., and Hogan, A.G. Congenital malformations as related to deficiencies of riboflavin and vitamin B$_{12}$ source of protein, calcium to phosphorus ratio and skeletal phosphorus metabolism. *J. Nutr. 54*:33–48, 1954.

58. Hale, F. The relation of maternal vitamin A deficiency to microphthalmia in pigs. *Tex. State Med. J. 33*:228–232, 1937.

59. Halver, J.E. Nutrition of salmonid fishes. III. Water soluble vitamin requirements of Chinook salmon. *J. Nutr. 62*:225–243, 1957.

60. Halwer, M. The photochemistry of riboflavin and related compounds. *J. Am. Chem. Soc. 73*:4870–4874, 1951.

61. Hamilton, J.B. Eyes and scurvy. *Trans. Ophthalmol. Soc. Aust. 18*:83–91, 1958.

62. Harwood, R., Grant, M.E., and Jackson, D.S. Influence of ascorbic acid on ribosomal patterns and collagen biosynthesis in healing wounds of scorbutic guinea pigs. *Biochem. J. 142*:641–651, 1974.

63. Hayes, K.C. Retinal degeneration in monkeys induced by deficiencies of vitamin E and A. *Invest. Ophthalmol. 13*:499–510, 1974.

64. Hayes, K.C. Pathophysiology of vitamin E deficiency in monkeys. *Am. J. Clin. Nutr. 27*:1130–1140, 1974.

65. Heath, H. The distribution and possible functions of ascorbic acid in the eye. *Exp. Eye Res. 1*:362–367, 1962.

66. Heaton, J.M., McCormick, A.J.A., and Freeman, A.G. Tobacco amblyopia: A clinical manifestation of vitamin B$_{12}$ deficiency. *Lancet 2*:286–290, 1958.

67. Heffley, J.D., and Williams, R.T. The nutritional teamwork approach: Prevention and regression of cataracts in rats. *Proc. Natl. Acad. Sci. USA 71*:4164–4168, 1974.

68. Helgerud, P., Peterson, L.B., and Norum, K.R. Acyl CoA:retinol acyltransferase in rat small intestine: Its activity and some properties of the enzymic reaction. *J. Lipid Res. 23*:609–618, 1982.

69. Helgerud, P., Peterson, L.B., and Norum, K.R. Retinol esterification by microsomes from the mucosa of human small intestine: Evidence for acyl-coenzyme a retinol acyltransferase activity. *J. Clin. Invest. 71*:747–753, 1983.

70. Hirsawa, K., and Yamada, E. The localization of the vitamin A in the mouse liver as revealed by electron microscope radioautography. *J. Electron Microsc. 22*:337–346, 1973.

71. Hirosawa, K., and Yamada, E. The localization of the vitamin A in the mouse retina as revealed by radioautography. In *The Structure of the Eye*, Third Symposium, Tokyo, Japan, E. Yamada and S. Mishima (Eds.). Jp. J. Ophthalmol. pp. 165–175, 1976.

72. Horwitt, M.K., and Witting, L.A. Riboflavin biochemical systems. In *The Vitamins*, Vol. 5, W.H. Sebrell and R.S. Harris (Eds.), Academic Press, New York, pp. 53–70, 1967.

73. Hubbard, R., and Kroft, A. The action of light on rhodopsin. *Proc. Natl. Acad. Sci. USA 44*:130–139, 1958.

74. Hubbard, R., and Wald, G. Cis-trans isomers of vitamin A and retinene in the rhodopsin system. *J. Gen. Physiol. 36*:269–315, 1952.

75. Irinoda, K., and Sato, S. Contribution to ocular manifestation of riboflavin deficiency. *Tohoku J. Exp. Med. 61*:93–104, 1954.

76. Jackson, B., and Kinsey, V.E. The relation between maternal vitamin-A intake blood level and ocular abnormalities in the offspring of the rat. *Am. J. Ophthalmol. 29*:1234–1242, 1946.

77. Jackson, S.F., and Fell, H.B. Epidermal fine structure in embryonic chicken skin during atypical differentiation induced by vitamin A in culture. *Dev. Biol. 7*:394–419, 1963.

78. Jacques, P.F., Hartz, S.C., Chylack, L.T., McGandy, R.B., and Sadowski, J.A. Nutritional status in persons with and without senile cataract: Blood vitamin and mineral levels. *Am. J. Clin. Nutr. 48*:152–158, 1988.

79. Jayaraj, A.P., Leela, R., and Rama Rao, P.B. Studies on corneal mucous metaplasia in vitamin A deficient rats. *Exp. Eye Res. 12*:1–15, 1971.

79a. Jernigan, H.M. Jr. Role of hydrogen peroxide in riboflavin-sensitized photodynamic damage to cultured rat lenses. *Exp. Eye Res. 41*:121–129, 1985.

80. Johnson, L., Quinn, G.E., Abbasi, S., Otis, C., Goldstein, D., Sacks, L., Porat, R., Fong, E., Delivoria-Papadopoulos, M., Peckham, G., Schaffer, D.B., and Bowen, F.W., Jr. Effect of sustained pharmacologic vitamin E levels on incidence and severity of retinopathy of prematurity: A controlled clinical trial. *J. Pediatr. 114*:827–838, 1989.

81. Kalter, H., and Warkany, J. Congenital malformations in inbred stains of mice induced by riboflavin-deficient galactoflavin containing diets. *J. Exp. Zool. 136*:531–565, 1957.

82. Katz, M.L., Kutryb, M.J., Norberg, M., Gao, C., White, R.H., and Stark, W.S. Maintenance of opsin density in photoreceptor outer segments of retinoid-deprived rats. *Invest. Ophthalmol. Vis. Sci. 32*:1966–1980, 1991.

83. Katz, M.L., Norberg, M., and Stientjes, H.J. Reduced phagosomal content of the retinal pigment epithelium in response to retinoid deprivation. *Invest. Ophthalmol. Vis. Sci.* *33*:2612–2618, 1992.
84. Kim, Y.C.L., and Wolf, G. Vitamin A deficiency and the glycoproteins of rat corneal epithelium. *J. Nutr.* *104*:710–718, 1974.
85. Kobayashi, K., Takahashi, Y., and Shibasaki, S. Cytological studies of fat-storing cells in the liver of rats given large doses of vitamin A. *Nature New Biol.* *243*:186–188, 1973.
86. Kroft, A., and Hubbard, R. The mechanism of bleaching rhodopsin. *Ann. N.Y. Acad. Sci.* *74*:266–280, 1958.
87. Lamming, G.E., Salisbury, G.W., Hays, R.L., and Kendall, K.A. The effect of incipient vitamin A deficiency on reproduction in the rabbit. II. Embryonic and fetal development. *J. Nutr.* *52*:227–239, 1954.
88. LaRosa, G.J., and Gudas, L.J. Early retinoic acid induced F9 teratocarcinoma stem cell gene ERA-1: Alternate splicing creates transcripts for homeobox-containing protein and one lacking the homeobox. *Mol. Cell. Biol.* *8*:3906–3917, 1988.
89. Leuenberger, P.M., and Novikoff, A.B. Studies on microperoxisomes. VII. Pigment epithelial cells and other cell types in the retina of rodents. *J. Cell Biol.* *65*:324–334, 1975.
90. Levij, I.S., and Polliack, A. Potentiating effect of vitamin A on 9-10 dimethyl 1-2 benzanthracene-carcinogenesis in the hamster cheek pouch. *Cancer* *22*:300–306, 1968.
91. Lippincott, S.W., and Morris, H.P. Pathologic changes associated with riboflavin deficiency in the mouse. *J. Natl. Cancer Inst.* *2*:601–610, 1942.
92. McCormick, D.B. The fate of riboflavin in the mammal. *Nutr. Rev.* *30*:75–79, 1972.
93. McDonald, P.N., and Ong, D.E. Evidence for a lecithin-retinol acyltransferase activity in the rat small intestine. *J. Biol. Chem.* *263*:12478–12482, 1988.
94. Maynard, R.B. Blindness among prisoners of war. *Trans. Ophthalmol. Soc. Aust.* *6*:92–103, 1946.
95. Merrill, A.H., Lambeth, J.D., Edmondson, D.E., and McCormick, D.B. Formation and mode of action of flavoproteins. *Annu. Rev. Nutr.* *1*:281–317, 1981.
96. Meyer, A. The Wernicke syndrome; with special reference to manic syndromes associated with hypothalamic lesions. *J. Neurol. Psychiatry* *7*:66–75, 1944.
97. Miller, P.J., Johnston, R.L., Hoefer, J.A., and Luecke, R.W. The riboflavin requirement of the baby pig. *J. Nutr.* *52*:405–413, 1954.
98. Molenaar, I., Vox, J., and Hommes, F.A. Effect of vitamin E deficiency on cellular membranes. *Vitam. Horm.* *30*:45–82, 1972.
99. Moon, R.C., and Itri, L.M. Retinoids and cancer. In *The Retinoids*, Vol. 2, M.B. Sporn, A.B. Roberts, and D.S. Goodman (Eds.), Academic Press, Orlando, FL, pp. 327–371, 1984.
100. Moore, L.A. Relationship between carotene, blindness due to constriction of the optic nerve, papillary edema and nyctalopia in calves. *J. Nutr.* *17*:443–459, 1939.
101. Muller, F. Flavin radicals: Chemistry and biochemistry. *Free Radic. Biol. Med.* *3*:215–230, 1987.
102. Muto, Y., Smith, J.E., Milch, P.O., and Goodman, D.S. Regulation of retinol-binding protein metabolism by vitamin A status in the rat. *J. Biol. Chem.* *247*:2542–2550, 1972.
103. Nelson, M.M., Baird, C.D.C., Wright, H.V., and Evans, H.M. Multiple congenital abnormalities in the rat resulting from riboflavin deficiency induced by the antimetabolite galactoflavin. *J. Nutr.* *58*:125–134, 1956.
104. Nelson, M.M., Wright, H.V., Baird, C.D.C., and Evans, H.M. Teratogenic effects of pantothenic acid deficiency in the rat. *J. Nutr.* *62*:395–405, 1957.
105. Nilsson, J.L.G., Daves, G.D., Jr., and Folkers, K. The oxidative dimerization of alpha-, beta-, gamma-, and delta tocopherols. *Acta Chem. Scand.* *22*:207–218, 1968.
106. Noell, W.K., Delmelle, M.C., and Albrecht, R. Vitamin A deficiency effect on retina: Dependence of light. *Science* *172*:72–75, 1971.
107. Olson, J.A. Some aspects of vitamin A metabolism. *Vitam. Horm.* *26*:1–63, 1968.
108. Ong, D.E., and Chytil, F. Retinoic acid-binding protein in rat tissues: Partial purification and comparison to rat tissue retinal-binding protein. *J. Biol. Chem.* *250*:6113–6117, 1975.
109. Ong, D.E., Kakkad, B., and MacDonald, P.N. Acyl-CoA-independent esterification of retinol bound to cellular retinol-binding protein (type II) by microsomes from rat small intestine. *J. Biol. Chem.* *262*:2729–2736, 1987.
110. Owens, W.C., and Owens, E.U. Retrolental fibroplasia in premature infants. II. Studies on the prophylaxis of the disease: The use of alpha tocopheryl acetate. *Am. J. Ophthalmol.* *32*:1631–1637, 1949.
111. Peterson, P.A., and Berggard, I. Isolation and properties of a human retinol-transporting protein. *J. Biol. Chem.* *246*:25–33, 1971.
112. Pfister, R.R., and Renner, M.E. The corneal and conjunctival surface in vitamin A deficiency: A scanning electron microscope study. *Invest. Ophthalmol. Vis. Sci.* *17*:874–883, 1978.
113. Philpot, F.J., and Pirie, A. Riboflavin and riboflavin adenine dinucleotide in ox ocular tissues. *Biochem. J.* *37*:250–254, 1943.
114. Pirie, A. Xerophthalmia. *Invest. Ophthalmol.* *15*:417–422, 1976.
115. Pirie, A., Werb, Z., and Burleigh, M.C. Collagenase and other proteinase in the cornea of the retinol deficient rat. *Br. J. Nutr.* *34*:297–309, 1975.
116. Polliak, A., and Sasson, Z.B. Enhancing effect of excess topical vitamin A on Rous sarcoma in chicken. *J. Natl. Cancer Inst.* *48*:407–416, 1972.

117. Poswillo, D. The pathogenesis of the Treacher Collins syndrome (mandibulofacial dysostosis). *Br. J. Oral Surg.* 13:1–26, 1975.
118. Poswillo, D. Mechanisms and pathogenesis of malformations. *Br. Med. Bull.* 32:59–64, 1976.
119. Powell, S.R., and Schwab, I.R. Nutritional disorders affecting the peripheral cornea. *Int. Ophthalmol. Clin.* 26(4):137–146, 1986.
120. Pray, L.G., McKeown, H.S., and Pokard, W.E. Hemorrhagic diathesis of the newborn effect of vitamin A prophylaxis and therapy. *Am. J. Obstet. Gynecol.* 42:836–845, 1941.
121. Prchal, J.T., Conrad, M.E., and Skalda, H.W. Association of presenile cataracts with heterozygosity for galactosaemic states and with riboflavin deficiency. *Lancet* 1:12–13, 1978.
122. Prutkin, L. The effect of vitamin A acid on tumorigenesis and protein production. *Cancer Res.* 28:1021–1030, 1968.
123. Ramalingaswami, V., Leach, E.H., and Sriramachari, S. Ocular structure in vitamin A deficiency in the monkey. *Q. J. Exp. Physiol.* 40:337–347, 1955.
124. Robertson, W. van B. The biochemical role of ascorbic acid in connective tissue. *Ann. N.Y. Acad. Sci.* 92:159–167, 1961.
125. Robison, W.G., Jr., and Kuwabara, T. Vitamin A storage and peroxisomes in retinal pigment epithelium and liver. *Invest. Ophthalmol. Vis. Sci.* 16:1110–1117, 1977.
126. Robison, W.G., Jr., Kuwabara, T., and Bieri, J.G. Vitamin E deficiency and the retina: Photoreceptor and pigment epithelial changes. *Invest. Ophthalmol. Vis. Sci.* 19:1030–1037, 1980.
127. Rodger, F.C. Experimental thiamin deficiency as a cause of degeneration in the visual pathway of the rat. *Br. J. Ophthalmol.* 37:11–29, 1953.
128. Saari, J.C. Enzymes proteins of the visual cycle. In *Progress in Retinal Research*, Vol. 8, N.N. Osborne and G.J. Chader (Eds.), Pergamon Press, Oxford, pp. 363–381, 1989.
129. Shenefelt, R.E. Morphogenesis of malformations in hamsters caused by retinoic acid: Relation to dose and stage at treatment. *Teratology* 5:103–118, 1972.
130. Sklan, D. Vitamin A in human nutrition. *Prog. Food Nutr. Sci.* 11:39–55, 1987.
131. Smith, E.C., and Metzler, D.E. The photochemical degradation of riboflavin. *J. Am. Chem. Soc.* 85:3285–3288, 1963.
132. Smith, F.R., Goodman, D.S., Zaklama, M.S., Gabr, M.K., El Maraghy, S., and Patwardhan, V.N. Serum vitamin A, retinol-binding protein and prealbumin concentrations in protein-calorie malnutrition. I. A functional defect in hepatic retinol release. *Am. J. Clin. Nutr.* 26:973–981, 1973.
133. Smith, F.R., Suskind, R., Thanangkul, O., Leitzmann, C., Goodman, D.S., and Olson, R.E. Plasma vitamin A, retinol-binding protein and prealbumin concentration in protein-calorie malnutrition. III. Response to varying dietary treatments. *Am. J. Clin. Nutr.* 28:732–738, 1975.
134. Sommer, A. Vitamin A deficiency today: Conjunctival xerosis in cystic fibrosis. *J. R. Soc. Med.* 82:1–2, 1989.
135. Sommer, A. Xerophthalmia, keratomalacia and nutritional blindness. *Int. Ophthalmol.* 14:195–199, 1990.
136. Sporn, M.B., Dunlop, N.M., Newton, D.L., and Smith, J.M. Prevention of chemical carcinogenesis by vitamin A and its synthetic analogs (retinoids). *Fed. Proc.* 35:1332–1338, 1976.
137. Sporn, M.B., Dunlop, N.M., and Yuspa, S.H. Retinyl acetate: Effect on cellular content of RNA in epidermis in cell culture in chemically defined medium. *Science* 182:722–723, 1973.
138. Sporn, M.B., and Roberts, A.B. Biological methods for analysis and assay of retinoids: Relationship between structure and activity. In *The Retinoids*, Vol. 1, Chap. 5, M.B. Sporn, A.B. Roberts, and D.S. Goodman (Eds.), Academic Press, Orlando, FL, pp. 235–279, 1984.
139. Stenflo, J. A new vitamin K-dependent protein. *J. Biol. Chem.* 251:355–363, 1976.
140. Sulkin, D.F., Sulkin, N.M., and Nushan, H. Corneal fine structure in experimental scorbutus. *Invest. Ophthalmol.* 11:633–643, 1972.
141. Sullivan, W.R., McCulley, J.P., and Dohlman, C.H. Return of goblet cells after vitamin A therapy in xerosis of the conjunctiva. *Am. J. Ophthalmol.* 75:720–725, 1973.
142. Tielsch, J.M., and Sommer, A. The epidemiology of vitamin A deficiency and xerophthalmia. *Annu. Rev. Nutr.* 4:183–205, 1984.
143. Tripathi, B.J., and Tripathi, R.C. Cellular and subcellular events in retinopathy of oxygen toxicity with a preliminary report on the preventive role of vitamin E and gamma-aminobutyric acid: A study in vitro. *Curr. Eye Res.* 3:193–208, 1984.
144. Vahlquist, A., and Peterson, P.A. Comparative studies on the vitamin A transporting protein complex in human and cynomolgus plasma. *Biochemistry* 11:4526–4532, 1972.
145. Waisman, H. Production of riboflavin deficiency in the monkey. *Proc. Soc. Exp. Biol. Med.* 55:69–71, 1944.
146. Wake, K. Development of vitamin-A-rich lipid droplets in multivesicular bodies of rat liver stellate cells. *J. Cell Biol.* 63:683–691, 1974.
147. Wald, G., Molecular basis of visual excitation. *Science* 162:230–239, 1968.
148. Wald, G., Jeghers, H., and Arminio, J. An experiment in human dietary night blindness. *Am. J. Physiol.* 123:732–746, 1938.
149. Warkany, J., and Roth, C.B. Congenital malformations induced in rats by maternal vitamin A deficiency. II. Effects of varying preparatory diet upon yield of abnormal young. *J. Nutr.* 35:1–11, 1948.

150. Warkany, J., and Schraffenberger, E. Congenital malformations induced in rats by maternal vitamin A deficiency. I. Defects of the eye. *Arch. Ophthalmol. 35*:150–169, 1946.

151. Weissman, G., and Thomas, L. Studies on lysosomes. II. The effect of cortisone on the release of acid hydrolases from a large granule fraction of rabbit liver induced by an excess of vitamin A. *J. Clin. Invest. 42*:661–669, 1963.

152. Wiggert, B., Masterson, E., Israel, P., and Chader, G.J. Differential retinoid binding in chick pigment epithelium and choroid. *Invest. Ophthalmol. Vis. Sci. 18*:306–310, 1979.

153. Wiggert, B.O., Bergsma, D.R., and Chader, G.J. Retinol receptors of the retina and pigment epithelium: Further characterization and species variation. *Exp. Eye Res. 22*:411–418, 1976.

154. Wille, H. Investigations in the influence of K avitaminosis on the occurrence of retinal hemorrhages in the newborn: A preliminary report. *Acta Ophthalmol. (Copenh.) 22*:261–269, 1944.

155. Wilson, J., and Langman, M.J.S. Relation of subacute combined degeneration of the cord to vitamin B_{12} deficiency. *Nature (Lond.) 212*:787–789, 1966.

156. Wilson, J., and Matthews, D.M. Metabolic interrelationships between cyanide, thiocyanate and vitamin B_{12} in smokers and non-smokers. *Clin. Sci. 31*:1–7, 1966.

157. Wilson, J.G., Roth, C.B., and Warkany, J. An analysis of the syndrome of malformations induced by maternal vitamin A deficiency: Effects of restoration of vitamin A at various times during gestation. *Am. J. Anat. 92*: 189–217, 1953.

158. Wiss, O., and Weber, F. The liver and vitamins. In *The Liver, Morphology, Biochemistry, Physiology*, Vol. 2, C. Rouiller (Ed.), Academic Press, New York, pp. 133–176, 1964.

159. Witkovsky, P., Gallin, E., Hollyfield, J.G., Ripps, H., and Bridges, C.D.B. Photoreceptor thresholds and visual pigment levels in normal and vitamin A-deprived *Xenopus laevis* tadpoles. *J. Neurophysiol. 39*:1272–1287, 1976.

160. Wolbach, S.B., and Howe, P.R. Tissue changes following deprivation of fat-soluble A vitamin. *J. Exp. Med. 42*:753–778, 1925.

161. Wolf, G. Multiple functions of vitamin A. *Physiol. Rev. 64*:873–937, 1984.

162. Young, R.W., and Bok, D. Autoradiographic studies on the metabolism of retinal pigment epithelium. *Invest. Ophthalmol. 9*:524–536, 1970.

39
Drugs and Toxins

Mark W. Scroggs
Duke University School of Medicine, Durham, North Carolina

Gordon K. Klintworth
Duke University Medical Center, Durham, North Carolina

I. INTRODUCTION

Certain chemicals, detergents, cosmetics, and animal toxins have a deleterious effect upon the eye and its adjacent structures. Some drugs administered for systemic diseases also evoke ocular toxicological complications. Local and generalized toxic reactions to drugs used in the treatment of ophthalmological disorders are also occasionally encountered.

Adverse reactions to toxic agents are mediated by a variety of mechanisms. Toxins possess intrinsic biochemical characteristics that are directly responsible for adverse tissue reactions, and their reaction often occurs in a dose-related manner. This is in contrast to drugs or chemicals that incite an immunological response in which minute quantities of the compound may cause a significant response.

An extensive literature on ocular toxicology has accumulated. This chapter provides an overview of medications and other chemicals associated with toxic effects on ocular structures. For more detailed information the reader should consult one of the several excellent texts on this subject [75,91,105,163]. Immunologically mediated adverse reactions to drugs, such as drug allergy and hypersensitivity, are considered in Chapter 5. Chemical injuries due to acids and alkalis are discussed in Chapter 14.

II. FACTORS PREDISPOSING TO DRUG TOXICITY

Individual ocular responses to particular toxic agents often vary considerably because of many factors, including the route of administration of the toxin, the age of the individual, the presence of underlying disease, and sometimes a genetic predisposition.

Numerous variables influence the absorption of medications applied topically to the eye and hence possible adverse reactions. Certain pathological conditions of ocular structures influence drug bio-availability. For example, conjunctivitis, keratitis, focal defects in the integrity of the ocular surface epithelium, a dry eye, or a decreased tear film may increase drug absorption. The position of the head of the patient as medication is administered to the eye may also enhance drug delivery [86,207]. Impaired blinking, which may result in less drug dilution by tears, may also increase the amount of drug absorbed. Any condition that decreases lacrimation, such as anesthesia, increases the likelihood of toxic reactions to certain topically applied drugs [195].

Factors that influence drug absorption and metabolism predispose infants and the elderly to drug toxicities. In the pediatric population, adult doses of topically applied ocular medication potentially increase the risk of adverse effects [174,175]. Enzyme systems in the liver and kidney are responsible for the detoxification and excretion of many drugs, and such mechanisms are frequently poorly developed in infants, predisposing them to the untoward effects of many therapeutic agents. The elderly are prone to drug toxicity because of potential underlying renal, hepatic, and/or cardiac diseases, as well as drug-drug interactions, since they are frequently receiving multiple medications.

Systemic uptake of certain topically applied ocular medications can cause adverse generalized manifestations. Drug absorption through the nasal mucosa and other parts of the nasolacrimal system may follow drainage of medications from the ocular surface. Absorption may occur through the gastrointestinal tract if the drug is eventually swallowed. Topically applied drugs may reach the systemic circulation in sufficient quantities through the ocular vasculature, especially in the conjunctiva and episclera, and can induce systemic side effects. Once such ocular medications reach the systemic circulation, toxic complications may be enhanced by impaired detoxification or excretion as a result of renal or liver disease.

Medications administered systemically for nonocular conditions that lead to significant toxic ocular manifestations usually enter the eye via the circulatory system. The blood-aqueous and the blood-retinal barriers, however, normally prevent many drugs from gaining access to the eye by way of the vasculature. The absorption of systemically administered drugs by the eye may increase when these blood-ocular barriers are impaired, as during inflammation, and in such settings drugs may reach toxic levels. For example, several reports suggest that a compromised blood-retinal barrier may enhance the entry of chloroquine [183] and vincristine [190] into the eye and exacerbate undesirable side effects.

Individual toxic reactions to medicines in acceptable therapeutic doses are well known and have been attributed to genetically controlled mechanisms, but few studies have addressed this issue. The influence of heredity on steroid-induced glaucoma has been known for some time [10]. The development of penicillamine-induced ocular myasthenia gravis in patients with rheumatoid arthritis may also have a genetic basis: several studies have disclosed an association of this form of myesthenia gravis with a distinct major histocompatibility haplotype. Almost half of patients who develop myasthenia gravis spontaneously bear the HLA-DR3 antigen [222]. Several independent studies of penicillamine-induced myasthenia gravis in patients with rheumatoid arthritis indicate that only 4.0% (1 of 25 patients) possess the HLA-DR3 haplotype; most (68.0%; 17 of 25 patients) have the HLA-DR1 haplotype [35,63,64,128,139,150,171].

The influence of genetics on acetaminophen-induced cataracts has been demonstrated experimentally in mice [204]. The metabolism of acetaminophen involves several cytochrome P_{450}-mediated monooxygenases [205]. Mice that express the genes for this P_{450} system develop lenticular opacities more frequently than animals deficient in such genes, suggesting that acetaminophen-induced cataracts are a sequel to a metabolite of the drug caused by a genetic capacity to express the P_{450} system [204]. Animals lacking such metabolic capabilities are free of cataracts, presumably because of an inability to generate the toxic metabolite.

III. ROLE OF ACTIVATED OXYGEN SPECIES IN OCULAR TOXICITY

The mechanisms by which many drugs and toxins exert their harmful effects on the eye remain poorly understood. Activated oxygen species probably play a role in the toxicity of certain compounds, including acetaminophen and bromobenzene [79]. Energy is derived from intracellular oxygen as it is converted to water. During this process, reactive oxygen molecules, such as the superoxide anion (O_2^-) and the hydroxyl radical (HO·), are formed, which may cause cell injury by peroxidation of the phospholipids present in cellular membranes. Fortunately, the body possesses enzymes, such as superoxide dismutase, catalase, and glutathione peroxidase, that limit the damage of superoxide radicals and other excited oxygen species. For example, superoxide dismutase catalyzes the formation of oxygen (O_2) and hydrogen peroxide (H_2O_2) from superoxide radicals. Also, hydrogen peroxide is reduced to water by glutathione peroxidase and catalase (Figs. 1 and 2).

Reactive oxygen molecules putatively affect different ocular structures adversely in several species. Reactive oxygen species affect proteins, such as the crystallins, which aggregate and precipitate. They are implicated in cataract formation [32,212]. Reactive oxygen molecules are also released by stimulated mononuclear phagocytes and neutrophils during the inflammatory response and probably play a role in the toxic effects on the cornea during inflammation [115,117,189], increased iris vascular permeability [116], experimental allergic uveitis [186], and hypoxic retinal damage as measured in tissue homogenates [68]. The toxic effect of some drugs, such as acetaminophen, results from the conjugation of the drug or its metabolites with components of major antioxidant defense mechanisms, like glutathione reductase.

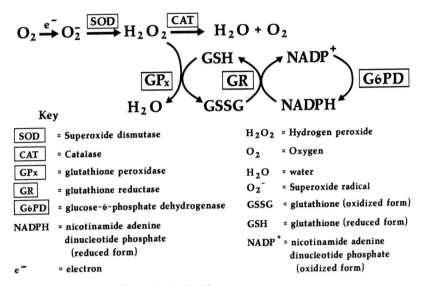

Figure 1   Antioxidant enzyme system.

Consequently, the cellular defenses against oxidative damage may be overwhelmed as membranes and other cellular constituents become subjected to oxidative damage [79].

The role of activated oxygen species in cataractogenesis has been extensively investigated [95,98, 213,226,229]. Exposure of the lens to hydrogen peroxide causes it to become cataractous. Cataracts can also be induced in rabbits by supplementing their diet with the catalase inhibitor 3-aminotriazole [32]. Such cataracts are associated with an increased hydrogen peroxide content of the aqueous and vitreous and decreased superoxide dismutase activity in the lens. Superoxide dismutase activity is also diminished in extracts of rabbit lenses incubated with hydrogen peroxide, and this inhibition is potentiated by 3-aminotriazole [32].

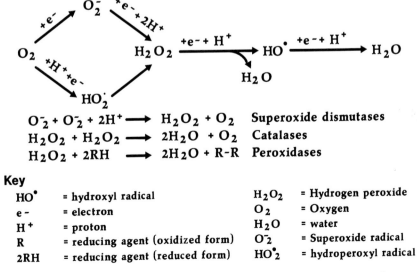

Figure 2   Pathway of oxygen reduction and catalytic scavenging of intermediates.

Hydrogen peroxide is routinely used in certain contact lens disinfectants, but its role in corneal toxicity via the generation of superoxide radicals is unknown. However, exposure of cultured human and rat corneal epithelial cells to hydrogen peroxide or superoxide radicals causes morphological abnormalities and decreased DNA synthesis as reflected by decreased thymidine incorporation, as well as lysis of these cells [110]. Pretreatment of corneal epithelial cell cultures with superoxide dismutase and catalase partially counteracts these toxic effects of the superoxide radicals. Exposure of cultured corneal endothelial cells to hydrogen peroxide results in morphological changes that are blocked by the addition of catalase [115].

IV. TOXICOLOGICAL REACTIONS AT DIFFERENT ANATOMICAL SITES

Drugs and toxins may incite adverse reactions in virtually any part of the eye and its adnexa, and such alterations may be restricted to one or multiple ocular structures.

A. Ocular Surface Membrane

Following exposure to one of numerous chemical agents, including drugs, air pollutants, and detergents [Figs. 3–4 (for Fig. 4 see plate following p. 1436); Tables 1 and 2], the ocular surface membrane may undergo a toxic reaction, especially a nonspecific conjunctivitis or keratoconjunctivitis.

Subconjunctival injections of 5-fluorouracil have been administered to patients with glaucoma to prevent scar formation following filtering procedures. In related studies, decreased cell growth and numerous morphological changes (including nuclear and cytoplasmic vacuolization, abnormal chromatin clumping, and reduction in the number of microvilli) have been observed in human cultured conjunctival cells incubated with 5-fluorouracil [223].

Various agents may discolor the conjunctiva and cornea. For example, after prolonged exposure to heavy metals, such as silver, gold, and mercury, these tissues become pigmented from tissue deposition. Oxidation of topically applied epinephrine to adrenochrome may result in pigmentation of both the cornea and conjunctiva.

Adverse corneal responses to toxins or certain therapeutic agents may occur immediately but frequently become manifest only after chronic exposure [90]. To penetrate the normal cornea, topically applied toxic agents must possess particular solubility characteristics. Water-soluble compounds enter the corneal stroma, but lipid-soluble agents are more likely to enter the lipid-rich epithelium. Conditions that disrupt the integrity of the corneal epithelium, as well as viscous drugs that prolong contact time with the cornea, may predispose this tissue to adverse toxic reactions.

Gentamicin, an aminoglycoside antibiotic, is frequently used in the treatment of ocular bacterial infections and is also sometimes a component of transport media for donor corneas [3]. This agent accumulates in lysosomes, where it binds to membrane phospholipids, leading to cell membrane instability and lysosomal rupture [113]. Gentamicin may thus have deleterious effects upon tissues, such as the cornea, conjunctiva [3,4], and the retina [54]. Indeed, gentamicin is toxic to both the corneal epithelium and endothelium of rabbits in culture [3,177]. Morphological abnormalities (including intralysosomal lamellated bodies) appear in cultured conjunctival and renal tubular epithelial cells following exposure to 50 μg/ml or more of gentamicin without preservatives [3]. High concentrations (1000 mg in 1 ml) of gentamicin with preservatives result in endothelial cell swelling and intracytoplasmic granules, but not lamellated bodies.

Preservatives may also incite toxic reactions in the ocular surface membranes. Some evidence supports the notion that preservatives account for the toxicity of topical gentamicin [4]. During reepithelialization of large corneal wounds, conjunctival epithelium migrates over the surface of the injured cornea, and topical gentamicin is often used in such settings to prevent bacterial infection. In an attempt to study persistent epithelial defects in rabbits, Alfonso and colleagues [4] examined the effects of gentamicin on healing conjunctival epithelium. The corneal and conjunctival epithelia were reinjured by gentle debridement 28 days following initial epithelial injury with n-heptanol. In these animals, treatment with either topical gentamicin or its preservative (benzalkonium chloride) significantly retarded epithelial healing rates in rabbits subjected to corneal and conjunctival reinjury compared to controls receiving only topical saline.

The ocular surface membrane may be adversely affected by certain chemical contaminants of contact lenses. For example, chlorbutanol and chlorhexidine are used as preservatives in some contact lens cleaning

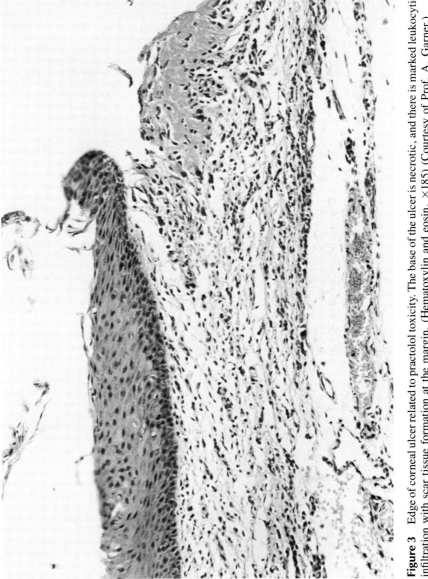

Figure 3 Edge of corneal ulcer related to practolol toxicity. The base of the ulcer is necrotic, and there is marked leukocytic infiltration with scar tissue formation at the margin. (Hematoxylin and eosin, ×185) (Courtesy of Prof. A. Garner.)

Table 1   Toxins Affecting the Conjunctiva

Reaction	Toxin	Reference
Conjunctivitis	Acetylcysteine	237
	Bacitracin, fortified	237
	Benzalkonium chloride	237
	Boric acid	237
	Carbachol	237
	Cyclophosphamide	118
	Cytosine arabinoside	118
	Doxorubicin	118
	5-Fluorouracil	118
	Idoxuridine	237
	Ketoprofen	169
	Methotrexate	118
	Neomycin, fortified	237
	Pilocarpine	237
	Silver nitrate	237
	Thimerosal	45
	Tobramycin	45
Follicular conjunctivitis	Apraclonidine	235
	Dipivefrin	149
Edema	Marijuana	162
	Nitrosureas	118
Pigmentation	Atabrine	216
	Chlorpromazine	216
	Cosmetics (mascara or eyeliner)	237
	Epinephrine	237
	Gold	129
	Mercury	237
	Silver	215
	Tetracycline	39
Ocular cicatrization	Demecarium	83
	Echothiophate	83
	Epinephrine	83
	Idoxuridine	83
	Pilocarpine	83
	Timolol	83
Decreased epithelial mitosis	5-Fluorouracil	203
Defective wound healing	Gentamicin	4
Concretions in conjunctival cysts	Sulfadiazine	237

solutions. These chemicals may bind to soft lenses and result in a mild conjunctivitis when the lens is placed on the eye [146]. For unknown reasons, systemically administered isotretinoin is associated with contact lens intolerance in some patients [88].

B. Lacrimal System

A normally functioning lacrimal system protects the eye from topically applied noxious agents. Tears dilute toxins and serve as a buffer to counteract the extreme tonicity and pH ranges of certain topically applied drugs. Hence inadequate tearing and blinking may enhance drug availability to the ocular surface and increase the risk of reactions to these agents. Certain drugs directly affect the lacrimal system (Table 3). For example, topical anesthetics suppress the tearing and blinking reflexes and decrease lacrimation [195].

Some systemically administered drugs that are transported to the lacrimal gland and secreted into the tears may be toxic to the ocular surface. An example is isotretinoin, an oral drug used in the treatment of

Table 2 Toxins Affecting the Cornea

Reaction	Toxin	References
Epithelial toxicity	Adenine arabinoside	45
	Amphotericin B	45
	Anesthetics, topical	195
	Benoxinate	45
	Benzalkonium chloride	178
	Carabachol	134
	Chloramphenicol	45
	Cocaine	45
	Echothiophate	134
	Epinephrine	134
	Fluorescein	178
	5-Fluorouracil	203
	Gentamicin	3
	Hibiclens	154, 230
	Hydrogen peroxide	110
	Idoxuridine	45, 237
	Lidocaine	45
	Miconazole	240
	Neomycin-gramicidin-polymyxin	237
	Neostigmine	134
	Povidone iodine scrub	154
	Tetracaine	45
	Trifluorothymidine	45
Calcific band keratopathy	Mercurial vapors	237
	Phenylmercuric nitrate	237
Opacities	Amantadine	92
	Indomethacin	44
	Isotretinoin	88
	Nitrosureas	118
	Tamoxifen	118
	Tilorone	118
Decreased stromal wound healing	Ara-A	140
	Ara AMP	140
	Cytosine arabinoside	45
	Idoxuridine	140
	Trifluridine	140
	Vidarabine	45
Edema	Acetylcysteine, 20%	221
	EDTA	45
Haze	Calcium EDTA (0.2 M)	221
	Cysteine (0.2 M)	221
Endothelial toxicity	Amphotericin B	45
	Epinephrine	233
	Gentamicin	177
	Methylparaben	234
	Phenylephrine	74
	Propylparaben	234
	Silicone oil	84
	Sodium bisulfite	234
Pigmentation	Amiodarone	61
	Chloroquine	26
	Chlorpromazine	157
	Epinephrine (adrenochrome)	81
	Gold	129

Table 3 Toxins Affecting the Lacrimal System

Reaction	Toxin	References
Shortened tear breakup time	Anesthetics	195
	Benzalkonium chloride	195
	Chlorbutanol	195
	Methylcellulose	45
	Polyvinyl alcohol	45
	Retinoids	88, 141
Decreased tear secretion/reflex	Anesthetics	195
	Methotrexate	118
Excessive lacrimation	Cytosine arabinoside	118
	Doxorubicin	106
	Formaldehyde	152
	5-Fluorouracil	106
Decreased lipid film stability	Benzalkonium chloride	45
	Retinoids	88, 145
Nasolacrimal duct obstruction	Epinephrine	106
		188
Tear duct fibrosis	5-Fluorouracil	106
Increased tear evaporation	Retinoids	85, 141
Decreased meibomian gland tissue	Retinoids	137
Pigmentation of lacrimal sac	Silver	151

severe cystic acne [191]. This medication commonly causes toxic ocular reactions, such as blepharoconjunctivitis, keratoconjunctivitis sicca, blurred vision, and corneal opacities [88]. A decreased lipid content of the tear film may account for the isotretinoin-induced dry eye and the associated lower tear breakup time (time between a complete blink and the appearance of the first randomly distributed corneal dry spot) [76]. Isotretinoin may also influence the amount of lipid that reaches the ocular surface by affecting the meibomian glands. In experimental animals (hamsters), orally administered isotretinoin markedly decreases the amount of acinar tissue in these sebaceous glands [137].

C. Sclera

Toxic reactions in the sclera are uncommon, which may reflect anatomical characteristics of this tissue. Topically applied agents are more likely to be absorbed by the more anteriorly located cornea and conjunctiva than the sclera. Hematogenous exposure to toxins probably affects the sclera insignificantly because of this tissue's relative avascularity. The prolonged administration of systemic, but not topical, corticosteroids has been associated with scleral thinning and darkening [59,111]. This discoloration probably results from visualization of the underlying uvea through the thinned sclera.

Plaques that are usually located just anterior to the insertion of one of the rectus muscles (senile scleral plaques) form especially in elderly individuals [201]. Such lesions may darken following prolonged topical epinephrine, as in the treatment of glaucoma, and the discolored tissue may lead to a clinical suspicion of a melanoma [210]. Darkening of the sclera also occurs in ochronosis due to quinacrine and hydroquinone [7].

D. Lens

Numerous drugs cause cataracts, reversible myopia (attributed to abnormalities in lens hydration), lens pigmentation, or transient lenticular opacities in experimental animals (Table 4).

Corticosteroids are among the drugs most frequently implicated in cataract formation. Cataracts, which are typically subcapsular in type, are associated with long-term corticosteroid therapy. They are widely used in many clinical settings and are cataractogenic following topical application to the skin [56] or eye [71], as well as after administration in nasal aerosols or in an inhalation form [93] or orally [20,33].

Table 4 Toxins Affecting the Lens

Reaction	Toxin	Reference
Cataract	Allopurinol	89
	Busulfan	118
	Corticosteroids	33
	Dinitrophenol	170
	Echothiophate	12
	Ethylene oxide	67
	Naphthalene	231
	Phenmetrazine	162
	Phenothiazines	206
	Psoralen and UV light	147
	Triparanol	232
Pigmentation	Chlorpromazine	17
	Phenylmercuric nitrate	1
Transient lenticular opacities	Ketamine	49
	Xylazine	49

Without corticosteroids, posterior subcapsular cataracts form in less than 8% of individuals with rheumatoid arthritis and in 0.2–4% of normal individuals. However, in patients with rheumatoid arthritis subjected to 10 mg prednisone (or equivalent) for at least 2 years, the incidence of posterior subcapsular cataracts rises to 30–40%. With higher doses (>15 mg prednisone) and more prolonged therapy (>4 years), the incidence of cataracts approaches 80–100% [20]. An increased incidence of cataracts in other systemic diseases has also been noted after corticosteroid therapy [99]. The lens changes develop at all ages and relate to the dose and time of administration. When corticosteroid therapy is withdrawn these cataracts do not regress [38]. Experimental studies suggest that prednisone has an additive or synergistic effect on other cataractogenic toxic agents [30,31,57]. Several mechanisms of corticosteroid-induced cataract have been proposed and include drug-induced biochemical changes in the lens epithelium as well as binding of drugs to lens crystallins.

Following its incubation in medium containing dexamethasone, levels of sodium and certain other cations increase within the lens and potassium decreases in this structure, possibly as a sequel to an effect on the sodium-potassium-ATPase pump within the lens epithelium [108,130,131,159]. These abnormalities of ion flow may increase lens hydration, which may account at least in part for lens opacification.

Nonenzymatic reactions between prednisolone and lysine residues of lens crystallins result in steric changes within the crystallins, which exposes their sulfhydryl residues and hence increases their likelihood of oxidation [41,42,156]. The formation of disulfide bonds between crystallin molecules may result in insoluble high-molecular-weight complexes capable of scattering light. That the creation of disulfide bonds plays a role in cataractogenesis is supported by the observation that the reducing agent, dithiotreitol, reverses corticosteroid-induced lens opacities [42].

Some therapeutic agents administered to reduce serum lipid and cholesterol levels may produce cataracts [14,51,96], putatively because of an inhibition of cholesterol synthesis in lens epithelial cells [196], which normally migrate toward the center of the lens as they increase the surface area of their cholesterol-containing plasma membranes. Triparanol, which inhibits cholesterol biosynthesis by blocking the enzymatic reduction of desmosterol (24-dehydrocholesterol) to cholesterol, induces cataracts in humans and experimental animals [232]. The high incidence of cataracts produced by this drug resulted in its withdrawal from clinical use. When young rats are maintained on a diet containing triparanol for 3–4 months, cataracts resembling those in humans on prolonged triparanol therapy develop. The cataract is characterized by a feathery radial arrangement of fine gray dots in the anterior lens cortex.

The interaction of ultraviolet light with certain drugs may also lead to lens opacities. For example, granular lenticular deposits occasionally form in patients after the chronic ingestion of phenothiazines, such as chlorpromazine [17], but these deposits do not appear to lead to progressive opacification of the lens

E. Anterior Chamber, Ciliary Body, and Intraocular Pressure

Drugs may induce adverse consequences in the anterior chamber. Tissue plasminogen activator has been used to decrease intraocular fibrin formation following vitrectomy for proliferative vitreoretinopathy and retinal detachment in humans or following experimentally induced hyphema in rabbits [121,138]. In rabbits with experimentally produced hyphemas, the incidence of rebleeding into the anterior chamber from the original injury site increases following the intraocular injection of tissue plasminogen activator [236]. This adverse effect of tissue plasminogen activator is not the result of a toxic effect of the enzyme but rather of an overdosage.

Other therapeutic agents capable of deleterious effects upon the anterior chamber include amphotericin B and topical phenylephrine. The intravitreal administration of amphotericin B in the monkey may lead to the formation of transient fibrin clots in the anterior chamber [18]. Some therapeutic agents, such as corticosteroids, certain mydriatic and cycloplegic drugs, and, rarely, tricyclic antidepressants, elevate the intraocular pressure [21,29,53,72,91,143]. Viscous solutions introduced into the anterior chamber may also elevate intraocular pressure [101].

For poorly understood reasons, systemic and topically administered corticosteroids precipitate glaucoma in susceptible individuals [211]. The trabecular meshwork is sometimes histologically normal in steroid-induced glaucoma, but a fibrillar material may be present in the area immediately surrounding the canal of Schlemm [192,211]. Cell culture studies of animal and human trabecular meshwork have detected corticosteroid-induced alterations of the glycosaminoglycan (GAG) and proteoglycan composition of the trabecular meshwork [85,112,123,132,193], but it remains uncertain whether increased amounts of GAG impair aqueous drainage and lead to steroid-induced glaucoma. The incubation of trabecular meshwork explants with corticosteroids results in an increased DNA content of trabecular meshwork cells [228] and the induction of some soluble proteins [173,227]. The contribution, if any, of these aberrant proteins to steroid-induced glaucoma remains unknown.

Drugs, such as cocaine, opiates, marijuana, amphetamines, and diazepam, may result in defective accommodation [162].

F. Retina and Vitreous

Different toxic agents have deleterious effects upon the retina and vitreous (Figs. 5 and 6; Table 5). Visual disturbances attributed to retinal dysfunction following toxin exposure include decreased visual acuity, impaired color perception, visual field defects, scotomata, night blindness, visual perseveration beyond the physiological afterimage (palinopsia), and an illusory movement of the physical environment (oscillopsia). Long-term administration of some drugs results in a pigmentary retinopathy, whereas short-term exposure to other toxins results in retinal degeneration, hemorrhage, ischemia, and necrosis. Macular edema, retinal pigment epithelium defects, and a compromised blood-retinal barrier are also consequences of some drug toxicities affecting the retina.

Chloroquine, which is used in the treatment of malaria and connective tissue disorders, such as rheumatoid arthritis and systemic lupus erythematosus, may adversely affect the retina, causing decreased visual acuity, blurred vision, diplopia, decreased color and night vision, and visual field defects [26]. Chloroquine retinopathy develops insidiously and is characterized by a fine mottling of the macula, arteriolar narrowing, peripheral retinal pigmentation, and loss of the foveal reflex and, in advanced cases, by a depigmented macula surrounded by a pigmented ring (bull's-eye macular pigmentation; Fig. 5). As a consequence of the retinopathy, both the electroretinogram and electrooculogram are frequently abnormal. Chloroquine retinopathy is clinically serious and irreversible with no effective therapy. This toxic retinopathy is dose related, most cases occurring only after a cumulative dose of 300 g or more [26]. Chloroquine retinopathy is characterized morphologically by curvilinear intracytoplasmic bodies within the retinal pigment epithelium (RPE) and clumping of these cells, as well as focal destruction of the photoreceptors [185]. The mechanism by which chloroquine damages the retina is poorly understood, but this drug has an affinity for melanin-containing cells, such as the RPE. In rats, chloroquine inhibits protein synthesis in the RPE [102]. Most investigators contend that RPE damage is the first manifestation of chloroquine retinopathy and that the rods and cones are damaged subsequently [28,185].

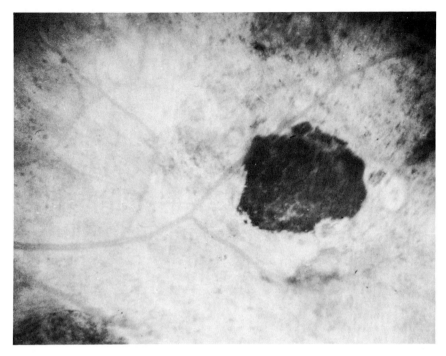

Figure 5   Pseudoretinitis pigmentosa following the use of thioridazine (Mellaril) showing pigment deposits throughout the retina. (Courtesy of Drs. C. Hanna and F. T. Fraunfelder.)

Phenothiazines, such as chlorpromazine and thioridazine, are commonly used in the treatment of certain psychiatric illnesses. They may result in a clinically significant retinopathy as well as corneal, conjunctival, lenticular, and periocular dermatological abnormalities. Affected patients commonly have blurred vision, difficulty with night vision, and visual field defects, as well as abnormalities in color vision and in the electroretinogram. Fundus changes include macular and peripheral retinal pigmentation. Phenothiazine retinopathy is dose related, but in contrast to chloroquine retinopathy, visual acuity, color vision, visual fields, and the electroretinograms return to normal when the drug is no longer administered. In phenothiazine retinopathy individual RPE cells are larger than normal and contain increased amounts of lipofuscin, melanolysosomes, and curvilinear bodies [166].

Phenothiazines are absorbed onto melanin granules and accumulate within the uvea and RPE [180]. Their toxic effects upon the retina may be secondary to RPE damage [166]. Support for the view that phenothiazines affect RPE function is found in the observation that phenothiazines inhibit the phagocytosis of latex particles by cultured chick RPE cells in a dose-dependent manner [158] and that chlorpromazine causes morphological abnormalities in the RPE in culture [158].

Various drugs, including antibacterial, antifungal, and antiviral agents, as well as tissue plasminogen activator, are injected into the vitreous cavity in several clinical settings, and many of these agents incite a transient inflammatory response [18,69,124,219].

G.   Iris

Toxins rarely affect the iris or other uveal structures. Quinine is administered in the treatment of nocturnal leg cramps and malaria but is also used to dilute abused drugs, such as heroin [162]. In quinine toxicity the iris may atrophy for unknown reasons (Table 6) [133]. Echothiophate, an anticholinesterase agent used in the therapy of open-angle glaucoma, may cause cysts at the pupillary margin of the iris [209]. The cysts and the associated miosis may decrease visual acuity by occluding the visual axis.

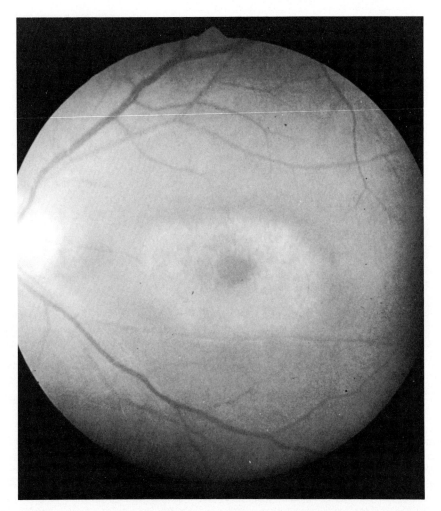

Figure 6   Retinal changes following the long-term use of high doses of chloroquine. Macular degeneration has developed in the form of a bull's-eye. (Courtesy of Drs. C. Hanna and F. T. Fraunfelder.)

The aperture of the pupil is controlled by the dilator and sphincter muscles of the iris and is under the regulation of the central nervous system (CNS). Many toxins affect pupil size, but such changes are not necessarily due to a direct effect on the sphincter or dilator pupillae. For example, the miosis associated with morphine reflects a CNS effect since it is abolished by severing the optic nerve [160].

Melanosomes are occasionally released into the aqueous from the iris after topical phenylephrine [167], presumably following rupture of iris epithelial cells [136]. The released pigment may be associated with a transient increase in intraocular pressure, putatively due to a blockage of aqueous outflow at the trabecular meshwork [135].

H.   Choroid

Relatively few agents are associated with unexpected and deleterious effects upon the choroid. In the eye, thioridazine toxicity primarily involves the retina (see page 1173), but focal chorioretinal atrophy and associated focal absence of the choriocapillaris occur in some cases of progressive thioridazine toxicity [165,166]. Illicit intravenously administered drugs are often contaminated with foreign particles (talc or cornstarch) that occasionally accumulate in choroidal and other ocular blood vessels in drug addicts [142].

Table 5 Toxins Affecting Retina and Vitreous

Reaction	Toxin	Reference
Retinopathy	Amikacin	224
	Amphotericin B	18
	Chloroquine	26
	Chlorpromazine	158
	Cis-platinum	118
	Gentamicin	54
	Indomethacin	104
	Moxolactam	82
	Netilmicin	60
	Nitrosureas	118
	Quinine	13
	Silicone	103
	Tamoxifen	118
	Tobramycin	60
	Thioridazine	166
	Tilorone	118
	Tissue plasminogen activator	124
	Vincristine	190
Transient vitritis	Amphotericin B	18
	Interferon-α	69
	Tissue plasminogen activator	219

An isolated example of a necrotizing choroiditis due to intracarotid nitrogen mustard administered for a brain tumor was confirmed at autopsy [8].

I. Optic Nerve

Certain drugs and toxins may result in optic atrophy, optic neuritis, and optic nerve head edema (Table 7). Most of these compounds exert their toxic effect on the optic nerve only after prolonged administration, but methanol is a notable exception.

The visual symptoms of methanol intoxification include blurred vision, loss of central vision, and complete blindness some 18–48 h after ingestion [25]. In an investigation of 320 individuals who ingested a mixture containing 35% methanol and 15% ethanol, Benton and Calhoun [25] found hyperemia and edema of the optic disk and surrounding retina in some patients who later manifested permanent impairment of

Table 6 Toxins Affecting the Uvea

Reaction	Toxin	Reference
Iris atrophy	Quinine	162
Release of iris pigment into anterior chamber	Phenylephrine	167
Cyclitis	Cyclophosphamide (in rats)	106
Abnormal accommodation	Amitriptyline	100
	Amphetamines	162
	Cocaine	162
	Diazepam	162
	Marijuana	162
	Opiates	162
Choroidal atrophy and choriocapillaris degeneration	Thioridazine	166
	Talc	162
Necrotizing choroiditis	Nitrogen mustard	118

Table 7 Toxins Affecting the Optic Nerve

Reaction	Toxin	References
Optic neuritis	Arsenic	217
	Barbiturates	162
	Chloramphenicol	52
	Chlorpropamide	217
	Cis-platinum	118
	Digitalis	217
	Ethambutol	47, 58
	Ibuprofen	100, 169
	Isoniazid	217
	Methanol	25
	Nitrosureas	118
	Pantopaque (contrast agent)	125
	Penicillamine	62, 217
	Quinine	217
	Streptomycin	217
	Sulfonamides	217
Optic neuropathy	Barbiturates	162
	Chloramphenicol	62
	Chlorpropamide	62
	Cytosine arabinoside	118
	Disulfiram	168
	Ethambutol	62
	Ethchlorvynol	162
	Isoniazid	62
	Methotrexate	118
	Nitrosureas	118
	Streptomycin	62
	Sulfonamides	62
	Tolbutamide	62
	Vincristine	106, 118
Papilledema	Barbiturates	162
	Cis-platinum	106
	Corticosteroids	118
	Gold	106
	Isotretinoin	88
	Lead	106
	Mercury	106
	Mitotane	118
	Thallium	106

vision. In persons with marked acidosis, optic atrophy sometimes followed severe retinal edema. A central scotoma was a common visual field defect. Vision recovered partially or completely if improvement began during the first week. In the rhesus monkey methanol intoxification produces edema of the optic disk as a result of intracytoplasmic swelling in the axons [19] and mydriasis and a poor pupillary response to light [19]. In this primate, the disk and intraorbital part of the optic nerve are conspicuously affected instead of the retina.

Patients with cystic fibrosis are frequently treated with several grams of chloramphenicol for years because they are extremely prone to pulmonary infections. After such prolonged treatment, they sometimes manifest an optic and peripheral neuropathy [27,40,145,238]. Atrophy and demyelination of both optic nerves, as well as loss of ganglion cells and gliosis of the nerve fiber layers of the corresponding retinas, have been observed in autopsy studies of eyes from chloramphenicol-treated children with cystic fibrosis [107,238]. Improvement in visual acuity after cessation of chloramphenicol in affected patients suggests that the nerve damage is secondary to the drug, not to cystic fibrosis [107].

Ethambutol suppresses the growth of *Mycobacterium tuberculosis*, including those resistant to isoniazid and streptomycin. This orally administered drug readily accumulates in persons with impaired renal function [58]. Blurred vision, edema of the optic nerve head and macula, visual field defects, and abnormal color vision may occur in individuals receiving this drug. Optic atrophy and blindness may also occur [37]. If the drug is discontinued at the first sign of visual loss, recovery may occur; however, it may take years if it is slowly withdrawn [16]. The visual abnormalities have been attributed to (1) dysfunction of the central fibers of the optic nerve (loss of central vision associated with a central scotoma and a marked decrease in color discrimination, usually with loss of ability to recognize green and sometimes red) and (2) less commonly, impaired function of the peripheral fibers of the optic nerve (defects in the peripheral field isopters) [144]. Both the duration and the incidence of visual changes appear to be dose related [66]. Although uncommon, some patients on high doses of ethambutol develop an irreversible optic neuropathy [197].

Ethambutol (high doses for prolonged periods) depigments the tapetum lucidum in laboratory animals [199]. In several animals (rat, rabbit, dog, and monkey) ethambutol causes a focal swelling of the axons in the optic chiasm [144]. Ethambutol is the only drug known to create chiasmal lesions experimentally, and a few examples of primary chiasmal lesions have been documented in humans with toxic amblyopia [144].

J. Orbit

The orbital tissue most frequently affected by toxic reactions is the extraocular muscle (Table 8). Disorders of ocular motility and diplopia are occasional manifestations of drug toxicity. Antineoplastic agents, such as vincristine, 5-fluorouracil and fludarabine, the antimalarials chloroquine and hydroxychloroquine, and commonly abused drugs, such as marijuana and barbiturates, may result in diplopia and extraocular muscle dysfunction. Phenytoin and the contrast agent iopamidol (used in myelography) sometimes cause an abducens nerve palsy [22,200].

Retrobulbar injections of anesthetics rarely cause diplopia [184] or an inability to elevate the eye in the adducted position, by both voluntary and passive forced ductions (Brown's syndrome) [77]. Retrobulbar anesthesia is more likely to cause complications if the drug is injected directly into one of the rectus muscles or into the optic nerve [184]. In a study of the lateral rectus muscle of rats given a single retrobulbar injection of mepivacaine, ultrastructural analysis disclosed destruction of muscle fibers, activation of myoblasts, phagocytosis, and regeneration of muscle fibers [172]. Okland and colleagues [172] suggest that this local anesthetic affects the sarcolemma and membranes of the sarcoplasmic reticulum and that nuclear and mitochondrial membranes become damaged subsequently. Biochemical studies indicate that disturbances in calcium distribution may account for the membrane abnormalities detected morphologically [23,218]. Myoblasts and motor nerve terminals are not significantly affected morphologically by injections of local anesthetics [122,208].

K. Central Visual Sensory System

Toxins affecting the CNS may involve visual processing and result in different clinically significant abnormalities. For example, transient cortical blindness occasionally follows the administration of antineoplastic agents, such as intravenous vincristine [48] and intravenous cis-platinum [70,179], as well as intrathecal metrizamide used in vertebral arteriography [125]. Also, fetal exposure to isotretinoin may cause cortical blindness [88]. Lesions in the parietooccipital or temporoparietal areas of the cerebral hemispheres can result in visual illusions and may account for disturbances in individuals taking illicit drugs [148].

Ophthalmoplegia has been associated with some antineoplastic drugs (nitrosureas, vincristine, and methotrexate) [118], anticonvulsants (phenytoin and carbamazepine) [200,214], and antidepressants (imipramine) [181]. The mechanism of drug-induced ophthalmoplegia is poorly understood, but the total external ophthalmoplegia induced by phenytoin may reflect a vestibulooculomotor disturbance [214]. Phenytoin is thought to potentiate inhibitory synapses in the vestibulooculomotor system, as well as to increase neural discharge in Purkinje's cells, which exert an inhibitory influence on the same structures [214].

Table 8 Toxins Affecting the Orbital Tissues

Reaction	Toxin	Reference
Orbital vasodilatation	Nitrosoureas	118
Brown's syndrome	Lidocaine/bupivacaine/hyaluronidase	77
Diplopia, Extraocular muscle abnormalities	Barbiturates	162
	Bupivacaine	172
	Carbamazepine	187
	Diazepam	162
	Fludarabine	118
	5-Fluorouracil	118
	Glutethimide	162
	Laetrile	106
	Lidocaine	172
	Marijuana	162
	Mepivacaine	172
	Metrizamide	125
	Mitotane	118
	Nitrosoureas	118
	Opiates	162
	Phenytoin	187
	Quinine	162
	Vincristine	106

Atypical ocular movements attributed to CNS dysfunction may accompany the use of some drugs. Ocular dyskinesias, such as ocular skew deviation and nystagmus (downbeating and horizontal), are occasionally associated with the administration of carbamazepine but do not correlate with serum levels of the drug [200]. Increased catecholaminergic activity in the central nervous system may account for the carbamazepine-induced ocular dyskinesias [200]. Lithium toxicity sometimes may evoke a wide range of ocular motility disturbances (downbeating or horizontal nystagmus, saccadic pursuit or dysmetria, unilateral gaze palsy, oculogyric crisis, and opsoclonus) [55]. Studies of the brain postmortem in rhesus monkeys, as well as in a single human case, suggest that lithium causes neuronal degeneration and loss, as well as gliosis in neuronal groups beneath the fourth ventricle (medial vestibular and propositus hypoglossi nuclei) that connect to the vestibular nuclei, cerebellum, cerebral cortex, and cranial nerve nuclei that innervate the extraocular muscles [55]. Other abnormal ocular movements evoked by drugs or toxins include an abnormal spontaneous and rapid conjugate movement of the eyes in the vertical plane with a slow return to the midposition (atypical ocular bobbing), as documented in acute poisoning with organophosphate pesticides [109].

L. Eyelids

Certain toxic reactions culminate in blepharitis, blepharospasm, ptosis, scarring in the eyelid, or pigmentation of this tissue (Table 9). The phenothiazines, particularly thioridazine [157,206], as well as silver and some other heavy metals [215], deposit in the skin, discoloring the eyelids. Hyperpigmentation of the eyelids may also follow industrial exposure to tars, oils rich in hydrocarbon, and phenols [73]. Depigmentation of the eyelid margins in black patients has been attributed to topical eserine ointment, possibly secondary to contact allergy [120]. Blepharitis complicates the topical application of many agents, and with some compounds, such as 5-fluorouracil, this also follows their systemic administration [119,220]. In addition to blepharitis, 5-fluorouracil may produce blepharospasm [198]. Solar radiation potentiates the toxic effects of several agents, and such phototoxic reactions may result in blepharitis in patients treated with isotretinoin, sulfonamides, barbiturates, phenothiazines, and dimethylchlortetracycline [80,88,237].

Table 9 Toxins Affecting the Eyelids

Reaction	Toxin	Reference
Blepharitis	Barbiturates	237
	Demethylchlortetracycline	237
	5-Fluorouracil	106
	Isotretinoin	88
	Phenothiazines	237
	Sulfonamides	237
Blepharospasm	Carbamazepine	200
	Marijuana	162
	5-Fluorouracil	118
Ptosis	Barbiturates	162
	Guanethedine	237
	Laetrile	118
	Opiates	162
	Phenycyclidine	162
	Steroids	237
	Vincristine	118
Pigmentation	Chlorpromazine	237
	Hydrocarbon oils	237
	Mercury	237
	5-Methoxypsoralen	237
	Phenols	237
	Phenothiazines	36
	Silver	237
	Tars	237
Scarring	Amphetamine, topical	162
	Cocaine, topical	162
	5-Fluorouracil	118
Ocular myasthenia gravis	D-Penicillamine	127

perfumes and colognes [43]. Eversion (ectropion) or fusion (ankyloblepharon) of the eyelid margins may follow the intravenous use of 5-fluorouracil [119]. Retraction of the upper eyelids has been associated with amphetamine and cocaine abuse [91,105].

The eyelashes may also be subject to deleterious drug effects. In some patients treated with thiotepa (triethylenethiophosphoramide) to decrease corneal neovascularization or to prevent recurrence of pterygium, the eyelashes become depigmented (poliosis) [11,114]. In an isolated report, loss of the eyelashes (madarosis) complicated long-term topical epinephrine administration [126], but this may have been due to compulsive pulling and removal of the lashes (trichotillomania).

V. INTRAOCULAR TUMORS

The chemical induction of tumors is well documented in non-ocular tissues, but there is little evidence to implicate toxins in ocular carcinogenesis. However, squamous cell carcinoma of the conjunctiva, harderian gland adenocarcinoma, unspecified malignant iris tumors, choroidal melanomas, and orbital sarcomas have followed intraocular methylcholanthrene in mice [176]. A single intravenous injection of radium apparently induced ciliary body melanomas in 24 of 169 dogs [225]. An intraocular melanoma developed in an experimental animal following prolonged intraperitoneal ethionine and oral N-2-fluorenylacetamide [24]. In a population of current or former workers at a chemical plant that produced a variety of suspected carcinogens, more workers developed choroidal melanoma (5 of 847) than one would expect by chance in a population of this size [2].

VI. SYSTEMIC COMPLICATIONS OF OCULAR MEDICATIONS

Systemic side effects of medications administered for ocular disease are uncommon but may be life threatening (Fig. 7). Indeed, topical ocular anesthetics, such as cocaine and tetracaine, have been fatal on rare occasions [195]. Many reported systemic side effects of ocular medications are due to mydriatic and cycloplegic agents used to facilitate ocular examination or to treat glaucoma.

Some topical antiglaucoma agents (epinephrine, phenylephrine, and anticholinergic drugs) may cause tachycardia and arrhythmias, but β-adrenergic antagonists (timolol and betaxolol) may result in bradycardia [164,239]. In patients with preexisting heart disease, these drugs may cause congestive heart failure and exacerbate conduction defects, leading to cardiac arrest.

Pulmonary complications of topically applied ocular medications are also potentially life threatening. Bronchospasm may follow ocular administration of β-adrenergic blocking agents (timolol and betaxolol), cholinergic drugs (pilocarpine and carbachol), and cholinesterase inhibitors (echothiophate) and other drugs [6,87,97,182,194]. Status asthmaticus, which can be fatal, may follow the topical application of timolol to the eye in asthmatics [87]. Respiratory arrest may complicate retrobulbar injections of the local anesthetics bupivacaine or lidocaine [161].

CNS side effects of ophthalmic medications are well documented. Confusion, hallucinations, and other psychotic symptoms may follow the application of anticholinergic drugs, such as scopolamine, homatropine, or cyclopentolate, to the eye [202]. Echothiophate may result in confusion, slurred speech, and ataxia [202]. As a consequence of drug-induced hypertension, rupture of intracranial aneurysms and subarachnoid hemorrhage may follow the topical instillation of phenylephrine [50,94].

Untoward reactions to ophthalmic medications may affect several organ systems. Anorexia, nausea, and abdominal discomfort sometimes follow treatment with the carbonic anhydrase inhibitors, tropicamide, pilocarpine, timolol, epinephrine, and atropine [89,202]. Aplastic anemia or pancytopenia may accompany topical ocular chloramphenicol therapy or administration of the carbonic anhydrase inhibitors acetazolamide and methazolamide [89]. Carbonic anhydrase inhibitors may also cause metabolic acidosis.

VII. EFFECT OF OCULAR MEDICATIONS ON FETUS AND NEONATE

Pregnant women are generally not treated with topical ophthalmic medications, because they may adversely affect the fetus or neonate following systemic absorption. The teratogenic effects of certain drugs upon the developing fetus are discussed in Chapter 43. Systemically absorbed ocular medications, such as timolol, may be excreted into the milk of lactating mothers [153].

Several drugs used in the treatment of ophthalmic disorders may have adverse effects on the fetus or neonate if administered during pregnancy. The mydriatic agent scopolamine can cause fetal tachycardia and dysrhythmias, and in the newborn the scopolamine toxicity is manifested by fever, tachycardia, and lethargy [78]. Pilocarpine may cause hyperthermia, restlessness, seizures, and diaphoresis in the neonate [5]. Treatment of myasthenia gravis with cholinesterase inhibitors produces temporary muscle weakness in newborns [34].

VIII. TOXICITY OF INACTIVE AGENTS PRESENT IN OCULAR MEDICATIONS

Inactive compounds, such as preservatives, antioxidants, and buffers, as well as viscosity-increasing, wetting, and tonicity agents, are often present in ocular medications. Although generally safe, some of these chemicals incite responses in the eye. Most toxic reactions due to these ingredients follow topical therapy and therefore most often affect the cornea and conjunctiva.

Subconjunctival injections of the preservatives sodium bisulfite, methylparaben, and propylparaben [234] cause a dose-dependent intercellular vacuolization and thickening of the corneal endothelium in rabbits. Benzalkonium chloride, another preservative frequently used in ocular medications, induces loss of microvilli and desquamation of rabbit corneal epithelial cells when applied topically and causes corneal edema with swelling and rupture of the corneal endothelium when injected into the anterior chamber [45]. Thimerosal and chlorbutanol, preservatives found in soft contact lens solutions, increase corneal epithelial permeability in isolated rabbit corneas [46]. This toxic effect is not detected in corneas from living rabbits, however, perhaps because of dilution by tears.

IX. POTENTIATION OF TOXICITY BY MULTIPLE AGENTS

The ocular side effects of some medications are potentiated by other therapeutic agents. The synergistic toxic effect of multiple agents on the eye is most frequently encountered when multiple antineoplastic agents are administered in association with radiotherapy. For example, the combination of intravenous azathioprine or cyclophosphamide, together with local irradiation, accentuates the severity of corticosteroid-induced cataracts [118]. Intravenous methotrexate, cytosine arabinoside, lomustine, and 5-fluorouracil may all potentiate radiation-induced optic neuropathy [118].

The systemic toxicity of certain medications may be exacerbated by drugs used in the therapy of ocular disorders. For example, treatment of glaucoma with carbonic anhydrase inhibitors, such as acetazolamide and methazolamide, increases the serum level of nonionized salicylate and therefore increases the risk of salicylate toxicity in patients concurrently receiving high doses of aspirin [9]. At least one other carbonic anhydrase inhibitor, acetazolamide, worsens osteomalacia in patients who are also ingesting phenytoin [155].

REFERENCES

1. Abrams, J.D. Iatrogenic mercurialentis. *Trans. Ophthalmol. Soc. UK 83*:263–269, 1963.
2. Albert, D.M., Robinson, N.L., Fulton, A.B., Zakov, Z.N., Dryja, T.P., Puliafito, C.A., Smith, A.B., and Egan, E.A. Epidemiological investigation of increased incidence of choroidal melanoma in a single population of chemical workers. *Int. Ophthalmol. Clin. 20*:71–92, 1980.
3. Alfonso, E.C., Albert, D.M., Kenyon, K.R., Robinson, B.S., Hanninen, L., and D'Amico, D.J. In vitro toxicity of gentamicin to corneal epithelial cells. *Cornea 9*:55–61, 1990.
4. Alfonso, E., Kenyon, K.R., D'Amico, D.J., Saulenas, A.M., and Albert, D.M. Effects of gentamicin on healing of transdifferentiating conjunctival epithelium in rabbit eyes. *Am. J. Ophthalmol. 105*:198–202, 1988.
5. Altman, B. Ocular effects in the newborn from maternal drugs. In *Symposium on Ocular Therapy*, 11th ed., I.H. Leopold and R.P. Burns (Eds.), John Wiley & Sons, New York, pp. 97–99, 1979.
6. Anand, K.B., and Eschmann, E. Systemic effects of ophthalmic medications in the elderly. *NY State J. Med. 89*:134–136, 1988.
7. Anderson, B. Corneal and conjunctival pigmentation among workers engaged in manufacture of hydroquinone. *Arch. Ophthalmol. 38*:812–826, 1947.
8. Anderson, B., and Anderson, B., Jr. Necrotizing uveitis incident to perfusion of intracranial malignancies with nitrogen mustard or related compounds. *Trans. Am. Ophthalmol. Soc. 58*:95–105, 1960.
9. Anderson, B., Kaufman, P.L., and Sturm, R.J. Toxicity of combined therapy with carbonic anhydrase inhibitors and aspirin. *Am. J. Ophthalmol. 86*:516–519, 1978.
10. Armaly, M.F. Effect of corticosteroids on intraocular pressure and fluid dynamics. I. The effect of dexamethasone in the normal eye. *Arch. Ophthalmol. 70*:492–499, 1963.
11. Asregadoo, E.R. Surgery, thio-tepa and corticosteroid in the treatment of pterygium. *Am. J. Ophthalmol. 74*:960–963, 1972.
12. Axelsson, V. Glaucoma, miotic therapy and cataract. *Acta Ophthalmol. (Copenh.) 47*:1049–1059, 1969.
13. Bacon, P., Spalton, D.J., and Smith, S.E. Blindness from quinine toxicity. *Br. J. Ophthalmol. 72*:219–224, 1988.
14. Bagdon, R.E., Engstrom, R.G., Kelly, L.A., Hartman, H.A., Robison, R.L., and Visscher, G.E. Hypolipidemic activity and toxicity studies of a styrl-hexahydroindolinol 34-250. *Toxicol. Appl. Pharmacol. 69*:12–28, 1983.
15. Barrada, A., Peyman, G.A., Case, J., Fishman, G., Thomas, A., and Fiscella, R. Evaluation of intravitreal 5-fluorouracil, vincristine, VP 16, doxorubicin, and thiotepa in primate eyes. *Ophthalmic Surg. 15*:767–769, 1984.
16. Barron, G.J., Tepper, L., and Iovine, G. Ocular toxicity from ethambutol. *Am. J. Ophthalmol. 77*:256–260, 1974.
17. Barsa, J.A., Newton, J.C., and Saunders, J.C. Lenticular and corneal opacities during phenothiazine therapy. *JAMA 193*:98–100, 1965.
18. Barza, M., Baum, J., Tremblay, C., Szoka, F., and D'Amico, D.J. Ocular toxicity of intravitreally injected liposomal amphotericin B in rhesus monkeys. *Am. J. Ophthalmol. 100*:259–263, 1985.
19. Baumbach, G.L., Cancilla, P.A., Martin-Amat, G., Tephly, T.R., McMartin, K.E., Makar, A.B., Hayreh, M.S., and Hayreh, S.S. Methyl alcohol poisoning, IV. Alterations of the morphologic findings of the retina and optic nerve. *Arch. Ophthalmol. 95*:1859–1865, 1977.
20. Becker, B. The side effects of corticosteroids. *Invest. Ophthalmol. 3*:492–497, 1964.
21. Becker, B., Podos, S.M., Assef, C., and Cooper, D.G. Plasma cortisol suppression in glaucoma. *Am. J. Ophthalmol. 75*:73–76, 1973.
22. Bell, J.A., Dowd, T.C., McIlwaine, G.G., and Brittain, G.P.H. Postmyelographic abducent nerve palsy in association with the contrast agent iopamidol. *J. Clin. Neuro. Ophthalmol. 10*:115–117, 1990.

23. Benoit, P.W., Yagiela, J.A., and Fort, N.F. Pharmacologic correlation between local anesthetic-induced myotoxicity and disturbances of intercellular calcium distribution. *Toxicol. Appl. Pharmacol.* 52:187–198, 1990.

24. Benson, W.R. Intraocular tumor after ethionine and N-2-fluorenylacetamide. *Arch. Pathol.* 73:404–406, 1962.

25. Benton, C.D., and Calhoun, F.P., Jr. The ocular effects of methyl alcohol poisoning: Report of a catastrophe involving 320 persons. *Am. J. Ophthalmol.* 36:1677–1689, 1953.

26. Bernstein, H.N. Ocular toxicity of chloroquine. *Surv. Ophthalmol.* 12:415–419, 1968.

27. Bernstein, H.N. Some iatrogenic ocular diseases from systemically administered drugs. *Int. Ophthalmol. Clin.* 10:614–616, 1970.

28. Bernstein, H.N., and Ginsberg, G. The pathology of chloroquine retinopathy. *Arch. Ophthalmol.* 71:238–245, 1964.

29. Bernstein, H.N., Mills, D.W., and Becker, B. Steroid induced elevation of intraocular pressure. *Arch. Ophthalmol.* 70:15–18, 1963.

30. Bettman, J.W., Fung, W.E., and Noyes, P.O. Potentiating action of prednisolone on galactose cataracts in rats. *Invest. Ophthalmol.* 3:678–679, 1964.

31. Bettman, J.W., Noyes, P., and Debaskey, R. The potentiating action of steroids in cataractogenesis. *Invest. Ophthalmol.* 3:459, 1964.

32. Bhuyan, K.C., and Bhuyan, D.K. Superoxide dismutase of the eye: Relative functions of superoxide dismutase and catalase in protecting the ocular lens from oxidative damage. *Biochim. Biophys. Acta.* 542:28–38, 1978.

33. Black, R.L., Oglesby, R.B., and von Sallman, L. Posterior subcapsular cataract induced by corticosteroids in patients with rheumatoid arthritis. *JAMA* 174:166–171, 1960.

34. Blackhall, M.I., Buckley, G.A., Roberts, D.V., Roberts, J.B., Thomas, B.H., and Wilson, A. Drug-induced neonatal myasthenia. *J. Obstet. Gynaecol. Br. Commonw.* 76:157–162, 1969.

35. Bocanegra, T., Espinoza, L.R., Vasey, F.B., and Germain, B.F. Myasthenia gravis and penicillamine therapy of rheumatoid arthritis. *JAMA* 244:1822–1823, 1980.

36. Bond, W.S., and Yee, G.C. Ocular and cutaneous effects of chronic phenothiazine therapy. *Am. J. Hosp. Pharm.* 37:74–78, 1980.

37. Bowman, G., and Calissendorf, B. A case of irreversible bilateral optic damage after ethambutol toxicity. *Scand. J. Respir. Dis.* 55:176–180, 1974.

38. Braver, D.A., Richards, R.D., and Good, T.A. Posterior subcapsular cataracts in corticosteroid-treated children. *J. Pediatr.* 69:735–737, 1966.

39. Brothers, D.M., and Hidayat, A.A. Conjunctival pigmentation associated with tetracycline medication. *Ophthalmology* 88:1212–1215, 1981.

40. Bruce, G., Denning, C., and Spalter, H. Ocular findings in cystic fibrosis of the pancreas. *Arch. Ophthalmol.* 63:391–396, 1960.

41. Bucala, R., Fishman, J., and Cerami, A. Formation of covalent adducts between cortisol and 16 alpha-hydroxyestrone and protein: Possible role in the pathogenesis of cortisol toxicity and systemic lupus erythematosus. *Proc. Natl. Acad. Sci. USA* 79:3320–3324, 1982.

42. Bucala, R., Manabe, S., Urban, R.C., Jr., and Cerami, A. Nonenzymatic modification of lens crystallins by prednisolone induces sulfhydryl oxidation and aggregate formation: In vitro and in vivo studies. *Exp. Eye Res.* 41:353–363, 1985.

43. Burdick, K.H., and Hanover, N.H. Phototoxicity of Shalimar perfume. *Arch. Dermatol.* 93:424–425, 1966.

44. Burns, C.A. Indomethacin, reduced retinal sensitivity and corneal deposits. *Am. J. Ophthalmol.* 66:825–835, 1968.

45. Burstein, N.L. Corneal cytotoxicity of topically applied drugs, vehicles and preservatives. *Surv. Ophthalmol.* 25:15–30, 1980.

46. Burstein, N.L., and Klyce, S.D. Electrophysiologic and morphologic effects of ophthalmic preparations on rabbit cornea endothelium. *Invest. Ophthalmol.* 16:988–1011, 1977.

47. Buyske, D.A., Sterling, W., and Peets, E. Pharmacological and biochemical studies on ethambutol in laboratory animals. *Ann. NY Acad. Sci.* 135:711–725, 1966.

48. Byrd, R.L., Rohrbaugh, T.M., Raney, R.B., Jr., and Norris, D.G. Transient cortical blindness secondary to vincristine therapy in childhood malignancies. *Cancer* 47:37–40, 1981.

49. Calderone, L., Grimes, P., and Shalev, M. Acute reversible cataract induced by xylazine and by ketamine-xylazine anesthesia in rats and mice. *Exp. Eye Res.* 42:331–337, 1986.

50. Cass, E., Kadar, D., and Stein, H.A. Hazards of phenylephrine topical medication in persons taking propranol. *Can. Med. Assoc. J.* 120:1261–1262, 1979.

51. Cendella, R.J., and Bierkamper, G.G. Mechanism of cataract production by 3 beta (2-diethylaminoethox)-androst-5-en 17-one-hydrochloride, UL86 66A: An inhibitor of cholesterol biosynthesis. *Exp. Eye Res.* 28:673–688, 1979.

52. Chang, N., Giles, C.L., and Gregg, R.H. Optic neuritis and chloramphenicol. *Am. J. Dis. Child.* 112:46–48, 1966.

53. Christensen, R.E., and Pearce, I. Homatropine hydrobromide. *Arch. Ophthalmol.* 770:376–380, 1963.

54. Conway, B.P., Tabatabay, C.A., Campochiaro, P.A., D'Amico, D.J., Hanninen, L.A., and Kenyon, K.R. Gentamicin toxicity in the primate retina. *Arch. Ophthalmol.* 107:107–112, 1989.

55. Corbett, J.J., Jacobson, D.M., Thompson, H.S., Hart, M.N., and Albert, D.W. Downbeating nystagmus and other ocular motor defects caused by lithium toxicity. *Neurology 39*:481–487, 1989.
56. Costagliola, C., Cati-Giovannelli, B., and Picirillo, A. Cataracts associated with long-term steroids. *Br. J. Dermatol. 120*:472–473, 1989.
57. Cotlier, E., and Becker, B. Topical corticosteroids and galactose cataracts. *Invest. Ophthalmol. 4*:806–814, 1965.
58. Courty, G., Martre, P., LeRebeller, M.J., Verin, P., and Tessier, R. Bilateral optic neuritis caused by ethambutol in patient with renal insufficiency. *Board Med. 4*:1193–1200, 1971.
59. Crews, S.J. Adverse reaction to corticosteroid therapy in the eye. *Proc. R. Soc. Med. 58*:533–535, 1963.
60. D'Amico, D.J., Caspers-Velu, L., Libert, J., Shanks, E., Schrooyen, M., Hanninen, L.A., and Kenyon, K.R. Comparative toxicity of intravitreal aminoglycoside antibiotics. *Am. J. Ophthalmol. 100*:264–275, 1985.
61. D'Amico, D.J., Kenyon, K.R., and Rushkin, J.N. Amiodarone keratopathy: Drug induced lipid storage disease. *Arch. Ophthalmol. 99*:257–261, 1981.
62. Davidson, S.I. Drug-induced disorders of the eye. *Br. J. Hosp. Med. 24*:24–28, 1980.
63. Dawkins, R.L., Garlepp, M.J., McDonald, B.L., Williamson, J., Zilko, P.J., and Carrano, J. Myasthenia gravis and D-penicillamine. *J. Rheumatol. 8*(Suppl. 7):169–172, 1981.
64. Delamere, J.P., Jobson, S., Mackintosh, L.P., Wells, L., and Walton, K.W. Penicillamine-induced myasthenia in rheumatoid arthritis: Its clinical and genetic features. *Ann. Rheum. Dis. 42*:500–504, 1983.
65. Delong, S.L., Poley, B.J., and McFarlane, J.R. Ocular changes associated with long-term chlorpromazine therapy. *Arch. Ophthalmol. 73*:611–617, 1965.
66. Derka, H. Besteht korrelation zwischen der hohe der myambutoldosis und der häufigkeit der neuritis nervi optici? *Ophthalmologica 171*:123–131, 1975.
67. Deschamps, D., Leport, M., Laurent, A.M., Cordier, S., Festy, B., and Conso, F. Toxicity of ethylene oxide on the lens and on leukocytes: An epidemiological study in hospital sterilization installations. *Br. J. Ind. Med. 47*:308–313, 1990.
68. Desrochers, P.E., and Hoffert, J.R. Superoxide dismutase provides protection against the hyperoxia in the retina of the rainbow trout (*Salmo gairdneri*). *Comp. Biochem. Physiol. 76*:241–247, 1983.
69. Dharma, S.K., Peyman, G.A., Vernot, J., and Fiscella, R. Toxicity of intravitreally administered alpha-interferon. *Ophthalmic Surg. 18*:51–54, 1987.
70. Diamond, S.B., Rudolph, S.H., Lubicz, S.S., and Cohen, C.J. Cerebral blindness in association with cis-platinum chemotherapy for advanced carcinoma of the fallopian tube. *Obstet. Gynecol. 59*:845–865, 1982.
71. Donshik, P.C., Cavanaugh, D., and Boruchoff, S.A. Posterior subcapsular cataracts induced by topical corticosteroids following keratoplasty for keratoconus. *Ann. Ophthalmol. 13*:29–32, 1981.
72. Drance, S.M., and Ross, R.A. The ocular effects of epinephrine. *Surv. Ophthalmol. 14*:330–335, 1970.
73. Duke-Elder, S., and MacFaul, P.A. The ocular adnexa. Diseases of the eyelids. In *System of Ophthalmology*, Duke-Elder, S. (Ed.), C.V. Mosby, St. Louis, p. 367, 1974.
74. Edelhauser, H.F., Hine, J.E., Pederson, H., Van Horn, D.L., and Schultz, R.O. The effect of phenylephrine on the cornea. *Arch. Ophthalmol. 97*:937–947, 1979.
75. Ellis, P.P. *Ocular Therapeutics and Pharmacology*, 7th ed., C.V. Mosby, St. Louis, 1985.
76. Ensink, B.W., and van Voorst Vader, P.C. Ophthalmologic side effects of 13-cis-retinoic acid therapy. *Br. J. Dermatol. 108*:627, 1983.
77. Erie, J.C. Acquired Brown's syndrome after peribulbar anesthesia. *Am. J. Ophthalmol. 109*:349–350, 1990.
78. Evens, R.P., and Leopold, J.C. Scopolamine toxicity in a newborn. *Pediatrics 66*:329–330, 1980.
79. Farber, J.L. Biochemical mechanisms of toxic cell injury. *Klin. Wochenschr. 64*(Suppl. 7):142–143, 1986.
80. Ferguson, J., and Johnson, B.E. Photosensitivity due to retinoids: Clinical and laboratory studies. *Br. J. Dermatol. 115*:275–283, 1986.
81. Ferry, A.P., and Zimmerman, L.E. Black cornea: A complication of topical use of epinephrine. *Am. J. Ophthalmol. 58*:205–210, 1964.
82. Fett, D.R., Silverman, C.A., and Yoshizumi, M.O. Moxalactam retinal toxicity. *Arch. Ophthalmol. 102*:435–438, 1984.
83. Fiore, P.M. Drug-induced ocular cicatrization. *Int. Ophthalmol. Clin. 29*:147–150, 1989.
84. Foulks, G.N., Hatchell, D.L., Proia, A.D., and Klintworth, G.K. Histopathology of silicone oil keratopathy in humans. *Cornea 10*:29–37, 1991.
85. Francois, J. The importance of the mucopolysaccharides in intraocular pressure regulation. *Invest. Ophthalmol. 14*:173–176, 1975.
86. Fraunfelder, F.T. Extraocular fluid dynamics: How best to apply topical ocular medication. *Trans. Am. Ophthalmol. Soc. 74*:457–487, 1976.
87. Fraunfelder, F.T., and Barker, A.F. Respiratory effects of timolol (letter to the editor). *N. Engl. J. Med. 311*:1441, 1984.
88. Fraunfelder, F.T., LaBraico, J.M., and Meyer, S.M. Adverse ocular reactions possibly associated with isotretinoin. *Am. J. Ophthalmol. 100*:534–537, 1985.
89. Fraunfelder, F.T., and Meyer, S.M. Ocular toxicology update. *Aust. J. Ophthalmol. 12*:391–394, 1984.
90. Fraunfelder, F.T., and Meyer, S.M. Corneal complications of ocular medications. *Cornea 5*:55–59, 1986.

91. Fraunfelder, F.T., and Meyer, S.M. *Drug-Induced Ocular Side Effects and Drug Interactions*, Lea and Febiger, Philadelphia, 1989.
92. Fraunfelder, F.T., and Meyer, S.M. Amantadine and corneal deposits. *Am. J. Ophthalmol. 110*:96–97, 1990.
93. Fraunfelder, F.T., and Meyer, S.M. Posterior subcapsular cataracts associated with nasal or inhalation corticosteroids. *Am. J. Ophthalmol. 109*:489–490, 1990.
94. Fraunfelder, F.T., and Scafidi, A.F. Possible adverse effects from topical ocular 10% phenylephrine. *Am. J. Ophthalmol. 85*:447–453, 1978.
95. Garner, M.H., Garner, W.H., and Spector, A. H_2O_2-modification of Na,K-ATPase. *Invest. Ophthalmol. Vis. Sci. 27*:103–107, 1986.
96. Gerson, R.J., MacDonald, J.S., Alberts, A.W., Chen, J., Yudkovitz, J.B., Greenspan, M.D., Rubin, L.F., and Bokelmann, D.L. On the etiology of subcapsular lenticular opacities produced in dogs receiving HMG-CoA reductase inhibitors. *Exp. Eye Res. 50*:65–78, 1990.
97. Gesztes, T. Prolonged apnoea after suxamethonium injection associated with eye drops containing an anticholinesterase agent: A case report. *Br. J. Anaesth. 38*:408–409, 1966.
98. Giblin, F.J., McCready, J.P., and Reddy, V.N. The role of glutathione metabolism in the detoxification of H_2O_2 in rabbit lens. *Invest. Ophthalmol. Vis. Sci. 22*:330–335, 1982.
99. Giles, C., Mason, G.L., Duff, I.F., and McLean, I.A. The association of cataract formation and systemic corticosteroid therapy. *JAMA 182*:719–722, 1962.
100. Gilmartin, B. Ocular manifestations of systemic medications. *Ophthalmic Physiol. Optics 7*:449–459, 1987.
101. Glasser, D.B., Matsuda, M., and Edelhauser, H.F. A comparison of the efficacy and toxicity of and intraocular pressure response to viscous solutions in the anterior chamber. *Arch. Ophthalmol. 104*:1819–1824, 1986.
102. Gonasun, L.M., and Potts, A.M. In vitro inhibition of protein synthesis in the retinal pigment epithelium by chloroquine. *Invest. Ophthalmol. 13*:107–115, 1974.
103. Gonvers, M., Hornung, J.P., and de Courten, C. The effect of liquid silicone in the rabbit retina. *Arch. Ophthalmol. 104*:1057–1062, 1986.
104. Graham, C.M., and Blach, R.K. Indomethacin retinopathy: Case report and review. *Br. J. Ophthalmol. 72*:434–438, 1990.
105. Grant, W.M. *Toxicology of the Eye*, 2nd ed., Charles C. Thomas, Springfield, IL, 1974.
106. Griffin, J.D., and Garnick, M.B. Eye toxicity of cancer chemotherapy. *Cancer 48*:1539–1549, 1981.
107. Harley, R.D., Huang, N.N., Macri, C.H., and Green, W.R. Optic neuritis and optic atrophy following chloramphenicol in cystic fibrosis patients. *Trans. Am. Acad. Ophthalmol. Otolaryngol. 74*:1011–1031, 1970.
108. Harris, J.E., and Gruber, L. The electrolyte and water balance of the lens. *Exp. Eye Res. 1*:372–384, 1962.
109. Hata, S., Bernstein, E., and Davis, L.E. Atypical ocular bobbing in acute organophosphate poisoning. *Arch. Neurol. 43*:185–186, 1986.
110. Hayden, B.J., Zhu, L., Sens, D., Tapert, M.J., and Crouch, R.K. Cytolysis of corneal epithelial cells by hydrogen peroxide. *Exp. Eye Res. 50*:11–16, 1990.
111. Henderson, R.P., and Lander, R. Scleral discoloration associated with long-term prednisone administration. *Cutis 34*:76–77, 1984.
112. Hernandez, M.R., Weinstein, B.I., Wenk, E.J., Gordon, G.G., Dunn, M.W., and Southren, A.L. The effect of dexamethasone on the in vitro incorporation of precursors of extracellular matrix components in the outflow pathway region of the rabbit eye. *Invest. Ophthalmol. Vis. Sci. 24*:704–709, 1983.
113. Hodges, G.R. Aminoglycoside toxicity. In *The Aminoglycoside Antibiotics: A Guide to Therapy*, W.G. Barnes and G.R. Hodges (Eds.), CRC Press, Boca Raton, FL, pp. 153–179, 1984.
114. Howitt, D., and Karp, E.J. Side effects of topical thio-tepa. *Am. J. Ophthalmol. 63*:473–474, 1969.
115. Hull, D.S., Csukas, S., Green, K., and Livingston, V. Hydrogen peroxide and corneal endothelium. *Acta Ophthalmol. (Copenh.) 59*:409–421, 1981.
116. Hull, D.S., Green, K., and Elijah, R.D. Effect of oxygen free radical products on rabbit iris vascular permeability. *Acta Ophthalmol. (Copenh.) 63*:513–518, 1985.
117. Hull, D.S., Green, K., Thomas, L., and Alderman, N. Hydrogen peroxide-mediated corneal endothelial damage. *Invest. Ophthalmol. Vis. Sci. 25*:1246–1253, 1984.
118. Imperia, P.S., Lazarus, H.M., and Lass, J.H. Ocular complications of systemic cancer chemotherapy. *Surv. Ophthalmol. 34*:209–230, 1989.
119. Insler, M.S., and Helm, C.J. Ankyloblepharon associated with systemic 5-fluorouracil treatment. *Ann. Ophthalmol. 19*:374–375, 1987.
120. Jacklin, H.N. Depigmentation of the eyelids in eserine allergy. *Am. J. Ophthalmol. 59*:89–92, 1964.
121. Jaffe, G.J., Lewis, H., Han, D.P., Williams, G.A., and Abrams, G.W. Treatment of postvitrectomy fibrin pupillary block with tissue plasminogen activator. *Am. J. Ophthalmol. 108*:170–175, 1989.
122. Jirmanova I. Ultrastructure of motor end-plates during pharmacologically-induced degeneration and subsequent regeneration of skeletal muscle. *J. Neurocytol. 4*:141–151, 1975.
123. Johnson, D.H., Bradley, J.M.B., and Acott, T.S. The effect of dexamethasone on glycosaminoglycans of human trabecular meshwork in perfusion organ culture. *Invest. Ophthalmol. Vis. Sci. 31*:2569–2571, 1990.
124. Johnson, M.W., Olsen, K.R., Hernandez, E., Irvine, W.D., and Johnson, R.N. Retinal toxicity of recombinant tissue plasminogen activator in the rabbit. *Arch. Ophthalmol. 108*:259–263, 1990.

125. Junck, L., and Marshall, W.H. Neurotoxicity of radiological contrast agents. *Ann. Neurol. 13*:469–484, 1983.

126. Kass, M.A., Stamper, R.L., and Becker, B. Madarosis in chronic epinephrine therapy. *Arch. Ophthalmol. 88*:429–431, 1972.

127. Katz, I.J., Lesser, R.L., Merikangas, J.R., and Silverman, J.P. Ocular myasthenia gravis after D-penicillamine administration. *Br. J. Ophthalmol. 73*:1015–1018, 1989.

128. Keesey, J., and Novom, S. HLA antigens in penicillamine induced myasthenia gravis. *Neurology 29*:528–529, 1979.

129. Kincaid, M.C., Green, W.R., Hoover, R.E., and Schenck, P.H. Ocular chrysiasis. *Arch. Ophthalmol. 100*:1791–1794, 1982.

130. Kinoshita, J.H. Mechanisms initiating cataract formation. *Invest. Ophthalmol. 13*:713–724, 1974.

131. Kinsey, V.E. Amino acid transport in the lens. *Invest. Ophthalmol. 4*:691–699, 1965.

132. Knepper, P.A., Breen, M., Weinstein, H.G., and Blacik, L.J. Intraocular pressure and glycosaminoglycan distribution in the rabbit eye: Effect of age and dexamethasone. *Exp. Eye Res. 27*:567–575, 1978.

133. Knox, D.L., Palmer, C.A.L., and English, F. Iris atrophy after quinine amblyopia. *Arch. Ophthalmol. 76*:359–362, 1966.

134. Krecji, L., and Harrison, R. Antiglaucoma drug effects on corneal epithelium: A comparative study in tissue culture. *Arch. Ophthalmol. 84*:766–769, 1970.

135. Kristensen, P. Mydriasis-induced pigment liberation in the anterior chamber associated with acute rise in intraocular pressure in open-angle glaucoma. *Acta Ophthalmol. (Copenh.) 43*:714–724, 1965.

136. Kubo, D.J., Wing, T.W., Polse, K.A., and Jauregui, M.J. Mydriatic effects using low concentrations of phenylephrine hydrochloride. *J. Am. Optom. Assoc. 46*:817–822, 1975.

137. Lambert, R.W., and Smith, R.E. Effects of 13-cis-retinoic acid on the hamster meibomian gland. *J. Invest. Dermatol. 92*:321–325, 1989.

138. Lambrou, F.H., Snyder, R.W., Williams, G.A., and Lewandowski, M. Treatment of intra-vitreal fibrin with tissue plasminogen activator. *Am. J. Ophthalmol. 104*:619–623, 1987.

139. Lang, A.E., Humphrey, J.G., and Gordon, D.A. Plasma exchange therapy for severe penicillamine induced myasthenia gravis. *J. Rheumatol. 8*:303–307, 1981.

140. Lass, J.H., Langston, R.H.S., Foster, C.S., and Pavan-Langston, D. Antiviral medications and corneal wound healing. *Antiviral Res. 4*:143–157, 1984.

141. Lebowitz, M.A., and Berson, D.S. Ocular effects of oral retinoids. *J. Am. Acad. Dermatol. 19*:209–211, 1988.

142. Lederer, C.M., Jr., and Sabates, F.N. Ocular findings in the intravenous drug abuser. *Ann. Ophthalmol. 14*:436–438, 1982.

143. Lee, P.F. The influence of epinephrine and phenylephrine on intraocular pressure. *Arch. Ophthalmol. 60*:863–867, 1958.

144. Leibold, J.E. The ocular toxicity of ethambutol and its relation to dose. *Ann. NY Acad. Sci. 135*:904–909, 1966.

145. Leitman, P.D., De Santagnes, P.A., and Wong, V. Optic neuritis in cystic fibrosis of the pancreas-role of chloramphenicol therapy. *JAMA 189*:924–927, 1964.

146. Lemp, M.A., and Holly, F.J. Ophthalmic polymers as ocular wetting agents. *Ann. Ophthalmol. 4*:15–20, 1972.

147. Lerman, S. Ocular phototoxicity and psoralen plus ultraviolet radiation (320–400 nm) therapy: An experimental and clinical evaluation. *J. Natl. Cancer Inst. 69*:287–302, 1982.

148. Levi, L., and Miller, N.R. Visual illusions associated with previous drug abuse. *J. Clin. Neuro. Ophthalmol. 102*:103–110, 1990.

149. Liesegang, T.J. Bulbar conjunctival follicles associated with dipivefrin therapy. *Ophthalmology 92*:228–233, 1985.

150. Liu, G.T., and Bienfang, D.C. Penicillamine-induced ocular myasthenia gravis in rheumatoid arthritis. *J. Clin. Neuro. Ophthalmol. 10*:201–205, 1990.

151. Loeffler, K.U., and Lee, W.R. Argyrosis of the lacrimal sac. *Graefes Arch. Clin. Exp. Ophthalmol. 225*:146–150, 1987.

152. Loomis, T.A. Formaldehyde toxicity. *Arch. Pathol. Lab. Med. 103*:321–324, 1979.

153. Lustgarten, J.S., and Podos, S.M. Topical timolol and the nursing mother. *Arch. Ophthalmol. 101*:1381–1382, 1983.

154. MacRae, S.M., Brown, B., and Edelhauser, H.F. The corneal-toxicity of presurgical skin antiseptics. *Am. J. Ophthalmol. 97*:221–232, 1984.

155. Mallette, L.E. Acetazolamide-accelerated anticonvulsant osteomalacia. *Arch. Intern. Med. 137*:1013–1017, 1977.

156. Manabe, S., Bucala, R., and Cerami, A. Nonenzymatic addition of glucocorticoids to lens proteins in steroid-induced cataracts. *J. Clin. Invest. 74*:1803–1810, 1984.

157. Mathalone, M.B.R. Eye and skin changes in psychiatric patients treated with chlorpromazine. *Br. J. Ophthalmol. 51*:86–93, 1967.

158. Matsumura, M., Yamakawa, R., Shirakawa, H., and Ogino, N. Effects of phenothiazines on cultured retinal pigment epithelial cells. *Ophthalmic Res. 18*:47–54, 1986.

159. Mayman, C.I., Miller, D., and Tijerina, M.L. In vitro production of steroid cataract in bovine lens. II.

Measurement of sodium-potassium adenosine triphosphate activity. *Acta Ophthalmol. (Copenh.) 57*:1197–1116, 1979.

160. McCrea, F.D., Eadie, G.S., and Morgan, J.E. The mechanism of morphine miosis. *J. Pharmacol. Exp. Ther. 74*:239–246, 1942.

161. McGalliard, J.N. Respiratory arrest after two retrobulbar injections. *Am. J. Ophthalmol. 105*:90–91, 1988.

162. McLane, N.J., and Carrol, D.M. Ocular manifestations of drug abuse. *Surv. Ophthalmol. 30*:298–313, 1986.

163. McLaren, D.S. Age-dependent changes in the effects of food toxins and other dietary factors on the eye. *Pharmacol. Ther. 16*:103–142, 1982.

164. McMahon, C.D., Shaffer, R.N., Hoskins, H.D., Jr., and Heterington, J., Jr. Adverse effects experienced by patients taking timolol. *Am. J. Ophthalmol. 88*:736–738, 1979.

165. Meredith, T.A., Aaberg, T.M., and Willerson, W.D. Progressive chorioretinopathy after receiving thioridazine. *Arch. Ophthalmol. 96*:1172–1176, 1978.

166. Miller, F.S., III, Bunt-Milam, A.H., and Kalina, R.E. Clinical-ultrastructural study of thioridazine retinopathy. *Ophthalmology 89*:1478–1488, 1982.

167. Mitsui, Y., and Takagi, Y. Nature of aqueous floaters due to sympathomimetic mydriatics. *Arch. Ophthalmol. 65*:626–631, 1961.

168. Norton, A.L., and Walsh, F.B. Disulfiram-induced optic neuritis. *Trans. Am. Acad. Ophthalmol. Otolaryngol. 72*:1263–1264, 1972.

169. O'Brien, W.M., and Bagby, G.F. Rare adverse reactions to nonsteroidal antiinflammatory drugs. *J. Rheumatol. 12*:785–790, 1985.

170. Ogino, S., and Ichihara, T. Biochemical studies on cataract. *Am. J. Ophthalmol. 43*:754–764, 1957.

171. O'Keefe, M., Morley, K.D., Haining, W.M., and Smith, A. Penicillamine-induced ocular myasthenia gravis. *Am. J. Ophthalmol. 99*:66–67, 1985.

172. Okland, S., Komorowski, T.E., and Carlson, B.M. Ultrastructure of mepivacaine-induced damage and regeneration in rat extraocular muscle. *Invest. Ophthalmol. Vis. Sci. 30*:1643–1651, 1989.

173. Partridge, C.A., Weinstein, B.L., Southern, A.L., and Gerritsen, M.E. Dexamethasone induces specific proteins in human trabecular meshwork cells. *Invest. Ophthalmol. Vis. Sci. 30*:1843–1847, 1989.

174. Patton, T.F. Pediatric dosing considerations in ophthalmology—dosage adjustments based on aqueous humor volume ratio. *J. Pediatr. Ophthalmol. 14*:254–256, 1977.

175. Patton, T.F., and Robinson, J.R. Pediatric dosing considerations in ophthalmology. *J. Pediatr. Ophthalmol. 13*:171–178, 1976.

176. Patz, A., Wulff, L.B., and Rogers, S.W. Experimental production of ocular tumors. *Am. J. Ophthalmol. 48*:98–117, 1959.

177. Petroutsos, G., Savoldelli, M., and Pouliquen, Y. The effect of gentamicin on the corneal endothelium: An experimental study. *Cornea 9*:62–65, 1990.

178. Pfister, R.R., and Burstein, N. The effects of ophthalmic drugs, vehicles, and preservatives on corneal epithelium: A scanning electron microscope study. *Invest. Ophthalmol. Vis. Sci. 15*:246–259, 1976.

179. Pippitt, C.H., Muss, H.B., Homesley, H.D., and Jobson, V.W. Cisplatin associated cortical blindness. *Gynecol. Oncol. 12*:253–255, 1981.

180. Potts, A.M. Uveal pigment and phenothiazine compounds. *Trans. Am. Ophthalmol. Soc. 60*:517–552, 1962.

181. Pulst, S.M., and Lombroso, C.T. External ophthalmoplegia, alpha and spindle coma in imipramine overdose: Case report and review of the literature. *Ann. Neurol. 14*:587–590, 1983.

182. Radius, R.L., Diamond, G.R., Pollack, I.P., and Langham, M.E. Timolol: A new drug for management of chronic simple glaucoma. *Arch. Ophthalmol. 96*:1003–1008, 1978.

183. Raines, M.F., Bhargava, S.K., and Rosen, E.S. The blood-brain barrier in chloroquine retinopathy. *Invest. Ophthalmol. Vis. Sci. 30*:1726–1731, 1989.

184. Rainin, E.A., and Carlson, B.M. Postoperative diplopia and ptosis: A clinical hypothesis based on the myotoxicity of local anesthetics. *Arch. Ophthalmol. 103*:1337–1339, 1985.

185. Ramsey, M.S., and Fine, B.S. Chloroquine toxicity in the human eye: Histopathologic observations by electron microscopy. *Am. J. Ophthalmol. 73*:229–235, 1972.

186. Rao, N.A., Sevanian, A., Fernandez, M.A.S., Romero, J.L., Faure, J.P., de Kozak, Y., Till, G.O., and Marak, G.E., Jr. Role of oxygen radicals in experimental allergic uveitis. *Invest. Ophthalmol. Vis. Sci. 28*:886–892, 1987.

187. Remler, B.F., Leigh, R.J., Osorio, I., and Tomsak, R.L. The characteristics and mechanisms of visual disturbance associated with anticonvulsant therapy. *Neurology 40*:791–796, 1990.

188. Rengstorff, R.H., and Doughty, C.B. Mydriatic and cycloplegic drugs: A review of ocular and systemic complications. *Am. J. Optom. Physiol. Optics 59*:162–177, 1982.

189. Riley, M.V., and Giblin, F.J. Toxic effects of hydrogen peroxide on corneal endothelium. *Curr. Eye Res. 2*:451–458, 1982/1983.

190. Ripps, H., Mehaffey, L., III, Siegel, I.M., and Niemeyer, G. Vincristine-induced changes in the retina of the isolated arterially-perfused cat eye. *Exp. Eye Res. 48*:771–790, 1989.

191. Rismondo, V., and Ubels, J.L. Isotretinoin in lacrimal gland fluid and tears. *Arch. Ophthalmol. 105*:416–420, 1987.

192. Rohen, J.W., Linner, E., and Witmer, R. Electron microscopic studies on the trabecular meshwork in two cases of corticosteroid-glaucoma. *Exp. Eye Res. 17*:19–31, 1973.

193. Rohen, J.W., Schachtechabel, D.O., and Berghoff, K. Histoautoradiographic and biochemical studies on human and monkey trabecular meshwork and ciliary body in short-term explant cultures. *Graefes Arch. Clin. Exp. Ophthalmol. 221*:199–206, 1984.

194. Roholt, P.C. Betaxolol and restrictive airway disease (letter to the editor). *Arch. Ophthalmol. 105*:1172, 1987.

195. Rosenwasser, G.O.D. Complications of topical ocular anesthetics. *Int. Ophthalmol. Clin. 29*:153–158, 1989.

196. Rothstein, H., Worgul, B.V., Medvedovsky, C., and Merriah, G.R., Jr. G_0/G_1 arrest of cell proliferation in the ocular lens prevents development of radiation cataract. *Ophthalmic Res. 14*:215–220, 1982.

197. Roussos, T., and Tsolkas, A. The toxicity of myambutol on the human eye. *Ann. Ophthalmol. 2*:578–580, 1970.

198. Salminen, L., Jantti, V., and Brontross, M. Blepharospasm associated with tegafur combination chemotherapy (letter to the editor). *Am. J. Ophthalmol. 97*:649–650, 1984.

199. Schmidt, I.G., and Schmidt, L.H. Studies of the neurotoxicity of ethambutol and its racemate for the rhesus monkey. *J. Neuropathol. Exp. Neurol. 25*:40–67, 1966.

200. Schwartzman, M.J., and Leppik, I.E. Carbamazepine-induced dyskinesia and ophthalmoplegia. *Cleve. Clin. J. Med. 57*:367–372, 1990.

201. Scroggs, M.W., and Klintworth, G.K. Senile scleral plaques: A histopathologic study employing energy dispersive x-ray microanalysis. *Hum. Pathol. 22*:557–562, 1991.

202. Selvin, B.L. Systemic effects of topical ophthalmic medications. *South. Med. J. 76*:349–358, 1983.

203. Shapiro, M.S., Thoft, R.A., Friend, J., Parrish, R.K., and Gresse, M.G. 5-Fluorouracil toxicity to the ocular surface epithelium. *Invest. Ophthalmol. Vis. Sci. 26*:580–583, 1985.

204. Shichi, H., and Nebert, D.W. Genetic differences in drug metabolism associated with ocular toxicity. *Environ. Health Perspect. 44*:107–117, 1982.

205. Shichi, H., Tanaka, M., Jensen, N.M., and Nebert, D.W. Genetic differences in cataract and other ocular abnormalities induced by paracetamol and naphthalene. *Pharmacology 20*:229–241, 1980.

206. Siddal, J.R. The ocular toxic findings with prolonged and high dosage chlorpromazine intake. *Arch. Ophthalmol. 74*:460–464, 1965.

207. Sieg, J.W., and Robinson, J.R. Corneal absorption of fluorometholone in rabbits. *Arch. Ophthalmol. 92*:240–243, 1974.

208. Snow, M.H. Myogenic cell formation in regenerating rat skeletal muscle injured by mincing. II. An autoradiographic study. *Anat. Rec. 188*:201–218, 1977.

209. Soll, D.B. Glaucoma. *Am. Fam. Physician 9*:125–133, 1974.

210. Soong, H.K., McKenney, M.J., and Wolter, J.R. Adrenochrome staining of senile plaque resembling malignant melanoma. *Am. J. Ophthalmol. 101*:380, 1986.

211. Spaeth, G.L., Rodrigues, M.M., and Weinreb, S. Steroid-induced glaucoma: A persistent elevation of intraocular pressure. B. Histopathological aspects. *Trans. Am. Ophthalmol. Soc. 75*:353–381, 1977.

212. Spector, A., and Garner, W.H. Hydrogen peroxide and human cataract. *Exp. Eye Res. 33*:673–681, 1981.

213. Spector, A., Huang, R.R.C., Wang, G.M., Schmidt, C., Yan, G.Z., and Chifflet, S. Does elevated glutathione protect the cell from H_2O_2 insult? *Exp. Eye Res. 45*:453–465, 1987.

214. Spector, R.H., Davidoff, R.A., and Schwartzman, R.J. Phenytoin-induced ophthalmoplegia. *Neurology 26*:1031–1034, 1976.

215. Spencer, W.H., Garron, L.K., Contreras, F., Hayes, T.L., and Lai, C. Endogenous and exogenous ocular and systemic silver deposition. *Trans. Ophthalmol. Soc. UK 100*:171–178, 1980.

216. Spencer, W.H., and Zimmerman, L.E. Conjunctiva. In *Ophthalmic Pathology. An Atlas and Textbook*, 3rd ed., W.H. Spencer (Ed.), W.B. Saunders, Philadelphia, pp. 167–168, 1985.

217. Spiteri, M.A., and James, D.G. Adverse ocular reactions to drugs. *Postgrad. Med. J. 59*:343–349, 1983.

218. Steer, J.H., Mastaglia, F.L., Papimitriou, J.M., and van Bruggen, I. Bupivaine-induced muscle injury: The role of extracellular calcium. *J. Neurol. Sci. 73*:205–217, 1986.

219. Sternberg, P., Aguilar, H.E., Drews, C., and Aaberg, T.M. The effect of tissue plasminogen activator on retinal bleeding. *Arch. Ophthalmol. 108*:720–722, 1990.

220. Straus, D.J., Mausolf, F.A., Ellerby, R.A., and McCracken, J.D. Cicatrical ectropion secondary to 5-fluorouracil therapy. *Med. Pediatr. Oncol. 3*:15–19, 1977.

221. Sugar, A., and Waltman, S.R. Corneal toxicity of collagenase inhibitors. *Invest. Ophthalmol. 12*:779–782, 1973.

222. Svejgaard, A., Platz, P., and Ryder, L.P. HLA and disease 1982. *Immunol. Rev. 70*:193–218, 1983.

223. Takahashi, N., and Ikoma, N. The cytotoxic effect of 5-fluorouracil on cultured human conjunctival cells. In *Ocular Toxicology*, Proceedings of the First Congress of the International Society of Ocular Toxicology, S. Lerman and R.C. Tripathi (Eds.), Marcel Dekker, New York, pp. 157–166, 1988.

224. Talamo, J.H., D'Amico, D.J., Hanninen, L.A., Kenyon, K.R., and Shanks, E.T. The influence of aphakia and vitrectomy on experimental retinal toxicity of aminoglycoside antibiotics. *Am. J. Ophthalmol. 100*:840–847, 1985.

225. Taylor, G.N., Dougherty, T.F., Mays, C.W., Lloyd, R.D., Atherton, D.R., and Jee, W.S.S. Radium-induced eye melanomas in dogs. *Radiat. Res. 51*:361–373, 1972.

226. Thomas, D.M., Mahendroo, P.P., and Lou, M.F. Phosphorus-31 NMR study of the effects of hydrogen peroxide on young and old rat lenses. *Exp. Eye Res. 51*:233–239, 1990.

227. Tripathi, B.J., Millard, C.B., and Tripathi, R.C. Corticosteroids induce a sialated glycoprotein (Cort-GP) in trabecular cells in vitro. *Exp. Eye Res. 51*:735–737, 1990.

228. Tripathi, B.J., Tripathi, R.C., and Swift, H.H. Hydrocortisone-induced DNA endoreplication in human trabecular cells in vitro. *Exp. Eye Res. 49*:259–270, 1989.

229. Truscott, R.J.W., and Augusteyn, R.C. Oxidative changes in human lens proteins during senile nuclear cataract formation. *Biochim. Biophys. Acta 492*:43–50, 1977.

230. Varley, G.A., Meisler, D.M., Benes, S.C., McMahon, J.T., Zakov, Z.N., and Fryczkowski, A. Hibiclens keratopathy: A clinicopathologic case report. *Cornea 9*:341–346, 1990.

231. Van Heyningen, R. Experimental studies on cataract. *Invest. Ophthalmol. 15*:685–697, 1976.

232. Von Sallman, L., Grimes, P., and Collins, E. Triparanol induced cataract in rats. *Arch. Ophthalmol. 70*:522–530, 1963.

233. Waltman, S.R., Yarian, D., Hart, W., and Mecker, B. Corneal endothelial changes with long-term topical epinephrine therapy. *Arch. Ophthalmol. 95*:1357–1358, 1977.

234. Weinreb, R.N., Wood, I., Tomazzoli, L., and Alvarado, J. Subconjunctival injections: Preservative-related changes in the corneal endothelium. *Invest. Ophthalmol. Vis. Sci. 27*:525–531, 1986.

235. Wilkerson, M., Lewis, R.A., and Shields, M.B. Follicular conjunctivitis associated with apraclonidine. *Am. J. Ophthalmol. 111*:105–106, 1991.

236. Williams, D.F., Han, D.P., and Abrams, G.W. Rebleeding in experimental traumatic hyphema treated with intraocular tissue plasminogen activator. *Arch. Ophthalmol. 108*:264–266, 1990.

237. Wilson, F.M., II. Adverse external ocular effects of topical ophthalmic medications. *Surv. Ophthalmol. 24*:57–88, 1979.

238. Wong, V., and Collins, E. Optic atrophy in cystic fibrosis. *Am. J. Ophthalmol. 59*:763–769, 1965.

239. Zabel, R.W., and MacDonald, I.M. Sinus-arrest associated with betaxolol ophthalmic drops. *Am. J. Ophthalmol. 104*:431, 1987.

240. Zaidman, G.W. Miconazole corneal toxicity. *Cornea 10*:90–91, 1991.

40
Anterior and Posterior Corneal Dystrophies

Merlyn M. Rodrigues, Sankaran Rajagopalan, and Kelly A. Jones
University of Maryland at Baltimore, Baltimore, Maryland

I. ANTERIOR CORNEAL DYSTROPHIES

The superficial corneal dystrophies comprise Meesmann's dystrophy, Reis-Bücklers' dystrophy, and familial subepithelial corneal amyloidosis (primary gelatinous drop dystrophy). The third member of this group is discussed in Chap. 32. Epithelial basement membrane dystrophy, alternatively referred to as map-dot-fingerprint or Cogan's microcystic dystrophy, is not considered a true dystrophy but rather a non-specific reaction to a variety of corneal insults (see Chap. 23).

Anterior (superficial) corneal dystrophies primarily affect the corneal epithelium, the basement membrane of the epithelium, and Bowman's layer. Vision is less affected in these dystrophies than in the major stromal and endothelial dystrophies, with one exception—Reis-Bücklers' dystrophy.

A. Meesmann's Juvenile Epithelial Dystrophy

Meesmann and Wilke first documented the histological appearance of this bilaterally symmetrical corneal dystrophy with an autosomal dominant mode of inheritance in 1939 [31]. The disorder becomes evident in the first few years of life as bilateral, small, punctate epithelial vesicular opacities, but the patient remains asymptomatic until about middle age, when the opacities involve the entire corneal epithelium. The vesicles create irregular astigmatism, which transiently causes blurred vision, and breaks through the epithelial surface result in intermittent irritation and photophobia. These tiny, round, or oval bubblelike blebs appear as discrete gray dots by slit lamp examination and as transparent dewdrops in retroillumination. The lesions are extremely difficult to see without a slit lamp, since the intervening cornea is unaffected. Occasionally, the cysts take up topically applied fluorescein, but most of them fail to stain because they are usually intraepithelial and do not open to the surface. In more severe cases, scarring in the central subepithelial cornea produces a slight grayish opacification requiring keratoplasty. Simple removal of the corneal epithelium is of only temporary benefit, since the vesicles gradually recur in the regenerated epithelium. The corneal sensitivity is normal and the stroma is not involved.

The clinical appearance of Meesmann's dystrophy is distinctive, but must be differentiated from other cystic disorders of the epithelium, such as bleb pattern of epithelial basement membrane dystrophy, vapor spray keratitis, and mild epithelial edema.

Histopathology

A major morphological abnormality in Meesmann's dystrophy is the formation of intraepithelial cysts that gradually become displaced anteriorly to the surface. The clear clinical appearance of the epithelial microcysts is probably related to the marked degeneration of epithelial cells with scant residual cell debris.

The intraepithelial microcysts (Fig. 1A) contain periodic acid-Schiff–positive and diastase- and neuraminidase-resistant material. The contents of the cysts also stain with Hale's colloidal iron technique for negatively charged substances, such as glycosaminoglycans, and manifest autofluorescence when

1189

viewed in ultraviolet light [10]. In addition, a homogeneous substance with areas of vacuolation is usually located within the epithelial cysts and, less commonly, within the epithelial cells themselves [10].

Several transmission electron microscope (TEM) reports have described collections of amorphous electron-dense fibrillogranular material, termed peculiar substance by Kuwabara and Ciccarelli [25], since its nature is unknown [5,10,25]. This substance (Fig. 1B), which is surrounded by cytoplasmic filaments and vacuoles, has been observed in all TEM studies of the dystrophy, except for the report by Nakanishi and Brown, which postulated that their 7-year-old patient might have manifested an earlier stage of the disease, with electron-dense lysosomelike bodies in basal epithelial cells [33].

Pathogenesis

The specific genetic locus for this dystrophy and its underlying metabolic or enzymatic alteration is unknown. Although increased glycogen deposition has been described within the cytoplasm of epithelial cells of a single case [25], an ultramicrofluorimetric assay disclosed no increase in glycogen in the corneal epithelium in Meesmann's dystrophy compared with normal corneas with a regenerating epithelium [5]. The epithelial basement membrane is variably thickened in this dystrophy as a nonspecific change [10].

B. Reis-Bücklers' Ring-Shaped Dystrophy

A corneal dystrophy that forms a superficial reticular corneal opacity at about 4–5 years of age was described by Reis [36] and Bücklers [4]. This bilaterally symmetrical, central corneal dystrophy with an autosomal dominant mode of inheritance becomes clinically apparent in the first few years of life as a reticular superficial corneal opacification that progressively assumes a central ring-shaped pattern [4,35]. The irregularly shaped rings or discrete gray-white spots and lines focally elevate the epithelium, producing an irregular corneal surface and reducing corneal sensitivity. The dystrophy usually remains asymptomatic until spontaneous epithelial erosions produce acute episodes of pain, photophobia, and

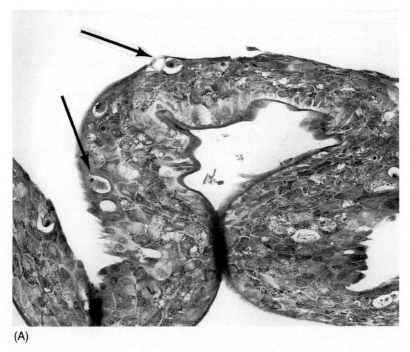

(A)

Figure 1 Meesmann's dystrophy. (A) Numerous epithelial microcysts (arrows) are present. (Periodic acid–Schiff, ×330) (B) Transmission electron micrograph showing electron-dense "peculiar substance"* in the cytoplasm of epithelial cells (E). (×30,000)

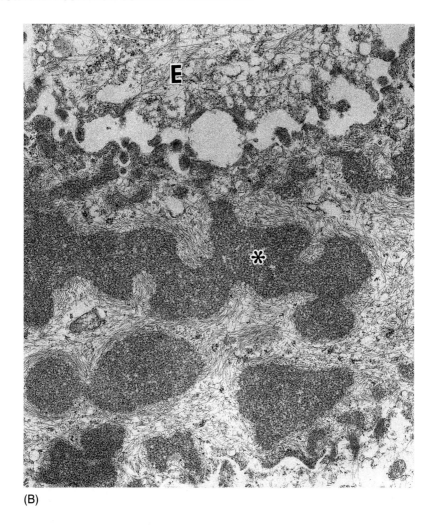

(B)

ocular hyperemia. Increasing superficial stromal haze and the irregular corneal surface combine to reduce visual acuity in the second and third decades of life. Superficial keratectomy may improve visual acuity, but in more advanced cases lamellar keratoplasty or penetrating keratoplasty may be necessary.

Clinically similar conditions but with infrequent epithelial erosions, normal corneal sensation, and visual acuity were described by Grayson and Wilbrandt [12]. Thiel and Behnke described another clinical "honeycomb" variant, involving 55 members of a family over 11 generations, with a similar clinical course, but less severe deterioration of vision than the usual cases of Reis-Bücklers' dystrophy [45]. Some confusion exists concerning the classification of these entities. The condition referred to as Reis-Bücklers' dystrophy is the same as Thiel-Behnke's honeycomb corneal dystrophy [54].

Reis-Bücklers' dystrophy may be confused clinically and histopathologically with a superficial type of granular corneal dystrophy (GCD) [41]. Some cases of what has been diagnosed clinically as Reis-Bücklers' dystrophy correspond to the superficial variant of GCD [32,55]. However, as discussed next, these deposits can be distinguished by their different TEM and histochemical staining features [32,42,54].

Histopathology

Bowman's layer, the basal corneal epithelium, and the epithelial basement membrane display varying amounts of degeneration and replacement with irregular subepithelial collagen (Fig. 2, inset). The corneal epithelium varies in thickness, the individual epithelial cells displaying cytoplasmic vacuolation, mitochondrial swelling, and pyknotic nuclei. These changes are nonspecific degenerative changes and hence

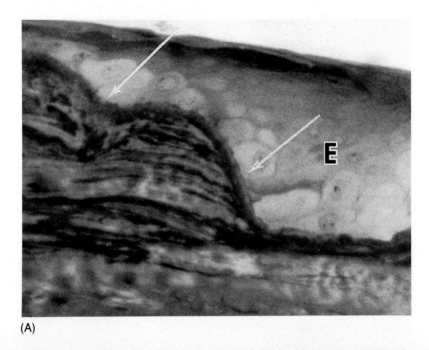

(A)

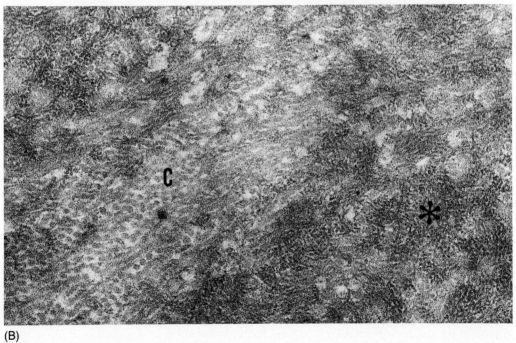

(B)

Figure 2   Reis-Bücklers dystrophy. (A) Irregular dense filamentous aggregates (arrows) are present beneath the epithelium (E). (Toluidine blue, ×500) (B) Electron micrograph showing short curly filamentous structures* between the collagen fibrils (C). (×30,000)

probably secondary to the pathological alterations in Bowman's layer and the superficial stroma. When viewed by TEM, characteristic short, curled filaments (Fig. 2A) replace Bowman's layer and measure approximately 8–10 nm in diameter. These filaments, which appear to be specific for Reis-Bücklers' dystrophy [35,49], are thicker in the central regions, taper in the periphery, and form electron-dense aggregates interspersed among normal collagen fibrils. It is uncertain whether they represent a collagen precursor, a product of collagen degeneration, or some other substance. In the later stages of Reis-Bücklers' dystrophy, there is considerable disorganization of the anterior stromal collagen, and Bowman's layer may be partially or totally replaced by masses of these filaments and connective tissue. The posterior stroma, Descemet's membrane, and endothelium are normal.

In Reis-Bücklers' dystrophy, TEM shows typical short curly filaments, whereas in GCD, there are electron-dense rod-shaped structures that stain for proteins (see Chap. 32) [42]. Immunofluorescent localization of laminin and bullous pemphigoid antigen has been described in the aberrant subepithelial region, suggesting that Reis-Bücklers' dystrophy may have an epithelial origin [27]. However, the nature of the material is unknown in both Reis-Bücklers' dystrophy and GCD.

Pathogenesis

It is possible that an abnormality of the epithelium and basement membrane is associated with the synthesis of abnormal curly filaments and collagen, in which case the involvement of the Bowman's layer and superficial stroma is secondary to the primary epithelial alteration. The precise mechanism is unknown.

II. ENDOTHELIAL CORNEAL DYSTROPHIES

The endothelial corneal dystrophies have three factors in common:

1. The endothelial cells become more irregular, as demonstrated by TEM or clinical specular microscopy.
2. The abnormal endothelial cells produce excess collagen posterior to Descemet's membrane, resulting in a multilaminar structure. This tissue appears clinically as a thickened Descemet's membrane, forming mushroom-shaped or anvillike excrescences on Descemet's membrane (guttata) or gray sheets.
3. The barrier functions of the endothelium break down, with resultant stromal and epithelial edema sufficient to reduce visual acuity. The normal corneal endothelium appears capable of pumping water and electrolytes out of the stroma toward the anterior chamber [29]. This active fluid transport prevents edema of the normal corneal stroma [29], and in the endothelial corneal dystrophies this physiological activity is presumably impaired [50].

A. Fuchs' Dystrophy

Fuchs' dystrophy is a bilateral, but commonly asymmetrical endothelial dystrophy, which gradually progresses to stromal and epithelial edema with subepithelial fibrosis. The cause is unknown, and although the disorder is sometimes familial, its exact mode of inheritance is uncertain [24]. Because females are affected three times more often than males, a simple autosomal dominant pattern is unlikely [24].

Three phases characterize the clinical course of Fuchs' dystrophy, a course that usually spans 10–20 years. In the first phase, the patient remains asymptomatic and the posterior cornea manifests central, irregularly distributed excrescences on Descemet's membrane (cornea guttata) and a fine dusting with pigment. On slit lamp examination, cornea guttata have a glittering golden brown appearance and in retroillumination light up like small dewdrops. Gradually, a grayish apparent thickening of Descemet's membrane occurs, often ringed by pigment dots.

In the second phase, the patient experiences hazy visual acuity and symptoms of glare as stromal and epithelial edema develop. Early stromal edema produces a blue-gray haze in front of Descemet's membrane and in the anterior stroma, but gradually the entire stroma develops a ground-glass appearance with thickening. Epithelial edema occurs with a characteristic fine pigskin texture, commonly called bedewing, and wrinkles in Descemet's membrane. Large subepithelial and intraepithelial lakes of fluid burst to produce a painful cornea.

In the third phase, subepithelial connective tissue, associated with decreased epithelial edema, appears and the patient becomes more comfortable, even though visual acuity is worse. Stromal scarring occurs, and the dystrophic process that began centrally spreads to the corneoscleral limbus. Secondary complications, such as epithelial erosion, may complicate this end stage. Microbial keratitis and peripheral vascularization are extremely rare sequelae.

Guttate excrescences on Descemet's membrane are not specific for Fuchs' dystrophy and may occur as part of corneal aging or after the inflammatory stage of interstitial keratitis [51].

Histopathology

The characteristic changes of Fuchs' dystrophy occur posterior to the normal Descemet's membrane, where the production of new collagen by abnormal endothelial cells results in a multilaminar pattern, in which layers stain with variable intensity with the periodic acid–Schiff stain. Focal thickening of the new collagenous tissue forms excrescences or warts that correspond to clinically detectable cornea guttata. Four morphological types of excrescences occur on Descemet's membrane [14]:

1. Mushroom-shaped or anvillike warts that protrude into the anterior chamber (Fig. 3, inset)
2. Multilaminar warts
3. Warts buried in the multilaminar tissue (Fig. 3A) and multilaminar tissue without warts

The surface distribution of the guttata can be visualized by flat preparations of Descemet's membrane, phase-contrast microscopy, and scanning electron microscopy (SEM) (Fig. 3B). The endothelium overlying the warts is attenuated. Histologically, the marked thickening of Descemet's membrane and abnormal corneal endothelium correspond to areas of severe clinical edema and are usually located in the central and paracentral regions [43]. Descemet's membrane displays multiple prominent guttata of varying sizes and shapes, either facing the anterior chamber or buried within multilaminar Descemet's membrane. The endothelium underlying the guttata is often attenuated. Clinical edema is accompanied by marked thickening of Descemet's membrane, with multiple guttata and attenuation of corneal endothelium [14]. In a histochemical study, oxytalan, a component of the elastic fiber, has been demonstrated around but not within the guttate excrescences of Fuchs' dystrophy [1].

TEM reveals a normal 3 μm thick anterior (100–110 nm) banded layer of Descemet's membrane and a normal layer of nonbanded basement membrane. Posterior to this is the abnormal tissue, characterized by fusiform bundles and sheets of wide-spacing (100 nm) collagen with interspersed amorphous basement material. This wide-spacing collagen has a macroperiodicity of 55 or 100 nm and manifests subbands with a periodicity of about 30–40 nm. Within this material, horizontal fibrils (Fig. 3C) run perpendicular to the vertical bands [16]. In tangential section, the wide-spacing collagen forms a hexagonal pattern similar to that seen in horizontal section of the normal anterior-banded Descemet's membrane. Adjacent to the wide-spacing bundles are groups of 10–20 nm diameter collagen fibrils that may fuse with the horizontal fibrils of the wide-spacing collagen. Interspersed accumulation of amorphous basement membrane-like material forms focal posterior protrusions (cornea guttata).

In some areas, fissures containing cellular debris penetrate the guttata excrescences, giving an appearance similar to the focal thickenings that form on the periphery of Descemet's membrane with aging (Hassall-Henle bodies). The latter posterior excrescences of Descemet's membrane involve the peripheral cornea of normal elderly individuals. They can usually be differentiated from cornea guttata by their dome-shaped configuration, fissured appearance [11,16], and lack of multilaminar pattern. Although fissures similar to those in the Hassall-Henle bodies are occasionally present in some cornea guttata, they are more abundant and prominent in Hassall-Henle bodies.

In more advanced cases, an additional layer of fibrillar collagen appears, consisting of a loose feltwork of collagen fibrils with a diameter of 20 nm, scattered within basement membrane-like material. Occasionally, collagen fibrils (20–30 nm in diameter) with 64 nm banding are present.

The abnormal endothelial cells show widened intercellular spaces, swollen mitochondria, dilated rough endoplasmic reticulum, and melanin pigment. Some cells display morphological features of fibroblasts [34].

In milder cases epithelial edema involves only the basal layer, but in the advanced stages the more superficial layers are also affected, with separation of the epithelium from the underlying basement membrane and Bowman's layer (bullous keratopathy). This is accompanied by patchy loss of hemidesmosomes and fragmentation of the epithelial basement membrane. Bowman's layer is usually intact, except for focal breaks adjacent to subepithelial connective tissue. Pathological studies suggest that abnormalities in endothelial function develop much earlier than the symptoms, which are delayed until middle age [53].

A histochemical study of cytochrome oxidase activity in corneal endothelium from Fuchs' dystrophy patients showed that regional differences in endothelial energy metabolism may be related to decreased numbers of mitochondria in the diseased cells [47].

Recent biochemical characterization of the Descemet's membrane and posterior collagenous layer from Fuchs' dystrophy corneas has shown collagen types similar to those of age-matched controls [3,21]. However, immunofluorescence showed a staining response consistent with fibrinogen/fibrin in the posterior collagenous layer in Fuchs' dystrophy that was not detected in normal Descemet's membrane. In Fuchs' dystrophy, in addition to the endothelial changes, it is possible that there is involvement of the fibrinolytic system, since the antifibrinolytic agent tranexamic acid, which has been found to diminish corneal edema and the aqueous humor in Fuchs' patients, contains elevated levels of substances associated with the fibrinolytic system [3].

Pathogenesis

In Fuchs' dystrophy, altered assembly of collagen molecules and a possible defect in the fibrinolytic system have been postulated [3,21]. That a virus is the causal agent has been postulated on the presumption of ultrastructurally identified "viral" nucleocapsids within the cytoplasm of endothelial cells in a patient with Fuchs' dystrophy [44]. Others have observed similar structures corresponding to distorted mitochondria in a variety of diseases, however, including keratoconus and Fuchs' dystrophy [15].

Several TEM reports have shown that production of the banded posterior collagenous layer begins within the first two decades of life, even though the clinical effects are not experienced until much later. Corneal edema is a consequence of progressive decrease in endothelial barrier function.

The basic endothelial abnormality is unknown, but abnormal corneal endothelial cells may undergo fibroblastlike transformation and produce collagenous tissue posterior to the normal Descemet's membrane [52]. This corresponds to an accumulation of multilaminar abnormal basement membrane and loosely arranged fibrillary tissue that corresponds clinically to thickened Descemet's membrane. Impaired endothelial cell function allows aqueous penetration of the endothelial barrier, with resulting stromal and epithelial edema. Pathological studies suggest that the abnormality in endothelial function occurs much earlier than the onset of symptoms in middle age [53].

B.   Posterior Polymorphous Dystrophy

Posterior polymorphous dystrophy is an autosomal dominant disorder with an extremely variable expression [9]. It generally occurs bilaterally but may be unilateral or asymmetrical. Although the disorder is probably congenital—some cases have corneal edema at birth—the exact age of onset is difficult to determine because most patients remain asymptomatic.

On slit lamp examination, posterior polymorphous dystrophy manifests a variety of configurations at the level of Descemet's membrane, including small groups of apparent vesicles surrounded by a gray haze, larger gray geographical lesions that sometimes appear nodular and contain round or elliptical vesicular zones, creating a Swiss cheese pattern, broad bands with roughly parallel edges, and sheets of gray material that appear as thickenings of Descemet's membrane. In retroillumination, these alterations have a striking refractile quality. In contrast to Fuchs' dystrophy, cornea guttata are absent.

In some instances, stromal and epithelial edema occur, sometimes complicated by anterior corneal scarring and band keratopathy. In other instances, broad iridocorneal adhesions occupy the peripheral 1 mm of the posterior cornea, sometimes accompanied by a membrane that extends down the adhesions onto the surface of the iris. This may account for the glaucoma that occasionally develops. These have a different appearance from the fine strands that attach to a prominent Schwalbe's ring in Axenfeld's and Rieger's anomalies.

Posterior polymorphous dystrophy can be distinguished from an acquired posterior corneal opacification following recurrent uveitis and keratitis (confusingly called posterior polymorphous keratopathy) [26] by its typical bilateral vesicular opacities and autosomal dominant transmission.

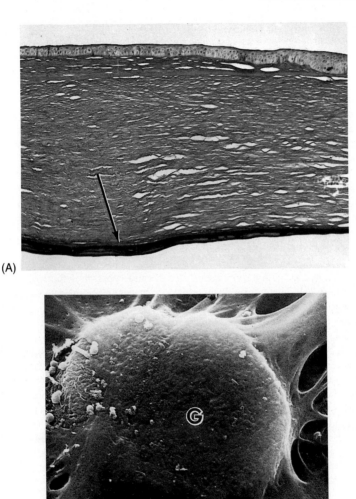

(A)

(B)

Figure 3 Fuchs' dystrophy. (A) Corneal changes are related to the degree of corneal edema. Thickened Descemet's membrane shows interlaminar guttata, most pronounced in the most edematous area (arrow). (Periodic acid–Schiff, ×330) (B) Scanning electron micrograph in which cells seem to overlie guttata (G). (×2000) (C) Transmission electron micrograph showing guttate excrescence (G) with abnormal 110 nm long-spacing collagen covered by attenuated corneal endothelial cells. (×5850)

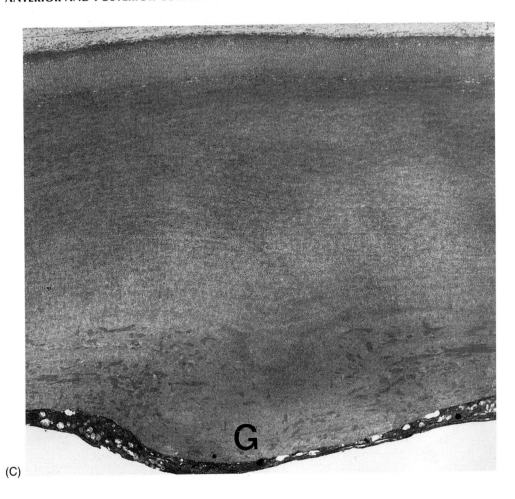

(C)

Histopathology

Tissue examinations have been limited to material obtained at penetrating keratoplasty from severe symptomatic cases. In these cases Descemet's membrane is multilaminar and irregular in thickness, sometimes with focal nodular excrescences [13,17]. TEM reveals anterior 3 μm thick, 110 nm banded and extremely thin posterior nonbanded layers, comprising the normal Descemet's membrane (Fig. 4A). Collagen fibrils of two varieties occur in this layer: loosely packed collagen fibrils 10–20 nm in diameter interspersed with basement membrane-like material and fusiform bundles of 55–110 nm banded wide-spacing collagen. When viewed by TEM the cells lining the posterior cornea usually exhibit features like epithelium, including numerous villous projections, keratofibrils, desmosomal junctions, tonofilaments, and sparse mitochondria (Fig. 4A) [2,17,46], but may have fibroblastlike features [17]. Scanning electron microscopy (SEM) discloses cells with numerous microvilli [13].

In more advanced stages, epithelial and stromal edema may be present, but Bowman's layer is usually intact.

That the 110 nm banded anterior layer of Descemet's membrane is not only present but of normal thickness suggests that the abnormality of the corneal endothelium does not become manifest until late gestation. The cells similar to epithelium on the posterior cornea are a prominent feature of cases with clinical corneal edema and may represent an advanced stage of the disease [2,13,46]. This view is supported by the case report of Johnson and Brown [17], in which both corneal edema and posterior epitheliallike cells were absent. By SEM, the abnormal cells lining the posterior surface of the cornea can be seen to have numerous microvilli (Fig. 4B). The cells contain abundant filaments (10 nm thick) and express keratin protein (Fig. 4C) [38,39].

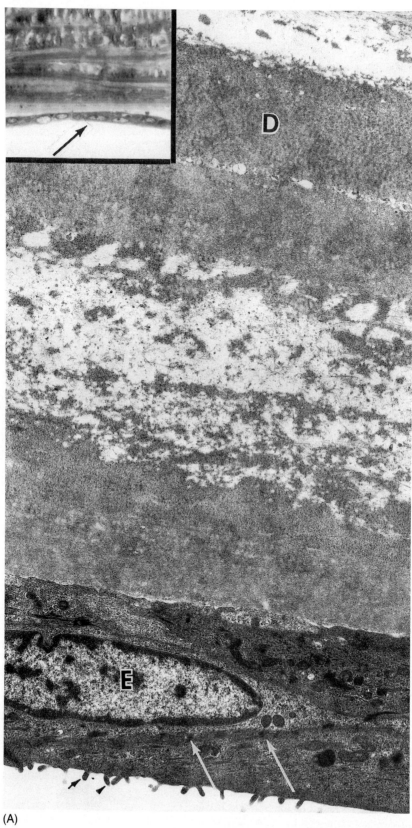

(A)

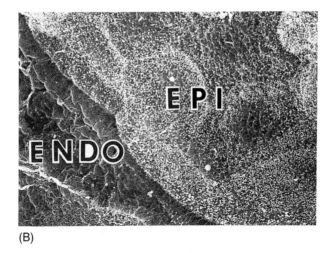

(B)

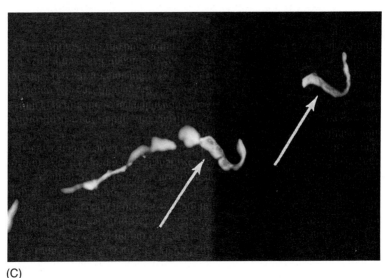

(C)

Figure 4 Posterior polymorphous dystrophy. (A) Inset: irregular double-layered corneal endothelium (arrow). (Toluidine blue, ×500) Transmission electron micrograph shows multilaminar Descemet's membrane (D) with abnormal "endothelium" (E) showing epitheliumlike features, including multiple desmosomal attachments (arrows) and microvillous projections (curved arrows). (×12,900) (B) Scanning electron micrograph of the posterior cornea showing abnormal "epitheliumlike" cells (EPI) with myriad microvilli adjacent to endothelial cells. (×2200) (C) Abnormal expression of keratin by some of the endothelial cells with epitheliumlike features (arrows). (Immunofluorescent stain for keratin AE3, ×500)

In the normal cornea, keratin is expressed only in the epithelium, vimentin constituting the more usual intermediate filaments of the endothelium and keratocytes [37].

Pathogenesis

The origin of the abnormal epitheliumlike layer on the posterior corneal surface is uncertain. Possibilities that have been raised include an embryonal displacement of cells of unknown origin [2] and an epithelial transformation of corneal endothelium [39,40]. Occasionally, desmosomelike junctions have been observed in normal human corneal endothelium [16]. Thus, it is possible that the endothelium may transform to cells with epitheliumlike features. This has been documented in tissue culture studies of corneal endothelium [28]. In culture, rabbit corneal endothelium can form desmosomes and intracytoplasmic fibrils [28].

C. Hereditary Corneal Edema

An entity characterized by a congenital diffuse ground-glass clouding of the cornea has been termed hereditary corneal edema [20]. In this disorder, a moderately dense corneal opacification occupies the entire stroma, with minimal corneal thickening, distinguishing it from the markedly thick cornea in congenital hereditary endothelial dystrophy and from the edema with breaks in Descemet's membrane that accompanies infantile glaucoma.

D. Congenital Hereditary Endothelial Dystrophy

In the entity designated congenital hereditary endothelial dystrophy (CHED), the corneas manifest a diffuse ground-glass appearance and are two to three times thicker than normal. CHED is inherited in a more common autosomal recessive or a less frequent autosomal dominant pattern [19]. Since the disorder is rare, further studies are needed to clarify the clinical distinctions between these two genetic forms. The autosomal recessive type is present at birth, remains stationary and asymptomatic, and is accompanied by nystagmus; the autosomal dominant type appears in the first or second year with photophobia and tearing, progresses slowly over 5–10 years, and lacks nystagmus.

The diffuse corneal edema of posterior polymorphous dystrophy may simulate CHED, but the corneas are thicker in the latter condition [48].

In cases of CHED in whom bilateral corneal opacification is severe, penetrating keratoplasty is the only hope for improved vision.

Histopathology

In CHED, Descemet's membrane consists of the normal anterior 110 nm banded portion and a narrow zone of posterior nonbanded material. In addition, there is a fibrous connective tissue layer posterior to Descemet's membrane, which is composed of an admixture of fibrils measuring 20–40 nm in diameter and small amounts of basement membrane-like material [22]. In some foci, the latter becomes densely packed, resembling an additional layer of Descemet's membrane [22]. The entire multilaminar zone varies from 2.0 to 35.0 μm in thickness and corresponds to the gray thickening observed clinically. The endothelial cells are scant or degenerated when present (Fig. 5) [48].

The stroma shows marked edema with some enlargement of collagen fibrils [20]. These changes, together with the decreased fibril density, produced scattering of light, resulting in the clinical ground-glass appearance. The keratocytes and Bowman's layer are usually unremarkable.

Histologically, a subtle difference in the thickness of collagen in Descemet's membrane between dominant and recessive cases has been described [23]. The recessive cases show an increased tendency for the abnormal endothelium to synthesize a homogenous, posterior, nonbanded Descemet's, with an accelerated rate of deposition. In the dominant cases, a posterior collagenous layer of fibrillary collagen contributes to the thickness of Descemet's membrane [23].

Pathogenesis

It is possible that in cases with thinned Descemet's membrane, total endothelial damage occurred in utero, whereas thickened Descemet's membrane probably results from production of a posterior collagenous layer at a later stage of development.

There is some controversy regarding the spectrum of changes in posterior polymorphous dystrophy and CHED, some reports suggesting a common mechanistic process [6,30]. However, there are distinct histological, ultrastructural, and immunohistochemical differences between these entities. Posterior polymorphous dystrophy is characterized by patchy epitheliumlike alterations of corneal endothelium, whereas these changes are absent in CHED.

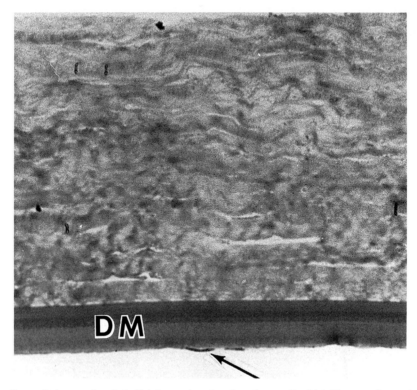

Figure 5   Congenital corneal endothelial dystrophy, showing abnormally thick Descemet's membrane (DM) with scant endothelium (arrow). (×500)

III.   POSTERIOR AMORPHOUS CORNEAL DYSTROPHY

Posterior amorphous corneal dystrophy is a rare autosomal dominant heritable disorder characterized clinically by irregular sheetlike opacities in the deep corneal stroma and Descemet's membrane and is distinct from pre-Descemet's dystrophy, posterior polymorphous dystrophy, and CHED [7,9,18]. Histopathology of a corneal button has shown disorganized posterior stromal collagen lamellae and attenuated endothelium. Descemet's membrane was interrupted by a zone of collagen fibers beneath the anterior banded layer [18].

Since these changes have been observed in infancy and childhood, a developmental abnormality has been postulated. Additional pathological material needs to be evaluated since histological examination of only one case has been reported.

REFERENCES

1. Alexander, R.A., Grierson, I., and Garner, A. Oxytalan fibers in Fuchs' endothelial dystrophy. *Arch. Ophthalmol. 99*:1622–1627, 1981.
2. Boruchoff, S., and Kuwabara, T. Electron microscopy of posterior polymorphous degenerations. *Am. J. Ophthalmol. 72*:879–887, 1971.
3. Bramsen, I., and Ehlers, N. Bullous keratopathy (Fuchs' endothelial dystrophy) treated systemically with 4-transaminocyclohexano-carboxylic acid. *Acta Ophthalmol. (Copenh.) 55*:665–673, 1977.
4. Bücklers, M. Über eine weitere familiär Hornhautdystrophie (Reis). *Klin. Monatsbl. Augenheilkd. 114*:386–387, 1949.
5. Burns, P.R. Meesmann's corneal dystrophy. *Trans. Am. Ophthalmol. Soc. 66*:530–635, 1968.
6. Chan, C.C., Green, W.R., Barraquer, J., Barraquer-Somers, E., and de la Gruz, Z. Similarities between posterior polymorphous and congenital hereditary endothelial dystrophies: A study of 14 buttons of 11 cases. *Cornea 1*:155–172, 1982.

7. Carpel, E.F., Sigelman, R.J., and Doughman, D.J. Posterior amorphous corneal dystrophy. *Am. J. Ophthalmol.* *83*:629–632, 1977.

8. Cibis, G., Krachmer, J., Phelps, C., and Weingeist, T. The clinical spectrum of posterior polymorphous dystrophy. *Trans. Am. Acad. Ophthalmol. Otolaryngol.* *81*:770–777, 1976.

9. Dunn, S.P., Krachmer, J.H., and Ching, S.S.T. New findings in posterior amorphous corneal dystrophy. *Arch. Ophthalmol.* *102*:236–239, 1984.

10. Fine, B.S., Yanoff, M., Pitts, E., and Slaughter, F.D. Meesmann's epithelial dystrophy of the cornea. *Am. J. Ophthalmol.* *83*:633–642, 1977.

11. Fine, B.S., and Yanoff, M. *Ocular Histology. A Text and Atlas*, 2nd ed., Harper and Row, New York, pp. 171–176, 1979.

12. Grayson, M., and Wilbrandt, H. Dystrophy of the anterior limiting membrane of the cornea (Reis-Bücklers' type). *Am. J. Ophthalmol.* *61*:345–349, 1966.

13. Grayson, M. The nature of hereditary deep polymorphous dystrophy of the cornea: Its association with iris and anterior chamber dysgenesis. *Trans. Am. Ophthalmol. Soc.* *72*:516–559, 1974.

14. Hogan, M., Wood, I., and Fine, M. Fuchs' endothelial dystrophy of the cornea. *Am. J. Ophthalmol.* *78*:363–383, 1974.

15. Humayun, M.S., and Pepose, J.S. A viral etiology in Fuchs' corneal dystrophy. *Hum. Pathol.* *19*:245, 1988.

16. Iwamoto, T., and DeVoe, A.G. Electron microscopic studies on Fuchs' combined dystrophy. I. Posterior portion of the cornea. *Invest. Ophthalmol.* *10*:9–28, 1971.

17. Johnson, B.L., and Brown, S.I. Posterior polymorphous dystrophy: A light and electron microscopic study. *Br. J. Ophthalmol.* *62*:89–96, 1978.

18. Johnson, A.T., Folberg, F., Vrabec, M.P., Florakis, G.J., Stone, E.M., and Krachmer, J.H. The pathology of posterior amorphous corneal dystrophy. *Ophthalmology* *97*:104–109, 1990.

19. Judisch, G.F., and Maumenee, I.H. Clinical differentiation of recessive congenital hereditary endothelial dystrophy and dominant hereditary endothelial dystrophy. *Am. J. Ophthalmol.* *85*:606–612, 1978.

20. Kanai, A., Waltman, S., Polack, F.M., and Kaufmann, H.E. Electron microscopic study of hereditary corneal edema. *Invest. Ophthalmol.* *10*:89–95, 1971.

21. Kenney, M.C., Labermeier, U., Hinds, D., and Waring, G.O., III. Characterization of the Descemet's membrane/ posterior, collagenous layer isolated from Fuchs' endothelial dystrophy corneas. *Exp. Eye Res.* *39*:267–277, 1984.

22. Kenyon, K., and Maumenee, A.E. Further studies of congenital hereditary endothelial dystrophy of the cornea. *Am. J. Ophthalmol.* *76*:419–430, 1973.

23. Kirkness, C.M., McCartney, D., Rice, N.S., Garner, A., and Steele, A.D. Congenital hereditary corneal oedema of Maumenee: Its clinical features management and pathology. *Br. J. Ophthalmol.* *71*:130–144, 1987.

24. Krachmer, J.H., Purcell, J.J., Young, C.W., and Bucher, A. Study of sixty-four families with corneal endothelial dystrophy. *Arch. Ophthalmol.* *96*:2036–2039, 1978.

25. Kuwabara, T., and Ciccarelli, E.C. Meesmann's corneal dystrophy: A pathological study. *Arch. Ophthalmol.* *71*:676–682, 1964.

26. Liakos, G.M., and Casey, T.A. Posterior polymorphous keratopathy. *Br. J. Ophthalmol.* *62*:39–45, 1978.

27. Lohse, E., Stock, E.L., Jones, J.C.R., Brande, L.S., O'Grady, R.B., and Roth, S.I. Reis-Bückler's corneal dystrophy: Immunofluorescent and electron microscopic studies. *Cornea* 8:200–209, 1989.

28. Lowry, G.M., Corneal endothelium in vitro: Characterization by ultrastructure and histochemistry. *Invest. Ophthalmol.* *5*:355–361, 1966.

29. Maurice, D.M. The location of the fluid pump in the cornea. *J. Physiol.* *221*:43–54, 1972.

30. McCartney, A.C.E., and Kirkness, C.M. Comparison between posterior polymorphous dystrophy and congenital hereditary endothelial dystrophy of the cornea. *Eye* 2:63–70, 1988.

31. Meesmann, A., and Wilke, F. Klinische und anatomische Utersuchungen über eine bisher unbekannte, dominant verebte Epitheldystrophie der Hornhaut. *Klin. Monatsbl. Augenheilkd.* *103*:361–391, 1939.

32. Møller, H.U. Granular dystrophy Groenouw type I and Reis-Bücklers' corneal dystrophy. *Acta Ophthalmol. (Copenh.)* *67*:678–684, 1989.

33. Nakanishi, I., and Brown, S.I. Ultrastructure of the epithelial dystrophy of Meesmann. *Arch. Ophthalmol.* *93*:259–263, 1975.

34. Polack, F.M. Contributions of electron microscopy to the study of corneal pathology. *Surv. Ophthalmol.* 20: 375–414, 1976.

35. Perry, H.D., Fine, B.S., and Caldwell, D.R. Reis-Bücklers' dystrophy: A study of eight cases. *Arch. Ophthalmol.* *97*:664–670, 1979.

36. Reis, W. Familiäre fleckige Horhautentartung. *Dtsch. Med. Wochenschr.* *43*:575, 1917.

37. Risen, L.A., Binder, P.S., and Nayak, S.K. Intermediate filaments and their organization in human corneal endothelium. *Invest. Ophthalmol. Vis. Sci.* 28:1933–1938, 1987.

38. Rodrigues, M., Waring, G., Laibson, R., and Weinreb, S. Endothelial alterations in congenital corneal dystrophies. *Am. J. Ophthalmol.* *80*:678–689, 1975.

39. Rodrigues, M.M., Sun, T.-T., Krachmer, J., and Newsome, D. Epithelialization of the corneal endothelium in posterior polymorphous dystrophy. *Invest. Ophthalmol. Vis. Sci.* *19*:832–835, 1980.

40. Rodrigues, M.M., Sun, T.-T., and Krachmer, J. Posterior polymorphous dystrophy: Recent developments. *Birth Defects 18*:479–491, 1982.
41. Rodrigues, M.M., Gaster, R.N., and Pratt, M.V. Unusual superficial confluent form of granular corneal dystrophy. *Ophthalmology 90*:1507–1511, 1983.
42. Rodrigues, M.M., Streeten, B.W., Krachmer, J.H., Laibson, P.R., Salem, N., Passonneau, J., and Chock, S. Microfibrillar protein and phospholipid in granular corneal dystrophy. *Arch. Ophthalmol. 101*:802–810, 1983.
43. Rodrigues, M.M., Krachmer, J.H., Hackett, J., Gaskins, R., and Halkias, A. Fuchs' corneal dystrophy: A clinicopathologic study of the variation in corneal edema. *Ophthalmology 93*:789–796, 1986.
44. Roth, S.I., Stock, E.L., and Jutabha, R. Endothelial viral inclusions in Fuchs' corneal dystrophy. *Hum. Pathol. 18*:338–341, 1987.
45. Thiel, H.J., and Behnke, H. Ein bisher unbekannte subepitheliale hereditäre Hornhautdystrophie. *Klin. Monatsbl. Augenheilkd. 150*:862–847, 1967.
46. Tripathi, R., Casey, T., and Wise, G. Hereditary posterior polymorphous dystrophy: An ultrastructural and clinical report. *Trans. Ophthalmol. Soc. UK 94*:211–225, 1974.
47. Tuberville, A.W., Wood, T.O., and McLaughlin, B.J. Cytochrome oxidase activity of Fuchs' endothelial dystrophy. *Curr. Eye Res. 5*:939–947, 1986.
48. Waring, G.O., Rodrigues, M.M., and Laibson, P.R. Corneal dystrophies. II. Endothelial dystrophies. *Surv. Ophthalmol. 23*:147–168, 1978.
49. Waring, G.O., Rodrigues, M.M., and Laibson, P.R. Corneal dystrophies. I. Dystrophies of the epithelium, Bowman's layer and stroma. *Surv. Ophthalmol. 23*:71–122, 1978.
50. Waring, G.O., Bourne, W.M., Edelhauser, H.F., and Kenyon, K.R. The corneal endothelium: Normal and pathologic structure and function. *Ophthalmology 89*:531–590, 1982.
51. Waring, G.O., Font, R.L., Rodrigues, M.M., and Mulberger, R.D. Alterations of Descemet's membrane in interstitial keratitis. *Am. J. Ophthalmol. 81*:773–785, 1976.
52. Waring, G.O., Laibson, P., and Rodrigues, M. Clinical and pathologic alteration of Descemet's membrane with emphasis on endothelial metaplasia. *Surv. Ophthalmol. 18*:325–368, 1974.
53. Wilson, S.E., and Bourne, W.M. Fuchs' dystrophy. *Cornea 7*:2–18, 1988.
54. Weidle, E.G. Differential diagnose der Hornhautdystrophien vom Typ Groenouw I, Reis-Bücklers and Thiel-Behnke. *Fortschr. Ophthalmol. 86*:265–271, 1989.
55. Wittebol-Post, D., and Pels, E. The dystrophy described by Reis-Bücklers': Separate entity of the granular dystrophy. *Ophthalmologica 199*:1–9, 1989.

41

Retinal Photoreceptor Disorders

Alan C. Bird and Barrie Jay
Institute of Ophthalmology, University of London, London, England

Ali Aijaz Hussain and John Marshall
United Medical and Dental Schools of Guy's and St. Thomas's Hospitals, London, England

I. RETINAL PHOTORECEPTOR DYSTROPHIES

Retinal receptor dystrophies comprise a variety of disparate genetically determined conditions that differ from one to another in their mode of inheritance, their pattern of visual loss, and their ophthalmoscopic appearances. Over the past few years, as a result of research by clinicians, biochemists, cell biologists, and molecular biologists, an increasing number of distinct disorders has been recognized within this heterogeneous group, and in some a clue to their pathogenesis has started to emerge. It is possible to subdivide patients with photoreceptor dystrophies into groups depending on their clinical features. Some patients have symptoms early in the disease, indicating primary loss of rod function, and examination reveals defective vision in the midzone of the visual field and morphological changes in the postequatorial fundus; most of the diseases in this category are known collectively as retinitis pigmentosa (RP). Other disorders, with loss of cone function and morphological changes in the central fundus, are known as macular dystrophies or cone dystrophies. This subdivision into "peripheral dystrophies," in which the rods may be the primary target of disease, and "central dystrophies," in which the cones may be the cells initially affected, is superficially attractive. It is tempting to assume that the pathogenesis of conditions within the RP group are related to a disorder of a metabolic function or structural protein peculiar to rods and, conversely, that macular dystrophies are due to defects of cones. Many patients have a combined disorder of both rods and cones, however, even in the early stages of the disease, and all patients with RP have some degree of cone loss. The retinal photoreceptor dystrophies therefore comprise a spectrum of disorders ranging from pure rod dystrophies to pure cone dystrophies, with disorders intermediate between the two in which there is varying involvement of both rod and cone systems. Despite these reservations, photoreceptor dystrophies are considered in two broad categories: peripheral photoreceptor dystrophies, typified by RP, and central dystrophies.

A. Peripheral Receptor Dystrophies

Differences in phenotype may reflect the effect of different genes or different mutations in the same gene, but in some instances the differences may be due to observation of the same disorder at different stages of evolution or different phenotypic expression of the same genetic disorder. Identification of genetic heterogeneity depends on studies in which comparison is made of inter- and intrafamilial variation in disease. If a characteristic is identified consistently in one family but is absent in another, it is reasonable to assume genetic heterogeneity. This has limited most clinical studies to large families with autosomal dominant and X-linked disease.

Retinitis Pigmentosa

RP is a solitary manifestation of several genetically determined disorders characterized by loss of dark adaptation and progressive reduction in peripheral visual fields early in the disease, leading eventually to impairment of central vision. It is becoming increasingly clear that each disease within this family of disorders has a different fundamental genetic defect.

Clinical Genetic Studies. RP may be inherited as an autosomal dominant, an autosomal recessive, or an X-linked trait. When transmission has occurred through several generations the recognition of X-linked or autosomal dominant inheritance is usually simple. As with other disorders, parental consanguinity may indicate the possibility of autosomal recessive inheritance. When faced with a sporadic case, however, the problem of identifying the genetic form of the disease may be more difficult. In the large series of cases at Moorfields Eye Hospital, London, the frequency of simplex (sporadic) cases in families with RP is at present 52%, a figure a little larger than that published 10 years previously (42%) [229]. Other authors have found a similar high frequency of simplex cases [56,132,191,212,357]. Autosomal dominant RP (adRP) causes between 10 and 25% of cases and X-linked RP (xRP) 5–18% in different series [56,132, 191,212,229,357].

Until fairly recently it was commonly assumed that patients with simplex RP had autosomal recessive RP (arRP), but there is increasing clinical evidence that some of these patients do not express RP in the same manner as patients with proven arRP [192]. There is an excess of males, implying the presence of xRP within this group [229]. Simplex cases may be X-linked if heterozygous females are asymptomatic and affected male relatives are not known to the proband, or the disease may be adRP as a result of a new mutation.

Further genetic information may be obtained by examining asymptomatic relatives. In particular, it is useful to examine the mothers of severely affected males because they may show mild retinal involvement, indicating the heterozygous state of xRP [47].

The severity of RP may be used as a guide to the likely inheritance [228]. In general, xRP and arRP cause severe disease of early onset, but adRP is milder. Severe disease in a female may indicate arRP and mild disease in a male, adRP. Mild RP in a female is compatible with the heterozygous state of either xRP or adRP, whereas severe disease in a male suggests xRP or arRP.

Functional Studies. By careful studies of visual function considerable success has been achieved in establishing a subdivision of RP. In some disorders, the target cells have been identified, and the characteristics of functional loss indicate the nature of the disease mechanism.

Autosomal dominant retinitis pigmentosa. Two broad categories of adRP have been identified that are designated type I (diffuse) and type II (regional) forms [16,286,309]. The functional characteristics are consistent within families, indicating genetic heterogeneity. In families with diffuse RP, affected members manifest widespread loss of rod function with relatively well preserved cone function at some stage in the evolution of the disease. Those with regional RP show variation in the state of rod and cone function, with severe losses of both systems in some regions and nearly normal function in others. In regional RP the loss of rhodopsin accounts for the reduction in sensitivity, but in diffuse RP there is more rhodopsin than would be predicted if reduced light absorption by visual pigment were responsible for sensitivity loss [240]. These findings suggest that in regional RP loss of rod function is due to photoreceptor cell death, short outer segments, or a combination of the two, but in diffuse RP this cannot be the case. These two subtypes can be distinguished clinically by history alone [286]. In the diffuse form, night blindness is consistently reported within the first decade of life and symptoms of visual field loss by day follow some 20 years later. Pigmentation is often sparse until late in the disease, which may reflect the lack of cell death, at least in the first few years of disease. By contrast, in the regional form night blindness and trouble by day occur simultaneously, and the age of onset is variable even within the same family. Pigmentation is seen much earlier in regional RP than in the diffuse form.

Additional variants have been identified in adRP in which the distribution is different from the usual pattern of preferential involvement in the midperiphery throughout 360° of the fundus.

Variants of Retinitis Pigmentosa. *Sector retinitis pigmentosa.* Sector RP [46,177] is characterized by retinal atrophy restricted to part of the fundus, and gross field loss is confined to the area of visual field corresponding to the involved retina. The lower half of the fundus is usually affected (Fig. 1), with loss of visual function in the upper field [137], but rarely the disease affects only the superior [373], nasal [475], or temporal fundus [4,454]. In most reported cases with limited sector involvement, the inheritance is

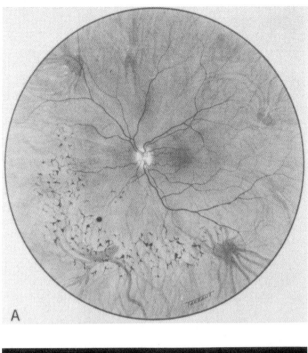

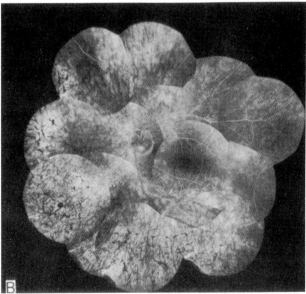

Figure 1 (A) Fundus painting of an X-linked heterozygote showing apparent sectorial retinitis pigmentosa affecting the inferior and nasal retina. (B) Fluorescein angiography confirms the regional nature of the changes but demonstrates retinal pigment epithelial atrophy in the superior fundus.

autosomal dominant and the distribution of disease is common to affected members of the family [137, 177,209,261,281]. However, a similar pattern of disease also appears in patients with relatives who have involvement of the whole fundus [256], and some are heterozygous for xRP [47,256]. By fluorescein angiography minor changes are often found to be more widespread than might be appreciated by ophthalmoscopy with white light, and the sector of RP may be an area of maximum disease rather than of exclusive involvement [47,256]. In typical sector RP, rod and cone electroretinograms (ERG) show mild reduction in amplitude with normal cone implicit times [42,157,309]. This pattern of disease is common to all affected members within a family irrespective of age, suggesting that the disease, in contrast to other forms of adRP, is nonprogressive or progresses very slowly.

No good explanation exists for the regional predilection for disease. It is tempting to ascribe the inferior involvement to higher lighting levels of the inferior retina than the superior retina [193], but this is unproven and it does not account for the different distribution of disease between families.

Slow dark adaptation. In some families with RP recovery of bleachable rhodopsin is slow [3,323]. Cone adaptation and the early part of the recovery of rod sensitivity follow the normal time course, but the later phase of rod adaptation is markedly prolonged.

Paravenous pigmented chorioretinal atrophy. Paravenous pigmented chorioretinal atrophy has been described in several reports, with atrophy of the RPE beneath the retinal veins that usually extends from the optic disk with pigment around the retinal veins [140]. In most cases the disorder is described as an isolated phenomenon, possibly of inflammatory origin [140,185,335]. However, reports exist with familial involvement [335,405,432]. It may vary considerably in severity within a family such that affected relatives cannot be excluded without a family survey. Rapid or slow progression and stable visual function have been described [276,335,405]. The disorder may also be asymmetrical [80,432]. Most authors believe that this condition may be genetically determined but that phenocopies exist.

Choroiditis striata (helicoid peripapillary chorioretinal degeneration). Well-defined atrophy radiating from the optic disk but not following the blood vessels has also been described as an autosomal dominant disorder. This was first described in an Icelandic family [427] and was called choroiditis striata. In a further report on the same family the term "helicoid peripapillary chorioretinal degeneration" was used [428]. Several reports have followed that appear to concern families exclusively from Iceland and Switzerland, implying the possibility that only two families exist [59,141,294,389]. The disorder is believed to be slowly progressive, causes few visual symptoms, and is associated with a refractive error that is usually the reason for ascertainment [294,428].

Variable expressivity. The expressivity in some families is highly variable, such that about 70% of members with the abnormal gene have moderate to severe disease and the remainder are asymptomatic but with mild fundus abnormalities and electrophysiological changes indicating the presence of the abnormal gene [122]. In some families there appears to be bimodal expression of disease, although the factors that modulate gene expression are unknown.

Autosomal recessive retinitis pigmentosa. Specific clinical subtypes of arRP have also been recognized. One form has preservation of the RPE adjacent to the retinal arterioles, and unlike most other forms of RP they are consistently hypermetropic [191,369].

A further variant comprises night blindness and variably reduced visual acuity associated with restricted pigmentation in the ocular fundus, cystoid macular changes resembling macular schisis, and distinctive ERG abnormalities [301]. The rod ERG is unrecordable, maximal stimulus evokes a large response with very prolonged implicit time of the b wave, photopic and scotopic responses are of similar magnitude, and the response is much greater when produced by short- than by long-wavelength light. The last attribute is known as the enhanced S cone response. At least in some respects this disorder resembles the Goldmann-Favré syndrome [129], and it is not yet clear whether this represents a single disorder with variable expressivity.

X-linked retinitis pigmentosa. As early as 1914, Diem reported abnormal fundus reflexes in females heterozygous for xRP [109], but during subsequent years similar phenomena were reported in other genetic forms of RP and were referred to as "tapetal reflexes" [298] (Fig. 2). An abnormal tapetal reflex has been claimed to be the most common expression of the heterozygous state in xRP [123,147,217,248,254,379, 458,461]. Ricci and his colleagues [379] reported that this reflex could not be seen after exposure of the fundus to light but reappeared after a period of darkness; they called this the *phénomène de Mizuo inverse*. Schappert Kimmijser could identify this abnormal reflex in females in only one family of eight, however, and concluded that although this sign is useful when present, its absence does not indicate a normal genotype [397].

Attempts have been made to subdivide xRP on the basis of differential affection of heterozygotes. In only a few of the early reports of families with xRP was retinal degeneration in females described [227,292], but profound visual loss in heterozygotes was recorded by McKenzie in New Zealand [290]. In 1960 Kobayashi described a family with even more severe involvement of the female members, five

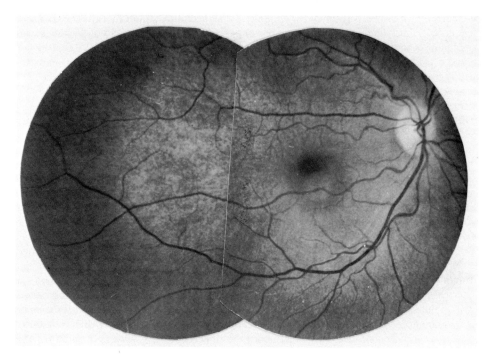

Figure 2 Punctate reflex in the posterior fundus of an X-linked heterozygote.

heterozygous females having manifest RP, 11 having some stigmata of the disease, and at least 4 being normal [248]. No accurate comparison was made of the severity of the disease between affected men and women, although it was stated that the females were more mildly affected than the males. From this information, he concluded that there were three separate types of xRP: recessive, intermediate, and dominant. However, subsequent experience indicates that there is considerable intrafamilial variation in the severity of the disease in heterozygotes and that there is no justification for separating xRP into different categories on the basis of the severity of the disease in women [39,47].

The presence of a tapetal reflex in women heterozygous for the abnormal gene in some families, but not others [397], may serve to differentiate xRP into two categories on clinical grounds, an observation in keeping with recent genomic studies that indicate the existence of at least two loci for xRP.

Unilateral retinitis pigmentosa. Unilateral RP was reported as early as 1865 by Pedralgia [360], and the ophthalmoscopic observations were corroborated by histological examination 25 years later [108]. In 1952, François and Verriest reviewed the 56 unilateral cases reported until that time and concluded that only 10 cases had the typical ophthalmoscopic appearance of RP and were strictly unilateral [150]. Subsequent reports have shown that, in some cases, minor changes can be demonstrated in the unaffected fellow eye by sophisticated examination [76,250]. Furthermore, Carr and Siegel thought that the disease in cases described by them and by some previous authors was due to vascular disease and was not heritable [76]. To illustrate the difficulty in assessing the significance of such cases, Pearlman and colleagues described a patient with mild but widespread unilateral outer retinal disease, but they presented no evidence about the inheritance of the disease [359]. In no case of unilateral RP has a family history of eye disease been identified, although in one patient the parents were consanguineous [91]. Most workers take the view that there is no good evidence that unilateral RP represents a heritable condition.

Electrophysiological Studies. Soon after the introduction of the ERG into clinical practice, its amplitude was found to be reduced in RP [19,48,110,146], and some patients with relatively good visual function had unrecordable ERG [110,382]. Riggs believed that photoreceptor cell death alone was insufficient to account for the absence of the ERG and suggested that peripheral photoreceptor degeneration caused short-circuiting between the retina and the choroid so that potentials generated in the retina could not be recorded by a distant corneal electrode [382]. He quoted observations by Bush [65] in support of this hypothesis, namely that multiple perforations of the retina cause extinction of the ERG by electrical short-circuiting without causing massive retinal destruction.

It is now evident that with better recording systems and averaging techniques, ERG potentials can be recorded in many cases [20,198]. These observations suggest that the reduction of the ERG in RP is due to retinal dysfunction alone.

Using a homogeneous light stimulus and an adapting background illumination, qualitative analyses of the ERG in different forms of RP have been undertaken. It has been postulated that diminution of the ERG potential in the presence of normal latency implies a reduced population of normal photoreceptors, whereas a prolonged implicit time implies widespread receptor dysfunction [41]. The ERG varies in different families with RP. For example, in patients of a single pedigree with adRP the rod ERG component was reduced in amplitude and latency but the cone component was normal. In another family with adRP with reduced penetrance, the cone responses were also abnormal [40]. This finding supports the concept that the difference in penetrance signifies distinct forms of adRP, and the difference in the influence of the diseases on retinal function implies the presence of different pathogenetic mechanisms within this genetic group of RP. In xRP, both cone and rod responses are delayed and reduced [40].

The early receptor potential (ERP), which has a short latent period [17,64,85], results from the photochemical reaction induced by light falling on the outer segments [63,86] and depends upon the concentration of visual pigment [85], the orientation of the outer segments [62,86], and their morphology [17]. The ERP potential is reduced early in xRP, and adRP [36,37] and is considered to be caused by a reduction in the visual pigment content of the outer segments in the early stages of these conditions.

The light-induced rise in ocular potential as recorded by electrooculography (EOG) has also been shown to be reduced or abolished early in RP, when the clinical diagnosis may be in doubt [15,18]. The response is believed to be due to ion movement by the retinal pigment epithelium (RPE) in response to changes in the ionic content of the extracellular space of the outer retina that occur with changes in the state of the photoreceptor cation channels. No variation has been recorded between one form of RP and another, and the EOG changes merely reflect the severity of the photoreceptor defect.

Genomic Studies. *X-linked retinitis pigmentosa.* The first RP gene to be localized was one for xRP using a probe L1.28 [44] that maps to the short arm near the centromere at Xp11. Subsequent studies have supported the original observation [156,325,477]. The first indication of a second locus resulted from the identification of a deletion at Xp21 in a child with xRP, Duchenne muscular dystrophy, and X-linked chronic granulomatous disease [145]; this locus is telomeric to that of L1.28. Localization of a gene linked with RP to this distal site was confirmed by other studies [103,341]. There is no wide agreement on the clinical differences between xRP transmitted at the two loci, although all heterozygotes in whom a tapetal reflex is seen seem to belong to families in which the gene is at the more telomeric locus. The possibility of more than one abnormal allele at each locus has not been excluded; that not all families with disease transmitted at the telomeric site have a tapetal reflex supports this view.

Autosomal dominant retinitis pigmentosa. In 1989 a locus for adRP was identified on the long arm of chromosome 3 [293]. Three candidate genes exist close to the proposed site, and within a short time a proline/histidine mutation was detected at codon 23 of the rhodopsin molecule [116]. Since then more than 40 genomic defects have been detected on the rhodopsin gene, and it appears that this gene accounts for between 25 and 30% of adRP [114,115,219,239,423]. Most of the substitutions appear to be peculiar to a single family, although some, notably a mutation at codon 347, have been found in many parts of the world. The proline/histidine mutation at codon 23 was identified in a proportion of apparently unrelated subjects in the United States but not in other countries. There is now some evidence that the adRP patients with this mutation may form part of one large pedigree.

In several families with adRP, there is no linkage with markers on the long arm of chromosome 3 [277], confirming heterogeneity of adRP, and it has now been shown that genes other than that for rhodopsin may be responsible for adRP [50,51,127,128,231]. One of these is the gene for the glycoprotein peripherin/rds that is of particular interest since a mutation in this gene is responsible for the retinal degeneration in the rds mouse [87,433]. Peripherin/rds is localized to the outer segment disk membranes of both rods and cones and is thought to be essential for the assembly, orientation, and physical stability of the outer segment disks of the retinal photoreceptors [21,88,436].

Histopathological Studies.   With few exceptions, all histological reports of the retinal dystrophies are based on inadequately preserved material and describe the most advanced stages of these disorders. These diseases are not life threatening, and because visual difficulties are usually apparent in early adult life, the microscopic examination of material 20 years or more after the onset of severe visual handicap or total blindness gives little information about the underlying cause. However, recently established eye donor schemes for patients with retinal dystrophies have provided relatively fresh eyes for the investigation of pathological mechanisms [125,207,384,430].

The retina has a limited spectrum of response to injurious agents, and it is not surprising that the histological appearance of advanced cases of RP is remarkably similar regardless of the genotype of the disease [82,108,118,169,251,274,285,318,327,429,447,476]. In essence, the primary abnormality is the disappearance of both the rods and cones; the inner retinal layers may appear relatively normal, except for some gliosis and the appearance of variable amounts of pigment-containing cells concentrated around blood vessels. There may be depigmentation, atrophy, degeneration, or proliferation of the RPE, such changes usually being most pronounced toward the periphery of the retina.

Electron microscopic studies have revealed that in advanced adRP [251,429], and possibly in others [318], the only remaining photoreceptor cells in the retina are cones. The surviving cones are located in the posterior pole, are few in number, and have an atypical appearance. Clearly, with any insidious disease process the degree of cellular change is unique to a given individual at a particular time, and therefore care must be exercised in interpreting the cytopathology of a limited number of specimens. However, in all the eyes just described except one [125], only the foveal cones had outer segments, and these were truncated and composed of small groups of disoriented disk membranes, many of which had degenerated into a vesicular form. The outer segments were connected to abnormally wide and short inner segments via an apparently normal cilium. Many of the cells contained autophagic vacuoles [377]. The cone nuclei were also swollen to a diameter 30% larger than normal [447]. In the macula, cone remnants became progressively more degenerate with increasing distance from the fovea. These changes occurred first as a loss of the outer segment, with subsequent swelling of the inner segment and, finally, a loss of both inner and outer segments to leave a residual photoreceptor cell of spherical shape with little cytoplasm. These changes are morphologically identical to those exhibited by cones in areas of retinal detachment [260] or those exposed to mild light damage [308]. In most eyes in the advanced stages of RP, photoreceptor cells have not been observed beyond 5 mm from the macula. In the peripheral regions, proliferated glial tissue is in direct contact with the RPE.

Knowledge of photoreceptor changes associated with the early stages of RP is limited to two specimens, one from a 23-year-old male with xRP and the other a 17 year old with adRP [125,430]. The sufferer with xRP had a typical annular zone of pigment distributed in the bone spicule pattern between about 45° and 60° from the fovea. Although all the remaining photoreceptor cells in this patient exhibited abnormalities, there were marked differences between the center and the periphery. Central foveal cones were reduced in number by about 50% and had shortened and severely distorted outer segments containing vesiculated and disrupted disk membranes similar to the remnants seen in advanced disease. A further similarity was noted in the parafoveal region, where cones first lost their outer segments and then became progressively more disorganized as the distance from the fovea increased. In the major portion of the zone showing bone spicule formation, only occasional vestiges of cones were noted, these being identified by their swollen tigroid nuclei and, in some cases, tiny ellipsoids protruding through the outer limiting membrane. On the outermost border of this zone, inner and outer segments of both rods and cones were apparent, and these became progressively more organized toward the periphery. Both rods and cones had outer segments at least 25% shorter than those in a comparable location in a normal eye. However, whereas the disk membranes of the rods were well ordered and nearly normal in appearance, those of the cones were both disorientated and vesiculated. Thus, the cones in this young patient were similar to those of the very elderly [306].

The adRP specimen was obtained from a 17-year-old motorcycle accident victim and was enucleated within 1 h of death [125]. His visual acuity was normal 2 years before the accident, rod thresholds were raised about 4 log units, scotopic and photopic electrical responses were barely detectable, and he displayed the characteristic features of RP. Eyes were used for both histopathological and biochemical investigations. Within the fovea, cone cells were less densely packed but maintained good structural integrity of their slightly shortened outer segments. Extrafoveal regions showed an increasing number of both rod and cone photoreceptors devoid of an outer segment. The equatorial and peripheral parts of the central regions were severely affected, with a total absence of receptors. Progress toward the peripheral retina showed an increasing number of both rods and cones. Rather surprisingly, the RPE layer showed little morphological abnormality even in the equatorial region. It therefore appears that in this young eye, the RPE has sufficient capacity to remove and degrade the degenerate mass of retinal tissue without undue damage to its own structural integrity. Aged RPE may not be as efficient, leading to gross changes as documented in more advanced stages of the disease.

Both retinal protein and the activity of the photoreceptor-specific cGMP-phosphodiesterase (PDE) mirrored the changes in photoreceptor density across the entire retina. In the peripheral part of the superior temporal quadrant, PDE activity was only slightly reduced (10%). Unlike the PDE complex from the rd animal model of retinal degeneration, that in the human dystrophy could be partially activated by the polycation, histone. The most important finding of this biochemical study was an elevation in the level of cyclic guanosine 5'-monophosphate (cGMP) when expressed as content per photoreceptor cell. In the postequatorial regions, photoreceptors devoid of outer segments showed a 40- to 100-fold increase in cGMP. Peripheral and parafoveal areas, where complete photoreceptors were present, showed a 2- to 3-fold increase in cGMP. It is surprising that human photoreceptors can tolerate such a toxic level of cGMP for extended periods, whereas the cells in the rd mouse and affected Irish setter degenerate quickly following the rise in cGMP. Mechanisms of cGMP toxicity and possibilities for therapeutic intervention are discussed later in the section on cyclic nucleotide metabolism.

In RP, changes in the RPE may be divided into three main classes, which roughly correspond to the degree of retinal eccentricity (Fig. 3):

1. Cells from the central region are typically tall with apically displaced nuclei and a cytoplasm crammed with electron-dense inclusions interpreted as lipofuscin [251] or melanolysosomes [429,430]. They contain few melanin granules and occasional phagosomes, the latter having been found only in cells associated with cones possessing vestigial outer segments. Where extensive photoreceptor degeneration has occurred, the RPE has been identified in various stages of budding or migration from Bruch's membrane.
2. Cells from the central region may be flattened or devoid of either melanin granules or lipofuscin. These cells may occur in more than one layer and are often found with macrophagelike cells whose processes often penetrate to the midlayers of Bruch's membrane.
3. In the periphery, in contrast to the center, the RPE cell contains little lipofuscin but many melanosomes. In some specimens, particularly on the peripheral edge of the bone spicule zone, localized circular regions of epithelial loss with sharply demarcated borders are found, although similar findings have also been reported in the eyes of the elderly [306].

One of the most striking features of the RP is the presence of pigment in the retina associated with photoreceptor degeneration (Fig. 4). This is seen as free granules and granules within Müller cells and macrophages and within the cytoplasm of displaced RPE cells. These cells are most commonly found in clumps or masses around the retinal vessels and the basement membrane complexes of atrophic vessels, but in some patients they become oriented beneath the inner limiting membrane [169,447]. Fluorescence microscopy gives a strong indication that the pigmented cells responsible for bone spicule formation in the neural retina emanate solely from the peripheral RPE, which is relatively devoid of lipofuscin and is hence nonfluorescent, as opposed to the fluorescing lipofuscin-rich RPE near the fovea [251]. However, transmission electron microscopy reveals that the melanin granules within these cells are predominantly spheroidal, not fusiform like those of normal RPE [429].

Degenerative changes in the neural retina are highly variable, with retention of relatively unchanged ganglion cell and nerve fiber layers in some eyes long after the eye has become blind (Fig. 5); in others it is frequently impossible to recognize any retinal architecture. In all cases, the retinal vessels are atrophic,

---

Figure 3 Light micrographs of flat preparations of pigment epithelium from the macular region (A), the "bone spicule" zone (B), and the peripheral retina (C) of an 80-year-old female heterozygous for X-linked retinitis pigmentosa. Although the cells appear relatively normal, there are large sharply demarcated holes in the bone spicule zone and "fibroblastlike" cells in the periphery. (Toluidine blue, ×350)

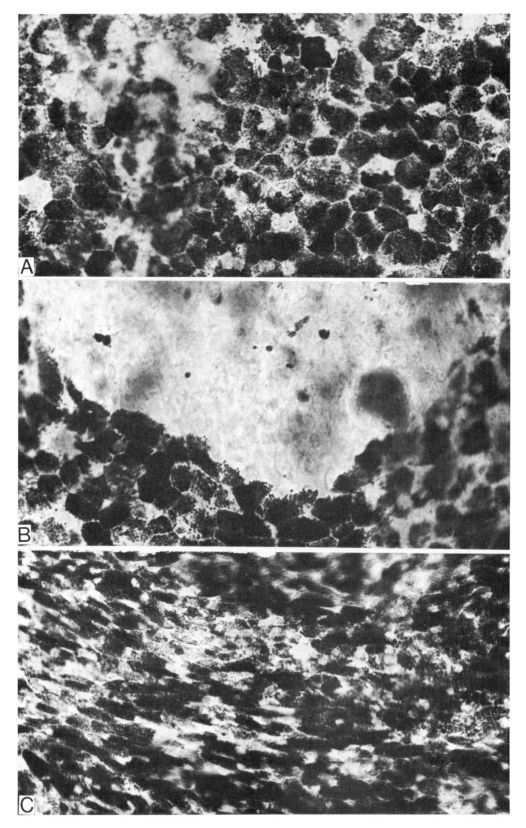

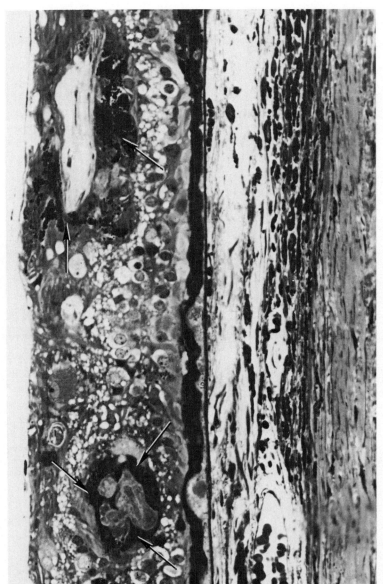

Figure 4 Light micrograph of a nonmacular area of atrophic retina from the eye of an 80-year-old female heterozygous for X-linked retinitis pigmentosa. The photoreceptor cells are lost, but the inner nuclear, inner plexiform, and ganglion cells remain. Large numbers of pigmented cells (arrows) can be seen aggregated around atrophied blood vessels. (Toluidine blue, ×370)

with loss of endothelium and invasion of basement membrane tubes by both macrophages and glial elements.

With the increasing loss of neurons, secondary changes take place in the retinal glia. In areas of photoreceptor loss, the Müller fibers increase in size and come to lie in contact with the RPE. At such regions the complex villi of the Müller cells interdigitate with those of the apical surface of the RPE, a phenomenon that has been reported in a variety of conditions in which photoreceptor degeneration has been induced [263]. The outer limiting membrane of the retina is preserved long after photoreceptor cells are lost but becomes less clear in areas where Bruch's membrane is covered by nonpigmented epithelial cells or cells that look like macrophages. There is often a displacement of the nuclei of Müller cells into regions between the inner nuclear layer and the RPE. In some eyes thin preretinal membranes thought to be composed of glia have been described forming a single layer of cells with long, thin overlapping processes [429].

Considerable variation has been noted in the condition of the choroid and its vessels, but most studies indicate that any atrophic changes are secondary [14,71,82,274,448] and that the loss of choriocapillaris occurs after the loss of photoreceptor cells. As such, in the young eye with adRP described earlier, only localized attenuation of choroidal capillaries was seen in areas where severe degeneration of the photoreceptor layer was apparent.

Lack of human material in the early stages of dystrophic disease severely handicaps investigation of the pathogenesis of these conditions, and it should be emphasized that many late changes, such as RPE migration and gliosis, are secondary and may obscure previous pathological changes.

Choroideremia

Choroideremia, a diffuse photoreceptor dystrophy that may be difficult to distinguish from RP, particularly in young males, was recorded as a distinct condition by Mauthner in 1871 [311], and the inheritance was recognized as X linked in 1942 [168,455]. Apart from its inheritance the distinctive feature of this disorder is diffuse progressive atrophy of the RPE and choriocapillaris.

The symptoms in affected men are identical to those of RP, with early loss of dark adaptation and peripheral fields that progresses to leave a small central field. Visual acuity is maintained at a good level until late in the disorder, often well into the sixth decade of life. Electrophysiological responses are severely depressed in early disease, as they are in RP.

In males the fundus manifests a generalized loss of the RPE pigment, resulting in a blond fundus as early as 2 years of age, followed by the appearance of fine granular subretinal pigment deposits in the ocular midequatorial region. By the third decade of life multifocal areas of the RPE are lost, with concurrent underlying choriocapillaris atrophy in a typically scalloped pattern, becoming more widespread and slowly progressing to a generalized confluent loss of the RPE and choriocapillaris. The disease progresses until a small area of choriocapillaris and RPE survives at the fovea [288], and even this is eventually lost. Fluorescein angiographic studies disclose well the loss of pigment in the RPE and the associated loss of the choriocapillaris.

Histopathological examinations confirm the extensive chorioretinal atrophy [66,287,372], as well as epiretinal membrane formation and vascular endothelial cell abnormalities [66].

Heterozygous females almost always have abnormal fundi with changes in the RPE, but functional loss is unusual in the young and mild later in life. The most common appearance is of midperipheral pigmentation localized deep in the retina and associated with patchy depigmentation of the RPE. Pigment clumping that may be linear in distribution sometimes develops. Occasionally, focal areas of choroidal atrophy occur around the optic disk or in the midperiphery. These fundus changes are usually stationary, but progression has been noted [66]. Microscopic examination disclosed abnormalities of the RPE only [255], widespread malformation of the outer photoreceptor segments and patches of retinal atrophy [163], short or absent photoreceptor outer segments in much of the ocular equatorial region, irregular thickness and pigmentation of the RPE, and areas of profound atrophy in the equatorial region [136].

Choroideremia is a distinct entity within the group of outer retinal dystrophies, in which the RPE appears primarily to be affected, rather than the choroid as the name implies. The choroideremia locus has been mapped to band q21 on the X chromosome [342], and DNA clones that span Xq21 deletions in patients with the disease have been isolated [94]. In some patients with microdeletions, mental retardation

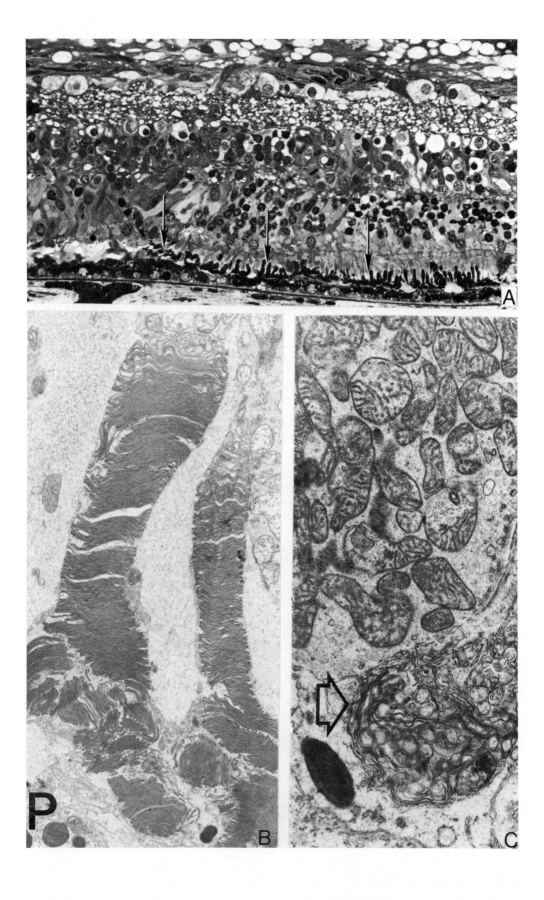

and/or deafness has been reported [95,202,312,387], but despite the size of the deletion, choroideremia remains remarkably constant in clinical expression.

The prominent choroidal atrophy is probably a secondary response to RPE loss. It cannot even be assumed that the primary metabolic abnormality resides within the RPE. Choroidal atrophy is not unique to choroideremia, since it has been identified in about half the eyes with RP subject to histopathological study, but profound early atrophy is unlike RP and signifies a pathogenic process different from those in other outer retinal diseases.

Bietti's Crystalline Dystrophy

A unique fundus appearance was reported by Bietti in three patients, two of whom were brothers, who had crystals in the retina and in the peripheral cornea [45,46]. There is progressive atrophy of the retina with prominent atrophy of the RPE and choroid. As the atrophy supervenes, the intraretinal crystals disappear. The pattern of retinal functional loss is similar to that of RP, the initial symptoms usually appearing in the third or fourth decade of life. Autosomal recessive inheritance was established in this condition by Hu [213], although crystals have been described in patients heterozygous for the abnormal gene [380]. Patients with a similar fundus appearance but without corneal changes have been described and are considered to represent the same disorder [149,187,464]. No systemic biochemical disorder has been identified, although the corneal crystals resemble cholesterol, suggesting that Bietti's crystalline dystrophy may be due to a systemic abnormality of lipid metabolism [473]. This conclusion is supported by the finding of crystals in lymphocytes [473].

B. Central Retinal Dystrophies

A number of genetically determined disorders cause progressive loss of visual functions associated with cones, namely loss of visual acuity, impaired color vision and central visual field defects, and diffuse, poor vision in bright light. These patients also remark upon difficulty with night vision, but on closer questioning this often relates to a short transient period on first entering a dark environment.

Specific disorders, such as Best's disease and Sorsby's fundus dystrophy, can be identified as single nosological entities, but the remainder include groups of disorders that cannot be clearly distinguished one from another. They have been subdivided with respect to inheritance and the appearance of the fundus, but no satisfactory categorization has been devised, and it is likely that each subdivision contains more than one condition. Most disorders fall into two broad subdivisions, fundus flavimaculatus and bull's-eye maculopathy, which can be identified on fundus appearances although the distinction may not be absolute. In some disorders both clinical and histopathological observations imply that the major changes occur at the level of the RPE, with good visual function at least for a period, whereas in others the photoreceptor cells appear to be affected initially.

Dystrophies with Retinal Pigment Epithelial Changes

Vitelliform Macular Dystrophy (Best's Disease).   The typical lesion of Best's disease is a round yellow deposit at the macula [43] (Fig. 6A) that may be identified within a short time of birth [25] or that may develop later in a previously normal fundus [26,106]. Rarely the macular disease is not seen until later life [14]; the lesion may be extramacular, the disease may be asymmetrical, or the fundus may be entirely normal [26,106,167,320]. Godel and colleagues state that about half of those with the abnormal gene have a normal or nearly normal fundus appearance and normal vision [167]. Although flicker fusion studies indicate cone dysfunction much earlier [310], central cone function remains relatively good in most patients until the second decade of life, at which time there may be progressive loss of central vision

---

Figure 5   (A) Light micrograph of an area of nasal retina from an 80-year-old female heterozygous for X-linked retinitis pigmentosa, showing a region of surviving but atypical photoreceptor cells (arrows). ($\times$390) (B and C) Electron micrographs of rod (B) and cone (C) from the area shown in (A). The rod outer segments were shorter and contain fewer disks with a somewhat larger diameter than those of rods in an age-matched normal eye. All the surviving rods exhibited a disorientation of disks adjacent to the pigment epithelium (P). Cone outer segments (arrow) were only seen as disorganized vesiculated remnants of membranes. (B, $\times$95,000; C, $\times$116,000)

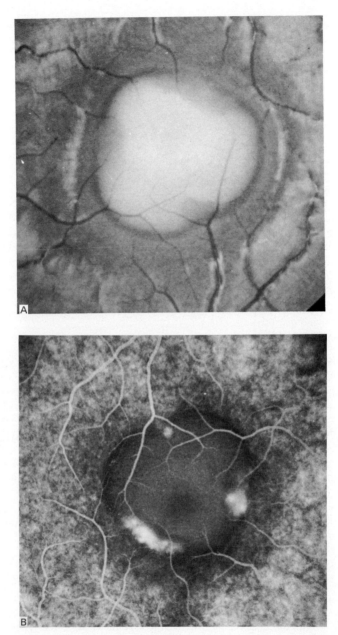

Figure 6 Best's disease with a well-defined submacular deposit of yellow material (A) with invasion of the material with new vessels (B). The other eye of the same patient has subretinal fibrosis in which there was vascular tissue (C, D).

associated with disintegration of the central yellow area. The evolution of the lesion during this period is determined by whether or not new blood vessels invade the abnormal deposit from the choroid (Fig. 6B). If new vessels invade the lesion, there may be subretinal hemorrhages and fibrosis (disciform response), and the visual outcome is poor [315] (Figs. 6C–D). In other patients the yellow material may become partially liquefied, forming fluid levels within the subretinal space, and eventually the material resorbs, leaving confluent atrophy of the central RPE and choriocapillaris. The appearance of patients with a normal

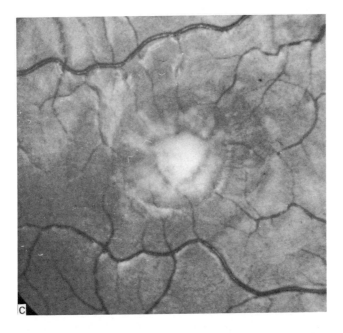

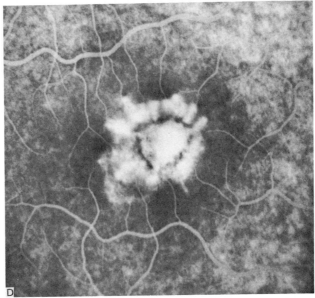

macula, minimal RPE changes, atrophic macula, or fibrous macular scars tended not to change; those with vitelliform or pseudohypopyon lesions progress to later atrophic macular stages [320].

The autosomal dominant mode of inheritance of this disorder was first suggested by Best [43] and was substantiated later by further observations of the same family [230,453,463].

The rise in ocular potential induced by light is always reduced in patients with the abnormal gene for Best's disease, whatever their clinical status, but ERG potentials are normal [105,106]. The universal reduction in the light-induced rise in ocular potential, even in those patients with normal fundi, indicates a widespread dysfunction of the photoreceptor-RPE complex that has possibly been present from birth.

Histopathological studies imply that the abnormal material accumulates initially at the level of the RPE and that the deposits seen clinically are probably between Bruch's membrane and the RPE [346]. In patients with advanced disease, the histopathology included extensive atrophy of the photoreceptors in the macular area [10,289]. In slightly less advanced cases, a widespread abnormality of the RPE in which an excessive amount of lipofuscin accumulates also occurs [153,346,462]. In one case, an accumulation of heterogeneous material between Bruch's membrane and the RPE at the fovea was believed to represent the location of a previtelliform lesion. This material appeared to be derived from degenerating RPE [346]. Despite that two abnormalities of structure and electrical response to light have been clearly defined over many years, the pathogenetic relationship between the two is unknown.

The locus of the gene for vitelliform macular dystrophy has been linked to chromosome 11 (11q13), but the gene has yet to be characterized [421].

Adult Vitelliform Macular Dystrophy.   Adult vitelliform macular dystrophy was first described by Gass [160]. It is characterized by a focal, round or oval, subretinal yellowish foveal lesion, often with one or more pigment spots on the anterior surface at the level of the RPE. The lesions may vary in size but are typically one-third to one-half of a disk diameter and are usually bilateral and symmetrical. Patients usually present in the fourth or fifth decade of life and tend to have minimal visual symptoms [60].

The disorder differs from vitelliform macular dystrophy (Best's disease) in several respects: (1) the foveal lesions are smaller, (2) it presents at a later age, (3) often there is no progression of the foveal lesion, and (4) the light-induced rise in ocular potential is rarely absent.

Although nonfamilial cases have been documented [248], adult vitelliform macular dystrophy is regarded as an autosomal dominant trait [60,160,244,449].

The histopathological studies in this condition have disclosed a loss of RPE and disruption of photoreceptors at the fovea [160,354]. Perhaps of greater significance is the intense autofluorescence seen in the intact RPE outside the fovea, implying that the accumulation of lipofuscin at this site is central to the pathogenesis of the disorder.

It is noteworthy that a mutation in the peripherin gene resulting in a stop codon at position 258 has been found in one patient with a retinal lesion typical of adult vitelliform macular dystrophy [467].

Pattern Dystrophy.   In 1970, five members of a family from Holland were described with a unique fundus appearance consisting of patterned hyperpigmentation at the macula [107]. The pigment appeared to be in the RPE, and fluorescein angiography showed granular hyperpigmentation of the remaining RPE at the posterior pole. The disorder caused few symptoms since the worst visual acuity was 0.8. The most striking feature was the universal reduction in the light-induced rise in ocular potential to 130% or lower in the presence of good visual function. It was concluded that there was diffuse dysfunction of the RPE with little associated visual deficit since there was no indication of rod disease as gauged by the ERG and no abnormality of color vision was apparent. In this respect butterfly-shaped dystrophy is similar to Best's disease. The original pedigree is suggestive of autosomal dominant inheritance; in the original communication the disease was identified in only two generations, but large pedigrees have been published subsequently [370].

A number of families have been described with autosomal dominant disease characterized by linear or irregular changes of pigment at the level of the RPE, with considerable variability in each family [101,460]. Members had "macroreticular change," "fundus pulverilentus," or an appearance of butterfly dystrophy as described by Deutmann [101,174–176]. The deposits at the level of the RPE may be pale or dark and may or may not be linear [92]. In all families the light-induced rise in ocular potential may be depressed, and the condition is compatible with retention of good acuity throughout life. Pattern dystrophy is now believed to represent one or more than one nosological entity with variable expressivity. Comparisons between families or genomic analyses would resolve the question.

Sorsby's Fundus Dystrophy (Pseudoinflammatory Macular Dystrophy)

Sorsby and his colleagues [411] first reported an autosomal dominant disorder in which there is bilateral central visual loss in the fifth decade of life due to subretinal scarring and loss of ambulatory vision during the seventh decade. Three of the original families reported by Sorsby have been extensively studied more recently [69,179,211,368,411]. Before any reduction in central vision, fine drusen or a confluent deposit of yellow subretinal material may be seen [211]. Early in the course of the disease there is delayed filling of the choriocapillaris. Loss of central vision may result from atrophy of the outer retina or ingrowth of subretinal new vessels. Peripheral retinal dysfunction occurs, with a deposit of a yellow subretinal material throughout the fundus, and in late life the subjects may lose all vision.

Electrophysiological responses were originally thought to be usually within normal limits, suggesting that the disorder was localized to the macular region [453], although a reduced light rise on electro-oculography was reported recently [72,113].

A light and electron microscopic study of the eyes of one patient disclosed a 30 μm thick deposit in the inner portion of Bruch's membrane. In addition, there was pronounced loss of the outer retina, a discontinuous RPE, and atrophy of the choriocapillaris [68].

It is believed that the angiographic finding of a slow filling phase indicates a change in blood flow and that there may be a causal relationship between the abnormal deposits and the choroidal changes [69,211,368]. It has been suggested that the abnormal deposits in Bruch's membrane may impair normal metabolic exchange between the choriocapillaris and RPE, as in age-related maculopathy [78,355]. This hypothesis finds support in several laboratory and clinical observations. There is strong circumstantial evidence that diffusible substances produced by the RPE govern the behavior of the choroid [11,165,252]. Failure of these agents to diffuse toward the choroid may cause the choriocapillaris to change from a sinusoidal system to the tubular arrangement of most capillary beds [349], a process also associated with age-related change in Bruch's membrane [395,438]. The preservation of choroidal arterioles makes it unlikely that this is due to primary vascular disease, such as hypertension [154,155,313]. The diffusion barrier may also impair retinal function. Patients with age-related maculopathy, Sorsby's macular disease, and slow filling of the choroid on angiography may have severely depressed scotopic thresholds in the presence of good visual acuity [78,119,418,419,425,426]. The pattern of functional loss simulates very closely that seen in patients deficient in vitamin A [457], which would impair photopigment regeneration and with time cause progressive loss of outer segment mass as a consequence of increasing metabolic impairment [236]. The metabolic needs of the retina other than vitamin A might also be compromised.

Central Areolar Choroidal Sclerosis

A dominantly inherited dystrophy with well-defined atrophy of the outer retina RPE and inner choroid causing loss of central vision was described by Sorsby [409]. Initially, the choriocapillaris was thought to be primarily affected in this so-called central areolar choroidal atrophy [333,409,410] because atrophy of choroid at the macula was the most prominent ophthalmoscopic change when the patient was first seen. However, Ashton [23] demonstrated that the major choroidal blood vessels were normal in a case of central areolar choroidal sclerosis by histopathological examination, such that the target cell of disease was uncertain.

Recently, two mutations in the rds gene at codon 172 were identified as causing a macular dystrophy most closely resembling central areolar choroidal sclerosis [467]. In two families arginine replaces tryptophan, and in another family glutamine replaces the arginine. Each is associated with difficulty in passing from light to dark in the third decade of life, and RPE changes centered at the fovea that extend outside the posterior pole are identifiable by this time. Profound atrophy of the outer retina and inner choroid occurs during the next three decades at a variable rate. Peripheral rod function is normal. The diseases are qualitatively similar, but the mutations with the Arg-172-Trp substitution is more severe. This finding implies that the primary defect lies in the photoreceptor cell, at least in these families, and that losses of RPE and choriocapillaris are secondary phenomena.

Fundus Flavimaculatus (Stargardt's Disease)

This broad category comprises diseases in which white material is deposited at the level of the RPE. Fundus flavimaculatus [142,144] and Stargardt's disease [414,415] have been used to denote these disorders, but evidence that these two terms describe separate conditions is lacking. Most cases have autosomal recessive inheritance, although autosomal dominant forms have been described [81,441]. These conditions usually cause rapid loss of central vision during a 6 month period in the first 15 years of life, although in some cases good visual acuity is maintained until the age of 50 years.

At the time of visual loss confluent atrophy of the RPE and choriocapillaris occurs at the fovea, and this area grows slowly during the rest of the patient's life. The white "fishtail" flecks occupy the remaining part of the posterior pole, with characteristic sparing of the peripapillary region. These lesions can be identified at the time of the initial visual loss and resolve as additional lesions appear elsewhere [178].

On fluorescein angiography the choroid appears normal in some patients, but most lack background choroidal fluorescence [55,131,133]. It seems likely that the nonappearance of the choroid signifies an even deposition of abnormal material at the level of the RPE that absorbs blue-green light [441]. This conclusion has been supported by the detection in histopathological studies of RPE packed with lipofuscin and melanolipofuscin [117,133,247,284]; these changes start to develop in childhood [417]. At the site of previous white lesions, depigmentation of the RPE occurs and fluorescein angiography discloses multifocal hyperfluorescence, corresponding to the areas of pigment loss [178].

All patients have a significant abnormality of cone function on ERG, and many have abnormal rod function [322]. The EOG is initially normal but frequently becomes subnormal late in the disease [322,334].

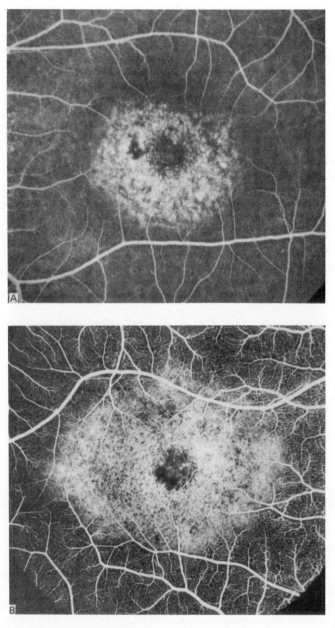

Figure 7   Fluorescein angiography in bull's-eye dystrophy may show retinal capillary dilation and a "dark choroid" (A), or the choroid and retinal capillaries may be normal (B).

Bull's-Eye Dystrophies (Including Cone and Cone-Rod Dystrophies)

The typical fundus changes in this group of cone and cone-rod dystrophies consist of one or more concentric rings of pigment epithelial change around the fovea that give rise to a characteristic appearance on fluorescein angiography. Visual loss may occur at any time during the second to the fifth decades of life and, once started, progresses slowly [173]. There may or may not be white deposits at the level of the RPE. A dark choroid is also seen in some families [131] (Fig. 7).

The heterogeneity of this group is indicated by the inheritance in different families, which may be autosomal dominant, autosomal recessive, or X linked. This group of disorders includes the progressive cone dystrophies, which usually present in adolescence or early adult life with reduced vision, photophobia, and defects of color vision that usually precede the macular changes. These macular changes result from atrophy of the RPE, giving rise to a bull's-eye appearance.

The cone dystrophies are currently classified by their mode of inheritance, which may be autosomal dominant [38,61,170,257,358,446,468], autosomal recessive [172,478], or X linked [194,222,376,445]. Even within these different genetic forms of cone dystrophy there is heterogeneity. The dominant cone dystrophies include a recently described form with early and nearly complete absence of blue cone function [61,446,468]. A family with X-linked cone dystrophy accompanied by loss of red cone function contains a 6.5 kb deletion within the red cone pigment gene [445].

Heterogeneity is further indicated by the presence of peripheral retinal degeneration in some cases, and these cone-rod dystrophies must be distinguished from cone dystrophies, in which rod function is normal as shown by electrophysiological tests. Many patients with each of the genetic forms of RP (rod-cone dystrophies) also have a bull's-eye appearance at the macula [371]. Drug-induced phenocopies occur [238,259], and comparable dystrophies have also been described in the Pierre-Marie type of hereditary ataxia [49], in fucosidosis [408], and in amelanogenesis imperfecta [225].

There is considerable doubt about whether the fundus changes of fundus flavimaculatus and bull's-eye dystrophy indicate that the disorders are clearly separated into two distinct groups. Studies of the fundus appearance show that in some families the changes are constant, but in others bull's-eye dystrophy may be seen in early disease whereas flavimaculatus lesions are seen later.

II. CONGENITAL PHOTORECEPTOR DEFECTS

A series of conditions is recognized in which there is a genetically determined nonprogressive visual defect that may be related to either the cone or the rod systems.

A. Cone Defects

Defective Color Vision

Defects in color vision have been classified on the basis of the concept that color vision is determined by three classes of cones: red sensitive, green sensitive, and blue sensitive. The basis for this classification has been confirmed by the sequencing of the three cone pigment genes [332]. If color-matching tests demonstrate that one of the three systems is defective but present (*trichromats*), the terms "protanomaly" (red), "deuteranomaly" (green), and "tritanomaly" (blue) are used. If one is functionally absent (*dichromats*), the suffix *anopia* replaces the suffix *anomaly*.

Deuteranomaly, deuteranopia, protanopia, and protanomaly are X-linked conditions: deuteranomaly is found in about 5% of the population of Western Europe and North America and deuteranopia, protanomaly, and protanopia in about 1% each [456]. Tritanomaly and tritanopia, which are inherited as autosomal dominant disorders, are much less common, affecting between 0.002 and 0.007% of the population [448].

Individuals with these abnormalities of color vision have normal visual acuity, and anomalous trichromats are often unaware of the condition. Apart from the color defect, the eye is normal.

The molecular genetic basis of the red and green color defects has now been demonstrated. Abnormalities of the red and green pigment genes occur to differing degrees in deuteranopia, deuteranomaly, protanopia, and protanomaly. People with deuteranopia have a normal red pigment gene but no green pigment gene(s). Those with protanopia lack a normal red pigment gene, which is replaced by a hybrid red-green pigment gene. Deuteranomalous and protanomalous trichromats had hybrid red-green genes [6,331,452].

Monochromatism.   Patients suffering from monochromatism have absent or markedly impaired color vision. In complete rod monochromatism there is little evidence of cone function, so that visual acuity is poor, color vision absent, the patient has nystagmus, and extreme photophobia is characteristic. No obvious abnormality of the fundus is apparent, although the foveola may appear abnormal and changes in the central RPE are sometimes identified [456]. The dark adaptation curve is typically monophasic, with elevated final threshold, fusion frequency is very low, and the photopic (cone) ERG is absent but the scotopic (rod) ERG is normal. Rod monochromatism is an autosomal recessive trait.

Blue cone monochromatism presents in a fashion similar to complete rod monochromatism, except that there appears to be an intact blue cone system and the inheritance is X linked [6]. The gene for this form of monochromatism has been mapped to the long arm of the X chromosome (Xq28), and it is possible that this rare disorder results from alterations of the red and green pigment genes or from their deletion [279].

An incomplete form of rod monochromatism has been described in which the symptoms are less severe, visual acuity is better, and photophobia and nystagmus may be absent [255,403,406]. In another form of monochromatism the central cones are absent [255].

Four eyes from individuals with monochromatism have been examined histopathologically [124,166, 183,269]. These showed a change at the fovea with a reduced number of cones and an abnormality of those that remained.

B. Rod Defects

Congenital Stationary Night Blindness

Congenital stationary night blindness (CSNB) is characterized by night blindness, a normal fundus appearance, the absence of rod dark adaptation (monophasic dark adaptation curve), and lack of progression. It may be inherited as an autosomal dominant, an autosomal recessive, or an X-linked trait.

The most widely reported form of CSNB is an autosomal dominant disorder [100]. These patients appear to have normal cone function but little rod function. Visual acuity, color vision, and photopic visual fields are normal or are at most mildly abnormal, and dark adaptation shows only a cone segment that may be abnormally prolonged [258]; there is no shift from cone to rod characteristics in the dark adaptation curve, and the ERG discloses no prolongation of the b wave implicit time between the photopic and scotopic records. However, fundus reflectometry indicated a normal concentration of bleachable rhodopsin in one case [74], and histological studies have shown no structural abnormalities either in the retina as a whole or in the rods in particular [444].

Most patients with autosomal recessive and X-linked CSNB and occasional patients with autosomal dominant CSNB have an ERG with a nearly normal a wave and a substantially reduced b wave on testing under scotopic conditions (negative ERG) [336,400]. With increasing intensity of the test stimulus the amplitude of the a wave increases but that of the b wave is unchanged [398]. These patients can be further divided into two groups: one group lacks rod function (complete type), and the other has some rod function (incomplete type) [317]. Patients with the complete type are myopic; those with the incomplete type may be hyperopic or myopic [243]. Although complete and incomplete CSNB did not coexist in any of the families reported by Miyake and colleagues [317], others have found patients with both complete and incomplete CSNB within the same X-linked pedigrees [243,356]. This led Pearce and others [356] to propose that X-linked CSNB is a single clinical entity manifesting a wide variation in clinical expression. It has also been suggested that incomplete CSNB and Åland Island eye disease may be the same condition [5,465].

Myopia is almost always associated with the X-linked form of CSNB in which visual acuity is reduced and nystagmus may be present. Carriers of X-linked CSNB do not suffer from night blindness but may manifest abnormal oscillatory potentials on ERG [316,482]. Myopia also occurs in those cases of autosomal recessive CSNB who have abnormal vision, and again, these patients may have nystagmus [466]. These forms of CSNB may present in infancy with apparent blindness [466].

The complete form of X-linked CSNB has been assigned to the Xp11.3 [158,329] or Xp11.22 [32] region of the short arm of the X chromosome.

Light and electron microscopic studies of one eye with CSNB and a negative ERG showed a normal arrangement of disks of rod outer segments and normal synaptic ends of the photoreceptors. The cause in this case of CSNB may be related to mechanisms inhibitory to cells of the bipolar layer [459]. The absence of rod-cone interaction, together with an absent scotopic b wave, also implies that the defect is in the midretinal layers [404].

Prolonged Dark Adaptation

Three distinct conditions have been described in which the final threshold of dark adaptation is normal but the rod phase is abnormally prolonged; the defect in each appears to be static.

Oguchi's Disease. An autosomal recessively inherited disorder with prolonged dark adaptation was first reported in Japan in 1907 by Oguchi [347], and most subsequent reported cases have come from the same country, although non-Japanese patients have been described [246,475]. In most patients defective night vision is the only complaint, visual acuity being normal. The characteristic feature of this condition is the abnormal coloration of the light-adapted fundus, the abnormal white or cream-colored appearance being derived from the inner limiting membrane and, presumably, from the foot plates of Müller cells. The abnormal color resolves over a period of 30 minutes to 8 h in darkness and has been termed the Mizuo-Nakamura phenomenon after the authors who initially described it [319,330]. A similar phenomenon has been described in X-linked cone dystrophy [194] and X-linked retinoschisis [102]. Dark adaptation is characteristically slow, and a final rod threshold may be attained only after several hours and even then may be slightly elevated [151].

Histopathological examination has been undertaken on three eyes with prolonged dark adaptation. An excess of cones compared with rods, together with an abnormal layer of material between the photo-receptors and the RPE, was reported by Oguchi [348]. Parallel histological studies on the other half of the same eye by another investigator [479] failed to confirm this additional layer. An abundance of round lipofuscin granules confined to the apical portion of the RPE was then regarded as a characteristic feature. A light and electron microscopic study of another eye [264] was claimed to show an abnormal layer between the outer segments of the photoreceptors and the RPE. The constituents were normal components of the retina, however, consisting of lipofuscin granules and protrusions of the RPE with complex interdigitations of the outer segments. There was no abnormal cone distribution. Another histological study [480] is open to question because the patient had reduced vision with a pigmentary retinopathy and both parents had RP. On electrophysiological testing, both the a wave of the ERG and the light rise in the standing potential of the eye are normal, but the scotopic b wave of the ERG is severely depressed even in the fully dark-adapted eye [74].

The pathogenesis of Oguchi's disease is not understood. Rhodopsin regeneration is normal [73,74]. These observations imply that the primary abnormality is unrelated to light catch and rhodopsin bleaching but is related to other systems of visual transduction. Electrophysiological observations indicate that the region of bipolar cells appears to be the earliest stage in the visual pathway exhibiting signs of defective function. Because the abnormal reflex arises from the inner limiting membrane, at which site the major cellular component is the foot plate of Müller cells, and that Müller cells are the source of the b wave, it is likely that these cells are primarily at fault, as suggested by de Jong and colleagues [102]. Unfortunately, the histopathological studies did not report on the state of Müller cells.

Fundus Albipunctatus Fundus albipunctatus is a static autosomal recessive condition in which the only symptoms are related to defective dark adaptation [270]. The condition should not be confused with the progressive albipunctate dystrophy (retinitis punctata albescens) that represents a variant of RP.

Uniformly sized, almost white dots at the level of the RPE are distributed throughout the fundus but are most dense in the postequatorial region; the macula may or may not be involved. Changes in the distribution of the white dots have been described [299], as have their change from flecks in childhood to relatively permanent punctate dots that become more numerous over years [300]. Diffuse pigmentary alterations in the RPE are unusual. Fluorescein angiography shows punctate hyperfluorescence that does not correspond, however, with the punctate white dots [159]. Although fundus albipunctatus usually involves both eyes, unilateral disease has been reported [197].

Typically, the visual acuity and visual fields are normal, but minor loss of visual fields has been described [299]. In most cases the dark adaptation of both cones and rods is markedly prolonged [74,258,298,299,400], and the acquisition of scotopic ERG thresholds is delayed [258,298,299,407]. Variation from this pattern has been described in which the dark adaptation and the ERG are normal [143,152] or dark adaptation discloses a cone segment only [295]. It is not clear whether this variation implies various degrees of severity of a single disease or several disorders share this fundus abnormality.

Studies of rhodopsin kinetics show slow rhodopsin regeneration that parallel dark adaptation [74]. This implies that, by contrast with Oguchi's disease, the sensory defect in fundus albipunctatus is due to abnormal photopigment kinetics.

Fleck Retina of Kandori

A rare condition in which a prolonged dark adaptation gives rise to difficulty with night vision but no other symptoms has been described only in Japan [233]. Dark adaptation shows a prolonged rod phase, reaching normal thresholds within 40 minutes in this entity, known as the fleck retina of Kandori. The fundus presents large, irregular white lesions at the level of the RPE that are most concentrated in the equatorial region. The photopic ERG is normal, and a prolonged interval of dark adaptation is needed to reach scotopic potentials.

III. PATHOGENESIS OF PHOTORECEPTOR DYSTROPHIES

A. General Considerations

Hereditary disorders are caused by defects in the genetic code, which in turn result in an abnormal amino acid composition of specific proteins. If the defective protein encoded by a gene is confined to a single cell type, the primary effect of the mutation is localized in that cell type, even though secondary effects may occur in other cells. For example, the mutation may either reside in the photoreceptor cell, giving rise to the observed degeneration, or it may be expressed in a support tissue, leading to the same consequences. Alternatively, a systemic metabolic abnormality may result in the degeneration of a specific cell type, such as visual cells, by depriving them of vital metabolites.

In recent years there have been considerable advances in the understanding of the micrometabolism of retinal cells, particularly with regard to the interactions between the photoreceptor cells and the RPE [343]. However, perhaps the most significant finding pertinent to the cause and pathogenesis of the receptor dystrophies is that the light-sensitive disk membranes in the outer segments of the photoreceptor cells are constantly being renewed throughout life [485,486,488]. This process involves multiple steps, each of which may require specific proteins and enzyme systems. Because each of these processes must be integrated with the next, abundant opportunities exist for defects in the genetic code to disturb renewal mechanisms and lead to cell abnormalities or death (Fig. 8).

That a defect in cell support systems may cause retinal dystrophies is not a new concept, but recent work has served to identify some of the specific metabolic attributes of photoreceptor cells that may be involved in the pathogenesis of these disorders.

During photoreceptor maintenance, blood-borne metabolites within the choriocapillaris are free to diffuse out of the vessel lumen through fenestrations in the endothelial lining. They pass through Bruch's membrane and into the extracellular spaces both beneath and between the RPE. Free diffusion into the neural retina is prevented by junctional complexes, zonulae occludentes, which occur between the apical portion of the lateral membranes of adjacent RPE. These junctions constitute a blood-retina barrier [366]. In contrast, the basal membranes of the RPE are highly convoluted and contain specific receptors [54,195] that enable metabolites to accumulate actively within the cell [267]. Inside the cell, those molecules required by the photoreceptor cells are transported by special intracellular carrier proteins [52,196, 390,469] to the apical surfaces. It seems that rapid transport could be achieved by transfer from these sheaths directly into the outer segments, but autoradiographic evidence from animals shows that metabolites actively accumulate in the inner segments of the photoreceptor cells following diffusion through the interphotoreceptor matrix [344,386]. Uptake by the photoreceptor also requires the presence of specific receptor sites.

The necessary molecular moieties accumulate within the inner segments of the photoreceptor cells and are then utilized in the metabolic processes essential for both cellular renewal and integrity [490]. After synthesis, the proteins, glycoproteins, and phospholipids begin to move to various cellular locations. A considerable portion of the protein, much of it now complexed with carbohydrate and possibly lipid, moves through the cilium to reach the photoreceptor outer segments [484]. At this point the renewal systems in rods and cones differ strikingly. In rods the newly formed proteins are incorporated into small membranous outgrowths in the outer segment portion of the cilium. By a complex mechanism of membrane fusion and migration, these outgrowths are eventually incorporated into the rod outer segments and form the hollow, coinlike disk membranes. Each disk is a discrete structure, isolated from both its neighbors and the boundary membrane of the rod. With successive disk production, units are progressively displaced toward the RPE. In monkeys the outer segment transit time for a disk is 9–13 days [487], and because each rod contains approximately 1000 disks, between 30 and 100 new disks are made each day. In normal eyes there

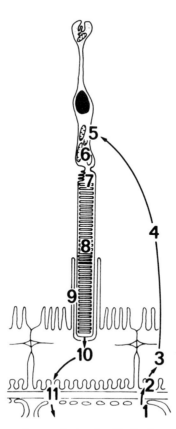

Figure 8   Diagram of the mechanisms that may be involved in the degeneration of photoreceptor cells: (1) uptake or transport defect, (2) abnormal membrane receptor sites (retinal pigment epithelium), (3) transepithelial transport defect, (4) epithelial to photoreceptor donor defect, (5) abnormal sites (photoreceptor cell), (6) micro-metabolism malfunctions, (7) faulty membranogenesis, (8) inability to stabilize membranes, (9) malfunction in phagocytosis, (10) malfunction in lysis, and (11) inability to void lytic products. For a detailed explanation, see the text.

is a high degree of membrane stability in the disks, and no structural differences can be detected between new and old structures. To prevent large fluctuations in rod length, old disks are lost from the tips of the outer segment by the phagocytic action of the RPE [304] (Fig. 9). This process seems to be initiated by the onset of light [29,271] but may also be mediated by hormones because a diurnal rhythm of disk shedding is exhibited even in prolonged periods of darkness [271,345]. The exact mechanism whereby rod disks are shed is subject to debate, some workers believing that there is active ingression of the RPE sheath into the tips of the rod cells [413] and others suggesting a passive role for the RPE in response to an active shedding of spent disks by the rods [487]. Whatever the mechanism, phagocytosis of the disks is dependent upon triggering of membrane recognition sites within the apical membrane of the RPE [98,205,208,375].

Experimental studies of cones are more difficult to interpret because the light-sensitive membranes in the cone outer segments do not form discrete disks but constitute a continuum [83]. Thus, as newly formed proteins are free to diffuse to any part of the cone outer segment membrane, radioactive tracer studies on cones express a random and diffuse distribution of the label [366]. Nevertheless, there is increasing morphological evidence of cone renewal [29,416,489], with cone shedding at night. It seems, however, from studies of cone function after detachment surgery [139] and of cone morphology during aging [306] that the capacity for membrane replacement in cones is less well developed than that in rods.

Once inside the RPE, the group of disks, engulfed in phagosomes, undergoes lysis, which results in their progressive degradation [221,303,307]. Some of the breakdown products of this process may be

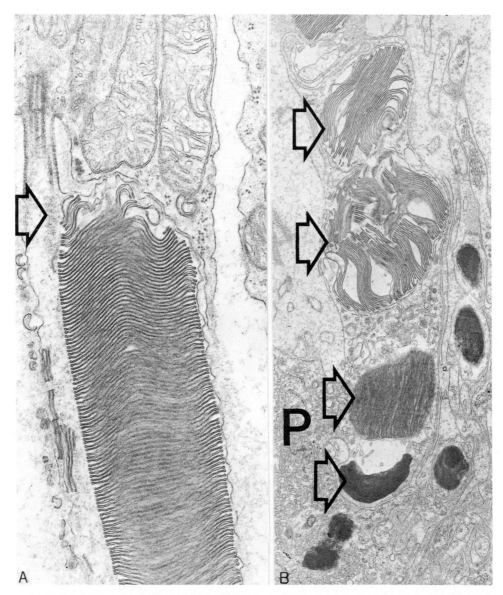

Figure 9   Electron micrographs of the junctions between the inner and outer segments of a rod cell (A) and the rod cell and the pigment epithelium (B) from a normal human retina. Newly formed "disk" membranes can be seen (arrows) adjacent to the cilium, while multiple phagosomes can be seen entering the pigment epithelium (P). (A, ×39,000; B, ×15,000).

recycled back to the photoreceptor cells, but others are voided into the choriocapillaris via Bruch's membrane.

The lipofuscin granules seen within the RPE cells of the elderly [130,422] have been attributed to the retention of incompletely degraded remnants of phagocytosed photoreceptor outer segments [203,221]. They are comparable to the lipofuscin granules described in many other parts of the body, such as the central nervous system and the myocardium, which are considered the oxidized and polymerized residues of inadequate lysosomal hydrolysis [162]. In nonocular tissues the evidence suggests that they originate from the catabolism of mitochondria and various forms of intracellular lipid [437]. In ocular tissues, the spectral properties of the pigment granules imply that they arise from an interaction of light with vitamin A [120,121]. The presence of oxygen and light in the vicinity of high concentrations of unsaturated fatty acids of disk membranes may lead to peroxidative attack, leading to cross-linking and formation of proteolipid aggregates. These products do not form good degradative substrates for the normal lysosomal enzymes of the RPE, and their accumulation complexed with vitamin A accounts for the changes seen. However, the retina contains a protective mechanism against peroxidation [361–365]. Since lipofuscin is not extruded from the cell but slowly accumulates with the passing years, it is most prominent in the tissues of older individuals. In the context of the RPE, the heavy demands on lysosomal activity caused by the need to dispose of engulfed photoreceptor material increase the predisposition to lipofuscin formation. In the RPE, the situation is complicated by the presence of melanin, which, although apparently exposed to lysosomal enzymes [278], appears to be little affected by them [302]. In some instances, particles of melanin pigment and lipofuscin granules occur in the same organelle [30]. In consequence, several terms describe the various types of residual body seen in the RPE [8]:

1. *Lipofuscin granules* are golden brown autofluorescent residues of incomplete lysosomal hydrolysis of phagocytosed and endogenous lipid.
2. *Melanolysosomes* are formed by the fusion of melanosomes with primary lysosomes.
3. *Melanolipofuscin* presents as melanin with a surrounding rim of lipofuscin and represents a residual body formed by the fusion of the partially degraded products of a melanolysosome with one or more lipofuscin granules.

In a number of conditions involving degeneration of visual cells, it is now possible to identify specific malfunctions in the maintenance cycle. Although numerous mutations are now recognized in rhodopsin in patients with adRP, clues to the underlying biochemical events that lead ultimately to photoreceptor cell death remain obscure.

B. Systemic Disorders and Environmental Factors in Retinal Dystrophies

Systemic disorders may result in a secondary degeneration of visual cells. The efficient transfer of essential metabolites requires the presence of normal concentrations in plasma, together with their appropriate carriers, transporters in the epithelial processes, carrier proteins in the interphotoreceptor matrix, and receptors in the final target tissue. Even mild alterations in these parameters could be detrimental to an already stressed cell. However, there is little experimental evidence that a deficit in the supply of metabolites is responsible for visual cell loss, although the isolation of the photoreceptor cells from their metabolic input is presumed to be fundamental to the degenerative changes seen in retinal detachment [139]. Investigations of receptor sites in the basal membranes of RPE in animals with inherited retinal dystrophies indicate that such sites are similar to those of unaffected animals [195]. Little is known of mechanisms of transepithelial transport [52,390,469], but a failure in this system may give rise in part to the photoreceptor degeneration of Refsum disease (see Chap. 37). This is an autosomal recessive disease in which there is absence or deficiency of the enzyme that oxidizes phytanic acid, so that abnormally high levels of this substrate build up in the blood [30]. Phytanic acid is similar to palmitic acid (branched); furthermore, experimental studies have shown that rod outersegment renewal systems become disorganized if fatty acids (polyunsaturated) are withheld from the diet [8] (but see Anderson [7]). In Refsum disease the earliest symptom is night blindness, and this is followed by other symptoms reminiscent of RP [148]. Receptor degeneration is associated with lipid deposits rich in phytanic acid within the RPE [97,431]. Such findings may be interpreted as indicating either a failure in the transepithelial transport of fatty acids or a limited ability to degrade phagocytosed particles of rod outer segments containing abnormal lipid components.

The metabolism of vitamin A, taurine, and plasma lipids has been intensely studied with reference to RP. Vitamin A deficiency induced in animals has been compared with the disease process in certain forms of RP. The important role of taurine in photoreceptor maintenance was established following the discovery that cats fed diets free of taurine developed retinal degeneration. Photoreceptor outer segments contain a high concentration of polyunsaturated fatty acids, and a disturbance of the delivery system is expected to compromise severely the processes of cellular renewal. The potential value of these studies to the understanding of possible pathological mechanisms in RP is not established. In the past, that environmental factors cause retinal degeneration was assumed to provide important clues concerning the pathogenesis of inherited disease. A large body of investigative work has been driven by this concept, but little of it has been fruitful to date. There has also been a tendency to draw conclusions concerning RP as a whole from data from a limited number of observations. Since RP is comprised of many different disorders, data from one patient may be relevant only to individuals with the same disease but not to others. This is not to deny the potential value of these observations, but each conclusion must be treated with caution when generalizations are made.

Vitamin A

After release from opsin, all-*trans*-retinal is reduced to all-*trans*-retinol by a retinal reductase within the photoreceptor cell (see also Chap. 38) [220]. It is then transported to the RPE for storage in an esterified form. The retinoid is isomerized to the 11-cis form before transportation to the outer segment [27,34]. Interstitial retinol binding protein is synthesized by the photoreceptor cell and transported into the interphotoreceptor matrix to facilitate the intertissue transportation of retinoids [206]. Intracellular retinaldehyde binding proteins have also been identified [93]. Similarly, the transport of retinol from liver storage compartments occurs via a plasma retinol binding protein. There are therefore many possible targets for the disruption of the visual cycle. Many attempts have been made to correlate disturbances in the vitamin A cycle with various disease processes in RP. Certainly, a deficiency of vitamin A leads to photoreceptor degeneration in animals [188]. The presence of light is essential for the lethal effects since animals reared in the dark show fairly normal outer segment structure [339].

The similarities of symptoms in vitamin A deficiency and the RP group of diseases has led to extensive investigations of vitamin A levels in the blood of the latter, with a profusion of claims and counterclaims in the literature. No convincing relationships have been discovered [67,253], however, and no beneficial results have been obtained by administering this vitamin to RP sufferers [33,77,275,328].

A deficiency or abnormality in the plasma retinol binding protein itself has also been ruled out in some forms of RP [62,191,297]. Reductions in RPE 11-*cis*-retinol content and interphotoreceptor retinoid binding protein in the interphotoreceptor matrix have been reported in some donated eyes of RP sufferers, but these are most likely to reflect secondary changes due to photoreceptor loss [62,385].

The most persuasive evidence against vitamin A deficiency as a cause of RP is derived from the work of Ripps and colleagues [383], who demonstrated that the rhodopsin concentration in the rods differed markedly between a limited number of patients with RP and one patient with vitamin A deficiency. These findings imply that investigation of vitamin A metabolism is unlikely to reveal an abnormality in a patient with RP unless it can be demonstrated that rod sensitivity is reduced below that of cones with a small reduction in rhodopsin concentration only. Similarly, Kemp and colleagues [240,241] have shown markedly different effects of vitamin A deficiency and RP on visual parameters, such as dark adaptation and rhodopsin regeneration following a bleach.

Nevertheless, caution should be exercised when investigating 11-*cis*-retinal interactions with the mutant forms of opsin in patients with autosomal dominant RP.

Taurine

The relative contribution of a taurine deficiency in the pathogenetic mechanisms remains unsettled (see also Chap. 31). Taurine is the largest amino acid pool in photoreceptors, and in vitro experiments have shown its protective actions against light damage [353]. In cats a dietary deficiency of this amino acid leads to photoreceptor degeneration [189]. Although other mammalian species are more resistent to dietary manipulations, an induced deficiency using the taurine analog guanidinium ethane sulfonic acid leads to photoreceptor damage [266]. In the human, also, under pathological conditions of total parenteral nutrition in children and intestinal bacterial overgrowth in adults, a generalized deficiency is induced and is accompanied by disturbances in visual function [161,402].

In RP, an assessment of a possible taurine deficiency would require investigation of plasma levels, integrity of taurine carriers in the RPE and retina, and an estimation of retinal levels before the onset of photoreceptor loss. Plasma levels have not been found to be reduced in any type of RP [215]. The transport properties of carriers in the retina and RPE have not been undertaken, but some work on peripheral carriers has been performed. The transport of taurine by platelets (in autologous plasma) from patients with R-type autosomal dominant and X-hemizygotic disease was indeed reduced [450]. The consequences for transport across the blood-retina barrier has not been addressed.

Lipids

Photoreceptor membranes contain a high level of polyunsaturated fatty acids (PUFA), among which docosohexanoic acid constitutes about 50% [31,138]. The high levels of PUFA in the phospholipid moiety of disk membranes leads to increased fluidity and rapid diffusion pathways for intrinsic proteins. This facilitates conformational change, and photoexcited rhodopsin can interact quickly with many transducin molecules, thereby increasing the amplification factor for subsequent visual transduction. There is an inner lipid transport loop between the photoreceptor cell and the RPE for recycling of shed outer segment material, which may explain the resistance to depletion following dietary deficiencies. Reduced levels of plasma docosohexanoic and arachidonic acids and hypercholesterolemia and an increase in low-density lipoproteins have been noted in some forms of RP [9,31,89,90,138,224,451]. However, the relevance of these mild changes in lipid composition to the pathogenesis of RP is not clear.

A systemic defect resulting in degeneration of visual cells is seen in Bassen-Kornzweig syndrome, a condition in which the primary defect seems to interfere with the synthesis of the protein component of serum lipoproteins in the liver (see Chap. 35). Because these serum lipoproteins normally transport lipids through the blood, plasma lipid fractions, including vitamin A, are markedly reduced in this disease. Visual cell degeneration probably ensues as a result of a derangement in the renewal of lipids in the disk membranes or of vitamin A deficiency [171]. It has been shown that the degeneration can be halted by diet and supplementation with vitamins A and E.

Light Damage

Even in cells with a normal metabolic support mechanism, the light-sensitive membranes contained within the visual cell outer segments may be induced to undergo degenerative changes by relatively mild changes in their environment. Thus the continuous exposure of animals to environmental levels of light leads to photoreceptor degeneration [268,340,362,399]. The rate of degeneration can be altered by changing either the duration of the light exposure or the level of illuminance. Similar results are obtained with intermittent exposures to high-intensity light, although the primary lesion may reside in different tissue compartments.

A dietary deficiency of vitamin A reduced the damaging effects of light exposure [338,339]. Similarly, it was demonstrated that if dystrophic rats (Royal College of Surgeons, RCS, strain) are deprived of light, the rate of degeneration is retarded [112,483] and that a similar decrease in degeneration occurs if the animals are deprived of vitamin A [199,200]. These findings have resulted in the suggestion that RP sufferers should occlude one eye in the hope that such light deprivation would extend their visual life [35]. Cones are more sensitive to light-induced damage than rods [184,308,412,440], however, and this sensitivity may not represent a different threshold for damage but may be related to differences in membrane replacement mechanisms [305]. Rods have an incremental repair system, making 10–100 disks per day, so that if some of their outer segments are damaged by phototoxic substances, they can rapidly resynthesize and replace damaged membranes by disk replacement. The confluent nature of cone membranes means that the entire unit must be replaced if it is damaged. This difference may also explain the differences in aging of the two types of photoreceptor cells: it has been observed that after the fifth decade, degenerative changes are increasingly apparent in the outer segments of cone cells [262,306]. Perhaps there is a synergistic relationship between the light history of an eye and aging processes; if so, a limited light input to the eyes of sufferers of retinal dystrophies can only be beneficial.

The mechanisms of light damage are only now emerging. When albino rats were exposed to light of differing wavelengths at constant photon fluxes, the degree of damage as a function of wavelength was analogous to the action spectrum of rhodopsin [471]. The results suggest that rhodopsin is the primary instigator of light damage under the luminance used. It was shown that free radicals are produced as by-products following bleaching of rhodopsin, which interact with molecular oxygen to produce oxygen radicals, such as the superoxide ion. Oxygen radicals are very active and lead to peroxidation of the unsaturated fatty acids present in the disk membrane [180,439]. Thus a decrease in docosohexanoic acid and an increase in lipid peroxides is observed following light injury [351]. The consequences are membrane vesiculation and, depending on the degree of damage, eventual cell death.

The photoreceptors possess several protective mechanisms to counteract light damage. Vitamin E is the principal scavenger of free radicals and serves to terminate the propagating chain reactions induced by the formation of free radicals. A deficiency of vitamin E leads to photoreceptor degeneration, although the levels of this protectant are not reduced in light-damaged retinas [237]. Vitamin C can accept electrons from vitamin E to set up a cycle for the regeneration of "spent" vitamin E. Taurine is present in photo-receptors at very high concentrations and functions as a stabilizer of membranes. It is not clear whether taurine also acts as a scavenger of free radicals or protects against the consequences of membrane damage. In taurine deficiency, the threshold for light damage is greatly reduced [374]. Other protective systems against peroxidation in the retina-RPE complex include glutathione peroxidase, catalase, and superoxide dismutase [180].

It also appears that the photoreceptor cells change in structure and protective mechanisms with variations in light exposure [360a–365]. In rats brought up in low light levels, the outer segments contain high quantities of long-chain unsaturated fatty acids in the outer segments, and the levels of free radical scavenging systems are low. These animals show considerable damage when exposed to even moderate lighting. By contrast, rats brought up in high lighting levels have largely unsaturated fatty acids in the outer segments that are relatively resistant to photic injury, and the levels of free radical scavengers are high.

Two aspects of light damage are worth considering in relation to RP. First, there appears to be a good spatial correlation between the funduscopic areas receiving the greatest amounts of light and the severity of pigmentary changes in the major classes of RP. Second is the observation that in normal retinas, intense light exposure damages the rhodopsin molecule, preventing regeneration [96]. This may arise from conformational changes induced by covalent modifications of the chains or formation of aberrant disulfide bridges or by damage to the intrinsic lipids linked to the molecule. Visual contribution is then dependent on the formation of new disks. Some of the rhodopsin mutations in autosomal dominant patients may increase the susceptibility of these molecules to light damage.

C. Animal Models of Retinal Degeneration

Much of our knowledge regarding the disturbance of the maintenance cycle of the photoreceptors is derived from studies of animals with inherited retinal dystrophies, particularly the rd and rds mice. These animal models provide the opportunity to study the temporal basis of genetically induced biochemical lesions and simultaneously target appropriate sites for future therapeutic intervention. The introduction of mutant human genes into steps between the expression of the abnormal rhodopsin and the ensuing death of the cell. An analogous situation exists with the peripherin defects, but the investigation of the rds mouse model (carrying a similar peripherin defect) should prove highly informative regarding the mechanism of degeneration.

rds Mouse

A mutation in the peripherin molecule was first documented in an animal model, namely the "retinal degeneration slow" (rds) mouse [391]. Mice homozygous for the defect do not form an outer segment but nevertheless produce an ERG signal [378]. Presumably, a form of the transduction machinery is housed within the inner segment. Peripherin is normally found localized to the outer segment disks and is presumed to stabilize the structure during both morphogenesis and subsequent maintenance. It may also participate in holding the disk against the outer plasma membrane [321]. Mice heterozygous for the peripherin defect produce an outer segment, albeit abnormal, but some cellular loss occurs over a period of 12–18 months. The mechanism of cell death is not known, although it is possible that unstable disks severely disturb the sequestration of key cytoplasmic components, for example calcium. Further studies are underway to elucidate the underlying abnormalities.

Mutations in Phosphodiesterase

Phosphodiesterase is a tetrameric protein complex. The α (molecular weight 88 kD) and β (molecular weight 84 kD) subunits contain the catalytic and noncatalytic cGMP binding sites [24,164,481], and the γ subunit interacts to provide an inhibitory constraint on enzymic activity. Following light stimulation and activation of transducin, the GTP-T-α of transducin dissociates and interacts with the γ-inhibitory subunit of PDE, thereby activating the hydrolysis of cGMP [104]. The physiological role of the noncatalytic binding sites is not clear. It is thought that these sites act as cGMP "sensors." A reduction in cGMP, for example during continuous background illumination, is therefore sensed by the PDE, and this information may regulate the GTP lifetime on GTP-α transducin. Shortening of lifetime hydrolyzes GTP and inhibits the PDE. These changes are important for the processes of light adaptation [22]. The ensuing reduction in cGMP following PDE activation closes the cGMP-dependent conductance of outer segments, leading to the initial hyperpolarization phase of the ERG [481].

Disturbances in cyclic nucleotide metabolism have been reported in both animal models of inherited retinal degeneration (rd mouse, Rdy kitten, and Irish setter) and in a donor retina of a patient with adRP [1,125,126,214]. The mechanism of cell death is not known, but it has been shown that exposure of both developing animal and mature human cells to high levels of cGMP are detrimental to photoreceptor survival [283,442,470]. Defective PDE activity leads to an accumulation of total and free cGMP. Increased cGMP binds to and opens the cGMP-gated ionic conductance in the outer segment membrane, which leads to an increase in the inflow of sodium and calcium down an electrochemical gradient. The cell is therefore committed to a metabolic stress from which it may never recover.

In the rd mouse, a mutation has been identified in the gene for the β portion of phosphodiesterase [58]. The insertion of both a virallike sequence and a stop codon has been identified consistently [57,367]. The position of the mutation is such that the catalytic subunit is lost, and hence a defective enzyme is produced that leads to the ensuing toxic accumulation of cGMP [337]. The rd mouse also presents an interesting anomaly in that despite the absence of a functional PDE-β unit and the presence of elevated levels of cGMP, the developing photoreceptor produces a good ERG response. It is possible that the PDE-α unit has some functional activity so that it can respond to light stimulation but that the regulation of basal levels is disturbed.

If the lethal insult is due to an increased metabolic work load against the incessant entry of ions through the cGMP-gated channel, then a possible therapeutic regimen would be to block this channel. Preliminary experiments with the specific channel blocker 1-*cis*-diltiazem using a perfused cat eye preparation were unsuccessful [352]. These authors used isobutylmethylxanthine to elevate the level of cGMP, but this compound also interferes with both protein synthesis and the noncatalytic binding sites on the PDE molecule [481]. More appropriate would be to monitor directly the dark current with suction electrodes using perhaps the isolated photoreceptor from rd/rd retinas and then assess the effects of 1-*cis*-diltiazem under a defined pathological situation.

The persistence of high levels of cGMP in the donor eye of the adRP patient discussed earlier is also puzzling. However, it is becoming increasingly apparent that major species differences exist in the differential toxicity of this compound [216].

D.   Functional Consequences of Mutations

Many questions are amenable to investigation. In adRP the abnormality is produced in the heterozygous state. It is not known whether the disease is due to the product of the abnormal gene or to a shortage of the product from the normal gene; both mechanisms may be exist. That mice transfected with a mutant rhodopsin gene develop retinal degeneration is evidence for the first mechanism. The second possibility is illustrated in the rds mouse [87,433], in which transgenic rescue has been achieved by insertion of a normal peripherin gene on a rhodopsin promotor [435]. Retinal changes in the heterozygous rds mouse are compatible with this concept [186]. The relevance of this model to human disease is illustrated by the finding of mutations on the peripherin gene in adRP [127,128,231,467].

Rhodopsin

Rhodopsin is an intrinsic protein of rod disk membranes, and its activation by light to the photoexcited form R* is the first step in the enzymatic amplification cascade of vertebrate phototransduction. Thus specific functional and structural domains are inherent in the three-dimensional topography of the molecule to enable (1) effective quantum capture and (2) appropriate energy transfer kinetics and pathways for conformational alterations, thereby leading to (3) the unmasking of receptor sites for information transfer to cytoplasmic proteins. More generalized considerations include appropriate folding and incorporation into membranes during synthesis and stabilization on transfer to the disk membrane.

The basic membrane topography of the rhodopsin molecule is known, but details of structural reorganization during photostimulation and understanding of the consequent alterations in receptor sites are rudimentary. Therefore it is not possible to predict at present the subtle alterations in function that should be induced by a mutational change in amino acid residues. Generalizations can be made, however. The rhodopsin molecule consists of 348 amino acid residues with two asparagine-linked oligosaccharide side chains. Peptide folding results in seven α helices being embedded in the disk bilayer with interconnecting hydrophilic segments protruding from the membranous surface [2,13,99,181,182,314,388]. A lysine residue (position 296) situated at the midpoint of the seventh helix is the attachment site for the 11-*cis*-retinal chromophore. 11-*cis*-retinal also interacts with the other helixes, and since all seven are aligned in a plane perpendicular to the disk surface, they effectively form a cage around the chromophore [210, 232,388]. Photon absorption by 11-*cis*-retinal causes isomerization of the chromophore to the all-trans form with simultaneous rearrangement of the helices. This conformational change in rhodopsin exposes a binding site for the G protein, transducin, on the cytoplasmic surface (residues 231–252) [249]. This is the first step in signal amplification and activation of the enzymatic cascade leading to visual transduction [291]. On the cytoplasmic surface, the carboxyl terminus contains many serines and threonines, which on formation of R* are phosphorylated by a rhodopsin kinase. The ensuing binding of arrestin to phosphory-lated rhodopsin blocks the further activation of transducin, which is one of the termination steps in visual transduction. Also important for the structural stability of rhodopsin are the two highly conserved cysteines on the intradiskal surface [13].

In excess of 40 specific rhodopsin mutations have now been documented in adRP [114–116,218, 239,293,401,423]. We cannot as yet predict how a specific mutation might alter the dynamic stability of the resting molecule or its effects on cytoplasmic interactions of photoexcited rhodopsin. Nevertheless, certain generalizations are legitimate. Mutations in the hydrophobic regions or near the oligosaccharide attach-ment sites may interfere with initial folding and glycosylation to disturb membrane incorporation of the newly synthesized protein severely. Thus it is expected that newly formed rhodopsin accumulates in the inner segment.

In families with adRP showing mutations in the rhodopsin gene, different patterns of retinal dysfunc-tion have been demonstrated with the various mutations [134,135,193,223,242,323,424]. In three muta-tions, proline to leucine at codon 347, lysine to glutamic acid at codon 296 (which is the binding site for retinal), and an isoleucine deletion at codon 255 or 256, functional loss compatible with diffuse (type I) adRP was identified. With all three mutations poor night vision was consistently identified in early life, and rod ERG were severely reduced or unmeasurable. In those with measurable visual function, psychophysi-cal testing showed rod function to be severely affected throughout the retina (with threshold elevations of more than 3 log units), even in younger individuals, but loss of cone function varied widely between families and was less widespread and less severe than loss of rod function. In the most severely affected family (Lys-296-Glu) there was little visual function after the age of 30 years in most members [239]. With the isoleucine deletion at codon 256, cone function was limited to the central 10° by the age of 25 years, but little further loss occurred thereafter. Cone function was retained over most of the visual field until middle life in the 347 mutation despite widespread and severe early loss of rod function.

The functional abnormality in families with mutations Thr-17-Arg, Pro-23-His, Thr-58-Arg, Gly-106-Arg, and Gua-182-Ade is qualitatively similar, with altitudinal distribution of disease, and this attribute appears to be constant within the families [134,135,223,242,323,381,420]. These characteristics are in marked contrast with those seen in patients with other rhodopsin mutations. Rod sensitivity is severely depressed in the superior field but is nearly normal in the inferior field. Loss of cone sensitivity closely follows that of the rods. In this respect the pattern of disease resembles regional (type II) RP. An addi-tional striking finding in these families with sectorial RP is a characteristic abnormality in one compo-nent of the kinetics of dark adaptation following exposure to a bright light. Before bleaching, measure-ments made in the relatively intact portion of the visual field show mild threshold elevations of approximately 1 log unit. Following light adaptation there is a marked delay in the recovery of sensitivity. The initial portion of recovery mediated by cones and rods is normal. By 1 h, however, when in normal subjects the recovery of sensitivity is complete, these patients showed residual threshold elevations of 1–2 log units from the prebleach values. Even after nearly 2 h thresholds are still elevated by more than 1.0 log unit. In two subjects it was found that the time course of this slow recovery of sensitivity was of the order at least 80–120 [323]. Using a model based upon primate data of rod outer segment length and turnover, it has been calculated that the delayed phase of the recovery of rod sensitivity following strong light adaptation could be due in part to the formation of new disk membranes with a normal concentration of rhodopsin rather than in situ regeneration of photopigment [323]. The model requires that the outer segments are short as a result of RP and that a major portion of the outer segment is shed following strong light adaptation.

These observations show that there are both quantitative and qualitative differences in the RP con-sequent upon different mutations in the rhodopsin gene. Also important is that is has been shown for the first time that some forms of RP are due to defects of metabolic systems that are limited to rod photoreceptors, and yet it is evident that loss of photopic function is consistently found in these disorders. No explanation exists to account for cone cell death. It is possible that cone loss occurs either as a result of a release of toxins by dying rods or because cones are metabolically dependent upon the presence of rods. It follows that loss of cone function, although important to the patient, is a secondary effect.

The mechanism by which alteration of the amino acid sequence of the rhodopsin molecule may influence rod photoreceptor function is unclear. Some observations on the behavior of the abnormal protein made in the laboratory allow predictions to be made concerning the possible effects of the mutation on metabolic systems. More general concepts can be formulated on the basis of recently identified mechanism of protein formation and the cellular handling of abnormal proteins produced by mutant genes. It is known that abnormal proteins may or may not pass from the rough endoplasmic reticulum to the Golgi apparatus and that this depends on the influence of the mutation upon molecular folding [282]. Those proteins that do not pass on may be destroyed or may accumulate in the rough endoplasmic reticulum, which in turn may interfere with cell function [70,79,245,280].

From these considerations it is predictable that the nature of cell dysfunction depends upon the site of expression of the abnormal protein. For example, if it is incorporated into the outer segment it may generate physical instability of the membrane if either glycosylation on the N-terminal or the disulfide bond between the cysteine residues 110 and 187 are abnormal [234,235]. Transduction efficiency may be reduced by mutations near the C terminus, causing a reduction in sensitivity due to a reduced signal. It has been shown that rhodopsin with a mutation at the 296 amino acid, which is the binding site for retinal, fails to form a complex with 11-cis-retinal and reacts constantly with transducin. It can be predicted from this observation that the retina may act as if it is in constant lighting and does not dark adapt. These possibilities could be distinguished one from another by clinical testing. The interaction of the abnormal with the normal protein may also influence function.

The fate of protein produced by rhodopsin genes with mutations found in human RP has been investigated [111,424] by transfecting COS and 293S cells with various mutant rhodopsin genes. The abnormal proteins could be divided into distinct classes according to their behavior compared with normal [424]. In class I mutations rhodopsin was expressed normally on the plasma membrane and bound 11-cis-retinal, creating a chromophore with an absorbance spectrum similar to that of rhodopsin. Class II mutations showed little if any ability to form a pigment when exposed to 11-cis-retinal, inefficient transport to the plasma membrane, and low levels of cell surface localization. However, in no instance was expression on the plasma membrane absent.

Several of the mutations were identical to those found in forms of RP in which the functional deficit has been characterized. Pro-347-Leu was designated as biochemical class I, and the same mutation in the human causes diffuse RP. The mutations Pro-23-His, Thr-58-Arg, and Gly-106-Trp were designated biochemical class II, and in the human are associated with regional RP with altitudinal distribution of disease and slow recovery from strong light adaptation. The information to date shows striking confirmation that there are fundamental differences of disease mechanisms in RP types.

Peripherin

Even more striking is the recognition that both RP and macular dystrophy may be due to mutations in the rds gene [127,128,231,467]. Two families with a form of macular dystrophy have been shown to have a tryptophan substitution for arginine at codon 172, and another family with almost identical disease has a glutamine substitution for arginine at the same codon. A mutation resulting in a stop codon at position 258 has been identified in another family with a retinal degeneration similar in appearance to adult vitelliform macular dystrophy. These findings demonstrate that some forms of adRP and dominantly inherited macular dystrophies are caused by mutations in the same (rds) gene. The variability of phenotype caused by mutations at different codons suggests that the functional significance of certain amino acids for cones and rods may be different.

The current knowledge of the putative function of peripherin-rds provide an explanation for the disease being different with the various mutations in the rds gene. Peripherin has an amino acid sequence of 346 amino acids, with four transmembrane hydrophobic domains and two putative N-linked glycosylation sites [88], one of which is conserved across four species, and is thought to be important to the protein's function in stabilizing the parallel array of photoreceptor outer segment membranes [21,434,436]. Immuno-cytochemical studies have shown that the protein is limited to the membranes of outer segments of both rods and cones, although there is disagreement over its precise localization. One study using a polyvalent antibody to a short peptide sequence near the carboxyl terminus implied that the protein was distributed over the entire length of the outer segment disk membrane [436]. Covalent bonding between peripherin molecules has been suggested as responsible for the maintenance of the parallel arrangement of the outer segment membranes [436]. By contrast, a separate study using a monoclonal antibody to purified photoreceptor disks showed that labeling was confined to the rims of the outer segment, implying that the primary function of the protein was to stabilize the unfavorable thermodynamic bend at the disk rim [21]. A difference in the epitopes available for antibody binding at the disk rim compared with other parts of the disk membrane has been hypothesized to explain these different findings [436]. Regardless of the precise distribution of the protein, the general belief is that peripherin-rds is important to the structural stability of the outer segment disk membrane. Studies of the *rds* mouse support this belief. In the homozygous *rds/rds* genotype, outer segment disks are not formed, the disk membrane being discharged as small vesicles into the subretinal space [84,226,393,443]. In the heterozygous *rds/+* mouse outer segments disk membranes are long and distorted [186,392].

Peripherin may be noncovalently associated with ROM1, a protein structurally related to peripherin [28]. ROM1 has been localized to the disk rims of rod outer segments but has not been identified in cones [28]. It has been suggested that the formation and stability of the bend in the disk membrane in rods are dependent upon the noncovalent bonding between peripherin-rds and ROM1. However, the absence of ROM1 in cones implies that there are differences in the precise mechanisms by which peripherin-rds stabilizes outer segment membranes in the two classes of photoreceptor. In rods the association between peripherin-rds and ROM1 may be important, whereas in cones peripherin may bind to a different membrane protein or act alone. If the binding sites are different in rods and cones, constancy of one amino acid of the peripherin-rds molecule may be important to rods only, and a mutation causing an abnormality at this site would cause a dystrophy falling within the category of RP in which rods are the target cell of disease with relative preservation of cones. Conversely, different mutation on the *rds* gene may disrupt the metabolism or structure of either cones alone, causing macular dystrophy, or of both rods and cones. It appears that the presence of arginine at position 172 is important to the structure and function of cones but not rods [467]. It is noteworthy that a disorder in which the photoreceptors are the primary site of dysfunction may cause the profound atrophy of the choroid characteristic of late disease.

The disorder associated with a stop sequence at codon 258 is different from the others with mutations in the *rds* gene in that there is little evidence of functional loss, and the changes in the ocular fundus are apparently at the level of the RPE. This mutation possibly produces changes similar to those in the mouse heterozygous for the abnormal *rds* gene in which there is a 10 kb insert at codon 238 [436]. In the homozygous *rds* mouse a relatively high molecular weight mRNA is produced, demonstrating that the entire insert is transcribed [436]. On the other hand, the abnormal gene may not express the protein in the photoreceptor outer segment since the mRNA appears not to leave the nucleus. If this is the case only half the normal amount of protein is available in the heterozygous state as a result of expression of the normal gene. In the heterozygous *rds/+* mouse, the photoreceptor outer segments develop but contain long disk membranes [392], which is compatible with less peripherin-rds than normal. The ERG is well preserved, however, and 50% of the photoreceptors survive after 18 months of life [186,392], which is close to the life expectancy of the mouse. The outer segments appear to be unstable, and the RPE contains large and abnormal phagosomes [392]. Such a situation may exist in some patients with adult vitelliform macular degeneration since the gene with a stop codon may not be expressed. As in the heterozygous *rds* mouse, the photoreceptors probably receive only half the normal quantity of peripherin-rds, and the abnormal protein does not pass into the outer segment. If the homology is close, it is understandable that excessive shedding of the photoreceptor outer segments over many years causes change in the RPE but little photoreceptor dysfunction. If this reasoning is correct, a primary photoreceptor disease causes changes that are recognizable at the level of the RPE.

IV. PHOTORECEPTOR-RETINAL PIGMENT EPITHELIAL INTERACTION

Failure of the phagocytic relationship between the photoreceptor cells and the RPE leads to degenerative changes in the former. Such a situation arises in the RCS strain of rat, in which the RPE manifests an inability to phagocytose the disks shed from the overlying rod cells. The spent disks accumulate pro

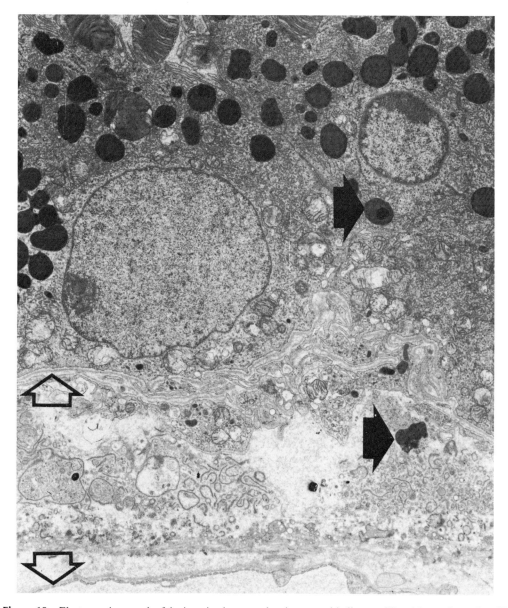

Figure 10 Electron micrograph of the junction between the pigment epithelium and Bruch's membrane in a 57-year-old normal human eye. Lipofuscin granules (solid arrows) can be seen both within the epithelial cells and in Bruch's membrane (open arrows). (×8000)

gressively between the outer segments of the photoreceptor cells and the apical surface of the RPE [53, 199,201,273]. There are four primary mechanisms by which such a development could occur [98].

1. The RPE lacks some component necessary for phagocytosis.
2. The rod outer segment either lacks an essential inducing agent or possesses an inhibiting agent that precludes phagocytosis.
3. Both the preceding mechanisms are present in combination and contribute collectively.
4. Complementary defects are present in the rod outer segment and the RPE such that disease manifestations are expressed only when both defects are combined.

Initially, most of the experimental evidence seemed to indicate that the primary abnormality was in the outer segments of the photoreceptor cell [12,98,375]. However, that the fault occurs solely within the RPE was elegantly demonstrated in a series of experiments by Mullen and LaVail [326]. Chimeric rats were created by flushing eight-cell embryos from the oviducts of both normal and dystrophic animals and then aggregating them in culture overnight before implanting the fused blastocytes into the uteri of pregnant or pseudopregnant females. By using albino dystrophic animals and combining them with pigmented normals, the distribution of the RPE in the resultant chimera represented a mosaic of both genotypes. Degeneration of the photoreceptor cells occurred only in areas of nonpigmented RPE. Given the complex and separate sequences of invagination and differentiation undertaken by the RPE and neural retina during their embryonic development, it is unlikely that areas of dystrophic retina would always come to lie adjacent to dystrophic RPE [326]. This led the authors to conclude that in RCS rats, the genetic defect is expressed solely within the RPE.

Although there is no direct evidence of such a failure of the phagocytic mechanism in any of the human dystrophies, subretinal membranous deposits could account for both the small white dots seen in the fundus of many sufferers of retinal dystrophies and for the masking of the choroidal circulation in bull's-eye dystrophies or Stargardt's disease. It is difficult to determine the boundaries between physiological and pathological processes in the age-related changes associated with the phagosome degradation and voiding mechanisms of the RPE. In all human eyes intracellular lipofuscin accumulates progressively with increasing age [130,474]. In addition, aging changes also occur in both the basement membrane of the RPE and in other components of Bruch's membrane [394]. These changes include an increase in the amount and complexity of the fibrous content of the various layers [204]. Such changes may both impede metabolic input to the RPE and obstruct the voiding processes. Thus, whereas accumulation of lipofuscin may reflect an increasing inability to effect total degradation of ingested outer segment material on the part of the RPE, it may in part also be an expression of a progressive resistance to the passage of waste products across Bruch's membrane. Such a concept is supported by the observations that increasing amounts of debris become trapped within Bruch's membrane with age (Fig. 10). These waste products are probably the precursors of drusen [203], and in most eyes over the age of 40 years some accumulation may be observed. The observations of both lipofuscin and debris within Bruch's membrane in several dystrophic human retinas [251,265,422,429] suggest that phagocytic processes are occurring within these eyes but do not exclude some quantitative fault. For example, the lipofuscin content within some of the RPE cells of a 24-year-old patient with xRP [429] was comparable to that of a 70- or 80-year-old normal individual. However, whether this represents an inundation of the degradative capacity of the RPE by prematurely degenerating photoreceptor cells or whether the photoreceptor cell degeneration is secondary to reduced metabolic exchange by prematurely aged RPE cannot currently be determined. That a patient with a mutation on the *rds* gene has adult vitelliform degeneration implies that a primary defect in the photoreceptors may cause disease that presents with dysfunction.

V. CONCLUSIONS

The recent advances in molecular biology whereby specific genomic defects have been identified, combined with those in cell biology that demonstrate the influence of genomic defects on cell function, render the findings of clinical investigation much more intelligible. In the past the functional deficits in RP were of value in distinguishing one disorder from another or at least identifying categories of disease. It is now possible to relate these characteristics to putative disease mechanisms and to generate hypotheses that are amenable to testing in the laboratory. It is also the case that observations are possible in the human, particularly with respect to detailed recording of functional loss in those with retinal dystrophies, that cannot be made in animals. Thus the results of clinical and laboratory studies are mutually relevant.

Although functional loss differs both quantitatively and qualitatively between families, the severity of disease varies considerably within families. The impression exists that there is more concordance of affection within sibships than might be expected by chance alone, at least in some families. If this is true it has implications about the determination of the phenotype in adRP in which disease appears in the heterozygous state, and it would allow investigation of the potential influence of such mechanisms as genomic imprinting and allelic competition on phenotypic expression [324,472].

The initial subdivision of RP was achieved on the basis of its inheritance; functional studies added to our understanding of this complex group of disorders. The recent identification of different mutations in the rhodopsin and peripherin genes are at present being correlated with clinical and functional abnormalities, and in the near future we can expect to find other genes responsible for further members of this group of disorders.

The mechanism by which an alteration of the amino acid sequence in rhodopsin or peripherin molecules may influence photoreceptor function is unclear, but much may depend upon the site of expression of the abnormal protein. Further studies should clarify this aspect of the problem. More sophisticated visual testing is required to correlate the genotype with the phenotypic expression of the disease. The recruitment of transgenic mice carrying a specific human mutation would accelerate our understanding of functional aberrations and, more importantly, the mechanisms leading to eventual death of the photoreceptor. Suction electrode techniques recording from single photoreceptors would allow the detection of subtle functional changes due to specific mutations. These studies could then be extended, using current mathematical models of phototransduction, to predict functional changes in the retina.

The considerable advances achieved so far have not yet brought any great advance in therapy, although some effect on clinical management is already evident. Genetic counseling in a family is undoubtedly simplified if the genomic abnormality is known, and advice about visual prognosis may be made on a firmer basis if single nosological entities are identified by genomic studies. In addition, it is hoped that with the knowledge that will result from the extension of current studies, it may eventually be possible to offer effective treatment to the patient with RP.

REFERENCES

1. Aguirre, G., Farber, D.B., Lolley, R.N., O'Brien, P., Aligood, J., Fletcher, R.T., and Chader, G. Retinal degeneration in the dog. III. Abnormal cyclic nucleotide metabolism in rod-cone dysplasia. *Exp. Eye Res.* 35:625–642, 1982.
2. Albert, A.D., and Litman, B.J. Independent structural domains in the membrane protein bovine rhodopsin. *Biochemistry* 17:3893–3900, 1978.
3. Alexander, K.R., and Fishman, G.A. Prolonged rod adaptation in retinitis pigmentosa. *Br. J. Ophthalmol.* 68:561–569, 1984.
4. Alezzandrini, A. Retinitis pigmentosa in symmetric quadrants. *Am. J. Ophthalmol.* 60:1160, 1965.
5. Alitalo, T., Kruse, T.A., Forsius, H., Eriksson, A.W., and de la Chapelle, A. Localization of the Åland Island eye disease locus to the pericentromeric region of the X chromosome by linkage analysis. *Am. J. Hum Genet.* 48:31–38, 1991.
6. Alpern, M., Lee, G.B., and Spivey, B.E. Pi cone monochromatism. *Arch. Ophthalmol.* 74:334–337, 1965.
7. Anderson, R.E. Essential fatty acid deficiency and photoreceptor membrane renewal: A reappraisal. *Invest. Ophthalmol. Vis. Sci.* 17:1102–1104, 1978.
8. Anderson, R.E., Benolken, R.M., Dudley, P.A., Landis, D.J., and Wheeler, T.G. Polyunsaturated fatty acids of photoreceptor membranes. *Exp. Eye Res.* 18:205–213, 1974.
9. Anderson, R.E., Maude, M.B., Lewis, R.A., Newsome, D.A., and Fishman, G.A. Abnormal plasma levels of polyunsaturated fatty acid in autosomal dominant retinitis pigmentosa. *Exp. Eye Res.* 44:155–159, 1987.
10. Anderson, S. Quoted in Krill, A.E. *Hereditary and Choroidal Diseases*, Harper & Row, New York, p. 697, 1977.
11. Andracchi, S., and Korte, G.E. Expression of plasma membrane alkaline phosphatase in normal and regenerating choriocapillaris of the rabbit. *Invest. Ophthalmol. Vis. Sci. (Suppl)* 32:1081, 1991.
12. Ansell, P.L., and Marshall, J. Laser induced phagocytosis in the pigment epithelium of the Hunter dystrophic rat. *Br. J. Ophthalmol.* 60:819–828, 1976.
13. Applebury, M.L., and Hargrave, P.A. Molecular biology of the visual pigments. *Vision Res.* 26:1881–1895, 1986.
14. Archer, D.B., Krill, A.E., and Ernest, J.T. Choroidal vascular aspects of degenerations of the retinal pigment epithelium. *Trans. Ophthalmol. Soc. UK* 92:187–207, 1972.
15. Arden, G.B., and Barrada, A. Analysis of the electro-oculograms of a series of normal subjects. *Br. J. Ophthalmol.* 46:468–482, 1962.
16. Arden, G.B., Carter, R.M., Hogg, C.R., Powell, D.J., Ernst, W.J.K., Clover, G.M., Lyness, A.L., and Quinlan, M.P. Rod and cone activity in patients with dominantly inherited retinitis pigmentosa: Comparison between psychophysical and electroretinographic measurements. *Br. J. Ophthalmol.* 67:405–418, 1983.
17. Arden, G.B., and Ikeda, H. Effects of hereditary degeneration of the retina on the early receptor potential and the corneo-fundal potential of the rat eye. *Vis. Res.* 6:121–184, 1966.
18. Arden, G.B., and Kolb, H. Electrophysiological investigations in retinal metabolic disease: Their range and application. *Exp. Eye Res.* 3:334–347, 1964.
19. Armington, J.C. Electrical responses of the light adapted eye. *J. Opt. Soc. Am.* 43:450–456, 1953.

20. Armington, J.C., Gouras, P., Tepas, D.L., and Gunkel, R. Detection of the electroretinogram in retinitis pigmentosa. *Exp. Eye Res. 1*:74–80, 1961.

21. Arokawa, K., Molday, M.M., Molday, R.S., and Williams, D.S. Localization of peripherin/rds in the disk membranes of cone and rod photoreceptors: Relationship to disk membrane morphogenesis and retinal degeneration. *J. Cell Biol. 116*:659–667, 1992.

22. Arshavsky, V.Y., Gray-Keller, M.P., and Bownds, M.D. cGMP suppresses GTPase activity of a portion of transducin equimolar to phosphodiesterase in frog rod outer segments. *J. Biol. Chem. 266*:18530–18537, 1991.

23. Ashton, N. Central areolar choroidal sclerosis. A histopathological study. *Br. J. Ophthalmol. 37*:140–147, 1953.

24. Baehr, W., Devlin, M.J., and Applebury, M.L. Isolation and characterization of cGMP phosphodiesterase from bovine rod outer segments. *J. Biol. Chem. 254*:11669–11677, 1979.

25. Barkman, Y. A clinical study of a central tapeoretinal degeneration. *Acta Ophthalmol. (Copenh.) 39*:663–671, 1961.

26. Barricks, M.E. Vitelliform lesions developing in normal fundi. *Am. J. Ophthalmol. 83*:324–327, 1977.

27. Barry, R.J., Canada, F.J., and Rando, R.R. Solubilisation and partial purification of retinyl ester synthetase and retinoid isomerase from bovine ocular pigment epithelium. *J. Biol. Chem. 264*:9231–9238, 1989.

28. Bascom, R.A., Manara, S., Collins, L., Molday, R.S., Kalnins, V.I., and McInnes, R.R. Cloning of the cDNA for a novel photoreceptor membrane (rom-1) identifies a disk rim protein family implicated in human retinopathies. *Neuron 8*:1171–1184, 1992.

29. Basinger, S., Hoffman, R., and Matthes, M. Photoreceptor shedding is initiated by light in the frog retina. *Science 194*:1074–1076, 1976.

30. Baum, J.L., Tannenbaum, M., and Kolodny, E.H. Refsum's syndrome with corneal involvement. *Am. J. Ophthalmol. 60*:699–708, 1965.

31. Bazan, N.G. The identification of a new biochemical alteration early in the differentiation of visual cells in inherited retinal degeneration. In *Inherited and Environmentally Induced Retinal Degenerations*, M.M. LaVail, R.E. Anderson, and J.G. Hollyfield (Eds.), Alan R. Liss, New York, pp. 191–215, 1989.

32. Bech-Hansen, N.T., Field, L.L., Schramm, A.M., Reedyk, M., Craig, I.W., Fraser, N.J., and Pearce, W.G. A locus for X-linked congenital stationary night blindness is located on the proximal portion of the short arm of the X chromosome. *Hum. Genet. 84*:406–408, 1990.

33. Bergsma, D.R., and Wolf, M.L. A therapeutic trial of vitamin A in patients with pigmentary retinal degenerations: A negative study. *Adv. Exp. Med. Biol. 77*:197–209, 1977.

34. Bernstein, P.S., Law, W.C., and Rando, R.R. Biochemical characterization of the retinoid isomerase system in the eye. *J. Biol. Chem. 262*:16848–16857, 1987.

35. Berson, E.L. Light deprivation for early retinitis pigmentosa: A hypothesis. *Arch. Ophthalmol. 85*:521–529, 1971.

36. Berson, E.L., and Goldstein, E.B. The early receptor potential in sex-linked retinitis pigmentosa. *Invest. Ophthalmol. 9*:58–63, 1970.

37. Berson, E.L., and Goldstein, E.B. Recovery of the human early receptor potential during dark adaptation in hereditary retinal disease. *Vis. Res. 10*:219–226, 1970.

38. Berson, E.L., Gouras, P., and Gunkel, R.D. Progressive cone degeneration, dominantly inherited. *Arch. Ophthalmol. 80*:77–83, 1968.

39. Berson, E.L., Gouras, P., Gunkel, R.D., and Myrianthopoulos, N.C. Rod and cone responses in sex-linked retinitis pigmentosa. *Arch. Ophthalmol. 81*:215–225, 1969.

40. Berson, E.L., Gouras, P., Gunkel, R.D., and Myrianthopoulos, N.C. Dominant retinitis pigmentosa with reduced penetrance. *Arch. Ophthalmol. 81*:226–235, 1969.

41. Berson, E.L., Gouras, P., and Hoff, M. Temporal aspects of the electroretinogram. *Arch. Ophthalmol. 81*: 207–214, 1969.

42. Berson, E.L., and Howard, J. Temporal aspects of the electroretinogram in sector retinitis pigmentosa. *Arch. Ophthalmol. 48*:653–665, 1971.

43. Best, F. Über eine hereditäre Maculaaffektion: Beitrag zur Vererbungslehre. *Z. Augenheilkd. 13*:199–212, 1905.

44. Bhattacharya, S.S., Wright, A.F., Clayton, J.F., Price, W.H., Phillips, C.T., McKeown, C.M.E., Jay, M., Bird, A.C., Pearson, P.L., and Southern, E.M. Close genetic linkage between X-linked retinitis pigmentosa and a restriction fragment length polymorphism identified by recombinant DNA probe L1.28. *Nature 309*:253–255, 1984.

45. Bietti, G. Ueber familiares vorkommen von "retinitis punctata albascens" (verbunden mit "dystrophia marginalis cristallinea cornea"), glitzern des glascorpers und anderen degenerativen augenveranderungen. *Klin. Monastbl. Augenheilkd. 99*:737–756, 1937.

46. Bietti, G.B. Su alcune forme atipiche o rare di degenerazione retinica (degenerazioni tappeto-retiniche e quadri morbosi similari). *Boll. Ocul. 16*:1159–1241, 1937.

47. Bird, A.C. X-linked retinitis pigmentosa. *Br. J. Ophthalmol. 59*:177–199, 1975.

48. Bjork, A., and Karp, G. The electroretinogram in retinitis pigmentosa. *Acta Ophthalmol. (Copenh.) 29*:361–371, 1951.

49. Bjork, A., Lindbalm, V., and Wadanstein, L. Retinal degeneration in hereditary ataxia. *Neurol. Neurosurg. Psychiatr. 19*:186–193, 1956.

50. Blanton, S.H., Cottingham, A.W., Giesenschlag, N., Heckenlively, J.R., Humphries, P., and Daiger, S.P. Further evidence of exclusion of linkage between type II autosomal dominant retinitis pigmentosa (ADRP) and D3S47 on 3q. *Genomics 8*:179–181, 1990.

51. Blanton, S.H., Heckenlively, J.R., Cottingham, A.W., Friedman, J., Sadler, L.A., and Wagner, M. Linkage mapping of autosomal dominant retinitis pigmentosa (RP1) to the pericentric region of human chromosome 8. *Genomics 11*:857–869, 1991.

52. Bok, D. Retinal photoreceptor-pigment epithelium interactions. *Invest. Ophthalmol. Vis. Sci. 26*:169, 1985.

53. Bok, D., and Hall, M.O. The role of the pigment epithelium in the etiology of inherited retinal dystrophy in the rat. *J. Cell Biol. 49*:664–682, 1971.

54. Bok, D., and Heller, J. Transport of retinol from the blood to the retina: An autoradiographic study of the pigment epithelium cell surface receptor for plasma retinol binding protein. *Exp. Eye Res. 22*:395–402, 1976.

55. Bonin, P. Le signe du silence choroidien dans les dégénérescences tapéto-rétiniennes centrales examinées sous fluorescéine. *Bull. Soc. Ophtalmol. Fr. 71*:348–351, 1971.

56. Boughman, J.A., and Fishman, G.A. A genetic analysis of retinitis pigmentosa. *Br. J. Ophthalmol. 66*:405–416, 1983.

57. Bowes, C., Li, T., Danciger, M., Baxter, L.C., Applebury, M.L., and Farber, D.B. Retinal degeneration of the rd mouse is caused by a defect in the beta subunit of rod cGMP-phosphodiesterase. *Nature 347*:677–680, 1990.

58. Bowes, C., Danciger, M., Kozak, C.A., and Farber, D.B. Isolation of a candidate cDNA for the gene causing retinal degeneration in the rd mouse. *Proc. Natl. Acad. Sci. USA 86*:9722–97226, 199 .

59. Brazitikos, P.D., and Safran, A.B. Helicoid peripapillary chorioretinal degeneration. *Am. J. Ophthalmol. 109*:290–294, 1990.

60. Brecher, R., and Bird, A.C. Adult vitelliform macular dystrophy. *Eye 4*:210–215, 1990.

61. Bresnick, G.H., Smith, V.C., and Pokorny, J. Autosomal dominantly inherited macular dystrophy with preferential short wavelength sensitive cone involvement. *Am. J. Ophthalmol. 108*:265–276, 1989.

62. Bridges, C.D., Liou, G.I., Gonzalez-Fernandez, F., Alvarez, R.A., and Fong, S.L. Vitamin A: Utilization, metabolism and role in retinal disease. In *Retinal Diseases: Biomedical Foundations and Clinical Management*, M.O.M. T'so (Ed.), J.B. Lippincott, Philadelphia, pp. 49–59, 1988.

63. Brindley, G.A., and Gardner-Medwin, A.R. The origin of the early receptor potential of the retina. *J. Physiol. (Lond.) 182*:105–191, 1966.

64. Brown, K.T., and Murakami, M.A. A new receptor potential of the monkey retina with no detectable latency. *Nature 201*:626–628, 1964.

65. Bush, N.R. The electrical responses of the eye before and after perforation of the retina, M.D. thesis, Brown University, 1951.

66. Cameron, J.D., Fine, B.S., and Shapiro, I. Histopathological observations in choroideremia with emphasis on vascular changes of the uveal tract. *Ophthalmology 94*:187–196, 1987.

67. Campbell, D.A., and Tonks, E.L. Biochemical findings in human retinitis pigmentosa with particular relation to vitamin A deficiency. *Br. J. Ophthalmol. 46*:151–164, 1962.

68. Capon, M.R.C., Marshall, J., Krafft, J.I., Alexander, R.A., Hiscott, P.S., and Bird, A.C. Sorsby's fundus dystrophy: A light and electron microscopic study. *Ophthalmology 96*:1769–1777, 1989.

69. Capon, M.R.C., Polkinghorne, P.J., Fitzke, F.W., and Bird, A.C. Sorsby's pseudoinflammatory macula dystrophy: Sorsby's fundus dystrophies. *Eye 2*:114–122, 1988.

70. Carlson, J.A., Rogers, B.B., Sifers, R.N., Hawkins, H.K., Finegold, M.J., and Woo, S.L. Multiple tissues express alpha 1-antitrypsin in transgenic mice and man. *J. Clin. Invest. 82*:26–36, 1988.

71. Carr, R.E. Symposium: Pigmentary retinopathy. Summing-up. *Trans. Ophthalmol. Soc. UK 92*:289–301, 1972.

72. Carr, R.E., Mittl, R.N., and Noble, K.G. Choroidal abiotrophies. *Trans. Am. Acad. Ophthalmol. Otolaryngol. 79*:796–816, 1975.

73. Carr, R.E., and Ripps, H. Rhodopsin kinetics and rod adaptation in Oguchi's disease. *Invest. Ophthalmol. 6*:426–436, 1967.

74. Carr, R.E., Ripps, H., and Siegel, I.M. Visual pigment kinetics and adaptation in fundus albipunctatus. *Doc. Ophthalmol. 4*:193–204, 1974.

75. Carr, R.E., Ripps, H., Siegel, I.M., and Weale, R.A. Rhodopsin and the electrical activity of the retina in congenital night blindness. *Invest. Ophthalmol. 5*:497–507, 1966.

76. Carr, R.E., and Siegel, I.M. Unilateral retinitis pigmentosa. *Arch. Ophthalmol. 90*:21–26, 1973.

77. Chatzinoff, A., Nelson, E., Stahl, N., and Clahane, M.S. Eleven-cis vitamin A in the treatment of retinitis pigmentosa: A negative study. *Arch. Ophthalmol. 80*:417–419, 1968.

78. Chen, J.C., Fitzke, F.W., Pauleikhoff, D., and Bird, A.C. Functional loss in age-related Bruch's membrane change with choroidal perfusion defect. *Invest. Ophthalmol. Vis. Sci. 33*:334–340, 1992.

79. Cheng, S.H., Gregory, R.J., Marshall, J., Paul, S. Souza, S.W., White, G.A., and O'Riodan, C.R. Defective intracellular transport and processing of CFT is the molecular basis of most cystic fibrosis. *Cell 63*:827–834, 1990.

80. Cheung, D.S. Pigmented paravenous chorioretinal atrophy. *Am. J. Ophthalmol.* 97:113, 1984.
81. Cibis, G.N., Morey, M., and Harris, D.J. Dominantly inherited macular dystrophy with flecks (Stargardt). *Arch. Ophthalmol.* 98:1785–1789, 1980.
82. Cogan, D.G. Symposium: Primary chorioretinal aberrations with night blindness. Pathology. *Trans. Am. Acad. Ophthalmol. Otolaryngol.* 54:629–661, 1950.
83. Cohen, A.I. Further studies on the question of the patency of saccules in outer segments of vertebrate photoreceptors. *Vis. Res.* 10:445–453, 1970.
84. Cohen, A.I. Some cytological and initial biochemical observations on photoreceptors in retinas of rds mice. *Invest. Ophthalmol. Vis. Sci.* 24:832–843, 1983.
85. Cone, R.A. Early receptor potentials of the vertebrate retina. *Nature* 204:736–739, 1964.
86. Cone, R.A., and Brown, P.K. Dependence of the early receptor potential on the orientation of rhodopsin. *Science* 156:536, 1967.
87. Connell, G., Bascom, R., Molday, L., Reid, D. McInnes, R.R., and Molday, R.S. Photoreceptor peripherin is the normal product of the gene responsible for retinal degeneration in the rds mouse. *Proc. Natl. Acad. Sci. USA* 88:723–726, 1991.
88. Connell, G., and Molday, R.S. Molecular cloning, primary structure and orientation of the vertebrate photoreceptor cell protein peripherin in the rod disc membrane. *Biochemistry* 29:4691–4698, 1990.
89. Converse, C.A., Hammer, H.M., Packard, C.J., and Shepherd, J. Plasma lipid abnormalities in retinitis pigmentosa and related conditions. *Trans. Ophthalmol. Soc. UK* 103:508–512, 1983.
90. Converse, C.A., Huq, L., McLachlan, T., Bow, A.C., and Alvares, E. Apolipoprotein E isotypes in retinitis pigmentosa. *Invest. Ophthalmol. Vis. Sci.* 29:169, 1988.
91. Cordier, J., Reny, A., and Seigneur, J.-B. Rétinite pigmentaire unilatérale. *Bull. Soc. Ophtalmol. Fr.* 66:224–227, 1966.
92. Cortin, P., Archer, D., and Maumennee, I.H. A patterned macular dystrophy with yellow plaques and atrophic changes. *Br. J. Ophthalmol.* 64:127–134, 1980.
93. Crabb, J.W., Heinzmann, C., Mohandas, T., Goldflam, S. Saari, J.C., and Sparkes, R.S. Assignment of the gene for cellular retinaldehyde-binding protein to human chromosome 15. *Invest. Ophthalmol. Vis. Sci. (Suppl.)* 30:115, 1989.
94. Cremers, F.P.M., van de Pol, D.J., Diergaarde, P.J., Wieringa, B., Nussbaum, R.L., Schwartz, M., and Ropers, H.-H. Physical fine mapping of the choroideremia locus using Xq21 deletions associated with complex syndromes. *Genomics* 4:41–46, 1989.
95. Cremers, F.P.M., van de Pol, D.J.R., van Kerkhoff, L.P.M., Wieringa, B., and Ropers, H.-H. Cloning of a gene that is rearranged in patients with choroideremia. *Nature* 347:674–677, 1990.
96. Crouch, R.K., and Coffman, M. The effect of visible light on the regeneration of rhodopsin. *Biochem. Biophys. Res. Commun.* 73:428–433, 1976.
97. Cumings, J.N. Inborn errors of metabolism in neurology (Wilson's disease, Refsum's disease and lipidoses). *Trans. R. Soc. Med.* 64:313–322, 1971.
98. Custer, N.V., and Bok, D. Pigment epithelium photoreceptor interactions in normal and dystrophic rats. *Exp. Eye Res.* 21:153–166, 1975.
99. Davison, M.D., and Findlay, J.B.C. Modification of ovine opsin with the photosensitive hydrophobic probe 1-azido-4-[^{125}I]iodobenzene. *Biochem. J.* 234:413–420, 1986.
100. Dejean, C., and Gassenc, R. Note sur la généalogie de la famille Nougaret, Vendémian. *Bull. Soc. Ophtalmol.* 1:96–99, 1949.
101. De Jong, P.T.V.M., and Delleman, J.W. Pigment epithelial pattern dystrophy. *Arch. Ophthalmol.* 3:1416–1421, 1982.
102. De Jong, P.T., Zrenner, E., van Meel, G.J., Keunen, J.E., and van Norren, D. Mizuo phenomenon in X-linked retinoschisis: Pathogenesis of the Mizuo phenomenon. *Arch. Ophthalmol.* 109:1104–1108, 1991.
103. Denton, M.J., Chen, J.-D., Serravalle, S., Colley, P., Halliday, F.B., and Donald, J. Analysis of linkage relationships of X-linked retinitis pigmentosa with the following Xp loci: L1.28, OTC, 754, XJ1.1, pERT 87 and C7. *Hum. Genet.* 78:60–64, 1988.
104. Deterre, P., Bigay, J., Robert, M., Pfister, C., Kuhn, H., and Chabre, M. Activation of retinal rod cyclic GMP-phosphodiesterase by transducin: Characterization of the complex formed by phosphodiesterase inhibitor and transducin Á-transducin. *Proteins Structure Function Genet.* 1:188–193, 1986.
105. Deutman, A.F. Electro-oculography in families with vitelliform dystrophy of the fovea. *Arch. Ophthalmol.* 81:305–316, 1969.
106. Deutman, A.F. *The Hereditary Dystrophies of the Posterior Pole of the Eye*, Van Gorcum, Assen, 1971.
107. Deutman, A.F., van Blommestein, J.D.A., Henkes, H.E., Waardenburg, P.J., and Solleveld-van Dreist, E. Butterfly shaped pigment dystrophy of the fovea. *Arch. Ophthalmol.* 83:558–569, 1970.
108. Deutschmann, R. Einseitige typische Retinitis Pigmentosa mit pathologish anatomischem Befund. *Beitr. Augenheilkd.* 1:69–80, 1891.
109. Diem, M. Retinitis punctata albescens et pigmentosa. *Klin. Monatsbl. Augenheilkd.* 53:371–379, 1914.
110. Dodt, F., and Wadenstein, L. The use of flicker electroretinography in the human eye. *Acta Ophthalmol. (Copenh.)* 32:165–180, 1954.

111. Doi, T., Molday, R.S., and Khorana, H.G. Role of the intradiscal domain in rhodopsin assembly and function. *Proc. Natl. Acad. Sci. USA* 87:4991–4995, 1990.

112. Dowling, J.E., and Sidman, R.L. Inherited retinal dystrophy in the rat. *J. Cell Biol.* 14:73–109, 1962.

113. Dreyer, R.F., and Hidayat, A.A. Pseudoinflammatory macular dystrophy. *Am. J. Ophthalmol.* 106:154–161, 1988.

114. Dryja, T.P., Hahn, L.B., Cowley, G.S., McGee, T.L., and Berson, E.L. Mutation spectrum of the rhodopsin gene among patients with autosomal dominant retinitis pigmentosa. *Proc. Natl. Acad. Sci. USA* 88:9370–9374, 1991.

115. Dryja, T.P., McGee, T., Hahn, L.B., Cowley, G.S., Olsson, J.E., Reichel, E., Sandberg, M.A., and Berson, E.L. Mutations within the rhodopsin gene in patients with autosomal dominant retinitis pigmentosa. *N. Engl. J. Med.* 323:1302–1307, 1990.

116. Dryja, T.P., McGee, T., Reichel, E. Hahn, L.B., Cowley, G.S., Yandell, D.W., Sandberg, M.A., and Berson, E.L. A point mutation of the rhodopsin gene in one form of retinitis pigmentosa. *Nature 343*:364–366, 1990.

117. Eagle, R.C., Lucier, A.C., Bernardino, J.R., and Yanoff, M. Retinal pigment epithelial abnormalities in fundus flavimaculatus: A light and electron microscopic study. *Ophthalmology 87*:1189–1200, 1980.

118. Eicholtz, W. Histologie der Retinopathia pigmentosa cum et sine Pigmento. *Klin. Monatsbl. Augenheilkd.* 164:467–475, 1974.

119. Eisner, A., Stoumbos, V.D., Klein, M.L., and Fleming, S.A. Relations between fundus appearance and function; eyes whose fellow eye has exudative age-related macular degeneration. *Invest. Ophthalmol. Vis. Sci. (Suppl.)* 32:1507, 1991.

120. Eldred, G.E., and Katz, M.L. Fluophores of the human retinal pigment epithelium: Separation and spectral characterization. *Exp. Eye Res.* 47:71–86, 1988.

121. Eldred, G.E. Vitamins A and E in RPE lipofuscin formation and implications for age-related macular degenerations. In *Inherited and Environmentally Induced Retinal Degenerations*, M.M. LaVail, R.E. Anderson, and J.G. Hollyfield (Eds.), Alan R. Liss, New York, pp. 113–129, 1989.

122. Ernst, W., and Moore, A.T. Heterogeneity, anomalous adaptation and incomplete penetrance in autosomal dominant retinitis pigmentosa. In *Research in Retinitis Pigmentosa*, E. Zrenner, H. Krastel, and H.-H. Goebel (Eds.), Pergamon Press, Oxford, pp. 115–120, 1988.

123. Falls, H.F., and Cotterman, C.W. Choroido-retinal degeneration: A sex-linked form in which heterozygous women exhibit a tapetal-like reflex. *Arch. Ophthalmol.* 40:685–703, 1948.

124. Falls, H.F., Wolter, J.R., and Alpern, M. Typical total monochromacy. *Arch. Ophthalmol.* 74:610–616, 1965.

125. Farber, D.B., Flannery, J.G., Bird, A.C., Shuster, T., and Bok, D. Histopathological and biochemical studies of donor eyes affected with retinitis pigmentosa. In *Degenerative Retinal Disorders. Clinical and Laboratory Investigations*, J.G. Hollyfield, R.E. Anderson, and M.M. LaVail (Eds.), Alan R. Liss, New York, pp. 53–67, 1987.

126. Farber, D.B., and Lolley, R.N. Cyclic guanosine monophosphate: Elevation in degenerating photoreceptor cells of the C3H mouse retina. *Science 186*:449–451, 1974.

127. Farrar, G.J., Jordan, S.A., Kenna, P., Lawler, M., Jordan, S.A., and Humphries, P. Autosomal dominant retinitis pigmentosa: Localization of a disease gene (RP6) to the short arm of chromosome 6. *Genomics 11*:870–874, 1991.

128. Farrar, G.J., Kenna, P., Jordan, S.A., Kumar-Singh, R., Humphries, M.M., and Sharp, E.M. A three-base-pair deletion in the peripherin-RDS gene in one form of retinitis pigmentosa. *Nature 354*:478–480, 1991.

129. Favre, M. A propos de deux cas de dégénérescence hyaloïdéo-rétinienne. *Ophthalmologica 135*:604–609, 1958.

130. Feeney, L. Lipofuscin and melanin of human retinal pigment epithelium: Fluorescence, enzyme cytochemical and ultrastructural studies. *Invest. Ophthalmol. Vis. Sci.* 17:583–600, 1978.

131. Fish, G., Grey, R.H.B., Sehmi, K.S., and Bird, A.C. The dark choroid in posterior retinal dystrophies. *Br. J. Ophthalmol.* 65:359–363, 1981.

132. Fishman, G.A. Retinitis pigmentosa: Genetic percentages. *Arch. Ophthalmol.* 96:822–926, 1978.

133. Fishman, G.A., Farber, M., Patel, B.S., and Derlacki, D.J. Visual acuity loss in patients with Stargardt's macular dystrophy. *Ophthalmology 94*:809–814, 1987.

134. Fishman, G.A., Stone, E.M., Gilbert, L.D., Kenna, P., and Sheffield, V.C. Ocular findings associated with a rhodopsin gene codon 58 transversion mutation in autosomal dominant retinitis pigmentosa. *Arch. Ophthalmol.* 109:1387–1393, 1991.

135. Fishman, G.A., Stone, E.M., Sheffield, V.C., Gilbert, L.D., and Kimura, A.E. Ocular findings associated with rhodopsin gene codon 17 and codon 182 transition mutations in dominant retinitis pigmentosa. *Arch. Ophthalmol.* 110:54–62, 1992.

136. Flannery, J.G., Bird, A.C., Farber, D.B., Weleber, G.R., and Bok, D. A histopathologic study of a choroideremia carrier. *Invest. Ophthalmol. Vis. Sci.* 31:229–236, 1990.

137. Fledelius, H., and Simonsen, S.E. A family with bilateral symmetrical sectorial pigmentary retinal lesion. *Acta Ophthalmol (Copenh.)* 48:14–22, 1970.

138. Fliesler, S.J., and Anderson, R.E. Chemistry and metabolism of lipids in the vertebrate retina. *Prog. Lipid Res.* 22:79–131, 1983.

139. Foulds, W.S. The retinal pigment epithelial surface. *Br. J. Ophthalmol.* 63:71–84, 1979.

140. Foxman, S.G., Heckenlively, J.R., Sinclair, S.H. Rubeola retinopathy and pigmented paravenous retinochoroidal atrophy. *Am. J. Ophthalmol. 99*:605–606, 1985.

141. Franceschetti, A. A curious affection of the ocular fundus. Helicoid peripapillary chorioretinal degeneration: Its relation to pigmented paravenous chorioretinal degeneration. *Doc. Ophthalmol. 16*:18–109, 1962.

142. Franceschetti, A. Über Tapeto-retinale degeneration in Kindesalter. In *Entwicklung ud Fortschritt in der Augenheilkhunde*, Enke Verlag, Stuttgart, p. 107, 1963.

143. Franceschetti, A., Dieterle, P., Amman, P., and Marty, F. Une nouvelle forme de fundus albipunctatus cum hemeralopia. *Ophthalmologica 145*:403–410, 1963.

144. Franceschetti, A., and François, J. Fundus flavimaculatus. *Arch. Ophtalmol. (Paris) 25*:505–530, 1965.

145. Francke, U., Ochs, H.D., DeMartinville, B., Giacalone, J., Lindergren, V., Disteche, C., Pagon, B.A., Hofker, M.H., and van Ommen, G.J. Minor Xp21 chromosome deletion in a male associated with expression of Duchenne muscular dystrophy and McLeod syndrome. *Am. J. Hum. Genet. 37*:250–267, 1985.

146. François, J. L'électrorétinigraphie dans les dégénérescences tapéto-rétiniennes périphériques et centrales. *Ann. Ocul. 185*:842–856, 1952.

147. François, J. Chorioretinal degeneration of retinitis pigmentosa of intermediate sex-linked heredity. *Doc. Ophthalmol. 16*:111–127, 1962.

148. François, J. Ocular manifestations of inborn errors of carbohydrates and lipid metabolism. IV. Familial lipoprotein deficiencies. *Bibl. Ophthalmol. 84*:138–149, 1975.

149. François, J., and De Laey, J.J. Bietti's crystalline fundus dystrophy. *Klin. Monatsbl. Augenheilkd. 170*:353–362, 1970.

150. François, J., and Verriest, G. Rétinopathie pigmentaire unilatérale. *Ophthalmologica 124*:65–88, 1952.

151. François, J., and Verriest, G. La Maladie d'Oguchi. *Bull. Soc. Belg. Ophthalmol. 108*:465–506, 1954.

152. François, J., Verriest, G., and De Rouck, A. Les fonctions visuelles dans les dégénérescences tapéto-rétiniennes. *Ophthalmologica 131 (Suppl. 43)*:1–40, 1956.

153. Frangieh, G.T., Green, R., and Fine, S.L. A histopathological study of Best's macular dystrophy. *Arch. Ophthalmol. 100*:1115–1121, 1982.

154. Friedman, E., Smith, T.R., and Kuwabara, T. Senile choroidal vascular patterns and drusen. *Arch. Ophthalmol. 69*:220, 1963.

155. Friedman, E., Smith, T.R., Kuwabara, T., and Beyer, C.K. Choroidal vascular patterns in hypertension. *Arch. Ophthalmol. 71*:842, 1964.

156. Friedrich, U., Warburg, M., Wieacker, P., Wienker, T.F., Gal, A., and Ropers, H.-H. X-linked retinitis pigmentosa: Linkage with the centromere and a cloned DNA sequence from the proximal short arm of the X chromosome. *Hum. Genet. 71*:93–99, 1985.

157. Fulton, A.B., and Hansen, R.M. The relationship of rhodopsin and scotopic retinal sensitivity in sector retinitis pigmentosa. *Am. J. Ophthalmol. 105*:132–140, 1988.

158. Gal, A., Schinzel, A., Orth, U., Fraser, N.A., Mollica, F., Craig, I.W., Kruse, T., Machler, M., Neugebauer, M., and Bleeker-Wagemakers, L.M. Gene of X-chromosomal congenital stationary night blindness is closely linked to DXS7 on Xp. *Hum. Genet. 81*:315–318, 1989.

159. Gass, J.D.M. *Stereoscopic Atlas of Macular Diseases*, C.V. Mosby, St. Louis, p. 124, 1970.

160. Gass, J.D.M. A clinicopathologic study of a peculiar foveomacular dystrophy. *Trans. Am. Ophthalmol. Soc. 72*:139–156, 1974.

161. Geggel, H.S., Ament, M.E., Heckenlively, J.R., Martin, P.A., and Kopple, J.D. Nutritional requirement for taurine in patients receiving long-termparenteral nutrition. *N. Engl. J. Med. 312*:142–146, 1985.

162. Ghadially, F.N. *Ultrastructural Pathology of the Cell. A Text and Atlas of Physiological and Pathological Alterations in Cell Fine Structure*, Butterworths, London, pp. 306–308, 1975.

163. Ghosh, M., McCulloch, C., and Parker, J.A. Pathological study in a female carrier of choroideremia. *Can. J. Ophthalmol. 23*:181–186, 1988.

164. Gillespie, P.G., and Beavo, J.A. cGMP is tightly bound to bovine retinal rod phosphodiesterase. *Proc. Natl. Acad. Sci. USA 86*:4311–4315, 1989.

165. Glaser, B.M., Campochiaro, P.A., Davis, J.L., and Sato, M. Retinal pigment epithelial cells release an inhibitor of neovascularization. *Arch. Ophthalmol. 103*:1870–1875, 1985.

166. Glickstein, M., and Heath, G.G. Receptors in the monochromat eye. *Vis. Res. 15*:633–636, 1975.

167. Godel, V., Chaine, G., Regenbogen, L., and Coscas, G. Best's vitelliform macular dystrophy. *Acta Ophthalmol. Suppl. (Copenh.) 175*:1–31, 1986.

168. Goedbloed, J. Mode of inheritance in choroideraemia. *Ophthalmologica 104*:308–315, 1942.

169. Gonin, J. Examen anatomique d'un oeil atteint de retinite pigmentaire avec scotome zonulaire. *Ann. Ocul. 129*:24–48, 1903.

170. Goodman, G., Ripps, H., and Siegel, I.M. Cone dysfunction syndromes. *Arch. Ophthalmol. 70*:214–231, 1963.

171. Gouras, P., Carr, E.E., and Gunkel, R.D. Retinitis pigmentosa in abetalipoproteinemia: Effects of vitamin A. *Invest. Ophthalmol. 10*:784–793, 1971.

172. Gouras, P., Eggars, H.M., and MacKay, C.J. Cone dystrophy, nyctalopia and supernormal rod responses: A new retinal degeneration. *Arch. Ophthalmol. 101*:718–724, 1983.

173. Grey, R.H.B., Blach, R.K., and Barnard, W.M. Bull's eye maculopathy with early cone degeneration. *Br. J. Ophthalmol. 61*:702–718, 1977.
174. Guiffre, G. Autosomal dominant pattern dystrophy of the retinal pigment epithelium. *Retina 8*:169–173, 1988.
175. Guiffre, G., and Lodato, G. Vitelliform dystrophy and pattern dystrophy of the retinal pigment epithelium: Concomitant presence in a family. *Br. J. Ophthalmol. 70*:526–532, 1988.
176. Gutman, I., Walsh, J.B., and Henkind, P. Vitelliform macular dystrophy and butterfly-shaped epithelial dystrophy. *Br. J. Ophthalmol. 66*:170–173, 1982.
177. Haase, W., and Hellner, K.A. Über familiäre bilaterale sektorenformige Retinopathia pigmentosa. *Klin. Monatsbl. Augenheilkd. 147*:365–375, 1965.
178. Hadden, O.B., and Gass, J.D.M. Fundus flavimaculatus and Stargardt's disease. *Am. J. Ophthalmol. 82*:527–539, 1976.
179. Hamilton, W.K., Ewing, C.C., Ives, E.J., and Carruthers, J.D. Sorsby's fundus dystrophy. *Ophthalmology 96*:1755–1762, 1989.
180. Handelman, G.J., and Dratz, E.A. The role of antioxidants in the retina and retinal pigment epithelium and the nature of proxidant-induced damage. *Adv. Free Radic. Biol. Med. 2*:1–89, 1986.
181. Hargrave, P.A. Rhodopsin chemistry, structure and topography. *Prog. Retinal Res. 1*:1–51, 1982.
182. Hargrave, P.A., Fong, S.L., McDowell, J.H., Mas, M.T., Curtis, D.R., Wang, J.K., Juszczak, E., and Smith, D.P. The partial primary structure of bovine rhodopsin and its topography in the retinal rod cell disc membrane. *Neurochem. Int. 1*:231–244, 1980.
183. Harrison, R., Hoeffnagel, D., and Hayward, J.N. Congenital total color blindness: A clinicopathological report. *Arch. Ophthalmol. 64*:685–692, 1960.
184. Harwerth, R.S., and Sperling, H.G. Prolonged color blindness induced by intense spectral lights in rhesus monkeys. *Science 174*:520–523, 1971.
185. Haustrate, F.M., and Oosterhuis, J.A. Pigmented paravenous retinochoroidal atrophy (PPRA). *Doc. Ophthalmol. 63*:209–237, 1986.
186. Hawkins, R.K., Jansen, H.G., and Sanyal, S. Development and degeneration of retina in rds mutant mice: Photoreceptor abnormalities in the heterozygotes. *Exp. Eye Res. 41*:701–720, 1985.
187. Hayasaka, S., and Okoyuma, S. Crystalline retinopathy. *Retina 4*:177–181, 1984.
188. Hayes, K.C. Retinal degeneration in monkeys induced by deficiencies of vitamins E or A. *Invest. Ophthalmol. 13*:499–510, 1974.
189. Hayes, K.C., Carey, S.Y., and Schmidt, S.Y. Retinal degeneration associated with taurine deficiency in the cat. *Science 188*:949–951, 1975.
190. Heckenlively, J.R. Preserved para-arteriole retinal pigment epithelium (PPRPE) in retinitis pigmentosa. *Br. J. Ophthalmol. 66*:26–31, 1982.
191. Heckenlively, J.R. Quoted in Heckenlively, J.R. *Retinitis Pigmentosa*, J.B. Lippincott, Philadelphia, p. 21, 1988.
192. Heckenlively, J.R. *Retinitis Pigmentosa*, J.B. Lippincott, Philadelphia, p. 21, 1988.
193. Heckenlively, J.R., Rodriguez, J.A., and Daiger, S.P. Autosomal dominant sectoral retinitis pigmentosa: Two families with transversion mutation in codon 23 of rhodopsin. *Arch. Ophthalmol. 109*:84–91, 1991.
194. Heckenlively, J.R., and Weleber, R.G. X-linked recessive cone dystrophy with tapetal like sheen: A newly recognized entity with Mizuo-Nakamura phenomenon. *Arch. Ophthalmol. 104*:1322–1328, 1986.
195. Heller, J. Interactions of plasma retinol-binding protein with its receptor: Specific binding of bovine and human retinol binding protein to pigment epithelium cells from bovine eyes. *J. Biol. Chem. 250*:3613–3619, 1975.
196. Heller, J., and Bok, D. Transport of retinol from the blood to the retina: The involvement of high molecular weight lipoproteins as intracellular carriers. *Exp. Eye Res. 22*:403–410, 1976.
197. Henkes, H.E. Unilateral fundus albipunctatus. *Ophthalmologica 145*:470–480, 1963.
198. Henkes, H.E., van der Tweel, L., and van der Gon, J.J. Selective amplication of the electroretinogram. *Ophthalmologica 132*:140–150, 1956.
199. Herron, W.L., Jr., and Riegel, B.W. Production rate and removal of rod outer segment material in vitamin A deficiency. *Invest. Ophthalmol. 13*:46–53, 1974.
200. Herron, W.L., Jr., and Riegel, B.W. Vitamin A deficiency-induced "rod thinning" to permanently decrease the production of rod outer segment material. *Invest. Ophthalmol. 13*:54–59, 1974.
201. Herron, W.L., Jr., Riegel, B.W., Myers, O.E., and Rubin, M.L. Retinal dystrophy in the rat: A pigment epithelial disease. *Invest. Ophthalmol. 8*:595–604, 1969.
202. Hodgson, S.V., Robertson, M.E., Fear, C.N., Goodship, J., Malcolm, S., and Jay, B. Prenatal diagnosis of X-linked choroideremia with mental retardation, associated with a cytologically detectable chromosome deletion. *Hum. Genet. 75*:286–290, 1987.
203. Hogan, M.J. Role of the retinal pigment epithelium in macular disease. *Trans. Am. Acad. Ophthalmol. Otolaryngol. 76*:64–80, 1972.
204. Hogan, M.J., Alvardo, J.A., and Weddell, J.E. *Histology of the Human Eye. An Atlas and Textbook*, W.B. Saunders, Philadelphia, 1971.
205. Hollyfield, J.G. Phagocytic capabilities of the pigment epithelium. *Exp. Eye Res. 22*:457–469, 1976.
206. Hollyfield, J.G., Fliesler, S.J., Rayborn, M.E., Fong, S.L., Landers, R.A., and Bridges, C.D.B. Synthesis and

secretion of interstitial retinol-binding protein by the human retina. *Invest. Ophthalmol. Vis. Sci.* 26:58–67, 1985.

207. Hollyfield, J.G., Frederick, J.M., Tabor, G.A., and Ulshafer, R.J. Metabolic studies on retinal tissue from a donor with a dominantly inherited chorioretinal sectoral retinitis pigmentosa. *Ophthalmology* 91:191–196, 1984.

208. Hollyfield, J.G., and Ward, A. Phagocytic activity in the retinal pigment epithelium of the frog *Rana pipiens.* I. Uptake of polystyrene spheres. *J. Ultrastruct. Res.* 46:327–338, 1974.

209. Hommer, K. Das Elektroretinogramm bei sektorenförmiger Retinitis pigmentosa (retinopathia pigmentosa). *Graefes Arch. Klin. Exp. Ophthalmol.* 161:16–26, 1959.

210. Honig, B., Dinur, U., Nakanishi, K., Balogh-Nair, V., Gawinowicz, M.A., Arnaboldi, M., and Motto, M.G. An external point-charge model for wavelength regulation in visual pigments. *J. Am. Chem. Soc.* 101:7084–7086, 1979.

211. Hoskin, A., Bird, A.C., and Sehmi, K. Sorsby's pseudoinflammatory macular dystrophy. *Br. J. Ophthalmol.* 65:859–865, 1981.

212. Hu, D. Genetic aspects of retinitis pigmentosa in China. *Am. J. Med. Genet.* 12:51–56, 1982.

213. Hu, D.-N. Ophthalmic genetics in China. *Ophthalmic Paediatr. Genet.* 2:39–45, 1983.

214. Hussain, A.A., Leon, A., Curtis, R., and Barnett, K.C. Photoreceptor dysplasia in the Abyssinian cat: Biochemical and electrophysiological evidence for abnormal cyclic nucleotide metabolism. *Biochem. Soc. Trans.* 17:221–222, 1980.

215. Hussain, A.A., and Voaden, M.J. Some observations on taurine homeostasis in patients with retinitis pigmentosa. In *Degenerative Retinal Disorders: Clinical and Laboratory Investigations*, J.G. Hollyfield, R.E. Anderson, and M.M. LaVail (Eds.), Alan R. Liss, New York, pp. 119–129, 1987.

216. Hussain, A.A., Willmott, N.J., and Voaden, M.J. Species differences in the response of mammalian photoreceptor cGMP and PIII to a reduction in calcium. *Vis. Res.* 32:809–813, 1992.

217. Hussels, I. Une famille atteinte de rétinopathie pigmentaire liée au sexe, de maladie de Parkinson et d'autres troubles neuro-psychiatriques. *J. Genet. Hum.* 16:106–155, 1967.

218. Inglehearn, C.F., Bashir, R., Lester, D.H., Jay, M., Bird, A.C., and Bhattacharya, S.S. A 3-bp deletion in the rhodopsin gene in a family with autosomal dominant retinitis pigmentosa. *Am. J. Hum. Genet.* 48:26–30, 1991.

219. Inglehearn, C.F., Keen, T.J., Bashir, R., Jay, M., Fitzke, F., and Bird, A.C. A completed screen for mutations of the rhodopsin gene in a panel of patients with autosomal dominant retinitis pigmentosa. *Hum. Mol. Genet.* 1:41–45, 1992.

220. Ishiguro, S.I., Mizuno, K., and Tamai, M. Solubilization and partial purification of retinol dehydrogenase from bovine rod outer segments. *Invest. Ophthalmol. Vis. Sci. (Suppl.)* 30:288, 1989.

221. Ishikawa, T., and Yamada, E. The degradation of the photoreceptor outer segments within the pigment epithelial cell of rat retina. *J. Electron Microsc. (Tokyo)* 19:85–91, 1970.

222. Jacobson, D.M., Thompson, H.S., and Bartley, J.A. X-linked progressive cone dystrophy: Clinical characteristics of affected males and female carriers. *Ophthalmology* 96:885–895, 1989.

223. Jacobson, S.G., Kemp, C.M., Sung, C.H., and Nathans, J. Retinal function and rhodopsin levels in autosomal dominant retinitis pigmentosa with rhodopsin mutations. *Am. J. Ophthalmol.* 112:256–271, 1991.

224. Jahn, C.E., Leiss, O., Bergmann, K.V., and Schafer, K. Serum lipoprotein concentrations in patients with retinitis pigmentosa. In *Research in Retinitis Pigmentosa*, E. Zrenner, H. Krastel, and H.H. Goebel (Eds.), Pergamon Press, Oxford, pp. 571–574, 1987.

225. Jalili, I.K., and Smith, N.J.D. A progressive cone rod dystrophy and amelanogenesis imperfecta: A new syndrome. *J. Med. Genet.* 25:738–740, 1988.

226. Jansen, H.G., and Sanyal, S. Development and degeneration of retina in rds mutant mice: Electron microscopy. *J. Comp. Neurol.* 224:71–84, 1984.

227. Janssen, O. Zur Erbbiologie der Retinitis pigmentosa, Inaugural dissertation, Munster in Westfalen, 1938.

228. Jay, B., and Bird, A.C. X-linked retinitis pigmentosa. *Trans. Am. Acad. Ophthalmol. Otolaryngol.* 77:641–651, 1973.

229. Jay, M. On the hereditary of retinitis pigmentosa. *Br. J. Ophthalmol.* 7:405–416, 1982.

230. Jung, E.E. (1936). Quoted in Duke-Elder, S. *System of Ophthalmology*, Vol. 10, Henry Kimpton, London, p. 632.

231. Kajiwara, K., Hahn, L.B., Mukai, S., Travis, G.H., Berson, E.L., and Dryja, T.P. Mutations in the human retinal degeneration slow gene in autosomal dominant retinitis pigmentosa. *Nature* 354:480–483, 1991.

232. Kakitani, H., Kakitani, T., Rodman, H., and Honig, B. On the mechanism of wavelength regulation in visual pigments. *Photochem. Photobiol.* 41:471–479, 1985.

233. Kandori, F., Tamai, A. Kurimoto, S., and Fukunaga, K. Fleck retina. *Am. J. Ophthalmol.* 73:673–685, 1972.

234. Karnik, S.S., and Khorana, H.G. Assembly and functional rhodopsin requires a disulfide bond between cysteine residues 110 and 187. *J. Biol. Chem.* 265:17520–17524, 1990.

235. Karnik, S.S., Sakmar, T.P., Chen, H.B., and Khorana, H.G. Cysteine residues 110 and 187 are essential for the formation of correct structure in bovine rhodopsin. *Proc. Natl. Acad. Sci. USA* 85:8459–8463, 1988.

236. Katz, M.L., Kutryb, M.J., Norberg, M., Gao, C.L., White, R.H., and Stark, W.S. Maintenance of opsin density in photoreceptor outer segments of retinoid-deprived rats. *Invest. Ophthalmol. Vis. Sci.* 32:1968–1980, 1991.

237. Katz, M.L., and Robinson, W.G. Light and aging effects on vitamin E in the retina and retinal pigment epithelium. *Vision Res. 27*:1875–1879, 1987.
238. Kearns, T.P., and Hollenhorst, R.W. Chloroquine retinopathy: Evaluation by fluorescein angiography. *Arch. Ophthalmol. 76*:378–384, 1966.
239. Keen, T.J., Inglehearn, C.F., Lester, D.H., Bashir, R., Jay, M., Bird, A.C., Jay, B., and Bhattacharya, S.S. Autosomal dominant retinitis pigmentosa: Four new mutations in rhodopsin, one of them in the retinal attachment site. *Genomics 11*:199–205, 1991.
240. Kemp, C.M., Jacobson, S.G., and Faulkner, D.J. Two types of visual dysfunction in autosomal dominant retinitis pigmentosa. *Invest. Ophthalmol. Vis. Sci. 29*:1235–1241, 1988.
241. Kemp, C.M., Jacobson, S.G., Faulkner, D.J., and Walt, R.W. Visual function and rhodopsin levels in humans with vitamin A deficiency. *Exp. Eye Res. 46*:185–197, 1988.
242. Kemp, C.M., Jacobson, S.G., Roman, A.J., Sung, C.H., and Nathans, J. Abnormal rod adaptation in autosomal dominant retinitis pigmentosa with Pro-23-His rhodopsin mutation. *Am. J. Ophthalmol. 113*:165–174, 1992.
243. Khouri, G., Mets, M.B., Smith, V.C., Wendell, M., and Pass, A.S. X-linked congenital stationary night blindness: Review and report of a family with hyperopia. *Arch. Ophthalmol. 106*:1417–1422, 1988.
244. Kingham, J.D., and Lochen, G.P. Vitelliform macular degeneration. *Am. J. Ophthalmol. 84*:526–531, 1977.
245. Klausner, R.D., and Sitia, R. Protein degradation in the endoplamic reticulum. *Cell 62*:611–614, 1990.
246. Klein, B.A. A case of so-called Oguchi's disease in the USA. *Am. J. Ophthalmol. 22*:953–955, 1939.
247. Klein, B.A., and Krill, A.E. Fundus flavimaculatus: Clinical, functional and histologic observations. *Am. J. Ophthalmol. 64*:3–23, 1967.
248. Kobayashi, V.A. Genetic study on retinitis pigmentosa. *Jpn. J. Ophthalmol. 7*:82–88, 1960.
249. Kohn, H., and Hargrave, P.A. Light-induced binding of guanosinetriphosphate to bovine photoreceptor membranes: Effect of limited proteolysis of the membranes. *Biochemistry 20*:2410–2417, 1981.
250. Kolb, H., and Galloway, N.R. Three cases of unilateral pigmentary degeneration. *Br. J. Ophthalmol. 48*:471–479, 1964.
251. Kolb, H., and Gouras, P. Electron microscopic observations of human retinitis pigmentosa, dominantly inherited. *Invest. Ophthalmol. 13*:489–498, 1974.
252. Korte, G.E., Repucci, V., and Henkind, P. RPE destruction causes choriocapillary atrophy. *Invest. Ophthalmol. Vis. Sci. 25*:1135–1145, 1984.
253. Krachmer, J.H., Smith, J.L., and Tocci, P.M. Laboratory studies in retinitis pigmentosa. *Arch. Ophthalmol. 75*:661–673, 1966.
254. Krill, A.E. X-chromosomal linked diseases affecting the eye: Status of the heterozygote female. *Trans. Am. Ophthalmol. Soc. 67*:535–608, 1969.
255. Krill, A.E. Incomplete rod-cone degenerations. In *Hereditary Retinal and Choroidal Diseases*, A.E. Krill and D. Archer (Eds.), Harper Row, Hagerstown, MD, pp. 625–636, 1977.
256. Krill, A.E., Archer, D.B., and Martin, D. Sector retinitis pigmentosa. *Am. J. Ophthalmol. 69*:977–987, 1970.
257. Krill, A.E., and Deutman, A.F. Dominant macular degenerations: The cone dystrophies. *Am. J. Ophthalmol. 73*:352–369, 1972.
258. Krill, A.E., and Martin, D. Photopic abnormalities in congenital stationary night blindness. *Invest. Ophthalmol. 10*:625–636, 1971.
259. Krill, A.E., Potts, A.M., and Johanson, C.E. Chloroquine retinopathy: Investigation of discrepancy between dark adaptation and electroretinographic findings in advanced stages. *Am. J. Ophthalmol. 71*:530–543, 1971.
260. Kroll, A.J., and Machemer, R. Experimental retinal detachment in the owl monkey. III. Electron microscopy of retina and pigment epithelium. *Am. J. Ophthalmol. 66*:410–427, 1968.
261. Kuper, J. Familiäre sektorenförmige retinitis pigmentosa. *Klin. Monatsbl. Augenheilkd. 136*:97–102, 1960.
262. Kuwabara, T. Photic damage to the retina. In *Ophthalmology*, Proceedings of the 23rd International Congress of Ophthalmology, Kyoto 1978, K. Shimizu and J.A. Oosterhuis (Eds.), Excerpta Medica, Amsterdam, pp. 369–374, 1979.
263. Kuwabara, T., and Gorn, R.A. Retinal damage by visible light: An electron microscopic study. *Arch. Ophthalmol. 79*:69–78, 1968.
264. Kuwabara, Y., Ishikara, K., and Akiyas, S. Histologic and electron microscopic studies of the retina in Oguchi's disease. *Acta Soc. Ophthalmol. Jpn. 67*:1323–1351, 1963.
265. Lahav, M., Albert, D.M., Buyukmihci, N., Jampol, L., McLean, E.B., Howard, R., and Craft, J. Ocular changes in Laurence Moon Bardet Biedl syndrome: A clinical and histopathologic study of a case. *Adv. Exp. Biol. 77*:51–84, 1977.
266. Lake, N. Abnormal visual function induced by treatment with guanidinethylsulfonate. *Life Sci. 29*:445–448, 1981.
267. Lake, N., Marshall, J., and Voaden, M.J. The entry of taurine into the neural retina and pigment epithelium of the frog. *Brain Res. 128*:497–503, 1977.
268. Lanum, J. The damaging effects of light on the retina: Empirical findings, theoretical and practical implications. *Surv. Ophthalmol. 22*:221–249, 1987.
269. Larsen, H. Demonstration mikroskopischer Präparate von einem monochromatischen Auge. *Klin. Monatsbl. Augenheilkd. 67*:301–302, 1921.

270. Lauber, H. The origin of hyalin formations within the eye. *Berl. Dtsch. Ophthalmol. Ges. 44*:216–220, 1924.

271. LaVail, M.M. Rod outer segment disc shedding in rat retina: Relationship to cyclic lighting. *Science 194*:1071–1074, 1976.

272. LaVail, M.M., and Mullen, R.J. Experimental chimeras: A new approach to the study of inherited retinal degeneration in laboratory animals. *Adv. Exp. Med. Biol. 77*:153–173, 1977.

273. LaVail, M.M., Sidman, R.L., and O'Neil, D. Photoreceptor pigment epithelial cell relationships in rats with inherited retinal degeneration. *J. Cell Biol. 53*:185–209, 1972.

274. Leber, T. Die Pigmentdegeneration der Netzhaut und die mit ihr verwandte Erkrankungen. In *Graefe-Saemisch Handbuch der gesamten Augenheilkunde*, Vol. 5, A. Wagenmann (Ed.), Wilhelm Engelmann, Leipzig, p. 1125, 1915.

275. Levine, J. Is retinitis pigmentosa due to vitamin deficiency? *Arch. Ophthalmol. 9*:453–458, 1933.

276. Lessel, M.R., Thaler, A., and Heilig, P. ERG and EOG in progressive paravenous retinochoroidal atrophy. *Doc. Ophthalmol. 62*:25–30, 1986.

277. Lester, D.H., Inglehearn, C.F., Bashir, R., Ackford, H., Esakowitz, L., Jay, M., Bird, A.C., Wright, A.F., Papiha, S.S., and Bhattacharya, S.S. Linkage to D3S47 (C17) in one large dominant retinitis family and exclusion in another: Confirmation of genetic heterogeneity. *Am. J. Hum. Genet. 47*:536–541, 1990.

278. Leuenberger, P.M., and Novikoff, A.B. Studies on microperoxisomes. VII. Pigment epithelial cells and other cell types in the retina of rodents. *J. Cell Biol. 65*:324–335, 1975.

279. Lewis, R.A., Holcomb, J.D., Bromley, W.C., Wilson, M.C., Roderisk, T.H., and Hejtmancik, J.F. Mapping X-linked ophthalmic diseases. III. Provisional assignment of the locus for blue cone monochromacy to Xq28. *Arch. Ophthalmol. 105*:1055–1059, 1987.

280. Lippincott-Shwartz, J.L., Bonifacio, J.S., Yuan, L.C., and Klausner, R.D. Degradation from the endoplasmic reticulum: Disposing of newly synthesized protein. *Cell 54*:209–220, 1988.

281. Lisch, K. Isolierte Entwicklungsstorungen. *Med. Wochenschr. 14*:720–725, 1960.

282. Lodish, H.F. Transport of secretory and membrane glycoproteins form the rough endoplasmic reticulum to the Golgi. *J. Biol. Chem. 263*:2107–2110, 1988.

283. Lolley, R.N., Farber, D.B., Rayborn, M., and Hollyfield, J. Cyclic GMP accumulation causes degeneration of photoreceptor cells: Simulation of an inherited disease. *Science 196*:664–665, 1977.

284. Lopez, P.F., Maumenee, I.H., de la Cruz, Z., and Green, W.R. Autosomal-dominant fundus flavimaculatus: Clinicopathologic correlation. *Ophthalmology 97*:798–809, 1990.

285. Lucas, D.R. Retinitis pigmentosa: Pathological findings in two cases. *Br. J. Ophthalmol. 40*:14–23, 1956.

286. Lyness, A.L., Ernst, W., Quinlan, M.P., Clover, G.M., Arden, G.B., Carter, R., Bird, A.C., and Parker, J.A. A clinical, psychophysical, and electroretinographic survey of patients with autosomal dominant retinitis pigmentosa. *Br. J. Ophthalmol. 69*:326–339, 1985.

287. McCulloch, C. Choroideraemia: A clinical and pathological review. *Trans. Am. Ophthalmol. Soc. 67*:142–195, 1969.

288. McCulloch, C., and McCulloch, R.J.P. A hereditary and clinical study of choroideremia. *Trans. Am. Acad. Ophthalmol. Oto-laryngol. 52*:160–190, 1948.

289. McFarland, C.B. Heredodegeneration of macula lutea; study of clinical and pathological aspects. *Arch. Ophthalmol. 53*:224–228, 1955.

290. McKenzie, D.S. The inheritance of retinitis pigmentosa in one family. *Trans. Ophthalmol. Soc. NZ 5*:79–82, 1951.

291. McNaughton, P.A. Light response of vertebrate photoreceptors. *Physiol. Rev. 70*:847–883, 1990.

292. McQuarrie, M.D. Two pedigrees of hereditary blindness in man. *J. Genet. 30*:147–153, 1935.

293. McWilliams, P., Farrar, G.J., Kenna, P., Bradley, D.G., Humphries, M.M., Sharp, E.M. McConnell, D.J., Lawler, M., Sheils, D., Ruan, C., Stevens, K.J., Daiger, S.P., and Humphries, P. Autosomal dominant retinitis pigmentosa (ADRP) localization of an ADRP gene to the long arm of chromosome 3. *Genomics 5*:619–620, 1989.

294. Magnusson, L. Atrophia areata, a variant of peripapillary chorioretinal degeneration. *Acta Ophthalmol. (Copenh.) 59*:659–664, 1981.

295. Mandelbaum, J. Dark adaptation: Some physiologic and clinical observations. *Arch. Ophthalmol. 26*:203–239, 1941.

296. Mann, I. *Developmental Abnormalities of the Eye*, Cambridge University Press, Cambridge, 1937.

297. Maraini, G., Fadda, G., and Gozzoli, F. Serum levels of retinol-binding protein in different genetic types of retinitis pigmentosa. *Invest. Ophthalmol. 13*:236–237, 1975.

298. Margolis, S., Siegel, I.M., and Ripps, H. Variable expressivity in fundus albipunctatus. *Ophthalmology 94*:1416–1422, 1987.

299. Marmor, M.F. Defining fundus albipunctatus. *Doc. Ophthalmol. 13*:227–234, 1977.

300. Marmor, M.F. Long-term follow-up of the physiologic abnormalities and fundus changes in fundus albipunctatus. *Ophthalmology 97*:380–384, 1990.

301. Marmor, M.F., Jacobson, S.G., Foerster, M.H., Kellner, U., and Weleber, R.G. Diagnostic findings of new syndrome with night blindness, maculopathy, and enhanced s-cone sensitivity. *Am. J. Ophthalmol. 110*:124–134, 1990.

302. Marsden, C.D. Brain melanin. In *Pigments in Pathology*, M. Wolman (Ed.), Academic Press, New York, pp. 396–420, 1969.
303. Marshall, J. Acid phosphatase activity in the retinal pigment epithelium. *Vis. Res. 10*:821–824, 1970.
304. Marshall, J. The retinal receptors and the retinal pigment epithelium. In *Scientific Foundations of Ophthalmology*, E.S. Perkins and D. W. Hill (Eds.), William Heinemann, London, pp. 8–17, 1977.
305. Marshall, J. Retinal injury from chronic exposure to light and the delayed effects from retinal exposure to intense light sources. In *Current Concepts in Ergophthalmology*, B. Tengroth (Eds.), Societes Ergophthalmologica Internationalis, Stockholm.
306. Marshall, J. Aging changes in human cones. In *Proceedings of the 23rd International Congress of Ophthalmology* (Kyote 1978), K. Shimizu (Ed.), Excerpta Medica, Amsterdam, pp. 375–378, 1979.
307. Marshall, J., and Ansell, P.L. Membranous inclusions in the retinal pigment epithelium: Phagosomes and myeloid bodies. *J. Anat. 110*:91–104, 1971.
308. Marshall, J., Mellerio, J., and Palmer, D.A. Damage to pigeon retinae by moderate illumination from fluorescent lamps. *Exp. Eye Res. 14*:164–169, 1972.
309. Massof, R.W., and Finkelstein, D. Two forms of autosomal dominant primary retinitis pigmentosa. *Doc. Ophthalmol. 51*:289–346, 1981.
310. Massof, R.W., Fleishman, J.A., Fine, S.L., and Yoder, F. Flicker fusion thresholds in Best's macular dystrophy. *Arch. Ophthalmol. 95*:991–994, 1977.
311. Mauthner, L. (1871). Quoted in Duke-Elder, S. *System of Ophthalmology*, Vol. III, Part 2, Henry Kimpton, London, p. 619, 1964.
312. Merry, D.E., Lesko, J.G., Sosnoski, D.M., Lewis, R.A., Lubinsky, M., and Trask, B. Choroideremia and deafness with stapes fixation: A contiguous gene deletion syndrome in Xq21. *Am. J. Hum. Genet. 45*:530–540, 1989.
313. Meves, H. Die pathologisch-anatomischen gefassveranderungen des Auges bei der beningen und malingen Nephrosklerose. *Graefes Arch. Ophthalmol. 148*:287–317, 1948.
314. Michel-Villaz, M., Saibil, H.R., and Chabre, M. Orientation of rhodopsin Á-helices in retinal rod outer segment membranes studied by infrared linear dichroism. *Proc. Natl. Acad. Sci. USA 76*:4405–4408, 1979.
315. Miller, S.A., Bresnik, G.H., and Chandra, S.R. Choroidal neovascular membrane in Best's vitelliform macular dystrophy. *Am. J. Ophthalmol. 82*:252–255, 1976.
316. Miyake, Y., and Kawase, Y. Reduced amplitude of oscillatory potentials in female carriers of X-linked recessive congenital stationary night blindness. *Am. J. Ophthalmol. 98*:208– 215, 1984.
317. Miyake, Y., Yagasaki, K., Horiguchi, M., Kawase, Y., and Kanda, T. Congenital stationary night blindness with negative electroretinogram: A new classification. *Arch. Ophthalmol. 104*:1013–1020, 1986.
318. Mizuno, K., and Nashida, S. Electron microscopic studies of human retinitis pigmentosa. *Am. J. Ophthalmol. 63*:791–803, 1967.
319. Mizuo, A. On new discovery in dark adaptation in Oguchi's disease. *Acta Soc. Ophthalmol. Jpn. 17*:1148–1150, 1913.
320. Mohler, C.W., and Fine, S.L. Long-term evaluation of patients with Best's vitelliform dystrophy. *Ophthalmology 88*:688–692, 1981.
321. Molday, R., Hicks, D., and Molday, L. Peripherin: A rim-specific membrane of the rod outer segment discs. *Invest. Ophthalmol. Vis. Sci. 28*:50–61, 1987.
322. Moloney, J.B., Mooney, D.J., and O'Connor, M.A. Retinal function in Stargardt's disease and fundus flavimaculatus. *Am. J. Ophthalmol. 96*:57–65, 1983.
323. Moore, A.T., Fitzke, F.W., Kemp, C.M., Arden, G.B., Keen, T.J., Inglehearn, C.F., Jay, M., and Bird, A.C. Abnormal dark adaptation kinetics in autosomal dominant sector retinitis pigmentosa due to rod opsin mutation. *Br. J. Ophthalmol. 76*:465–469, 1992.
324. Moore, T., and Haig, D. Genomic imprinting in mammalian development: A parental tug of war. *Trend. Genet. 7*:45–49, 1991.
325. Mukai, S. Dryja, T.P., Bruns, G.A.P., Alridge, J.F., and Berson, E.L. Linkage between the X-linked retinitis pigmentosa locus and the L1.28 locus. *Am. J. Ophthalmol. 100*:225–229, 1985.
326. Mullen, R.J., and LaVail, M.M. Inherited retinal dystrophy: Primary defect in pigment epithelium determined with experimental rat chimeras. *Science 192*:799–801, 1976.
327. Müller, H. Anatomische Beitrage zur Ophthalmologie. *Graefes Arch. Ophthalmol. 4*:1–54, 1858.
328. Müller-Limmroth, W., and Kuper, J. Über den Einfluss des-Adaptinols auf dac elektroretinogramm bei tapetoretinalen Degenerationem. *Klin. Monatsbl. Augenheilkd. 138*:37–41, 1961.
329. Musarella, M.A., Weleber, R.G., Murphey, W.H., Young, R.S., Anson-Cartwright, L., Mets, M., Kraft, S.P., Polemeno, R., Litt, M., and Worton, R.G. Assignment of the gene for complete X-linked congenital stationary night blindness (CSNB1) to Xp11.3. *Genomics 5*:727–737, 1989.
330. Nakamura, B. Über ein neues Phänomen der Farberverndrung des menschlichen Augenhintergrundes im Zusammenhang mit der fortschreitenden Dunkeladaptation. *Klin. Monatsbl. Augenheilkd. 65*:83–85, 1920.
331. Nathans, J., Piantandida, T.P., Eddy, R.L., Shows, T.B., and Hogness, D.S. Molecular genetics of inherited variation in human color vision. *Science 232*:203–210, 1986.

332. Nathans, J., Thomas, D., and Hogness, D.S. Molecular genetics of human color vision: The genes encoding blue, green, and red pigments. *Science 232*:193–202, 1986.

333. Noble, K.G. Central areolar choroidal dystrophy. *Am. J. Ophthalmol. 84*:310–318, 1977.

334. Noble, K.G., and Carr, R.E. Stargardt's disease and fundus flavimaculatus. *Arch. Ophthalmol. 97*:1281–1285, 1979.

335. Noble, K.G., and Carr, R.E. Pigmented paravenous chorioretinal atrophy. *Am. J. Ophthalmol. 90*:338–344, 1983.

336. Noble, K.G., Carr, R.E., and Siegel, I.M. Autosomal dominant congenital stationary night blindness and normal fundus with an electronegative electroretinogram. *Am. J. Ophthalmol. 109*:44–48, 1990.

337. Noell, W.K. Aspects of experimental and hereditary retinal degeneration. In *Biochemistry of the Retina*, C.N. Graymore (Ed.), Academic Press, New York, pp. 51–72, 1965.

338. Noell, W.K., and Albrecht, R. Irreversible effects of visible light on the retina: Role of vitamin A. *Science 172*:76–80, 1971.

339. Noell, W.K., Delmelle, M.C., and Albrecht, R. Vitamin A deficiency effect on the retina: Dependence on light. *Science 172*:72–75, 1971.

340. Noell, W.K., Organisciak, D.T., Ando, H., Braniecki, M.A., and Durlin, C. Ascorbate and dietary V:F7 protective mechanisms in retinal light damage of rats: Electrophysiological, histological and DNA measurements. In *Degenerative Retinal Disorders: Clinical and Laboratory Investigations*, J.G. Hollyfield, R.E. Anderson, and M.M. LaVail (Eds.), Alan R. Liss, New York, pp. 469–483, 1987.

341. Nussbaum, R.L., Lewis, R.A., Lesko, J.G., and Ferrell, R. Mapping ophthalmological disease. II. Linkage of relationship of X-linked retinitis pigmentosa to X chromosome short arm markers. *Hum. Genet. 70*:45–50, 1985.

342. Nussbaum, R.L., Lewis, R.A., Lesko, J.G., and Ferrell, R. Choroideremia is linked to the restriction fragment length polymorphism DXYS1 at Xq13–21. *Am. J. Hum. Genet. 37*:473–481, 1985.

343. O'Brien, P.J. (Ed.). Symposium on the pigment epithelium: its relationship to the retina in health and disease. I. *Exp. Eye Res. 22*:395–568, 1976.

344. Ocumpaugh, D.E., and Young, R.W. Distribution and synthesis of sulphated mucopolysaccharides in the retina of the rat. *Invest. Ophthalmol. 5*:196–203, 1966.

345. O'Day, W.T., and Young, R.W. Rhythmic daily shedding of outer segment membranes by visual cells in the gold fish. *J. Cell Biol. 76*:593–604, 1978.

346. O'Gorman, S., Flaherty, W.A., Fishman, G.A., and Berson, E.L. Histopathologic findings in Best's vitelliform macular dystrophy. *Arch. Ophthalmol. 106*:1261–1268, 1988.

347. Oguchi, C. Über einen Fall von eigenartiger Hemeralopie. *Nippon Ganka Gakkai Zasshi 11*:123, 1907.

348. Oguchi, C. Zur Anatomie der sogenannten. Oguchi'schen Krankheit. *Graefes Arch. Klin. Exp. Ophthalmol. 115*:234–245, 1925.

349. Olver, J., Pauleikhoff, D., and Bird, A.C. Morphometric analysis of age-changes in the choriocapillaris. *Invest. Ophthalmol. Vis. Sci. (Suppl.) 31*:47, 1991.

350. O'Malley, P., Allen, R.A., Straatsma, B.R., and O'Malley, C.C. Pavingstone degeneration of the retina. *Arch. Ophthalmol. 73*:169–182, 1965.

351. Organisciak, D.T., Wang, H.M., Xie, A., Reeves, D.S., and Donoso, L.A. Intense-light mediated changes in rat rod outer segment lipids and proteins. In *Inherited and Environmentally Induced Retinal Degenerations*, M.M. LaVail, R.E. Anderson, and J.G. Hollyfield (Eds.), Alan R. Liss, New York, pp. 493–512, 1989.

352. Pawlyk, B.S., Sandberg, M.A., and Berson, E.L. Effects of IBMX on the rod ERG of the perfused cat eye: Antagonism with light, calcium or L-cis-diltiazem. *Vis. Res. 31*:1093–1097, 1991.

353. Pasantes-Morales, H., Ademe, R.M., and Quesada, O. Protective effect of taurine on the light induced disruption of isolated frog rod outer segments. *J. Neurosci. Res. 6*:337–348, 1981.

354. Patrinely, J.R., Lewis, R.A., and Font, R.L. Foveomacular vitelliform macular dystrophy, adult type: A clinicopathological study including electron microscopic observations. *Ophthalmology 92*:1712–1718, 1985.

355. Pauleikhoff, D., Chen, J.C., Chisholm, I.H., and Bird, A.C. Choroidal perfusion abnormality with age-related Bruch's membrane change. *Am. J. Ophthalmol. 109*:211–217, 1990.

356. Pearce, W.G., Reedyk, M., and Coupland, S.G. Variable expressivity in X-linked congenital stationary night blindness. *Can. J. Ophthalmol. 25*:3–10, 1990.

357. Pearlman, J.T. Mathematical models of retinitis pigmentosa: A study of the rate of progress in the different genetic forms. *Trans. Am. Ophthalmol. Soc. 77*:643–656, 1979.

358. Pearlman, J.T., Owen, G.W., Brounley, D.W., and Sheppard, J.J. Cone dystrophy with dominant inheritance. *Am. J. Ophthalmol. 77*:293–303, 1974.

359. Pearlman, J.T., Saxton, J., Hoffman, G., and Carson, S. Unilateral retinitis pigmentosa sine pigmento. *Br. J. Ophthalmol. 60*:354–360, 1976.

360. Pedralgia, C. Klinische Beobachtungen. Retinitis pigmentosa. *Klin. Monatsbl. Augenheilkd. 3*:114–117, 1865.

360a. Penn, J.S., Baker, B.N., Howard, A.G., and Williams, T.P. Retinal light damage in albino rats: Lysosomal enzymes, rhodopsin, and age. *Exp. Eye Res. 41*:275–284, 1985.

361. Penn, J.S., Naash, M.I., and Anderson, R.E. Effect of light history on retinal antioxidants and light damage susceptibility in the rat. *Exp. Eye Res. 44*:779–788, 1987.

362. Penn, J.S., and Thum, L.A. A comparison of the retinal effects of light damage and high illuminance light history. *Prog. Clin. Biol. Res.* *247*:425–438, 1987.

363. Penn, J.S., Thum, L.A., and Naash, M.I. Photoreceptor physiology in the rat is governed by the light environment. *Exp. Eye Res.* *49*:205–215, 1989.

364. Penn, J.S., Wiegand, R.D., Thum, L.A., and Anderson, R.E. Light environment affects the metabolism of docosohexanoate-containing molecular species of glycerophospholipids in rat rod outer segments. *Invest. Ophthalmol. Vis. Sci. (Suppl.)* *31*:471, 1990.

365. Penn, J.S., and Williams, T.P. Photostasis: Regulation of daily photon-catch by rat retinas in response to various cyclic illuminances. *Exp. Eye Res.* *43*:915–92, 1986.

366. Peyman, G.A., Spitznas, M., and Straatsma, B.R. Peroxidase diffusion in the normal and photocoagulated retina. *Invest. Ophthalmol.* *10*:181–189, 1971.

367. Pittler, S.J., and Baehr, W. Identification of a nonsense mutation in the rod photoreceptor cGMP phosphodiesterase Á-subunit gene of the rd mouse. *Proc. Natl. Acad. Sci. USA* *88*:8322–8326, 1991.

368. Polkinghorne, P.J., Capon, M.R.C., Berninger, T., Lyness, A.L., Sehmi, K., and Bird, A.C. Sorsby's fundus dystrophy: A clinical study. *Ophthalmology* *96*:1763–1768, 1989.

369. Porta, A., Pierrottet, C., Aschero, M., and Orzalesi, N. Preserved para-arteriole retinal pigment epithelium retinitis pigmentosa. *Am. J. Ophthalmol.* *113*:161–164, 1992.

370. Prensky, J.G., and Bresnic, G.H. Butterfly-shaped macular dystrophy in four generations. *Arch. Ophthalmol.* *101*:1198–1203, 1983.

371. Pruett, R.C. Retinitis pigmentosa: Clinical observations and correlations. *Trans. Am. Ophthalmol. Soc.* *81*:693–735, 1983.

372. Rafuse, E.V., and McCulloch, C. Choroideremia, a pathological report. *Can. J. Ophthalmol.* *3*:347–352, 1968.

373. Ragnetti, E. An atypical form of retinitis pigmentosa. *Boll. Ocul.* *41*:617–625, 1962.

374. Rapp, L.M., Thum, L.A., and Anderson, R.E. Synergism between environmental lighting and taurine depletion in causing photoreceptor cell degeneration. *Exp. Eye Res.* *46*:229–238, 1988.

375. Reich-d'Almeida, F.B., and Hockley, D.J. In situ reactivity of the retinal pigment epithelium. II. Phagocytosis in the dystrophic rat. *Exp. Eye Res.* *21*:347–357, 1975.

376. Reichel, E., Bruce, A.M., Sandberg, M.A., and Berson, E.L. An electroretinographic and molecular genetic study of X-linked cone degeneration. *Am. J. Ophthalmol.* *108*:540–547, 1989.

377. Reme, C.E. Autophagy in visual cells and pigment epithelium. *Invest. Ophthalmol. Vis. Sci.* *16*:807–815, 1977.

378. Reuter, J.H., and Sanyal, S. Development and degeneration of retina in rds mutant mice: The electroretinogram. *Neurosci. Lett.* *45*:231–237, 1984.

379. Ricci, A., Ammann, F., and Franceschetti, A. Reflet tapétoïde reversible (phénomène de Mizuo inverse) chez des conductrices de rétinopathie pigmentaire récessive liée au sexe. *Bull. Mem. Soc. Fr. Ophtalmol.* *76*:31–35, 1963.

380. Richards, B.W., Brodstein, D.E., Nussbaum, J.J., Ferencz, J.R., Maeda, K., and Weiss, L. Autosomal dominant crystalline dystrophy. *Ophthalmology* *98*:568–665, 1991.

381. Richards, J.E., Kuo, C.Y., Boehnke, M., and Sieving, P.A. Rhodopsin Thr58Arg mutation in a family with autosomal dominant retinitis pigmentosa. *Ophthalmology* *98*:1797–1805, 1991.

382. Riggs, L.A. Electroretinography in cases of night blindness. *Am. J. Ophthalmol.* *38*:70–78, 1954.

383. Ripps, H., Brin, K.P., and Weale, R.A. Rhodopsin and visual threshold in retinitis pigmentosa. *Invest. Ophthalmol. Vis. Sci.* *17*:735–745, 1978.

384. Rodrigues, M.M., Bardenstein, D., Wiggert, B., Lee, L., Fletcher, R.T., and Chader, G. Retinitis pigmentosa with segmental massive retinal gliosis. *Ophthalmology* *94*:180–186, 1987.

385. Rodrigues, M.M., Wiggert, B., and Hackett, J. Dominantly inherited retinitis pigmentosa: Ultrastructure and biochemical analysis. *Ophthalmology* *92*:1165–1172, 1985.

386. Rohlich, P. The interphotoreceptor matrix: Electron microscopic and histochemical observations on the vertebrate retina. *Exp. Eye Res.* *10*:80–96, 1970.

387. Rosenberg, T., Niebuhr, E., Yang, H.M., Parving, A., and Schwartz, M. Choroideremia, congenital deafness and mental retardation in a family with an X chromosomal deletion. *Ophthalmic Paediatr. Genet.* *8*:139–143, 1987.

388. Rothschild, K.J., Sanches, R., Hsiao, T.L., and Clark, N.A. A spectroscopic study of rhodopsin alpha-helix orientation. *Biophys. J.* *31*:53–64, 1980.

389. Rubino, A. Suuna paraticolarae anomalia bilaterale alle e simmetica dello stratato pigmento retinico. *Bull. Ocul.* *19*:318, 1940.

390. Saari, J.C., and Futterman, S. An intracellular retinol binding protein isolated from bovine retina: Isolation and partial characterization. *Exp. Eye Res.* *22*:425–433, 1976.

391. Sanyal, S., De Ruiter, A., and Hawkins, R.K. Development and degeneration of retina in rds mutant mice: Light microscopy. *J. Comp. Neurol.* *194*:193–207, 1980.

392. Sanyal, S., and Hawkins, R.K. Development and degeneration of retina in rds mutant mice: Altered disc shedding pattern in the albino heterozygotes and its relation to light exposure. *Vis. Res.* *28*:1171–1178, 1988.

393. Sanyal, S., and Jansen, H. Absence of receptor outer segments in the retina of rds mutant mice. *Neurosci. Lett.* *21*:23–26, 1981.

394. Sarks, S.H. Aging and degeneration in the macular region: A clinicopathological study. *Br. J. Ophthalmol. 60*:324–341, 1976.
395. Sarks, S.H. Changes in the region of the choriocapillaris in aging and degeneration. In *XXIII Concilium Ophthalmologicum*, K. Shimizu and J.A. Oosterhuis (Eds.), Excerpta Medica, Kyoto, pp. 228–238, 1979.
396. Sarks, S.H., Sarks, J., and Killingsworth, C. Evolution of geographic atrophy of the retinal pigment epithelium. *Eye 2*:552, 1988.
397. Schappert-Kimmijser, J. Les dégénérescences tapéto-rétiniennes du type X chromosomal aux Pays-Bas. *Bull. Mem. Soc. Fr. Ophthalmol. 76*:122–129, 1963.
398. Schubert, G., and Bornschein, H. Beitrag zur Analyse des menschlichen Elektroretinogramms. *Ophthalmologica 123*:396–412, 1952.
399. Semple-Rowland, S.L., and Dawson, W.W. Cyclic light intensity threshold for retinal damage in albino rats raised under 6 lux. *Exp. Eye Res. 44*:643–661, 1987.
400. Sharp, D.M., Arden, G.B., Kemp, C.R., Hogg, C.R., and Bird, A.C. Mechanisms and sites of loss of scotopic sensitivity: A clinical analysis of congenital night blindness. *Clin. Vis. Sci. 5*:217–230, 1990.
401. Sheffield, V.C., Fishman, G.A., and Kimura, A. Identification of novel rhodopsin mutations associated with retinitis pigmentosa using GC-clemped denaturing gradient gel electrophoresis. *Am. J. Hum. Genet. 49*:699–706, 1991.
402. Sheikh, K., Toskes, P., and Dawson, W. Taurine deficiency and retinal defects with small intestine bacterial overgrowth. *Gasteroenterology 80*:1363, 1981.
403. Siegel, I.M., Graham, C.H., Ripps, H., and Hsia, Y. Analysis of photopic and scotopic function in an incomplete achromat. *J. Opt. Soc. Am. 56*:699–704, 1966.
404. Siegel, I.M., Greenstein, V.C., Seiple, W.H., and Carr, R.E. Cone function in congenital nyctalopia. *Doc. Ophthalmol. 65*:307–318, 1987.
405. Skalka, H.W., Hereditary pigmented paravenous retinochoroidal atrophy. *Am. J. Ophthalmol. 87*:286–291, 1979.
406. Sloan, L.L., and Newhall, S.M. Comparison of cases of atypical and typical achromatopsia. *Am. J. Ophthalmol. 25*:945–961, 1942.
407. Smith, B.F., Ripps, H.A., and Goodman, G. Retinitis punctata albescens: A functional and diagnostic evaluation. *Arch. Ophthalmol. 61*:93–101, 1959.
408. Snodgrass, N.B. Ocular findings in fucosidosis. *Br. J. Ophthalmol. 60*:508–511, 1976.
409. Sorsby, A. Choroidal angiosclerosis with special reference to its hereditary character. *Br. J. Ophthalmol. 23*:433–444, 1939.
410. Sorsby, A., and Crick, R.P. Central areolar choroidal sclerosis. *Br. J. Ophthalmol. 37*:129–139, 1953.
411. Sorsby, A., Mason, M.E.J., and Gardener, N. A fundus dystrophy with unusual features. *Br. J. Ophthalmol. 33*:67–97, 1949.
412. Sperling, H.G., and Johnson, C. Histological findings in the receptor layer of primate retina associated with light-induced dichromacy. *Mod. Probl. Ophthalmol. 84*:810–819, 1974.
413. Spitznas, M., and Hogan, M.J. Outer segments of photoreceptors and the pigment epithelium: Interrelationship in the human eye. *Arch. Ophthalmol. 84*:810–819, 1970.
414. Stargardt, K. Über familiäre, progressive Degeneration in der Makulagegend des Auges. *Graefes Arch. Klin. Exp. Ophthalmol. 71*:534–550, 1909.
415. Stargardt, K., Über familiäre, progressive Degeneration in der Maculagegend des Auges. *Z. Augenheilkd. 30*:95–116, 1913.
416. Steinberg, R.H., Wood, I., and Hogan, M.J. Pigment epithelium ensheathment and phagocytosis of extrafoveal cones in human retina. *Proc. R. Soc. Lond [Biol.] 277*:459–471, 1977.
417. Steinmetz, R.L., Garner, A., Maguire, J.I., and Bird, A.C. Histopathology of incipient fundus flavimaculatus. *Ophthalmology 98*:953–956, 1991.
418. Steinmetz, R.L., Polkinghorne, P.C., Fitzke, F.W., Kemp, C.M., and Bird, A.C. Abnormal dark adaptation and rhodopsin kinetics in Sorsby's fundus dystrophy. *Invest. Ophthalmol. Vis. Sci. 33*:1633–1636, 1992.
419. Steinmetz, R.L., Walker, D., Fitzke, F., and Bird, A.C. Prolonged dark adaptation in patients with age-related macular degeneration. *Invest. Ophthalmol. Vis. Sci. (Suppl.) 32*:711, 1991.
420. Stone, E.M., Kimura, A.E., Nichols, B.E., Khadivi, P., Fishman, G.A., and Sheffield, V.C. Regional distribution of retinal degeneration in patients with the proline to histidine mutation in codon 23 of the rhodopsin gene. *Ophthalmology 98*:1806–1813, 1991.
421. Stone, E.M., Nichols, B.E., Streb, L.M., Kimura, A.E., and Sheffield, V.C. Genetic linkage of vitelliform macular degeneration (Best's disease) to chromosome 11q13. *Nature Genet. 1(29)*:42–44, 1992.
422. Streeten, B.W. The sudanophilic granules of the retinal pigment epithelium. *Arch. Ophthalmol. 66*:125–132, 1961.
423. Sung, C.-H., Davenport, C.M., Hennessey, J.C., Maumenee, I.H., Jacobson, S.G., Heckenlively, J.R., Nowakowski, R., Fishman, G., Gouras, P., and Nathans, J. Rhodopsin mutations in autosomal dominant retinitis pigmentosa. *Proc. Natl. Acad. Sci. USA 88*:6481–6485, 1991.
424. Sung, C.H., Schneider, B.G., Agerwal, N., Papermaster, D.S., and Nathans, J. Functional heterogeneity on mutant rhodopsins responsible for autosomal retinitis pigmentosa. *Proc. Natl. Acad. Sci. USA 88*:8840–8844, 1991.

425. Sunness, J.S., Johnson, M.A., Massof, R.W., and Marcus, S. Retinal sensitivity over drusen and nondrusen areas: A study using fundus perimetry. *Arch. Ophthalmol. 106*:1081–1084, 1988.

426. Sunness, J.S. Massof, R.W. Johnson, M.A., Finkelstein, D., and Fine, S.L. Peripheral retinal function in age-related macular degeneration. *Arch. Ophthalmol. 103*:811–816, 1985.

427. Sveinsson, K. Choroiditis areata. *Acta Ophthalmol. (Copenh.) 17*:73–79, 1939.

428. Sveinsson, K. Helicoid peripapillary chorio-retinal degeneration. *Acta Ophthalmol (Copenh.) 57*:69–75, 1979.

429. Szamier, R.B., and Berson, E.L. Retinal ultrastructure in advanced retinitis pigmentosa. *Invest. Ophthalmol. Vis. Sci. 16*:947–962, 1977.

430. Szamier, R.B., Berson, E.L., Klein, R., and Myers, S. Sex-linked retinitis pigmentosa: Ultrastructure of photoreceptors and pigment epithelium. *Invest. Ophthalmol. Vis. Sci. 18*:145–160, 1971.

431. Toussaint, D., and Danis, P. An ocular pathology study of Refsum's syndrome. *Am. J. Ophthalmol. 72*:342–347, 1971.

432. Traboulsi, E.I., and Maumenee, I.H. Hereditary pigmented paravenous chorioretinal atrophy. *Arch. Ophthalmol. 104*:1636–1640, 1986.

433. Travis, G.H., Brennan, M.B., Danielson, P.E., Kozak, C.A., and Sutcliffe, J.G. Identification of a photoreceptor-specific mRNA encoded by the gene responsible for retinal degeneration slow (rds). *Nature 338*:70–73, 1989.

434. Travis, G.H., Christerson, L. Danielson, P.E., Klisak, I., Sparkes, R.S., and Hahn, L.B. The human retinal degeneration slow (rds) gene: Chromosome assignment and structure of the mRNA. *Genomics 10*:733–739, 1991.

435. Travis, G., Lloyd, M., and Bok, D. Complete reversal of photoreceptor dysplasia in transgenic retinal degeneration slow (rds) mice. *Neuron 9*:113–120, 1992.

436. Travis, G., Sutcliffe, J.G., and Bok, D. The retinal degeneration slow (rds) gene product is a photoreceptor disc membrane associated glycoprotein. *Neuron 6*:61–70, 1991.

437. Travis, D.F., and Travis, A. Ultrastructural changes in the left ventricular rat myocardial cells with age. *J. Ultrastruct. Res. 39*:124–148, 1972.

438. Tso, M.O.M. Pathogenetic factors of aging macular degeneration. *Ophthalmology 92*:628, 1985.

439. Tso, M.O.M. Photic injury to the retina and pathogenesis of age-related macular degeneration. In *Retinal Diseases: Biomedical Foundations and Clinical Management*, M.O.M. T'so (Ed.), J.B. Lippincott, Philadelphia, pp. 187–214, 1988.

440. Tso, M.O.M., Wallow, I.H.L., and Powell, J.O. Differential susceptibility of rod and cone cells to argon laser. *Arch. Ophthalmol. 89*:228–234, 1973.

441. Uliss, A.E., Moore, A.T., and Bird, A.C. The dark choroid in posterior retinal dystrophies. *Ophthalmology 95*:1423–1427, 1987.

442. Ulshafer, R.J., Garcia, C.A., and Hollyfield, J.G. Sensitivity of photoreceptors to elevated levels of cGMP in the human retina. *Invest. Ophthalmol. Vis. Sci. 119*:1236–1241, 1980.

443. Usukura, J., and Bok, D. Changes in the localization and content of opsin during retinal development in the rds mutant mouse: Immunocytochemistry and immunoassay. *Exp. Eye Res. 45*:501–515, 1987.

444. Vaghefi, H.A., Green, R., Kelly, J.S., Sloane, L.L., and Patz, A. Correlation of clinicopathological findings in a patient: Congenital night blindness, branch retinal vein occlusion, cilioretinal artery, drusen of the nerve head and intraretinal pigmented lesion. *Arch. Ophthalmol. 96*:2079–2104, 1978.

445. Van Everdingen, J.A.M., Went, L.N., Keunen, J.E.E., and Oosterhuis, J.A. X linked progressive cone dystrophy with specific attention to carrier detection. *J. Med. Genet. 29*:291–294, 1992.

446. Van Schooneveld, M.J., Went, L.N., and Oosterhuis, J.A. Dominant cone dystrophy starting with blue cone involvement. *Br. J. Ophthalmol. 75*:332–336, 1991.

447. Verhoeff, F.H. Microscopic observations in a case of retinitis pigmentosa. *Arch. Ophthalmol. 5*:392–407, 1931.

448. Verriest, M.G. Recent progress in the study of acquired deficiencies of colour vision. *Bull. Soc. Ophtalmol. Fr. 74*:595–620, 1974.

449. Vine, A.K., and Schatz, H. Adult-onset foveomacular pigment epithelial dystrophy. *Am. J. Ophthalmol. 89*: 680–691, 1980.

450. Voaden, M.J., Hussain, A.A., and Chan, I.P.R. Studies on retinitis pigmentosa in man. I. Taurine and blood platelets. *Br. J. Ophthalmol. 66*:771–775, 1982.

451. Voaden, M.J., Polkinghorne, P.J., Belin, J., and Smith, A.D. Studies on blood from patients with dominantly-inherited retinitis pigmentosa. In *Inherited and Environmentally Induced Retinal Degenerations*, M.M. LaVail, R.E. Anderson, and J.G. Hollyfield (Eds.), Alan R. Liss, New York, pp. 57–68, 1989.

452. Vollrath, D., Nathans, J., and Davis, R.W. Tandem array of human visual pigment genes at Xq28. *Science 240*:1669–1672, 1988.

453. Vossius, A. Über die Bestsche Familiäre Maculadegeneration. *Graefes Arch. Ophthalmol. 105*:643, 1921. Quoted in Duke-Elder, S. *System of Ophthalmology*, Vol. 10, Henry Kimpton, London, p. 632.

454. Vukovich, V. Das ERG bei Retinitis pigmentosa (retinopathia pigmentosa) mit bitemporalen Gesichstfeld ausfall. *Graefes Arch. Klin. Exp. Ophthalmol. 161*:27–32, 1959.

455. Waardenburg, P.J. Choroideremia als Erbmerkmal. *Acta Ophthalmol. (Copenh.) 20*:235–274, 1942.

456. Waardenburg, P.J., Franceschetti, A., and Klein, D. *Genetics and Ophthalmology*, Vol. 2, Charles C. Thomas, Springfield, IL, p. 1736, 1963.

457. Walt, R.P., Kemp, C.M., Lyness, A.L., Bird, A.C., and Sherlock, S. Vitamin A treatment for night blindness in primary biliary cirrhosis. *Br. Med. J.* 288:1030–1031, 1984.

458. Warburg, M., and Simonsen, S.E. Sex-linked recessive retinitis pigmentosa. *Acta Ophthalmol. (Copenh.)* 46:494–499, 1968.

459. Watanabe, I., Taniguchi, Y., Morioka, K., and Kato, M. Congenital stationary night blindness with myopia: A clinicopathologic study. *Doc. Ophthalmol.* 63:55–62, 1986.

460. Watzke, R.C., Folk, J.C., and Lang, R.M. Pattern dystrophy of the retinal pigment epithelium. *Ophthalmology* 66:1400–1406, 1982.

461. Weiner, R.L., and Falls, H.F. Intermediate sex-linked retinitis pigmentosa. *Arch. Ophthalmol.* 53:539–553, 1955.

462. Weingeist, T.A., Kobrin, J.L., and Watzke, R.C. Histopathology of Best's macular dystrophy. *Arch. Ophthalmol.* 100:1108–1114, 1982.

463. Weisel, G. Quoted in Duke-Elder, S. *System of Ophthalmology*, Vol. 10, Henry Kimpton, London, p. 643, 1922.

464. Welch, R.B. Bietti's tapetoretinal degeneration with marginal corneal dystrophy. *Crystalline retinopathy. Trans. Am. Ophthalmol. Soc.* 75:164–179, 1977.

465. Weleber, R.G., Pillers, D.A., Powell, B.R., Hanna, C.E., Magenis, R.E., and Buist, N.R. Åland Island eye disease (Forsius-Eriksson syndrome) associated with contiguous deletion syndrome at Xp21: Similarity to incomplete congenital stationary night blindness. *Arch. Ophthalmol.* 107:1170–1179, 1989.

466. Weleber, R.G., and Tongue, A.C. Congenital stationary night blindness presenting as Leber's congenital amaurosis. *Arch. Ophthalmol.* 105:360–365, 1987.

467. Wells, J., Wroblewski, J., Keen, J., Inglehearn, C., Jubb, C., and Eckstein, A. Mutations in the human retinal degeneration slow (rds) gene can cause either retinitis pigmentosa or macular dystrophy. *Nature Genet.*: in press, 1993.

468. Went, L.N., van Schooneveld, M.J., and Oosterhuis, J.A. Late onset dominant cone dystrophy with early blue cone involvement. *J. Med. Genet.* 29:295–298, 1992.

469. Wiggert, B.D., Bergsma, R., and Chader, G.J. Studies on the intracellular binding of retinol in the retina and pigment epithelium. *Exp. Eye Res.* 22:411–418, 1976.

470. Williams, D.S., Colley, N.J., and Farber, D.B. Photoreceptor degeneration in a pure cone retina. *Invest. Ophthalmol. Vis. Sci.* 28:1059–1069, 1987.

471. Williams, T.P., and Howell, W.L. Action spectrum of retinal light damage in albino rats. *Invest. Ophthalmol. Vis. Sci.* 24:285–287, 1983.

472. Willison, K. Opposite imprinting of the mouse Igf2 and Igf2r genes. *Trends Genet.* 7:107–109, 1991.

473. Wilson, D.J., Weleber, R.G., Klein, M.L., Welch, R.B., and Green, W.R. Bietti's crystalline dystrophy: A clinicopathologic correlative study. *Arch. Ophthalmol.* 107:213–221, 1989.

474. Wing, G.L., Blanchard, G.L., and Weiter, J.J. The topography and age relationship of lipofuscin concentration in the retinal pigment epithelium. *Invest. Ophthalmol. Vis. Sci.* 17:601–607, 1978.

475. Winn, S., Tasman, W., Spaeth, G., McDonald, P.R., and Justice, J. Oguchi's disease in Negroes. *Arch. Ophthalmol.* 81:501–507, 1969.

476. Wolter, J.R. Retinitis pigmentosa. *Arch. Ophthalmol.* 57:539–553, 1957.

477. Wright, A.F., Bhattacharya, S.S., Clayton, J.F., Dempster, M., Tippett, P., McKeown, C.M.E., Jay, M., Jay, B., and Bird, A.C. Linkage relationships between X-linked retinitis pigmentosa and six short arm markers: Exclusion of the disease locus from Xp21. *Am. J. Hum. Gen.* 41:635–644, 1987.

478. Yagasaki, Y., and Jacobson, S.G. Cone-rod dystrophy: Phenotypic diversity by retinal function testing. *Arch. Ophthalmol.* 107:701–708, 1989.

479. Yamanaka, J. Existiert die Pigmentverschiebung im Retinalepithel im menschlichen Auge? Der erste Sektionsfall von sogenannter Oguchischer Krankheit. *Klin. Monatsbl. Augenheilkd.* 73:742–752, 1924.

480. Yamanaka, M. Histologic study of Oguchi's disease: Its relationship to pigmentary degeneration of the retina. *Am. J. Ophthalmol.* 68:19–26, 1969.

481. Yamazaki, A., Sen, I., and Bitensky, M.W. Cyclic GMP-specific, high affinity, noncatalytic binding sites on light activated phosphodiesterase. *J. Biol. Chem.* 256:11619–11624, 1980.

482. Young, R.S., Chaparro, A., Price, J., and Walters, J. Oscillatory potentials of X-linked carriers of congenital stationary night blindness. *Invest. Ophthalmol. Vis. Sci.* 30:806–812, 1989.

483. Young, R.W. The renewal of photoreceptor outer segments. *J. Cell Biol.* 33:61–72, 1967.

484. Young, R.W. Passage of newly formed protein through the connecting cilium of retinal rods. *J. Ultrastruct. Res.* 23:462–473, 1968.

485. Young, R.W. Visual cells. *Sci. Am.* 223:80–91, 1970.

486. Young, R.W. Shedding of discs from rod outer segments in the rhesus monkey. *J. Ultrastruct. Res.* 34:190–203, 1971.

487. Young, R.W. The renewal of rod and cone outer segments in the rhesus monkey. *J. Cell Biol.* 49:303–318, 1971.

488. Young, R.W. Visual cells and the concept of renewal. *Invest. Ophthalmol.* 15:700–725, 1976.

489. Young, R.W. The daily rhythm of shedding and degradation of cone outer segment membranes. *J. Ultrastruct. Res.* 61:172–185, 1977.

490. Young, R.W. Visual cell renewal systems and the problem of retinitis pigmentosa: Clinical implications of current research. *Adv. Med. Biol.* 77:93–113, 1977.

42
Embryological Development of the Eye

Alison C. E. McCartney
United Medical and Dental Schools of Guy's and St. Thomas's Hospitals, London, England

I. INTRODUCTION

As detailed in Chapter 43, many congenital malformations can affect the eye. They may be confined to the eye or may reflect a wider disorder of growth patterns within the developing brain or entire body that can be inherited or acquired. An example of disordered growth mediated by an inherited genetic defect can be seen in neurofibromatosis. Neurofibromatosis type 1 gene has been mapped to chromosome 17 and lies just upstream of the gene for nerve growth factor (NGF). The widespread but variable effects within the eye and adnexa arise as a result of disordered transcriptive control of the cephalic neural crest and its derivatives. A similar sequence has also been ascribed to other postulated neurocristopathies (see Chap. 45) [88].

Conversely noninherited congenital abnormalities of the eye can arise as a result of toxicity at critical stages of embryogenesis [138], an apposite example being the widespread ocular abnormalities seen in the fetal alcohol syndrome, which occur in concert with abnormalities of other organs being formed at 21 days gestation, such as the heart [138]. If the toxic insults occur later in embryogenesis the effects are different even though the teratogen remains the same.

Interest in the development of the eye began in the time of Aristotle and restarted in the scientific academic revival in the seventeenth century with the work of Stoli and Malpighi [77]. In this century, the painstaking histological investigations of Mann [78], initially prompted by Frazer, on a series of human embryos established the value of such studies in understanding the role of morphogenesis in congenital malformations.

The most impressive features of embryogenesis have been described as complexity coupled with reliability [33], and a trio of growth, differentiation, and morphogenesis underlies the development of the entire adult from the fertilized ovum. The development of the eye, which follows a series of complex interactions [152], depends on an ordered sequence of morphogenic events, which themselves rely on processes of both growth and programmed selective cell death [1].

In humans much of this development takes place during the first 8 weeks of postovulatory life, the embryonic period that was divided into 23 stages by O'Rahilly (Table 1) [101–103]. The sequence of events in this period is governed by genetic transcription and modulated by diffusible growth factors and mechanical mass effects generated by structures developing within and alongside the eye. Postembryonic and postnatal growth also occurs within the eye, especially in the development of the retinal vasculature and orbital and adnexal structures. The final wave of migration of the cells of the neural crest that form melanocytes does not reach the eye or skin until 18 weeks of gestation, and retinal modeling continues after birth.

Formed structures also can be deformed and remodeled for awhile after birth, an example being the buphthalmic cornea, and postnatal growth of the orbit depends on the presence and retention of an intact globe of normal size. Physiological "modeling" also occurs: for example, the development of binocular vision depends on the inherent plasticity of the developing central nervous system (CNS) and its response

Table 1 Embryology of Normal Ocular Development

Months	Weeks	Days	Length (mm)	Developmental Changes
1	3	22	2–3.5	Optic primordium in forebrain
	4	24	2.4–4.5	Formation of optic vesicles (OV)
				Contact of OV with surface ectoderm
		25		Lens placode thickens
		26	3–5	Neural crest mesenchyme surrounds OV
2	5	28	4–6	OV starts to invaginate,
				Lens placode invaginates
				Retinal cells start to divide at OLM
		32	5–7	Optic vesicle forms cup
				Optic fissure formed
				Nerve III present
		33	7–9	RPE pigmented
				Hyaloid artery grows through optic fissure
				Lens vesicle and capsule present
				Lens fiber formation
				Nerves IV and VI appear
	6	37	8–11	Optic fissure edges oppose
				Tunica vasculosa lentis develops from hyaloid
				Ciliary ganglion present
		41	11–14	Lids present as folds
				Retina has inner and outer nuclear layers
				Secondary lens fibers
	7	44	13–17	Obliteration of lens vesicle cavity by fibers
				Anterior chamber forming
		48	16–18	Ganglion cells and formation of nerve fiber layer
				Corneal endothelium present
	8	51	18–22	Optic nerve fibers reach brain
				Lens suture appears
				Stroma of cornea appears acellular
		54	23–28	Scleral condensation of neural crest mesenchyme
3	9	57	27–31	Secondary vitreous
	10			Ciliary processes and iris start to form
				Eyelids fuse
	12			Photoreceptors appear
				Atrophy of hyaloid artery, growth of central retinal artery
				Ciliary muscle appears
4				Axis changed to front, sphincter pupillae differentiates
				Tunica vasculosa lentis atrophies
				Cilia appear
5			320	Layers of the choroid completed
6			385	Eyelids open
7			435	Pupillary membrane atrophies
8			475	Retinal layers all developed (except macula)
9			500	Regression of pupillary membrane and hyaloid artery
				Canalization of lacrimal duct

Source: After Strömland et al. [138].

to retinal output, and myopia can be induced by rapid changes in accommodation even late in child-hood [11,36].

Young [158] described the normal processes of multiplication, differentiation, and renewal of retinal cells as empirical laws, or paradigms explicable in terms of developmental genetics, molecular biology, and biological renewal. His excellent review covers the competence of cells and their receptivity to different categories of genes at certain times in development, resulting in commitment after the action of integrator genes. These regulatory genes are especially important in early retinal development, in which there is no ingrowth of axons to deliver signals for growth. This is in contrast to the situation in other structures within the eye, such as the iris, where the input generated by the sympathetic axons regulates the development of uveal pigmentation [68,84]. The process of retinal vascularization, which occurs toward the end of fetal life, is also too late to initiate normal retinal development, although it may influence pathological changes [4,5].

Both normal and abnormal development and pathological changes are underscored by a series of molecular recognitions [135,152], including base pairing of DNA and RNA, that result in protein transcription and differentiation. Retinal differentiation depends on the interaction of receptor proteins on cells on the inner surface of the invaginated outpouching of the optic vesicle, which have similarities to ventricular cells elsewhere within the developing CNS. These cells are receptors for a range of inducing molecules, resulting in specific binding to DNA and subsequent RNA transcription. In retinal cells a steady state of intracellular renewal is required since the cells have lost the ability to divide and renew themselves. This is in marked contrast to the endless renewal of cells destined to be shed, such as those produced from epithelial stem cells at the corneoscleral limbus. Young [158] postulates that liberation from the stereo-typic, repetitive pathway achieved by terminally differentiated end-stage cells, such as those in the retina, allows them greater chemical, physiological, and anatomical diversity.

II. NORMAL EMBRYOGENESIS OF THE EYE AND THE OPTIC STALK

Three distinct parts of the primitive embryo contribute to the development of the human eye: the neuroectoderm, the neural crest [9,10,12,13,23,27,35,41,55,57,105], and the surface ectoderm. The true mesodermal component [76] is limited to the formation of the striated extraocular muscles [122] and the endothelium of the vessels.

A. Role of the Neural Crest in the Formation of Mesenchyme of Head and Neck

The neural crest as a potential source of mesenchymal elements has been recognized since 1888, when Kastschenko [62] claimed that some of the mesenchyme of the head in selachians originates from the neural crest. Parallel findings were described in telosts, salamanders, and birds [38,54,107], and Platt proposed the name "mesectoderm" for such tissues [108]. The work of these early embryologists has since been confirmed in birds and mammals using nuclear markers [59,69,107]. Hörstadius [55] and Starck [137] originally reviewed the concept that the mesenchyme is a functional entity rather than an anatomical structure derived from one particular blastodermic or embryonic layer (the mesoderm).

The vertebrate neural crest not only gives rise to melanocytes, Schwann cells, neuroblasts, and ganglion cells of the peripheral nervous system but also contributes extensively to the formation of facial cartilage, bone, and teeth. Holtfreter [54] observed that cells from the neural crest produce cartilage when grown in the presence of endodermal cells from the pharyngeal area. Johnston and colleagues [59,60], commenting on extant literature concerning amphibian and avian embryos, considered that "apparently, the only major components of the face not of crest origin are the retina and lens, epithelial tissues, vascular endothelia, and skeletal (voluntary) muscle cells," a pioneering statement that has not yet been disproven.

From studies of normal human embryos it has been claimed that neural crest cells from the outer surface of the primary optic vesicle in the 15- to 16-somite stage begin to migrate into the axial mesoderm to form a sheath known as the "optic neural crest" around the optic vesicle. This migration reaches its peak in a 22- to 23-somite embryo (week 4), and after several cell divisions, such neural crest cells lose their distinctive characteristics and cannot be distinguished from other mesenchymal cells derived from the axial mesenchyme. It was concluded that the optic crest cells give rise to the uveal melanocytes in humans in a manner comparable to that demonstrated by others in amphibians and birds. The reason for the expanded role of the neural crest in the cephalic region may be the absence of somites in this area in humans and other animals.

B. Role of Neuroectoderm in the Formation of the Eye and Optic Vesicle

The human optic primordium forms as a thickening within the developing neural folds before the closure of the forebrain at somite 8, 2 mm stage at about day 18 of gestation. As the sulcus enlarges, optic evaginations and subsequently optic pits appear in the region of the developing forebrain and the mesencephalic neural crest develops from the region adjacent to the midbrain (Figs. 1 and 2). At the 3 mm (24 day) stage, the neural tube closes and the optic pits are pushed outward toward the surface ectoderm [90,92].

All mammalian eyes develop from this outpouching of the neuroectoderm of the diencephalon, which then forms the optic vesicle. This subsequently invaginates but remains connected to the cavity within the diencephalon, the third ventricle, by the optic stalk. The optic vesicle becomes sheathed with neural crest cells, except for a small central area where the attachment to the surface occurs and the lens and cornea develop (Fig. 3).

C. Induction of Lens

At the same time as the optic vesicle approaches the surface epithelium, before its apposition, these cells on the surface alter to become the lens placode [78]. This alteration is typified morphologically by thickening of the surface epithelium to form the lens placode, a disklike thickening separated by its basal lamina from the basal lamina of the optic vesicle. This mesenchyme eventually undergoes necrosis and resorption but acts as a temporary channel for communication for subsequent interaction between the surface and neuroectodermal components. This is evidenced by studies that show that the development of the lens is crucial for eye growth. Without a lens or with a delay in lens migration, retinal development and fissure formation are impaired because invagination may not occur.

The normal optic vesicle, which is lined by ciliated cells, invaginates, a process achieved by a buckling and a variation in cellular growth that results in the optic cup. The outer layer of the cup is destined to become the melanin-containing retinal pigment epithelium (RPE), and the inner layer differentiates toward the neural retina. The tubular optic stalk is grooved in its ventral portion by the optic fissure. Cell death also contributes to the formation of the fissure [129–131].

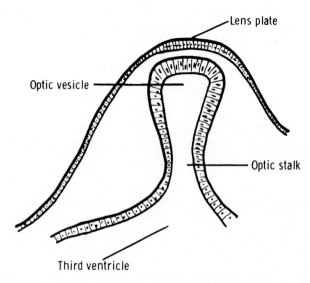

Figure 1   Original outpouching of neuroectoderm to form optic vesicle at 24 days gestation in human embryo.

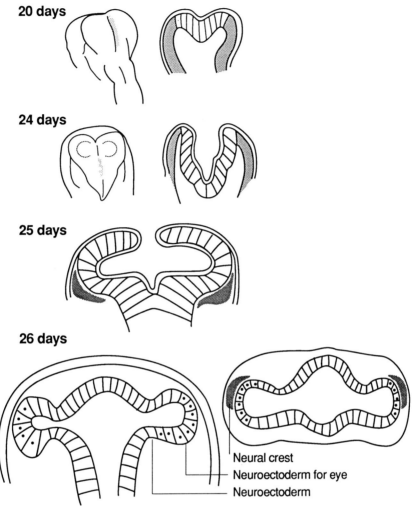

Figure 2 Early development of optic vesicle. At 20 days the neuroectodermal plate has a central depression or groove. The lateral ridges grow and converge, and by 24 days the central portion of the groove closes and the ridges become centrally depressed, forming the optic pits and allowing the convex edge of the neuroectoderm to become opposed to the surface ectoderm. At 25 days the anterior neuropore is rapidly closing, and by 26 days the optic vesicles are well formed, with defined neuroectoderm separated from the rest of the neural tube. There is rapid apposition of neural crest elements.

D. Formation of Optic Stalk and Fissure

The optic stalk is tubular and divided, as is the mammalian embryo, into ventral and dorsal tiers. Sidedness originally developed during evolution as a result of primitive tubular organisms flopping over so that the right side became the ventral side and the left side (facing upward) became the dorsal. This process of dexiothetism occurred in a primitive ancestor of vertebrates 500 million years ago. The development of the head region also arose in primitive forms [118], and the role of the active peptide described and sequenced [79].

The grooving of the ventral portion of the optic stalk forms the optic fissure as a process of invagination. This fissure eventually disappears to leave only the small aperture occupied by the hyaloid artery (Figs. 3 and 4). In cross section the stalk has, like the optic cup, a thick inner and thin outer layer. The distal portion is grooved by the optic fissure, and the proximal section is added to by the diencephalon and

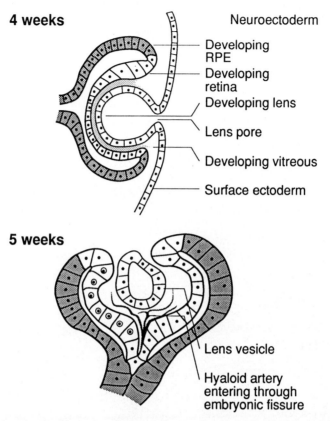

Figure 3 By 4 weeks gestation the surface ectoderm has invaginated to form the lens but the lens pore is still open. By 5 weeks the lens vesicle has closed and the hyaloid artery invading from beneath starts to envelope it posteriorly. The embryonic fissure is starting to close. In both diagrams the increasing pigmentation of the RPE is seen as it differentiates; the inner sensory neuroretina remains unpigmented.

forms a cylinder that is subsequently invaded by the retinal axonal projections. The epithelial cells forming the walls of the stalk differentiate into the neuroglia of the optic nerve, and the cavity, which is initially crescentic, becomes progressively filled. The stalk remains connected to the third ventricle until its lumen is obliterated by the axons growing from the developing retina. In its initial phases the dorsal part of the optic stalk remains continuous with the pigment epithelium and the ventral is continuous with the neural retina.

The processes arising from the developing ganglion cells grow along the optic stalk, after traversing the optic disk, in channels that are predetermined by the surrounding neuroepithelial cells, which also modulate their growth along the walls of the optic stalk. Their exit from the optic disk may be determined by the presence of pigmented cells at this site. Silver and Sapiro [130] suggested that melanin in dorsal cells may prevent the outgrowth of neurites in their vicinity and, in previous work, also commented on the varying roles of necrosis and the effect of the intercellular spaces. This loss of topographical precision with the consequent bending and centripetal migration of the previously straight columns of optic axons results in the clusters of axons that form the optic nerve as it heads toward the brain. Myelination of the axons of the optic nerve starts late in gestation, beginning at the optic chiasm and progressing distally to cease at the lamina cribrosa 1 month after birth. Redistribution of the fatty components of the myelin sheaths and increase in the number of layers occurs after birth [29,61]. The position of the ophthalmic artery (with its temporal ventral axis) and glial septa also adds to the modeling of the optic nerve: the glial processes in particular mold the development of the axons by deforming the temporal side of the optic nerve. Astrocytes encircle the hyaloid artery to envelop it, forming Bergmeister's papilla as it protrudes into the vitreous

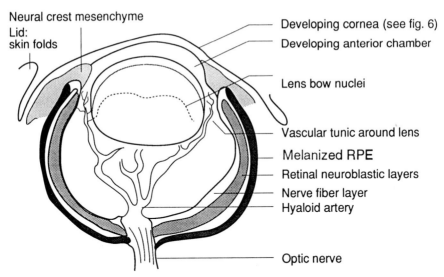

Neural crest mesenchyme
Lid:
skin folds

Developing cornea (see fig. 6)
Developing anterior chamber

Lens bow nuclei

Vascular tunic around lens
Melanized RPE
Retinal neuroblastic layers
Nerve fiber layer
Hyaloid artery

Optic nerve

Figure 4   By 45 days the ciliary portion of the optic cup is relatively undifferentiated compared to the sensory neuroretina (divided into nerve fiber and neuroblastic layers) and the RPE; it extends to the equatorial region of the lens, where the lens bow is developing and the anterior chamber can be discerned. The cornea is at this stage multilayered (see Fig. 5). The hyaloid artery is well developed, and the optic nerve is starting to form as axons extend toward the brain. The skin folds that form the lids are seen encroaching on the developing eye.

cavity. These have usually regressed by the time the lamina cribrosa is formed in the last month of gestation, as myelination is established.

The separation of the pathways of the stem cells committed to neuronal or glial differentiation and the further development of the two main precursors of macroglial cells into either astrocytic or oligodendrocytic lineage [113] are probably determined before the formation of the optic cup, when the neural tube is forming, so that the paraventricular cells become neuronal, with a limited potential for division, and the glial precursors retain the potential for mitosis longer, as discussed later. The glial cells form a radial network and scaffold for migrating nerve cells, and during this phase, mitosis within the glial cells is diminished or even inhibited. After migration of neuronal cells has ceased (see later), there is population of the developing optic nerve by type 1 astrocytes, and their density decreases from the eye toward the brain end of the optic nerve. These cells are thought to provide platelet-derived growth factor (PDGF), a proliferative and chemotactic factor that induces the formation of the type 2 lineage cells that form the oligodendrocytic cells [113]. Type 2 cells form the bulk of the cells within the optic nerve, migrating out from around the optic chiasm but not differentiating until the time of birth, when myelination is at its zenith [14,29].

Vertebrate eyes evolved as underwater visual organs, and in fish the capacity to grow during life is retained, as it is to a lesser extent in amphibious animals [35]. Even in fish, however, the density of the rod photoreceptors remains constant and the density of other cell types drops with age, leading to the hypothesis that rods arise from cell divisions in the outer nuclear layer. The concept that cell death underlies the modeling of the CNS, in particular the eye, is relatively recent. This is in contrast to the numerous comparative studies [89,110] that outlined the initial development of the eye, recording the emergence of cell populations [53,125] rather than the process of apoptosis [1,109,160].

Much of the understanding of the nonuniform distribution of ganglion cells with their consequent retinal sequelae has resulted from studying the development of the visual system within marsupials [7] using horseradish peroxidase labeling. This technique has underscored the importance of this concept of preprogrammed cell death in the development of the human retina [109,111]. This is especially important in the modeling of the peripheral retina. The contraction of the potentially spherical population of retinal cells to the retained hemispherical distribution leads to dilation of the retinal margin so that flattening and diminution of the peripheral cell density occurs. This sequence of events may arise as a result of changing elasticity, with consequent stretching as the globe enlarges, or spatial gradients in neurogenesis [109,11].

E.   Growth Factors and the Eye

All the changes detailed here in the morphology of the developing eye are to a certain extent under the control of diffusible growth factors [81]. Those implicated in this development include fibroblast growth factor (FGF), insulin and insulinlike growth factor (IGF), transforming growth factors α and β (TGF-α and TGF-β), PDGF, NGF, epidermal growth factor (EGF), and a granulocyte-macrophage colony-stimulating factor (GM-CSF) [19]. In addition specific gradients of cell surface-expressed ganglioside-related compounds can control retinal development [135].

Specialized eye development factors have been shown in vitro to have mitogenic and inductive morphogenic powers. FGF has been shown to have effects on the proliferation of lens fiber-producing and corneal epithelial cells [81]. In the bovine eye the nerve fiber layer has been shown to be rich in acid FGF (αFGF), which induces ganglion cell development; it has also been shown to be important in the differentiation of photoreceptors, whereas basic FGF (βFGF) appears to determine lens development as well as retinal development [81]. Different concentrations of FGF have been demonstrated on either side of the developing lens: the much higher concentrations in the posterior chamber have been postulated to account for the increased fiber-producing ability of the posterior lens epithelial cells [81].

The lens cells are also responsive to the insulin and insulin-type growth factors. In vitro experiments have shown their fiber-inducing properties to be age dependent. An active component of the developing vitreous, lentropin, belongs to this family of growth factors. In the rat retina IGF type I is localized to Müller cells in the postnatal development phase, but receptors for this factor have been shown in mature bovine retina and IGF-I may act in a paracrine and/or autocrine manner in older animals [81].

Transforming growth factors can elicit both stimulatory and regulatory responses: TGF-β is implicated in the modulation of growth of retinal capillaries and is thought to be released by pericytes. This growth factor is a strong stimulator of the formation of extracellular matrix and can induce fibrosis. TGF may also act synergistically with the fibroblast growth factors and with epithelial growth factors.

PDGF may initiate gliogenesis in the optic nerve and the induction of the two lineages of type 1 astrocytes and 02A oligodendrocyte precursors that form both the oligodendrocytes and type 2 astrocytes [113]. PGDF may also be involved in lens induction. Cultured RPE can also secrete PDGF-like proteins that may initiate the formation of the choroid and Bruch's membrane, acting as modulators of fibroblast growth.

NGF is important in the modulation of growth in the peripheral nervous system and may be implicated in retinal modeling. NGF receptors have been demonstrated in both avian and mammal eyes, including monkeys and it is likely that the effects of the NF-1 gene on the developing neural crest structures in the eye may also depend on the uncoordinated action of NGF, which may in addition to its inductive role act as a suppressor of neuroectodermal growth. This observation is akin to the role of tumor suppressor genes, which may paradoxically promote growth when one allele is deleted [148].

EGF acts as a mitogen, has been shown in studies in vitro to affect corneal epithelial and endothelial proliferation, and may be involved in lens induction.

The role of the CSF in the eye is unclear, but GM-CSF has been postulated to be involved in the process of ocular remodeling in transgenic mice [19], particularly in the resorption of the vitreous.

Angiogenic growth factors regulate endothelial cell proliferation, which also varies under differing conditions. This proliferation includes both vasculogenesis, giving rise to immature vascular plexuses arising from in situ differentiation of angioblasts in the embryo and, alternatively, new capillary growth from existing vessels (angiogenesis). In the embryo the development of the vascular system predates the requirement for or onset of circulation [114].

III.   HISTOGENESIS AND MORPHOGENESIS OF THE RETINA AND RETINAL PIGMENT EPITHELIUM

As outlined earlier, the retina is formed as part of the outgrowth of the neural tube, and its original histogenesis echoes that of the rest of the CNS. A cycle of multiplication, differentiation, and renewal is set in train; however, the retinal primordium is present in the optic pit stage even before the neural tube is closed at the 3 mm stage and before the outpouchings become grooved and subsequently erupt out from the surface of the neural tube as the optic vesicles.

By the end of the embryonic period the retina consists of a pigmented outer layer and a primitive sensory retina, with external limiting membrane, a proliferative zone, an external neuroblastic layer, a transient layer, and an internal neuroblastic layer covered by the nerve fiber layer and the internal limiting membrane. The rapid evolution of the thick inner layer and the thin RPE layer is well documented in several species, including rats, chicks, cats, marsupials, and, to a lesser extent, humans [78]. All have developed from the primitive two-layered optic vesicle. Much of the comparative data refer to work on the cat [109,151], which has a gestation time of 64–65 days, and the ferret (gestation 42 days), in contrast to the human gestation of 9 months. Nevertheless, the information gained in these dynamic studies of cell production and differentiation is relevant, since studies in humans and even in other primates are limited in number.

The primitive optic vesicle consists of elongated, fusiform, ventricular cells arranged in a pseudo-stratified columnar epithelium. These ventricular cells are capped by a single layer of more spherical cells undergoing mitosis [158] that have formed from the ventricular cells.

Precursor ventricular cells are joined by junctional complexes forming the inner and outer limiting membranes, and there are appositional lateral junctions [109]. Before each division by mitosis, the ventricular cells, having replicated their DNA, release their attachments to the inner limiting membrane (ILM) [109].

The untethered cells become rounder and come to lie against the outer limiting membrane (OLM) and divide, leaving the daughter cell in the inner position. The OLM is the equivalent to the ventricular zone elsewhere in the developing CNS. Cells destined to become photoreceptors or Müller glial cells remain attached to the OLM, and the other daughter cells detach and migrate to the appropriate level within the retina, closer to the ILM [53,109]. Müller cells remain as bridges from OLM to ILM. All cells in the ventricular layer are capable of division, but they are not synchronized. In early embryogenesis there is no evidence of differentiation.

In the early stages, mitoses takes place throughout the retinal neuroblast layer, but some loci begin to differentiate into ganglion cells [151]; these are seen as rounded cells with plump clear nuclei and prominent nucleoli, from which axons begin to develop. This expanding "front" of ganglion cell neurogenesis and differentiation travels as a wave from the center to the periphery. In early development there is dorsal-ventral asymmetry, more cells being present above the optic stalk than below. The temporal side also has more cells than the nasal side of the retina [78,109].

Cell mitosis ceases first in the central area, but growth continues at the periphery until late fetal life. Cessation of mitosis heralds the onset of differentiation.

Retinal ganglion cells can be distinguished by their rounded appearance, vesicular nuclei, and prominent nucleoli, as well as their closeness to the ILM. They first appear above and temporal to the optic stalk in an area that may correspond to the area centralis in the cat [109]. In human studies retinal cell mitosis is similarly initiated and ceases first in the center, followed by differentiation [112,136], which occurs in a front sweeping from the center to the periphery.

Axon outgrowths from the medium-sized retinal ganglion cells form an optic nerve fiber layer that stretches back to the optic stalk. At this stage, therefore, there are ganglion and neuroblast layers but no definable inner plexiform layers.

Retinal cells of dissimilar classes undergoing concurrent neurogenesis are referred to as cohorts, capable of different rates of differentiation and migration. Using thymidine labeling and autoradiography [109], it has been shown that the birth of retinal ganglion cells, type A horizontal cells, and cone photoreceptors occurs at the same embryological stage, but although the latter two lineages are committed, they do not immediately proceed to differentiate. Mitosis usually ceases in the central retina and is completed by 15 weeks gestation (120 mm stage) [136].

Axon development and the pathways that they take to the brain (retinal projections) appear to depend heavily on the degree of melanin pigmentation [147]. Albino mutations in all species studied, including humans [31], reduce ipsilateral projection by allowing more axons to cross at the optic chiasm. In humans and other albino primates, this lack of pigmentation leads to a failure of normal foveal development (see Chap. 31). In some albinoid animals there may be abnormally large ganglion cells in the central retina. Müller cells also appear at about the time of ganglion cell differentiation, and they also show a spatio-temporal gradient of cell birth [109].

Before considering further sensory retinal development, the evolution of the monolayer on the outside of the vesicle, which forms the RPE, will be discussed.

A. Development of the Retinal Pigment Epithelium

In albinism lack of melanin within the RPE [31] may also control the laterality of the retinal ganglion cells. RPE cells are derived from the outer layer of the invaginated optic vesicle and normally become pigmented in week 5 (6–7 mm) at the same stage as the ganglion cells leave the mitotic cycle.

RPE cells at this stage lose their erstwhile immature gap [30,46] and desmosomal junctions [66] and become extensively interdigitated, possibly as a result of the chelating effect of the melanin granules. These granules allow the cells to have enormous calcium-buffering potential [21], and because many intercellular junctional communications are recognized as affected by calcium [32] the lack of such buffering pigment in albino animals may underlie the abnormal spatial distribution of cell proliferation, lead to disruption of maturation, and result in anomalous organization [40,94]. At the same time as melanogenesis is instigated, the cilia present on the inner surface disappear. The original two- to three-layered pseudostratified columnar epithelium becomes a monolayer of cuboidal cells with the apices oriented internally, joined by tight junctions instead of a pseudostratified columnar epithelium [52]. Stubby cell extensions project from the apices of the cells in the monolayer to lie alongside the photoreceptor outer segments, which developed from the cilia of the sensory retinal layer. These two cell layers must be opposed for normal growth to occur. The RPE precursor cells have a prominent endoplasmic reticulum [15].

The developing RPE cells slowly increase in number throughout fetal development, but after birth the cells hypertrophy to cover the increased surface area of 800 mm^2 [105] and mitoses are not seen. The sequence of neuroectodermal melanogenesis is similar to that seen in neural crest melanocytes, although the melanin-containing organelles (melanosomes) of all the pigment epithelia are much larger than uveal or dermal melanocyte melanosomes [82]. The pigment forms as electron-dense deposits on ovoid shuttle-shaped organelles (the premelanosomes), which emerge from the outer nuclear membrane or Golgi apparatus as folded vesicles at 3 weeks gestation (6–7 mm stage) and is the earliest pigment to form in the body.

The basal surface of the developing pigment epithelium is enveloped by a thin but continuous basal lamina that develops from the mesectoderm of neural crest origin.

Bruch's membrane appears as a basal lamina at the optic cup stage [105] and in the 6 week embryo consists of collagen fibrils without well-defined elastic tissue. The basal lamina of the epithelium is well defined but that of the choriocapillaris is indistinct. Initially there is apposition of the choroidal collagen fibrils against the RPE basement membrane, until first the capillary basement membrane and then a fenestrated elastic sheet derived from the neural crest-derived fibroblasts are interposed from 13 weeks [120] and Bruch's membrane starts to resemble its mature form. The choriocapillaris arises, after induction by the pigment epithelium, in week 4–5 of gestation, so that by week 6 there is a primitive capillary network surrounding the whole developing eye. Fenestrations appear within the walls of the vessels as the endothelium flattens. Pericytes are present at 6 weeks, and these also have been postulated to be derived from the surrounding mesenchyme and are probably of neural crest origin. They have been implicated as possible sources of basement membrane material [120,121].

B. Further Differentiation of the Sensory Retinal Cells

As discussed, the lateral connecting neurons (A-type horizontal cells) [80] and cone photoreceptors have delayed morphological differentiation and migration although they are already committed to differentiate after the final wave of mitosis, which also produces the faster differentiating ganglion cells [7,52,53,90, 91,109–111,119,135,144,158].

Sequential waves of neuroblastic activity can be recognized, and at least three waves of ganglion cell neurogenesis occur [109]. The definitive layers in the retina are formed as ganglion cells migrate into the neuroblastic layer along with amacrine cell precursors (of which there are at least 30 different subtypes [80]), leaving cellular processes in the transient layer of Chievitz. The final arrangement of nuclear layers evolves as cell nuclei are squeezed and manipulated into position by cell processes.

Differentiation of the photoreceptor cells varies between species. The migration of the rods depends on the guidance of the radial Müller cells, which are produced at the same time as the cone precursors at about

9 weeks. Both Müller cells and cone precursors are developed after the migration of the ganglion cells and the emergence of amacrine cells. The photoreceptor outer segments are derived from the cilia that sprout from the outermost layer of cells and project toward the contracting outer layer, which will form the RPE. Müller cells, in addition to acting as guides, probably contribute to the thickening of the inner limiting membrane and the outmost part of the vitreous. Although their nuclei lie in the inner nuclear layer, their radial processes add to the basement membrane of the ILM. Together the combination of basement membrane glycoproteins and reticulin fibers and the branching expanded processes of Müller cells produce a smooth inner surface to which the vitreous gel is attached [129].

In humans, the outer segments of the rod photoreceptors develop late in gestation, at 23 weeks, and by week 36 stacked lamellar sacs formed from invaginated plasma membranes are present, adding to the components derived from the ciliary tubules [28,109,126].

During earlier human embryogenesis, development is most advanced at the posterior pole, and although outer neuroblastic proliferation ceases early at 15–17 weeks (103–120 mm), further differentiation continues, especially in the macula, where, having started in month 8, it persists until month 4 of postnatal life [17,18].

C. Development of the Fovea

The fovea can be recognized in both primate and human retina originating after 26–30% of the length of gestation as a region containing all adult layers of the retina and only cone photoreceptors [17,18,109]. The foveal pit and the outer segments of the cones are visible at 63–65% gestation [48–50]. There is species variation. In the monkey prenatal development continues so that at birth there is a single layer of inner retinal neurons accompanied by cones stacked three cells deep and having elongated inner segments. This stage is not reached in humans until several months after birth [49]. Postnatal foveal development continues for much longer in the human, starting to become mature at about 1 year and continuing for 4 years more. The monkey fovea does not develop further after 12 weeks of postnatal life [17,18,49,74]. This further development and maturation of the fovea is the principle reason for the dramatic increase in visual function in childhood [74], since the fovea mediates color vision and high resolution and also underlies the development of amblyopia in eyes that do not for a variety of reasons mature in this way [149].

Specification of the fovea occurs early in gestation, and division of cells ceases first in this region at about 14 weeks gestation. The formation of the foveal pit, where the inner retinal layers are absent, is accompanied by an accumulation of ganglion cells at its periphery, on the foveal slope, where the highest concentration of these cells in the retina is to be found [16]; the highest concentration of cones is within the center of the fovea in the region called the foveola [17,18]. In the human there are no rods within an area measuring 350μm in diameter, and the incidence of cones in the human fovea has been variably reported as between 100,000 and 300,000 mm^{-2} [17] and can be demonstrated in the living eye [150].

Each cone signals to at least two ganglion cells via several bipolar cells, and this accounts for the high visual acuity and color perception of this region. The development of the fovea involves the longest period of maturation of any part of the retina, starting first and finishing last but resulting in an exquisitely discriminative and sensitive region [50].

Retinal development is therefore determined by three distinct processes, those of differentiation, lamination, and the emergence of cellular cohorts. The initial mitotic division of the ventricular cells is followed by a process of renewal and proliferation. After these mitoses cease, the postmitotic cells follow patterns of neurogenesis, migration, differentiation, and maturation [109–111]. Although in other parts of the CNS the existence of multiple committed lineages of cells is postulated, within the eye the ventricular cells appear to be multipotential but unidirectional. In any given period of neurogenesis, more than one cell type may emerge and these cells form a cohort. Local environmental factors appear to govern postmitotic commitment. The initial period of neurogenesis is followed by a pattern of preprogrammed cell death that results in the organized adult retina. The distribution and maturation of any cell within the retina therefore depends on five separate processes or events, as discussed by Young [158]:

1. Time and location of the final mitotic division
2. Morphological differentiation and the extent of surface development of the retina at the time of formation and placement (insertion) of the postmitotic cell

3. Subsequent growth and development after insertion of the postmitotic cell (a process known as dilution)
4. Intercellular trophic effects and cell death leading to refinement
5. Nonuniform expansion of the growing retina

Within the retina, division of cells occurs early and differentiation is initiated at the inner and outer limiting membranes into primitive photoreceptors and ganglion cells. Processes from postmitotic cells grow throughout the retina, and the movement of nuclei is a secondary event resulting from rearrangement rather than migration of the cells. Postnatal retinal cell metabolic activity is directed toward a continual cycle of reconstruction not always regulated or instigated by vision per se.

The entire outer segment of a rod, about 1000 double membrane disks, is replaced every 2 weeks, the shed disks being phagocytosed by the RPE because the photoreceptor has lost the ability to disassemble them as a result of its terminal differentiation and specialization [158].

D. Development of Retinal Vasculature

The blood supply to the retina is derived from a branch of the internal carotid artery forming the tip of the primitive ophthalmic artery. This sprig invades the embryonic fissure, passing upward from below at the 5 mm stage of the human embryo. As the optic cup closes the vessel remains trapped within it and is referred to thereafter as the hyaloid artery [4,5]. As is described later in Section III.N, the branches that sprout within the cavity form the network that covers the region from the marginal zone of the retina to the lens vesicle. These together with small vessels from the ophthalmic artery close to the optic disk supply nutrients to the developing retina. Such blood flow continues until primitive retinal vessels start to develop in month 4 from spindle-shaped mesenchymal cells from the vascular plexus at the optic disk that invade the nerve fiber layer. The intraneural portions of the hyaloid vessels later become the definitive central retinal artery and vein, the branches of which reach out toward the ocular equator. The solid cores, developing from the spindle cells within the buds, become patent at month 5 of gestation and contain erythrocytes. At the same time as this network is emerging, the hyaloid artery is regressing, enveloped in a coat of glial cells. The primitive vessels proceed toward the peripheral parts of the retina and are seen at the ora serrata by month 8 of gestation [87]. The rate of growth of these vessels in humans is 0.1 mm per day [58]. There is substantial postnatal maturation, and Ashton [4,5] has postulated that endothelial cell growth is promoted by the relative anoxia of venous blood. Pericytes are present in small numbers from month 5 of gestation, but they rapidly become more numerous also at or about the time of birth. The vascular endothelial and mural cells (both fibroblasts and pericytes) have been postulated to have a common cell of origin after tissue culture experiments that showed multipotentiality [105]. At birth retinal vessels have a continuous endothelial cell lining. The vasculature of the fovea has been described in other primates [26], and the avascular zone is developed by 125 days gestation, which is comparable with 7 months in the human. Henkind and colleagues thought that in humans the avascular zone developed after obliteration of previously extant vessels [51].

E. Formation of the Lens

The formation of the lens can be divided into four stages: (1) induction and formation of the lens plate, (2) formation of the vesicle, (3) formation of primary fibers, and (4) formation of secondary fibers.

The lens is regarded by embryologists as a classic example of a cascade of intercellular interactions. Current theories [35,65,66] support a staged theory of lens induction, with initial dependence on surface ectodermal competence to respond to lens inducers during the period of gastrulation of the embryo. This is followed almost immediately by an intermediate stage in which the designated area of head ectoderm develops a lens-forming bias before moving into a period of autonomy such that the lens ectoderm is able to differentiate on its own, a process known as speciation. The continued presence of the optic vesicle ensures the final stage of differentiation at the specified site and suppression of lens-forming bias in adjacent sites.

The cells that form the lens are derived from a region of head surface ectoderm that was previously in contact with the developing neuroectoderm of optic vesicle [39,106]. The varying responses to experiments in differing species have led to controversy, however. The subject was reviewed by Saha and others [115,116], and the consensus is that although this interaction is a normal requirement, the lens develops in the absence of the optic vesicle in some species by a phenomenon known as "double assurance," resulting from fleeting contacts with foregut endodermal derivatives and heart mesoderm. These lenses, induced without the final input from the optic vesicle, are very rudimentary, but it is not certain whether the influence of the optic vesicle is directly positive and inductive or permissive in the nature of a removal of inhibition. It has been suggested that the neural crest inhibits lens differentiation and that the lens placode is sheltered for awhile from the influence of the crest by the vesicle [39,127].

Stage 1

In humans the lens placode arises after induction of the surface ectoderm to form a thickening over the area between the encroaching edges of the optic vesicle; it subsequently becomes covered by two cell layers from the surface ectoderm. As described later, there is a narrow space filled with mesenchyme, derived from the cephalic neural crest, bordered on each side by the basal laminae of the neuroectodermal outgrowth and the surface ectoderm, respectively. The thickening occurs at 27 days gestation in the human embryo, and by 29 days there has been sufficient transfer of inductive substances, probably in both directions [106], to cause movement of the lens placode so that it comes to lie within the lips of the invaginating optic vesicle, although the inducing properties of the neuroectoderm are thought to be even more powerful.

Stage 2

The invagination of the lens placode initially to form a pit and subsequently a cup and finally a vesicle is achieved by processes of elongation of the cells at the same time as the apices contract [153], producing a series of interlocked cone-shaped cells, each bordered by a basal lamina [131]. Separation from the surface ectoderm is complete by 33 days. The basal lamina thickens with substantial deposition of type IV collagen and becomes the lens capsule [73]. Evanescent fibers add considerably to the posterior part of the developing lens capsule, which appears much thicker than the anterior at this stage. Part of this thickening is due to a component thought to develop from the mesectodermal components arising from the developing hyaloid vascular network [73]. The separation of the lens and its closure result from zonal necrosis and contracture of the apical filamentous network [105].

Stage 3

The posterior lens cells start to produce the specific lens proteins at this stage after the onset of decreased DNA synthesis [157]. This allows the cells to lengthen and start to produce the lens fibers at the expense of other cell organelles [105]. The formation of these primary lens fibers, which progressively fill the vesicle, is soon succeeded by the production of secondary fibers.

These secondary fibers originate in the anterior lens cells, which migrate centrally toward the equator of the lens, their retained nuclei producing the lens bow. The planes of the mature lens are laid down at about 7 weeks of gestation [132].

Stage 4

The evolution of successive waves of secondary fibers and loss of their nuclei results in an inverted Y-shaped suture replacing a previously observed posterior horizontal suture present at the end of month 2. An anterior Y-shaped suture is also present at this stage and after birth, when branching occurs and both sutures become star shaped [65].

The lens capsule is formed at 5 weeks (Fig. 5) from the basement membrane of the invaginated surface epithelium, and a contribution from the tunica vasculosa also occurs. The zonules appear in month 4. Modification of the shape of the developing lens is thought to be under both neural retinal and neural ectomesenchymal control [106]. The lens becomes progressively more ellipsoid, as intracytoplasmic fibers are laid down at the expense of the nuclei of the developing lens cells. At the end of 3 months of gestation, no nuclei are visible in the innermost cells of the lens nucleus and no mitoses are seen in cells apart from those in the capsule. The number of lamellae within the lens increases from about 400 in the 45 mm fetus to about 1450 in the newborn and postnatal increase in the ellipsoid shape brings the final total to about 2000 lamellae in the adult lens [24]. The normal lens epithelial cover remains appropriate and is never buckled or stretched.

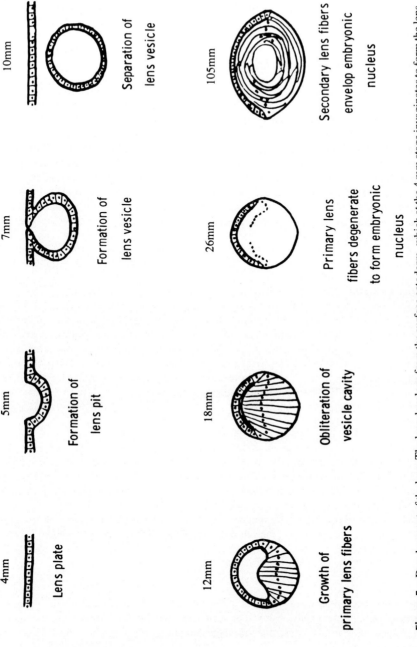

Figure 5   Development of the lens. The lens develops from the surface ectoderm, which at the 4 mm stage invaginates to form the lens pit and successively the lens vesicle by the 7 mm stage. Separation is achieved by the 10 mm stage, and subsequently the primary lens fibers fill the cavity until they degenerate and are succeeded by the secondary lens fibers, which continue to grow throughout life.

F. Development of the Cornea

The cornea develops from both the surface ectoderm, which gives rise to the epithelial layer and its basement membrane, and the neural crest, from which originate the stroma, Descemet's membrane, and the endothelial (posterior epithelial) cells (Fig. 6). In contrast to the developing avian embryo, Bowman's layer (which is not present in all species) in primates is thought to develop from the neural crest rather than the anterior stroma secreted by surface epithelium in birds. Avian corneal studies have disclosed subtle differences in the sequencing of stromal development in birds compared to mammals, especially in the anterior stroma [43–45]. Understanding of the contribution of the cephalic neuroectomesenchyme, derived from the neural crest, has come from the use of tritiated thymidine incorporation into neural crest cells. Dilution of the radiolabel as the cells divided meant that not all the ultimate destinations of migrating cells could be ascertained. A characteristic marker within the nucleus of quail cells was exploited by the group led by Le Douarin in a series of elegant transplantation experiments producing chimeric chick-quail embryos [70,71]. This has allowed the final destinations and the tissues derived from the transplanted neural crest cells to be determined and has led to the realization that most of the connective tissue of the head and neck, including the bones of the skull, except for the squamosal bone, in birds are of neural crest, not mesodermal origin as was previously thought [97–99]. These data have been extrapolated to mammals, including humans, and have led to greater understanding of complex anomalies; however, direct evidence is still largely derived from avian work [41,42], although the effect of generalized failure of neural crest migration is thought to underlie the diseases classified as neurocristopathies (see also Chap. 45) [59,60,88].

Ectomesenchymal cells are seen as rests at the lip of the optic cup, beneath the basal lamina of the surface ectodermal component, at the 7 mm stage. At the same time as the surface ectodermally derived

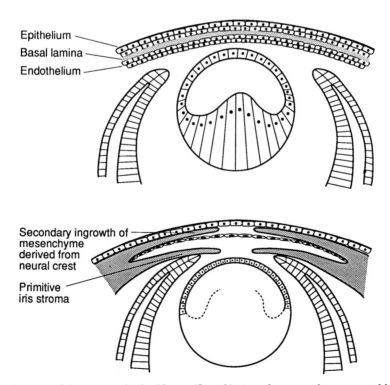

Figure 6   Development of the cornea. At the 10 mm (5 week) stage the cornea is represented by a double-layered epithelium, derived from the surface epithelium, separated from the layer of mesenchymal cells derived from the neural crest. The neural crest forms the corneal endothelial cells. By 20 mm (45 days) the cornea is better developed and the primitive iris stromal component and pupillary membrane are also growing inward; this mesenchyme is also developed from the neural crest.

lens epithelial cells start to form the lens fibers, a double layer of cuboidal cells, derived from these neural crest rests, forms the precursor of the corneal endothelium. At the 24 mm stage, a further wave of migration of neural crest cells occurs, to both the developing corneal stroma and the area where scleral condensation will occur. By 8 weeks gestation there are 8–10 layers of these cells, surrounded by primitive collagen fibrils. At the scleral level the true mesenchymal derivatives that eventually form the extraocular muscles also start to form from spindle-shaped precursors.

The diverse morphological expression of neural crest-derived tissues depends on the ability of these cells to migrate and disperse, on their invasive characteristics, and on the precision of their localization. The age-old conflict of nature versus nurture has been reevoked by studies of the neural crest. Some neural crest elements of caudal distribution are precommitted and produce their characteristics wherever transplanted, but conversely, when trunk neural crest cells are transplanted caudally they are capable of differentiating into appropriate structures for that position without further instruction [12,13,35,76,97–99,140,141]. Neural crest cells are not generally contact inhibited until they reach their final resting place and assume the terminal structural mode [12].

So that migration from the neural crest through other embryological structures can occur, the leading cells of the migrating neural crest cells pour out a carpet of fibronectin and other extracellular matrix proteins [12,13]. This acts both as a guiding pathway for the cells in the wake of the leading edge and as a scaffold for subsequent connective tissue elements. The fibronectin in the extracellular matrix, at the point of entry of the corneal neural crest cells at the corneoscleral limbus, can be seen with the transmission electron microscope to consist of a series of 3–5 nm filaments interspersed with spherical structures, known as interstitial bodies, also composed of fibronectin covered with a glycoprotein [12]. The adjacent epithelial cells of ectodermal origin cannot be invaded by the crest cells because they secrete a barrier of their own fibronectin, as well as laminin, type IV collagen, and proteoglycans on microfibrils. Migration of neural crest cells is also modified by the bulk of other adjacent developing structures [146]. Caudal neural crest cells at the level of the optic vesicles and optic placodes are thought to be obstructed by these cell masses and puddles of fibronectin accumulate around these structures, and the rate of migration is slowed from 70 μm per hour.

The surface ectoderm that forms the corneal epithelium is probably determined by induction or interaction with the neuroectodermal outgrowth early in embryogenesis [86], but under the influence of the developing lens this ectoderm becomes columnar. In birds, but not in mammals or primates, including humans, these cells secrete the primary corneal stroma [8,22,43,49]. In humans two rows of cells rest on a thin basal lamina at the 33 mm stage. The outer layer is squamous and the inner basal layer is columnar. At this stage the eyelids are fused and the developing cornea is protected from the amniotic fluid. The epithelium of the cornea is much more regular than that of the conjunctiva [124]. Wing cells appear in month 4 of gestation, by which time the stroma has 15 lamellae secreted by the invading neural crest cells. When the eyelids separate at the 210 mm stage, the epithelium is four to five cell layers thick, but the central corneal stroma is attenuated so that the curve of the developing cornea resembles that of the developing lens. Condensation of keratocytes is more prominent in the anterior third than elsewhere in the stroma, and the parallel arrangement of the cornea, when the collagen fiber layers are compared to the corkscrew array of the scleral fibers, is established by week 7 of gestation.

In avian corneal development, the invading first wave of neural crest cells, which forms the endothelial cell layer, accumulates posterior to the primary stroma [22], which has been secreted by the epithelial cells and contains types I and II collagen and glycosaminoglycans (GAG) but not fibronectin [43–45]. This primary stroma also acts as a scaffold for the architecture of the secondary stroma laid down by the second wave of migrating neural crest cells (characterized by filopods and lamellopods) after they have arrived. To facilitate the ingress of the migrating neural crest cells, the stroma becomes greatly hydrated, probably by the secretion of large amounts of hyaluronic acid [43–45]. Subsequently compression of the stromal lamellae occurs posteriorly. At least part of this compression is because hyaluronic acid production ceases [46]. Neural crest cells in the corneal stroma secrete a higher proportion of sulfated GAG than cells in the neural tube or ectoderm. The endothelial cells also produce chondroitin-4-sulfate, keratan sulfate, and heparan sulfate [45].

Laying down of the corneal stroma in an ordered array is of paramount importance to the subsequent successful transmission of light [142]. Before fibril formation can occur, the stellate fibroblasts, which are randomly scattered through the ground substance of the developing stroma, must become more spindle shaped, with their long axes aligned parallel to the surface. This orientation starts from the posterior layers and progresses forward. Once aligned, the cells start to produce collagen fibrils and there is appositional growth as well as the continued evolution of additional lamellae until there are about 30 layers by the end of gestation. As with all collagen networks, postsecretional modeling and rearrangements are the norm, and the cornea remains plastic until about the age of 3 years. This plasticity allows postnatal normal growth, and in cases with raised intraocular pressure, as in buphthalmic eyes, increased bowing can be seen. In normal human embryos the corneal diameter increases from 2 mm at 12 weeks of gestation to 9.3 mm at birth.

The structural collagens are laid down in a spiral orthogonal fashion, with diminishing angles as the posterior lamellae are created. The spiral has the same clockwise twist in both eyes [124]. The GAG are fitted into the interstices. The composition of the collagen matrix varies between species, young birds having types I and II whereas humans have no type II but at least during embryological life have some type III (see Chap. 33). The translucency of the stroma that occurs at the beginning of secretion of Descemet's membrane has been shown in the chick to be under the influence of thyroxine [15]. The resulting transparent cornea is in part due to the completion of the endothelial cell monolayer and the switching on of the pump functions of these cells once they become contact inhibited.

A striking difference between the development of mammalian and avian stroma is the greater speed in the latter at which the second wave of migrating mammalian neural crest arrives and starts to secrete stroma. In the absence in nonavians of a primary scaffold, this speed may be essential to maintain the separation of the ectodermal and endothelial layers [44]. Posterior compaction of stromal layers also occurs relatively earlier in mammals than in birds. Collagen fibrils are not demonstrable in human embryos using silver stains and light microscopy until the 87 mm stage [124]. The human embryonic cornea is translucent in the embryo [161]. This translucency is observable as compaction occurs, starting in the posterior stroma, and is completed as the most anterior layers are secreted; at this point a concomitant "adult" level of corneal hydration is reached [44,104]. The thinning of the central part of the corneal stroma in early fetal life has been attributed to its distance from the corneoscleral limbus and the time incoming cells take to migrate there in sufficient numbers. An alternative rationale postulates that the central thinning arises as a result of the impingement of the lens mass against the developing corneal stroma [124]. This impingement also encourages curvature of the cornea around the lens.

Little is known of the long-term history of the stromal keratocyte, but DNA synthesis is stable in the chick just before hatching and it may be that keratocytes form a static population of cells, not normally capable of reproduction. This may explain the slight decrease in keratocyte numbers with age, as is the case for other ocular neural crest-derived cells, including the corneal endothelium, thought not to reproduce in the human [143].

G.   Descemet's Membrane

The posterior basement membrane of the cornea was described by Duddell [23], 29 years before Descemet's account in 1758 [20], and was subsequently recognized as of endothelial (posterior epithelial) origin. Development of Descemet's membrane in the human at the 36 mm stage has been shown to start as a patchy condensation of basement membrane fibers that become progressively thickened and confluent [58,145,154,155]. The evolution of this complex basement membrane [117] shows variation in constituent collagens and rates of growth [95,145], which allows dating of pathophysiological insults in a manner akin to tree ring dating techniques [82]. There is a continuous membrane by 12 weeks of gestation, consisting of a 37 nm electron-lucent zone next to the endothelial cells, which secrete the membrane, and a more electron dense zone of similar thickness adjacent to the stroma. This double-layered structure is succeeded by serial secretion of further layers, so that 10 layers are present by the end of the second trimester and 30 layers or more at birth [124]. At the same time there is a secretion of short and thin collagen fibrils perpendicular to the original fibrils, starting at about 16 weeks. This results in a cross-linked striated anterior banded zone, which becomes compacted by contraction of these bridging links. Initially the bridging links are between 110 and 120 nm apart, giving rise to the characteristic banded pattern, but later in gestation they become more closely compacted. This pattern of secretion and banding ceases at about the time of birth, and thereafter nonstriated, amorphous, and nonlamellar type IV collagen is laid down for the most part, with only occasional randomly oriented fibrillar or wide-spaced elements, which are infrequent except in dystrophic corneas [64,83]. Microfibrillary components have been shown by immunogold techniques to include fibronectin, laminin, and tenascin, and in addition to predicted collagen subtypes there is also type

VIII collagen in long-spacing areas [75]. Although the membrane is widely supposed to have been secreted by the endothelial cells, the emergence of the highly organized anterior banded zone and its segmentation could result from mesenchymal stromal cell secretion, the close adherence to the stroma being cited in evidence [145]. Although this is possible, recapitulation of rather grotesque parodies of the segmental pattern [83] can be demonstrated in both congenital posterior polymorphous dystrophy and in the iridocorneal endothelial syndrome in association with acquired endothelial cell abnormalities. These membrane abnormalities can occur in the presence of ostensibly normal stromal cells, an intact anterior banded zone, and posterior non-banded zone, secreted postnatally before the syndrome becomes manifest.

Schwalbe's ring (a visible circumvallate structure) is present at the periphery of the cornea and marks the transition zone from Descemet's membrane to the trabecular meshwork. Flat-topped elevations—Hassall-Henle warts—appear in this position with increasing age. These capstanlike structures are composed of type IV and some type III collagen and have a peripheral ring of oxytalan, an elastin precursor, as well as long-spaced collagen. The structure of the guttate excrescences in Fuchs' dystrophy is similar.

H. Corneal Endothelial Cells

Endothelial cells of the cornea are originally double layered, first appearing at about 40 days of gestation (17–18 mm) [78]. Initially these cells have ill-defined junctions. Maculae occludens develop at about 8 weeks, and by the 3 month stage there is a single layer of cells with apical zonulae occludens. These cells are still widely held to be responsible for the secretion of Descemet's membrane, as just described. In human eyes the number of endothelial cells stabilizes at birth at about 500,000, with up to 7500 cells mm^{-2}. Normally mitoses were not thought to be present in humans but have occasionally been seen using the specular microscope. Cells are lost during life at the rate of 0.52% per year [96,143,155], and the remainder spread to negate the deficiency as long as this is feasible. In the adult the endothelial cells are 5–6 μm thick and 18–20 μm in width, linked by both zonulae and maculae occludentes and the rare desmosome. The development of zonulae occludentes also coincides with the onset of secretion of the aqueous humor from the developing ciliary body.

I. Development of the Ciliary Body

The ciliary body develops from the outermost tip of the optic cup. Development of the ciliary body lags behind that of the retina. It has been postulated that there must be contact between the optic cup tip and the lens for the ciliary body to develop [105]. An essential input of mesenchyme of neural crest origin is also required. Two masses of mesenchyme are seen in 20 mm human embryos, and by the 36 mm stage these resolve into a triangular wedge that forms the trabecular meshwork and another mass of mesenchymal cells lateral to this mass. The outer lip of the optic cup lies inside and next to this.

By the 54 mm stage [105] the outer pigmented cells start to create folds, and by 12 weeks ridges arranged as meridians are in place. These folds, lined on the inner surface by the cuboidal nonpigmented epithelial cells, become the ciliary processes. A triangular wave of mesenchyme, seen as a tip in profile, grows forward, dragging a mass of folded double-layered epithelium in its wake. This area becomes increasingly indented and forms the ciliary processes, and the forward arching wave forms part of the iris. There is at the same time a smoothing of the curve of the part of the region that becomes the pars plana. The apical surfaces of the nonpigmented epithelial cells develop microvilli, and primitive oligocilia are present in these early stages, as is an intermittent basal lamina [105]. The surface features are lost as the secretion of aqueous is switched on but may persist at the apices of the pigmented epithelial cells.

The mesenchymal cells outside these epithelial elements give rise to the stromal components of the ciliary body. In the week 7 embryo primitive myoblasts are seen in the ciliary muscle anlage in the form of cells with large nuclei and prominent eosinophilic cytoplasm, in continuity with the meshwork but with an attachment to the scleral spur. Differentiation into tendons and muscle fibers and strands is not initiated until 7 months gestation [78] and is completed postpartum.

Penetration of the developing stroma by vessels growing inward from an anterior vascular network occurs by month 4 [105] to give rise to an annular series of tufts of feathery interconnected venules and capillaries. At 5 months the arterial component forms a distinct circle with recurrent branches to the ciliary stroma. At 8 months the anastomoses with the choroidal circulation [100] with branches to each of the ciliary processes are completely formed [70]. The capillaries of the ciliary process have fenestrated endothelia and those present within the muscles do not [105].

J. Formation of the Iris

The iris has both neuroectodermal and neural crest-derived components arising on a mesodermal vascular template. The formation of the lower part of the iris is dependent on the closure of the optic fissure. The neuroectoderm gives rise to the very dark pigment epithelium and the sphincter and dilator muscles, which arise from less pigmented epithelium [105], and the neural crest contributes the stroma and anterior border. The vessels enveloping the lens provide the scaffolding around which the iris develops. At the 6 week stage of embryogenesis, the anterior chamber is delineated by the emerging corneal endothelial cells on one side and a lamina formed by the connective tissue associated with vessels cuffing the lens (tunica vasculosa lentis) on the other. At the same time as the wavelike extension of the optic cup moves forward to form the ciliary processes, a further extension of neuroectoderm slides in front of the developing lens and the sphincter pupillae starts to form at its farthest limit, as it creeps into the lamina. So that the pupil can form, the central portion of the lamina, derived from the tunica vasculosa lentis, is remodeled, the membranous parts becoming interdigitated with melanocytes of neural crest origin that migrate and become pigmented under the influence of the emerging sympathetic nervous system [84]. The anterior border of the developing iris therefore contains mesenchymal elements, some derived from the lamina of blood vessels and others of neural crest origin, as are the melanocytes. The stroma also contains an admixture of components with fibroblasts and melanocytes arranged around the vascular arcades.

The development of the sphincter pupillae follows reduced melanogenesis in the anterior epithelial layer and a switch toward production of extracellular basement membranelike material and myofibrils within slender extensions of the epithelial cells. The peripheral limit of the sphincter muscle is defined anatomically by a short cuff of pigmented epithelium (von Michel's spur). Separation of the sphincter muscle from the pigment epithelium occurs after the invasion of capillaries and the establishment of a cell-to-cell signaling network, which develops at about the same time as the muscle becomes innervated, at about 7½ months gestation (250 mm stage) [105]. The radial vessels of the iris also develop within this plane; separation of the sphincter from the epithelial layer is achieved by insinuating connective tissue elements.

The dilator muscle fibers arise after the appearance of fibrils within the columnar anterior epithelial cells of the developing iris, lying peripheral to von Michel's spur, which acts as a watershed between development of the sphincter and dilator muscles. The fibrils alter the shape of the cells, so that they become longer and slimmer, with displacement of the nucleus and melanosomes toward the apex. A basement membrane separates the cytoplasm of these altered neuroectodermal cells from the stromal cells of neural crest origin. Innervation of the muscles of the iris follows their anatomical differentiation, adrenergic terminals forming a loose network within the stroma by 5 months gestation [68].

The iris stroma consists of fibroblastic and melanocytic neural crest cells arranged around vessels. The vessels are arranged as a series of elegant arcades during the time that the pupillary membrane is in existence [105], but as this is resorbed, the remnants come to form a frill or ruff (the so-called collarette) around the pupillary margin that persists as the lesser circle of the iris circulation [100]. The anterior border cells of the iris migrate in from the neural crest. Pigmentation of the iris depends on an intact sympathetic innervation [68]. Migration of these cells is late in human gestation and continues in the stroma after birth. Melanosomes within stromal melanocytes have been reported to be mature at birth [93], having passed beyond the stage of the premelanosomal shuttle-shaped organelle, and become filled with electron-dense melanin. At the light microscopic level this maturity of organelles does not confer obvious pigmentation, and at birth the iris is flat, the stroma being thin and almost transparent except close to the collarette [105]. Nonmigration of melanocytes has been implicated in the wider remit of a "neurocristopathy" in cases of Potter's syndrome in which there is also generalized posterior axial corneal malformation and uveoretinal angiodysgenesis [88].

K. Development of the Anterior Chamber Angle and Trabecular Meshwork

The structures forming the filtration meshwork derive from the rim of ectomesenchyme, which accumulates as a roll around the lip of the optic cup and, as described earlier, gives rise to the corneal stroma as well as most of the development of the sclera (see later) [104,105]. The angle and meshwork arise from the second wave of migrating neural crest cells, and the iridocorneal angle is absent before 12–13 weeks gestation [85]. In sections of 4-month-old embryos the angle is seen as a triangular mass [105,124]. The peripheral corneal endothelium sweeps over the lower face of the developing meshwork, and the single layer of flattened endothelial cells merges into the meshwork. Contiguous with the meshwork is a circumferential channel (Schlemm's canal), which is destined to facilitate the drainage of aqueous humor from the anterior chamber when fully formed. The canal of Schlemm is also continuous with the meshwork. By the 210 mm stage the canal is seen to have a vascular endothelial lining, having been preceded by an ill-defined plexus of vessels [105]. Some authors believe that the corneal endothelial cells also contribute to Schlemm's canal [133] and that the canal develops from several foci and eventually becomes continuous.

The collagen cores within the trabecular meshwork develop during month 7 and are laid down alongside the basement membrane surrounding the canal. The endothelial cells of the canal are vacuolated during month 4 of gestation and thin out, to become joined by tight junctions [105,133]. The angle is represented by a loose reticulum into which the uveal elements interdigitate. Molding of the meshwork and the increasing growth of the ciliary body, plus the extension of the iris tissue, mean that the canal eventually comes to rest at the apex of the angle. The formation of the anterior chamber angle was previously ascribed to a cleavage phenomenon and to atrophy, but it seems more likely, from transmission electron microscopy studies [84,133], to result from rearrangement and tectonic shifts. A progressive rise in the outflow of aqueous from the anterior chamber is facilitated by splitting and rearrangement of Descemet's membrane as it crosses the face of the meshwork. In the normal human fetus no permanent endothelial cell covering of the face of the meshwork can be distinguished, although in some instances membranous extensions of trabecular meshwork epithelial cells rather than endothelial cells appear to have developed [85].

L. Development of the Choroid

The choroid is one of the most vascular tissues of the body. Injection studies by Heimann and Terheggen [47] and others have shown that endothelially lined blood spaces appear to arise around the outer margin of the optic cup after pigmentation of the outer layer, developing as the RPE is initiated. These channels converge and coalesce at the annular vessel encircling the lip of the cup [105] and drain into the supraorbital and infraorbital venous plexus. At the 10 mm stage, during month 2 of gestation, the plexus forms a palisade around the cup. Later in the same month, at the 30 mm stage, it anastomoses, with twigs developing as spurs from the posterior ciliary arteries. The vortex veins form from collecting channels draining the plexus. A second venous layer is defined after the initial stretching of the network, and the closed channels of the choriocapillaris develop beneath this layer. Formation of the choriocapillaris is dependent on contact with the RPE [78].

The posterior ciliary arteries sprout branches that reach the macular region by the beginning of month 4. Haller's layer of larger choroidal arteriovenous vessels forms during month 4 [120,121], and the second venous layer becomes linked to the vortex veins. The arborizing vessels that radiate from the short posterior ciliary arteries extend through this vascular bed and eventually pierce the capillary network of the choriocapillaris. This gives rise to the characteristic dual arterial and venous systems that extend from the optic nerve head to the ocular equator. Distal to the ocular equator, the vasculature remains more primitive, in line with the relatively slower development delay of the anterior optic cup as opposed to the posterior. The circle of Zinn-Haller around the optic nerve head is derived from the posterior short ciliary arteries. The short posterior ciliary arteries also give rise to the third arterial layer of the choroid, extending toward the ocular equator in the plane lying between the choriocapillaris and the scleral vessels. At the same time the network is completed to form the venous component of the middle layer of the choroid, named after Sattler. These veins arise as arcades from the choriocapillaris. The final components to be added are the recurrent arterial branches in the anterior choroid, at the same time as the circle of Zinn-Haller is completed. The structure of venules and arterioles in the human choroid is established between 15 and 22 weeks of gestation [120,121].

The stromal elements of the choroid arise after the sclera has enveloped the optic cup and begin as a loose mesenchymal matrix, within which fibroblasts start to secrete collagen fibrils. Muscle elements and elastic tissue are also present by month 4 of gestation. Distinct layers within the choroid are distinguishable at this stage, with the emergence of the loose lamellae of the suprachoroidal layer [105]. Neural crest-derived pigmentation of the choroid occurs late in gestation as elsewhere, and the melanosomes are not usually visible before month 7, having migrated late from the neural crest. The presence of pigmentation depends on the integrity of the neural tube and starts in the outermost layers of the choroid [25]. Adrenergic nerve fibers are present throughout the uvea, and they probably play a role in induction and maintenance of pigmentation, as is thought to be the case in the iris [68,139].

M. Development of the Sclera

The sclera also forms from the neural crest. It initially presents as a mesenchymal condensation at the region of the corneoscleral limbus, and growth proceeds in a posterior direction. In contrast to the cornea, where there is a need for transparency, the scleral fibroblasts do not become realigned in a parallel array and the subsequent secretion and appositional growth is more random and has been likened to a corkscrew [104,142]. Appositional growth of fibrils is also more marked than in the cornea, and although the fibrils are slimmer than corneal fibrils early in their development, by the middle of the first trimester they are much thicker. Also, in contrast to the cornea, there is secretion of elastic moieties. In humans there is no cartilaginous element to the sclera as there is in birds. Birds also have scleral ossicles. In the series of human embryos examined by Sevel and Isaacs [124], it was possible to distinguish a superficial spongy area and a deeper, more compact area, corresponding to the episclera and the true sclera, respectively, by the 28 mm stage of embryogenesis.

By month 4 of gestation the scleral connective tissue fibrils have penetrated the optic nerve, where they run between the neuroglia surrounding the axons, forming the cup-shaped sieve of the lamina cribrosa, which is completed by month 8, and condensing around the axon bundles, where they provide a scaffold by month 5. They then merge with the adventitia of the hyaloid vessels.

N. Development of the Vitreous and Hyaloid System

The primary transitory vascular vitreous is of immense importance in the development of the eye. A survey [105] shows that the main development of the arborizing vascular elements of the primary vitreous arises as a result of the outgrowth of the hyaloid artery from the primitive dorsal ophthalmic artery at the 5 mm stage as it passes through the embryonic fissure. From the centrally placed hyaloid artery develops a vascular network that fills the cavity of the primary optic vesicle (vasa hyaloidea propria). This network comes to lie behind the developing lens vesicle and its fibrotic capsule, which also contains vasoformative elements. A capillary mesh joins the central hyaloid system and the perilenticular mesenchyme to form the lenticular vascular tunic, and other vessels form a palisade around the lens. Further branches arc around the lens to communicate with the annular vessel, which forms after curved outgrowths of the hyaloid artery reach the edge of the optic cup. These arcing vessels anastomose with vascular sinuses lying outside the cup. The annular vessel also sends branches forward to form the anterior vascular lens capsule and intercommunicates with sinusoids in the developing choroid.

The development of the hyaloid vasculature reaches its zenith in week 9 of gestation (40 mm), and at that time the annular vessel appears to function as both artery and vein, communicating with both the hyaloid artery and choroidal sinusoids. A network of small vessels, draining from the anterior lens capsule, the pupillary membrane, and the developing vitreous, centers on the region where the ciliary body develops. These vessels eventually connect with and drain into the choroidal vascular plexus [146].

The connective tissue of the vitreous evolves through a primary phase, first observable at 13 weeks gestation as a mass of fibrillary material, mesenchymal cells, and primitive blood vessels. Some authorities consider that at least part of the primary vitreous is of surface ectodermal origin, carried into the cavity with the invaginating lens placode; others suggest that the bulk of the mesenchyme is derived from cells of neural crest origin migrating in from the ventral rim and that in addition a substantial component from the mesenchyme accompanies the hyaloid vasculature [6,72,105]. It is also possible, since the footplates of the Müller cells at the posterior pole of the vitreous are continuous with the vitreous fibers, that there is a contribution from the neuroectoderm of the optic cup from the inner neuroblastic layer. Fibroblastic, filamentous, and macrophagelike cells have all been described within the primary vitreous, and the number of macrophages increases as the vascular system develops. In the beginning there is no discernible orientation of the fibrils, but as part of the development of the secondary (permanent) vitreous between the

13 and 70 mm stages a more ordered and often parallel fibrillary network eventually replaces the primary loose meshwork (Fig. 7) [105].

The fully developed hyaloid vasculature at 2 months consists of nonfenestrated endothelial cells lying on a basement membrane, partially surrounded by connective tissue elements. Regression begins in the vasa hyaloidea propria, when the vessels become choked and occluded with macrophages. Resolution continues as the capillaries surrounding the lens atrophy in a sequential centrifugal fashion, followed last by the regression of the hyaloid artery. This process is initiated very early at the 13 mm stage and is almost complete by the end of the first trimester. Loss of the capillary network leads to atrophy of the perilenticular fibrotic capsule, especially in the central portion. The pitlike opening becomes part of a funnel-shaped structure formed from the media of the hyaloid artery and its arterioles. Known as the canal of Cloquet, this structure eventually contains remnants of both the hyaloid artery (in which flow ceases in month 7) and the primary vitreous, which retracts as its blood supply fails. At birth Cloquet's canal persists, running from the patellar fossa of the lens to the optic disk. In most cases resorption of almost all primary vitreous elements and those of the hyaloid artery has occurred.

In the rabbit [6] existing evidence suggests that the secondary vitreous is formed from specialized cells, dubbed hyalocytes, which are thought to derive from the immigration and entrapment of blood-borne monocytes that have migrated from the ciliary body. Such cells may also act as facultative phagocytes, engulfing all other elements of the primary vitreous before passing into a secretory mode in which they manufacture hyaluronic acid in addition to laying down the collagen fibrils of the secondary vitreous. These secondary vitreous fibrils are thicker and have a greater tendency to aggregate at the edge of the optic cup than those of the primary vitreous. They merge into the neuroectodermally derived mesenchyme at the lip of the optic cup. The vitreous base develops from this merger, seen at the 65 mm stage as a marginal bundle (of Druault) firmly anchoring the vitreous to the internal limiting membrane of the retina (Fig. 8).

Development of the zonular fibers (Fig. 9) has been credited to both lens epithelial and neural crest cells, but the studies of Bronner-Fraser [12,13] on tenascin appear to support the contention that they develop from the neural crest with a possible contribution from the tunica vasculosa lentis, with which the immature fibers connect. Other investigators consider that incorporation of vitreal fibrils is involved [105].

By month 5 of development (170 mm), with regression of the vitreous to its pars plana base, attachment to the lens by Wiegert's ligament is complete. Zonular fibrils traverse the posterior chamber from the ciliary body to form a fused structure. Zonules are added to by basement membrane-like material secreted by the columnar cells of the ciliary body. There is also some incorporation of the internal limiting membrane of the neuroectodermally derived ciliary body. This fusion of neuroectoderm and neural crest,

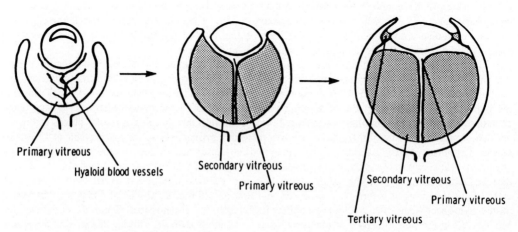

Figure 7   Development of the vitreous. The vascular tissue that forms the primary vitreous is first apparent at the 13 mm (6 week) stage and continues to grow for a further 3 weeks, until it dies back to be replaced by the connective tissue moieties that form the secondary vitreous. The development of the tertiary vitreous starts at the 65 mm (12 week) stage.

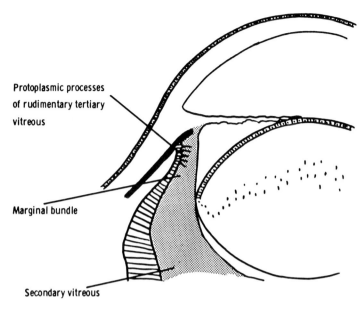

Figure 8   Formation of the tertiary vitreous. From the 65 mm, protoplasmic processes emerge from the rim of the optic cup and extend toward the lens. Initially such fibrillar processes run through the margins of the secondary vitreous.

with a possible contribution from both surface ectoderm and vascular mesenchyme, is eloquent testimony to the complexity of the orchestration involved in ocular development.

O.   Formation of the Adnexal Structures

The formation of the adnexa also involve complex interactions between surface ectodermal derivatives and mesenchyme, mostly of neural crest type but also of the normal, nonneural crest type.

The eyelids are derived from the frontonasal and maxillary processes. At the 4–5 week (12 mm) stage there is a proliferation of the skin ectoderm at the outer canthus, and by the 20 mm stage the eyelids are clearly seen as prominences. At this stage the mesenchymal proliferation starts, with proliferation of blood vessels and the influx of macrophages [2,3]. After the basal lamina thickens nerve fibers invade the developing eyelids and the amount of subepithelial collagen increases. As the underlying eye develops the eyelids grow both above and below the globe and elongate laterally until the margins contact one another at the 3 month (35–40 mm) stage [105,123]; fusion is complete by the 45 mm stage.

Fusion of the eyelids with the isolation of the developing conjunctiva and cornea from the amniotic fluid is contingent on the formation of desmosomal attachments, which remain intact until month 5 (150–170 mm) in the anterior portion and month 6 posteriorly. Subsequent separation is mediated by the keratinization of the eyelash follicles and the secretion of lipid within them, which serves to disrupt desmosomes uniting the two eyelids [2,3]. This time span of separation from initiation to completion is 2 months [123] and experimentally can be hastened by enhanced keratinization of epithelium under the influence of EGF, which is present in amniotic fluid from 20 weeks gestation.

The musculature of the eyelids develops from the second branchial arch mesoderm. These somatically derived muscles, which form the orbicularis palpebrae, differ structurally from oculomotor muscles, although both are innervated by cranial nerves.

The lacrimal gland is derived from the conjunctiva (see later). It is first perceived at the 25 mm stage as a bud from the conjunctiva in the temporal upper fornix [105]. This is subsequently divided by the tendon of the levator muscle to produce the palpebral lobe and orbital lacrimal gland. The gland develops as cores of secretory cells within which lumina appear, separated by connective tissue. The gland continues to grow until the age of 3 or 4 years [24]. Lymphoid aggregates occur with increasing frequency in age but are rare

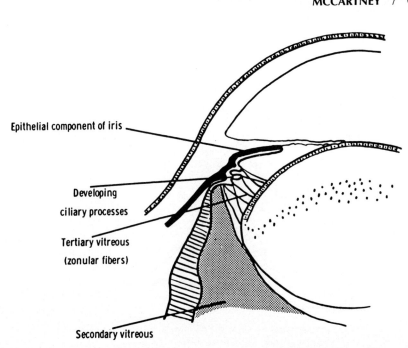

Epithelial component of iris

Developing
ciliary processes

Tertiary vitreous
(zonular fibers)

Secondary vitreous

Figure 9   Formation of the lens zonular fibers. During month 4 of gestation, the fibers of the tertiary vitreous become distinct and separate from the surrounding secondary vitreous, which is subsequently resorbed in their vicinity. Before their atrophy this annular region is known as the marginal bundle of Drualt.

in the young. The lacrimal passages also form as epithelial cores 15 mm beneath the nasal and maxillary processes. Canalization begins in month 3, and communication between the eye and nose is complete after 6 months gestation [105].

The eyelashes are first seen at the 40 mm stage as epithelial buds extending backward into the underlying mesenchyme. They are oriented in the anterior posterior plane with the upper eyelid cilia in two rows, and soon afterward the mucus-producing goblet cells are formed, being fully differentiated at the 52 mm stage [105]. These cells, which are present first in the apical part of the eyelid, are succeeded by the meibomian (holocrine) sebaceous gland anlage and the apocrine glands of Moll, associated with the hair shafts at the 80 mm stage. The sebaceous glands of Zeis are formed later at the 90–100 mm stage, and lipid production starts soon afterward, followed by the production of keratin within the walls of the shafts at the 110–120 mm stage. The lipid secretion within the shafts causes eruptions through the surface epithelium, and the hair-forming cells penetrate down through these lipid-filled shafts to produce the entire pilosebaceous complex, which becomes completely keratinized by 5 months (170 mm stage). The tarsus is formed from the condensation of basal laminae around the developing glands, with incorporation of the adjacent collagen. The eyelid is innervated with periadventitial fibers present at 3 months, and motor endings are also seen at this stage. Sensory innervation occurs later, at the 6 month stage, but the development of specialized endings, Krause's corpuscles, is delayed until the end of month 7 [105,123].

The development of the orbit is dependent on the formation of the optic cup, which develops before any bony formation. Enchondral ossification of the base of the skull in the lesser wing of the sphenoid bone is accompanied by membranous ossification of its greater wing and the rest of the bony orbit at the 6 month stage, with fusion at about 7 months. These latter bones are neural crest derived. The mesenchymal cells derived from the crest interact with extracellular matrix (ECM) formed from epithelial cells. Without this interaction with ECM, ossification cannot occur. There is condensation of mesenchymal cells into compact nodules to produce osteoblasts, which become arrayed along the matrix, which then becomes progressively calcified. This is achieved by secretion of GAG and collagen to form an osteoid matrix [67], and at the same time calcium salts are relayed to the region by the capillaries. Some osteoblasts become entrapped within the matrix [56,134]. Calcification radiates out from the center until the whole region of developing spicules becomes enveloped in a compact band of mesenchymal cells that form the periosteum. All flat diploic bones of the head and neck follow this sequence, including those bones developed from the frontonasal and maxillary processes. The maxillary process forms the floor and lateral wall of the orbit and the nasal, the lacrimal and ethmoid bones. The ethmoid bone is the first membranous bone of the orbit, formed at 6–8 weeks gestation, and the fibrous trochlea is present at 40 mm. In concert with other membranous bone, ossification is not complete at birth: the angle of the orbital axes slowly closes so that the eyes become more frontally oriented, changing from almost 180° to the 105° position at 3 months and 71° at birth; 68° is the adult angle [105]. Reorientation is due to accumulation of connective tissues behind and lateral to the globes.

The enchondral ossification of the lesser wing of the sphenoid bone follows a different sequence as the cartilaginous model that forms from the aggregates of non–neural crest-derived mesenchymal cells is progressively remodeled into bone [56].

The connective tissue of the orbit includes fat as well as fibrous septa. Both of these are of neural crest origin, and the fat is of the primitive brown cell type, with characteristic polygonal cell shape and prominent nuclei. The brown color seen macroscopically is due to the high mitochondrial cytochrome content of the cells. This type of fat is associated with the process of hibernation in lower animals when energy is conserved in these cells.

The oculomotor muscles are of mesodermal origin and arise as vesicles in conjunction with cranial nerves III, IV, and VI in the absence of segmental development in the head. Ozanics and Jakobiec [105] reviewed the work of Gilbert [34], who showed a prechordal mass giving rise to the premandibular condensation and four oculomotor muscles associated with cranial nerve III at 26 days, whereas the other two oculomotor primordia arise in the maxillomandibular mesoderm [at 27 days for nerve VI innervated lateral rectus and on day 29 for the superior oblique (cranial nerve IV)]. Sevel [122], however, has suggested that the development of the extraocular muscles is a result of differentiation within the orbital (neural crest-derived) connective tissues. He contends that there is no ingrowth of mesodermal muscle precursors with anterior growth but that all the muscle parts develop contemporaneously and pass through a sequence of myoblastic induction from indistinguishable mesenchyme into recognizable myotubular elements following fusion of the myoblasts.

The growth of the orbit is dependent on the growth of the globe, and its shape changes from a hemisphere to a more conical shape as the globe becomes more mature. Although growth of the eye ceases at about 3 years, the orbit continues to grow with the rest of the faciomaxillary bones until the final stages of puberty are over

ACKNOWLEDGMENTS

I thank Prof. Peter Thorogood, Dr. Glen Jeffries, Dr. M. Andy Parsons, and Mrs. Sarah Lawrence for their help in the initial preparation of this chapter and acknowledge the seminal role of Drs. Ozanics and Jakobiec. Portions of the material included in this chapter were originally presented in the chapter in the first edition authored by Dr. Joan Mullaney.

REFERENCES

1. Alison, M.R., and Sarraf, C.E. Apoptosis: A gene directed programme of cell death. *J. R. Coll. Physicians Lond.* 26:25–35, 1992.
2. Andersen, H., Ehlers, N., and Matthiessen, M.E. Histochemistry and development of the human eyelids. *Acta Ophthalmol. (Copenh.)* 45:642–668, 1965.
3. Andersen, H., Ehlers, N., and Mattiessen, M.E. Histochemistry and development of the human eyelids II. *Acta Ophthalmol. (Copenh.)* 47:288–293, 1967.
4. Ashton, N. The mode of development of the retinal vessels in man. In *William MacKensie Centenary Symposium on the Ocular Circulation in Health and Disease*, J.S. Cant (Ed.), C.V. Mosby, St. Louis, pp. 7–17, 1969.
5. Ashton, N. Retinal angiogenesis in the human embryo. *Br. Med. Bull.* 26:103–106, 1970.
6. Balazs, E.A., Toth, L.Z., and Ozanics, V. Cytological studies on the developing vitreous as related to the hyaloid vessel system. *Graefes Arch. Clin. Exp. Ophthalmol.* 213:71–85, 1980.
7. Beazley, L.D., Dunlop, S.A., Harman, A.M., and Coleman, L.-A. Development of cell density gradients in the retinal ganglion cell layer of amphibians and marsupials. Two solutions to one problem. In *Development of the*

Vertebrate Retina, B.L. Finlay and D.R. Segelaub (Eds.), Perspectives in Vision Research, C. Blakemore (Ed.), Plenum Press, New York, pp. 199–226, 1989.

8. Bee, J.A. Development and pattern of innervation of the avian cornea. *Dev. Biol. 92*:5–15, 1982.
9. Bee, J., and Thorogood, P. The role of tissue interactions in the skeletogenic differentiation of avian neural crest cells. *Dev. Biol. 78*:47–62, 1980.
10. Bellairs, R. The primitive streak and the neural crest: comparable regions of cell migration. In *Developmental and Evolutionary Aspects of the Neural Crest*, P.F.A. Maderson (Ed.), John Wiley & Sons, New York, pp. 124–139, 1987.
11. Bock, G., and Widdows, K. (Eds.). *Myopia and the Control of Eye Growth*, Ciba Foundation Symposium 155, John Wiley & Sons, Chichester, pp. 1–256, 1990.
12. Bronner-Fraser, M. Adhesive interactions in neural crest development. In *Developmental and Evolutionary Aspects of the Neural Crest*, P.F.A. Maderson (Ed.), John Wiley, New York, pp. 11–32, 1987.
13. Bronner-Fraser, M. Distribution and function of tenascin during cranial neural crest development in the chick. *J. Neurosurg. Res. 21*:135–147, 1988.
14. Compston, A. Cellular organisation of the optic nerve and the implications for optic neuritis. *Eye 6*:123–128, 1992.
15. Coulombre, A.J. Regulation of ocular morphogenesis. *Invest. Ophthalmol. 8*:25–30, 1969.
16. Curcio, C.A., and Allen, K.A. Topography of ganglion cells in human retina. *J. Comp. Neurol. 300*:5–25, 1990.
17. Curcio, C.A., Sloan, K.R., Packer, O., Hendrickson, A.E., and Kalina, R.E. Distribution of cones in monkey and human retina: Individual variability and radial asymmetry. *Science 236*:579–582, 1987.
18. Curcio, C.A., and Hendrickson, A. Organisation and development of the primate photoreceptor mosaic. In *Progress in Retinal Research*, Vol. 10, N.N. Osborne and G.J. Chader (Eds.), Pergamon Press, Oxford, pp. 90–120, 1991.
19. Cuthbertson, R.A., and Lang, R.A. Developmental ocular disease in GM-CSF transgenic mice is mediated by autostimulated macrophages. *Dev. Biol. 134*:119–129, 1989.
20. Descemet, J. An sola lens crystallina cataracte sedes? (Praes. C.F. Theroulde) 1758.
21. Drager, U.C. Calcium binding in pigmented and albino eyes. *Proc. Natl. Acad. Sci. USA 82*:6716–6720, 1985.
22. Duband, J.L., and Thiery, J.P. Distribution of fibronectin in the early phase of avian cephalic neural crest cell migration. *Dev. Biol. 93*:308–323, 1982.
23. Duddell, B.A. Treatise of the diseases of the horney-coat of the eye. J. Clark & J. Roberts, London, 1729.
24. Duke-Elder, S. Normal and abnormal development, Part 1. *System of Ophthalmology*, Vol. 3, Kimpton, London, pp. 1–312, 1964.
25. Endo, H., and Hu, F. Pigment cell development in rhesus monkey eyes: An electron microscopic and histo-chemical study. *Dev. Biol. 32*:69–81, 1973.
26. Engerman, R.L. Development of macular circulation. *Invest. Ophthalmol. Vis. Sci. 15*:835–843, 1976.
27. Erickson, C.A. Role of the extracellular matrix in neural crest and mesenchyme cell migration. In *Developmental and Evolutionary Aspects of the Neural Crest*, P.F.A. Maderson (Ed.), John Wiley & Sons, New York, pp. 39–55, 1987.
28. Fernald, R.D. Retinal rod neurogenesis. In *Development of the Vertebrate Retina*, B.L. Finlay and D.R. Sengelaub (Eds.), Plenum Press, New York, pp. 31–42, 1989.
29. Friede, R.L., and Hu, K.H. Proximo-distal differences in myelin development in human optic fibers. *Z. Zellforsh. 79*:259–264, 1967.
30. Fujisawa, H., Morioka, H., Wanatabe, H., and Nakamura, H. A decay in gap junctions associated with cell differentiation of neural retina in chick embryonic development. *J. Cell Sci. 22*:585–596, 1976.
31. Fulton, A.B., Albert, D.M., and Craft, J.L. Human albinism. Light and electron microscopy study. *Arch. Ophthalmol. 96*:305–310, 1978.
32. Garrod, P.R. Desmosomes, cell adhesion markers and the adhesive properties of cells in tissues. *J. Cell Sci. (Suppl.) 4*:221–237, 1986.
33. Gierer, A. Regulation and reproducibility of morphogenesis. *Dev. Biol. 2*:89–93, 1991.
34. Gilbert, P.W. The origin and development of the human extrinsic ocular muscles. *Contrib. Embryol.*, Vol. 36, Carnagie Inst. Publication 416; *246*:59–78, 1957.
35. Gilbert, S.F. *Developmental Biology*, 3rd ed. Sinauer Associates, Sunderland, MA, pp. 176–661, 1991.
36. Goldschmidt, E. Myopia in humans: Can progression be arrested? In *Myopia and the Control of Eye Growth*, G. Bock and K. Widdows (Eds.), John Wiley & Sons, Chichester, Ciba Foundation Symposium 155, pp. 222–233, 1990.
37. Goldstein, J.E., and Cogan D.G. Sclerocornea and associated congenital abnormalities. *Arch. Ophthalmol. 67*: 761–768, 1962.
38. Goronowitsch, N. Untersuchungen über die Entwicklung der sogenannten Ganglienleisten im Kopfe der Vögel-embryonen. *Morphol. Jahrb. 20*:187–259, 1893.
39. Grainger, R.M., Henry, J.J., Saha, M.S., and Servetnick, M. Recent progress on the mechanisms of embryonic lens formation. *Eye 6*:117–122, 1992.
40. Guillery, R.W., Jeffrey, G., and Cattenach, B.M. The number of uncrossed retinofugal fibers in mice that show albino mosaicism: High variability indicates that a small cell group determines the albino abnormality. *Soc. Neurosci. Abstr. 12*:122, 1986.

41. Hall, B.K. Tissue interactions in the development and evolution of the vertebrate head. In *Developmental and Evolutionary Aspects of the Neural Crest*, P.F.A. Maderson (Ed.), John Wiley & Sons, New York, pp. 230–257, 1987.

42. Hall, B.K. The embryonic development of bone. *Am. Sci. 76*:174–181, 1988.

43. Hay, E.D., and Revel, J.-P. Fine structure of the developing avian cornea. *Monographs in Developmental Biology* No. 1, A. Wolsky and P.S. Chen (Eds.), Basel Karger, Basel, 1–144, 1969.

44. Hay, E. Development of the vertebrate cornea. *Int. Rev. Cytol. 63*:263–322, 1980.

45. Hay, E.D., Linsenmayer, T.F., Trelsted, R.L., and von der Mark, K. Origins and distribution of collagens in the developing avian cornea. *Curr. Top. Eye Res. 1*:1–35, 1982.

46. Hayes, B.P. The distribution of intercellular gap junctions in the developing retina and retinal pigment epithelium of *Xenopus laevis*. *Anat. Embryol. 150*:99–111, 1976.

47. Heimann, K., and Terheggen, G. Über das Vorkommen von choroidalen Blubildungsherden bei Embryonne und Feten. *Ber, Zusammenkunft Dtsch. Ophthalmol. Ges. 70*:467–472, 1969.

48. Hendrickson, A. A morphological comparison of foveal development in man and monkey. *Eye 6*:136–142, 1992.

49. Hendrickson, A., and Kupfer, C. The histogenesis of the fovea in the macaque monkey. *Invest. Ophthalmol. Vis. Sci. 15*:746–756, 1976.

50. Hendrickson, A., and Yuodelis, C. The morphological development of the human fovea. *Ophthalmology 91*:603–612, 1984.

51. Henkind, P., Bellhorn, R.W., Murphy, M.E., and Roa, N. Development of macular vessels in monkey and cat. *Br. J. Ophthalmol. 59*:703–709, 1975.

52. Hilfer, S.R., and Yang, J-J.W. Accumulation of CPC-precipitable material at apical cell surfaces during formation of the optic cup. *Anat. Rec. 197*:423–433, 1980.

53. Hinds, J.W., and Hinds, P.L. Development of retinal amacrine cells in the mouse embryo: Evidence for two modes of formation. *J. Comp. Neurol. 213*:1–23, 1983.

54. Holtfreter, J. Mesenchyme and epithelia in inductive and morphogenetic processes. In *Epithelial-Mesenchymal Interactions*, 18th Hahnemann Symposium, R. Fleischmajer and R. Billingham (Eds.), Williams & Wilkins, Baltimore, pp. 1–30, 1968.

55. Hörstadius, S. *The Neural Crest, Its Properties and Derivatives in the Light of Experimental Research*, Oxford University Press, London, 1950.

56. Horton, W.A. The biology of bone growth. *Growth Genet. Horm. 6*:1–3, 1990.

57. Jacobson, A.G. Determination and morphogenesis of axial structure: mesodermal metamerism, shaping of the neural plate and tube, and segregation and functions of the neural crest. In *Developmental and Evolutionary Aspects of the Neural Crest*, P.F.A. Maderson (Ed.), 148–180, John Wiley & Sons, New York, 1987.

58. Johnson, D.H., Bourne, W.M., and Campbell, R.J. The ultrastructure of Descemet's membrane. I. Changes with age in normal corneas. *Arch. Ophthalmol. 100*:1942–1947, 1982.

59. Johnston, M.C. The neural crest in abnormalities of the face and brain. In *Morphogenesis and Malformation of Face and Brain*, D. Bergsma (Ed.), Liss, New York, pp. 1–18, 1975 (*Birth Defects* Original article Series XI, Vol. 7).

60. Johnston, M.C., Morriss, G.M., Kushner, D.C., and Bingle, G.J. Abnormal organogenesis of facial structures. In *Handbook of Teratology*, Vol. 2, J.G. Wilson and F. Clarke Frazer (Eds.), Plenum Press, New York, pp. 421–451, 1977.

61. Kanasawa, S. Electron microscopic study of the human foetal optic nerve. *Nippon Ganka Gakkai Zasshi 73*:1330–1353, 1969.

62. Kastschenko, N. Zur Entwicklungsgeschichte der Selachierembryos. *Anat. Anz. 3*:445–467, 1888.

63. Kessel, M., and Gruss, P. Murine development control genes. *Science 249*:374–379, 1990.

64. Kirkness, C.M., McCartney, A., Rice, N.S.C., Garner, A., and Steele, A.D.McG. Congenital hereditary corneal oedema of Maumenee; its clinical features, management and pathology. *Br. J. Ophthalmol. 71*:130–144, 1987.

65. Kuwabara, T. The maturation of lens cells: A morphological study. *Exp. Eye Res. 20*:427–443, 1975.

66. Kuwabara, T., and Weidman, T.A. Development of the prenatal rat retina. *Invest. Ophthalmol. Vis. Sci. 3*:725–739, 1974.

67. Langman, J. *Medical Embryology*, 4th ed., Williams & Wilkins, Baltimore, pp. 1–212, 1981.

68. Laties, A.M. Ocular melanin and the adrenergic innervation to the eye. *Trans. Am. Ophthalmol. Soc. 72*:560–605, 1974.

69. Le Douarin, N.M. Cell recognition based on natural morphological nuclear markers. *Med. Biol. 52*:281–319, 1974.

70. Le Douarin, N.M. Cell line segregation during peripheral nervous system ontogeny. *Science 231*:1515–1522, 1986.

71. Le Douarin, N.M., Cochard, P., Vincent, M., Duband, J.L., Tucker, G.C., Teillet, M.-A., and Thiery, J.-P. Nuclear, cytoplasmic, and membrane markers to follow neural crest migration. A comparative study. In *The Role of the Extracellular Matrix in Development*, R.L. Trelsted (Ed.), Alan R. Liss, New York, pp. 373–398, 1984.

72. Lerche, W., and Wulle, K.-G. Zur Feinstruktur des embryonalen menischlichenen Glakörpers unter besonder

Berucksichtigung seiner Beziehung zu Linse und retina. *Ber Zusammenkunft Dtsch. Ophthalmol. Ges. 68*:82–92, 1967.

73. Lerche, W., and Wülle, K.-G. Electron microscopic studies on the development of the human lens. *Ophthalmologica 158*:296–309, 1969.

74. Leventhal, A.G., and Schall, J.D. Extrinsic determinants of retinal ganglion cell development in cats and monkeys. In *Development of the Vertebrate Retina*, B.L. Finlay and D.R. Sengelaub (Eds.), Plenum Press, New York, pp. 173–195, 1989.

75. Levy, S.G., Moss, J., and McCartney, A.C.E. Abnormal Descemet's membrane in the iridoendothelial syndrome: An electron microscopic immunocytochemical study. *Invest. Ophthalmol. Vis. Sci. (Suppl.) 32*:771, 1992.

76. Maderson, P.F.A. Historical background and our hopes for an interdisciplinary consideration of the neural crest. In *Development and Evolutionary Aspects of the Neural Crest*, P.F.A. Maderson (Ed.), Wiley, New York, pp. 3–7, 1987.

77. Malpighi, M. Opera omnia. Lugduni, Batav, 1687.

78. Mann, I. *The Development of the Human Eye*, 2nd ed., British Medical Association, London, pp. 1–312, 1949.

79. Marx, J. How embryos tell heads from tails. *Science 254*:1586–1588, 1991.

80. Masland, R.H. The functional architecture of the retina. In *The Biology of the Brain: From Neurons to Networks* (readings from *Scientific American*), R.R. Llinas (Ed.), W.H. Freeman, New York, pp. 131–145, 1989.

81. McAvoy, J.W., and Chamberlain, C.G. Growth factors in the eye. *Prog. Growth Factor Res. 2*:29–43, 1990.

82. McCartney, A.C.E., Bull, T.B., and Spalton, D.J. Fuchs' heterochromic cyclitis: An electron microscopic study. *Trans. Ophthalmol. Soc. UK 116*:324–329, 1985.

83. McCartney, A.C.E., and Kirkness, C.M. Comparison between posterior polymorphous dystrophy and congenital hereditary endothelial dystrophy of the cornea. *Eye 2*:63–70, 1988.

84. McCartney, A.C.E., Riordan-Eva, P., Howes, R., and Spalton, D.J. Electron microscopy of the iris in Horner's syndrome. *Br. J. Ophthalmol. 76*:746–749, 1992.

85. McMenamin, P.G. A morphological study of the inner surface of the anterior chamber angle in pre and postnatal eyes. *Curr. Eye Res. 8*:727–739, 1989.

86. Meier, S. Initiation of corneal differentiation prior to cornea-lens association. *Cell Tissue Res. 184*:255–267, 1977.

87. Michaelson, I.C. The mode of development of the vascular system of the retina with some observations on its significance for certain retinal diseases. *Trans. Ophthalmol. Soc. UK 68*:137–180, 1948.

88. Mooy, C.M., Clark, B.J., and Lee, W.R. Posterior axial corneal malformation and uveoretinal angiodysgenesis—a neurocristopathy. *Graefes Arch. Clin. Exp. Ophthalmol. 228*:9–18, 1990.

89. Morest, D.K. The pattern of neurogenesis in the retina of the rat. *Z. Anat. Entwicklungsgesch. 131*:45–67, 1970.

90. Morriss-Kay, G.M. Growth and development of pattern in the cranial neuroepithelium of rat embryos during neurulation. *J. Embryol. Exp. Morphol. (Suppl.) 65*:225–241, 1981.

91. Morse, D.E., and McCann, P.S. Neuroectoderm of the early embryonic rat eye. *Invest. Ophthalmol. Vis. Sci. 25*:899–907, 1984.

92. Müller, F., and O'Rahilly, R. The development of the human brain, the closure of the caudal neuropore, and the beginning of secondary neurulation at stage 12. *Anat. Embryol. 176*:413–430, 1987.

93. Mund, M.L., Rodrigues, M.M., and Fine, B.S. Light and electron microscopic observations on the pigmented layers of the human eye. *Am. J. Ophthalmol. 73*:167–182, 1972.

94. Murakami, D., Sesma, M.A., and Rowe, M.H. Characteristics of nasal and temporal retina in Siamese and normally pigmented cats. *Brain Behav. Evol. 21*:67–113, 1982.

95. Murphy, C., Alvarado, J., and Juster, R. Prenatal and postnatal growth of the human Descemet's membrane. *Invest. Ophthalmol. Vis. Sci. 25*:1402–1415, 1984.

96. Murphy, C., Alvarado, J., Juster, R., and Maglio, M. Prenatal and postnatal cellularity of the human corneal endothelium: A quantitative histologic study. *Invest. Ophthalmol. Vis. Sci. 25*:312–320, 1984.

97. Noden, D.M. Periocular mesenchyme: Neural crest and mesodermal interactions. In *Ocular Anatomy, Embryology, and Teratology*, F.A. Jakobiec (Ed.), Harper and Row, Philadelphia, pp. 97–119, 1982.

98. Noden, D.M. Origins and patterning of craniofacial mesenchymal tissues. *J. Craniofac. Genet. Dev. Biol. Suppl. 2*:15–32, 1986.

99. Noden, D.M. Interactions between cephalic neural crest and mesodermal populations. In *Developmental and Evolutionary Aspects of the Neural Crest*, P.F.A. Maderson (Ed.), John Wiley & Sons, New York, pp. 90–119, 1987.

100. Olver, J.M., and McCartney, A.C.E. Anterior segment casting. *Eye 3*:302–307, 1989.

101. O'Rahilly, R. The early development of the eye in staged human embryos. *Contrib. Embryol. Carneg. Inst. 38*:1–42, 1966.

102. O'Rahilly, R. Developmental Stages in Human Embryos, Including a Survey of the Carnegie Collection, Part A. Embryos of the First Three Weeks (Stages 1–9). Carnegie Institution, Publication 631, Washington, DC, pp. 1–167, 1973.

103. O'Rahilly, R. The prenatal development of the human eye. *Exp. Eye Res. 21*:91–112, 1975.

104. Ozanics, V., Rayborn, M., and Sagun, D. Some aspects of corneal and scleral differentiation in the primate. *Exp. Eye Res. 22*:305–328, 1976.

105. Ozanics, V., and Jakobiec, F.A. Prenatal development of the eye and its adnexae. In *Ocular Anatomy, Embryology, and Teratology*, F.A. Jakobiec (Ed.), Harper and Row, Philadelphia, pp. 11–96, 1982.

106. Piatigorsky, J. Lens differentiation in vertebrates: A review of cellular and molecular features. *Differentiation 19*:134–153, 1981.

107. Platt, J.B. Ectodermic origin of the cartilages of the head. *Anat. Anz. 8*:506–509, 1893.

108. Platt, J.B. Ontogenetische Differentierung des Ectoderms in Necturus. *Arch. Mikro. Anat. 43*:911–966, 1894.

109. Polley, E.H., Zimmerman, R.P., and Fortney, R.L. Neurogenesis and maturation of cell morphology in the development of the mammalian retina. In *Development of the Vertebrate Retina*, B.L. Finlay and D.R. Sengelaub (Eds.), Plenum Press, New York, pp. 3–42, 1989.

110. Polyak, S.L. *The Retina*, University of Chicago Press, Chicago, 1941.

111. Provis, J.M. Patterns of cell death in the ganglion cell layer of the human retina. *J. Comp. Neurol. 259*:237–246, 1987.

112. Provis, J.M., van Driel, D., Bilson, F.A., and Russell, P. Development of the human retina: Patterns of cell distribution and redistribution in the ganglion cell layer. *J. Comp. Neurol. 233*:429–451, 1985.

113. Raff, M.C., Miller, R.H., and Noble, M. A glial progenitor cell that develops in vitro into an astrocyte or oligodendrocyte depending on culture medium. *Nature 303*:390–396, 1983.

114. Riseau, W. Angiogenic growth factors. *Prog. Growth Factor Res. 2*:71–79, 1990.

115. Saha, M., Spann, C.L., and Grainger, R.M. Embryonic lens induction: More than meets the optic vesicle. *Cell Differ. Dev. 28*:153–172, 1989.

116. Saha, M.S. Spelmann seen through a lens. In *A Conceptual History of Modern Embryology*, Vol. 7, S.F. Gilbert (Ed.), Plenum Press, New York, pp. 91–108, 1991.

117. Sawada, H., Konomi, H., and Hirosawa, K. Characterisation of the collagen in the hexagonal lattice of Descemet's membrane: Its relation to type VIII collagen. *J. Cell Biol. 110*:219–227, 1990.

118. Schaller, H.C., Hoffmeister, S.H., and Dübel, S. Role of the neuropeptide head activator for growth and development in *hydra* and mammals. *Development (Suppl.) 107*:99–100, 1989.

119. Schatz, C.J., and Sretavan, D.W. Interactions between retinal ganglion cells during the development of the mammalian visual system. *Annu. Rev. Neurosci. 9*:171–207, 1986.

120. Sellhayer, K. Development of the choroid and related structures. *Eye 4*:255–261, 1990.

121. Sellhayer, K., and Spitznas, M. Morphology of the developing choroidal vasculature in the human fetus. *Graefes Arch. Clin. Exp. Ophthalmol. 226*:461–467, 1988.

122. Sevel, D. Reappraisal of the origin of human extraocular muscles. *Ophthalmology 88*:1330–1338, 1988.

123. Sevel, D. A reappraisal of the development of the eyelids. *Eye 2*:123–129, 1988.

124. Sevel, D., and Issacs, R. A re-evaluation of corneal development. *Trans. Am. Ophthalmol. Soc. 34*:178–207, 1988.

125. Sidman, R.L. Histogenesis of mouse retina studied with thymidine-^{3}H. In *The Structure of the Eye*, G. Smelser (Ed.), Academic Press, New York, 1961.

126. Sigelman, J., and Ozanics, V. Retina. In *Ocular Anatomy and Teratology*, F.A. Jakobiec (Ed.), Harper and Row, Philadelphia, pp. 441–506, 1982.

127. Silver, J., and Hughes, A.F.W. The role of cell death during morphogenesis of the mammalian eye. *J. Morphol. 140*:159–170, 1973.

128. Silver, J., and Hughes, A.F.W. The relationship between morphogenetic cell death and the development of congenital anophthalmia. *J. Comp. Neurol. 157*:281–301, 1974.

129. Silver, J., and Robb, R.M. Studies on the development of the eye cup and optic nerve in normal mice and in mutants with congenital optic nerve aplasia. *Dev. Biol. 68*:175–190, 1979.

130. Silver, J., and Sapiro, J. Axonal guidance during development of the optic nerve: The role of the pigment epithelia and other extrinsic factors. *J. Comp. Neurol. 202*:521–538, 1981.

131. Silver, P.H.S., and Wakely, J. The initial stage in the development of the lens capsule in chick and mouse embryo. *Exp. Eye Res. 19*:73–77, 1974.

132. Smelser, G.K. Embryology and morphology of the lens. *Invest. Ophthalmol. Vis. Sci. 4*:398–410, 1965.

133. Smelser, G.K., and Ozanics, V. Development of the cornea. In *Symposium on the Cornea: Transactions of the New Orleans Academy of Ophthalmology*, Smelser, G.K. (Ed.), C.V. Mosby, St. Louis, pp. 20–29, 1972.

134. Smith, M.M. Putative skeletal neural crest cells in early late ordovician vertebrates from Colorado. *Science 251*:303–303, 1991.

135. Sparrow, J.R., and Barnstaple, C.J. A gradient molecule in developing rat retina: Expression of 9-O-acetyl GD_3 in relation to cell type, developmental age, and GD_3 ganglioside. *J. Neurosci. Res. 21*:398–409, 1988.

136. Spira, A.W., and Hollenberg, M.J. Human retinal development: Ultrastructural of the inner retinal layers. *Dev. Biol. 31*:1–21, 1973.

137. Starck, D. Embrylogie. *Ein Lehrbuch auf allgemein biologishcer Grundlage*, 2nd ed., G. Thieme, Stuttgart, pp. 1–562, 1965.

138. Strömland, K., Miller, M., and Cook, C. Ocular teratology. *Surv. Ophthalmol. 35*:429–446, 1991.

139. Stone, R.A., Ton, L.P., Iuvone, M., and Laties, A.M. Postnatal control of ocular growth: Dopaminergic mechanisms. In *Myopia and the Control of Eye Growth*, G. Bock and K. Widdows (Eds.), Ciba Foundation Symposium 155, John Wiley & Sons, Chichester, pp. 45–62, 1990.

140. Thorogood, P. Developmental and evolutionary aspects of the neural crest. *Trends Neurosci. 12*:38–39, 1989.

141. Thorogood, P., and Smith, L. Neural crest cells: The role of extracellular matrix in their differentiation. In *Matrices and Cell Differentiation*, R. Kemp and J.R. Hinchcliffe (Eds.), Liss, New York, pp. 171–185, 1984.

142. Trelsted, R.L. The bilaterally asymmetrical architecture of the submammalian corneal stroma resembles a cholesteric liquid crystal. *Dev. Biol. 92*:133–134, 1982.

143. Tuft, S.J., and Coster, D.J. The corneal endothelium. *Eye 4*:389–424, 1990.

144. Turner, D.L., and Cepko, C.L. A common progenitor for neurons and glia persists in rat retina late in development. *Nature 328*:131–136, 1987.

145. Waring, G.O. Posterior collagenous layer of the cornea. Ultrastructural classification of abnormal collagenous tissue posterior to Descemet's membrane in 30 cases. *Arch. Ophthalmol. 100*:122–134, 1982.

146. Webster, E.H., Silver, A.F., and Gonsalves, N.I. The extracellular matrix between the optic vesicle and the presumptive lens during lens morphogenesis in an anophthalmic strain of mice. *Dev. Biol. 103*:142–150, 1984.

147. Webster, M.J., Drager, U.C., and Silver, J. Development of the visual system in hypopigmented mutants. In *Development of the Vertebrate Retina*, B.L. Finlay and D.C. Sengelaub (Eds.), Plenum Press, New York, pp. 69–86, 1989.

148. Weinberg, R.L. Tumor suppressor genes. *Science 254*:1138–1146, 1991.

149. Whitmore, W.G. Congenital and developmental myopia. *Eye 6*:361–365, 1992.

150. Williams, D.R. Topography of the foveal cone mosaic in the living human eye. *Vision Res. 28*:43–454, 1988.

151. Williams, R.W., Bastiani, M.J., Lia, B., and Chalupa, L.M. Growth cones, dying axons and developmental fluctuations in the fiber population of the cat's optic nerve. *J. Comp. Neurol. 246*:32–69, 1986.

152. Wolpert, L. Positional information and pattern formation. *Curr. Top. Dev. 6*:183–223, 1971.

153. Wrenn, J.T., and Wessels, N.K. An ultrastructural study of lens invagination in the mouse. *J. Exp. Zool. 171*:359–367, 1969.

154. Wulle, K.-G., and Lerche, W. Electron microscopic observations of the early development of the human corneal endothelium and Descemet's membrane. *Ophthalmologica 157*:451–461, 1969.

155. Wulle, K.-G. Electron microscopy of the fetal development of the corneal endothelium and Descemet's membrane of the human eye. *Invest. Ophthalmol. Vis. Sci. 11*:897–904, 1972.

156. Wulle, K.-G., Ruprecht, K.W., and Windruth, L.C. Electron microscopy of the development of the cell junctions in the embryonic and fetal human corneal endothelium. *Invest. Ophthalmol. Vis. Sci. 13*:923–934, 1974.

157. Yamada, T. Morphological and biochemical aspects of cytodifferentiation: differentiation of lens cells. In *Experimental Biology and Medicine*, Vol. I, E. Hagen, W. Welchsler, P. Zilliken, and A.F. Gardner (Eds.), S. Karger, Basel, pp. 77–89, 1967.

158. Young, R.W. The life history of retinal cells. *Trans. Am. Ophthalmol. Soc. 81*:193–228, 1983.

159. Yuodelis, C., and Hendrickson, A. A qualitative and quantitative analysis of the human fovea during development. *Vision Res. 26*:847–855, 1986.

160. Zimmerman, R.P., Polley, E.H., and Fortney, R.L. Cell birthdays and rate of differentiation of ganglion and horizontal cells of the developing cat retina. *J. Comp. Neurol. 274*:77–90, 1988.

161. Zinn, K.M., and Mockel-Pohl, S. Fine structure of the developing cornea. *Int. Ophthalmol. Clin. 15*:19–37, 1975.

43

Developmental Anomalies of the Eye

Elise Torczynski
Rush Medical Center, Chicago, Illinois

I. INTRODUCTION

A wide variety of congenital malformations may arise during the formation of the eye. Anomalies may involve a single ocular tissue, a region of the eye, or the entire eye. Ocular anomalies may occur in association with a constellation of cranial, facial, or somatic abnormalities. When many tissues are affected, the significance of the associations is not always clear, but a chromosomal abnormality, an intrauterine infection, or a maternal toxin is often involved. The rapidly expanding information about genes and genetic mechanisms brings new insights to our understanding of congenital anomalies. Ocular malformations are not always bilateral: one eye is sometimes normal.

Some anomalies are clearly related to specific embryonic events. A typical coloboma results from failure of closure of the embryonic fissure [310], whereas others, such as retinal dysgenesis, reflect inaccurate timing of the sequential growth of the embryo.

II. TERATOGENESIS

That so much of what is initially induced as eye-forming tissue completes the entire program, resulting in normal, fully functioning eyes, attests to the strength of the basic program of eye formation found in the chromosomes and the inherent stability of the process of growth and development from conception to maturity.

Internal and external factors, called teratogens, may affect the process and result in a defective eye. A *teratogen* in an agent that produces a defect in the developing embryo or fetus, literally, an inducer of monsters. The template for development carried in the genes is relatively constant. The pathways to maldevelopment are many, and the same phenotype can result from a variety of teratogens. The phenotypic expression of a genetic defect can be highly variable, as in von Recklinghausen's neurofibromatosis, so that influences other than genetic alter the formation of the mature individual or part of the individual [236].

Two stimuli may be needed for teratogenesis: a predisposing gene and an environmental factor. Mice with the gene for cleft palate produce some affected offspring. The number of offspring with cleft palates increases if the genetically predisposed female is exposed to diphenylhydantoin, which independently produces cleft palate in the offspring. Even in this richly teratogenic milieu, not all offspring are affected. Further, the chronology of development can be key: a teratogen may be active only during a limited time in embryogenesis, as Gregg's study of rubella infection in the first trimester showed [129]. Pregnant women infected by the rubella virus in the first trimester produce infants with the rubella syndrome (cataracts, deafness, and mental retardation). If the infection occurs later in pregnancy, the infants are less likely to be affected and less severely damaged [234,352].

An abnormal karyotype may be identical in several members of a family, yet only one is affected [215]. Warburg [360], in analyzing the data on X-linked cataracts and X-linked microphthalmos, suggested that the variability seen may be due to submicroscopic deletions of variable sizes in the affected gene. Careful analysis of other pedigrees may reveal the same kind of data.

A. Teratogenetic Mechanisms

The intricacy of embryogenesis, as it is increasingly becoming understood at the ultrastructural, biochemical, and molecular biological levels, can be disrupted in a number of ways. Intrinsic factors contributing to dysgenesis include altered, defective, or imperfect genes, impaired cellular induction and proliferation [156], defective cell migration [156], cell death [272], abnormal extracellular substrates, inadequate differentiation [156], and physical constraint [202]. The extent of damage to the developing organism is further effected by external factors, namely the health and well-being of the mother and the nature of the teratogen, whether physical [44,307], chemical [233,294], or infectious, and its timing and degree.

Chromosomes

The human genome consists of 44 somatic chromosomes and 2 sex chromosomes (XX for females and XY for males), for a total of 46 chromosomes, half from each parent [145,235,389]. All are needed for the development of the human embryo. The chromosomes are paired, and one of each pair, a *chromatid*, is transmitted to each daughter cell, where it replicates.

To examine defects or alterations in the genetic material, preparations of isolated chromosomes are made from cells in metaphase. They may be stained with dyes, such as quinacrine or Giemsa, revealing specific banded patterns for each chromosome, termed Q bands for quinacrine [389] and G bands for Giemsa staining [389]. R bands, the reverse or nonstained bands in a typical Giemsa preparation, stain with Giemsa if the conventionally fixed chromosomes are warmed in saline before Giemsa is applied. The staining of chromosomes can reveal additions or deletions of chromosomes or major chromosomal parts. Structural changes noted in the banding patterns provide evidence of chromosomal alterations. However, this technique shows only gross alterations, involving regions in excess of 1,000,000 base pairs.

More specific information about gene defects may be obtained by studying restriction fragment length polymorphisms [41] and single-stranded conformational polymorphism (see Chap. 24) [2].

Bands, as well as DNA fragments and genes, are by convention [145] mapped on the chromosome starting at the *centromere*, the central constricted zone of attachment of the two chromatids. The short arm of the chromosome is designated p and the long arm, q. The bands or regions are numerically listed starting at the centromere and moving outward [145,388,389]. For example, the retinoblastoma gene has been mapped to region 14 from the centromere on the long arm of chromosome 13 (13q14) [388]. As smaller and smaller segments of DNA sequence are mapped, additional decimals are added to delineate their locations in a given band. Gene mapping is at present in progress in many countries. There are libraries and data banks of DNA sequences on file, yet less than 1% of the human genome has been mapped or sequenced [131,145,232a,327]. Maternal cytosomes transmit tiny pieces of DNA to the fetus [12,91,263].

Chromosomal Anomalies

Gross changes in the chromosomal structure include addition of one or more sets of chromosomes—triploidy [112] or tetraploidy; addition or duplication of a single chromosome or equivalent chromosomal material—trisomy [184]; deletion of a single chromosome—monosomy; inversions or reversal of a portion of a chromosome; translocation or repositioning of a significant fragment of DNA from one chromosome to another; *nondysjunction*, or failure of separation of chromosomal material during replication; and ring formation. Other defects include the loss of a centromere (acentric) or the duplication of a centromere (dicentric) in a chromosome [215]. A break in a chromosome followed by rearrangement of the DNA in an altered sequence may be stable; that is, the rearrangement may be replicated during cell division without changing. Alternatively, it may be unstable and be lost or changed with replication. Deletions, duplications, inversions, translocations, and isochromosomes (a chromosome with two short arms or two long arms) are examples of stable rearrangements; ring formation, loss of a centromere, and two centromeres are unstable configurations [164a].

Absence of a chromosome, deletion of a significant portion of a chromosome, duplication of a chromosome, and other aberrant formations usually result in mutilating and often lethal defects for the embryo. Spontaneously aborted infants in great measure show major chromosomal abnormalities [158]. Monosomy is a universally lethal defect, except for the monosomy of females with Turner's syndrome, in which one X chromosome is lost (X0), the only known monosomy compatible with life. Trisomies are relatively common, and although many are lethal, individuals with trisomies may lead long lives, although they are frequently retarded. The most common is trisomy 21, Down syndrome. In 1962 this syndrome, formerly called mongolism because of the downward slant of the lateral palpebral fissures, was the first syndrome in humans to be ascribed to a specific chromosome, chromosome 21 [180,283,297].

B. Genes

Genes control the development of an individual from conception to maturity. The precise turning on and turning off of a gene, allowing it to produce its desired effect and then stopping its influence, is not understood. Each cell contains a complete number of chromosomes, and yet most genes in the mature cell are inactive. In the embryo cells are pluripotent, having the potential to differentiate into several or many cell types upon further division. Genes direct the synthesis of proteins, which include enzymes and structural cellular and extracellular proteins. Specific cell types distinguish the tissues, organs, and, finally, the whole organism. With development, pluripotency is lost and a cell of given type limits its gene activity to produce only those proteins needed for its particular function. The retention of pluripotency is occasionally seen when choristomas are produced, although local factors may induce tissues in an abnormal location. The sequencing of microevents in the embryo is genetically directed and affected by the surrounding substrate.

Genetic Mutations

Modification of the genetic information carried by the chromosomes can be caused by a mutation occurring in a single or, less commonly, multiple gene loci (see Chap. 25).

Impaired Cellular Proliferation

Minor setbacks to the embryo and fetus that delay the proliferation of cells integral to the whole or to a particular structure can be corrected by a subsequent spurt in growth [272]. Malformations are prone to arise when the cellular damage occurs at a time or to such a degree that compensatory growth is incomplete before the next phase of development.

Cell Death

With development, cells that are part of the ongoing process of development early in embryogenesis may disappear as the organ develops. For example, cells in the stalk connecting the surface ectoderm to the lenticular vesicle disappear as the lenticular vesicle separates from the surface ectoderm [64,65]. If residual cells do not die, then the next phase of neural crest migration to produce the corneal stroma is impaired. The cell death that should take place as development proceeds may not occur, and the residual primitive cells then obstruct later phases of development. Cell death also relates to the loss of cells that are destined to produce all or part of a structure. In this case the loss of a significant number of cells may result in the absence or limited formation of that structure [272]. In consecutive anophthalmia evidence is found of the early development of an eye that subsequently degenerates. The causes of cell death are poorly understood.

Defective Cell Migration

The considerable movement of cells that occurs in embryogenesis is essential to normal development. Early in embryogenesis neural crest cells migrate to new positions distant from their origin on the crest of the neural folds. The contributions of these cells to the eye and its supporting structures are extensive, and interference with the migration of the cells into the new location can be expected to result in abnormalities. Neural crest cells migrate in an extracellular matrix, which if limited or defective alter migration [175, 176]. Many craniofacial anomalies are thought to result from faulty migration or abnormal fusion of the cranial neural crest processes.

In the arhinencephalic syndromes, a cleft lip and palate result when the frontal nasal and maxillary processes fail to meet and fuse inferior and nasal to the globe. The cranial neural crest cells contribute much of the mesenchyme of the eye and the upper face. Other cellular or tissue movements may be focally impeded as the tips of the optic vesicle grow anteriorly and interact with late waves of neural crest cells to develop the anterior segment of the eye [20].

Cellular migration within the tissue is noteworthy in the retina. The movement of cells from the marginal layer, a zone rich in dividing nuclei (see Chap. 42), in the developing retina toward the interior or molecular layer that is responsible for producing ganglion cells and, later, bipolar, horizontal, and glial cells can be interrupted. Teratogens throughout gestation may interfere with the formation of the normal retina because retinal differentiation continues until after birth.

Abnormal Extracellular Substrate

The extracellular matrix in the embryo has not been well studied, but deficiencies in it alter development.

Inadequate Differentiation

As multipotency is lost from the growing embryonic cells, the cells become committed to forming a particular tissue or organ. This is the process of *differentiation*. Fully differentiated cells are structurally and biochemically mature and functional. Cells that show only partial or aberrant development are dysgenetic or dysplastic. A tissue can be identified histologically because sufficient, but not all, mature features are present. For example, in the retina, one or more nuclear layers may be absent, nuclei can form circles or rosettes, manifest variations in density, or establish only a single layer; these changes constitute retinal dysplasia, better termed dysgenesis. Severely dysgenetic cells and tissues are not well differentiated and may function only to a limited extent or not at all [272].

Physical Constraint

Amniotic bands have been implicated in the formation of fissures and clefts that do not correspond to the closure of processes or developmental lines in the embryo. Peculiar indentations with adjacent folds, coupled with a malformed eye, ear, nose, or cheek, may result from pressure of an amniotic band on the fetal face.

C. Chemicals, Drugs, and Toxins

Although many drugs have been linked with developmental defects [26,54,233,294,303,319,334,350, 376], convincing evidence through rigorous testing has been presented in only a few: radioactive iodine [303], cyclophosphamide [303,315], coumarin anticoagulants [21,137,142,303,366], diphenylhydantoin [98,159,276,303], 13-*cis*-retinoic acid [29,75,141,303], lithium [303], and thalidomide [376]. A human fetus is most susceptible to teratogens during organogenesis (18–60 days of gestation).

The thalidomide story illustrates a number of important points in the effort to establish that an agent is teratogenic. In the early 1960s a number of infants, first in Germany and then elsewhere [184], were born with phocomelia, a rare congenital anomaly of absent or limited limb development [208]. Epidemiological studies implicated a recently released sedative, thalidomide. Maternal ingestion of thalidomide between days 27 and 40 of gestation resulted in complete or partial phocomelia in 20% of the offspring. Other defects, such as ear anomalies, occurred if the drug was ingested between days 21 and 27. Premarket testing of thalidomide in rats and mice did not reveal the teratogenic potency. It was later learned that rodents are relatively undisturbed by this teratogen; had rabbits or monkeys been used, the teratogenic potential would have been unmasked. This experience illustrates that the same defect is produced in those exposed to the teratogen, that a critical period of susceptibility is present, that a species variability in response to a teratogen exists, and that the individual ability to withstand the affects of the teratogen is remarkable [303]. Only 20% of those at risk were affected [184]. These principles are paramount to the understanding of teratogenesis and must be understood when any agent is implicated as a possible teratogen. Thalidomide-induced ocular defects were only occasionally found and included microphthalmos, anophthalmos, buphthalmos, lens anomalies, colobomas, disturbances of ocular motility, gaze paresis, facial palsy, and "crocodile" tears [69,119,208,239,390].

Fetal Alcohol Syndrome

In contrast to the detailed and rapidly completed epidemiological studies prompted by the severe and unusual teratogenic effect of thalidomide, many years were taken to uncover the teratogenesis of maternal alcohol ingestion. Although ethanol was suspected as a teratogen years ago, it was only in 1968 that Lemoine et al. first described the less dramatic but characteristic findings of the fetal alcohol syndrome

[207a]. The results of their study have been widely confirmed, and it is now recognized that the fetal alcohol syndrome is one of the most widespread teratogenetic disorders. Fetal alcohol syndrome occurs in 1–2 live births per 1000, and partial expressions may be found in as many as 5 per 1000 live births; one survey in British Columbia, Canada, disclosed that 190 of 1000 children age 1–18 years were affected [285].

A characteristic mild facial dysmorphia is seen in all patients with the full-blown syndrome and partially in those who are less affected. The features include short palpebral fissures in 80% of those affected, short upturned nose, hypoplastic philtrum with thin upper vermillion border of the lip, and retrognathia and micrognathia in infancy with a relative prognathia in later life [59,207a,336]. Facial appearance is only mildly modified by a relative prognathism as the infant grows into adulthood. Mental retardation is one of the most prominent and serious manifestations of the syndrome. Affected persons test lower than 2 standard deviations below the mean on intelligence tests; only occasionally does an affected person have an average or better than average mental ability. Pathological studies demonstrate a variety of alterations in the brain; the most common are cerebellar dysplasias, heterotopic cell clusters on the brain surface, failure or interruption of neuronal and glial migration, microcephaly, and hydrocephalus [230]. Behavioral features include irritability, hypotonia, hyperactivity, and poor coordination. The infants are small at birth, and the low weight and short stature continue throughout life (<2 standard deviations below normal for both). Affected individuals have a diminished amount of adipose tissue. Ocular findings include short palpebral fissures, poor vision, ptosis, esotropia, and epicanthal folds. Occasionally microphthalmia, myopia, blepharophimosis, hypoplasia of the optic nerve, and tortuous retinal veins [335,336] are found.

Infectious Agents

Many infectious agents have been labeled as teratogenetic for the developing human organism [89]. Only a few—cytomegalovirus [108,150,214], herpesvirus hominis [323], parvovirus B-19, rubella virus [129, 195,352], *Treponema pallidum* [62,134], *Toxoplasma gondii* [79,279], and Venezuelan equine encephalitis virus—have been unequivocally implicated as teratogens [303]. Varicella has been incriminated as a teratogen [40,55,201,299].

D. Radiation

Maternal exposure to high levels of various forms of radiation during the early stages of embryogenesis can result in severe damage to the fetus [44,93]. The earlier in pregnancy that radiation exposure occurs, the more likely is death or malformation to develop. Exposure up to week 11 is associated with malformations, and thereafter the number of anomalies decreases radically. Timing and dosage are critical [332,351]. Radiation damage to the ocular anlagen produces anophthalmia, microphthalmia, cataracts, coloboma, eyelid anomalies, and retinal pigmentary changes [44,74]. After week 11 little damage is produced in the eye, except cataracts or a predisposition to early cataracts. The most serious consequence of maternal radiation when it is not lethal is mental retardation.

Ophthalmic investigations in survivors of the atomic bombing of Hiroshima and Nagasaki, including those in utero, disclosed that only axial opacities in the posterior subcapsule (9% in Nagasaki and 5% in Hiroshima) and polychromatic changes in the posterior subcapsule were associated with ionizing radiation [250]. Similar findings were detected to a lesser extent in control populations not exposed to ionizing radiation [250]. Radiation following an atomic bomb explosion damages those closest to the center of the explosion. No increase in the number of infants with congenital defects attributable to chromosomal damage has been found in the children of survivors in Hiroshima exposed to ionizing radiation in excess of 200 rads [249,260].

Exposure at the current conservative standards for allowable doses of radiation does not increase fetal damage [249], but diagnostic and therapeutic radiation should be used cautiously in all women of childbearing age [93].

E. Maternal Nutrition

Maternal vitamin A deficiency may result in anophthalmia and xerophthalmia in the fetus. Hypervitaminosis A may be teratogenic by interfering with crest cell migration [272]. Deficiency of folic acid and the use of folate antagonists can produce anophthalmos, microphthalmos, cataract, and coloboma [15].

III. DEVELOPMENTAL ANOMALIES OF THE WHOLE EYE

A. Anencephaly

Suppression of development limited to the telencephalon results in anencephaly, with an infant without a forebrain but with eyes (Fig. 1). Glial nodules (Fig. 2) and intravitreal neovascularization, which may lead to partial retinal detachment (Figs. 3 and 4), may be seen in eyes of anencephaly.

B. Anophthalmia

Anophthalmia is the absence of the eye, but more often the orbit contains a microphthalmic globe and in those instances the term "clinical anophthalmia" is appropriate. True anophthalmia occurs when no rudiments of the neuroectoderm of the optic cup are present in the orbit [118]. True anophthalmia is a very rare event that occurs in week 3 or 4 of embryogenesis [13]. Anophthalmia may have autosomal recessive, autosomal dominant [28], and X-linked [48] patterns of inheritance [152,296].

The diagnosis of true anophthalmia is made histopathologically by serial sectioning of the orbital tissues, a technique almost never undertaken [296]. Primary anophthalmia results from the failure of the optic primordium in the earliest stages of embryogenesis. Either no optic anlagen or a limited ocular primordium is established and fails to grow. Secondary anophthalmia results from widespread failure of development of the anterior neural tube and is lethal because neither brain nor eyes result. The eyes arise from the diencephalon, caudal to the telencephalon on the neural tube. An ocular structure may be established and develop to some extent and then disintegrate (degenerative anophthalmia) [311].

Anophthalmia occurs in a variety of syndromes [226] and has been produced experimentally by a variety of techniques, including radiation to the developing embryo [311].

C. Microphthalmos

Microphthalmia, the small disorganized globe (Fig. 5), is a diverse condition with many causes [102,311]. Trisomies or abnormalities of virtually every chromosome [11,83,118,120,136,245,281,302,337,369], maternal radiation [44], infections, and toxins are associated with microphthalmia [67,97,361]. It can be inherited as an autosomal dominant [169], an autosomal recessive [161,169,216,325,347], or an X-linked [125,347,358,362] trait and may be an idiopathic phenomenon [43,192]. Microphthalmos is frequently associated with many systemic manifestations [106,123,151], most prominently mental retardation [6,66,151,183,198,248,347] and dwarfism [43,46,342,363]. The microphthalmic globe [192,274] has been associated with numerous ocular anomalies, including leukomas [90], anterior segment disorders [84], retinal dysplasia [84], colobomas [151,361], cysts [105,136,210,369,382], and marked internal ocular dysgenesis [106], to mention only a few. The associated adnexal abnormalities include a small orbit, shortened palpebral fissure, ptosis, and blepharophimosis (Fig. 5).

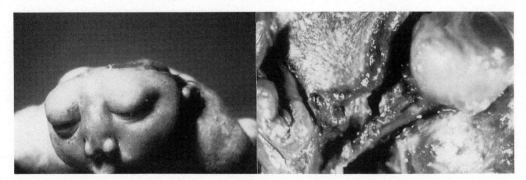

Figure 1   Anencephaly. (Left) Eyes and orbits are present despite failure of telencephalon. (Right) Globe of stillborn on left with well-developed nerve that tapers and fades in midline. Interior of globes was normal. (Courtesy S. Young, M.D.)

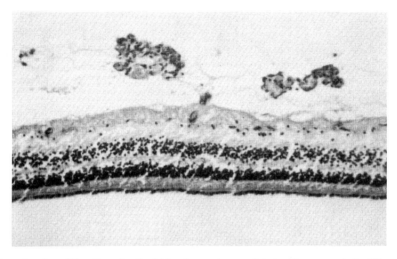

Figure 2 Intravitreal proliferation of retinal blood vessels associated with anencephaly. (Hematoxylin and eosin, ×100)

Chromosomal abnormalities, teratogens acting at any time during development [44], maternal infections [303], maternal nutrition, and other factors [183,361] may impinge on the developing eye in a variety of ways that result in microphthalmos. Microphthalmia is a constant feature of trisomy 13 (Fig. 6). The globes show anterior and posterior segment disorganization with a coloboma containing cartilage (Fig. 7).

Microphthalmia may simulate anophthalmia clinically [17] and is much more common than true anophthalmia. Weiss and coworkers [370,371] described findings in 62 of 6000 patients seen in a pediatric

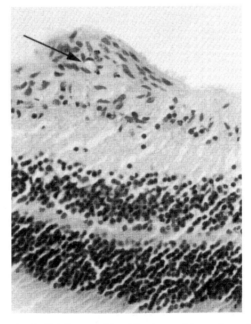

Figure 3 Anencephaly. Nodule of glial tissue, with a blood vessel (arrow), on the surface of the retina of an anencephalic fetus. (Hematoxylin and eosin, ×100)

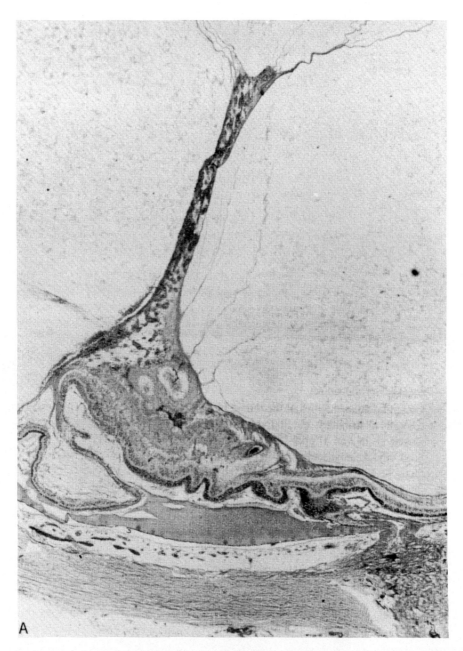

A

Figure 4   Anencephaly. (A) Intravitreal neovascularization has given rise to partial detachment of the retina. (Hematoxylin and eosin, ×16) (B) Higher magnification of the new vessels shows a focus of extramedullary erythropoiesis characterized by normoblasts and myelocytes. (Hematoxylin and eosin, ×500)

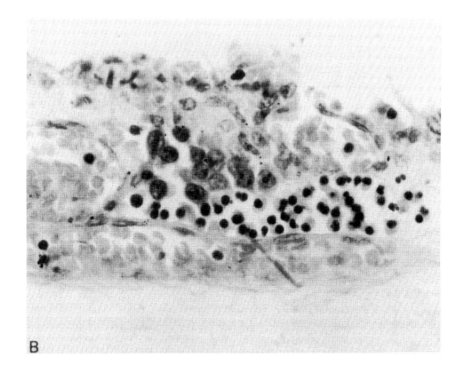

clinic over 6 years. A total of 40 patients had small globes with ocular malformations and associated systemic anomalies (complex microphthalmos) [371]. Simple microphthalmos occurred in 22 patients (0.36%) [370] who had normal-appearing eyes with an axial length of less than 2 standard deviations from the mean (Fig. 8) and vision in the 20/30–20/50 range. One patient with simple microphthalmos had vision of 20/100 [370]. All eyes were 3–4 mm shorter than globes of age-matched controls (Fig. 8). Only one eye of 20 children with growth hormone deficiency was microphthalmic. In the group with complex microphthalmia severe microcornea correlated with severe microphthalmia [371]. In those with simple microphthalmia, only 7 had microcornea (<10.5 mm in diameter); 6 had associated systemic disorders [370]. A single infant had nanophthalmos with an eye with an axial length of less than 18 mm, microcornea (10 mm),

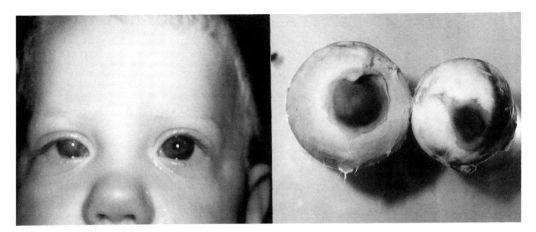

Figure 5   Unilateral microphthalmia. (Left) Clinical idiopathic microphthalmia of right eye. (Right) Normally sized left globe and microphthalmic right globe of individual with 13q syndrome. A small, opaque, irregular cornea hides internal disorganization.

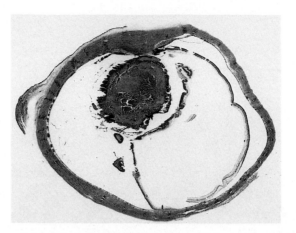

Figure 6   Microphthalmia in trisomy 13. Keratolenticular adhesion, persistent hyperplastic primary vitreous, retinal detachment, and dysgenesis.

and hyperopia of 9.00, in the absence of associated ocular or systemic disorders. The length of the posterior segment was consistently decreased in the eyes with both complex and simple microphthalmia (Figs. 9 and 10). In the complex microphthalmic group the anterior segment lengths were within or below normal range, whereas the posterior segment lengths were uniformly at least 2 standard deviations below the mean. All the simple microphthalmic eyes showed a posterior segment length of less than 2 standard deviations below the mean (Figs. 9 and 10). The mildest changes in the eyes with complex microphthalmia were microcornea and cataracts [371]. The more severely involved had colobomas, colobomatous cysts, severe microphthalmia, persistent hyperplastic primary vitreous (PHPV), facial malformations and the systemic disorders included the congenital rubella syndrome, Weill-Marchesani syndrome, deletion of 13q, trisomy 13, CHARGE

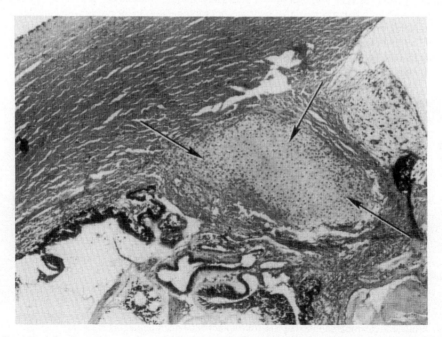

Figure 7   A nodule of cartilage (arrows) is present within the ciliary body of an eye removed from a case of trisomy 13–15. (Hematoxylin and eosin, ×50).

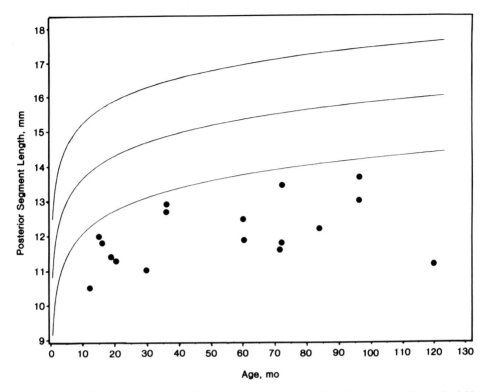

Figure 8 Total axial length in 21 patients with simple microphthalmos. Each dot represents the total axial length of one randomly selected eye of each patient. The mean total axial length values for normal subjects (middle curve) and upper and lower 95% confidence bands (outer curves) are shown for comparison. (Reproduced with permission from the American Medical Association and A.H. Weiss, B.G. Kousseff, E.A. Ross, and J. Longbottom. Simple microphthalmos. *Arch. Ophthalmol. 107*:1627–1628, 1989.)

(coloboma, heart defects, coanal atresia, mental retardation, genitourinary defects, and ear anomalies) and Lenz's syndromes, incontinentia pigmenti, and Norrie's disease [371].

High hyperopia accompanies almost all cases with simple microphthalmos [370], and the associated systemic diseases include achondroplasia, myotonic dystrophy, diabetic embryopathy, "pseudotrisomy 18," fetal alcohol syndrome, Maroteaux-Lamy syndrome, pseudo-Hurler syndrome, and isolated growth hormone deficiency. Vitreous development may be faulty in both simple and complex microphthalmos [370,371]. The postnatal lengthening of microphthalmic eye is similar to that of normal eyes [370,371].

D. Nanophthalmos

Nanophthalmos describes a small, functional eye with relatively normal internal structures, although the anterior chamber is crowded and the eye hyperopic [173,218,370]. Familial cases are reported [82,232]. Uveal effusion [73] and the exfoliation syndrome [82] may occur. Cataract extraction has been successful despite the small and crowded anterior segment [45].

E. Colobomas

A *coloboma* is defined as an absence of a part of an ocular structure [218]. Colobomas are divided into typical, those associated with the closure of the embryonic fissure of the optic vesicle (Fig. 11), and atypical, those not associated with the fissure closure [261].

As the optic vesicle invaginates, the embryonic fissure develops and fuses. Fusion begins in the equatorial region and proceeds anteriorly and posteriorly. The proliferation and ectropion of the inner layer

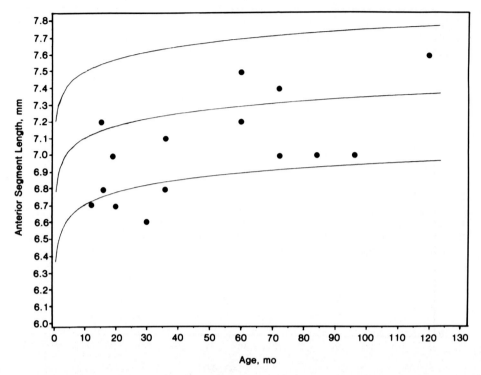

Figure 9 Anterior segment length in 17 patients. Each dot (except one) represents the anterior segment length of one randomly selected eye of each patient. Two pairs of patients with the same anterior segment length are represented by one dot each. The mean anterior segment length of age-similar normal subjects (middle curve) with upper and lower 95% confidence bands (outer curves) are shown for comparison. (Reproduced with permission from the American Medical Association and A.H. Weiss, B.G. Kousseff, E.A. Ross, and J. Long-bottom. Simple microphthalmos. *Arch. Ophthalmol. 107*:1627–1628, 1989.)

of neuroectodermal tissue displaces cells destined to become the retinal pigment epithelium (RPE) laterally. The inner edges of the fissure meet and close to form the neurosensory retina, nonpigmented ciliary epithelium, and posterior pigmented iridic epithelium; the outer lips form the pigment epithelium of the retina and ciliary body and the anterior pigmented iridic epithelium with the sphincter and dilator muscles of the iris. Hence, the primary defect in a typical coloboma involves these tissues. Because of the inductive influence of neuroectodermal tissues, especially the pigment epithelium on the subjacent mesenchyme, the associated uveal stroma, sclera, and optic nerve are involved; the ectodermal lens can be affected. Because the developing uveal tissue lacks focal stimulation by the RPE, growth and condensation of uveal tissue fail where the RPE is deficient [80].

Typical colobomas occur inferonasally from iris to optic nerve. In a complete coloboma there is no closure of the fissure, and this results in a microphthalmic or cystic eye (Fig. 12). Most typical colobomas are incomplete, being limited to a portion of the fissure. Intermittent closure results in bands of normal-appearing tissue, called skip areas, adjacent to the colobomas. Colobomas of the iris and optic nerve are frequently separated by a broad zone of normal fundus. In an otherwise unremarkable eye and individual, the edges of the coloboma end abruptly and normal tissue begins; a few pigmentary changes, clumps or thinning, and a little glial or fibrous tissue may mark the barely perceptible transition zone. In such eyes, even large colobomas are compatible with excellent vision, although an absolute scotoma corresponds to the retinal coloboma. Posterior pole colobomas are commonly termed chorioretinal colobomas because of their yellow-white scalloped appearance. Retinal and choroidal vessels can be seen traversing the coloboma. The associated mesenchymal coloboma includes an absence of the iris stroma, ciliary body muscles, and stroma, choroidal stroma, and vessels, as well as a thin ectatic underlying posterior sclera.

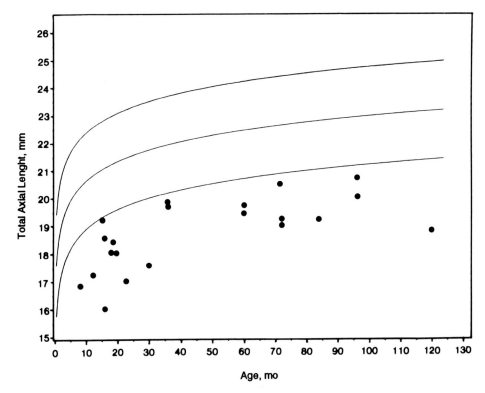

Figure 10   Posterior segment length in 17 patients. Each dot represents the posterior segment length of one randomly selected eye of each patient. The mean posterior segment length values for normal subjects (middle curve) and upper and lower 95% confidence bands (outer curves) are shown for comparison. (Reproduced with permission from the American Medical Association and A.H. Weiss, B.G., Kousseff, E.A. Ross, and J. Longbottom. Simple microphthalmos. *Arch. Ophthalmol. 107*:1627–1628, 1989.)

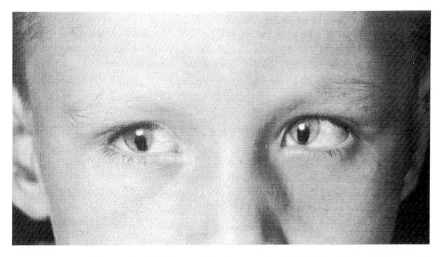

Figure 11   Bilateral iris colobomas in the inferonasal region associated with the embryonic fissure. (Reproduced with permission from G.K. Klintworth and M.B. Landers, III. *The Eye: Structure and Function in Disease*, Williams & Wilkins, Baltimore, 1976.)

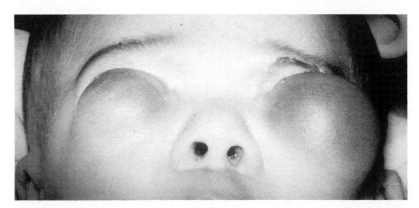

Figure 12   Bilateral cystic eyes. Histopathology showed limited dysgenetic neuroectodermal tissues. (Reproduced with permission from S. Foxman and J.D. Cameron. The clinical implications of bilateral microphthalmos with cyst. *Am. J. Ophthalmol. 97*:632–638, 1984.)

Delicate atrophic dysgenetic choroid, RPE, and neurosensory retina lie on the sclera in the affected area. The iris coloboma lacks all tissues, although a thinned wedge that can be transilluminated may be present. A notch in the equator of the lens is present (coloboma of the lens). Typical colobomas of the optic nerve vary from minimal thinning at the posterior termination of a chorioretinal coloboma to involvement of almost the entire nerve so that only a small portion of the superior pole of the nerve is identified as optic disk. The typical coloboma of the optic nerve is continuous with the white defect in the interior nasal fundus [80].

Colobomas, one of the more common clinically observed congenital ocular anomalies, are usually bilateral and are often asymmetrical [90]. Iris colobomas are the most frequent. Autosomal dominant inheritance with a high degree of penetrance is common [61]; recessive [163] and X-linked pedigrees [80,125] have also been reported. Even though one member of a family may have an isolated coloboma, other members of the pedigree may manifest microphthalmia, cataract, anterior segment dysgenesis [66], aniridia, PHPV, and other ocular malformations [51,85,90]. Teratogens [80] linked with colobomas include vitamin A deficiency, hypoxia, irradiation, lysergic acid diethylamide [54], thalidomide [208,239, 390], cytomegalovirus [108,214], and rubella virus [352], to mention only a few. Colobomas are frequently associated with systemic developmental anomalies [57,80,163,168] or craniofacial syndromes [273,339] and focal dermal dysplasia (Goltz syndrome) [358], as well as other intraocular malformations, like Rieger's anomaly, congenital cataract, corneal changes [321], retinal detachment, neovascular membranes [289], and retinal dysplasia, and occasionally with intraocular tumors (glioneuroma, medulloepithelioma, astrocytoma, and the 13q⁻ syndrome retinoblastoma) [9]. Cataracts can be successfully extracted in eyes with colobomas [167].

Some chromosomal defects [29,361] are associated with colobomas. In some, such as the CHARGE syndrome [1,10,151,292], colobomas of the iris are a constant feature, and in others, such as Klinefelter's [107,146], colobomas are found rarely. Cat-eye syndrome, known to result from chromosome 22 with incorporated fragments of chromosomes 13 or 14, was originally named because of the constant vertical uveal coloboma [120,215,267]. When associated with major chromosomal abnormalities, the infants are often stillborn or live only a short time [56,158,245], so the ocular defects have limited clinical significance and are not discussed here.

F. Cystic Colobomas

Cystic colobomas occur along the line of closure of the embryonic fissure [18] and are serious anomalies that usually occur in a blind eye. When the space within the ectopic, folded layers of inner neuroectoderm at the line of expected fusion remains open, either one or both tips of neuroectoderm may expand, one

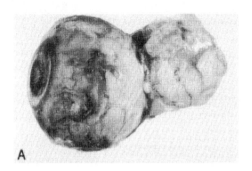

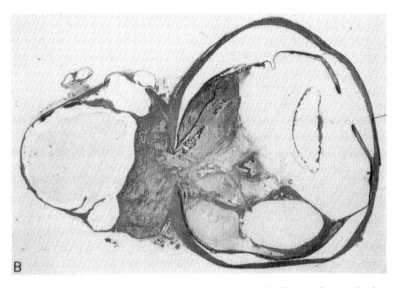

Figure 13 Microphthalmos with a colobomatous cyst. (A) A retrobulbar cystic mass is situated adjacent to a small malformed eye. (×1.86) (B) This horizontal section through specimen A demonstrates the cystic nature of the retrobulbar mass and the malformed retina within the microphthalmic eye. (Hematoxylin and eosin, ×3.2) (Reproduced with permission from G.K. Klintworth and M.B. Landers, III. *The Eye: Structure and Function in Disease*, Williams & Wilkins, Baltimore, 1976.)

edge into the globe, the other external to it [18]. The result may be a cystic eye, microphthalmos with cyst (Fig. 13), or coloboma with cyst, and the eyes have corneal leukomas, anterior segment dysgenesis, cataracts, PHPV, retinal nonattachment [104], and retinal dysplasia [132,201]. The cyst may be larger than the eye, approximately equal in size, or comprise only a small cavity near the optic nerve. Computed tomography and magnetic resonance imaging help to delineate these structures (Fig. 14) [380]. Cystic coloboma is associated with a deletion of the long arm of chromosome 13 (13q⁻) [371], a ring deletion of chromosome 18 [385], and trisomy 18 (Fig. 15) [136].

G.   Coloboma and Abnormal Intraocular Tissues

In trisomy 13 [152,192,257,274], the microphthalmic eyes often contain a large fibrous coloboma with cartilage, especially if the eyes are less than 10 mm in diameter (Figs. 6 and 7). Intraocular cartilage may be associated with the coloboma in individuals with a ring configuration of chromosome 18 [385], PHPV, and medulloepithelioma. Heterotopic tissues associated with colobomas include smooth muscle [247,385],

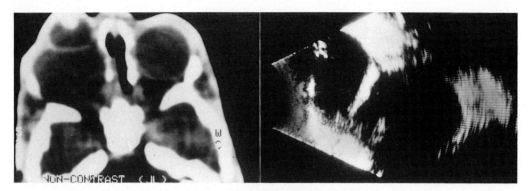

Figure 14 (Left) Computed tomographic scan shows small globe with large cyst on left. (Right) Ultrasound confirms microphthalmos with cyst in infant with trisomy 18. (Reproduced with permission from C. Guterman, E. Abboud, and M. Mets. Microphthalmos with cyst and Edwards' syndrome. *Am. J. Ophthalmol. 109*:228–230, 1990. Copyright by the Ophthalmic Publishing Company.)

bone [375], fibrous tissue, glial tissue [375], lacrimal gland [133], adipose tissue [375], and anterior chamber cyst [138]. Circumferential strands of smooth muscle are occasionally oriented concentrically around the optic disk (Fig. 16) [103,375]. Aberrant locations of pigmented ciliary processes are recorded at the margins of a coloboma [221,247]. Some of these are explained as heterotopic rests, but the abnormal generation of many of these disturbed tissues remains unexplained [248].

H. Atypical Colobomas

Focal defects in ocular tissues in regions distant to the embryonic fissure are called atypical colobomas. Atypical iris colobomas result from strands of the anterior hyaloid system and pupillary membrane that fail to regress spontaneously in late gestation. These exert traction on the edge of the developing iris and produce a notch or indentation. They may occur in any portion of the eye and usually are not as extensive as typical inferonasal colobomas. Macular colobomas [322], white, oval patches within the temporal arcade of vessels and sharply demarcated from the surrounding tissues, are associated with congenital toxoplasmosis, varicella [201], and syphilis and may have an autosomal dominant mode of inheritance [298, 322,341]. Leber's congenital amaurosis [227,240], skeletal defects [269], progeria with dwarfism [213], and keratoconus have been associated with macular colobomas. Markedly reduced vision is the rule in such cases.

All manner of deep, wide, elongated optic disks with vessels displaced to the rim edge and variable pigmentation are called optic disk colobomas, although many are not associated with the closure of the embryonic fissure. *Optic pits*, depressions within the optic nerve that usually do not extend to the rim of the disk, are generally included in atypical colobomas. The morning glory configuration (see optic disk colobomas and pits, discussed later) is called a coloboma. Many of these deformities are not strictly colobomatous, which by definition is an absence of a part of a structure but, rather, a maldevelopment of the whole optic disk and nerve.

I. Cystic Eye

The congenital cystic eye is diagnosed clinically rather than anatomically. A true cystic eye is rare and represents failure of the optic vesicle to invaginate, the most severe form of congenital nonattachment of the retina. A cystic blue mass, usually distending the eyelids, results from a cystic eye or from a coloboma with cyst (Fig. 12). Residual dysplastic neuroectodermal tissue forms the wall of the cyst.

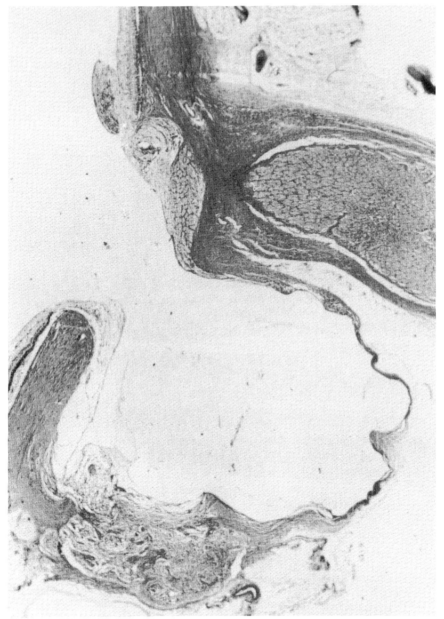

Figure 15 Colobomatous cyst in trisomy 18 in direct communication with the vitreous cavity. (Hematoxylin and eosin, ×16)

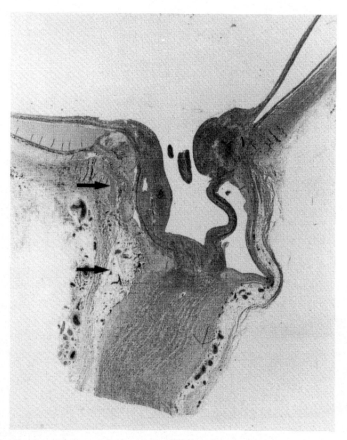

Figure 16   Optic disk malformation with striated muscle bundles (upper arrow) and mature adipose tissue (lower arrow). (Hematoxylin and eosin, ×8) (Courtesy of Dr. W. Lee.)

IV.   DEVELOPMENTAL ANOMALIES OF SPECIFIC OCULAR STRUCTURES

A.   Cornea, Sclera, and Conjunctiva

Sclerocornea

Scleral tissue replacing the peripheral cornea and obliterating the corneoscleral limbus is called scleralization of the cornea or sclerocornea (Fig. 17) [293,341,363]. It may be unilateral or bilateral, sporadic or inherited, and complete or incomplete. Sclerocornea is sporadic in half of the cases, but both dominant and recessive inheritance are reported [157,182,293]. The second neuroectodermal wave of neural crest tissue [20,147] destined for anterior segment development differentiates into tissue resembling sclera instead of clear cornea and is invaded by fine superficial vessels from the sclera, episclera, and conjunctiva [293]. The collagen has abnormally variable diameters throughout; Descemet's membrane and the endothelium are abnormal [182,381]. Aniridia, anterior segment dysgenesis, colobomas, cataract, glaucoma, and microphthalmos are associated [190,293,342]. Sclerocornea may be part of a systemic syndrome involving the skull and facial bones, ears, brain, digits, and testes [127,143,190,342]. It has been associated with osteogenesis imperfecta and blue sclera. Chromosomal abnormalities include an unbalanced chromosomal translocation (17p10q) [286]. Peripheral sclerocornea must be distinguished from microcornea and total scleralization from other conditions, such as secondary scarring involving the entire cornea.

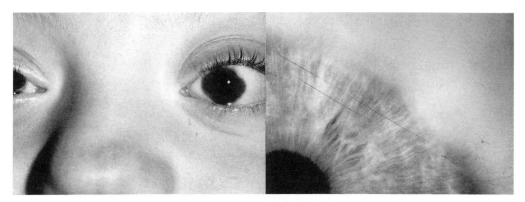

Figure 17 Partial sclerocornea, superior temporal quadrant. (Right) Above two lines, irregular scleral whitening of peripheral cornea of girl at left. (Courtesy of L.D. Perry, M.D.)

Microcornea

Microcornea may be found in a normally sized globe but most often is found in association with microphthalmos [371]. Simple or uncomplicated microcornea, a corneal diameter less than 10.5 mm [370], may arise from an overgrowth of the anterior tips of the optic cup so that it is smaller than normal but histologically orderly. A small clear cornea and otherwise normal growth is uncommon (Fig. 18); most commonly, microcornea is found with other anterior segment malformations or with nanophthalmos [370], hyperopia [370], cataract [293], and glaucoma. In a pedigree of 50 persons in five generations, Lambert and colleagues found sclerocornea, mesodermal dysgenesis, and cataract with microcornea, demonstrating the variability associated with faulty migration of neural crest cells [293].

Megalocornea

The corneal diameter is greater than 13 mm in megalocornea. This anomaly is usually bilateral:

1. It may be an isolated anomaly with autosomal or X-linked recessive inheritance.
2. It rarely coexists with other ocular malformations, such as persistent pupillary membrane.
3. It complicates Marfan syndrome, craniosynostosis, and lamellar ichthyosis.

Unilateral megalocornea and congenital glaucoma may occur in the same individual. In week 5–6 of embryonic life, the growing rim of the optic cup slows and may not bend axially, such that the ciliary ring and anterior segment of the globe become abnormally large. Because the cornea does not reach adult size until 1 year of age, megalocornea cannot be ruled out until after this age. The eyes are usually myopic and may show hypoplasia of the iris stroma, cataract, and ectopia lentis. Megalocornea [111] is often associated with mental retardation in the megalocornea-mental retardation syndrome, Del Giudice [76] or Neuhauser syndrome [76]. Other ocular and genetic abnormalities may be found.

Posterior Keratoconus

Posterior keratoconus is characterized by a normal anterior corneal surface, with the posterior stroma (Fig. 19) thinner than normal. The condition may be unilateral or bilateral and is usually nonfamilial. Other ocular anomalies may coexist [328]. The disorder may become manifest before month 5 or 6 of gestation [194]. Other corneal anomalies include a thickened Bowman's layer with leukoma [258] and a brittle cornea, one that easily perforates [290].

Dermoids

Epibulbar and bulbar dermoids are sequestrations or nests of primitive tissue [225]. Corneal (limbal) dermoids are white to tan, firm, usually solitary nodules often found in the lower temporal quadrant of the corneoscleral limbus. Histologically, they are covered by keratinized stratified squamous epithelium and contain adipose tissue, dense collagen, hair follicles, sweat and sebaceous glands, and even cartilage. In

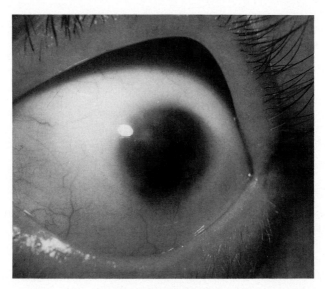

Figure 18 Microcornea.

complex choristomas smooth muscle, lacrimal glandular tissue, or brain tissue with myelin, neurofibrils, and neuroglia have been found. In one rare case a complete tooth was detected. Dermoids are usually sporadic and isolated lesions but may be a component of oculoauriculovertebral dysplasia (Goldenhar's syndrome) [25] and the epidermal nevus syndrome [33,128,225] and have been associated with microphthalmia [52a].

Episcleral Osseous Choristomas

Nonneoplastic masses of malformed tissue composed of mature compact bone surrounded by fibrous connective tissue are found on rare occasions in the episclera [225]. These so-called episcleral osseous choristomas are usually situated in the upper temporal quadrant of the orbit between the superior and lateral rectus muscles. This symptomless lesion is present at birth and is not associated with intraocular abnormalities [37].

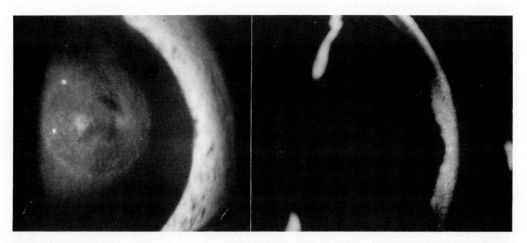

Figure 19 Posterior keratoconus. Amblyopic eye of 45-year-old man. (Left) Central opacified ring. (Right) Stromal whitening and posterior excavation of central opacity to right, iris at left. (Courtesy M. Mets, M.D.)

B. Uvea

Aniridia

Aniridia means the absence of the iris, but the term is widely used for a rudimentary iris and is nearly always bilateral [229,253]. The incidence is approximately 1 in 64,000–100,000 births [60,219,253]. The condition [31] may be sporadic [39] or familial [140], the familial form demonstrating autosomal dominant inheritance [301] and 85–90% penetrance.

Aniridia includes a variable combination and severity of the following abnormalities:

1. Ciliary body hypoplasia [229]
2. Cataracts with nuclear and peripheral degeneration [174,219,229,253,301]
3. Development of glaucoma due to angle closure secondary to peripheral anterior synechiae [219, 229,253]
4. Corneal pannus with variable disruption of Bowman's layer [60,219]
5. Mild optic disk hypoplasia [60,253]
6. Pendular nystagmus with macular hypoplasia [253]

The sporadic type is associated with deletion of the short arm of chromosome 11 (aniridia 2 locus of 11p13) [31,124,179]. The association of aniridia with Wilms' tumor was first reported by Miller et al. in 1964 [237] and is well documented. This mutation is frequently observed with WAGR syndrome (Wilms' tumor-aniridia-gonadoblastoma-mental retardation) [13,204,217,231,253]. Urogenital and anterior chamber angle abnormalities are also associated with sporadic type [32,219,229,231]. Although 1–3% of patients with Wilms' tumor have aniridia, approximately 25–33% of children with aniridia develop Wilms' tumor [31,34,219,253]. This relationship of Wilms' tumor and aniridia has also been reported in the familial, autosomal dominant mode of inheritance [179,191]. Loci on chromosome 1 linked to the Rh Duffy [101] locus and on chromosome 2 linked to the acid phosphatase 1 locus are found in aniridia [317]. Aniridia and deafness have been reported [68].

There are three morphological types of aniridia:

1. Stumps of iris may occlude the angle, although Schlemm's canal can be identified.
2. The mesenchyme may extend backward, curving around the pigment layer of the dwarf iris.
3. The blood vessels may ramify on the pigment layer of the iris, blocking further iris growth (Fig. 20).

A partial aniridia with absence of the iris stroma and sphincter central to the collarette has been associated with cerebellar ataxia and mental deficiency [378]. Many theories have been advanced to account for the occurrence of aniridia, but no unifying concept has emerged.

Hypoplasia of the Iris

Hypoplasia of either the stroma or the pigment layer of the iris is not uncommon. Segmental areas of poorly developed iris stroma permit the underlying sphincter and pigment epithelium to be seen easily. This abnormality may represent a potential coloboma [218] in which the iris has just succeeded in closing. Iris hypoplasia with changes in Descemet's membrane and congenital hereditary endothelial dystrophy have been found [264]. The pathogenesis of the defect, which must occur after month 4 of intrauterine life, is obscure, but it has been suggested that a persistent embryonic vessel prevents full development of the adjacent stroma [218]. Alternatively, the iris could develop normally and then atrophy.

Hyperplasia of the Iris

In a light-colored iris, focal hyperplasia at the surface of the iris stroma appears as white spots (Brushfield's spots), often seen in Down syndrome (Fig. 21). There may be an increase in thickness of the anterior leaf of the iris, representing the peripheral part of the pupillary membrane, which does not move readily with iris contraction and expansion. There is no hereditary element. Ectropion of the iris pigmented epithelium can simulate hyperplasia [377].

Hamartomas of the Iris

Hamartomas of the iris, namely the iris cyst [246], pigmented nevus, and angioma, are described in Chapter 48.

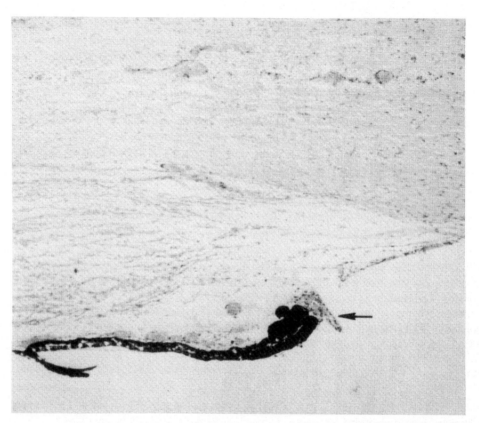

Figure 20   Aniridia with a persistent blood vessel extending over the edge of the pigment epithelium (arrow). (Hematoxylin and eosin, ×100)

Polycoria

More than one opening in the iris is called polycoria; most extrapupillary openings are colobomas or loci of atrophy. A true accessory pupil was first verified histologically in 1968 [104] by Foos, a sphincter muscle being identified in all sections of the iris in the accessory pupil. It was associated with a lens coloboma, which supports Mann's view [218] that accessory pupils are derived from partial iris colobomas in which mesectodermal hinges play a part.

Corectopia

Corectopia, an abnormal location of the pupil, is usually accompanied by ectopia lentis and rarely occurs alone. Corectopia is frequently inherited (autosomal dominant) and bilateral. The iris is normally formed, except for an increased thickness in the short segment, with thinning and attenuation in the long segment.

Microcoria

The tiny pupil is called microcoria. The pupil arises from myoblasts with cytoplasmic fibrils and features of smooth muscle cells [291]. Histologically the dilator myoepithelium is absent and the few myofibrils are disorganized [51,313]. Idiopathic microcoria with fibrous tissue at the pupil, which is slightly displaced, may be treated surgically, but despite clear lenses in all patients the visual outcome is poor [200].

Persistent Pupillary Membrane

After month 8 the iris-pupillary vascular membrane begins to atrophy, although remnants of it can frequently be seen in the newborn and occasionally in adults, arising from the anterior aspect of the iris in

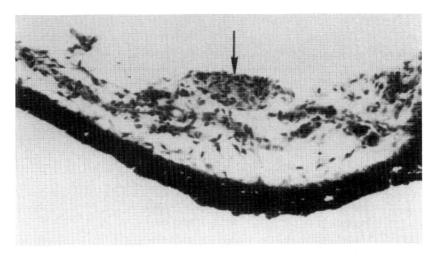

Figure 21   Brushfield's spot (arrow) on the anterior surface of the iris represents a focal overgrowth of stromal cells; the adjacent stroma is hypoplastic. (Hematoxylin and eosin, ×225)

the region of the iris collarette. The pupillary membrane may persist totally, but this is rare. Partial persistence, which is more common, presents many forms and can be classified as those attached to (1) the iris only, (2) the anterior capsule of the lens, where the adhesion may be marked by a white plaque (Fig. 22), and (3) the cornea. There does not seem to be an inherited predisposition [218].

C.   Anterior Chamber

Since 1920, when Axenfeld described a white line that represented a thickening of Schwalbe's line, many anomalies of the anterior segment have been reported [278]. These have been called by many names, including Axenfeld's syndrome, Rieger's anomaly [130], mesodermal dysgenesis, anterior segment cleavage syndrome, dysgenesis mesodermalis corneae et irides, and iridogoniodysgenesis [78,278,304–306,349,363]. Shields and collaborators suggest that these be listed under the title of Axenfeld-Rieger syndrome [304,306]. The latter term, or anterior segment dysgenesis, is used throughout this section. Infantile glaucoma is commonly found [77,197,278,304–306,364]. The phenotypic expression of this spectrum of disorders ranges from a simple thickening of Schwalbe's line, called posterior embryotoxon or Axenfeld's anomaly, through a major disorganization of the anterior segment, including leukomas and poorly formed anterior chamber angles [306,364]. The two eyes in a single individual may differ markedly in the expression of these anomalies [49,205]. In pedigrees [86,293], anterior segment dysgenesis involves the cornea, iris, and anterior chamber angle, either individually or collectively, and phenotypic variation in a family (Fig. 23) is common [205,293]. Ochratoxin A has induced anterior segment anomalies in mice [308].

The tissues that take part in the formation of the anterior segment include the ectoderm for the corneal and lenticular epithelium and neural crest cells for the corneal stroma, Descemet's membrane, and endothelium, as well as iris stroma and trabecular meshwork. The tissues that take part in the formation of the anterior segment include the ectoderm for the corneal and lenticular epithelium and neural crest cells for the corneal stroma, Descemet's membrane, and endothelium, as well as iris stroma and trabecular meshwork. The neuroectoderm contributes to the posterior iridic epithelium and dilator and sphincter muscles of the iris. The tissues now ascribed to neural crest origin were originally thought to come from mesoderm, and hence authors describing the previously listed conditions use the designation "mesoderm" [20,22,147,175,176,182,197,203,204,306,381]. The corneal epithelium is not involved primarily in these anomalies but is affected secondarily. Most of the malformations relate to the inappropriate growth and distribution of neural crest cells as amount, migration failure, histogenetic maturity, and misdirected or inappropriate tissue arrangements (Fig. 24) [20,203,293,304,306,349,377]. The lens, a surface ectodermal structure, may be involved in the condition called Peters' anomaly [139,144,190].

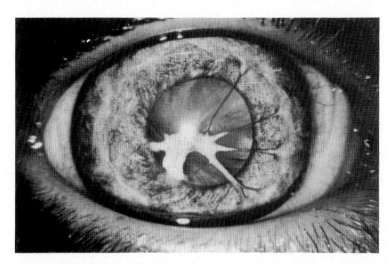

Figure 22 Persistent pupillary membrane extending from iris collarette to an anterior subcapsular cataract in a dog. (Courtesy of Dr. T.D. Grimes.)

Careful inspection of an infant's eye often reveals malformations, although these may be minimal. Findings in other family members indicate an autosomal dominant inheritance. Anomalies of the posterior segment and strabismus are occasionally reported but are not considered constant features of this syndrome [331]. Systemic features include developmental defects of the teeth and facial bones; odontoblasts are of neural crest origin [304,306]. Flattening of the midface, receding upper lip, maxillary hypoplasia, protrusion of the lower lip, hypertelorism, telocanthus, and a broad flat nose are characteristic of the anterior chamber dysgenesis syndrome [197,304,306]. Cardiac, otological, neurological, and dermatological changes occur with but are not specific features of the disorder [306].

Shields and his colleagues postulate that there is developmental arrest of anterior segment structures derived from neural crest cells [304,306]. Late in gestation, a layer of endothelial cells of crest origin normally covering or involved in the development of portions of the iris and angle fails to regress (Fig. 24). Some cells lay down abnormal basement membrane material. Cells originally crossing the anterior chamber angle fail to regress or regress incompletely, leaving residual strands of iridic tissue crossing the

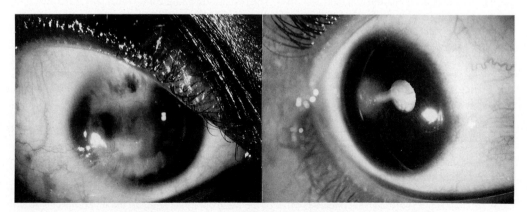

Figure 23 Axenfeld-Rieger anomaly, familial variation. (Left) Mother with corneal leukomas and anterior segment dysgenesis. (Right) Daughter with small corneal leukoma with stalk connected to anterior lens, Peters' anomaly.

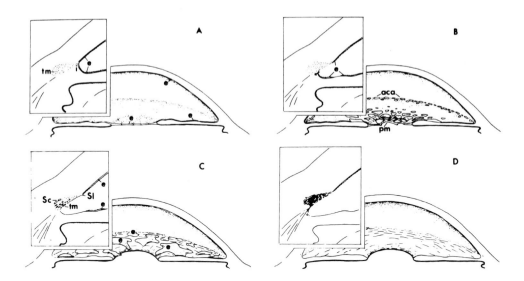

Figure 24 A concept of normal anterior segment development based on reported studies (insets show representative cross-sectional views of chamber angle). (A) At 5 months gestation, a continuous layer of endothelium (e) creates a closed cavity of the anterior chamber; anterior surface of iris (i) inserts in front of primordial trabecular meshwork (tm). (B) During the third trimester, endothelial layer progressively disappears from pupillary membrane (pm) and iris and cavitates over anterior chamber angle (aca), possibly becoming incorporated in trabecular meshwork. Peripheral uveal tissue begins to slide posteriorly in relation to chamber-angle structures. (arrow). (C) Development of trabecular lamellae and intertrabecular spaces begins in inner and posterior aspects of primordial tissue and progresses toward Schlemm's canal (Sc) and Schwalbe's line (Sl). (D) Normal anterior chamber angle is not fully developed until end of first year of life. (Reproduced with permission from M.B. Shields. Axenfeld-Rieger syndrome: A theory of mechanism and distinctions from the iridocorneal endothelial syndrome. *Trans. Am. Ophthalmol. Soc.* 81:736–784, 1983.)

chamber angle (Fig. 25) [304,306]]. The changes occur late in gestation and may continue through the first year of life until the chamber angle matures [304,306].

A number of malformations, occurring singly or in combination (Fig. 26), are recognized in the anterior chamber [349]. Undue prominence of the connective tissue bundles, which are located in Schwalbe's ring between the termination of Descemet's membrane and the beginning of trabecular meshwork (Fig. 27), may be seen. Known as posterior embryotoxon, this anomaly can occur in isolation [66], but not uncommonly strands of connective tissue extend from the ring across the anterior chamber to the iris (Axenfeld's anomaly; Figs. 28 and 29). Congenital ectropion of the iris pigment epithelium, recently added as part of the spectrum of Axenfeld-Rieger, consists of segments of iridic pigment epithelium over the iris in contact with retained primordial endothelial cells on the iris surface [114,377]. The combination of Axenfeld's anomaly and arteriohepatic dysplasia is found in Alagille's syndrome [277,282].

A severe anterior chamber deformity, in which prominent strands are associated with marked hypoplasia of the iris stroma, constitutes Rieger's anomaly. Dysgenetic endothelial cells and Descemet's membrane with changes similar to those found in the corneas of congenital hereditary endothelial dystrophy have been reported in a patient with Rieger's anomaly, adding to the spectrum of this condition [264]. Various abnormalities of the above-mentioned changes with dental and osseous deformities are known as Rieger's syndrome.

Persistence of mesenchymal tissue in the angle probably forms the prominent Schwalbe's ring and attached iris strands (Fig. 29) [304,305]. High insertion of the iris and dysgenesis of the aqueous drainage channel are causally related to the developmental glaucoma, which may have a delayed onset [304–306].

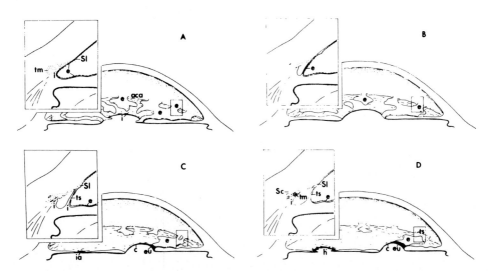

Figure 25   Theory of mechanism for ocular abnormalities of Axenfeld-Rieger syndrome (insets show cross-sectional views of anterior chamber angle corresponding to area within rectangle) (A) Late in gestation, a developmental arrest leads to retention of the primordial endothelium (e) over portions of iris (i) and anterior chamber angle (aca). Incomplete posterior recession of peripheral uvea produces high insertion of iris into posterior trabecular meshwork (tm). Zone of differentiation between corneal and chamber angle endothelium is abnormally forward and associated with excessive basement membrane deposition, causing prominence and anterior displacement of Schwalbe's line (SI). (B) Portions of retained endothelial layer crossing the anterior chamber angle, usually with a few strands of iridic tissue, are displaced centrally from the trabecular meshwork, presumably by contraction of cellular layer or differential growth rate of adjacent structures. (C) In most areas, endothelial layer disappears partially or completely, leaving uveal tissue strands (ts) of variable size extending from peripheral iris to prominent Schwalbe's line. Contraction of retained endothelium on iris in some cases leads to the progressive development of corectopia (c) and ectropion uveae (eu) toward the contracting tissue and iridic thinning and atrophy (ia) in the opposite quadrants, which may continue after birth. (D) Further endothelial contraction leads to hole formation (h) of iris in some eyes. Other factors, including secondary ischemia, are probably also involved in atrophic changes in the iris. Incomplete development of the trabecular meshwork and Schlemm's canal (Sc) is believed to be the mechanism of the glaucoma. (Reproduced with permission from M.B. Shields. Axenfeld-Rieger syndrome: A theory of mechanism and distinctions from the iridocorneal endothelial syndrome. *Trans. Am. Ophthalmol. Soc. 81*:736–784, 1983.)

Juvenile glaucoma develops in 50–70% of such eyes as a result of faulty development of the filtration angle [197,305,364].

Associated corneal anomalies are usually central abnormalities, termed clinically corneal leukomas [94,194,293,330,343–345]. A focal absence of the corneal endothelium and Descemet's membrane results in a gray to white corneal opacity. Ultrastructural examination of some cases show irregular basal epithelial cells, absence of Bowman's layer, stromal edema and scarring with derangement of the lamellar architecture, collagen fibrils with a larger than normal diameter in the posterior stroma, absence of Descemet's membrane, and endothelium in the central cornea. Fibrous tissue fills the defect.

The first main type of central corneal abnormalities is posterior corneal depression with minimal overlying opacity (posterior keratoconus) without contact to iris or lens [194,320,344,364].

Second is corneal leukoma with an adherent cataractous lens without inflammation (Peters' anomaly; Fig. 23, right) [139,144,364]. Peters' anomaly is bilateral in 80% of cases. Associated chromosomal aberrations [190] include partial trisomy 16q [99], the 18q$^-$ syndrome, and 13 deletion syndrome [326] and occasionally Wolf-Hirshhorn syndrome (due to a deletion of 4p16) [193].

Many theories have been proposed to explain Peters' anomaly, in which the lens is attached to the cornea (Fig. 30) [64,65,139,182,186,206]. The most convincing evidence comes from rat fetuses exposed

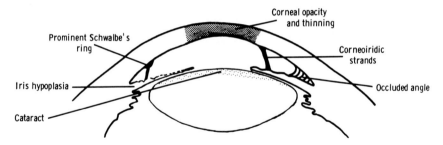

Figure 26   Composite diagram of developmental anomalies encountered in the anterior chamber.

to isoretinoin [64,65]. Histologically the ectodermal stalk from the corneal surface epithelium to the lens fails to disintegrate. The stalk prevents the complete migration of neural crest cells into the central cornea [64,65]. Isotretinoin administered during gastrulation to mice delays the production of extracellular matrix, laminin, and fibronectin and results in a condition similar to Peters' anomaly [64,65].

The third main type is corneal leukoma with strands from the iris adherent to the edge of the corneal opacity (von Hippel's internal corneal ulcer) [93,94,343–345,364]. Abnormal neural crest migration of the cells destined to become posterior corneal stroma, Descemet's membrane, and endothelium can result in this rare anomaly. Inflammation is not a feature of von Hippel's ulcer [345].

D. Lens

Aphakia

Aphakia, the absence of a lens, may be primary or secondary. Primary aphakia can occur when the lenticular placode fails to thicken from the surface ectoderm in response to the stimulus of the optic vesicle and no lens anlage develops. Aphakia in an otherwise normal eye is extremely rare and is usually associated with microphthalmos and trisomy 13 [180]. Secondary congenital aphakia may be found when a lens develops to some degree but is resorbed.

Ectopia Lentis

An abnormally located lens is not uncommon and is often related to defective zonular formation [251]. This frequently bilateral abnormality of the lens may occur with ectopic pupils [126] and is often associated with widespread systemic anomalies [107], as in the syndromes of Marfan [251], Weill-Marchesani [387], and

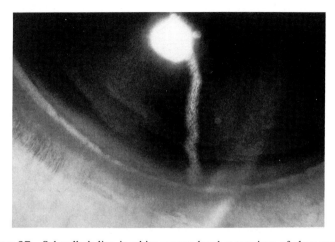

Figure 27   Schwalbe's line is white opaque band at terminus of clear cornea.

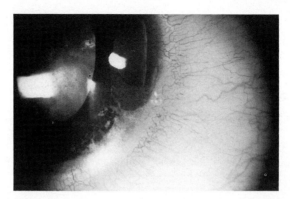

Figure 28   Axenfeld's anomaly with variable involvement of peripheral cornea.

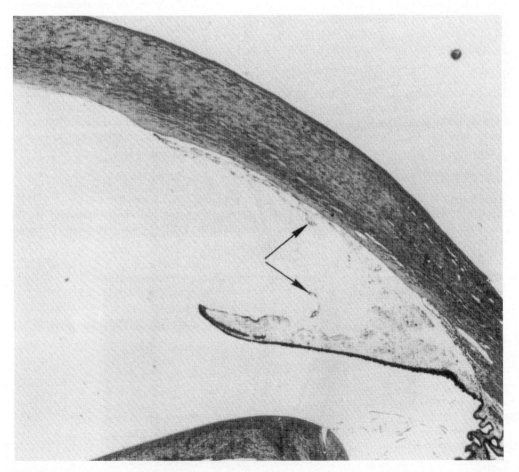

Figure 29   Anterior chamber dysgenesis manifested by delicate strands extending from a mildly atrophic iris stroma to the posterior surface of the cornea (arrows). Note absence of endothelium, centrally, in region of posterior keratoconus. (Hematoxylin and eosin, ×20)

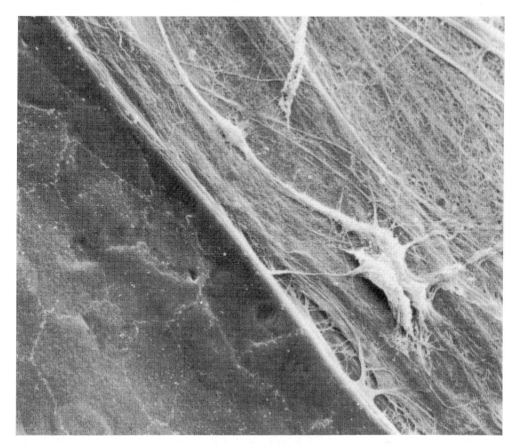

Figure 30 Peters' anomaly. Scanning electron micrograph of posterior corneal surface, showing normal endothelial cells on the left. The corneal endothelium and Descemet's membrane are missing over a crater in the central cornea (right side). (×1440) [Reproduced with permission from G.K. Klintworth and J.S. McCracken. Corneal diseases. In *Electron Microscopy in Human Medicine*, Vol. 6, Part 3, J.V. Johannessen (Ed.), McGraw-Hill, New York, pp. 239–266, 1979.]

Ehlers-Danlos [251], or an isolated dominant trait [171]. The lens may not dislocate until the second decade or later [27,251].

Extraocular ectopic lens tissue (with a normal intraocular lens) is a rare abnormality in the lower eyelids [225,392]. Histological studies suggest that a lens anlage lies in such tissue masses [392]. Zimmerman [392] speculated that an inductive factor causes the ectoderm to produce lens material and designated the entity phakomatous choristoma.

Biphakia

Biphakia, or reduplication of the lens, is extremely rare and is usually associated with a uveal coloboma. In one reported case [132], two well-formed circular clear lenses lay in the coronal plane behind a large cornea.

Microphakia (Spherophakia)

Microphakia, or spherophakia, refers to a lens that is smaller and more spherical than normal. The condition is usually bilateral. The anteroposterior axis of the lens is increased in relation to the diameter, and its anterior pole may be closely apposed to the cornea. Microphakia may be an isolated anomaly, although occasionally it is associated with irregularities of the angle of the anterior chamber. Families have been reported in which the condition was transmitted as a recessive trait. The combination of ectopic lens and pupil, persistent remnants of the vascular tunic of the lens, megalocornea, or disorders involving the anterior ocular segment, such as Marfan and Weill-Marchesani syndromes, are found with microphakia, and in these cases there is usually an autosomal dominant inheritance [252]. An uncomplicated microphakia is generally accepted as caused by an unexplained arrest in the lens development at about month 5 or 6 of development, when it is normally spherical. Actinomycin D administered to pregnant rats can produce microphakia in the offspring [350]. Microspherophakia is found in Alport's disease [270].

Anterior Lenticonus

Anterior lenticonus is usually an isolated ocular anomaly in which the anterior surface of the lens assumes an abnormal conical or spherical forward projection. It is associated with lens opacities, is usually bilateral, and is occasionally inherited as an autosomal recessive trait but predominately affects males. Ophthalmoscopic examination shows a dark area resembling the effect produced by an oil globule in water. The increased curvature of the central area causes high myopia.

Posterior Lenticonus

Posterior lenticonus, a spherical projection or ridge on the posterior surface of the lens, is more frequent than an anterior conical lens. This usually unilateral condition predominates in females and occurs as an isolated ocular anomaly.

Developmental or Congenital Cataracts

Lenses that are cataractous at birth can result from anomalous development [295] or from degenerative changes in normally formed lenticular tissue [218]. Different types of inheritance patterns [35,283,293, 362], maternal infections (Fig. 31), toxins [71], abnormal enzymes [209], and chromosomal abnormalities [245] have been associated. Moreover, animal experiments suggest that the abnormality involves either abnormal maturation of the lens epithelium and fibers or abnormal interaction of the secondary lens fibers in the suture areas.

The variable morphology of congenital cataracts [251] is determined largely by the timing of the insult during development, irrespective of its nature. Failure of the lens vesicle to close or to separate at the appropriate time has been linked with anterior polar cataract [218], and anomalous fusion of secondary lens fibers is possibly the basis of most sutural and axial cataracts. An insult occurring somewhat later would be expected to affect the fibers encircling the embryonic nucleus and produce a lamellar cataract: metabolic derangements, such as aminoaciduria [71] and hypoglycemia, are often associated with this type of opacity. Degeneration of the embryonic and, in some instances, the fetal nucleus is the cause of nuclear

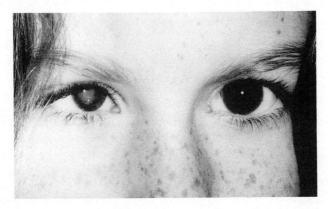

Figure 31   Congenital rubella syndrome. Although normal at birth, the eye grew more slowly and the cataract developed by age 10.

cataracts [72]. Cataractous changes affecting the whole of the lens (total cataract) represent an effect present throughout the development of the lens or one occurring toward the end of gestation. Congenital cataracts are discussed in Chapter 17.

E. Vitreous

Persistent Hyperplastic Primary Vitreous

Clinically, PHPV may produce leukocoria. This unilateral condition is recognized at birth and occurs in a small eye. The anterior chamber is shallow, and the posterior part of the tunica vasculosa lentis persists. Elongated ciliary processes run centrally to the back of the lens [90], where there is usually a break in the posterior capsule with or without a cataract (Fig. 32) or lens coloboma [53]. Retrolental tissue consisting of undifferentiated neural [90] and fibrous tissue sometimes contains fat, hyaline material, cartilage, and foci of calcification [220]. The cataract develops postnatally, suggesting that the tear in the capsule may be due to organization and contraction of the hyperplastic retrolental material. The lenticular capsular epithelium continues posteriorly and is probably associated with defective zonules, as well as adhesion of the ciliary processes to the fibrovascular sheath. A constant feature is the entry of the hyaloid artery into the posterior part of the retrolental mass. PHPV has been associated with maternal cocaine use [340], deficiency of protein C (a vitamin K-dependent inhibitor of the coagulation cascade) [148], and an autosomal dominant inheritance [211].

Persistence of the posterior hyperplastic primary vitreous is uncommon. Retinal folds and vitreoretinal adhesions may develop, leading to secondary retinal breaks and detachment [207]. Preretinal nodules growing into the vitreous are foci of glial tissue arising from Müller cells [207,220].

Miscellaneous Anomalies of the Vitreous

Remnants of the hyaloid artery may remain anteriorly or posteriorly. Normally the entire hyaloid system disintegrates, reabsorbed before birth [262]. The anterior portion of the hyaloid artery lies slightly

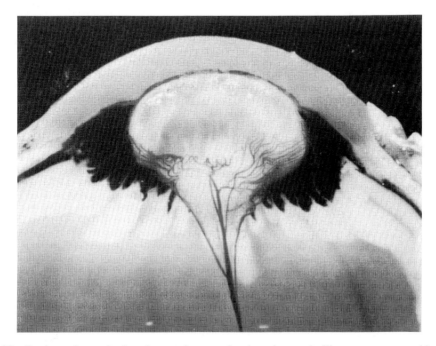

Figure 32 Persistent hyperplastic primary vitreous, showing elongated ciliary processes reaching to the surface of the lens and the persistence of the tunica vasculosa lentis. ($\times$10) (Courtesy of Dr. F. Stefani.)

nasal and inferior to the posterior pole of the lens. When a small remnant of the anterior hyaloid remains it can be seen as a black dot in the red reflex and is called Mittendorf's dot. Remnants of the hyaloid system on the optic disk are called Bergmeister's papilla and include a veil of glial or fibrosis tissue intermixed with remnants of the artery and surrounding glial tissue. Rarely, the hyaloid tissue may persist into adult life as a vascular loop or stalk, sometimes blood filled [80]. Vitreous cysts may occur [212].

Irregular vitreal neovascularization occurs with or without retinal detachment in anencephaly (Figs. 2 through 4) [3], hydranencephaly [222], and other conditions [3,207]. In Norrie's disease (see Chap. 25), the primary and secondary vitreous persists with many intravitreal blood vessels [14,165,254,391].

There is less vitreous than normal in microphthalmic eyes, as previously discussed [370,371].

F. Retina

Aplasia and Hypoplasia of the Retina

Total retinal aplasia occurs only in complete anophthalmia. The retinal anlage is essential to the development of the ocular structures. Complete anophthalmia represents a complete absence of the neuroectoderm destined to form the retina. Secondary aplasia of the retina may result from severe intraocular inflammation, degeneration, or other conditions. The retinal elements also fail to differentiate under the circumstances in which the optic vesicle neglects to invaginate, resulting in a cystic eye. Hypoplasia of the retina implies limited development of retinal tissue. Primary hypoplasia of the retina is difficult to identify clinically or pathologically. Foveal hypoplasia has been reported [90,259]. Secondary hypoplasia of the retina may occur in conjunction with anencephaly, microencephaly, and hydroencephaly [222,359]. The axons in the nerve fiber layer form normally but degenerate secondarily when they are unable to form synapses in the lateral geniculate body, where cerebral development is absent or limited.

Retinal Dysgenesis

Retinal dysgenesis (dysplasia) results from faulty embryogenesis of the retina. The term signifies a heterogeneous group of clinical and histopathological changes including disorderly cellular proliferation, a lack of cellular stratification, abnormal location of retinal elements, and the formation of rosettes [198,382]. Disturbances occur in the constituent cells, the retinal layers, retinal blood vessels, and supporting tissues. Retinal dysgenesis occurs often in abnormally developed eyes, especially microphthalmia, or as an isolated phenomenon, with or without systemic abnormalities [90]. Dysgenesis may coexist with retinoblastoma [257]. Healthy, normal RPE is necessary for the orderly growth and maturation of the retina [113]. Experimentally produced spaces between the photoreceptor layers and the RPE lead to the formation of rosettes [312]. Hence, where RPE is lacking or the neural retina is separated from it, dysgenetic development can be expected. Chromosome 13 carries a gene that controls normal retinal development, and one copy is needed to regulate maturation. When both genetic copies are absent in a cell, retinoblastoma can develop (see Chap. 49) [88,388,389]. Retinal dysgenesis is not an inevitable accompaniment of retinoblastoma because the tumorogenic somatic mutation(s) occur after retinal differentiation has ceased or is decreasing.

Rosettes vary in size and are circular to oval configurations of retinal nuclei and fibrils around a central opening (Figs. 33 and 34) and are seen histologically in most cases of retinal dysgenesis as well as in neuroectodermal tumors. Retinal features, such as the number of nuclear layers, fibrils, outer limiting membrane, photoreceptor elements, and cell junctions and the types of constituent cells (bipolar, photoreceptor, undifferentiated, and Müller), may be present, absent, or displaced, contributing to the disarray of rosettes. Müller cells have been identified in dysgenetic rosettes but not in those of retinoblastomas [113]. The better differentiated rosettes occur in association with systemic abnormalities: triploidy [113], trisomy 13 [169], Meckel's syndrome [216], and Norrie's disease [14]. Primitive single-layer rosettes are usually found as isolated abnormalities. Bipolar cells may be scattered through the inner and outer nuclear layers of the retina, with marked reduction in retinal width in retinal dysgenesis produced by certain viruses or chemicals [8]. In the case of cytosine arabinoside, this is due to its antimitotic activity [266]. The dysgenetic rosettes that result from experimentally induced herpetic infection are preceded by tissue necrosis, which suggests that, in some circumstances, the disturbed growth may be promoted by reparative factors. The degree of maturity of the retina seems to be of major importance in its susceptibility to retinal dysgenesis, since such changes do not follow retinal detachment or retinitis. Dysgenetic rosettes are also a

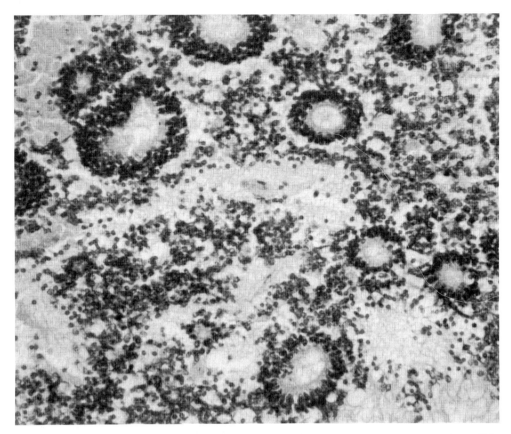

Figure 33   Rosettes in retinal dysgenesis, complicating trisomy 13. (Hematoxylin and eosin, ×100)

feature of the retina overlying foci of attached but unpigmented epithelium, so-called lacunae, in Aicardi's syndrome (Figs. 35 through 37) [5,160]. However, they may also be seen over normal RPE in Aicardi's syndrome [5]. The presence of pigment-containing cells in the center of some dysgenetic rosettes has been interpreted as attempted repair involving the phagocytosis of necrotic cell remnants [113,198].

The term "retinal dysgenesis" applies equally to a focal, single, isolated rosette in an otherwise normal eye as to the totally disorganized detached retina with large oval multi-layered rosettes as found in trisomy 13 [154,192,257,274].

The development of retinal tissue anterior to the ora serrata, indicating that the inner layer of the optic vesicle has differentiated into retinal tissue rather than into the nonpigmented ciliary epithelium or ciliary epithelium in the retina, can also be considered dysgenetic [90]. Abnormalities of intraretinal migration of primitive retinoblasts, as seen in Walker-Warburg syndrome (Fig. 38), manifest dysgenetic retinal stratification as well as lissencephaly, hydrocephalus, and muscular dystrophy [149,359,368]. In Walker-Warburg syndrome the photoreceptors were not found at 20 weeks of gestation. Infants at term with Walker-Warburg syndrome usually have retinal detachments that develop in the last trimester [359].

Retinoschisis

Retinoschisis, or splitting of the retina, involves division of the inner layers of the retina [63,223,384,393]. Isolated retinoschisis, probably sporadic, has been described in girls [393]; it can be inherited as an X chromosome-linked disease when it is found almost always in boys in the first years of life [384]. The large cavity that forms within the retina can reach the back of the lens and present clinically as leukocoria. Macular abnormalities, including cystoid edema and pigmentary changes, are present in about 50% of cases. Peripheral retinoschisis without macular abnormalities has been reported, although this is confined

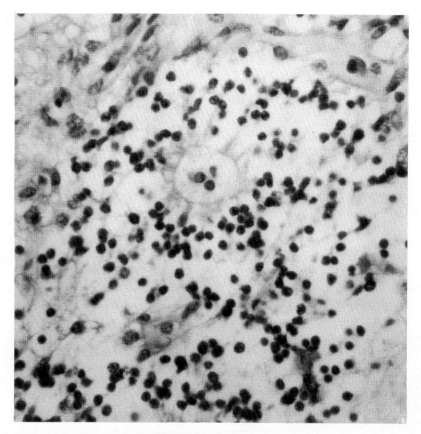

Figure 34 Retinal dysgenesis, showing a single-layered rosette with well-defined outer limiting membrane formation and central undifferentiated cells. (Hematoxylin and eosin, ×200)

to elderly patients in whom the foveal changes can disappear [80,223]. Early splitting, with or without rupture, within the nerve fiber layer may also be seen inferior to the cystic cavity. The wall of the cyst is reinforced by proliferated glial and connective tissue with condensed vitreous and remnants of the internal limiting membrane. Secondary glaucoma may develop in juvenile retinoschisis as a result of closure of the angles by anterior ballooning of the cyst. The microscopic findings of severe degeneration and atrophy of the nerve fiber layer, as well as the optic atrophy encountered clinically in some cases, suggests that the inherited defect may also involve the retinal nerve fibers. The RPE is abnormal in the macular area. Manschot [223] suggests that the limited evidence available at present points to an inherited defect primarily affecting the retinal nerve fiber layer. Whether the changes in the RPE at the posterior pole are primary or secondary to the changes in the sensory retina is uncertain, although Deutman [80] believes that they are acquired because the electrooculogram (which records the changes in the standing electrical potential across the retina under standardized conditions of darkness and light) is normal in young patients. On the basis of clinical examination, Conway and Welch [63] suggested that the splitting of the retinal nerve fiber layer begins in the region of the major retinal vessels: they found that as a vessel is traced centrifugally into an area of schisis, one branch may lie in the deep layer but another branch of the same vessel may run up to the elevated inner layer or travel unsupported in the space between the split retinal layers. In a similar manner, strands of what are probably nerve fibers may run obliquely between the separated retinal layers. These intact nerve fibers may explain why the peripheral visual field defects in these patients are often relative [63] compared with the more severe visual impairment of senile retinoschisis. The hemorrhagic tendency in this condition may be related to the absence of the vascular support usually provided by the surrounding nerve fibers and Müller cells [63,95].

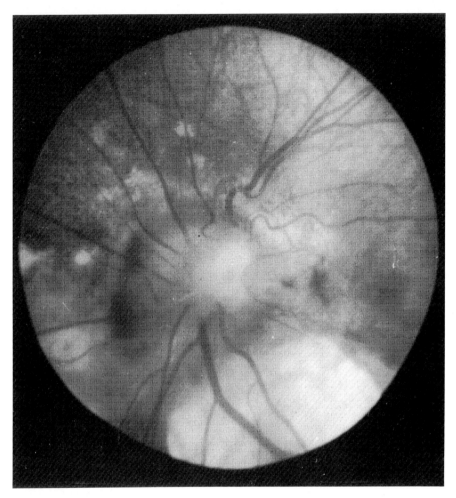

Figure 35 Aicardi's syndrome. Fundus photograph, showing several lacunae in the posterior retina, together with a choroidoretinal coloboma around the optic disk. (Courtesy of Professor D. Archer.)

Astrocytic Hamartomas

Hyperplastic nodular foci of astrocytes other than the specialized Müller cells are found on the inner surface of the retina in tuberous sclerosis as a glial hamartoma (see Chap. 45). The localization of astrocytic nodules over veins has led to the speculation that hamartomatous lesions may have a predilection for perivascular sites [115]: this association is obvious in such formations found occasionally in anencephalic retinas (Fig. 3).

Vascular Anomalies of the Retina

Numerous developmental abnormalities of the retinal blood vessels are recognized, some of which become apparent later in life. The vessel may be abnormally distributed and qualitatively defective as in Coats' disease [52], or quantitatively increased as in von Hippel-Lindau disease (discussed in Chap. 45). Non-oxygen-induced vitreal neovascularization occurs in such conditions as anencephaly, hydranencephaly, and Potter's syndrome [3,222,288a]. In anencephaly the unusual intraretinal neovascularization may be unilateral and of random distribution. The new vessels extend into the vitreous (Fig. 4) and are often associated with a retinal detachment that may be total, even at birth. The reactivation of dormant primitive vitreal vessels may account for some of the changes, but usually continuity between the neovascular

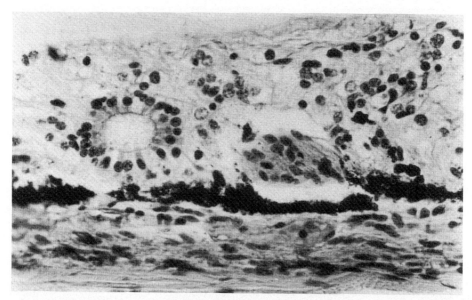

Figure 36   Aicardi's syndrome. Single-layered rosette in an immature retina overlying a partially deficient pigment epithelium. (Hematoxylin and eosin, ×400) (Courtesy of Dr. P. Dhermy.)

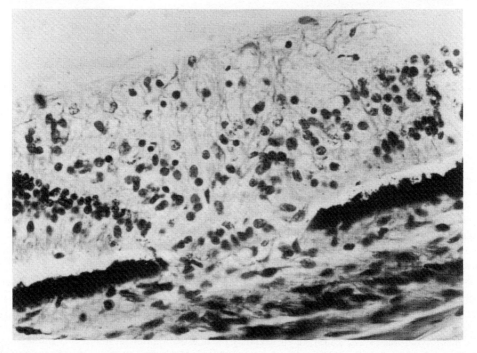

Figure 37   Aichardi's syndrome. Histology of a fundal lacuna shows focal absence of the retinal pigment epithelium with lack of normal differentiation and organization in the overlying neuroretina. (Hematoxylin and eosin, ×400) (Courtesy of Dr. P. Dhermy)

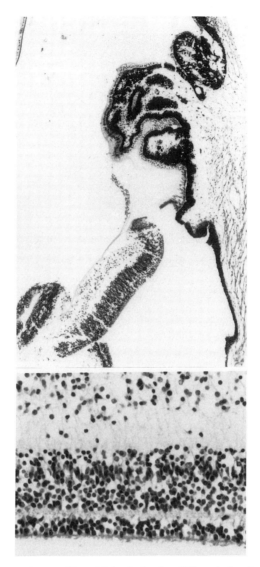

Figure 38 Walker-Warburg syndrome. (Upper) Island of retina differentiating from medullary epithelium of ciliary process. (Lower) Bizarre migration of differentiating retina and no phoreceptor development in 20-week-old fetus.

elements and the intraretinal vessels can be traced. The retina in premature infants is incompletely vascularized: the younger the infant, the greater the degree of avascularity. Postnatal growth of the vessels in immature infants is effected by the use of oxygen (see retinopathy of prematurity Chap. 52) [16]. Occasionally in the periphery of the immature retina vascularization is absent in an infant with multiple anomalies but normal chromosomes (Fig. 39).

Ectopic Retinal Tissue

Retinal tissue can be found outside the globe in association with colobomas. It has been seen along the optic nerve sheaths as far as the chiasm in Aicardi's syndrome [160] and in the hypothalamus in synophthalmia-cyclopia [346]. Retinal anlage tissue has been observed in tumors of the maxilla [138].

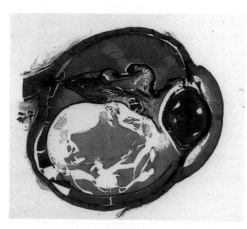

Figure 39 Globe with excessive vessels and folds on stalk from disk and avascular retina inferiorly. Hematoxylin and eosin, ×1)

Congenital Retinal Detachment

Congenital retinal detachment in the newborn is divided into developmental and secondary types. Developmental detachment is either total or focal, the latter termed retinal folds. The development of congenital nonattachment of the retina is part of the spectrum of the congenital cystic eye in which the stage of the optic vesicle persists. The continuous layer of neuroectoderm is dysgenetic and minimally differentiated, surrounding a fluid-filled space.

Incomplete invagination such that the neurosensory retina does not reach the RPE layer results in congenital nonattachment of the retina. Nonattachment of the retina is present normally through month 3 of intrauterine life, and thereafter the neurosensory layer, larger in area than the pigmented layer, forms shallow folds that gradually flatten with growth. Congenital nonattachment is found in eyes with other anomalies, such as congenital glaucoma [104], microphthalmos, PHPV, coloboma, and retinal dysgenesis. Congenital nonattachment may extend into the ciliary body. Nonattachment later in development occurs when the neurosensory retina is opposed to the pigmented layers but lacks photoreceptors. Without bonds to the RPE, the retina detaches later.

Complete or partial retinal nonattachment or detachment with retinal dysgenesis may be found in many syndromes with abnormal chromosomes and may be associated with maternal infections and toxins.

Bilateral cases of retinal detachment with giant retinal tears and nasal colobomas of the lens have been reported, the lens abnormality being related to a segmental failure of zonular development, with anteroposterior thickening of the lens edge in that area and, possibly, secondary flattening of the lens border [155].

In 1920, Gonin [127a] described and illustrated retinal disinsertions, and several years later Anderson [11a] suggested the importance of a congenital factor in the genesis of these dialyses at the ora serrata. The term "congenital retinal disinsertion syndrome" [36] was applied to cases with retinal detachment associated with other ocular abnormalities, such as unilateral microphthalmos, central anterior and posterior cortical cataracts, colobomas of the lens, and paving stone degeneration of the temporal retina [36].

Warburg [359] summarized the findings in 164 patients reported in the literature with congenital hydrocephalus, microphthalmos, and evidence of retinal separation or nonattachment at birth. She suggests that these cases constitute a nosological entity, probably with an autosomal recessive mode of inheritance.

The pathogenesis of the nonattachment is not clear, but retinal changes may be found in a wide variety of autosomal dominantly and recessive inherited syndromes. These include Meckel's [161,216] and Bloch-Sulzberger syndromes [34,324].

Congenital retinal detachment may be secondary to such conditions as toxoplasmosis, retinoblastoma, chromosomal anomalies, persistent hyperplastic primary vitreous, and Pierre Robin syndrome [359].

Retinal Folds

Persistence of an exuberant growth of the neurosensory retina in excess of the pigmented layer or tractional attachments from vessels or vitreous to the neurosensory retina may cause focal retinal folds, sometimes a total separation. Clinically folds appear to occur from a focus in the posterior pole in which the surrounding retina is attached. Alternatively, the adjacent retina may exhibit a lesser degree of tenting or detachment. Histologically folds usually show some degree of retinal dysgenesis, including the formation of rosettes. Proliferations of neural, glial, and vascular elements are associated. The vessels may be continuous with the hyaloid system or extend from the retina into the vitreous.

Retinal folds have many configurations. A peripheral retinal fold seen histologically only in eyes of infants and a few young people, called Lange's fold, is probably a fixation artifact. Kalina [181] could not find the fold in 370 eyes of infants, many premature, whom he examined. Falciform folds or retinal septa are folds, often bilateral, that extend from the disk to the ora serrata or ciliary body, often but not invariably in the inferotemporal quadrant. Remnants of the hyaloid system follow the ridge, which also manifests dysgenesis. The surrounding retina may be flat or tented, and the RPE is normal. Folds may occur in eyes with colobomas.

Tractional retinal folds occur from attachments to the hyaloid system and with PHPV. Vitreous adhesions may produce folds and traction on the retina. Experimentally, when drainage tubes are introduced through the wall of the embryonic eye, vitreous escapes and the neural retina progressively folds.

Anomalies of the Retinal Pigment Epithelium

The RPE may be absent from large colobomatous areas of or beneath dysgenetic retina. There may be no pigment in this epithelium in the lacunae seen ophthalmoscopically in the fundus in Aicardi's syndrome (Fig. 35), and hypopigmentation occurs in eyes from individuals with ocular albinism, trisomy 13 [158], trisomy 18 [287,353,385], and monosomy X-45 [158]. Depigmentation and vacuolization occur with retinal dysgenesis produced by experimental virus infection, such changes being related to the inflammatory foci in the choroid [7]. Numerous folds of RPE can be seen at the margins of uveal colobomas and thickening, and redundancy of this layer at the macula has been described in trisomy 18 [121].

Hypertrophy of the RPE can occur for no apparent reason and in individuals with the B ring chromosomal anomaly [122], and with familial adenomatous polyposis [288], including Gardner's syndrome [348]. Proliferation of primitive RPE occurs in medulloepitheliomas (see Chap. 47).

G. Optic Nerve

Optic nerve developmental anomalies represent a spectrum of malformations [72], including epipapillary fibrous and glial tissue, peripapillary pigmentary disturbance, optic disk colobomas, dysplasia of and variations in size of the optic nerve [100], and variable disk vessels with or without tufts of glial tissue [172].

Optic Nerve Aplasia

Human cases of true optic nerve aplasia are very rare [218,372]. The developmental anomaly usually occurs sporadically in only one eye of otherwise healthy individuals. Weiter and colleagues [372] discussed 13 cases with an age at enucleation from 1 week to 26 years (mean 2.5 years). Most of the eyes were microphthalmic, and the aplasia of the optic nerve was considered to result from abnormal invagination of the optic fissure, the other ocular changes being secondary. Aplasia was found in a mutant mouse following faulty closure of the embryonic fissure and cell death [284]. Bilateral aplasia of the optic system in a female infant with absence of the nose and extensive maldevelopment of the central nervous system (CNS); including partial agenesis of the medulla, pons, and cerebellum and poor development of the telencephalon and diencephalon, has been reported [386]. Except for the retina, however, which showed a diminution of the ganglion cell and nerve fiber layers, the eyes were unremarkable. Ultrastructural studies disclosed that the cells, believed to be ganglion cells, were undifferentiated and had not elaborated axons or dendrites, so that the nerve fiber layer was practically nonexistent. The first elements to be considered in the failure of the evolution of a normal optic nerve are the ganglion cells, the emergence of which does not take place until about the 10 mm stage. If these should fail to develop or, if once developed, there is failure to send out axons, the retinal nerve fiber layer, the optic nerve, the chiasm, and the optic tracts will be absent. Second, the role of the mesectodermal elements in the optic nerve stalk that will form the future blood supply of the optic nerve and retina, as well as the supportive tissues of the nerve fibers, may be abnormal. In a hypoplastic optic nerve supporting tissues are present. A third speculative factor is the importance of the proper sequence of the development of the optic vesicle and cup with that of the optic stalk.

Optic Nerve Hypoplasia

Underdevelopment or hypoplasia of the optic nerve is more common than total absence [110,199]. It may be bilateral or unilateral. A central retinal artery and vein are usually present at the disk (Fig. 40). The disk is small and encircled by a pigmented ring surrounded by a yellow mottling of the perineural tissues. Retinal ganglion cells are decreased [199]. Optic nerve hypoplasia is found with major intraocular and extraocular anomalies such as albinism, aniridia, colobomas, median cleft face, CNS and endocrine anomalies [316], anencephaly, hydranencephaly [359], and osteogenesis imperfecta and in septooptic dysplasia of de Morsier [46], to mention only a few of the associations [110]. Anticonvulsants [159] and varicella [201], a neurotropic virus, have been implicated as causes of hypoplasia of the optic nerve. Isolated cases confined to the eye have been reported clinically [46,244]. Partial hypoplasia has been noted [185]. Vision ranges from normal to blindness.

Optic Disk Colobomas and Pits

Bilateral congenital colobomas confined to the optic nerve can have an autosomal dominant mode of inheritance [383] and frequently result in macular or extramacular serous detachment of the retina with total blindness [241,300,338]. The defect in the disk may be associated with heterotopic adipose tissue and smooth muscle [375] or medullary epithelium [90]. The colobomas tend to remain asymptomatic until the second decade, and there is thus far no evidence to implicate cerebrospinal fluid as the source of the subretinal fluid [300]. Heterochromia iridis has been associated with a coloboma of the disk [84].

A minimal optic disk coloboma is the optic disk "pit" with a well-defined clinical appearance (Fig. 41), which is usually unilateral, although bilateral cases have been reported [47,188,338]. Macrodisks and pits are seen in the same eye [177,178]. The position is usually in the lower temporal quadrant, atypical for the usual ocular colobomas. Histological examination may reveal a herniation of the neural ectoderm dipping into the intermediary tissue near the junction of the lamina cribrosa with the sclera and extending along the sheath of the optic nerve [103]. The nature of the visual defects that can occur with these pits indicates interference with the transmission of normal impulses through the dysplastic herniated retina [241]. Macular detachment and subretinal neovascularization [170,320] may accompany an optic pit.

An optic nerve coloboma may be associated with a congenitally large scleral canal and posterior displacement of the optic disk. Under such circumstances the scleral ectasia may be associated with a

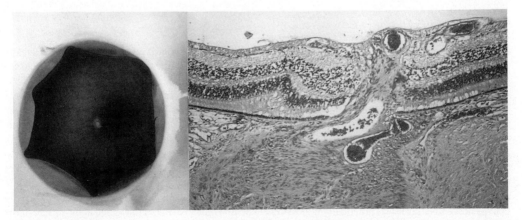

Figure 40 Hypoplasia of optic disk. (Left) Gross specimen. (Right) Small opening in pigment epithelium admits only retinal artery. No ganglion axons extend into nerve below. (Hematoxylin and eosin, ×100)

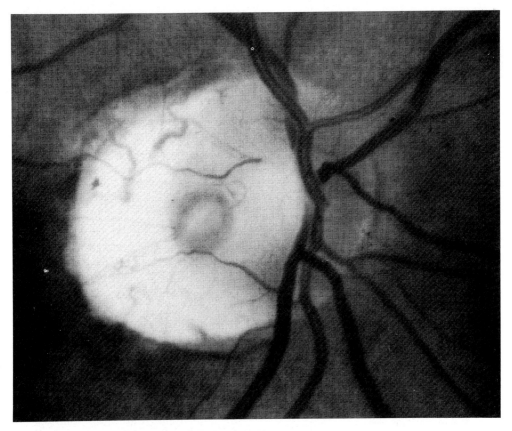

Figure 41   Optic disk pit.

peripapillary heaped retina, which may simulate a neoplasm [186]. Similarly, the condition called morning glory syndrome [186,320] is characterized by an enlarged, funnel-shaped nerve head surrounded by an elevated ring of chorioretinal tissue with pigmentary and vascular disturbances (Fig. 42). Pulsations may be observed [354]. The retinal vessels appear clinically as multiple narrow branches radiating at the edge of the disk. Lens colobomas and PHPV may be associated [53]. A marked diminution of visual acuity occurs in this entity, which needs to be distinguished clinically from a glioma of the optic nerve. In this regard very few histological examinations of eyes with the morning glory syndrome have been made [224]. Ultrasonography may disclose a cystic lesion of the optic nerve that communicates with the vitreous cavity, and computed axial tomography has shown an intraneural cyst of the optic nerve. Trisomy 4q has been reported with the morning glory disk [256]. The optic disk varies considerably in size when it is malformed and often shares features with the morning glory syndrome [172]. Some contend that optic nerve hypoplasia, megalopapilla, and optic disk colobomas represent a spectrum of anomalies of optic nerve development [19,172], because several variations have been reported in the same family [318]. Ultrasonography is useful in delineating the sclera and nerve posteriorly [100].

H.   Cranial-Facial-Ocular Abnormalities

Cyclopia, Synophthalmia, and Diophthalmos

Cyclopia [116], synophthalmia, and probably diophthalmos represent a continuum of regional upper facial, ocular, and cerebral [346] anomalies. The brain is holoprosencephalic, a cortical shell covering a single ventricle and lacking hemispheric development. The ocular structure in cyclopia is a single eye lacking an optic nerve (Fig. 43), whereas synophthalmos represents the fused parts of two eyes (Fig. 44) with a single

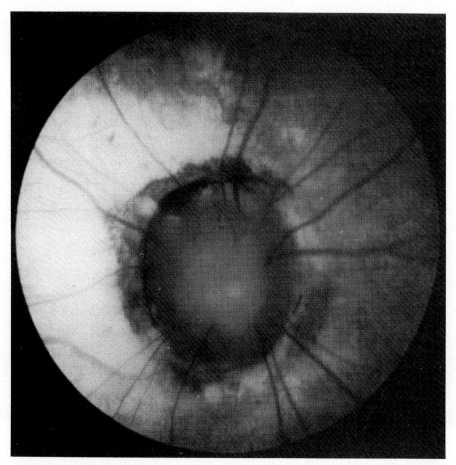

Figure 42 Optic disk in the morning glory syndrome. The disk is hyperemic, projects anteriorly in a dome-shaped manner, and is surrounded by a raised rim of grayish retina. (Courtesy of Professor D. Archer.)

optic nerve. The two eyes are barely separated in the midline in diophthalmos [92]. The nose is impeded in its descent from forehead to midface when the neural tube flexes in development and remains as aberrant nasal tissue above the eyes. It protrudes either as a flat stump or a proboscis. The pituitary gland is absent. The orbits, cranial bones, supporting soft tissues, eyelids, and ocular muscles are similarly absent in the midline, with the lateral structures fused centrally. The defect is organogenetic in that the structures that are correctly induced produce normal tissue components but the amount of tissue programmed initially is inadequate.

Cyclopia can be produced experimentally by excising the mesoderm underlying the anterior neural plate [176]. The mesoderm induces the ocular anlagen and provides growth support for the developing eyes. When a limited amount of midline neuroectoderm is induced by the mesoderm, the result is a symmetrical fused eye. Most cases are highly symmetrical and show differentiation of the lateral structures present with variable dysplasia in the midregion. The anterior and lateral parts show more complete differentiation than those that are medial and posterior [346].

In most cases, the lower face, although mildly hypoplastic, and the body are normal. Occasional cases are clearly associated with a genetic abnormality, as in certain chromosomal anomalies (18p deletion [196], balanced 3/7 translocations [50], and trisomy 13 [346]), all of which show the systemic and intraocular changes associated with the extra chromosome. Clinically the synophthalmic eye may blink and the pupils respond to light. Cyclopia is usually lethal in the first trimester; synophthalmics may be born alive but die within minutes because the maldevelopment of the nasopharynx is incompatible with life. Slightly more

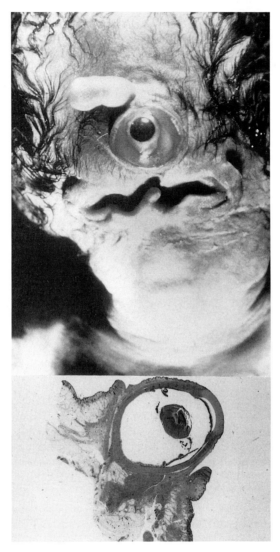

Figure 43   (Upper) Unusual cyclops with ears and mouth disfigured, proboscis above eye. (Lower) Cyclopic eye without optic nerve. (Courtesy of Dr. R. Tripathi.)

females than males are affected. Cases with a variety of abnormal karyotypes have been reported, but no consistent genetic pattern has yet emerged. Teratogens inducing cyclopia include veratrum alkaloids found in grass eaten by sheep, lithium, magnesium, vitamin A, and vinblastine. Cadmium, which destroys neural crest cells, does not produce cyclopia [346].

In cyclopia, the anterior tissues are usually orderly and well formed. The anterior retina shows three nuclear layers with the intervening plexiform layers, whereas posteriorly rosettes and dysplastic retinal formations occur in the area of the aborted optic nerve. There is no channel through the sclera for the optic nerve. The paired eyes in synophthalmia are symmetrical, even when somatic anomalies in the fetus suggest a concurrent chromosomal anomaly (Fig. 43). In one review only 1 of 34 cases of synophthalmia reviewed by the author were asymmetrical [346]. The cellular and tissue differentiation is mature, as indicated by functional response, blink, and movement in response to bright light. In synophthalmia, the optic nerve is single, often staphylomatous, with some axons and neural organization. The globes may have a single large vitreous cavity, or the cavity may be bifurcated by a band of sclera (Fig. 44).

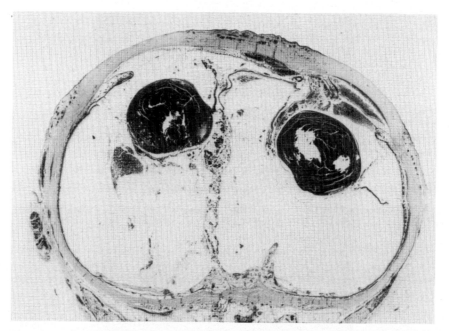

Figure 44   Synophthalmos showing duplication of the lens. (Hematoxylin and eosin, ×5.5)

The term "diophthalmos" refers to a condition in which two eyes develop on a single optic stalk [92]. A histopathological section of a very unusual case with bilateral microphthalmos and cyst has been documented [92], but the morphogenesis of diophthalmos has yet to be explained.

Cryptophthalmos

Cryptophthalmos (hidden eye) [357] is a very rare condition in which the anterior surface of the eye is fused with the overlying skin (Fig. 45). Multiple systemic [42,117,265,275] and other ocular anomalies [42] are commonly present. Although cryptophthalmos is usually bilateral, a few unilateral cases have also been described [135].

Isolated complete cryptophthalmos (ablepharon) is the most common form of the anomaly. A small horizontal line resembling a scar may be present where the palpebral fissure usually lies. As a rule the eyebrow and eyelashes are totally or partially absent [117]. Of all cases 20% are partial, the lateral portion of the eyelids being normal, whereas the facial skin is fused to an ectatic and vascularized cornea on the medial side. The conjunctiva, superior lacrimal punctum, and lacrimal gland are absent, so that xerosis of the globe occurs. Microscopically, the eye is rarely microphthalmic, but the anterior chamber may be small or nonexistent, and the lens may be present, absent, or represented by only a few abortive fragments. The iris is either missing or adherent to the back of the cornea, and the ciliary body is atrophic. Choroidal and retinal development range from normal to severe disorganization. Electroretinogram and flash VEP may be normal [162]. Cryptophthalmos may be associated with colobomatous cysts and microphthalmos. The overlying skin of the eyelids is keratinized, and the dermis is fused to fibrovascular tissue, which replaces the cornea. Hair follicles, meibomian glands, accessory lacrimal, and Zeis' glands are all absent [265]. The orbicularis oculi muscle is present, and a bright light provokes its constriction.

In Fraser syndrome, cryptophthalmos is associated with dyscephaly, syndactyly, and urogenital malformations [42,117,265,275,365]. Small bowel malrotation may also occur [379]. Ablepharon and macrostromia are linked [166]. There is autosomal recessive inheritance in 15% of cases of cryptophthalmos in general.

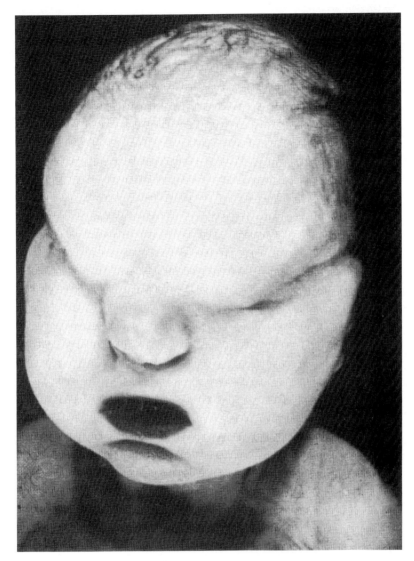

Figure 45   Cryptophthalmos. There is complete absence of palpebral structures and the globes are adherent to skin which is continuous between the cheeks and forehead. (Courtesy of Dr. J.W. Keeling.)

Facial Cleft and Other Anomalies

Disfiguring facial clefts of orbit, cheek, maxillary area, median face, nose, palate, teeth, and mouth are rare [187,190,329]. Because the profound facial malformations are not always lethal, early evaluation and prompt treatment must be instituted to preserve a useful eye. Facial asymmetry, lateral facial clefts, and midfacial clefts (Fig. 46) are among the more common [190]. Ocular anomalies, including colobomas, occur [273]. Exposure keratopathy and corneal ulcers may rapidly develop. Surgical repair may result in remarkable results [38,190,280]. Such infants should be referred to major treatment centers for long-term surgical and psychosocial rehabilitation. Amniotic bands [153,238], abnormalities of migration and fusion of neural crest processes, and chromosomal abnormalities have been implicated.

In cloverleaf skull, or Kleeblattschädel syndrome [243], severe proptosis with displacement of the globe results from shallow orbital fossae. Hypertelorism and exotropia with ear, nose, mouth, and limb deformities are associated [243].

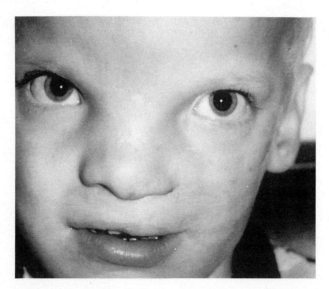

Figure 46   Median cleft face with marked hypertelorism.

Orbital teratomas [225] may be large orbital masses at birth and produce profound proptosis. The teratoma may contain brain tissue not connected to the brain, and mature germinal tissues [225].

The craniofacial syndromes of Crouzon [81], Apert [228], Michels [70], and others result from craniosynostosis, and many have proptosis, hypertelorism, eyelid colobomas, and irregular extraocular muscles [81] as presenting features. Dominant inheritance is common [190].

In trisomy 18, structures of the upper face are affected and the findings include short palpebral fissures, hypoplasia of the orbital ridges, epicanthal folds, blepharoptosis, corneal opacification, slanted palpebral fissures, hypertelorism, coloboma, cataract, and microphthalmos [245]. Colobomas of the eyelids occur in partial trisomy 2q and mandibulofacial dysostosis [66]. Hypertelorism and blepharoptosis occur in Aarskog syndrome [189].

I.   Eyelids and Lacrimal System

Colobomas of Eyelid

A deficiency of part of the eyelid may be unilateral or bilateral. The inner half of the upper eyelid and the outer half of the lower are the most common sites for colobomas. The experimental work of Poswillo [271,272] suggests that ischemia of the rapidly differentiating complex could cause infarction of that part of the developing upper eyelid that is farthest from the principal blood supply. Such an occurrence could also account for the colobomas of the eyelid in oculoauricular vertebral dysplasia (Goldenhar's syndrome) and mandibulofacial dysostosis (also called the Treacher Collins or Franceschetti syndrome), in which the lower eyelid coloboma involves the junction between the outer two-thirds and the inner third of the eyelid in a symmetrical manner. Some of the defects of mandibulofacial dysostosis have been produced experimentally in 100% of the offspring of pregnant rats given vitamin A at day 8.5 of gestation. Such treatment causes early destruction of the neural crest cells of the facial and auditory primordia that normally migrate to the first and second branchial arches. The otomandibular defects thus produced are the same as those in human cases of this syndrome, but details of the relationship between the vitamin A-induced models and the inherited human cases with Treacher Collins syndrome await elucidation [271].

Congenital Symblepharon

The upper eyelid may be fused with the globe but the lower eyelid is normal, a partial cryptophthalmos. In such cases there is no upper eyelid conjunctiva and the superior portion of the cornea is covered by a keratinized stratified squamous epithelium. The superior lacrimal punctum is absent and the eye is xerotic.

There may be no natural plane of tissue differentiation, with scar tissue adherent to an extensively disorganized globe.

Microblepharon

Microblepharon is a developmental shortening of the eyelids in the vertical plane. Limited tissue prevents closure of the eyelids, leaving the eyes exposed (Fig. 47).

Euryblepharon

Enlargement of the palpebral aperture, euryblepharon, may occur as an isolated abnormality of the eyelids or as bilaterally symmetrically large eyelids opening much more widely than normal. The anomaly may be familial, with an uncertain type of inheritance. Euryblepharon is thought to be due to a congenital hypoplasia or aplasia of the orbicularis oculi muscle.

Epicanthus

Epicanthus is a genetically determined half-moon–shaped fold of skin extending downward to the side of the nose, with its concavity directed to the inner canthus. Anatomically, epicanthus results from a Z-shaped kink in the fibers of the orbicularis oculi muscle produced by an insertion of the levator tendon nearer the eyelid margins than the usual upper border of the tarsus. Epicanthal folds have been reported in association with a number of syndromes, including Zellweger [325], cri-du-chat deletion of short arm of chromosome 5 (5p−) [156], partial deletion of chromosome D long arm (Dq−), trisomies 18 [72,245] and 21 [297], Klinefelter's [107,373], ring B [122], Rubinstein-Taybi with broad thumbs, hypertrichosis, and cataracts [96], Smith-Lemli-Opitz with ptosis and strabismus [143], and Waardenburg's [355].

Congenital Anomalies of the Eyelashes

Absence of the eyelashes is very unusual. Hypotrichosis, the partial absence of hair due to a congenital lack of most hair follicles, may be associated with some forms of ectodermal dysplasia [356] and abnormalities of the skin and its appendages. In hypertrichosis there is an excessive growth of hair and an increase in the number and the length of the eyelashes. When the eyelashes are found in regular rows, usually two, the disorder is called distichiasis and the meibomian glands are replaced by hair follicles. This condition may be inherited, usually as a dominant affliction, and the distichiasis may involve all eyelids and occur with partial ectropion of lower eyelids, chronic lymphedema of both lower extremities, and a connective tissue band from the mastoid to the clavicle. Distichiasis of the upper eyelid with no lashes on the lower eyelids is part of Setleis syndrome, which includes coarse facies, thick lips, and chronic conjunctivitis [58]. On the other hand, long eyelashes arranged in irregular rows are part of Schwartz syndrome. An association with cleft palate has been reported [24]. The eyebrows may be partially duplicated [30], joined medially in de Lange's syndrome (synophrys) [255], or absent laterally [309]. Arching eyebrows with hypertelorism are seen in the deletion of part of the short arm of chromosome 4 (4p16; the Wolf-Hirshhorn syndrome) [374].

J. Lacrimal Gland, Sac, and Duct

Agenesis of the lacrimal gland is a feature of cryptophthalmos. Ectopic lacrimal gland tissue has been reported intraocularly [242]. Congenital atresia of the nasolacrimal duct is common and may be familial [314]. The lumina of the canaliculi normally become patent during month 4 of intrauterine life, but the lacrimal puncta do not open onto the margins of the eyelids until just before the eyelids separate during month 7 of gestation. Atresia of the inferior opening of the nasolacrimal duct is very common and merely represents a lack of mucosal membrane perforation in the nose allied to a failure of canalization of the solid epithelial tract, the latter reaching the margins of the eyelids at 35 mm. The oculonasal connection usually takes place at the end of month 6 but may be delayed for several weeks or months after birth. The mucous membrane in the nose usually ruptures before tears begin to be secreted in the first weeks of life. Lacrimal drainage problems are part of mandibulofacial dysostosis [23]. Cysts of the nasolacrimal duct may enlarge [4,133]. Defects in the nasolacrimal system are frequently associated with medial facial and oblique clefts [109,333]. Atresias and aplasias of the lacrimal drainage system comprise part of the LADD syndrome of lacrimoauriculodentodigital anomalies [367].

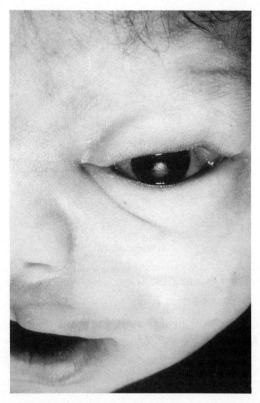

Figure 47 Microblepharon. Stillborn infant with staring look because upper eyelid is so short that it cannot forcibly be drawn downward to cover eye. Note eyelid notch of partial coloboma. (Courtesy of T. Baretta, M.D.)

K. Extraocular Muscles

Absence of the extraocular muscles has been reported [81,87,164].

ACKNOWLEDGMENTS

Portions of the material included in this chapter were originally presented in the first edition authored by Joan Mullaney.

REFERENCES

1. Abruzzo, M.A., and Erickson, R.P. Re-evaluation of new X-linked syndrome for evidence of CHARGE syndrome or association. *Am. J. Med. Genet. 34*:397–400, 1989.
2. Adams, M.D., Kelley, J.M., Gocayne, J.D., Dubnick, M., Polymeropoulos, M.H., Xiao, H., Merrill, C.R., Wu, A., Oeda, B., Moreno, R.F., Kerlavage, A.R., McCombe, W.R., and Venter, J.C. Complementary DNA sequencing: Expressed sequence tags and human genome project. *Science 252*:1651–1656, 1991.
3. Addison, D.J., Font, R.L., and Manschot, W.A. Proliferative retinopathy in anencephalic babies. *Am. J. Ophthalmol. 74*:67–69, 1972.
4. Aguirre-Vila-Coro, A., Mazow, M.L., Drtil, S.H., Robinson, L.K., and Arnoult, J.B. Lacrimal anomalies in Robinow's syndrome: Case report. *Arch. Ophthalmol. 116*:454, 1988.
5. Aicardi, J., Lefebvre, J., and Lerique-Koechlin, A. A new syndrome: Spasm in flexion, collosal agenesis and ocular abnormalities. *Electronencephalogr. Clin. Neurophysiol. 19*:606–612, 1965.
6. Aitchison, C., Easty, D.L., and Jancar, J. Eye abnormalities in the mentally handicapped. *J. Ment. Defic. Res. 34*:41–48, 1990.

7. Albert, D.M., Lahav, M., Carmichael, L.E., and Percy, D.H. Canine herpes-induced retinal dysplasia and associated ocular anomalies. *Invest. Ophthalmol. 15*:267–278, 1976.
8. Albert, D.M., Lahav, M., Colby, E.D., Shadduck, J.A., and Sang, D.N. Retinal neoplasia and dysplasia: Induction by feline leukemia virus. *Invest. Ophthalmol. Vis. Sci. 16*:325–338, 1977.
9. Allerdyce, P., David, J.G., Miller, O.J., Klinger, H.P., Warburton, D., Miller, D.A., Allen, F.H., Abrams, C.A.L., and McGilvray, E. The 13-q-deletion syndrome. *Am. J. Hum. Genet. 12*:499–512, 1969.
10. Allouche, C., Sarda, P., Tronc, F., Jalaguier, J., Montoya, F., and Bonnet, H. The CHARGE association. *Pediatrie 44*:391–395, 1989.
11. Alvarado, M., Bocian, M., and Walker, A.P. The interstitial deletion of the long arm of chromosome 3: Case report, review, and definition of a phenotype. *Am. J. Med. Genet. 27*:781–786, 1987.
13. Andersen, S.R., Geertinger, P., Larsen, H.W., Mikkelsen, M., Paving, A., Vestermark, S., and Warburg, M. Aniridia, cataract and gonadoblastoma in a mentally retarded girl with deletion of chromosome 11: A clinico-pathological case report. *Opthalmologica 176*:171–177, 1978.
14. Apple, D.J., Fishman, G.A., and Goldberg, M.F. Ocular histopathology of Norrie's disease. *Am. J. Ophthalmol. 78*:196–203, 1974.
15. Armstrong, R.C., and Monie, I.W. Congenital eye defects on rats following maternal folic-acid deficiency during pregnancy. *J. Embryol. Exp. Morphol. 16*:531–542, 1966.
16. Ashton, N. Oxygen and the growth and development of retinal vessels. *Am. J. Ophthalmol. 62*:412–435, 1966.
17. Aughton, D.J. Clinical anophthalmia, dextrocardia, and skeletal anomalies in an infant born to consanguineous parents. *Am. J. Med. Genet. 37*:178–181, 1990.
18. Awan, K.J. Intraocular and extraocular colobomatous cysts in adults. *Ophthalmologica 192*:76–81, 1986.
19. Badtke, G. Von. Uber die Grossenanomalien der Papilla nervi optici, unter besondrer Berucksichtigung der schwarzen Megalopapille. *Klin. Monatsbl. Augenheilkd. 135*:502–510, 1959.
20. Bahn, C.F., Falls, H.F., Varley, G.A., Meyer, R.F., Edelhauser, H.F., and Bourne, W.M. Classification of corneal endothelial disorders based on neural crest origin. *Ophthalmology 91*:558–563, 1984.
21. Baillie, M., Allen, E.D., and Elkington, A.R. The congenital warfarin syndrome: A case report. *Br. J. Ophthalmol. 64*:533–635, 1980.
22. Bartelmez, G.N., and Blount, M.P. The formation of neural crest from primary optic vesicle in man. *Contrib. Embryol. Carnegie Inst. 35*:55–71, 1954.
23. Bartley, G.B. Lacrimal drainage anomalies in mandibulofacial dysostosis. *Am. J. Ophthalmol. 109*:571–574, 1990.
24. Bartley, G.B., and Jackson, I.T. Distichiasis and cleft palate. *Plast. Reconstr. Surg. 84*:129–132, 1989.
25. Baum, J.L., and Feingold, M. Ocular aspects of Goldenhar's syndrome. *Am. J. Ophthalmol. 75*:250–257, 1973.
26. Beckman, D.A., and Brent, R.L. Mechanisms of known environmental teratogens: Drugs and chemicals. *Clin. Perinatol. 13*:649–687, 1986.
27. Behki, R., Noel, L.P., and Clarke, W.N. Limbal lensectomy in the management of ectopia lentis in children. *Arch. Ophthalmol. 108*:809–811, 1990.
28. BenEzra, D., Sela, M., and Pe'er, J. Bilateral anophthalmia and unilateral microphthalmia in two siblings. *Ophthalmologica 198*:140–144, 1989.
29. Benke, P.J. The isotretinoin teratogen syndromes. *JAMA 251*:3267–3269, 1984.
30. Berkenstadt, M., Zahavie, H., and Goodman, R.M. Partial duplication of the eyebrows with other congenital malformations: A new syndrome. *Clin. Genet. 33*:207–210, 1988.
31. Bickmore, W.A., and Hastie, N.D. Aniridia, Wilm's tumor and human chromosome 11. *Ophthalmic Paediatr. Genet. 10*:229–248, 1989.
32. Bickmore, W.A., Porteous, D.J., Christie, S., Seawright, A., Fletcher, J.M., Maule, J.C., Couillin, P., Junien, C., Hastie, N.D., and van-Heyningen, V. CpG islands surround a DNA segment located between translocation breakpoints associated with genitourinary dysplasia and aniridia. *Genomics 5*:685–693, 1989.
33. Binkley, G.W., and Johnson, H.H., Jr. Epithelioma adenoid cysticum: Basal cell nevi and agenesis of the corpus callosum and dental cysts. *Arch. Dermatol. Syphilol. 63*:73–84, 1951.
34. Blake, J., and Mullaney, J. Retinoblastoma in Bloch-Sulzberger syndrome *Ophthalmologica 172*:457–465, 1976.
35. Bodker, F.S., Lavery, M.A., Mitchell, T.N., Lovrien, E.W., and Maumenee, I.H. Microphthalmos in the presumed homozygous offspring of a first cousin marriage and linkage analysis of a locus in a family with autosomal dominant cerulean congenital cataracts. *Am. J. Med. Genet. 37*:54–59, 1990.
36. Boniuk, M., and Hittner, H.M. Congenital retinal disinsertion syndrome. *Trans. Am. Acad. Ophthalmol. Otolaryngol. 79*:827–834, 1975.
37. Boniuk, M., and Zimmerman, L.E. Epibulbar osteoma (episcleral osseous choristoma). *Am. J. Ophthalmol. 53*:290–296, 1962.
38. Boo-Chai, K. The oblique facial cleft: A 20-year-follow-up. *Br. J. Plast. Surg. 43*:355–358, 1990.
39. Bornstein, M.B. Aniridie bilaterale avec polydactylie. Relations des anomalies oculaires du type colobomateux associees a des malformations squelettiques avec les formes atypiques du syndrome de Bardet-Biedl. *J. Genet. Hum. 1*:211–226, 1952.

40. Borzyskowski, M., Harris, R.F., and Jones, R.W.A. The congenital varicella syndrome. *Eur. J. Pediatr.* *137*:335–338, 1981.
41. Botstein, D., White, R.L., Skolnick, M., and Davis, R.W. Construction of a genetic linkage map in man using restriction fragment length polymorphisms. *Am. J. Hum. Genet.* *32*:314–331, 1980.
42. Boyd, P.A., Keeling, J.W., and Lindenbaum, R.H. Fraser syndrome (cryptophthalmos-syndactyly syndrome): A review of eleven cases with postmortem findings. *Am. J. Med. Genet.* *31*:159–168, 1988.
43. Boyntow, J.R., Phesant, T.R., Johnson, B.L., Levin, D.B., and Streeten, B.W. Ocular findings in Kenny's syndrome. *Arch. Ophthalmol.* *97*:896–900, 1979.
44. Brent, R.L. Radiations and other physical agents. In *Handbook of Teratology*, F.C. Fraser and J.G., Wilson (Eds.), Plenum Press, New York, pp. 153–201, 1977.
45. Brockhurst, R.J. Cataract surgery in nanophthalmic eyes. *Arch. Ophthalmol.* *108*:965–967, 1990.
46. Brook, C.G., Sanders, M.D., and Hoare, R.D. Septo-optic dysplasia. *Br. Med. J.* *3*:811–813, 1972.
47. Brown, G.C., Shields, J.A., and Goldberg, R.E. Congenital pits of the optic nerve head. II. Clinical studies in humans. *Ophthalmalogy* *87*:51–65, 1980.
48. Brunquell, P.J., Papale, J.H., Horton, J.C., Williams, R.S., Zgrabik, M.J., Albert, D.M., and Hedley-Whyte, E.T. Sex-linked hereditary bilateral anophthalmos. Pathologic and radiologic correlation. *Arch. Ophthalmol.* *102*:108–113, 1984.
49. Bundy, W.E., Kaufman, P.L., Stainer, G.A., and Prensky, J.C. Unilateral Rieger's anomaly. *Am. J. Ophthalmol.* *90*:725–727, 1980.
50. Burrig, K.F., Gebauer, J., Terinde, R., and Pfitzer, P. Case of cyclopia with an unbalanced karyotype attributable to a balanced 3/7 translocation. *Clin. Genet.* *36*:262–265, 1989.
51. Butler, J.M., Raviola, G., Miller, C.D., and Friedmann, A.I. Fine structural defects in a case of congenital microcoria. *Graefes Arch. Clin. Exp. Ophthalmol.* *227*:88–94, 1989.
52. Cameron, J.D., Yanoff, M., and Frayer, W.C. Turner's syndrome and Coats' disease. *Am. J. Ophthalmol.* *78*:852–854, 974.
52a. Casey, R.J., and Garner, A. Epibulbar choristoma and microphthalmia: A report of two cases. *Br. J. Ophthalmol.* *75*:247–250, 1992.
53. Cennamo, G., Liguori, G., Pezone, A., and Iaccarino, G. Morning glory syndrome associated with marked persistent hyperplastic primary vitreous and lens colobomas. *Br. J. Ophthalmol.* *73*:684–686, 1989.
54. Chan, C.C., Fishman, M., and Egbert, P.R. Multiple ocular anomalies associated with maternal LSD ingestion. *Arch. Ophthalmol.* *96*:282–285, 1978.
55. Charles, N.C., Bennett, T.W., and Margolis, S. Ocular pathology of the congenital varicella syndrome. *Arch. Ophthalmol.* *95*:2034–2037, 1977.
56. Chemke, J., Czernobilsky, B., Mundel, G., and Barishak, Y.R. A familial syndrome of central nervous system and ocular malformations. *Clin. Genet.* *7*:1–7, 1975.
57. Chestler, R.J., and France, T.D. Ocular findings in CHARGE syndrome: Six case reports and a review. *Ophthalmology* *95*:1613–1619.
58. Clark, R.D., Golabi, M., Lacassie, Y., Hall, B., and Seto, S. Expanded phenotype and ethnicity in Setleis syndrome. *Am. J. Med. Genet.* *34*:354–357, 1989.
59. Clarren, S.K., and Smith, D.W. The fetal alcohol syndrome. *N. Engl. J. Med.* *298*:1063–1067, 1978.
60. Cohen, S.M., and Nelson, L.B. Aniridia with congenital ptosis and glaucoma: A family study. *Ann. Ophthalmol.* *20*:53–57, 1988.
61. Collum, L. Uveal colobomata and other anomalies in three generations of one family. *Br. J. Ophthalmol.* *55*:458–461, 1971.
62. Contreras, F., and Pereda, J. Congenital syphilis of the eye with lens involvement. *Arch. Ophthalmol.* *96*:1052–1053, 1978.
63. Conway, B.P., and Welch, R.B. Juvenile retinoschisis. *Am. J. Ophthalmol.* *83*:853–856, 1977.
64. Cook, C.S., and Sulik, K.K. Keratolenticluar dysgenesis (Peters' anomaly) as a result of acute embryonic insult during gastrulation. *J. Pediatr. Ophthalmol. Strabismus* *25*:60–66, 1988.
65. Cook, C.S., and Sulik, K.K. Laminin and fibronectin in retinoid-induced keratolenticular dysgenesis. *Invest. Ophthalmol. Vis. Sci.* *31*:751–757, 1990.
66. Cotlier, E., Reinglass, H., and Rosenthal, I. The eye in partial trisomy 2q syndrome. *Am. J. Ophthalmol.* *84*:251–259, 1977.
67. Cross, H.E., and Yoder, F. Familial nanophthalmos. *Am. J. Ophthalmol.* *81*:300–307, 1976.
68. Courteney-Harris, R.G., and Mills, R.P. Aniridia and deafness: An inherited disorder. *J. Laryngol. Otol.* *104*:419–420, 1990.
69. Cullen, B.A. Ocular defects in thalidomide babies. *Br. J. Ophthalmol.* *48*:151–153, 1964.
70. Cunniff, C., and Jones, K.L. Craniosynostosis and lid anomalies: Report of a girl with Michels syndrome. *Am. J. Med. Genet.* *37*:28–30, 1990.
71. Curtin, V.T., Joyce, E.E., and Ballin, N. Ocular pathology of the oculo-cerebral-renal syndrome of Lowe. *Am. J. Ophthalmol.* *64*:533–543, 1964.
72. Danis, L., DeGandt, D., Dodion, J., and Petit, P. Trisomie 16–18 et malformation congenitale juxta papillaire, étude anatomique. *Bull. Soc. Belge Ophtalmol.* *152*:497–506, 1969.

73. David, T., Chauvaud, D., and Pouliquen, Y. Nanophthalmos with uveal effusion. *Bull. Soc. Ophtalmol. Fr.* 90:263–265, 1990.
74. Dekaban, A.S. Abnormalities in children exposed to x-radiation during various stages of gestation: Tentative timetable of radiation injury to the human fetus, part 1. *J. Nucl. Med.* 9:471–477, 1968.
75. De La Cruz, M., Sun, S., Vangvanichyakorn, K., and Desposito, F. Multiple congenital malformations associated with maternal isotretinoin therapy. *Pediatrics* 74:428–430, 1984.
76. Del Giudice, E., Sartorio, R., Romano, A., Carrozzo, R., and Andria, G. Megalocornea and mental retardation syndrome: Two new cases. *Am. J. Med. Genet.* 26:417–420, 1987.
77. Deluise, V.P., and Anderson, D.R. Review primary infantile glaucoma (congenital glaucoma). *Surv. Ophthalmol.* 28:1–19, 1983.
78. Denis, D., Gabisson, P., and Saracco, J.B. Anterior chamber cleavage syndromes. *Bull. Soc. Ophtalmol. Fr. 90*: 557–560, 1990.
79. Dennehy, P.J., Warman, R., Flyn, J.T., Scott, G.B., and Mastrucci, M.T. Ocular manifestations in pediatric patients with acquired immunodeficiency syndrome. *Arch. Ophthalmol.* 107:978–982, 1989.
80. Deutman, A.F. Vitreoretinal dystrophies. In *Hereditary Retinal and Choroidal Diseases*, Vol. 2, A.E. Krill (Ed.), Harper and Row, New York, pp. 1043–1109, 1977.
81. Diamond, G.R., Katowitz, J.A., Whitaker, L.A., Quinn, G.E., and Schaffer, D.B. Variations in extraocular muscle number and structure in craniofacial dysostosis. *Am. J. Ophthalmol.* 90:416–418, 1980.
82. Diehl, D.L.C., Feldman, F., Tanzer, H., and Shea, M. Nanophthalmos in sisters, one with exfoliation syndrome. *Can. J. Ophthalmol.* 24:327–330, 1989.
83. Donnenfeld, A.E., Graham, J.M., Jr., Packer, R.J., Aquino, R., Berg, S.A., and Emanuel, B.S. Microphthalmia and chorioretinal lesions in a girl with an Xp22.2-pter deletion and partial 3p trisomy. *Am. J. Med. Genet.* 37:182–186, 1990.
84. Drews, R.C. Heterochromia iridum with coloboma of the optic disc. *Arch. Ophthalmol.* 90:437, 1973.
85. Drews, R.C., and Pico, G. Heterchromia associated with coloboma of the iris. *Am. J. Ophthalmol.* 72:827, 1971.
86. Drouilhet, J.H., Arbisser, A.I., and Mazow, M.L. Mesoectodermal dysgenesis: Familial iris anomaly. *J. Pediatr. Ophthalmol.* 14:368–372, 1977.
87. Drummond, G.T., and Keech, R.V. Absent and anomalous superior oblique and superior rectus muscles. *Can. J. Ophthalmol.* 24:275–279, 1989.
88. Dryja, T.P., Cavenee, W., White, R., Rapaport, J.M., Petersen, R., Albert, D.M., and Bruns, G.A.P. Homozygosity of chromosome 13 in retinoblastoma. *N. Engl. J. Med.* 310:550–553, 1984.
89. Dudgeon, J.A. Infective causes of human malformations. *Br. Med. Bull.* 32:77–83, 1976.
90. Duvall, J., Miller, S.L., Cheatle, E., and Tso, M.O. Histopathologic study of ocular changes in a syndrome of multiple congenital anomalies. *Am. J. Ophthalmol.* 103:701–705, 1987.
92. Emarah, M.H.H., Mousa, S.M., and Guthrie, W. Developmental anomalies in the organogenesis of the eyeball: Bilateral diophthalmos. *Trans. Ophthalmol. Soc. UK* 95:101–108, 1977.
93. EUROCAT Working Group. Preliminary evaluation of the impact of the Chernobyl radiological contamination on the frequency of central nervous system malformations in 18 regions of Europe. *Paediatr. Perinatol. Epidemiol.* 2:253–264, 1988.
94. Ewer, M.S. Sur fruhentwicklung des Stroma corneae und der Pupillarmembran beim menschen. *Acta Anat. (Basel)* 75:37–46, 1970.
95. Ewing, C.C., and Ives, E.J. Juvenile hereditary retinoschisis. *Trans. Ophthalmol. Soc. UK* 89:29–39, 1969.
96. Falbe-Hansen, J. A case of Rubinstein-Taybi syndrome. *Acta Ophthalmol. (Copenh.)* 47:33–38, 1969.
97. Falls, H.F. Chromosomal abnormalities in ophthalmology. In *Symposium on Surgical and Medical Management of Congenital Anomalies of the Eye*, Transactions of the New Orleans Academy of Ophthalmology, C. Beard, H.F. Falls, A. Franceschetti, J. François, G. Goodman, A.E. Krill, and H. Scheie (Eds.), C.V. Mosby, St. Louis, pp. 14–33, 1968.
98. Feldman, G.L., Weaver, D.D., and Lovrien, E.W. The fetal trimethadione syndrome. *Am. J. Dis. Child.* 131:1389–1392, 1977.
99. Ferguson, J.G., Hicks, E.L., Jr. Rieger's anomaly and glaucoma associated with partial trisomy 16q: Case report. *Arch. Ophthalmol.* 105:323, 1987.
100. Fernandez-Vigo, J., Castro, J., Diaz, A., and Cid, M.R. Ultrasonic forms of posterior staphyloma. *Ann. Ophthalmol.* 22:391–394, 1990.
101. Ferrel, R.E., Chakrovarte, A., Hittner, H.M., and Riccardi, V.M. Autosomal dominant aniridia: Probably linkage to acid phosphatase-1 locus on chromosome 2. *Proc. Natl. Acad. Sci. USA* 77:1580–1582, 1980.
102. Fischer, G. Abnorme Ciliarkoperanlage in einen Mikrophthalmos. *Graefes Arch. Ophthalmol.* 132:71–81, 1934.
103. Font, R.L., and Zimmerman, L.E. Optic disc coloboma. *Am. J. Ophthalmol.* 72:452–458, 1971.
104. Foos, F.Y., Kiechler, R.J., and Allen, R.A. Congenital nonattachment of the retina. *Am. J. Ophthalmol.* 65:202–211, 1968.
105. Foxman, S., and Cameron, J.D. The clinical implications of bilateral microphthalmos with cyst. *Am. J. Ophthalmol.* 97:632–638, 1984.

106.   François, J. A new syndrome, dyscephalia with birdface and dental anomalies, nanism, hypotrichosis, cutaneous atrophy, microphthalmia and congenital cataract. *Arch. Ophthalmol.* *60*:842–862, 1958.
107.   François, J., Matton-van-Leuven, M.T., and Gombault, P.H. Uveal colobomata and true Klinefelter syndrome. *J. Med. Genet.* *7*:215–223, 1970.
108.   Frenkel, L.D., Keys, M.P., Hefferen, S.J., Rola-Pleszcynski, M., and Bellanti, J.A. Unusual eye abnormalities associated with congenital cytomegalovirus infection. *Pediatrics 66*:763–765, 1980.
109.   Fries, P.D., and Katowitz, J.A. Congenital craniofacial anomalies of ophthalmic importance. *Surv. Ophthalmol.* *35*:87–119, 1990.
110.   Frisen, L., and Holmegaard, L. Spectrum of optic nerve hypoplasia. *Br. J. Ophthalmol.* *62*:7–15, 1978.
111.   Frydman, M., Berkenstadt, M., Raas-Rothschild, A., and Goodman, R.M. Megalocornea, macrocephaly, mental and motor retardation (MMMR). *Clin. Genet.* *38*:149–154, 1990.
112.   Fulton, A.B., Howard, R.O., Albert, D.M., Hsia, Y.E., and Packman, S. Ocular findings in triploidy. *Am. J. Ophthalmol.* *84*:859–867, 1977.
113.   Fulton, A.B., Craft, J.L., Howard, R.O., and Albert, D.M. Retinal dysplasia. *Am. J. Ophthalmol. 85*:690–699, 1978.
114.   Futterweit, W., Ritch, R., Teekhasaenee, C., and Nelson, E.S. Coexistence of Prader-Willi syndrome, congenital ectropion uvea with glaucoma, and factor XI deficiency. *JAMA 255*:3280–3292, 1986.
115.   Ganley, J.P., and Streeten, B.W. Glial nodules. *Am. J. Ophthalmol. 71*:1099–1104, 1971.
116.   Gartner, S. Cyclopia. *Arch. Ophthalmol. 37*:220–231, 1947.
117.   Gattuso, J., Patton, M.A., and Baraitser, M. The clinical spectrum of the Fraser syndrome: Report of three new cases and review. *J. Med. Genet. 24*:549–555, 1987.
118.   Gazali, L.I., Mueller, R.F., Caine, A., Antoniou, A., McCartney, A., Fitchett, M., and Dennis, N.R. Two 46,XX,t(X;Y) females with linear skin defects and congenital microphthalmia: A new syndrome at Xp22.3. *J. Med. Genet. 27*:59–63, 1990.
119.   Gilkes, M.J., and Strode, M. Ocular anomalies in association with developmental limb abnormalities of drug origin. *Lancet 1*:1026–1027, 1963.
120.   Ginsberg, J., Dignan, P., and Soukup, S. Ocular abnormality associated with an extra small chromosome. *Am. J. Ophthalmol. 65*:740–746, 1968.
121.   Ginsberg, J., Perrin, E.V., and Sueoka, W.T. Ocular manifestations in trisomy 18. *Am. J. Ophthalmol. 66*:59–67, 1968.
122.   Ginsberg, J., and Soukup, S. Ocular findings associated with ring B chromosome. *Am. J. Ophthalmol. 78*:624–629, 1974.
123.   Girard, B., Topouzis, F., and Saraux, H. Microphthalmos in Pierre Robin syndrome: Clinical and x-ray computed tomographic study. *Bull. Soc. Ophtalmol. Fr. 89*:1385–1390, 1989.
124.   Glaser, T., Rose, E., Morse, H., Housman, D., and Jones, C. A panel of irradiation- reduced hybrids selectively retaining human chromosome 11p13: Their structure and use to purify the WAGR gene complex. *Genomics 56*:48–64, 1990.
125.   Goldberg, M.F., and McKusick, V.A. X-linked colobomatous microphthalmos and other congenital anomalies, a disorder resembling Lenz's dysmorphogenetic syndrome. *Am. J. Ophthalmol. 71*:1128–1133, 1971.
126.   Goldberg, M.F. Clinical manifestations of ectopia lentis et pupillae in 16 patients. *Trans. Am. Ophthalmol. Soc. 86*:158–175, 1988.
127.   Goldstein, G.E., and Cogan, D.G. Sclerocornea and associated congenital anomalies. *Arch. Ophthalmol. 67*:761–768, 1962.
127a. Gonin, J. Pathogénie et anatomie pathologique des décollementes rétiniens. *Bull. Soc. Ophtalmol. 33*:1–18, 1920.
128.   Gorlin, R.J., and Goltz, R.W. Multiple nevoid basal cell epithelioma, jaw cysts and bifid rib. *N. Engl. J. Med. 262*:908–912, 1960.
129.   Gregg, N.M. Congenital cataract following German measles in the mother. *Trans. Ophthalmol. Soc. UK 3*:35–46, 1941.
130.   Gregor, Z., and Hitchings, R.A. Rieger's anomaly: 42 Year follow up. *Br. J. Ophthalmol. 64*:56–58, 1980.
131.   Green, E.D., and Waterston, R.H. The human genome project: Prospects and implications for clinical medicine. *JAMA 266*:1966–1975, 1991.
132.   Grey, R.H.B., and Rice, N.S.C. Congenital duplication of the lens. *Br. J. Ophthalmol. 60*:673–676, 1976.
133.   Grin, T.R., Mertz, J.S., and Stass-Isern, M. Congenital nasolacrimal duct cysts in dacryocystocele. *Ophthalmology 98*:1238–1242, 1991.
134.   Grossman, J. Congenital syphilis. *Teratology 16*:217–224, 1977.
135.   Gupta, V.P., and Sen, D.K. Unilateral cryptophthalmos. *Ind. J. Ophthalmol. 38*:97–99, 1990.
136.   Guterman, C., Abboud, E., and Mets, M. Microphthalmos with cyst and Edwards' syndrome. *Am. J. Ophthalmol. 109*:229–230, 1990.
137.   Hall, J.G., Pauli, R.M., and Wilson, K.M. Maternal and fetal sequelae of anticoagulation during pregnancy. *Am. J. Med. 68*:122–140, 1980.
138.   Halpert, B., and Patzer, R. Maxillary tumor of retinal anlage. *Surgery 22*:837–841, 1947.

139. Hamburg, A. Incomplete separation of the lens and related malformations. *Am. J. Ophthalmol. 64*:729–733, 1967.
140. Hamming, N.A., Miller, M.T., and Rabb, M. Unusual variant of familial aniridia. *J. Pediatr. Ophthalmol. Strabismus 23*:195–200, 1986.
141. Hansen, L.A., and Pearl, G.S. Isotretinoin teratogenicity. *Acta Neuropathol. (Berl.) 65*:335–337, 1985.
142. Hanson, J.W., Myrianthopoulos, N.C., Harvey, M.A.S., and Smith, D.W. Risks to the offspring of women treated with hydantoin anticonvulsants with emphasis on the fetal hydantoin syndrome. *J. Pediatr. 89*:662–668, 1976.
143. Harbin, R.L., Katz, J.I., Frias, J.L., Robinowicz, I.M., and Kaufman, H.E. Sclerocornea and Smith-Lemli-Optiz syndrome. *Am. J. Ophthalmol. 84*:72–75, 1977.
144. Harden, A., and Mooney, D. Congenital keratolenticular adhesion. *Am. J. Ophthalmol. 70*:975–977, 1970.
145. Harnden, D., and Klinger, H.P. (Eds.). *Chromosomal Nomenclature: International System for Human Cytogenic Nomenclature*, S. Karger, New York, 1985.
146. Hashmi, M.X., and Karseras, A.G. Uveal colobomata and Klinefelter syndrome. *Br. J. Ophthalmol. 60*:661–664, 1976.
147. Hay, E.D. Development of the vertebrate cornea. *Int. Rev. Cytol. 63*:263–322, 1980.
148. Hermsen, V.M., Conahan, J.B., Koops, B.L., and Cunningham, R.D. Persistent hyperplastic primary vitreous associated with protein C deficiency. *Am. J. Ophthalmol. 109*:608–609, 1990.
149. Heyer, R., Ehrich, J., Goebel, H.H., Christen, H.J., and Hanefeld, F. Congenital muscular dystrophy with cerebral and ocular malformations (cerebro-oculo-muscular syndrome). *Brain Dev. 8*:614–619, 1986.
150. Hittner, H., Desmond, M.M., and Montgomery, F.R. Optic nerve manifestations of human congenital cytomegalovirus infection. *Am. J. Ophthalmol. 83*:661–666, 1976.
151. Hittner, H.M., Hirsch, N.J., Kreh, G.M., and Rudolph, A.J. Colobomatous microphthalmos, heart disease, hearing loss and mental retardation: A syndrome. *J. Pediatr. Ophthalmol. Strabismus 16*:122–128, 1979.
152. Hoepner, J., and Yanoff, M. Ocular findings in trisomy 13–15. *Am. J. Ophthalmol. 74*:729–738, 1972.
153. Hollsten, D.A., and Katowitz, J.A. The ophthalmic manifestations and treatment of the amniotic band syndrome. *Ophthalmic Plast. Reconstr. Surg. 6*:1–15, 1990.
154. Hopkins, D.J., and Horan, E.C. Hallerman-Streiff syndrome. *Br. J. Ophthalmol. 54*:416–422, 1970.
155. Hovland, K.R., Schepens, C.L., and McKenzie-Freeman, H.M. Developmental giant retinal tears associated with lens coloboma. *Arch. Ophthalmol. 80*:325–331, 1968.
156. Howard, R.O. Ocular abnormalities in the "cri du chat" syndrome. *Am. J. Ophthalmol. 73*:949–954, 1972.
157. Howard, R.O., and Abrahams, I.W. Sclerocornea. *Am. J. Ophthalmol. 71*:1254–1260, 1971.
158. Howard, R.O., Boue, J., Deluchat, C., Albert, D.M., and Lahav, M. The eyes of embryos with chromosome abnormalities. *Am. J. Ophthalmol. 78*:167–188, 1974.
159. Hoyt, C.S., and Billson, F.S. Maternal anticonvulsants and optic nerve hypoplasia. *Br. J. Ophthalmol. 62*:3–6, 1978.
160. Hoyt, C.S., Billson, F., Ouvrier, R., and Wise, G. Ocular features of Aicardi's syndrome. *Arch. Ophthalmol. 96*:291–295, 1978.
161. Hsia, Y.E., Bratu, M., and Herbordt, A. Genetics of the Meckel syndrome (dysencephalia splanchnocystica). *Pediatrics 42*:237–247, 1971.
162. Hsing, S., Wilson-Holt, N., Kriss, A., Fleuler, U., and Taylor, D. Complete cryptophthalmos: Case report with normal flash-VEP and ERG. *J. Pediatr. Ophthalmol. Strabismus 27*:133–135, 1990.
163. Hunter, A.G.W., Rothman, S.J., Hwang, W.S., and Deckelbaum, R.J. Hepatic fibrosis, polycystic kidney, colobomata and encephalopathy in siblings. *Clin. Genet. 6*:82–89, 1974.
164. Ingham, P.N., McGovern, S.T., and Crompton, J.L. Congenital absence of the inferior rectus muscle. *Aust. NZ J. Ophthalmol. 14*:355–358, 1986.
164a. Isenberg, S.I. *The Eye in Infancy*, Yearbook Medical Publishers, Chicago, 1989.
165. Jacklin, H.N. Falciform fold, retinal detachment and Norrie's disease. *Am. J. Ophthalmol. 90*:76–80, 1980.
166. Jackson, I.T., Shaw, K.E., and del Pinal Matorras, F. A new feature of the ablepharon macrostomia syndrome: Zygomatic arch absence. *Br. J. Plast. Surg. 41*:410–416, 1988.
167. Jaffe, N.S., and Clayman, H.M. Cataract extraction in eyes with congenital colobomata. *J. Cataract Refract. Surg. 13*:54–58, 1987.
168. James, P.M., Karseras, A.G., and Wybar, K.C. Systemic association of uveal coloboma. *Br. J. Ophthalmol. 58*:917–921, 1974.
169. Jay, M. *The Eye in Chromosome Duplication and Deficiencies*, Ophthalmic Series 2, Marcel Dekker, New York, pp. 1–249, 1977.
170. Jay, W.M., Pope, J., and Riffle, J.E. Juxtapapillary subretinal neovascularization associated with congenital pit of the optic nerve. *Am. J. Ophthalmol. 97*:655–657, 1984.
171. Jaureguy, B.M., and Hall, J.G. Isolated congenital ectopia lentis with autosomal dominant inheritance. *Clin. Genet. 15*:97–109, 1979.
172. Jensen, P.E., and Kalina, R.E. Congenital anomalies of the optic disc. *Am. J. Ophthalmol. 82*:27–31, 1976.
173. Jin, J.C., and Anderson, D.R. Laser unsutured sclerotomy in nanophthlalmos. *Am. J. Ophthalmol. 109*:575–580, 1990.

174. Johns, K.J., and O'Day, D.M. Posterior chamber intraocular lenses after extracapsular cataract extraction in patients with aniridia. *Ophthalmology 98*:1698–1702, 1991.
175. Johnston, M.C., Bhakdinaronk, A., and Reid, Y.C. An expanded role of the neural crest in oral and pharyngeal development. In *Fourth Symposium on Oral Sensation and Perception*, J.F. Bosma (Ed.), U.S. Govt. Printing Office, Washington, D.C., pp. 37–52, 1973.
176. Johnston, M.C., Noden, D.M., Hazelton, R.D., Coulombre, J.L., and Coulombre, A.J. Origins of avian ocular and periocular tissues. *Exp. Eye Res. 29*:27–43, 1979.
177. Jonas, J.B. Pits of the optic papilla in large optic nerve papillae. Papillometric characteristics in 15 eyes. *Klin. Monatsbl. Augenheilkd. 191*:287–291, 1987.
178. Jonas, J.B., Koniszewski, G., and Naumann, G.O. "Morning glory syndrome" and "Handmann's anomaly" in congenital macropapilla. Extreme variants of "confluent optic pits"? *Klin. Monatsbl. Augenheilkd. 195*:371–374, 1989.
179. Jotterand, V., Boisjoly, H.M., Harnois, C., Bigonesse, P., Laframboise, R., Gagne, R., and St. Pierre, A. 11p13 deletion, Wilms' tumor, and aniridia: Unusual genetic, non-ocular and ocular features of three cases. *Br. J. Ophthalmol. 74*:568–570, 1990.
180. Journel, H., Urvoy, M., Baudet, D., Roussey, M., Varennes, B., and Le Marec, B. Manifestations oculaires de la trisomie 21. Etude de cinguante-trois cas et revue de la litérature. *Ann. Pediatr. (Paris) 33*:387–392, 1986.
181. Kalina, R.E. A histopathologic postmortem and clinical study of peripheral retinal folds in infant eyes. *Am. J. Ophthalmol. 71*:446–448, 1971.
182. Kanai, A., Wood, T.C., Polack, F.M., Kaufman, H.E. The fine structure of sclerocornea. *Invest. Ophthalmol. Vis. Sci. 10*:687–694, 1971.
183. Keppen, L.D., Brodsky, M.C., Michael, J.M., and Poindexter, A.R. Hypogonadotropic hypogonadism in mentally retarded adults with microphthalmia and clinical anophthalmia. *Am. J. Med. Genet. 36*:285–287, 1990.
184. Kida, M. *Thalidomide Embryopathy in Japan*, Kodansha, Tokyo, pp. 143–153, 1987.
185. Kim, R.Y., Hoyt, W.F., Lessell, S., and Narahara, M.H. Superior segmental optic hypoplasia. *Arch. Ophthalmol. 107*:1312–1315, 1989.
186. Kindler, P. Morning glory syndrome. *Am. J. Ophthalmol. 69*:376–384, 1970.
187. Kinsey, J.A., and Streeten, B.W. Ocular abnormalities in the median cleft face syndrome. *Am. J. Ophthalmol. 83*:261–266, 1977.
188. Kirchhof, B., Arnold, G., and Kirchhof, E. Zur Genese der Grubenpapille: Mikroscopische Untersung bei einem Neugeborenen. *Klin. Monatsbl. Augenheilkd. 188*:310–312, 1986.
189. Kirkham, T.H., Milot, J., and Berman, P. Ophthalmic manifestations of Aarskog syndrome. *Am. J. Ophthalmol. 79*:441–445, 1975.
190. Kivlin, J., Fineman, R.M., Crandall, A.S., and Olsen, R.J. Peters' anomaly as a consequence of genetic and nongenetic syndromes. *Arch. Ophthalmol. 104*:61–64, 1986.
191. Knudson, A.G., Jr., and Strong, L.C. Mutation and cancer: a model for Wilm's tumor of the kidney. *J. Natl. Cancer Inst. 48*:313–324, 1972.
192. Koole, F.D., Velzeboer, C.M., and van der Harten, J.J. Ocular abnormalities in Patau syndrome (chromosome 13 trisomy syndrome). *Ophthalmic Paediatr. Genet. 11*:15–21, 1990.
193. Kozma, C., Hunt, M., Meck, J., Traboulsi, E., and Scribanu, N. Familial Wolf-Hirschhorn syndrome associated with Rieger anomaly of the eye. *Ophthalmic Paediatr. Genet. 11*:23–30, 1990.
194. Krachmer, H.J., and Rodrigues, M.M. Posterior keratoconus. *Arch. Ophthalmol. 95*:1867–1873, 1978.
195. Krill, A.E. The retinal disease of rubella. *Arch. Ophthalmol. 77*:445–449, 1967.
196. Kuchle, M., Krauw, J., Rummelt, C., and Naumann, G.O. Synophthalmia and holoprosencephaly in chromosome in 18p deletion defect. *Arch. Ophthalmol. 109*:136–137, 1991.
197. Kupfer, C., and Kaiser-Kupfer, M.I. Observations on the development of the anterior chamber angle with reference to the pathogenesis of congenital glaucomas. *Am. J. Ophthalmol. 88*:424–426, 1979.
198. Lahav, M., Albert, P.M., and Wyand, S. Clinical and histopathologic classification of retinal dysplasia. *Am. J. Ophthalmol. 75*:648–667, 1973.
199. Lambert, S.R., Hoyt, C.S., and Narahara, M.H. Optic nerve hypoplasia. *Surv. Ophthalmol. 32*:1–9, 1987.
200. Lambert, S.R., Amaya, L., and Taylor, D. Congenital idiopathic microcoria. *Am. J. Ophthalmol. 106*:590–594, 1988.
201. Lambert, S.R., Taylor, D., Kriss, A., Holzel, H., and Heard, S. Ocular manifestations of the congenital varicella syndrome. *Arch. Ophthalmol. 107*:52–56, 1989.
202. Lammer, E.J., Chen, D.T., Hoar, R.M., Agnish, N.D., Benke, P.J., Braun, J.T., Curry, C.J., Fernhoff, P.M., Grix, A.W., Lott, I.T., Richard, J.M., and Sun, S.C. Retinoic acid embryopathy. *N. Engl. J. Med. 313*:837–841, 1985.
203. Lang, G.E., and Fleischer-Peters, A. Rieger syndrome as an expression of neural crest dysgenesis. *Fortschr. Ophthalmol. 86*:366–369, 1989.
204. Lavedan, C., Barichard, F., Azoulay, M., Couillin, P., Gomez, D.M., Nicholas, H., Quack, B., Rethore, M.O., Noel, B., and Junien, C. Molecular definition of de novo and genetically transmitted WAGR-associated rearrangements of 11p13. *Cytogenet. Cell Genet. 50*:70–74, 1989.

205. Lawin-Brussel, C., and Busse, H. Iridocorneotrabecular dysgenesis in a patient sample of the Munster University Eye Clinic. *Fortschr. Ophthalmol. 85*:101–104, 1988.
206. Lee, C.F., Yue, B.Y., Robin, J., Sawaguchi, S., and Sugar, J. Immunohistochemical studies of Peters' anomaly. *Ophthalmology 96*:958–964, 1989.
207. Lee, W.R., and Grierson, I. Posterior vitreo-retinal malformation: A clinic-pathological case report. *Ophthalmologica 171*:282–290, 1977.
207a. Lemoine, P., Harousseau, H., Borteyru, J.P., Menuet, J.C. Les enfants de parents alcooliques. Anomalies observees. A propos de 127 cas. *Ouest-Medical 21*:476–482, 1968.
208. Lenz, W. Thalidomide and congenital abnormalities. *Lancet 45*:2371–2372, 1962.
209. Levy, N.S., Krill, A.E., and Beutler, E. Galactokinase deficiency and cataracts. *Am. J. Ophthalmol. 74*:41–48, 1972.
210. Lieb, W., Rochels, R., and Gronemeyer, U. Microphthalmos with colobomatous orbital cyst: Clinical, histological, immunohistological, and electronmicroscopic findings. *Br. J. Ophthalmol. 75*:59–62, 1990.
211. Lin, A.E., Biglan, A.W., and Garver, K.L. Persistent hyperplastic primary vitreous with vertical transmission. *Ophthalmic Paediatr. Genet. 11*:121–122, 1990.
212. Lisch, W., and Rochels, R. Pathogenesis of congenital vitreous cysts. *Klin. Monatsbl. Augenheilkd. 195*:375–378, 1989.
213. Loh, R.C.K., and Tan, D.S.L. Unusual case of progeria-like dwarfism with bilateral macular coloboma. *Am. J. Ophthalmol. 70*:968–974, 1970.
214. Lonn, L. Neonatal cytomegalic inclusion disease chorioretinitis. *Arch. Ophthalmol. 88*:434–438, 1972.
215. Luleci, G., Bagci, G., Kivran, M., Luleci, E., Bektas, S., and Basaran, S. A hereditary bisatellite-dicentric supernumerary chromosome in a case of cat-eye syndrome. *Hereditas 111*:7–10, 1989.
216. MacRae, D.W., Howard, R.O., Albert, D.M., and Hsia, Y.E. Ocular manifestations of the Meckel syndrome. *Arch. Ophthalmol. 88*:106–133, 1972.
217. Margo, C.E. Congenital aniridia: A histopathologic study of the anterior segment in children. *J. Pediatr. Ophthalmol. Strabismus 20*:192–198, 1983.
218. Mann, I. *Developmental Abnormalities of the Human Eye*, Cambridge University Press, London, 1957.
219. Mannens, M., Bleeker-Wagemakers, E.M., Bliek, J., Hoovers, J., Mandies, I., van Tol, S., Frants, R.R., Heyting, C., Westerveld, A., and Slater, R.M. Autosomal dominant aniridia linked to the chromosome 11p13 markers catalase and D11S151 in a large Dutch family. *Cytogenet. Cell Genet. 52*:32–36, 1989.
220. Manschot, W.A. Persistent hyperplastic primary vitreous. *Arch. Ophthalmol. 59*:188–203, 1958.
221. Manschot, W.A. Primary congenital aphakia. *Arch. Ophthalmol. 69*:571–577, 1963.
222. Manschot, W.A. Eye findings in hydranencephaly. *Ophthalmologica 162*:151–159, 1971.
223. Manschot, W.A. Pathology of hereditary juvenile retinoschisis. *Arch. Ophthalmol. 88*:131–138, 1972.
224. Manschot, W.A. Morning glory syndrome: A histopathological study. *Br. J. Ophthalmol. 74*:560–580, 1990.
225. Mansour, A.M., Barber, J.C., Reinecke, R.D., and Wang, F.M. Ocular choristomas. *Surv. Ophthalmol. 33*:339–358, 1989.
226. Marcus, D.M., Shore, J.W., and Albert, D.M. Anophthalmia in the focal dermal hypoplasia syndrome. *Arch. Ophthalmol. 108*:96–100, 1990.
227. Margolis, S., Scher, B.M., and Char, R.E. Macular colobomas in Leber's congenital amaurosis. *Am. J. Ophthalmol. 83*:27–31, 1977.
228. Margolis, S., Siegel, I.M., Choy, A., and Bleinin, G.M. Oculocutaneous albinism associated with Apert's syndrome. *Am. J. Ophthalmol. 88*:27–31, 1977.
229. Margo, C.E. Congenital aniridia: A histopathological study of the anterior segment in children. *J. Pediatr. Ophthalmol. Strabismus 20*:192–198, 1983.
230. Martin, X.D., and Rabineau, P.A. Dysgenesis of the neural crest, ectoderm, mesoderm and fetal alcohol syndrome. *Klin. Monatsbl. Augenheilkd. 196*:279–284, 1990.
231. Martinez-Mora, J., Audi, L., Toran, N., Isnard, R., Castellvi, A., Iribarne, M.P., and Ecozcue, J. Ambiguous genitalia, gonadoblastoma, aniridia, and mental retardation with deletion of chromosome 11. *J. Urol. 142*:1298–1300, 1989.
232. Martorina, M. Familial nanophthalmos. *J. Fr. Ophthalmol. 11*:357–361, 1988.
232a. McKusick, V.A. *Mendelian Inheritance in Man: Catalogues of Autosomal Dominant, Autosomal Recessive, and X-linked Phenotypes*, 9th ed., Johns Hopkins University Press, Baltimore, 1990.
233. McLane, N.J., and Carroll, D.M. Ocular manifestations of drug abuse. *Surv. Ophthalmol. 30*:298–313, 1986.
234. Menser, M.A., Dods, L., and Harley, J.D. A twenty-five-year follow-up of congenital rubella. *Lancet 2*:1347–1350, 1967.
235. Mets, M.B. The eye and the chromosome. In *Goldberg's Genetic and Metabolic Eye Disease*, 2nd ed., W.A. Renie (Ed.), Little, Brown, Boston, pp. 81–99, 1986.
236. Miller, N.R. Optic nerve glioma and cerebellar astrocytoma in a patient with von Recklinghausen's neurofibromatosis. *Am. J. Ophthalmol. 79*:582–588, 1975.
237. Miller, R.W., Fraumeni, J.F., and Manning, M.D. Association of Wilm's tumor with aniridia, hemihypertrophy and other congenital malformations. *N. Engl. J. Med. 270*:922–927, 1964.

238. Miller, M.T., Deutsch, T.A., Cronin, C., and Keys, C.L. Amniotic bands as a cause of ocular anomalies. *Am. J. Ophthalmol. 104*:270–279, 1987.

239. Miller, M.T., and Stromland, K. Ocular motility in thalidomide embryopathy. *J. Pediatr. Ophthalmol. Strabismus 28*:47–54, 1991.

240. Mizuno, K., Takei, Y., Sears, M.L., Peterson, W.C., Char, R.E., and Jampal, C.M. Leber's congenital amaurosis. *Am. J. Ophthalmol. 83*:32–42, 1977.

241. Montenegro, M., and Bonnet, M. Optic nerve pits: Clinical and therapeutic review of 21 cases. *J. Fr. Ophtalmol. 12*:411–419, 1989.

242. Morgan, G., and Mushin, A. Ectopic intraocular lacrimal gland tissue. *Br. J. Ophthalmol. 56*:690–694, 1972.

243. Patterson, A., and Campbell, S. Kleeblatschadel syndrome. *Eye 3*:861–865, 1989.

244. Mosier, M.A., Lieberman, M.F., Green, W.R., and Knox, D.L. Hypoplasia of the optic nerve. *Arch. Ophthalmol. 96*:1437–1443, 1978.

245. Mullaney, J. Edwards' syndrome. *Am. J. Ophthalmol. 76*:246–254, 1972.

246. Mullaney, J., and Fitzpatrick, C. Idiopathic cyst of the iris stroma. *Am. J. Ophthalmol. 76*:64–68, 1973.

247. Mullaney, J. Complicated sporadic colobomata. *Br. J. Ophthalmol. 62*:384–385, 1978.

248. Mullaney, J. Curious colobomata. *Trans. Ophthalmol. Soc. UK 517*–522, 1978.

249. Neel, J.A. Update on the genetic effects of ionizing radiation. *JAMA 266*:698–701, 1991.

250. Nefzger, M.D., Miller, R.J., and Fujino, T. Eye findings in atomic bomb survivors of Hiroshima and Nagasaki: 1963–1964. *Am. J. Epidemiol. 89*:129–138, 1968.

251. Nelson, L.B. Diagnosis and management of congenital and developmental cataracts. *Semin. Ophthalmol. 5*: 154–165, 1990.

252. Nelson, L.B., and Maumenee, I.H. Ectopia lentis. *Surv. Ophthalmol. 27*:143–160, 1982.

253. Nelson, L.B., Spaeth, G.L., Nowinski, T.S., Margo, C.E., and Jackson, L. Aniridia: A review. *Surv. Ophthalmol. 28*:621–642, 1984.

254. Ngo, J.T., Bateman, J.B., Cortesis, V., Sparkes, R.S., Mohanda, T., Inana, G., and Spence, M.A. Norrie disease: Linkage analysis using a 4.2-kb RFLP detected by a human ornithine aminotransferase cDNA probe. *Genomics 4*:539–545, 1989.

255. Nicholson, D.A., and Goldberg, M.F. Ocular abnormalities in de Lange syndrome. *Arch. Ophthalmol. 76*:214–220, 1966.

256. Nucci, P., Mets, M.B., and Gabianelli, E.B. Trisomy 4q with morning glory disc anomaly. *Ophthalmic Paediatr. Genet. 11*:143–145, 1990.

257. O'Grady, R.B., Rothstein, T.B., and Romano, P.G. D-group deletion syndromes and retinoblastoma. *Am. J. Ophthalmol. 77*:40–45, 1974.

258. Ohrloff, C., Olson, R., and Apple, D. Angeborene Hornhauttrubung durch Verdickung der Bowmanschen Membran. *Klin. Monatsbl. Augenheilk. 191*:352–354, 1987.

259. Oliver, M.D., Dotan, S.A., Chemke, J., and Abraham, F.A. Isolated foveal hypoplasia. *Br. J. Ophthalmol. 71*:926–930, 1987.

260. Otake, M., and Schull, W.J. In utero exposure to A-bomb radiation and mental retardation: A reassessment. *Br. J. Radiol. 57*:409–411, 1984.

261. Pagon, R.A. Ocular coloboma. *Surv. Ophthalmol. 21*:223–236, 1981.

262. Pau, H. Die Strukturen des Glaskorpers in Bexiehung zu embryonalen Blutgeffasen und Glaskorperrindzellen. *Graefes Arch. Ophthalmol. 177*:261–270, 1969.

263. Phillips, C.I., and Gosden, C.M. Leber's hereditary optic neuropathy and Kearns-Sayre syndrome: Mitochondrial DNA mutations. *Surv. Ophthalmol. 35*:463–472, 1991.

264. Pedersen, O.O., Rushood, A., and Olsen, E.G. Anterior mesenchymal dysgenesis of the eye. *Acta Ophthalmol. (Copenh.) 67*:470–476, 1989.

265. Pe'er, J., BenEzra, D., Sela, M., and Hemo, I. Cryptophthalmos syndrome: Clinical and histopathological findings. *Ophthalmic Paediatr. Genet. 8*:177–182, 1987.

266. Percy, D.H., and Danylchuk, K.D. Retinal dysplasia and cytosine arabinoside. *Invest. Ophthalmol. Vis. Sci. 16*:353–364, 1977.

267. Petersen, R.A. Schmid-Fraccaro syndrome ("cat's eye" syndrome). *Arch. Ophthalmol. 90*:287–292, 1973.

268. Petersen, R.A., and Walton, D.S. Optic nerve hypoplasia with good visual acuity and visual field defects. *Arch. Ophthalmol. 95*:254–258, 1977.

269. Phillips, C.I., and Griffiths, D.L. Macular coloboma and skeletal abnormality. *Br. J. Ophthalmol. 53*:346–349, 1969.

270. Polak, B.C.P., and Hogewind, B.L. Alport's disease. *Am. J. Ophthalmol. 84*:532–536, 1977.

271. Poswillo, D. The pathogenesis of the Treacher-Collins syndrome (mandibulofacial dysostosis). *Br. J. Oral Surg. 13*:1–26, 1975.

272. Poswillo, D. Mechanisms and pathogenesis of malformations. *Br. Med. Bull. 32*:59–64, 1976.

273. Poswillo, D. Pathogenesis of craniofacial syndromes exhibiting colobomata. *Trans. Ophthalmol. Soc. UK 96*:69–72, 1976.

274. Raizman, M.B. Ocular abnormalities accompanying chromosome 13 defects (letter). *Arch. Ophthalmol.* *105*:744, 1987.
275. Ramsing, M., Rehder, H., Holzgreve, W., Meinecke, P., and Lenz, W. Fraser syndrome (cryptophthalmos with syndactyly) in the fetus and newborn. *Clin. Genet.* *37*:84–96, 1990.
276. Rating, D., Nau, H., Jäger-Roman, E., Göpfert, I., Koch, S., Mannagetta, G., Schmidt, D., and Helge, H. Teratogenic and pharmacokinetic studies of primidone during pregnancy and in the offspring of epileptic women. *Acta Paediatr. Scand.* *71*:301–311, 1982.
277. Raymond, W.R., Kearney, J.J., and Parmley, V.C. Ocular findings in arteriohepatic dysplasia (Alagille's syndrome). *Arch. Ophthalmol.* *107*:1077, 1989.
278. Reese, A.B., and Ellsworth, R.M. The anterior chamber cleavage syndrome. *Arch. Ophthalmol.* *75*:307–318, 1966.
279. Remington, J.S. Toxoplasmosis and congenital infection. *Birth Defects* *4*:47–56, 1968.
280. Resnick, J.I., and Kawamoto, H.K., Jr. Rare craniofacial clefts: Tessier no. 4 clefts. *Plast. Reconstr. Surg.* *85*:843–849, 1990.
281. Rethore, M.O., Dutrillaux, B., and Giovannelli, G. La trisomie 4p. *Ann. Genet.* *17*:125–128, 1974.
282. Riely, C.A., Cotlier, E., Jensen, P.S., and Klatskin, G. Arteriohepatic dysplasia: A benign syndrome of intrahepatic cholestasis with multiple organ involvement. *Ann Intern. Med.* *91*:520–527, 1979.
283. Robb, R.M., and Marchevsky, A. Pathology of the lens in Down's syndrome. *Arch. Ophthalmol.* *96*:1039–1043, 1978.
284. Robb, R.M., Silver, J., and Sullivan, R.T. Ocular retardation (or) in the mouse. *Invest. Ophthalmol. Vis. Sci.* *17*:468–473, 1978.
285. Robinson, G.C., Conry, J.L., and Conry, R.F. Clinical profile and prevalence of fetal alcohol syndrome in an isolated community in British Columbia. *Can. Med. Assoc. J.* *137*:203–207, 1987.
286. Rodrigues, M.M., Calhoun, J., and Weinreb, S. Sclerocornea with an unbalanced translocation (17p, 10q). *Am. J. Ophthalmol.* *78*:49–53, 1974.
287. Rodrigues, M.M., Punnett, H.H., Valdes-Dapena, M., and Martyn, L.J. Retinal pigment of epithelium in a case of trisomy 18. *Am. J. Ophthalmol.* *76*:265–268, 1973.
288. Romania, A., Zakov, Z.N., McGannon, E., Schroeder, T., Heyen, F., and Jagelman, D.G. Congenital hypertrophy of the retinal pigment epithelium in familial adenomatous polyposis. *Ophthalmology* *96*:879–884, 1989.
288a. Rotberg, M., Klintworth, G.K., and Crawford, J.B. Ocular dilation and angiogenesis in Potter's syndrome. *Am. J. Ophthalmol.* *97*:16–31, 1984.
289. Rouland, J.F., Hochart, G., and Constaninides, G. Chorioretinal coloboma and neovascular membrane. *Bull. Soc. Ophtalmol. Fr.* *90*:654–655, 1990.
290. Royce, P.M., Steinmann, B., Vogel, A., Steinhorst, U., and Kohlschuetter, A. Brittle cornea syndrome: An heritable connective tissue disorder distinct from Ehlers-Danlos syndrome type VI and fragilitas oculi, with spontaneous perforations of the eye, blue sclerae, red hair, and normal collagen lysyl hydroxylation. *Eur. J. Pediatr.* *179*:465–469, 1990.
291. Ruprecht, K.W., and Wulle, K.G. Licht und elektronenmikrospkopische Untersuchungen zur Entwicklung des menschlichen Musculus sphincter pupillae. *Graefes Arch. Ophthalmol.* *186*:117–130, 1973.
292. Russel-Eggit, I.M., Blake, K.D., Taylor, D.S., and Wyse, R.K. The eye in the CHARGE association. *Br. J. Ophthalmol.* *75*:421–426, 1990.
293. Salmon, J.F., Wallis, C.E., and Murray, A.D. Variable expressivity of autosomal dominant microcornea with cataract. *Arch. Ophthalmol.* *106*:505–510, 1988.
294. Samples, J.R., and Meyer, S.M. Use of ophthalmic medications in pregnant and nursing women. *Am. J. Ophthalmol.* *106*:616–623, 1988.
295. Sanyal, S., and Hawkins, R.K. Dysgenetic lens (dyl.) *Invest. Ophthalmol. Vis. Sci.* *18*:642–645, 1979.
296. Sassani, J.W., and Yanoff, M. Anophthalmos in an infant with multiple congenital anomalies. *Am. J. Ophthalmol.* *83*:43–51, 1977.
297. Saraux, J. Ocular manifestations of disease due to aberrations of non-sexual chromosomes. *J. Med. Genet.* *25*:227, 1970.
298. Satorre, J., Lopez, J.M., Martinez, J., and Pinera, P. Dominant macular colobomata. *J. Pediatr. Ophthalmol. Strabismus* *27*:148–152, 1990.
299. Savage, M.O., Moosa, A., and Gordon, R.R. Maternal varicella infection as a cause of fetal malformations. *Lancet* *1*:352–354, 1973.
300. Savell, J., and Cook, R., Jr. Optic nerve colobomas of autosomal dominant heredity. *Arch. Ophthalmol.* *94*:395–400, 1975.
301. Schanzlin, D.J., Goldberg, D.B., and Brown, S.I. Hallerman-Streiff syndrome associated with sclerocornea, aniridia and a chromosomal abnormality. *Am. J. Ophthalmol.* *90*:411–415, 1980.
302. Schinzel, A., and Dapuzzo, V. Anophthalmia in a retarded with partial trisomy 4p and 22 following a maternal translocation, rcp(4;22) (p15.2;911.2). *Ophthalmic Paediatr. Genet.* *11*:139–142, 1990.
303. Shepard, T.H. *Catalog of Teratogenic Agents*, 6th ed., Johns Hopkins University Press, Baltimore, 1989.
304. Shields, M.B. Axenfeld-Rieger syndrome: A theory of mechanism and distinctions from the iridocorneal endothelial syndrome. *Trans. Am. Ophthalmol. Soc.* *81*:736–784, 1983.

305. Shields, M.B. A common pathway for developmental glaucomas. *Trans. Am. Ophthalmol. Soc.* 85:222–237, 1987.
306. Shields, M.B., Buckley, E., Klintworth, G.K., and Thresher, R. Axenfeld-Rieger syndrome: A spectrum of developmental disorders. *Surv. Ophthalmol.* 29:387–409, 1985.
307. Shiota, K. Neural tube defects and maternal hyperthermia in early pregnancy: Epidemiology in a human embryo population. *Am. J. Med. Genet.* 12:281–288, 1982.
308. Shirai, S., Ohshika, S., Yuguchi, S., and Majima, A. Ochratoxin A. III. Developmental abnormalities of the anterior segment of the eye induced in mice by ochratoxin A. *Acta Soc. Ophthalmol. Jpn.* 89:753–760, 1985.
309. Sidransky, E., Feinstein, A., and Goodman, R.M. Ichthyosis-cheek-eyebrow (ICE) syndrome: A new autosomal dominant disorder. *Clin. Genet.* 31:137–142, 1987.
310. Silver, J., and Hughes, A. The role of cell death during morphogenesis of the mammalian eye. *J. Morphol.* 140:159–170, 1973.
311. Silver, J., and Hughes, A.F.W. The relationship between morphogenetic cell death and the development of congenital anophthalmia. *J. Comp. Neurol.* 157:281–301, 1974.
312. Silverstein, A.M. Dysplasia and rosettes. *Am. J. Ophthalmol.* 77:51–59, 1974.
313. Simpson, W.A., and Parsons, M.A. The ultrastructural pathological features on congenital microcoria: A case report. *Arch. Ophthalmol.* 107:99–102, 1989.
314. Singh, D., Daniel, R., Verma, M., Akhter, Z., and Beri, R.S. Split hand/split foot syndrome with atresia of nasolacrimal ducts and buphthalmos. *Indian Ped.* 26:1053–1055, 1989.
315. Singh, S., and Sanyal, A.K. Eye anomalies induced by cyclophosphamide in rat fetuses. *Acta Anat. (Basel)* 94:490–500, 1976.
316. Skarf, B., and Hoyt, C.S. Optic nerve hypoplasia in children: Association with anomalies of the endocrine and CNS. *Arch. Ophthalmol.* 102:62–67, 1984.
317. Sloderbeck, J.D., Maumenee, I.H., Elsas, F.E., Kenyon, K.R., Rivas, M.L., Hsu, S.H., Yoder, F.E., and Colleally, P.M. Linkage assignment of aniridia to chromosome 1. *Am. J. Hum. Genet.* 27:83A, 1975.
318. Slusher, M.M., Weaver, R.G., Jr., Greven, C.M., Mundorf, T.K., and Cashwell, L.F. The spectrum of cavitary optic disc anomalies in a family. *Ophthalmology* 96:342–347, 1989.
319. Smithells, R.W. Environmental teratogens of man. *Br. Med. Bull.* 32:27–33, 1976.
320. Sobol, W.M., Bratton, A.R., Rivers, M.B., and Weingeist, T.A. Morning glory disk syndrome associated with subretinal neovascular membrane formation. *Am. J. Ophthalmol.* 110:93–95, 1990.
321. Soong, H.K., and Raizman, M.B. Corneal changes in familial iris coloboma. *Ophthalmology* 93:335–339, 1986.
322. Sorsby, A. Congenital coloboma of the macula. *Br. J. Ophthalmol.* 19:65–74, 1935.
323. South, M.A., Tompkins, W.A.F., Morris, C.R., and Rawls, W.E. Congenital malformations of the central nervous system associated with genital type (type 2) herpes virus. *J. Pediatr.* 75:13–18, 1969.
324. Spallone, A. Incontinentia pigmenti (Bloch-Sulzberger syndrome): Seven case reports from one family. *Br. J. Ophthalmol.* 71:629–634, 1987.
325. Stanescu, B., and Dralands, L. Cerebrohepatorenal (Zellweger's) syndrome. *Arch. Ophthalmol.* 87:590–592, 1972.
326. Stathacopoulos, R.A., Bateman, J.B., Sparkes, R.S., and Hepler, R.S. The Rieger syndrome and a chromosome 13 deletion. *J. Pediatr. Ophthalmol. Strabismus* 24:198–203, 1987.
327. Stephens, J.C., Cavanaugh, M.L., Gradie, M.I., Mador, M.L., and Kidd, K.K. Mapping the human genome: Current status. *Science* 250:237–244, 1990.
328. Streeten, B.W., Karpik, A.G., and Spitzer, K.H. Posterior keratoconus associated with systemic abnormalities. *Arch. Ophthalmol.* 101:616–622, 1983.
329. Stevens, C.A., and Wilroy, R.S., Jr. The telecanthus-hypospadias syndrome. *J. Med. Genet.* 25:536–542, 1988.
330. Stone, D.L., Kenyon, K.R., Green, W.R., and Ryan, S.J. Congenital central corneal leukoma (Peters' anomaly). *Am. J. Ophthalmol.* 81:173–193, 1976.
331. Storimans, C.W., and Van Schooneveld, M.J. Rieger's eye anomaly and persistent hyperplastic primary vitreous. *Ophthalmic Paediatr. Genet.* 10:257–262, 1989.
332. Strange, J.R., and Murphree, R.L. Exposure-rate response in the prenatally irradiated rat: Effects of 100 R on day of gestation to the developing eye. *Radiat. Res.* 51:674–684, 1972.
333. Stretch, J.R., and Poole, M.D. Nasolacrimal abnormalities in oblique facial clefts. *Br. J. Plast. Surg.* 43:463–467, 1990.
334. Stromland, K. Ocular malformations in children exposed to drugs during gestation. *Clin. Pediatr.* 27:257–258, 1988.
335. Stromland, K., Miller, M., and Cook, D. Ocular teratology. *Surv. Ophthalmol.* 35:429–446, 1991.
336. Stromland, K. Ocular involvement in the fetal alcohol syndrome. *Surv. Ophthalmol.* 31:277–283, 1987.
337. Tarkkanen, A., Merenmies, L., and Rapola, J. Ocular pathology in triploidy (69/XXY). *Ophthalmologica* 163:90–97, 1971.
338. Taylor, D.S.I. The genetic implications of optic disc anomalies. *Trans. Ophthalmol. Soc. UK* 104:853–856, 1985.

339. Temple, I.K., Brunner, H., Jones, B., Burn, J., and Baraitser, M. Midline facial defects with ocular colobomata. *Am. J. Med. Genet. 37*:23–27, 1990.

340. Teske, M.P., and Trese, M.T. Retinopathy of prematurity-like fundus and persistent hyperplastic primary vitreous associated with maternal cocaine use. *Am. J. Ophthalmol. 103*:719–720, 1987.

341. Thompson, E.M., and Baraitser, M. Sorsby syndrome: A report on further generations of the original family. *J. Med. Genet. 25*:313–321, 1988.

342. Thompson, E.M., and Winter, R.M. A child with sclerocornea, short limbs, short stature, and distinct facial appearance. *Am. J. Med. Genet. 30*:719–724, 1988.

343. Townsend, W.M. Congenital corneal leukomas. 1. Central defect in Descemet's membrane. *Am. J. Ophthalmol. 77*:80–87, 1974.

344. Townsend, W.M., Font, R.L., and Zimmerman, L.E. Congenital corneal leukomas, 2. Histopathologic findings in 19 eyes with central defect in Descemet's membrane. *Am. J. Ophthalmol. 77*:192–206, 1974.

345. Townsend, W.M., Font, R.L., and Zimmerman, L.E. Histopathologic findings in 19 eyes with central defect in Descemet's membrane. *Am. J. Ophthalmol. 77*:192–206, 1974.

346. Torczynski, E., Jacobiec, F.A., Johnston, M.C., Font, R.L., and Madewell, J.A. Synophthalmia and cyclopia: A histopathologic, radiographic and organogenetic analysis. *Doc. Ophthalmol. 44*:311–378, 1977.

347. Traboulsi, E.I., Lenz, W., Gonzales-Ramos, M., Siegel, J., Macrae, W.G., and Maumenee, I.H. The Lenz microphthalmia syndrome. *Am. J. Ophthalmol. 105*:40–45, 1988.

348. Traboulsi, E.I., Maumenee, I.H., Krush, A.J., Alcorn, D., Giardiello, F.M., Burt, R.W., Hughes, J.P., and Hamilton, S.R. Congenital hypertrophy of the retinal pigment epithelium predicts colorectal polyposis in Gardner's syndrome. *Arch. Ophthalmol. 108*:525–526, 1990.

349. Troeber, R., and Rochels, R. Histologische Befunde bei Dysgenesis mesodermalis iridis et corneae Rieger. *Graefes Arch. Ophthalmol. 213*:169–174, 1980.

350. Tuchmann-Duplessis, H., and Mercier-Parot, L. The teratogenic action of the antibiotic actinomycin D. In *Ciba Foundation Symposium on Congenital Malformations*, G.E.W. Wolstenholme and C.M. O'Connor (Eds.), Little, Brown, Boston, pp. 115–133, 1960.

351. Tyndall, D.A. MRI effects on the teratogenicity of x-irradiation in the C57BL/6J mouse. *Magn. Reson. Imaging 8*:423–433, 1990.

352. Ueda, K., Nishida, Y., Oshima, K., and Shepard, T.H. Congenital rubella syndrome: Correlation of gestational age at time of maternal rubella with type of defect. *J. Pediatr. 94*:763–765, 1979.

353. Vilzeboer, C.M., van der Harten, J.J., and Koole, F.D. Ocular pathology in trisomy 18: A histopathological report of three cases. *Ophthalmic Paediatr. Genet. 10*:262–269, 1989.

354. Vuori, M.L. Morning glory disc anomaly with pulsating peripapillary staphyloma: A case history. *Acta Ophthalmol. (Copenh.) 65*:602–606, 1987.

355. Waardenburg, P.J. A new syndrome combining developmental anomalies of the eyelids, eyebrows and nose root with pigmentary defects of the iris and head, hair and with congenital deafness. *Am. J. Hum. Genet. 3*:195–253, 1951.

356. Wahl, J.W., and Ellis, R.P. Rothmund-Thomson syndrome. *Am. J. Ophthalmol. 60*:722–725, 1965.

357. Walton, W.T., Enzenauer, R.W., and Cornell, F.M. Abortive cryptophthalmos: A case report and a review of cryptophthalmos. *J. Pediatr. Ophthalmol. Strabismus 27*:129–132, 1990.

358. Warburg, M. Focal dermal hypoplasia: Ocular and general manifestations with a survey of the literature. *Acta Ophthalmol. (Copenh.) 48*:525–536, 1970.

359. Warburg, M. Hydrocephaly. *Am. J. Ophthalmol. 85*:88–95, 1978.

360. Warburg, M. X-linked cataract and X-linked microphthalmos: How many deletion families (letter to the editor).? *Am. J. Med. Genet. 34*:451–453, 1989.

361. Warburg, M., and Friedrich, U. Coloboma and microphthalmos in chromosomal aberrations: Chromosomal aberrations and neural crest cell developmental field. *Ophthalmic Paediatr. Genet. 81*:104–118, 1987.

362. Warburg, M. X-linked cataract and x-linked microphthalmos: How many deletion families? *Am. J. Med. Genet. 34*:451–453, 1989.

363. Waring, G.O., and Rodrigues, M.M. Ultrastructure and successful keratoplasty of sclerocornea of Mieten's syndrome. *Am. J. Ophthalmol. 90*:469–475, 1980.

364. Waring, G.O., and Rodrigues, M., and Laibson, P. Anterior chamber-cleavage syndrome: A stepladder classification. *Surv. Ophthalmol. 20*:3–27, 1975.

365. Waring, G.O., and Shields, J.A. Partial unilateral cryptophthalmos with syndactyly, brachycephaly and renal anomalies. *Am. J. Ophthalmol. 79*:437–440, 1975.

366. Warkany, J. Warfarin embryopathy. *Teratology 14*:205–210, 1976.

367. Wiedemann, H.R., and Drescher, J. LADD syndrome: Report of new cases and review of the clinical spectrum. *Eur. J. Pediatr. 144*:579–582, 1986.

368. Weinberg, A.G. Walker-Warburg syndrome. *Pediatr. Pathol. 9*:749–755, 1989.

369. Weiss, A., and Margo, C.F. Bilateral microphthalmos with cyst and 13q deletion syndrome. *Arch. Ophthalmol. 105*:29, 1987.

370. Weiss, A.H., Kousseff, B.G., Ross, E.A., and Longbottom, J. Simple microphthalmos. *Arch. Ophthalmol. 107*:1625–1630, 1989.

371. Weiss, A.H., Kousseff, B.G., Ross, E.A., and Longbottom, J. Complex microphthalmos. *Arch. Ophthalmol.* *107*:1619–1624, 1989.
372. Weiter, J.J., McLean, I.W., and Zimmerman, L.E. Aplasia of the optic nerve and disc. *Am. J. Ophthalmol.* *83*:569–576, 1977.
373. Welter, D.A., Lewis, L.W., Scharff, L., and Smith, W.S. Klinefelter's syndrome. *Am. J. Ophthalmol.* *77*:895–899, 1974.
374. Wilcox, L.M., Jr., Bercovitch, L., and Howard, R.O. Ophthalmic features of chromosome deletion 4p⁻ (Wolf-Hirschhorn syndrome). *Am. J. Ophthalmol.* *86*:834–839, 1978.
375. Willis, R., Zimmerman, L.E., O'Grady, R., Smith, R.S., and Crawford, B. Heterotopic adipose tissue and smooth muscle in the optic disc. *Arch. Ophthalmol.* *88*:139–146, 1972.
376. Wilson, J.G. Present status of drugs as teratogens in man. *Teratology* *7*:3–15, 1973.
377. Wilson, M.E. Congenital iris ectropion and a new classification for anterior segment dysgenesis. *J. Pediatr. Ophthalmol. Strabismus* *27*:48–55, 1990.
378. Wittig, E.O., Moreira, C.A., Freire-Maia, N., and Vianna-Morgante, A.M. Partial aniridia, cerebellar ataxia, and mental deficiency (Gillespie syndrome) in two brothers. *Am. J. Med. Genet.* *30*:703–708, 1988.
379. Woodhead, P., and Hall, C. Case report: Fraser syndrome, cryptophthalmos with small bowel malrotation. *Clin. Radiol.* *42*:362–363, 1990.
380. Wright, D.C., Yuh, W.T., Thompson, H.S., and Nerad, J.A. Bilateral microphthalmos with orbital cysts: MR findings. *J. Comput. Assist. Tomogr.* *11*:727–729, 1987.
381. Wulle, K.G. Fruhentwicklung der Ciliarfortsatze im menschlichen Auge. Phasenkontrast und elektron-mikrokopische Untersuchungen. *Z. Zellforsch.* *71*:545–571, 1976.
382. Yamada, E., and Ishikawa, T. Some observations on the submicroscopic morphogenesis of the human retina. In *The Structure of the Eye*, J.N. Rohen (Ed.), Schattauer, Stuttgart, 1965.
383. Yamshita, T., Kawano, K., and Ohba, N. Autosomal dominantly inherited optic nerve coloboma. *Ophthalmic Paediatr. Genet.* *9*:17–24, 1988.
384. Yanoff, M., Rahn, E.K., and Zimmerman, L.E. Histopathology of juvenile retinoschisis. *Arch. Ophthalmol.* *79*:49–53, 1968.
385. Yanoff, M. Rorke, L.B., and Niederer, B.S. Ocular and cerebral abnormalities in chromosome 18 deletion defect. *Am. J. Ophthalmol.* *70*:391–403, 1970.
386. Yanoff, M., Rorke, L.B., and Allman, M.I. Bilateral optic system aplasia with relatively normal eyes. *Arch. Ophthalmol.* *96*:97–101, 1978.
387. Young, I.D., Fielder, A.R., and Casey, T.A. Weill-Marchesani syndrome in mother and son. *Clin. Genet. 30*:475–480, 1986.
388. Yunis, J.J. *New Chromosomal Syndromes*, Academic Press, New York, 1977.
389. Yunis, J.J., and Chandler, M.E. The chromosomes of man: Clinical and biologic significance. *Am. J. Pathol.* *88*:466–495, 1977.
390. Zetterstrom, B. Ocular malformations caused by thalidomide. *Acta Ophthalmol. (Copenh.)* *44*:391–395, 1966.
391. Zhu, D.P., Antonarakis, S.E., Schmeckpeper, B.J., Diergaarde, P.J., Greb, A.E., and Maumenee, I.H. Micro-deletion in the X-chromosome and prenatal diagnosis in a family with Norrie disease. *Am. J. Med. Genet.* *33*:485–488, 1989.
392. Zimmerman, L.E. Phakomatous choristoma of the eyelid: A tumor of lenticular anlage. *Am. J. Ophthalmol.* *71*:169–177, 1971.
393. Zimmerman, L.E., and Naumann, G. The pathology of retinoschisis. In *New and Controversial Aspects of Retinal Detachment*, A McPherson (Ed.), Paul B. Hoeber, New York, pp. 400–423, 1968.

44

Overview of Oncogenesis

James G. Lewis

Duke University Medical Center, Durham, North Carolina

I. INTRODUCTION

Over the past 15 years there has been a virtual explosion of knowledge in the field of carcinogenesis. With each advance in cellular and molecular biology, there has been a corresponding advance in our understanding of the pathogenesis of neoplasia. Likewise, advances in the field of carcinogenesis have led to major advances in the comprehension of the molecular bases of many normal cell functions (see Sec. VI). Thus, as it has always been, the search for the molecular mechanisms of malignant transformation of the cell closely parallels the search for the molecular mechanisms that control the normal growth, development, differentiation, and adaptation of the cell. This overview deals with general concepts of carcinogenesis but, with the exception of retinoblastoma, does not discuss specific tumors of the eye. These are covered in subsequent chapters.

II. MULTISTEP NATURE OF CARCINOGENESIS

The pioneering experiments of Rous and coworkers in the 1920s demonstrated that the neoplastic process could be broken down experimentally into at least two stages, initiation and promotion [17]. These investigators noted that multiple applications of coal tar to rabbit ears induced skin tumors (complete carcinogenesis); single applications did not. If, however, following a single application of coal tar, the ears were subjected to chronic wounding, tumors were induced. No tumors were induced by the wounding alone. The application of coal tar was termed initiation, and the regimen of chronic wounding was termed promotion. Later investigations demonstrated that polycyclic hydrocarbons contained in coal tar, such as benzo[a]pyrene, were both potent complete carcinogens and initiating agents [23]. Other investigators in search of irritants that would serve as promoting agents discovered that the vesicant, croton oil, was a powerful promoting agent following application of polycyclic hydrocarbons to mouse skin [5]. It was later discovered that the phorbol ester 12-*O*-tetradecanoylphobol-13-acetate (TPA) was both the potent inflammatory agent and the tumor promoter in croton oil [7]. This simple model has been used extensively in the study of carcinogenesis and has remained a major model for studying its multistep process [50]. The induction of tumors in other organs, such as liver, lung, and bladder, has also been shown to be a multistep process [15].

Initiators are complete carcinogens that, if given repetitively, induce tumors. Most of them, or their metabolites, have been shown to covalently bind to DNA and are mutagens [1,35]. Many months can intervene between the application of the initiator and starting the promoting regimen [6]. In skin, this is sufficient time for several rounds of complete cell turnover. These observations strongly support the hypothesis that initiation is a somatic mutagenic event, and once a cell is initiated, all of that cell's progeny remain initiated cells.

In contrast to initiators, the mechanisms by which promoters act are not so clearly understood. Neither promoters nor their metabolites have been shown to bind to DNA, and they are not mutagenic [50]. They

1345

induce inflammation and cell replication in vivo and a wide array of biochemical alterations in cells in vitro [7]. Promotion is also thought to be a multistep process [49]. The initial lesions induced by the initiation-promotion sequence are benign growths, such as papillomas in skin, or foci of cells with altered morphology and enzymatic profiles as seen in the liver. Only after continued promotion do some of these benign lesions progress to carcinomas. The terms "conversion" and "progression" have been suggested for the later stages of promotion [49].

If the promotion regimen is discontinued before full malignant conversion occurs, the benign growths subside, suggesting that the early stages of promotion are reversible and thus epigenetic in nature [48]. A leading hypothesis explaining promotion is the selective or stimulated cell growth hypothesis. This theory contends that initiation is a rare, somatic mutational event that affects only a few cells in the tissue. Once initiated, these cells exhibit normal growth until the promotion regimen begins. The initiated cells are then selectively stimulated to grow or normal cells are selectively inhibited from growth, such that the initiated cells enjoy a significant growth advantage. Initiated cells then develop into benign tumors, thus explaining the monoclonal nature of many tumors. The final malignant transformation occurs when other rare genetic events occur. If promotion is stopped before malignant transformation occurs, the selective advantage disappears and the benign growths subside.

The mechanism(s) whereby additional genetic events required for conversion to the malignant phenotype occur is not well explained by the selective growth hypothesis. It has been shown that papillomas that develop as a result of TPA exposure can progress to carcinomas following exposure to additional genotoxic agents [22]. The means by which continued exposure to the apparently nongenotoxic compound TPA produces further genotoxicity is not certain. Because most agents that are active promoters in the mouse skin model are also potent inflammatory agents that cause inflammatory cells to migrate into the dermis, because these same agents stimulate inflammatory cells to release potentially genotoxic reactive oxygen intermediates (ROI), and because most agents that inhibit promotion are either antiinflammatory drugs or scavengers of ROI, it has been suggested that promoters may be indirectly genotoxic [13,30,50,56]. Fibroblasts cocultured with inflammatory cells, such as neutrophils or macrophages, and TPA have been shown to suffer significant levels of oxidative DNA damage [30]. Agents that are neither active promoters nor directly genotoxic, such as acetic acid, which can induce necrosis, inflammation, and cell replication, convert adenomas to carcinomas [41]. These studies suggest that chronic necrosis and inflammation involving expanded populations of initiated cells may provide the additional rare genetic events necessary for malignant transformation.

III. MOLECULAR MECHANISMS OF CARCINOGENESIS

The preceding is a general description of the multistage model of carcinogenesis. This section describes studies that have demonstrated tight correlations between specific molecular events and the development of neoplasms.

A. DNA Damage, Repair, and Replication

Since the discovery of DNA as the genetic substance, alterations in DNA have been suspected of being key events in carcinogenesis. It was hypothesized that carcinogens reacted with DNA, but this was difficult to demonstrate initially because most of the known carcinogens would not react with DNA in solution. The pioneering work of the Millers demonstrated that most carcinogens are fairly inert themselves and need to be metabolically activated to reactive species [35]. The principal site of metabolism occurs in the liver by the cytochrome P_{450} monooxygenase system.

Following this breakthrough and the advent of radiolabeled chemicals, the exact structures of reactive metabolites and their reactions with DNA have been determined for a number of carcinogens. Later studies indicated that some alterations in DNA were of little consequence, whereas others were highly mutagenic and correlated strongly with carcinogenesis. For example, simple alkylating (methylating) agents, such as dimethylnitrosamine (DMN) and dimethylsulfate (DMS), differ greatly in carcinogenic potency in vivo, DMN being much more potent than DMS. The most abundant alkylation product induced by both chemicals is methylation at the nitrogen atom in position 7 of guanine (^{7}MG). DMN induces a higher amount of oxygen alkylation, however, especially at position 6 of guanine (O^{6}MG) and the O^4 position of thymine (O^{4}MT) [40]. These oxygen atoms are involved with base pairing, whereas the nitrogen at position

7 in guanine is not. In vitro studies have shown that if O⁶MG or O⁴MT is contained in the template, mispairing occurs at a high frequency, resulting in the induction of point mutations [40].

Other forms of chemical and physical damage to DNA have been characterized, including large bulky adducts induced by covalent attachment of polycyclic hydrocarbons and aflatoxins; pyrimidine dimers and 5,6 photoproducts induced by ultraviolet (UV) irradiation; base alterations and strand breakage induced by ionizing radiation and oxygen radicals; production of thymine in DNA by the deamination of 5-methyl-cytosine; apurinic/apyrimidinic sties (AP sites) induced by both DNA damage and repair (AP sites are "holes" in the DNA backbone that lack an adenine or guanine—*apurinic*—and/or cytosine or thymine—*pyrimidinic*—base); DNA-DNA and DNA-protein cross-links induced by bifunctional agents; and the insertion of whole genes by viruses and proviruses [13,26,29,30,35,40]. The actual mechanisms by which many of these forms of damage induce mutations and tumors is not as well characterized as the simple alkylating agents just described. Frame shifts (see Chap. 24), gene deletions, gene inactivation, and gene rearrangements, in addition to point mutations, are some of the consequences of these forms of DNA damage. It is important to note that stubborn blocks to replication may be mutagenic. In some cases DNA polymerases bypass or replicate through a lesion. In these cases the polymerase most frequently places an adenine opposite the block [43]; this tendency is termed the A rule. Except in the case of damaged thymines, this represents a mutational event if it is not repaired by postreplication repair mechanisms before another round of DNA replication.

To maintain the integrity of the genome, the cell has evolved efficient methods of repairing DNA damage. The best understood DNA repair pathway is excision repair [19]. Damaged DNA is recognized in some uncharacterized manner, and an incision is made adjacent to the damaged site. An exonuclease then removes the damaged site along with a variable amount of normal DNA. Then, using the opposite strand as a template, polymerase fills in the gap and ligase seals the insert into place. This method is thought to repair bulky adducts and other alterations that make large disruptions of the secondary structure of DNA. Numerous other enzymes have been characterized that recognize specific types of DNA damage. The most common enzymes of this type are the glycosylases [31]. These enzymes recognize a specific altered base and remove it from the sugar, leaving an AP site in the DNA. Other enzymes, termed AP nucleases, then remove the AP site, leaving a gap with a 3' hydroxyl end. Polymerase then adds the appropriate nucleotides and the gap is sealed by ligase. Glycosylases specific for uracil, ⁷MG, 3-methyladenine, and oxidized pyrimidines have been detected in bacterial and eukaryotic cells [31].

The highly mutagenic O⁶MG mentioned earlier is repaired by a unique system. A protein called O⁶-methyltransferase actually removes the methyl group from the guanine and places it on a cysteine residue in the protein, leaving the unmodified guanine in the DNA [39]. The protein is not regenerated but is used in the process so it is not a classic enzyme. Other more complex mechanisms of repair have been characterized. In yeast over 10 proteins have been associated with the repair of UV-induced DNA damage [18]. It is probable that some of these proteins serve double duty and also participate in normal DNA replication. It has also been demonstrated that DNA repair does not occur at the same rate in all areas of the genome. Genes that are active in the cell and are being transcribed are repaired at a significantly faster rate than silent genes [32]. Thus, if genes critical for transformation are dormant, they may be repaired at a slower rate, which increases the probability that the damage is not repaired before cell replication (see later).

It is possible that DNA repair mechanisms themselves are prone to error and thus induce mutations or gene rearrangements. In bacteria, for example, when the level of DNA damage is so high that a reasonable amount of repair cannot take place before replication, the cell performs what is called SOS repair [59]. This is a complex recombination process involving several gene products in which the cell increases the chance for mutation as the price for enhancing the chance of survival and growth. The existence of this SOS system of repair in mammalian cells is still debatable. Clearly, recombination events occur or are increased in mammalian cells following DNA damage. For example, increases in sister chromatid exchanges have been observed in mammalian cells after exposure to DNA-damaging agents in vivo and in vitro [14].

Cell replication is also critical for carcinogenesis. The importance can easily be understood by observing the tissues commonly affected by tumors. Most cancers are carcinomas, tumors of the epithelial surfaces that are in a constant state of turnover. Other common tumors (leukemias and lymphomas) occur in the bone marrow, which has the highest rate of cell turnover in the body [37]. Sarcomas, tumors of the soft tissues, are relatively less common and the rate of cell replication is much less [37]. If cell division is induced in a normally quiescent tissue, it greatly enhances the chances for tumor formation. In adult rodent liver, for example, the rate of cell replication is very low. If a nonnecrogenic dose of a liver carcinogen is given once, very few tumors develop. If this same dose of carcinogen is given 24 h following a two-thirds partial hepatectomy, however, liver tumors are induced [8]. The time of maximal DNA synthesis, 24 h after partial hepatectomy, occurs during the regeneration of the original mass of the liver. Hepatocellular carcinoma is a relatively rare tumor in humans in the developed countries of the world but it is one of the most common tumors in underdeveloped nations [4]. The increased rates of hepatocellular carcinoma occur in populations in which viral hepatitis or other infections of the liver are endemic [4].

This issue of the role of cell replication, per se, in carcinogenesis has become a critical issue recently in the arena of safety evaluation for chemicals [2]. Most chemicals that test positive as carcinogens in rodent bioassays induce tumors of the liver as the main finding. Suspect carcinogens are administered at what is called the maximum tolerated dose, the highest dose that can be given without a significant percentage of the animals dying from acute toxicity. In many, if not most cases, necrosis, inflammation, and regenerative cell division are induced in the livers of these animals. Several investigators have questioned this practice, suggesting it is nothing more than the chronic toxicity in the liver inducing prolonged cell replication that is responsible for the tumors, not any specific carcinogenic or mutagenic action of the chemical [2]. The observation that over 40% of nonexposed control mice develop liver tumors eventually with age suggests that the toxicity of the chemicals is merely speeding the formation of tumors, not inducing tumors. Thus, undue attention is placed on manufactured chemicals and the risks are overstated. Proponents of maximal dose testing counter that this is the only way one can screen for carcinogens. If lower doses are used, some chemicals may slip through.

B. Viral Carcinogenesis

The existence of tumor viruses has been known since the initial work of Rous, who discovered the first tumor virus (Rous sarcoma virus) [42]. Since that time, numerous other viruses that induce tumors in animals and humans and transform cells in culture have been identified. They fall into two large categories, the DNA- and the RNA-containing viruses. The DNA-containing oncogenic viruses consist of six viral families: hepatitis B, herpesviruses, adenoviruses, simian virus 40 (SV40) and polyomavirus, papillomaviruses, and pox viruses. The RNA-containing oncogenic viruses comprise only one family, the retroviruses.

IV. DNA VIRUSES

Hepatitis B virus has been epidemiologically linked with human hepatocellular carcinoma. This tumor is rare in the developed countries, but in areas of the world where hepatitis B is endemic, hepatocellular carcinoma is the most common human cancer [4]. The mechanism of oncogenic transformation by hepatitis B is not known. The virus does not transform cells in culture, and no transforming genes have been identified. It is thought that the virus acts through nonspecific mechanisms, such as chronic hepatic necrosis, inflammation, and cell replication.

SV40 and polyomavirus transform cells only from species that are not permissive for viral replication. That is, the virus does not transform cells or induce tumors in the animal species the virus naturally infects, monkeys (SV40) or mice (polyomavirus). In permissive cells, the virus replicates and then kills the infected cells during the lytic cycle of virus release; thus, no cells are alive to become transformed. In nonpermissive cells (such as hamster cells) the virus is blocked from replication, and in a few cells the viral DNA becomes permanently integrated into the cellular genome and the viral gene products expressed. The viral genes expressed early during infection are the genes that are sufficient and necessary for transformation. They are called the large T (SV40) and large and middle T (polyomavirus) [11]. The function of these gene products is not known, but it has been suggested that the proteins interact with tumor suppressor genes and possibly protooncogenes (see later).

Papillomaviruses are known for neoplastic transformation in animals and humans. They are best known for the induction of benign papillomas of the skin, or the common wart. They are also implicated in the induction of cervical carcinoma. Two genes, termed E6 and E7, have been identified that induce transformation. The function of these genes remains to be established, but it is thought that they increase the activity of growth factor receptors and interact with tumor suppressor genes [11].

Adenoviruses are lytic for permissive cells but can transform nonpermissive cells. Two genes, E1A and E1B, which encode multiple proteins through alternative splicing, are responsible for transformation. Several of these proteins are thought to interact with the gene products of tumor suppressor genes [45].

Herpesviruses induce a number of malignant tumors in animals and possibly humans. The herpesviruses have larger and more complex genomes than many other viral families, but much less is known about the molecular mechanisms of transformation [24]. The Epstein-Barr virus is thought to induce both African Burkitt's lymphoma and nasopharyngeal carcinoma. The virus can transform human lymphocytes in culture.

Poxviruses induce benign neoplasms in rabbits and monkeys, but little is known about the mechanism of action.

V. RNA VIRUSES

The retroviruses have provided an immense amount of information about normal cell growth, differentiation, and transformation. Furthermore, studies of retroviruses have provided central unifying concepts and mechanisms for both viral and chemical carcinogenesis (see later). Retroviruses are the only family of the RNA viruses known to be oncogenic. These viruses replicate by making a DNA copy of the viral RNA genome using reverse transcriptase and actively inserting this provirus into the genome of the cell. There, under the influence of strong promoters, the gene products of the provirus are expressed. The provirus is replicated along with the cellular DNA, and in most cases the release of packaged virus proceeds in a nonlytic manner. These viruses are thus able to transform the cells of the natural host. Some of these viruses are the most potent cell transformation agents known. They induce a wide variety of tumors in numerous mammalian species, including the human. The human T cell leukemia viruses I and II are thought to induce human adult T cell leukemia and hairy cell leukemia, respectively. Another retrovirus, human immunodeficiency virus, causes the fatal disease known as the acquired immunodeficiency syndrome (AIDS). Because of the great importance of the retroviruses in our understanding of carcinogenesis through the discovery of oncogenes and protooncogenes, these agents are discussed in some detail in the next section.

VI. ONCOGENES AND PROTOONCOGENES

The oncogenic potential of retroviruses has been known for a long time. The retroviruses can be divided into two general classes, the acute transforming viruses (ATV) and the weak transforming viruses (WTV). ATV transform cells at a very high frequency and rapidly induce tumors in animals. One of the first and best examples of ATV is the Rous sarcoma virus (RSV), named after its discoverer [42]. The WTV transform cells poorly and induce tumors in animals only after extremely long latent periods. An example of WTV is the avian leukosis virus (ALV), which is very closely related to RSV.

ALV and RSV replicate in the same way in the same cells but, as mentioned, differ markedly in oncogenic potential. Some difference in the genetic makeup of the two viruses was hypothesized as responsible for this difference. The RNA genome of RSV was discovered to be larger than that of ALV, and it was hoped that the transformation capacity of RSV resided in the extra 1500 base pairs of RNA contained by RSV. By constructing nontransforming and temperature-sensitive mutants of RSV, this was found to be the case. The genome of both RSV and ALV consists of the long terminal repeat promoter regions followed by the *gag*, *pol*, and *env* genes. *gag* encodes the major structural proteins, *pol* the reverse transcriptase, and *env* the viral envelope glycoproteins. RSV has an extra gene called *src* (for sarcoma), which was solely responsible and sufficient for transformation [34].

src was the first known oncogene and gave science one of its greatest surprises. With the ability to construct molecular probes of the *src* gene came the discovery that the src gene was contained in all eukaryotic cells probed and was conserved over a large evolutionary range [54]. It was quickly recognized that *src* was not a viral gene at all but a eukaryotic gene picked up by the virus at some point. Quickly other retroviral oncogenes were tested, and all were found to have a normal cellular homolog. Numerous retroviral oncogenes have now been described. The viral oncogenes are not exact duplicates of the cellular gene but frequently are truncated, mutated, or gag-oncogene fusion proteins. Frequently the mutation confers the transforming ability of the expressed product. Nontransforming retroviruses picked up genes from normal cells that changed them into some of the most potent oncogenic agents known. For some of these viruses, there is almost 100% efficiency of transformation.

The studies described here greatly illuminated the mechanisms of viral carcinogenesis but shed little light on the cause and pathogenesis of chemical, physical, or inherited forms of cancer. A very simple experiment opened the door to another explosion in the fields of carcinogenesis, control of cell replication, and signal transduction. The DNA from tumor cells was transfected into NIH-3T3 fibroblasts [46]. These cells are immortal but not fully transformed and are contact inhibited in culture. Foci of piled-up transformed cells were noted in the exposed plates. A very low frequency of transformation was noted in plates exposed to DNA from normal cells. DNA from a human bladder tumor was then transfected [38]. DNA from foci was retransfected into NIH-3T3 cells, and a higher frequency of transformation was noted. This procedure was repeated until the frequency of transformation remained constant. The minimum amount of DNA necessary to transform the cells was assumed to be transferred. Because NIH-3T3 cells are murine and the tumor DNA was human, investigators could then search for human specific sequences and identify the exact stretch of DNA responsible for transformation. This was done, and when the DNA was sequenced, surprisingly the sequence was almost identical to the *ras* transforming gene of the Harvey sarcoma virus [38]. Of further importance was the presence of a single point mutation (G to T) in the *ras* gene from the tumor cells at codon 12, which caused a valine to be coded instead of a glycine [55]. Thus, for the first time, a specific alteration in a cellular gene was demonstrated to induce transformation. Further studies demonstrated that this specific mutation in *ras* occurred with a high frequency in animal tumors induced by chemical agents. It is now known that *ras* is a family of genes (H-*ras* and K-*ras*) and that mutations at a number of sites can activate these protooncogenes.

The next exciting question was whether this was the critical target gene in the cell mediating malignancy. Armed with the knowledge that the cellular homologs of retroviral oncogenes may be directly activated, the search for other oncogenes and the probing of tumors to see if they all had "activated" *ras* was begun. Other protooncogenes have been found, over 30 to date, and activated *ras* was not found in all tumors so the induction of tumors remained a more complicated issue.

Several different mechanisms of protooncogene activation have been discovered. Protooncogenes can be activated by gene amplification, gene rearrangements, chromosome translocations, and insertion of viral promoters adjacent to the protooncogene. The *myc* protooncogene, for example, has been shown to be activated by all these other mechanisms [12]. The *myc* gene is amplified in a number of tumor types, resulting in a higher than normal level of expression of the normal gene product. In some lymphomas and plasmacytomas the *myc* gene normally found on chromosome 8 has moved to a specific area of chromosome 14, where it comes under the control of the promoter of immunoglobulin G (IgG). This also results in abnormally high expression of the normal gene product. In bursal lymphomas in chickens, functional long terminal repeats of proviral promoters have become inserted upstream from the *myc* gene, causing an abnormally high level of expression of the normal gene product. Thus, a number of mechanisms, including abnormal expression of the normal gene product and normal expression of a mutated gene, have been shown to contribute significantly to cell transformation.

Fortunately for the basic scientist, these studies provided a wealth of data on the normal workings of the cell. By tracking down the functions of the proteins encoded by protooncogenes, much knowledge has been gained on how cells control replication and how they interact with the environment. The *ras* gene product was found to be located at the plasma membrane and to be a GTP binding protein thought to be involved in signal transduction pathways [44,57]. Interestingly, the specific point mutation described that results in activation of *ras* greatly reduces the ability of the protein to hydrolyze GTP to GDP [33]. This results in the protein remaining in the active state for a longer period of time. The *myc* gene product has been found to be located in the nucleus and to bind to DNA [12]. It is thought that *myc* has a role in regulation of transcription. The *erb*-B oncogene product has been shown to be a truncated version of the normal cellular homolog, which is a tyrosine kinase and is the epidermal growth factor receptor [36]. The viral oncogene lacks the receptor binding domain contained in the normal cellular gene but retains the tyrosine kinase domain. It is thought to function constitutively without the need for receptor binding. The *src* gene has been shown to be a nonreceptor tyrosine protein kinase. Thus, many oncogenes have been shown to be involved in gene regulation by either directly affecting transcription or altering signal transduction pathways.

Tumor Suppressor Genes

An alternative mechanism to oncogene activation for the transformation of cells is the loss of gene products that control and limit cell growth. Support for this concept has come from two lines of evidence. The first was the observation that if malignant cells are fused with normal cells, almost always the resulting hybrid cells initially lose the tumorigenic phenotype [51]. These hybrid cells may retain some characteristics of the transformed cell in vitro, but the hybrids cease to form tumors in animals. The observation that with time some of the cells revert to the tumorigenic phenotype and that this correlates with the loss of certain chromosomes from the nontransformed donor strongly suggested that some gene on the lost chromosome was responsible for the loss of tumorigenicity [53]. Loss of chromosomes 1, 4, and 11 in human tumor cell–normal fibroblast hybrids correlates with the reversion to tumorigenicity.

Retinoblastoma (see Chap. 49) has provided some of the best evidence for the existence of tumor suppressor genes. The disease exists in two forms, inherited and sporadic. Inherited retinoblastomas develop early in life and are frequently bilateral and multicentric. The sporadic form develops later, usually as a unilateral single tumor. Although multiple tumors occur in the hereditary form of retinoblastoma, the vast majority of retinal cells do not develop into tumors. These observations lead to the hypothesis that two mutations were required [25]. The first mutation was inherited, but the second occurred as a rare event in some of the cells over a period of time.

The concept of the loss of genes rather than the activation of an oncogene came from the observation that there was a specific deletion of a portion of chromosome 13 in both white blood cells and tumor cells from patients with the hereditary form of retinoblastoma [10]. Tumor cells from patients with the sporadic form of retinoblastoma had similar deletions, but blood cells did not. These large chromosomal deletions were not observed in all patients, but smaller deletions that could not be seen at the level of the light microscope were thought to occur. Further studies investigated genes known to map near the deleted locus. Two separable forms of esterase D are encoded by the two alleles contained on the two chromosomes 13. Normal cells contained both forms of esterase D, but tumor cells contained only one. Moreover, the lost gene was supplied by the unaffected parent, suggesting that the mutant retinoblastoma gene was retained and the normal gene was lost. Further studies cloned the candidate retinoblastoma gene and demonstrated that in the vast majority of tumors the gene is lost or partially deleted or when it is retained there is abnormal transcription. Thus, the complete loss of the activity of a gene occurred by inheritance of one mutant gene and secondary loss of the other normal functioning gene.

The product of the retinoblastoma gene (Rb) is located in the nucleus and binds to DNA. The retinoblastoma gene is considered either a repressor of transcription of genes that induce proliferation or a transactivator of other genes that repress genes involved in replication. Evidence for this is that several genes of oncogenic viruses that stimulate cell replication also complex with the retinoblastoma gene product and inhibit its binding to cell DNA [9,58].

The retinoblastoma gene was initially identified because of the hereditary nature and rarity of retinoblastoma. Recent studies, however, suggest a more general role of this gene in tumor development. Patients with inherited retinoblastoma have a high incidence of second tumors, such as osteosarcomas [20]. Studies of small cell carcinoma of the lung in particular have also implicated a mutated form or loss of the retinoblastoma gene product [21].

Another tumor suppressor gene candidate, p53, has been discovered. Its product is a nuclear protein that has been shown to bind to the SV40 transforming gene product (large T antigen) [28]. The p53 gene has been shown to be lost by deletion, rearranged, mutated, or inactivated by proviral insertion in a number of animal and human tumors. Its introduction into transformed cells can reverse the transformed phenotype [3,16]. Other cytogenetic studies of the loss of certain chromosomes or areas of chromosomes in childhood tumors, such as Wilms' tumor, neuroblastoma, and rhabdomyosarcoma, have identified areas in the genome that may contain other tumor suppressor genes [52]. Thus, the list of tumor suppressor genes may continue to grow.

The conversion of NIH-3T3 cells by a single oncogene superficially suggests a simple one-hit model of carcinogenesis. It is important to note, however, that although NIH-3T3 cells retain contact inhibition and are hence not fully transformed, they are immortal demonstrating preexisting genetic change(s). The observation that primary cultures of fibroblasts, without this preexisting change, could not be transformed by a single oncogene (activated *ras* or *myc*) but required the transfection of at least two (*ras* plus *myc*) is supportive of the multistage nature of carcinogenesis observed in vivo and suggests a more complicated model [59]. In this model at least two, but possibly more than two, rare genetic events must occur for stable malignant transformation of a cell. The interplay of numerous environmental and host factors, genetic and epigenetic, increases or decreases the probability of these events occurring. The existence of both dominant transforming oncogenes and tumor suppressor genes and multiple ways of activating or inactivating these genes, respectively, suggests a number of molecular changes that can result in transformation. The activation of multiple oncogenes, activation of oncogenes in combination with loss of suppressor genes, or the loss of more than one suppressor gene by mutation, deletion, rearrangement, or proviral insertion all have the potential for transforming the cell. Factors bearing on the chance that these events will occur include rates of xenobiotic exposure, metabolism, detoxification, viral exposure and immunity, radiation exposure, and DNA damage, repair, and replication.

Finally, it is important to add that the majority of the studies mentioned here deal with the control or loss of control of cell growth. The ability to metastasize is perhaps the worst feature of most tumors. Locally invasive tumors can frequently be cured, but those tumors that spread to distant sites while the primary tumor is still small and difficult to detect are the most lethal. Although not addressed in this overview, the development of the metastatic phenotype adds another layer of complexity to those phenotypic changes necessary for uncontrolled growth. Thus, understanding the complex process of the cell changing from normal, to initiated, to benign growth, to invasive growth, to the fully malignant cancer cell, in each of the different cells and tissues of the body, in specific molecular detail, is a monumental task that must be performed if we are to develop more specific and efficacious methods for the diagnosis and treatment of these diseases.

REFERENCES

1. Ames, B.N. Identifying environmental chemicals causing mutations and cancer. *Science 204*:587–593, 1979.
2. Ames, B.N., and Gold, L.S. Too many rodent carcinogens: Mitogenesis increases mutagenesis. *Science 249*:970–971, 1990.
3. Baker, S.J., Fearon, E.R., Nigro, J.M., Hamilton, S.R., Presinger, A.C., Jessup, J.M., Van Tuinen, P., Ledbetter, D.H., Barker, D.F., Nakamura, Y., White, R., and Vogelstein, B. Chromosome 17 deletion and p53 gene mutation in colorectal carcinomas. *Science 244*:217–221, 1989.
4. Beasley, R.P., and Hwang, L. Hepatocellular carcinoma and hepatitis B virus. *Semin. Liver Dis. 4*:113–121, 1984.
5. Berenblum, I. The cocarcinogenic action of croton resin. *Cancer Res. 1*:44–48, 1941.
6. Berenblum, I., and Shubik, P. The persistence of latent tumour cells induced in mouse skin by a single application of 9:10-dimethyl-1,2-benzanthracene. *Br. J. Cancer 3*:384–386, 1949.
7. Boutwell, R.K. Some biological aspects of skin carcinogenesis. *Prog. Exp. Tumor Res. 4*:207–250, 1964.
8. Craddock, V.M. Induction of liver tumors by a single treatment with nitroso compounds given after partial hepatectomy. *Nature 245*:386–388, 1973.
9. DeCaprio, T.A., Ludlow, J.W., Figge, J., Shew, J.Y., Huang, C.M., Lee, W.H., Marsilo, E., Paucha, E., and Livingston, D.M. SV40 large tumor antigen forms a stable complex with the product of the retinoblastoma susceptibility locus. *Cell 54*:275–283, 1988.
10. Dryja, T.P., Cavenee, R.L., White, J.M., Alberts, D.M., and Bruns, G.A.P. Homozygosity of chromosome 13 in retinoblastoma. *N. Engl. J. Med. 310*:550–554, 1984.
11. Eckart, W. Oncogenes of DNA tumor viruses: Papovaviruses. In *Oncogenes and the Molecular Origins of Cancer*, R.A. Weinberg (Ed.), Cold Spring Harbor Press, New York, pp. 223–238, 1989.
12. Eisenman, R.N. Nuclear oncogenes. In *Oncogenes and the Molecular Origins of Cancer*, R.A. Weinberg (Ed.), Cold Spring Harbor Press, New York, pp. 175–222, 1989.
13. Emerit, I., and Cerutti, P.A. Tumor promoter phorbol-12-myristate-13-acetate induces chromosomal damage via indirect action. *Nature 293*:144–146, 1981.
14. Erexson, G.L., Wilmer, J.L., Steinhegan, W.H., and Kligerman, A.D. Induction of cytogenetic damage in rodents after short-term inhalation of benzene. *Environ. Mutagen. 8*:29–40, 1986.
15. Farber, E. Chemical carcinogenesis: A biologic perspective. *Am. J. Pathol. 106*:271–296, 1982.
16. Finlay, C.A., Hinds, P.W., and Levine, A.J. The p53 proto-oncogene can act as a suppressor of transformation. *Cell 57*:1083–1093, 1989.
17. Friedwald, W.F., and Rous, P. The initiating and promoting elements in tumor production. *J. Exp. Med. 80*:101–144, 1944.
18. Game, J.C. Radiation-sensitive mutants and repair in yeast. In *Yeast Genetics*, D.H. Spencer, and A.P. Smith (Eds.), Springer-Verlag, New York, pp. 109–137, 1983.

19. Hanawalt, P.C., Cooper, P.K., Ganesan, A.K., and Smith, C.A. DNA repair in bacterial and mammalian cells. *Annu. Rev. Biochem.* 48:783–836, 1979.

20. Hansen, M.F., Koufos, A., Gallie, B.L., Phillips, R.A., Fodstad, O., Brogger, A., Gedde-Dahl, T., and Cavenee, W.K. Osteosarcoma and retinoblastoma: A shared chromosomal mechanism revealing recessive predisposition. *Proc. Natl. Acad. Sci. USA* 82:6216–6220, 1985.

21. Harbour, J.W., Lai, S.L., Whang-Peng, J., Gazdar, A.F., Minna, J.D., and Kaye, F.J. Abnormalities in structure and expression of the human retinoblastoma gene in SCLC. *Science* 241:353–357, 1988.

22. Hennings, H., Shores, R., Wenk, M.L., Spangler, E.F., Tarone, M.L., and Yuspa, S.H. Malignant conversion of mouse skin tumors is increased by tumor initiators and unaffected by tumor promoters. *Nature* 304:67–69, 1983.

23. Kennaway, E.I. The identification of a carcinogenic compound in coal tar. *BMJ* 2:749–752, 1955.

24. Kieff, E., and Liebowitz, D. Oncogenesis by herpesviruses. In *Oncogenes and the Molecular Origins of Cancer*, R.A. Weinberg (Ed.), Cold Spring Harbor Press, New York, pp. 259–280, 1989.

25. Knudson, A.G. Mutation and cancer: Statistical study of retinoblastoma. *Proc. Natl. Acad. Sci. USA* 68:820–823, 1971.

26. Kohn, K.W., Erickson, L.C., Ewig, R.A., and Friedman, C.A. Fractionation of DNA from mammalian cells by alkaline elution. *Biochemistry* 15:4629–4637, 1976.

27. Land, H., Parada, L.F., and Weinberg, R.A. Tumorigenic conversion of primary embryo fibroblasts requires at least two cooperating oncogenes. *Nature* 304:596–602, 1983.

28. Lane, D.P., and Crawford, L.V. T antigen is bound to a host protein in SV40-transformed cells. *Nature* 278:261–263, 1979.

29. Levin, J.D., Johnson, A.W., and Demple, B. Homogeneous *Escherichia coli* endonuclease IV. *J. Biol. Chem.* 263:8066–8071, 1988.

30. Lewis, J.G., and Adams, D.O. Inflammation, oxidative DNA damage, and carcinogenesis. *Environ. Health Perspect.* 76:19–27, 1987.

31. Lindahl, T. DNA glycosylases, endonucleases for apurinic/apyrimidinic sites, and base excision repair. *Prog. Nucleic Acid Res. Mol. Biol.* 22:135–192, 1979.

32. Madhani, H.D., Bohr, V.A., and Hanawalt, P.C. Differential repair in transcriptionally active and inactive protooncogenes c-*abl* and c-*mos*. *Cell* 45:417–423, 1985.

33. Manne, V., Bekesi, E., and Kung, H.F. Ha-ras proteins exhibit GTPase activity: Point mutations that activate Ha-ras gene products result in decreased GTPase activity. *Proc. Natl. Acad. Sci. USA* 82:376–380, 1985.

34. Martin, G.S., and Duesberg, P.H. The subunit in the RNA of transforming avian tumor viruses. I. Occurrence in different virus strains. II. Spontaneous loss resulting in nontransforming variants. *Virology* 47:494–497, 1972.

35. Miller, E.C., and Miller, J.A. Mechanisms of chemical carcinogenesis: Nature of proximate carcinogens and interactions with macromolecules. *Pharmacol. Rev.* 18:806–838, 1966.

36. Nilsen, T.W., Maroney, P.A., Goodwin, R.G., Rottman, F.M., Guttenden, L.B., Raines, M.A., and Kung, H.J. erb-B activation in ALV-induced erythroblastosis: Novel RNA processing and promoter insertion result in expression of an amino-truncated EGF receptor. *Cell* 41:719–726, 1985.

37. Oehlert, W. Cell proliferation in carcinogenesis. *Cell Tissue Kinetics* 6:325–335, 1973.

38. Parada, L.F., Tabin, C.J., Shih, C., and Weinberg, R.A. Human ET bladder carcinoma oncogene in homologue of Harvey sarcoma virus ras gene. *Nature* 297:474–478, 1982.

39. Pegg, A.E., and Perry, W. Stimulation of transfer of methyl groups from O_6-methylguanine in DNA to protein by rat liver extracts in response to hepatotoxins. *Carcinogenesis* 2:1195–1201, 1981.

40. Ridout, W.M., Coetzee, G.A., Olumi, A.F., and Jones, P.A. 5-Methylcytosine as an endogenous mutagen in the human LDL receptor and p53 genes. *Science* 249:1288–1290, 1990.

41. Rotstein, J.P., and Slaga, T.J. Acetic acid, a potent agent of tumor progression in the multistage mouse skin model for chemical carcinogenesis. *Cancer Lett.* 42:87–90, 1988.

42. Rous, P. Transmission of a malignant new growth by means of a cell-free filtrate. *JAMA* 56:198, 1911.

43. Sagher, D., and Strauss, B. Insertion of nucleotides opposite apurinic/apyrimidinic sites in deoxyribonucleic acid during in vitro synthesis: Uniqueness of adenine nucleotides. *Biochemistry* 22:4518–4523, 1983.

44. Scolnick, E.M., Papageorge, A.G., and Shik, T.Y. Guanine nucleotide-binding activity as an assay for ras protein of rat-derived murine sarcoma viruses. *Proc. Natl. Acad. Sci. USA* 76:5355–5359, 1979.

45. Shenk, T. Oncogenesis by DNA tumor viruses: Adenovirus. In *Oncogenes and the Molecular Origins of Cancer*, R.A. Weinberg (Ed.), Cold Spring Harbor Press, New York, pp. 239–258, 1989.

46. Shih, C., Shilo, B.Z., Goldfarb, M.P., Dannenberg, A., and Weinberg, R.A. Passage of phenotypes of chemically transformed cells via transfection of DNA and chromatin. *Proc. Natl. Acad. Sci. USA* 76:5714–5718, 1979.

47. Singer, B. Sites in nucleic acids reacting with alkylating agents of differing carcinogenicity or mutagenicity. *J. Toxicol. Environ. Health* 2:1279–1295, 1977.

48. Slaga, T.J. Overview of tumor promotion in animals. *Environ. Health Perspect.* 50:3–14, 1983.

49. Slaga, T.J., Fischer, S.M., Nelson, K., and Gleason, G.L. Studies on the mechanisms of skin tumor promotion: Evidence for several stages in promotion. *Proc. Natl. Acad. Sci. USA* 77:3659–3667, 1980.

50. Slaga, T., Fischer, S.M., Weeks, C.E., Nelson, K., Mamrack, M., and Klein-Santo, A.J.P. Specificity and

mechanisms of promoter inhibitors in multistage carcinogenesis. In *Carcinogenesis*, Vol. 7, E. Heckler, N.E. Fusenig, W. Kunz, F. Marks, and H.W. Theilmann (Eds.), Academic Press, New York, pp. 19–34, 1982.

51.   Stanbridge, E.J. Suppression of malignancy in human cells. *Nature 260*:17–20, 1976.

52.   Stanbridge, E.J., and Cavenee, W.K. Heritable cancer and tumor suppressor genes: A tentative connection. In *Oncogenes and the Molecular Origins of Cancer*, R.A. Weinberg (Ed.), Cold Spring Harbor Press, New York, pp. 281–306, 1989.

53.   Stanbridge, E.J., Flandemeyer, R.R., Daniels, D.W., and Nelson-Rees, W.A. Specific chromosome loss associated with the expression of tumorigenicity in human cell hybrids. *Somat. Cell Mol. Genet. 7*:699–712, 1981.

54.   Stehelin, D., Varmus, H.E., Bishop, J.M., and Vogt, P.K. DNA related to the transforming gene(s) of avian sarcoma viruses is present in normal avian DNA. *Nature 260*:170–173, 1976.

55.   Tabin, C.J., Bradley, S.M., Bergman, C.I., Weinberg, R.A., Papageorge, A.G., Scalnick, E.M., Dhar, R., Lowy, D.R., and Chang, E.H. Mechanisms of activation of a human oncogene. *Nature 300*:143–149, 1982.

56.   Weitzman, S., and Stossel, T.P. Effects of oxygen radical scavengers and antioxidants on phagocyte-induced mutagenesis. *J. Immunol. 128*:2770–2772, 1982.

57.   Wellingham, M.C., Pastin, I., Shik, T.Y., and Scolnick, E.M. Localization of the ras gene product of the Harvey strain of MSV to plasma membrane of transformed cells by electron microscopic immunocytochemistry. *Cell 19*:1005–1014, 1980.

58.   Whyte, P., Buchovich, K.J., Horowitz, J.M., Friend, S.H., Raybuck, M., Weinberg, R.A., and Harlow, E. Association between an oncogene and an anti-oncogene: The adenovirus EIA proteins bind to the retinoblastoma gene product. *Nature 334*:124–129, 1988.

59.   Witkin, E.M. Ultraviolet mutagenesis and inducible DNA repair in *Escherichia coli*. *Bacteriol. Rev. 40*:869–907, 1976.

45

Phakomatoses and Neurocristopathies

José A. Sahel
Clinique Ophtalmologique, Hôpitaux Universitaires, Strasbourg, France

Daniel M. Albert
University of Wisconsin—Madison, Madison, Wisconsin

I. INTRODUCTION

The phakomatoses are a varied group of diseases having in common disseminated tumorlike malformations [77,78] consisting of those tissues components normally found at the involved site (hamartomas) [2,83]. The hamartomas are usually congenital and involve particularly the central nervous system (CNS), retina, and skin. The label "phakomatoses" was introduced by van der Hoeve and derived from the Greek root for "mother spot," or birthmark. Van der Hoeve substituted the term "phakoma" in preference to the designation "nevus," which pathologists applied to these conditions until then [69,70]. Van der Hoeve included three entities under this designation: angiomatosis retinae, neurofibromatosis, and tuberous sclerosis.

Subsequently, encephalotrigeminal angiomatosis (Sturge-Weber syndrome), ataxia telangiectasia, and Wyburn-Mason syndrome were added to the phakomatoses. Other disorders, including Klippel-Trenaunay syndrome (a rare condition usually affecting one extremity, characterized by hypertrophy of the bone and related soft tissues, large cutaneous hemangiomas, nevus flammeus, and skin varices) and nevus sebaceous of Jadassohn, are included among the phakomatoses by some authors [1,51]. Except for Sturge-Weber syndrome, these disorders are transmitted as autosomal dominant or recessive (ataxia telangiectasia) traits.

Bolande [9] emphasized the wide distribution and multipotential nature of the migratory derivatives of the neural crest and their susceptibilities to teratogenic, oncogenic, and mutagenic influences. He has coined the term "neurocristopathies' to emphasize his conviction that neuroblastoma, von Recklinghausen's disease (neurofibromatosis), pheochromocytoma, medullary carcinoma of the thyroid, carcinoid tumors, Hirschprung's disease, and syndromes involving combinations of these abnormalities arise from aberrations in the early migration, growth, and differentiation of neural crest cells. He notes that because of the extremely variable and complex forms of Recklinghausen's disease, all of which can be pathogenetically related to primary dysontogenesis of the primitive neuroectoderm and its neural crest derivatives, Recklinghausen's neurofibromatosis represents "a most pivotal and dramatic representative" of the neurocristopathy concept [9].

II. VON HIPPEL-LINDAU DISEASE

Although ophthalmologists described the fundus appearance of angiomatosis retinae soon after the invention of the ophthalmoscope, von Hippel recognized angiomatosis retinae as a clinical entity in 1904 [73]. A Swedish neurologist, Lindau, in a subsequent neuropathological survey of cerebellar cysts, noted that many patients with hemangiomatous cysts of the cerebellum also had retinal angiomatosis [43]. The combination of retinal angiomatosis plus cerebellar hemangioblastomas has since been given the eponym von Hippel-Lindau disease, and the designation von Hippel's disease has been applied when only the retina is involved.

The average age at which the retinal lesions become apparent is 25 years, although one-fourth of cases have been described in the pediatric age group. About 20% of published cases have been familial, the disorder being transmitted in an autosomal dominant fashion with irregular penetrance [25]. Retinal angiomas are bilateral in 50% of cases, with cerebellar hemangioblastomas in 20% of affected individuals [77,78].

The typical lesion of the fundus is a two- to three-disk diameter, rounded, yellow to red mass usually associated with large dilated and tortuous feeder vessels. These lesions occur in any area of the retina but are most commonly located in the periphery. Fluorescein angiography distinguishes the vein from the arteriole and demonstrates continuous leakage from the angioma. This extravasation leads to retinal hemorrhages and exudates and, ultimately, the formation of organized fibroglial bands, gliosis, and retinal detachment [27]. Iris neovascularization, secondary angle-closure glaucoma, and eventually phthisis bulbi commonly develop. Systemic involvement includes most prominently the cerebellar "hemangioblastoma," which tends to become symptomatic during the fourth decade of life [80]. Less frequently, these vascular lesions occur in the medulla oblongata, upper spinal cord, and other parts of the CNS. Cysts of the kidney, pancreas, and epididymis may occur, and hypernephromas and pheochromocytomas have been described [15]. Melanocytic nevi and café-au-lait spots have been observed in some patients but are not considered an integral part of the disorder.

The basic vascular lesion in this disorder, whether in the retina or the cerebellum, is an angioma. By light microscopy it contains plump lipid-containing stromal cells surrounding capillaries. These cells appear vacuolated in routinely processed specimens and are regarded as endothelial cells, macrophages, nearoglia pseudoxanthomatous cells, or stromal cells. Solid lesions composed of masses of angioblastic cells occur as well and appear to have more growth potential than the lesions composed of capillary spaces [4]. The syndrome must be differentiated from Coats' disease, in which multifocal, sporadic unilateral telangiectases are present without systemic involvement. The mutant gene responsible for the von Hippel-Lindau syndrome has been localized to the short arm of chromosome 3 (3p26-p25) [30].

Of all of the phakomatoses von Hippel-Lindau syndrome is the most amenable to treatment, with regard to both CNS and ocular involvement. Goldberg and colleagues have described effective treatment of retinal lesions using photocoagulation, diathermy, cryocoagulation, and argon laser photocoagulation [4,31].

III. MULTIPLE NEUROFIBROMATOSIS (VON RECKLINGHAUSEN'S DISEASE OF NERVES)

Multiple neurofibromatosis (von Recklinghausen's disease of nerves) was described by the German pathologist von Recklinghausen in 1882 [74]. This systemic condition is characterized by a diffuse proliferation of the Schwann cells of the peripheral nerves and in many cases by astrocytes and/or meningeal cells of the CNS. Although most of the tumors are initially benign, a superimposed malignant change (fibrosarcoma, neurofibrosarcoma, or malignant schwannoma) may occur. Lesions may be present at birth or develop in infancy, although hamartomas do not usually become symptomatic until late in childhood or in adult life [23].

Neurofibromatosis is now subclassified into two different autosomal dominant disorders [48,52]. Neurofibromatosis type 1, or peripheral neurofibromatosis, has an incidence of 1 in 4000 births, the gene defect mapping to the long arm of chromosome 17 (17q11) [2,76]. Neurofibromatosis type 2 (central neurofibromatosis) has an incidence of 1 in 50,000 births, the gene defect mapping to chromosome 22. Neurofibromatosis type 2 is characterized by bilateral acoustic neuromas, multiple CNS tumors (meningiomas, gliomas, and schwannomas), and posterior subcapsular cataracts. Neurofibromatosis type 1 is seen more often than type 2 by ophthalmologists.

Ocular lesions may occur in the eyelid, the globe, the optic nerve, or the orbit. The complete triad of cutaneous manifestations consisting of café-au-lait spots, fibroma molluscum, and plexiform neuromas may affect the eyelids in neurofibromatosis type 1.

Café-au-lait spots are pigmented macular lesions of the skin with ill-defined, serrated edges caused by hyperpigmentation of the basal cell layer, which on histopathological examination corresponds to an increased number of melanocytes. Frecklelike spots, or pigmented nevi, are also frequently associated with the café-au-lait spots. Such lesions commonly occur on the trunk and may be the only clinical evidence of the disease (*forme fruste*). They develop in 10% of the population, but patients with six or more café-au-lait spots exceeding 1.5 cm in diameter usually have von Recklinghausen's disease type 1.

Fibroma molluscum, a common form of neurofibroma, is a pedunculated pigmented nodule composed of enlarged cutaneous nerves with a proliferation of Schwann cells and other connective tissue elements. The plexiform neuroma ("bag of worms") consists of enlarged nerves surrounded by thickened perineural sheaths. An additional cutaneous manifestation known as elephantiasis neuromatosa is characterized by a diffuse proliferation of the cellular elements of the nerve sheath, resulting in a marked thickening and folding of the skin.

Lesions of the globe include prominently thickened corneal and conjunctival nerves [71] and pigmented nodules of the iris. These so-called Lisch nodules are histologically indistinguishable from nevi located at the anterior border or deeper in the stroma of the iris [11,25,81].

Additional ocular lesions include diffuse neurofibromas of the uvea, particularly of the choroid (Fig. 1), localized or diffuse uveal melanocytosis, and astrocytomas of the retina and optic nerve [47,61]. An increased incidence of uveal melanomas among neurofibromatosis patients has been reported [63].

Hamartomas may occur in the trabecular meshwork, and Grant and Walton [32] observed unilateral congenital glaucoma in about 50% of patients with visible or palpable plexiform neuromas of the eyelid and ipsilateral hemihypertrophy of the face. Three mechanisms have been postulated to explain the glaucoma that may occur in Recklinghausen's disease: (1) obstruction to the outflow of aqueous humor by neurofibromatous tissue or by a developmental anomaly in the anterior chamber angle, (2) closure of the anterior chamber angle by a hamartoma involving the ciliary body and anterior choroid, and (3) a secondary fibrovascular membrane in the aqueous outflow angle and the formation of peripheral anterior synechiae secondary to iris neovascularization. The astrocytic hamartomas, which may occur in the retina, are localized to the ganglion cell and nerve fiber layers and do not extend beyond the internal limiting

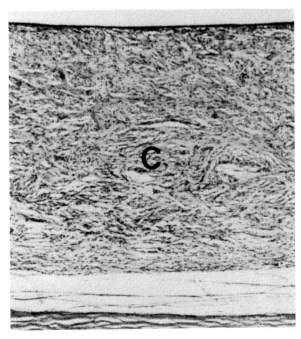

Figure 1 Diffuse choroidal lesion (C) from a patient with neurofibromatosis is composed of neural elements and melanocytes. (Hematoxylin and eosin, ×55)

membrane. They are benign and identical to the tumor seen in this location in patients with tuberous sclerosis. Approximately 10–15% of primary tumors of the optic nerve are associated with neuro-fibromatosis [25,77,78].

Orbital manifestations include plexiform neurofibromas, which may cause unilateral exophthalmos, as well as enlarge the orbit, and bony defects, such as an absence of the greater wing of the sphenoid or of the orbital roof. Intracranial tissue herniating into the orbit through a bony defect can produce a pulsating exophthalmos. More unusual is enophthalmos secondary to incomplete development of the orbital walls. Schwannomas (neurilemmomas) of the orbit sometimes develop, and enlargement of the optic foramen may accompany an astrocytoma of the optic nerve [27,77,78].

Systemic findings in neurofibromatosis include hamartomas of the brain, spinal cord, meninges, cranial and peripheral nerves, sympathetic nervous system, and gastrointestinal tract, as well as of other viscera. Occasionally, pheochromocytomas or medullary thyroid carcinomas may occur [51].

The neoplasms in the skin and orbit consist of a diffuse irregular proliferation of peripheral nerve elements, most notably Schwann cells, which results in encapsulated neurofibromas. Microscopically, these tumors are composed of cells with elongated basophilic nuclei and granular cytoplasm, associated with collagen fibers. Nerve fibers can frequently be distinguished with special stains.

IV. TUBEROUS SCLEROSIS (BOURNEVILLE'S DISEASE)

In 1880, Bourneville, a French physician, drew attention to a 15-year-old mentally retarded girl with epilepsy and the apparent cutaneous lesions of adenoma sebaceum (actually angiofibroma). At postmortem examination she was found to have multiple sclerotic nodules in the cerebral cortex and similar masses protruding into the ventricles. Noting the "potatolike" character of the lesions, Bourneville applied the term "tuberous sclerosis" to the disease [10].

Symptoms usually begin during the first 3 years of life, the triad of mental deficiency, seizures, and adenoma sebaceum being characteristic [19]. The disease occurs both in an autosomal dominant form and in a sporadic form, having a mutation rate of approximately 1:60,000 [19]. The gene responsible for one genetic form of tuberous sclerosis has been mapped to chromosomes 9 (9q34) close to the ABO blood group locus and 11 (11q22-23) [37,57,65,66]. There is no sex or racial predilection. Although the classic descriptions of tuberous sclerosis include mental deficiency, in some series, particularly those not based on patients from institutions for the mentally defective, as many as 38% of patients are of normal intelligence [40]. Tuberous sclerosis is transmitted as an irregular autosomal dominant trait with low penetrance, and approximately 75% of patients die before the third decade of life.

Among the systemic manifestations of tuberous sclerosis is the shagreen patch of the skin, usually located on the back. Congenital hypomelanotic macules ("ash leaf" lesions) are present on the trunk and limbs in 86% of patients. They can be demonstrated with a Wood's light and are an important early diagnostic sign of tuberous sclerosis [24]. Normal skin shows a uniform dark coloration under the Wood's light because of the absorption of blue light by melanin. The ash leaf lesions show a lighter coloration, presumably because of the lesser degree of melanization. Other cutaneous lesions include nevi, periungual fibromas, and café-au-lait spots. Hamartomas of the heart, thyroid, and kidney, as well as spina bifida, ectopic testes, and horseshoe kidneys, may develop. Subependymal giant cell astrocytomas can occur. Astrocytic hamartomas of the brain, which account for epilepsy and mental deficiency, calcify in more than half of the cases ("brain stones") and can be demonstrated radiologically.

Ocular findings [6,25,26,54,85] consist of angiofibromas of the eyelids, white pedunculated tumors of the palpebral conjunctiva, and yellowish red thickenings of the bulbar conjunctiva. Astrocytic hamartomas occur in the retina as gray-white tumors that with time and probably because of dystrophic calcification develop a nodular appearance like a mulberry [49]. Initially, when these lesions are smooth in appearance, they may resemble retinoblastomas. The tumors may be solitary or multiple and, although usually located near the nerve head, may occur anywhere in the retina [3,11,16,85].

In addition, glial hamartomas of the optic disk may develop anterior to the lamina cribrosa. Although referred to as giant drusen, these lesions should not be confused with the ordinary drusen of the optic disk or Bruch's membrane or with a true glioma [33,34,78].

The retinal and optic nerve astrocytic hamartomas are composed of elongated, fibrous astrocytes containing small, oval nuclei with fine, interlacing cytoplasmic processes. The retinal tumors are limited to the nerve fiber and ganglion cell layers and do not extend beyond the internal limiting membrane or infiltrate other structures [3,45,60]. The astrocytomas arising from the optic nerve tend to calcify, and osseous metaplasia of the adjacent pigment epithelium often occurs (Fig. 2). It should be noted that astrocytic hamartomas can occur as isolated lesions [3,16,33–36,45,55,58,59]. These lesions may be difficult to differentiate from localized forms of "massive" retinal gliosis and from retinoblastomas [17,62, 63,72,84].

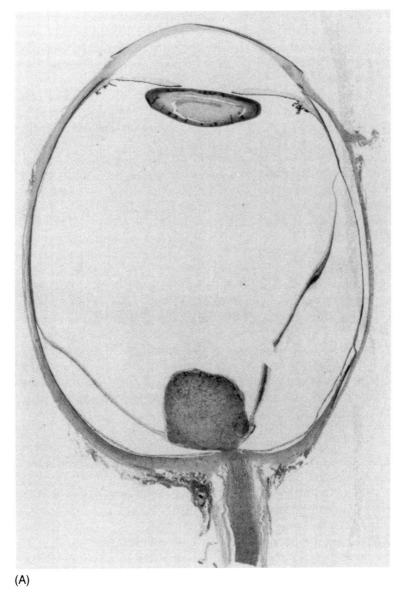

(A)

Figure 2   (A) Astrocytoma arising from the retina of a patient with tuberous sclerosis. (Hematoxylin and eosin, ×4.2) (B) Higher power view, showing pattern of growth of astrocytic hamartoma. (Hematoxylin and eosin, ×200) (C) Isolated astrocytoma of the retina. Note that the tumor is limited to the retina and remains within the confines of the internal limiting membrane. (Hematoxylin and eosin, ×40) (D) Higher power view showing elongated, fibrous astrocytes with small, oval nuclei and a delicate meshwork of interlacing cytoplasmic processes merging with normal retina. (Hematoxylin and eosin, ×40)

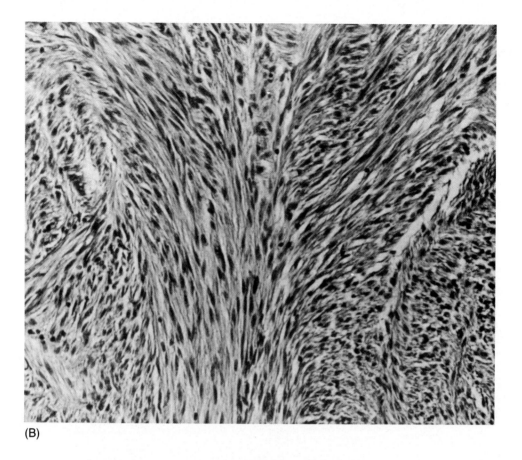

(B)

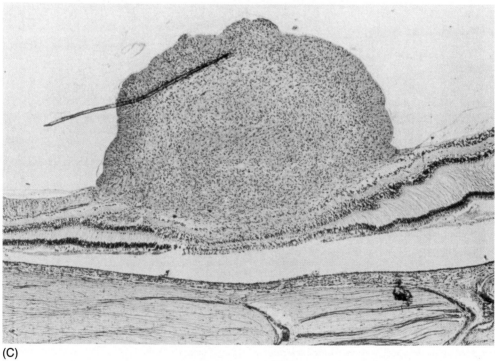

(C)

Figure 2 Continued

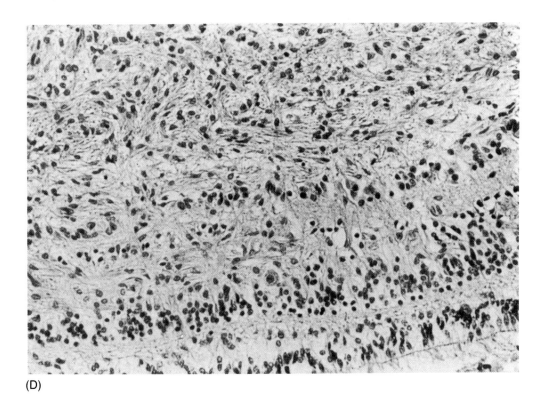

(D)

In the older literature, the symmetrically distributed, small reddish angiofibromas of the face were incorrectly referred to as "adenoma sebaceum" of Pringle. Nickel and Reed [53] demonstrated that the sebaceous glands in these lesions are generally atrophic, and the main findings are dermal fibrosis because of the large size and stellate shape of the fibroblasts. In older lesions, perifollicular proliferation of collagen may be seen, leading to the compression of atrophic hair follicles. Elastic tissue is lacking in angiofibromas.

V. ENCEPHALOTRIGEMINAL ANGIOMATOSIS (STURGE-WEBER SYNDROME)

In 1879, Sturge [67] described a clinical syndrome consisting of unilateral buphthalmos, homolateral facial hemangioma, and contralateral focal epilepsy. His postulate of an intracranial hemangioma was confirmed by Kalischer in 1897 [77,78], several years after choroidal hemangiomas became recognized by Jenning-Mills in 1884 [38]. The complete syndrome of encephalotrigeminal angiomatosis was described by Weber in 1922 [79] and, as now recognized, includes an intracranial and facial hemangioma with an ipsilateral choroidal hemangioma (Fig. 3) and congenital glaucoma. Incomplete forms of the syndrome are more frequently seen, however, but according to Reese [58], at least two of these lesions must be present to warrant the diagnosis.

Although instances of the entire triad of Sturge-Weber syndrome are not known to occur in more than one member of a family, familial examples of certain features of the syndrome have been reported [75]. There does not appear to be a significant sexual or racial predilection for this disease [26].

In about 40% of patients a choroidal hemangioma occurs on the side of the facial angioma, appearing as a yellowish, slightly elevated circular area with indiscrete margins [20,21,29]. Of all reported choroidal hemangiomas, about 50% have been in patients with Sturge-Weber syndrome [20,27]. Episcleral hemangioma is suggestive of uveal involvement. A cavernous hemangioma or telangiectasis of the eyelids on the side of the facial angioma is common and frequently associated with congenital glaucoma.

In about 30% of cases the glaucoma is associated with hemangiomas of the facial skin. Although the exact mechanism by which glaucoma develops is unknown, the following possibilities are listed by Font and Ferry [25]: (1) occlusion of the chamber angle by peripheral anterior synechiae, and (2) malformation

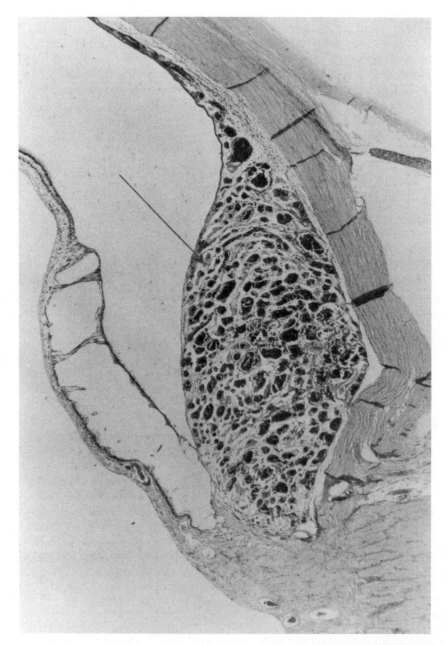

Figure 3   Juxtapapillary cavernous hemangioma arising in choroid. (Hematoxylin and eosin, ×60)

of the chamber angle with an anterior insertion of the longitudinal muscle of the ciliary body on the base of the trabecular meshwork and incomplete cleavage of the chamber angle with persistence of the uveal part on the meshwork. They also speculated concerning other possible causes: (1) vascular malformations in the episclera and limbal conjunctiva, which may impede the outflow of aqueous; (2) the "plethoric glaucoma" theory, which presumes that the elevated intraocular pressure results from the increased permeability of the thin-walled vessels of the choroidal tumor; and (3) hypersecretion of aqueous from the ciliary body associated with either the facial angioma or neural influences resulting from involvement of the trigeminal nerve. Other theories from the older literature are reviewed by Hogan and Zimmerman [32].

Systemic manifestations include disseminated angiomas and nevi, varices of the legs and arms, and café-au-lait spots [42]. Homolateral angiomas of the meninges may be associated with neurological signs, including epilepsy, hemiplegia, and mental retardation. The frequently occurring intracranial calcifications may be observed on roentgenographical examination of the skull ("railroad track sign").

Microscopic examination of the port-wine nevus of the skin reveals dilated capillaries in the epidermis, dermis, and subcutaneous tissue [42]. It should be noted that although the facial angioma is present at birth, telangiectases first become apparent histologically in patients at about 10 years of age. This may result from congenital weakness of the capillary walls. The intracranial hemangioma is characteristically of the racemose type and most often involves the meninges overlying the cerebral hemispheres [25]. Secondary changes, commonly observed in enucleated eyes, include microcystoid degeneration of the retina overlying a hemangioma, leakage of serous fluid into the subretinal space, and retinal detachment (Fig. 3) [25]. Cases of retinal cavernous hemangiomas with skin angiomas and seizures have been recognized by several authors as a different systemic hamartomatosis [50]. Isolated peripheral hemangiomas or telangiectases have been reported, but without histopathological documentation [13,64].

VI. ATAXIA-TELANGIECTASIA (LOUIS-BAR SYNDROME)

In 1941, Louis-Bar described a 9-year-old boy with progressive cerebellar ataxia and bilateral oculocutaneous telangiectasia. Boder and Sedgewick subsequently studied additional cases of this entity, documenting the clinical features and establishing it as one of the phakomatoses [7,8]. In the intervening 50 years the syndrome has been more fully elucidated [14]. Louis-Bar syndrome now includes (1) progressive cerebellar ataxia with degeneration of Purkinje's cells [56]; (2) hypersensitivity of fibroblasts and lymphocytes to ionizing radiation; (3) an extremely high cancer incidence [68] (61-fold in whites and 186-fold in blacks); (4) thymic hypoplasia with humoral immunodeficiencies involving IgA and IgG_2 [22]; (5) nonrandom chromosomal rearrangements in lymphocytes occurring at the sites responsible for the assembly of the genes required for the synthesis of antibodies and T cell antigen receptors [14]; (6) autosomal recessive transmission with gene (among possible multiple genes) located on the 11q22-23 chromosomal region [28]; (7) elevated serum level of α-fetoprotein; (8) premature aging; (9) endocrine disorders, such as insulin-resistant diabetes mellitus; (10) cutaneous telangiectasis (ears, face, and extensor surfaces of both extremities); and (11) bilateral bulbar conjunctival telangiectasis (all cases). Oculomotor apraxia and various abnormalities of ocular movements are frequent.

More than half the patients with this disease die from recurrent pulmonary infections. This disorder appears as a consequence of a defect in DNA repair.

VII. WYBURN-MASON SYNDROME

In 1943, Wyburn-Mason described markedly dilated and tortuous retinal vessels projecting forward from the retina in association with similar ipsilateral lesions of the midbrain [82]. The type of retinal arteriovenous malformations occurring in this syndrome were appreciated, however, long before Wyburn-Mason's report [85]. In a study of 27 known cases of retinal arteriovenous aneurysm, before the general use of cerebral angiography, Wyburn-Mason documented clinical evidence of a similar lesion within the brain of 22 patients (81%). Conversely, he found a retinal arteriovenous aneurysm in 14 of 20 cases (70%) with similar vascular anomalies in the midbrain. In a subsequent study (in which the diagnosis of intracranial hemagioma was accepted only when it could be demonstrated by angiography, operation, or autopsy), Beck and Jensen found an intracranial arteriovenous aneurysm coexisting with similar lesions in the retina in only 17% of patients [5]. The vascular lesion involving the retina and CNS in this disorder, which has been termed both a racemose hemangioma and a cirsoid aneurysm, is congenital and nonprogressive, with symptoms usually appearing before 30 years of age. The fully developed clinical picture accompanying the arteriovenous communication of the midbrain and retina is associated with pulsatile vascular lesions in the distribution of the trigeminal nerve and more rarely in other parts of the body. In addition, hemifacial hemangiomas have occasionally been associated (Bonnet-Duchaume-Blanc syndrome) [41]. Neurological signs and symptoms result from compression of structures by an intracranial arteriovenous malformation or from hemorrhage or infarction. Hydrocephalus from compression of the sylvian aqueduct, and occasionally visual symptoms, occur secondary to posterior cerebral artery involvement. Less frequently described manifestations have been seizures, delirium, disorientation, hallucinations, somnolence, sleep inversion, and mental retardation [41]. The ophthalmoscopic picture is that of dilated, tortuous retinal vessels projecting forward from the retina, the arterioles and veins being similar in appearance. Vision may be normal or severely impaired, depending on the location of the retinal vascular malformation.

Aside from these retinal vascular abnormalities and the associated visual impairment, strabismus, gaze palsies, diplopia, pulsating exophthalmos, ptosis, cutaneous hemangiomas of the face, epilepsy, intracranial hemorrhage, and intracranial calcification can occur [83].

VIII. NEVUS SEBACEUS OF JADASSOHN

The nevus sebaceus of Jadassohn [18,39] was recently added to the heterogeneous group of conditions included among the phakomatoses. This disorder has cerebral malformations (arachnoid cysts, hydrocephaly, and cortical atrophy), adnexal cutaneous tumors, and various ocular choristomas [46]. Uveal colobomas and hemangiomas within the sclera may be present.

REFERENCES

1. Adams, R.D., and Reed, W.B. Neurocutaneous diseases. In *Dermatology in General Medicine*, T.B. Fitzpatrick, K.A. Arndt, W.H. Clark, J.R., A.Z. Eisen, E.J. van Scott, and J.H. Vaughan (Eds.), McGraw-Hill, New York, pp. 1393–1396, 1971.
2. Albrecht-Munchen. Ueber Hamartome. *Verh. Dtsch. Pathol. Ges. Jena 7*:153–157, 1904.
3. Apple, D.J., and Boniuk, M. Clinical pathological review: Solitary retinal astrocytoma. *Surv. Ophthalmol. 30*:173–191, 1985.
4. Augsburger, J.J., Shields, J.A., and Goldberg, R.E. Classification and management of hereditary retinal angiomas. *Int. Ophthalmol. 4*:93–106, 1981.
5. Beck, K., Jensen, O.A. On the frequency of co-existing racemose haemangiomata of the retina and brain. *Acta Psychiatr. Scand. 36*:47–56, 1961.
6. Binaghi, M., Coscas, G., and Nucci, T. Les phacomes retiniens. *J. Fr. Ophtalmol. 6*:275–290, 1983.
7. Boder, E. and Sedgewick, R.P. Ataxia telangiectasis. *Univ. South. Calif. Med. Bull. 9*:15–27, 1957.
8. Boder, E., and Sedgewick, R.P. Ataxia telangiectasis. A familial syndrome of progressive cerebellar ataxia, oculocutaneous telangiectasia and frequent pulmonary infections. *Pediatrics 21*:525–554, 1958.
9. Bolande, R.P. The neurocristopathies. A unifying concept of disease arising in neural crest malformations. *Hum. Pathol. 5*:409–429, 1974.
10. Bourneville, D.M. Sclerose tubereuse des circonvolutions cerebrales: Idiotie et epilepsie hemiplegique. *Arch. Neurol. 1*:69–91, 1980.
11. Brini, A., Dhermy, P., and Sahel, J.A. *Oncology of the Eye and Adnexa*, Kluwer, Dordrecht NL, 1990.
12. Brown, G.C., and Shields, J.A. Tumors of the optic nerve head. *Surv. Ophthalmol. 29*:239–264, 1985.
13. Campochiaro, A., and Conway, B.P. Hemangiomalike masses of the retina. *Arch. Ophthalmol. 106*:1409–1413, 1988.
14. Carbonari, M., Cherchi, M., Paganelli, R., Giannini, G., Galli, E., Gaetano, C., Papetti, C., and Fiorilli, M. Relative increase of T cells expressing the gamma/delta rather than the alpha/beta receptor in ataxia-telangiectasia. *N. Engl. J. Med. 322*:73–6, 1990.
15. Chapman, R.C., and Diaz-Perez, R. Pheochromocytomas may be associated with cerebellar hemangioblastoma. *JAMA 182*:1014–1017, 1962.
16. Cleasby, G.W., Fung, W.E., and Shekter, W.B. Astrocytoma of the retina: Report of two cases. *Am. J. Ophthalmol. 64*:633–637, 1967.
17. Dejean, C. Le vrai gliome de la retine adulte. *Arch. Ophtalmol. (Paris) 51*:257–276, 1934.
18. Diven, D.G., Solomon, A.R., McNeeley, M.C., and Font, R.L. Nevus sebaceous associated with major ophthalmologic abnormalities. *Arch. Dermatol. 123*:383–386, 1987.
19. Donegi, G., Grattarola, F.R., and Wildie, H. Tuberous sclerosis: Bourneville disease. In *Handbook of Clinical Neurology*, Vol. 14, P.J. Vinken and G.W. Bruyn (Eds.), Elsevier, New York, pp. 340–349, 1972.
20. Duke-Elder, S. *Diseases of the Uveal Tract. System of Ophthalmology*, Vol. 9, C.V. Mosby, St. Louis, pp. 775–937, 1966.
21. Duke-Elser, S. *Diseases of the Lens and Vitreous: Glaucoma and Hypotony. System of Ophthalmology*, Vol. 11, C.V. Mosby, St. Louis, pp. 637–640, 1969.
22. Eisen, A.H., Karpati, G., Laszlo, T., Andermann, F., Robb, J.P., and Bacal, H.L. Immunologic deficiency in ataxia telangiectasia. *N. Engl. J. Med. 272*:18–22, 1965.
23. Fienman, N.L., and Yakovac, W.C. Neurofibromatosis in childhood. *J. Pediatr. 76*:339–346, 1970.

24. Fitzpatrick, T.B., Szabo, G., Hori, Y., Simone, A.A., Reed, W.B., and Greenberg, M.H. White leaf-shaped macules: Earliest sign of tuberous sclerosis. *Arch. Dermatol.* 98:1–6, 1968.

25. Font, F.R., and Ferry, A.P. The phakomatoses. *Int. Ophthalmol. Clin.* 12:1–50, 1972.

26. Francois, J. Ocular aspects of the phakomatoses. In *Handbook of Clinical Neurology*, Vol. 14, P.J. Vinken and G.W. Bruyn (Eds.), Elsevier, New York, pp. 689–732, 1972.

27. Gass, J.D., and Braunstein, R. Sessile and exophytic capillary angiomas of the juxtapapillary retina and optic nerve head. *Arch. Ophthalmol.* 98:1790–1797, 1980.

28. Gatti, R.A., Berkel, I., Boder, E., Braedt, G., Charmley, P., Connannon, P., Ersoy, F., Foroud, T., Jaspers, N.G.J., Lange, K., Lathrop, G.M., Leppert, M., Nakakuma, Y., O'Connell, P., Paterson, M., Salser, W., Sanal, O., Silver, J., Sparkes, R.S., Susi, E., Weeks, D.E., Wei, S., White, R., and Yoder, F. Localization of an ataxia-telangiectasia gene to chromosome 11q22-23. *Nature* 336:577–580, 1988.

29. Giuffre, G. Cavernous hemangioma of the retina and retinal telangiectasis. Distinct or related vascular malformations. *Retina* 5:221–224, 1985.

30. Glenn, G.M., Linehan, W.M., Hosoe, S., Latif, F., Yao, M., Choyke, P., Goria, M.B., Chew, E., Oldsfield, E., Manolatos, C., Orcutt, M.L., Walther, M.M., Weiss, G.H., Tory, K., Jensson, O., Lerman, M.I., and Zbar, B. Screening for von Hippel-Lindau by DNA polymorphism analysis. *JAMA* 267:1226–1231, 1992.

31. Goldberg, M.L. Clinico-pathologic correlation of von Hippel angiomas after xenon arc and argon laser photo-coagulation. In *Intraocular Tumors*, G.A. Peyman, J.D. Apple, and D.R. Saunders (Eds.), Appleton-Century-Crofts, New York, pp. 219–234, 1977.

32. Grant, W.M., and Walton, D.S. Distinctive findings in glaucoma due to neurofibromatosis. *Arch. Ophthalmol.* 79:127–134, 1968.

33. Green, W.R. The Retina. In *Ophthalmic Pathology: An Atlas and Textbook*, 3rd ed., W.H. Spencer (Ed.), W.B. Saunders, Philadelphia, pp. 589–1291, 1986.

34. Hogan, M.G., and Zimmerman, L.E. *Ophthalmic Pathology: An Atlas and Textbook*, 2nd ed., W.B. Saunders, Philadelphia, pp 433–607, 1962.

35. Huggert, A., and Hultquist, G.F. True glioma of the retina. *Ophthalmology* 113:193–202, 160.

36. Jakobiec, F.A., Brodie, S.E., Haik, B., and Iwamoto, T. Giant cell astrocytoma. A tumor of possible Mueller cell origin. *Ophthalmology* 90:1565–1575, 1983.

37. Janssen, L.A.J., Povey, S., Attwood, J., Sandkuyl, L.A., Lindout, D., Flodman, P., Smith, M., Sampson, J.R., Haines, J.L., Merkens, E.C., Flery, P., Short, P., Amos, J., and Halley, D.J.J. A comparative study on genetic heterogeneity in tuberous sclerosis: Evidence for one gene on 9q34 and a second on 11q22-23: Tuberous sclerosis an allied diseases. *Ann. NY Acad. Sci.* 615:306–315, 1991.

38. Jenning-Milles, W. Nevus of the right temporal and orbital region: Nevus of the choroid and detachment of the retina in the right eye. *Trans. Ophthalmol. Soc. UK* 4:168–171, 1884.

39. Katz, B., Wiley, C.A., and Lee, V.W. Optic nerve hypoplasia and the syndrome of nevus sebaceous of Jadassohn. *Ophthalmology* 94:1570–1576, 1987.

40. Lagos, J.C., and Gomez, M.R. Tuberous sclerosis. Reappraisal of a clinical entity. *Mayo Clin. Proc.* 42:26–49, 1967.

41. Lecuire, J., Duchaume, J.B., and Bret, P. Bonnet-Duchaume-Blanc syndrome. In *Handbook of Clinical Neurology*, 14 P.J. Vinken and G.W. Bruyn (Eds.), Elsevier, New York, pp. 280–315, 1978.

42. Lever, W.F., and Schumburg-Lever, G. *Histopathology of the Skin*, 5th ed., J.B. Lippincott, Philadelphia, 1975.

43. Lindau, A. Zur Frage der angiomatosis retinae und ihrer Hirnkomplikationen. *Acta Ophthalmol. (Copenh.)* 4:193–226, 1927.

44. Louis-Bar, D. Sur un syndrome progressif comprenant des telangiectasies capillaires cutanees et conjonctivales symetriques depostion navoide et des troubles cerebelleux. *Confina. Neurol.* 4:32–42, 1941.

45. McLean, J.M. Astrocytoma (true glioma) of the retina. *Arch. Ophthalmol.* 18:255–262, 1937.

46. Mansour, A.M., Laibson, P.D., Reinicke, R.D., Henkind, P., and Mikati, M. Bilateral total corneal and conjunctival choristomas associated with epidermal nevus. *Arch. Ophthalmol.* 104:245–248, 1986.

47. Marshall, D. Glioma of the optic nerve as a manifestation of von Recklinghausen's disease. *Trans. Am. Ophthalmol. Soc.* 51:117–155, 1953.

48. Martuza, R.L., and Elridge, R. Neurofromatosis 2 (bilateral acoustic neurofibromatosis). *N. Engl. J. Med.* 318:686, 1988.

49. Martyn, L. Tuberous sclerosis of Bourneville. In *Retinal Diseases of Children*, W. Tasman (Ed.), Harper and Row, New York, pp. 98–101, 1971.

50. Messmer, E., Laqua, H., Wessing, A., Spitznas, M., Weidle, E., Ruprecht, K., and Naumann, G. Nine cases of cavernous hemangioma of the retina. *Am. J. Ophthalmol.* 95:383–390, 1983.

51. Miller, N.R. The phakomatoses. In *Clinical Neuro-Ophthalmology*, 4th ed., Vol. II, Williams and Wilkins, Baltimore, pp. 1747–1827, 1988.

52. National Institutes of Health Consensus Development Conference. Neurofibromatosis conference statement. *Arch. Neurol.* 45:575–578, 1988.

53. Nickel, W.R., and Reed, W.B. Tuberous sclerosis. Special reference to microscopic alterations in cutaneous hamartomas. *Arch. Dermatol.* 89:209–226, 1962.

54. Nyboer, J.H., Robertson, D.M., and Gonney, M.R. Retinal lesions in tuberous sclerosis. *Arch. Ophthalmol.* 94:1277–1280, 1976.

55. Paufique, L., Audibert, J., and Laurent, C. Le gliome de la retine. Notions genetiques, anatomiques et cliniques. Etat actuel du traitement. *J. Med. Lyon 41*:1555–1560, 1960.
56. Perry, T.L., Kish, S.J., Hinton, D., Hansen, S., Becker, L.E., and Gelfand, W. Neurochemical abnormalities in a patient with ataxia-telangiectasia. *Neurology 34*:187–126, 1984.
57. Povey, S., Attwood, J., Janssen, L.A.J., Burley, M., Smith, M., Flodman, P., Morton, N.E., Edwards, J.H., Sampson, J.R., Yates, J.R.W., Haines, J.L., Amos, J., Short, M.P., Sandkuyl, L.A., Halley, D.J.J., Fryer, A.E., Bech-Hansen, T., Mueller, R., Al-Ghazali, L., Super, M., and Osborne, J. An attempt to map two genes for tuberous sclerosis using novel two-point methods. Tuberous sclerosis and allied diseases. *Ann. NY Acad. Sci. 615*:298–305, 1991.
58. Reese, A.B. *Tumors of the Eyes*, 3rd ed., Harper and Row, New York, pp. 89–132, 1976.
59. Rosa, D. Contributions to the study of so-called "glioma of the retina." *Boll. Ocul. 40*:492–505, 1961.
60. Rubinstein, L.J. Embryonal central neuroepithelial tumors and their differentiating potential—a cytogenetic view of a complex neurooncological problem. *J. Neurosurg. 62*:795–805, 1985.
61. Russell, D.S., and Rubenstein, L.J. *Pathology of the Nervous System*, 4th ed., Williams and Wilkins, Baltimore, pp. 299–330, 1977.
62. Sahel, J.A., Frederick, A.R., Pesavento, R., and Albert, D.M. Idiopathic retinal gliosis mimicking a choroidal melanoma. *Retina 8*:282–287, 1988.
63. Shields, J.A. *Diagnosis and Management of Intraocular Tumors*, C.V. Mosby, St. Louis, 1983.
64. Shields, J.A., Decker, W.L., Sandorn, G.E., Augsburger, J.J., and Goldberg, R.E. Presumed acquired retinal hemangiomas. *Ophthalmology 90*:1292–1300, 1983.
65. Smith, M., Smalley, S., Cantor, R., Pandolfo, M., Gomez, M.I., Baumann, R., Yoshiyama, K., Nakamura, Y., Julier, C., Dumars, K., Haines, J., Trofatter, M., Spence, A., Weeks, D., and Conneally, M. Mapping of a gene determining tuberous sclerosis to human chromosome 11q14-q23. *Genomics 6*:105–114, 1990.
66. Smith, M., Yoshiyama, K., Wagner, C., Flodman, P., and Smith, B. Genetic heterogeneity in tuberous sclerosis. Map position of the TSC2 locus on chromosome 11q and future prospects. Tuberous sclerosis and allied diseases. *Ann. NY Acad. Sci. 615*:274–283, 1991.
67. Sturge, W.A. A case of partial epilepsy, apparently due to a lesion of one of the vaso-motor centers of the brain. *Trans. Clin. Soc. Lond. 12*:162–167, 1879.
68. Swift, M., Reitnauer, P.J., Morrell, D., and Chase, C.L. Breast and other cancers in families with ataxia-telangiectasia. *N. Engl. J. Med. 316*:1289–94, 1987.
69. Van der Hoeve, T. Eye disease in tuberose sclerosis of the brain and in Recklinghausen's disease. *Trans. Ophthalmol. Soc. UK 43*:534–541, 1923.
70. Van der Hoeve, T. The Doyne Memorial Lecture: Eye symptoms in phakomatoses. *Trans. Ophthalmol. Soc. UK 52*:380–401, 1932.
71. Verhoeff, F.H. Discussion of Snell, S., and Collins, E.T. Plexiform neuroma (elephantiasis neuromatosis) of temporal region, orbit, eyelid and eyeball. Notes of three cases. *Trans. Ophthalmol. Soc. UK 23*:176–177, 1903.
72. Verhoeff, F.H. A rare tumor arising from the pars ciliaris retineas (teratoneuroma) of a nature hitherto unrecognized and its relation to the so-called glioma retinae. *Trans. Am. Ophthalmol. Soc. 10*:351–377, 1904.
73. Von Hippel, E. Uber eine sehr seltene Erkrankung der Netzhaut. *Graefes Arch. Ophthalmol. 59*:83–106, 1904.
74. Von Recklinghausen, F.D. Über die multiplin Fibrome der Haut und ihre Beziehung zu den multiplen Neuromen. Berlin Hirschwald, 1882.
75. Waardenburg, P.J., Franceschetti, A., and Klein, D. *Genetics and Ophthalmology*, Vol. 2, Charles C. Thomas, Springfield, IL, 1963.
76. Wallace, M.R., Marchuk, D.A., Andersen, L.B., Lechter, R., Brereton, A., Nicholson, J., Mitchell, A.L., Brownstein, B.H., and Collins, F.S. Type I neurofibromatosis gene: Identification of a large transcript disrupted in three NF 1 patients. *Science 249*:181–186, 1990.
77. Walsch, F.B., and Hoyt, W.F. *Clinical Neuro-Ophthalmology*, 3rd ed., Williams and Wilkins, Baltimore, pp 1939–1989, 1969.
78. Walsh, F.B., Hoyt, W.F., and Miller, N. *Clinical Neuro-Ophthalmology*, 4th ed., Williams and Wilkins, Baltimore, 1989.
79. Weber, F.P. Right-sided hemihypotrophy resulting from right sided congenital spastic hemiplegia, with a morbid condition of the brain revealed by radiograms. *J. Neurol Psychopathol. 3*:134–139, 1922.
80. Welch, R.B., Von Hippel-Lindau disease: The recognition and treatment of early angiomatosis retinae and the use of cryosurgery as an adjunct to therapy. *Trans. Am. Ophthalmol. Soc. 68*:367–424, 1970.
81. Williamson, T.H., Garner, A., and Moore, A.T. Structure of Lisch nodules in neurofibromatosis type 1. *Ophthal. Pediatr. Genet. 12*:11–17, 1991.
82. Wyburn-Mason, R. Arteriovenous aneurysm of mid-brain and retina, facial naevi and mental changes. *Brain 66*:163–203, 1943.
83. Yanoff, M., and Fine, B.S. *Ocular Pathology: A Text and Atlas*, Harper and Row, New York, pp. 686–698, 1989.
84. Zimmerman, L.E. Retinoblastoma and retinocytoma. In *Ophthalmic Pathology*, W.H. Spencer (Ed.), W.B. Saunders, Philadelphia, pp. 1292–1351, 1985.
85. Zion, V.M. Tuberous sclerosis, Bourneville's disease. In *Clinical Ophthalmology*, Vol. 5, T.D. Duane (Ed.), Harper and Row, New York, pp. 5–6, 1967.

46
Tumors of the Eyelids, Conjunctiva, and Cornea

R. Jean Campbell
Mayo Clinic and Mayo Foundation, and Mayo Medical School, Rochester, Minnesota

I. INTRODUCTION

The classification of tumors outlined here is adapted from the World Health Organization histological classification of tumors [229]. The staging of cancer at specific anatomical sites is as outlined by the American Joint Committee on Cancer [7].

II. TUMORS AND RELATED LESIONS OF THE EYELIDS

The more common tumors of the eyelid are listed in Table 1. Benign neoplasms are approximately three times more frequent than malignant tumors [9].

A. Tumors of the Epithelium

Epidermis

Benign. *Squamous cell papilloma.* This common benign tumor of the eyelid may be sessile or pedunculated. Fingerlike processes of vascularized connective tissue are covered by a hyperplastic epithelium with parakeratosis and variable degrees of hyperkeratosis. Clinically, the lesion may be confused with seborrheic keratosis, verruca vulgaris, and various other benign tumors.

Seborrheic keratosis (verruca senilis, basaloid cell papilloma). Seborrheic keratosis, a common, benign, hyperkeratotic, brownish, greasy lesion, develops most often on the face, trunk, and arms. This lesion, which is not associated with seborrhea, usually occurs in multiple numbers in patients older than 40 years and is generally soft and friable with a rough, craggy surface. On the eyelids, it is found most frequently along the line of the cilia and appears as a sharply demarcated slightly raised nodule, resembling a button stuck onto the skin. The amount of pigment in it varies, sometimes being so abundant that the lesion can be confused clinically with a melanoma. In the black population, a seborrheic keratosis that is pigmented is indistinguishable from dermatosis papulosa. The latter occurs almost exclusively in blacks and is benign.

Microscopically, both squamous and basal cells proliferate in an external direction with no encroachment on the dermis (Fig. 1). Hyperkeratosis, papillomatosis, and pseudohorn cysts are present in various degrees, and this feature has led to a subclassification into hyperkeratotic, acanthotic, and adenoid types [139]. In the adenoid type, the proliferating basal cells outnumber the squamous cells and the lesion may be confused with a basal cell carcinoma, but seborrheic keratosis does not undergo malignant change.

Chronic irritation of these lesions results in an inflammatory cell infiltration and pseudoepitheliomatous (pseudocarcinomatous) hyperplasia (discussed later in this section) with numerous cornified pearls. This picture may be misinterpreted as squamous cell carcinoma. Such an irritated seborrheic keratosis is also referred to as an inverted follicular keratosis. The latter designation, introduced by Helwig [95] in 1955 to describe a benign, usually solitary nodule or papule with a predilection for the face, is

Table 1   Common Tumors and Precancerous Lesions of Eyelid

Benign	Seborrheic keratosis
	Epithelial cyst
	Nevus
	Keratoacanthoma
	Pseudocarcinomatous hyperplasia
	Tumors of skin appendages
Precancerous and preinvasive lesions	Actinic keratosis
	Intraepithelial carcinoma
	Radiation dermatitis
	Xeroderma pigmentosum
Malignant	Basal cell carcinoma
	Squamous cell carcinoma
	Sebaceous carcinoma
	Malignant melanoma

merely a form of seborrheic keratosis with pseudocarcinomatous hyperplasia. The tumor may be flat and warty or papillomatous, and occasionally pigment is present. Clinically, it may be confused with a squamous cell carcinoma. Most lesions are smaller than 1 cm in diameter and involve the margin of the eyelid. They may be asymptomatic or be itchy and burning with seepage of serum [19].

Characteristically, there is an inverted configuration of the acanthotic epithelium, and the cells in the deepest portion of the epithelial mass resemble basal cells (Fig. 2); squamous eddies or small horned cysts may be present in the fingerlike extensions of tumor proliferation. Edema with vesicle formation may be intercellular or intracellular but is not necessarily a prominent feature. The lesion is sharply delineated from the underlying stroma, and the surface shows a variable degree of hyperkeratosis and parakeratosis. The lesion may resemble a keratoacanthoma both clinically and morphologically, and because of this resemblance and because viral particles have been described in keratoacanthoma [227], it is possible that a virus may be the causal agent for inverted follicular keratosis.

Keratoacanthoma (molluscum sebaceum, "self-healing carcinoma").   Usually, the keratoacanthoma is a solitary benign lesion developing in exposed areas in elderly people [27]. It also occurs after renal transplantation and in the immunosuppressed patient [209]. Rarely, multiple contiguous lesions involve the face, including the eyelids, and the extremities; this predisposition to multiple keratoacanthomas may be familial [205].

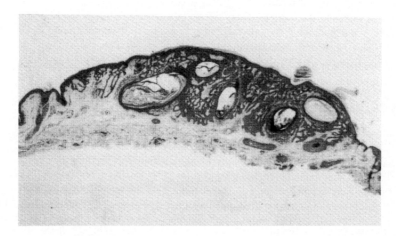

Figure 1   Seborrheic keratosis, adenoid type. Slender, lacelike proliferations of basal cells together with horn cysts. (Hematoxylin and eosin, ×20)

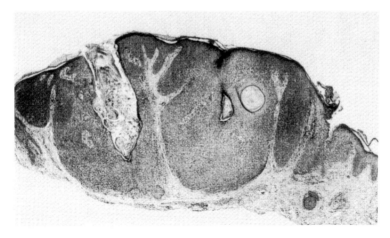

Figure 2 Inverted follicular keratosis. Note pronounced acanthosis with inverted papillary configuration. (Hematoxylin and eosin, ×40)

The tumor arises from the upper portion of a hyperplastic hair follicle, and the associated sebaceous gland manifests squamous metaplasia. In most instances, the lesion consists of a 1–2 cm dome-shaped nodule with a central keratin-filled crater. Two unusual giant palpebral keratoacanthomas have been reported [66]. Neither case had evidence of spontaneous regression, and the tumors were so large that skin grafts were required. Maximal size is reached within a few months, and if the tumor is left untreated, spontaneous regression may occur within 6 months, leaving a minimal scar; the spontaneous disappearance is unexplained, although an immunological process has been proposed [167].

The lesion must be distinguished from squamous cell carcinoma, which it may resemble both clinically and histopathologically [20]. Difficulties arise with the few keratoacanthomas that grow slowly for up to 12 months and reach a maximal diameter of 5 cm and with early squamous cell carcinomas that have a keratin-filled plug at the center. The lesion has also been confused clinically with a chalazion. In one report, a keratoacanthoma grew out of the eyelid margin and extended to the palpebral conjunctiva. The tumor disappeared 4 months after partial excision [160].

The characteristic cup shape with bordering acanthotic epithelium and elongated rete ridges can be appreciated best by complete excision of the lesion. Section through the center of the tumor is of the utmost importance, for only then can the architecture of the lesion be fully appreciated; a central keratin plug is embraced by an acanthotic epithelium (Fig. 3). Important histological guidelines in the differentiation from squamous cell carcinoma include the absence of cellular atypia at the margin of the epidermis in keratoacanthoma and the marked keratinization of the tumor cells. This distinction may be difficult, however, because a keratoacanthoma may occur in actinically damaged skin. Viral particles have been described within these lesions, but they are not present in all [227]. Section through the center of an early squamous cell carcinoma may show an architecture similar to that of keratoacanthoma, but a keratoacanthoma usually has marked keratinization, which gives an eosinophilic, glassy appearance to the cells. In sections of a keratoacanthoma that are "off center," the pseudocarcinomatous hyperplasia may be misinterpreted as an infiltrating squamous cell carcinoma; the presence of pseudoglandular formations, extensive dyskeratosis, and acantholysis favors a diagnosis of squamous cell carcinoma.

Pseudoepitheliomatous (Pseudocarcinomatous) Hyperplasia. "Pseudoepitheliomatous" and "pseudocarcinomatous" are synonymous terms and are applied to a reactive proliferation of the epithelium with dyskeratotic and pleomorphic cells that may occur in various conditions, including insect bites, reactions to drugs, and reactions to tumors, such as basal cell carcinoma and keratoacanthoma. It is important that the clinician be aware that this is a *benign* reaction; hence, many pathologists favor the term "pseudoepitheliomatous" rather than "pseudocarcinomatous" because the latter designation may mislead the clinician. A more descriptive term is "reactive hyperplasia with dysplasia."

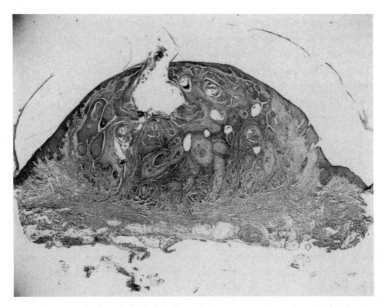

Figure 3   Keratoacanthoma. Cup-shaped tumor has a central ruptured plug of keratin. Adjacent epithelium shows pseudoepitheliomatous hyperplasia. (Hematoxylin and eosin, ×6)

Histologically, the picture may be confused with that of squamous cell carcinoma, but the squamous cells are well differentiated and nuclear hyperchromatism and individual cell keratinization are absent. The presence of inflammatory cells infiltrating the epithelium and disintegration of the latter are further supportive evidence of the reactive nature.

Precancerous Dermatoses and Preinvasive Carcinoma.   The designation of lesions as "precancerous" is a common practice. The term implies that they predispose to cancer, but in this heterogeneous group of conditions the risk of malignant transformation varies. In some it is inevitable; in others the risk of cancer is so low that it may be disregarded. This spectrum results, in part, from the fact that some of the lesions are not "precancerous" but are noninvasive carcinomas in which malignant transformation has already taken place at a cellular level [194].

The most common lesions in the eyelid that may, but do not necessarily, undergo malignant change include actinic keratosis, radiation dermatitis, and xeroderma pigmentosum. Bowen's disease is an in situ carcinoma of the epidermis [22].

Actinic keratosis (solar or senile keratosis).   The term "actinic keratosis" is more appropriate than "senile keratosis" because this lesion may be encountered over a wide age range. However, it occurs more commonly in sun-exposed skin of elderly fair-skinned persons. It is common on the dorsum of the hands but also develops on the eyelids. Multiple lesions commonly coexist and are frequently associated with other cutaneous neoplasms, such as squamous cell or basal cell carcinoma and intraepithelial squamous cell carcinomas.

The lesion has a red base and is slightly elevated, brownish, scaly, and usually smaller than 1 cm in diameter (Fig. 4). Keratin production may be marked, and a cutaneous horn sometimes develops on the surface. An essential component of the lesion is the dermal change known as actinic elastosis. Although most cutaneous horns are associated with actinic keratosis, they are also occasionally associated with seborrheic keratosis, intraepithelial squamous cell carcinoma, and verruca vulgaris. Actinic keratotic lesions may progress to squamous cell carcinoma, but usually these do not metastasize, except sun-induced carcinomas of the lip [210].

Microscopically, three types of actinic keratosis can be recognized: hypertrophic, atrophic, and bowenoid. All three are associated with actinic elastosis and a moderately dense, chronic, inflammatory infiltrate. The most frequent histological type is the hypertrophic variety, in which hyperkeratosis and

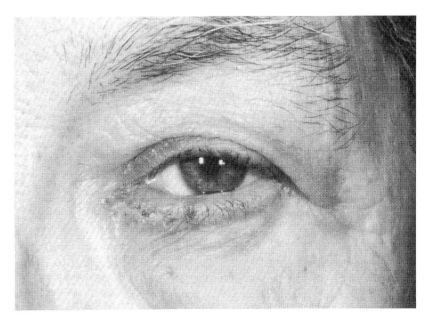

Figure 4   Localized patch of actinic (solar) keratosis on the left lower eyelid at the medial margin in a 60-year-old man. Note the loss of lower cilia.

parakeratosis are present with acanthosis, cellular pleomorphism, and disorientation. The limitation of pleomorphic cells to the deep layers of the epithelium differentiates this lesion from intraepithelial carcinoma (Bowen's disease), in which the whole epithelium is involved. Although anaplastic cells are present, the lesion is benign but premalignant. Squamous cell carcinoma is reported to develop in 12–13% of untreated lesions [90]. The epithelium is thin in some areas and thickened in others.

In the atrophic variety, the epidermis is atrophied and atypical basal cells proliferate into the dermis, forming buds and ductlike structures. Anaplastic cells lose their intracellular bridges, and as a result, collapse within the epidermis is common [139]. The epidermis above such clefts often appears normal. The "bowenoid" type of actinic keratosis is characterized by intraepithelial cellular atypia. The picture is indistinguishable from that of intraepithelial squamous cell carcinoma, but the lesions are smaller. Microinvasive carcinoma consists of invasion of malignant cells beyond the basement membrane.

When actinic keratosis progresses to a squamous cell carcinoma, the usual sharp demarcation line between the lesion and the adjacent normal skin disappears. Because this change can be focal and may not be evident in random sections through the lesion, it is difficult to exclude a squamous cell carcinoma in the absence of serial sections. This distinction is neither practical nor necessarily critical because squamous cell carcinoma arising in an actinic keratosis rarely metastasizes.

Intraepidermal squamous cell carcinoma (Bowen's disease).   In 1912, Bowen [22] first described the cutaneous lesions named eponymously in his honor. The condition may occur anywhere on the skin but is more common on nonexposed surfaces [22]. Although some pathologists consider the lesion precancerous, most regard the entity as an intraepithelial carcinoma. A high percentage (80%) of cases of Bowen's disease occurring in nonexposed skin are associated with other cancers of the skin or viscera [90,177].

Clinically, the usually solitary lesion appears as a flat, dark red, diffuse area with an irregular or indistinct outline. Serum may ooze from cracks within the crusted surface (Fig. 5). Growth occurs by slow, peripheral extension of the margins, leaving either a central ulcer or a fungating mass. The tumor is characterized by hyperkeratosis, parakeratosis, and acanthosis associated with elongation of the rete ridges. Pleomorphic epithelial cells with large hyperchromatic nuclei show complete loss of polarity, and multinucleated epidermal cells are occasionally present. Individual cell keratinization is a frequent and characteristic finding. Some cells, particularly those in the superficial epithelium, may show vacuolization of the cytoplasm. The dysplastic process occupies the full thickness of the epithelium. As a rule, there is a

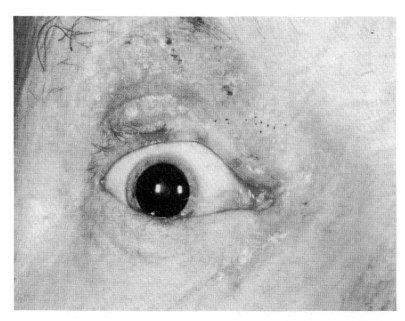

Figure 5   In situ carcinoma. Crusting and scaling of the right upper eyelid are associated with loss of cilia.

sharp transition between the zone of hyperplastic epithelium and the adjacent normal epithelium. Approximately 5% of cases progress to an invasive squamous cell carcinoma by breaking the integrity of the basement membrane at one or several points [90]; metastasis may then occur.

Radiation dermatitis.   A mild form of *acute* radiation dermatitis affecting the eyelids sometimes follows irradiation to the orbit, the globe, or the eyelids. Erythema occurs within a week of treatment, and telangiectasia, desquamation of surface epithelial cells, and eventually pigmentation develop. Less commonly blisters and ulcers may form, followed by healing with scarring. *Chronic* radiation dermatitis occurs months to years after treatment. Microscopically, an atrophic epithelium overlies a dermis with prominent actinic elastosis throughout its depth and contains numerous telangiectatic vessels with hyalinized walls. A dose of 4000 R or more produces severe atrophic changes, occlusion of vessels, and fibrosis, and in such areas squamous or basal cell carcinomas may develop. This malignant change takes place after many years. In the first well-documented patient with bilateral retinoblastoma cured by radiation and cared for by Verhoeff, basal cell carcinoma and squamous cell carcinoma developed in the eyelid 60 years later [3]. The authors of this report [3] questioned the relationship of irradiation and tumors in this patient and considered that the tumors may have been second primary lesions or coincidental.

Xeroderma pigmentosum.   Xeroderma pigmentosum is a rare, autosomal recessive inherited disease, and many affected patients are the offspring of consanguineous marriages [35]. Abnormalities affecting the eyelids, conjunctiva, and cornea, which are areas exposed to ultraviolet radiation, have been reported in 40% of published cases [128]. Heterogeneity of the molecular defect in xeroderma pigmentosum has been demonstrated [46]. A heterokaryon (a cell with nuclei from different donors in a common cytoplasm) is formed by fusion of fibroblasts from one patient with those of another patient. Each cell supplies the other with what is lacking, the implication being that each cell has different defects, and they are said to be in different complementation groups. The first five complementation groups were named A through E in the order of increasing residual DNA repair synthesis. Other groups have since been reported [64].

Mapping of the defective gene(s) has been studied by several research workers, and a defective gene locus has been identified in many of the individual complementation groups [154]. In xeroderma pigmentosum group A, the genetic determinant has been located on the long arm of chromosome 1 [118]. Others have located the defect in the same group A to chromosome 9 (9q22) [214]. Schwartz and coworkers [196] found that human chromosome 15 confers a partial complementation of phenotypes to xeroderma pigmentosum group F cells. An increased frequency of chromatin breaks and gaps after irradiation of G_2 phase peripheral blood lymphocytes and fibroblasts has been detected in carriers of xeroderma pigmentosum [173]. With further refinement of genetic studies, abnormalities in the individual xeroderma pigmentosum groups will no doubt be further identified.

Because the skin is profoundly sensitive to light, it becomes acutely erythematous in early childhood on exposure to sunlight, and increased pigmentation, telangiectasia, and actinic keratoses (solar keratoses) subsequently develop. In this disorder, there is a deficiency of ultraviolet endonuclease, an enzyme that cleaves thymidine dimers. In consequence, there is a defect in the repair of DNA damaged by ultraviolet light and a pronounced predisposition to sun-induced cancers [186]. Both the skin and the conjunctiva eventually develop many varieties of malignant tumor, including basal and squamous cell carcinoma and malignant melanoma [130]. The prevalence of cutaneous cancer in patients with xeroderma pigmentosum is much higher than that in the general population. The eyelids are frequently affected by one or more of the processes described (Fig. 6) and may manifest degenerative changes with atrophy, ectropion, and secondary inflammation. Most patients die before the age of 21 years from carcinomatous or melanomatous metastases. Clinically, the disease process may be divided into three stages. In the first stage, there is mild, diffuse erythema associated with dryness and increased pigmentation; in the second stage, atrophy with mottled pigmentation and telangiectasia occurs; and in the final stage, various types of malignant tumor appear in the skin.

Although the histological appearance is initially nonspecific, the combination of hyperkeratosis, atrophy of the stratum malpighii and rete ridges, and proliferation of adjacent rete ridges, accompanied by a chronic inflammatory infiltrate of the epidermis and accumulation of melanin in the basal layer, is suggestive of the disease. A combination of atrophy and acanthosis marks the second stage; these features are superimposed on the existing changes of hyperkeratosis and hyperpigmentation, but the latter are more pronounced. Finally, basal cell carcinomas, squamous carcinomas, and even malignant melanomas occur.

Malignant. *Basal cell carcinoma.* Basal cell carcinoma probably arises from the primordial epithelial germ cells in the deepest layer of the epidermis. This tumor is the most common malignant neoplasm of the eyelid (more than 90%) and occurs mainly on the lower lid in fair-skinned adults. Prolonged exposure to sunlight commonly precedes the lesion [23]. Immunohistochemical techniques have demonstrated an overexpression of a long-lived mutant form of p53 protein in basal cell carcinoma [156,157]. This overexpression is also demonstrable in the adjacent keratocytes but is not demonstrable in skin that is protected from sunlight [199]. Such findings suggest that the mutation of the tumor suppressor

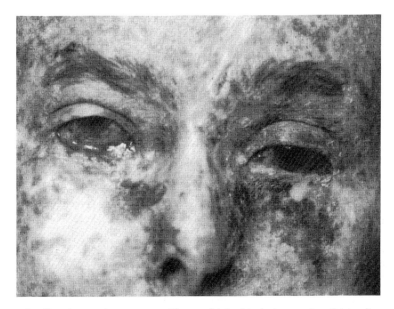

Figure 6 Xeroderma pigmentosum. Note multiple skin lesions and eyelid involvement.

gene p53 results from chronic exposure to ultraviolet light [199]. The mutant protein results from the point mutation of the p53 gene, which is located on chromosome 17 band p13. Usually, basal cell carcinoma is a tumor of the later decades of life, but one case has been reported in a 27-month-old girl without predisposing skin disease [121]. The tumor has also been reported in patients between 21 and 35 years old who are fair skinned or have the nevoid basal cell syndrome [163].

The nevoid basal cell syndrome, also known as Gorlin-Goltz syndrome [88], is inherited as an autosomal dominant disorder. Chromosome studies have shown a normal karyotype [157,199,207]. It consists of cysts of the jaw, pitting of the palms and soles, frontal bossing, skeletal abnormalities, ectopic calcification, and multiple basal cell carcinoma. The diagnosis can be made on the basis of the family history, clinical appearance, and radiographs [188]. The skin tumors appear in childhood or early adolescence and usually affect the upper lid [71]. This feature contrasts with the more common lower lid position in the elderly adult.

Initially a firm lesion, it subsequently ulcerates in the center to impart a pearly appearance with a rolled edge (Fig. 7). Various clinical appearances allow confusion with squamous and sebaceous carcinoma [131], as well as with keratoacanthoma [20]. It has also been reported to masquerade as an ectropion of the eyelid [15]. Important distinguishing features are the multicentricity of origin and the rapid surface spread rather than deep growth. When situated at the medial canthus, the tumor is more vicious in behavior than tumors located elsewhere. The recurrence rate at this site is high. The tumor appears to invade early, but this characteristic may be a consequence of an inadequate initial excision as a result of the proximity of the lacrimal drainage system.

Because the basal cell is pluripotential, the tumor has a propensity to differentiate toward a wide variety of cutaneous structures. Typically, the growth forms lobules that extend from the epithelium into the dermis (Fig. 8). The cells, with hyperchromatic nuclei and scanty cytoplasm, manifest a palisading around the periphery of the lobules [139]. Squamous differentiation or a cystic (adenocystic) pattern may develop in the tumor mass, yet the biological behavior has proved to be independent of such morphological variability. The tumor may also be pigmented and be misdiagnosed as a melanoma [98]. The behavior of this pigmented variant does not differ from that of the unpigmented basal cell carcinoma.

The morphea form of basal cell carcinoma is particularly aggressive. Clinically, this variety of the tumor forms a pale indurated plaque that is composed of compressed bands of basal cells entrenched in a dense fibrous matrix. This type of pattern often extends beyond the margins that are observed clinically and

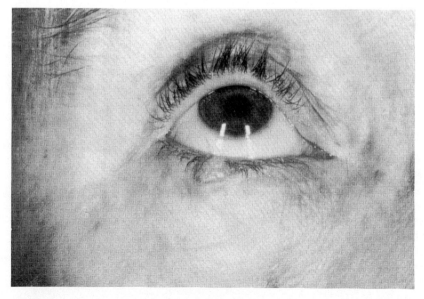

Figure 7   Basal cell carcinoma in a 70-year-old man. Note the ulcer nodule with pearly rolled edge on the right lower eyelid.

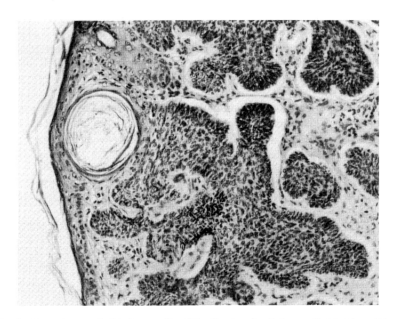

Figure 8 Basal cell carcinoma. Solid clumps of proliferating basal cells have a "picket fence" border of outer cells. Horn cyst is present at left. (Hematoxylin and eosin, ×200)

is more likely to be incompletely excised. Multifocality is often a feature, and it has been reported in 60% of patients with basal cell carcinoma of the morphea type [220]. Basal cell carcinoma, particularly of this type, often invades the orbit or the superficial part of the sclera, but intraocular invasion is most unusual. Aldred and colleagues [5] reported such atypical behavior of a basal cell carcinoma in a 53-year-old man with lepromatous leprosy. Although invasive, basal cell carcinomas rarely metastasize [39]. Meningeal carcinomatosis has followed a primary basal cell carcinoma of the upper eyelid [204]. Of 17 cases with metastatic basal cell carcinoma studied by Farmer and Helwig [59], one tumor was of the lower eyelid and one of the infraorbital region. Metastasis occurs to the lymph nodes, lungs, bone, liver, spleen, and adrenal gland.

Excision under frozen section control is effective therapy in 95% of cases [187]. The 5% that recur can be treated with radiation or other methods. Cryotherapy has proved valuable in some patients, such as those who are at a high surgical risk.

Squamous cell carcinoma. Several early studies indicated a high incidence of squamous cell carcinoma of the eyelid because of misinterpretation of other cutaneous tumors [53]. In the Western Hemisphere, this is an uncommon tumor of the palpebral tissue; it composes 9% of all eyelid malignancies [185]. At this site, the ratio of squamous cell carcinoma to basal cell carcinoma is 1:39 [131]. In Japan, squamous cell carcinoma is reported as the most frequent malignancy of the eyelid [1].

Elderly fair-skinned persons are particularly prone to this neoplasm. Its occurrence in the immunosuppressed patient with Graves' disease [74] and after renal transplantation [209] suggests that immunosuppressive therapy may enhance the growth of a preexisting malignancy. Its development is thought to progress through phases of intraepithelial squamous dysplasia and in situ carcinoma before invasion occurs [185]. When the tumor arises in actinic keratosis, metastasis is infrequent. The tumor also occurs after exposure to high doses of irradiation and, as previously mentioned, may occur at multiple sites in xeroderma pigmentosum [130].

The presence of human papillomavirus type 16 (HPV 160) viral DNA has been demonstrated in a recurrent squamous cell carcinoma of the lower eyelid with use of the polymerase chain reaction to amplify specific target DNA sequences. With primers specific for HPV 16 DNA, this procedure yielded a single band of amplified DNA product that was positive with radiolabeled HPV 16 dot-blot analysis. The implications of these findings in regard to the causative role of these viruses in the development of neoplasia and their management and prognosis were stressed by McDonnell and colleagues [151].

Clinically, the carcinoma begins in the lower eyelid as an indurated patch that becomes white as keratin accumulates on the surface; this eventually cracks to disclose an erythematous ulcer with hard edges. Of great significance are the slow growth and the relatively benign behavior, in contrast to squamous cell carcinoma at other sites of the body. With sun-induced cutaneous tumors, the skin in areas other than the eyelids often bears precancerous lesions and other malignant cutaneous tumors. Wide excision produces an effective 5 year cure rate; thus, the patient does not die of the disease if treated early and adequately. Late presentation allows metastasis to preauricular and submaxillary lymph nodes. A highly aggressive form of the tumor that is well differentiated microscopically has been termed "acute epithelioma" [65]. This variant is thought to be virally induced, but this hypothesis awaits confirmation. It requires close follow-up because of its lethal metastatic potential.

An adenoid form of squamous cell carcinoma is characterized histologically by acantholysis and a pseudoglandular pattern with alveolar and tubular structures. In a report of 15 such lesions of the eyelid in patients aged 43–85 years, local recurrence occurred in approximately one-third of patients, but none of the patients died of metastatic disease in an 8.8 year follow-up [31]. Among the lesions with which squamous cell carcinoma can be confused are actinic keratosis, keratoacanthoma, pseudoepitheliomatous hyperplasia, basal cell carcinoma, and sebaceous gland carcinoma.

Sweat Glands

Various tumors may arise from the sweat glands and their ducts [132,139]. Among the more common neoplasms of these eccrine glands are the syringoma, the eccrine spiradenoma, and the mixed tumor. Tumors of the apocrine glands of Moll also occur [111,133,192].

Benign.   *Syringoma.*   Histochemical and electron microscopic studies have shown that this benign adenoma arises from intraepidermal eccrine sweat glands. Enzymes of eccrine glands, such as phosphorylase, leucine aminopeptidase, and succinic dehydrogenase, are present in abundance [139]. The individual tumor cells have numerous short microvilli, abundant lysosomes, and tonofilaments arranged in a periluminal band, and it is by the coalescence of intracytoplasmic vacuoles that the lumen of the duct is formed. The presence of keratin within such ducts adjacent to the epidermis is evidence of the keratin-forming capacity of the cells lining the intraepidermal eccrine sweat glands.

Immunohistochemical studies support the theory that syringoma of the eyelids and eruptive syringoma of the neck and upper chest are similar tumors and are of eccrine duct origin [93]. The monoclonal antikeratin antibody EKH4, which predominantly labels the basal epithelial cells, also labels the cordlike epithelial structures of the syringoma and the peripheral cells of the cyst walls. The antibody EKH6, which recognizes normal eccrine secretory and ductal structures, is positive along the luminal border of the cyst walls. The antibody EKH5, which labels the eccrine secretory portion of the gland, is negative.

The syringoma occurs predominantly in the female at puberty or in late life. Single and multiple lesions of the axillae, abdomen, vulva, or cheeks form, and in many patients the lower eyelids alone are involved. The tumor is a pink or yellowish, 1–2 mm, soft nodule. Familial cases that involve the eyelids as well as the neck and body have been reported [93].

Microscopically, small ducts lined by two rows of epithelial cells are embedded in a fibrous stroma (Fig. 9). Many ducts have a taillike extension of epithelial cells and amorphous eosinophilic debris within the lumen. Keratin horn cysts immediately adjacent to the epithelium are a frequent finding. A clear cell variant that is frequently associated with diabetes mellitus cannot be distinguished clinically from the conventional syringoma. Glycogen that dissolves during tissue processing is responsible for the clear appearance. Transmission electron microscopy shows that intracytoplasmic and extracytoplasmic multivesicular bodies are present [6].

Eccrine spiradenoma.   The eyelids or other parts of the upper body may bear these solitary, benign, tender, flat pink lesions [2]. One or several demarcated lobules lie in the dermis and consist of two types of cells, one with a small hyperchromatic nucleus and the second with a large vesicular nucleus forming ductlike structures. Electron microscopic observations indicate differentiation toward dermal ducts as well as to the secretory segment of the gland [139]. In an immunohistochemical and ultrastructural study of an eccrine acrospiroma, Grossniklaus and Knight [91] showed that the tumor cells stained for cytokeratins of high molecular weight but were negative for those of low molecular weight. Epithelial membrane antigen was also demonstrable. Carcinoembryonic antigen and muscle-specific actin were focally positive. Negative staining was demonstrated with antibodies to S-100 protein, glial fibrillary protein, and desmin. It is

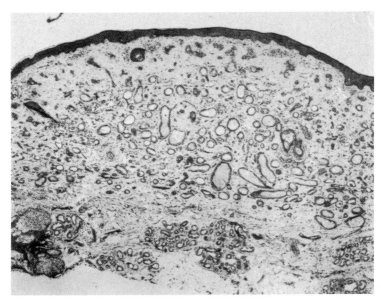

Figure 9   Syringoma. Numerous ducts lined by two rows of epithelial cells lie within the dermis. (Hematoxylin and eosin, ×40)

the presence of the epithelial markers that helps to distinguish eccrine tumors from other tumors that express S-100 protein. Ultrastructurally, tonofilaments were present in the polyhedral cells, clear cells contained glycogen granules, and microvilli were present on cells lining the lumen.

Mixed tumor.   This benign subcutaneous nodule, also known as a chondroid syringoma, frequently occurs in the skin of the eyelids, head, and neck. There are two histological types: a tubular cystic variety of apocrine origin and a small tubular type of eccrine origin.

Tumors of apocrine origin.   Tumors of apocrine origin occur at the eyelid margin, where only the apocrine glands of Moll are present. This group includes the hidrocystoma [133] and the syringocyst-adenoma papilliferum [111]. The origin of these tumors from the apocrine glands is supported by electron microscopy [111,192] and immunohistochemical studies [133]. The tumor may be single [111] or multiple [133,192]. Bilateral apocrine hidrocystomas occur as a feature of ectodermal dysplasia [72]. The hidradenoma papilliferum is also derived from the glands of Moll but more commonly it is from those of the anogenital region. It is a rare tumor of the eyelid [164,195]. The smooth surface contrasts with the verrucous surface of the syringocystadenoma. In the two cases described, the tumor has shown a central feature of either umbilication [195] or an epidermal poral opening [164]. It has been suggested that this opening represents an ectasia of the pilar canal of the cilia through which the secretions of the glands of Moll escape. Its identification may be of help in the diagnosis of tumors at this site. Histologically, the pattern is similar to that of intraductal papilloma of the breast, but the tumor cells have apical snouts. Ultrastructurally, there are apical secretory granules, and myofilaments are present in myoepithelial cells. The tumor is considered benign and has a low possibility of malignant progression.

Malignant.   *Malignant counterparts of benign sweat gland tumors.*   These tumors are rare, and each of the forms may be misinterpreted both clinically and histologically as squamous cell car-cinoma [38].

The malignant form of the syringoma is rare. It is a slow-growing tumor of the lower or upper lid and has been reported in patients of 18, 20, and 70 years of age [85,122]. Electron microscopy confirms the origin from the eccrine sweat gland [122]. The large size and evidence of muscle and nerve invasion are indications of malignancy.

Mucinous adenocarcinoma.   This rare tumor arises from the dark cells of the eccrine secretory coil. In a review of the literature, Wright and Font [224] found that almost half of the cases reported (21 of 45) were of the eyelid. The median age at presentation is 60 years (range 33–84 years), and the tumor is preponderant in the male. It occurs on the upper and lower lids as well as the inner canthus, and it presents in 1 month to 8 years as a bluish to red, papillomatous, pedunculated, or fungating lesion. Microscopically, strands of fibrous tissue divide the tumor into lobules of various sizes, and these contain an admixture of dark and light cells similar to those found in the eccrine coil. Collections of a nonsulfated sialic acid-containing mucosubstance are produced by the tumor cells, and an adenocystic pattern may be present. Enzymatic and electron microscopic studies are needed to make the diagnosis [142]. The tumor is of low-grade malignancy and has a slightly better prognosis than sweat gland carcinomas; the duration of survival is at least 8 years.

Malignant variants of apocrine tumors are commonly assumed to be of low-grade malignancy, but two patients have been reported with a highly malignant variant that progressed rapidly and was ultimately fatal [166].

A primary signet ring carcinoma of the eyelid may also occur [103]. The four cases reported have all occurred in elderly men who had diffusely indurated eyelids. Microscopically, the tumor resembles the "histiocytoid" variant of breast carcinoma metastatic to the eyelids. Ultrastructural studies give conflicting results. Some authors believe the tumor originates from the apocrine glands [103], whereas others believe it is of eccrine origin. The course is indolent, but regional and distant metastases occur with long-term follow-up.

Sebaceous Glands

The eyelid contains several types of sebaceous glands: the meibomian glands, which are unassociated with the hair follicles and have short ducts; the glands of Zeis; and sebaceous glands associated with the fine hair follicles that cover the cutaneous surface of the eyelids.

Torre [216] was the first to describe the association of sebaceous gland neoplasms with multiple visceral carcinomas. The syndrome usually manifests in both sexes between the fifth and sixth decades of life; the mean age at recognition is 46 years. The sebaceous gland tumor of the eyelid is usually benign and may be single [101], but more commonly multiple tumors occur. Other associated eyelid tumors include adenomatoid sebaceous hyperplasia, basal cell carcinoma with foci of sebaceous differentiation, kerato-acanthoma, and squamous cell carcinoma [112,216].

Most of the visceral carcinomas are low grade and affect the colon and stomach [32,63,101,215,216], but others affect the larynx, endometrium, urogenital system, breast, and hematological system [63]. The visceral carcinoma is usually the first to present clinically. A family history of carcinoma is usually apparent [63].

Benign. *Sebaceous adenoma.* Distinction between sebaceous adenoma and sebaceous gland hyperplasia may be difficult, if not impossible, because both consist of benign cells arranged in a lobular pattern. The solitary sebaceous adenoma is smooth, elevated, and smaller than 1 cm in diameter, and most reported examples have been situated on the scalp or face. Such a lesion is usually no more than a cosmetic problem, but it may masquerade as a chalazion.

The syndromes of Gardner [82] and Oldfield [169] are to be distinguished from Torre's syndrome [216]. Gardner's syndrome consists of multiple epidermal and "sebaceous" cysts and occurs in association with intestinal polyps, osteomas, and tumors of soft tissue [82]. In Oldfield's syndrome [169], multiple sebaceous cysts are found in association with familial polyposis and colonic carcinoma.

Malignant. *Sebaceous adenocarcinoma.* The meibomian glands are modified sebaceous glands present in both the upper and the lower eyelids, but they are more numerous in the former; this accounts for the greater number of tumors in the upper eyelid [52]. Occasionally, both eyelids may be involved simultaneously, and multicentric growth occurs [182]. The tumor usually occurs in elderly people (median age, 65 years), but it has been described in a 20 year old [16]. It is slightly more common in women than in men.

Most sebaceous gland carcinomas arise from meibomian glands, but it is frequently impossible histologically to determine the exact site of origin. The incidence varies from 1 to 5.5% of all malignant neoplasms of the eyelid [117]. Sebaceous carcinoma of the eyelid is a frequent tumor in Asian countries [172,212,226]. Although uncommon in Western countries, sebaceous carcinoma of the eyelid is important because it frequently masquerades as a chalazion or as unilateral chronic blepharoconjunctivitis [117,223,225]. Recurrent unilateral inflammatory disease must always, therefore, be suspected of indicating a carcinoma of the sebaceous glands. In a few instances, the tumor presents as an orbital neoplasm, the primary site having been ignored, and rare cases have followed radiation treatment of retino-blastoma [21].

Delay in recognition may vary from 5 months to 7 years, and this may account for the high mortality rate (reported as 30% after 5 year follow-up in Boniuk and Zimmerman's series [21]). When death occurs, metastasis is widespread. Spread may have occurred by the time the lesion is recognized, but in general metastasis is a late event. Lymphatic spread to ipsilateral lymph nodes is more frequent than orbital extension.

Clinically, the tumor usually presents as a circumscribed yellow nodule involving the tarsal plate (Fig. 10). It may also occur as a morpheic plaque. When the origin is from the glands of Zeis, the margin of the eyelid is involved, with thickening and loss of cilia. Occasionally, however, papillary forms develop and cause confusion with squamous cell carcinoma; basal cell carcinoma should be considered if ulceration occurs.

Various histological patterns may be seen. A common pattern consists of acinar structures arranged in lobules of various sizes and separated from the connective tissue by a basement membrane (Fig. 11). The individual polyhedral cells have vesicular nuclei with prominent nucleoli and foamy cytoplasm caused by the high lipid content, which is readily demonstrated in frozen sections by oil red O stains. The overlying epidermis, mucous membrane, or cornea may contain cells with abundant pale cytoplasm and hyperchromatic nuclei within the nonneoplastic epithelium. These cells resemble those found in some ductal carcinomas of the breast (Paget's disease of the breast), and this pagetoid phenomenon is of practical importance because it may be a presenting manifestation of the sebaceous carcinoma [191,223]. It is also a bad prognostic sign [181]. With growth and repeated surgical procedures, the tumor becomes undifferentiated, the original lobular pattern is lost, and clusters of more spindle-shaped cells show increased mitotic activity. Histologically, confusion with basal cell carcinoma or a high-grade squamous cell carcinoma is possible, but the cells of these tumors can be distinguished by the absence of fine intracellular droplets of fat.

Electron microscopically, the neoplastic cell is of epidermoid origin inasmuch as tonofibrils and desmosomes are present. This pattern suggests an origin from the sebaceous duct rather than the secretory cells.

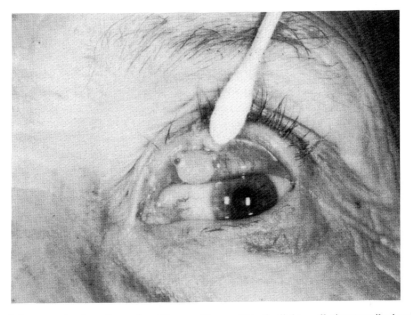

Figure 10 Sebaceous gland carcinoma in a 72-year-old man. Note the light, well-circumscribed nodule on the left upper eyelid.

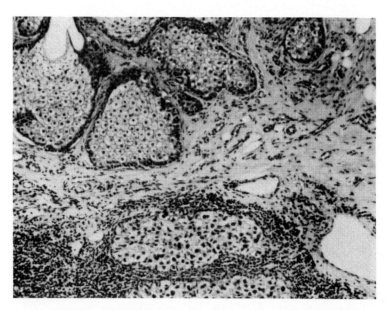

Figure 11　Sebaceous gland carcinoma. Note the normal sebaceous glands (above) and lobulated pleomorphic group of malignant cells with foamy cytoplasm (below). (Hematoxylin and eosin, ×100)

Hair Follicles

Benign eyelid tumors from hair follicles are rare. Frequently, they are misdiagnosed as basal cell carcinoma. Included in this group are trichoepithelioma, trichilemmoma, trichofolliculoma, and pilomatrixoma. In one large series, 117 such tumors were diagnosed over a 30 year period; in contrast, 2447 basal cell carcinomas were removed during the same period [203]. It is important to diagnose these benign tumors of hair follicles to avoid unnecessary extensive surgical treatment.

Trichoepithelioma.　This tumor occurs as a solitary lesion or as an inherited condition, when it is likely to be multiple. The solitary nodule is firm and elevated and appears in both men and women during the later decades of life. The multiple form (Brooke's tumor) is inherited in an autosomal dominant pattern. Microscopically, basaloid cells are arranged in strands and nests with multiple horn cysts, which represent immature hair follicles.

Trichilemmoma.　This benign tumor arises from the outer sheath of the hair follicle. The eyelid is the second most common site; the nose is the most common site. In a study of 31 such tumors of the eyelid (28) and eyebrow (3), the age range of the patients was 22–88 years (mean 53 years) [96]. Microscopically, glycogen-rich cells are arranged in lobules and show a palisade pattern at the periphery of the lobule; this pattern may lead to confusion with basal cell carcinoma. Multiple facial trichilemmomas, which may include the eyelid, are pathognomonic of Cowden's disease, a rare genodermatosis [11].

Trichofolliculoma.　A benign entity, the lesion is a hamartoma that consists of a large cystic follicle that represents a dilated hair follicle and contains immature hair structures. The appearance of white hairs growing from the central core may be distinctive, but this feature is not seen in all cases [30].

Pilomatrixoma (Calcifying Epithelioma of Malherbe).　This benign, solitary, cystic tumor favors the upper eyelid and eyebrow in children and young adults. In one study of 150 children 10 years of age or younger, 17% of these tumors were of the upper eyelid and brow [170]. Ashton [8] was the first to record this tumor of the eyelids in the ophthalmic literature. Clinically, it resembles a pilar cyst (sebaceous cyst) and arises from the primitive hair matrix. Histologically, the basaloid cell proliferation includes "ghost cells," and foci of calcification and foreign body giant cells are common in the supporting stroma. Reported complications are corneal ulceration secondary to an ectopic lesion in the tarsal plate [44] and necrosis with malignant degeneration [79].

B. Cysts of the Epithelium

Milia

These 1–2 mm white nodules are retention cysts caused by occlusion of a pilosebaceous follicle. Histologically, they resemble epidermal cysts.

Keratinous Cysts

Pilar ("Sebaceous") Cysts.   In the past, the pilar cyst was called a sebaceous cyst. Once it became apparent that the differentiation within these cysts was toward hair keratin, the terminology was changed. The cyst has an epithelial wall in which the cells lack easily visible bridges and the basal layer is distinctly palisaded. In contrast to the epidermal cyst, the epithelial lining lacks a granular layer (stratum granulosum). The innermost cells have increased numbers of filaments and fibrils, and it is these that are shed into the lumen. As they are shed, they lose their nuclei and cytoplasmic organelles. The contents of the cysts form an amorphous eosinophilic mass, which becomes calcified in approximately 25% of cases. In most instances the cyst is single, but multiple cysts may occur and form part of Gardner's or Oldfield's syndrome [82,169].

Epidermal Cysts.   Although clinically similar to the pilar cyst, the epidermal cyst lacks a palisade arrangement of the peripheral cells, and the luminal contents do not calcify. The epithelial wall contains a stratum granulosum, and the innermost cells are laminated. Growth is slow and is caused by the accumulation of keratin from the hornified cells of the epithelial lining. The lesion is round and firm and may enlarge to 3 cm in diameter. It is situated in the superficial or deep corium. On rupture, both pilar (sebaceous) and epidermal cysts excite a foreign body giant cell reaction. Clinically, the lesion becomes red and indurated.

C. Tumors and Related Lesions of Melanocytes

Nevocellular Nevi

Electron microscopy has shown that the nevus cell and the melanocyte of the epidermis are similar; both cells originate from the neural crest, contain melanosomes, and have pseudopodic cytoplasmic processes. However, the nevus cell differs from the epidermal melanocyte in two ways: (1) its pseudopodic cytoplasmic processes are shorter and are not visible by light microscopy, and (2) nevus cells are arranged in clusters.

Tumors may arise from nevus cells, melanocytes of the epidermis, and melanocytes of the dermis (Table 2).

Nevocellular nevi are benign tumors composed of nevus cells and may be divided into three main groups: intradermal, junctional, and compound. In practice, the range of possibilities encompasses a continuous spectrum such that individual cases, although compound lesions, have an overwhelming preponderance of nevus cells in either the junctional area or the dermis. The notion of *Abtropfung* (dropping off of melanocytes into the dermis) has long been accepted, but a recent concept, *Hochsteigerung*, is that melanocytes migrate from the dermis to the epidermis as a part of normal development and as a part of normal tissue maintenance [40]. A pleuripotential cell is considered to give rise to the melanocyte [40].

Microscopically, the low-power objective reveals the geographical distribution of the nevus cells. At higher magnification, the cells can be seen to have a tendency to be spindle shaped in the lower dermis and to become plumper as the epidermis is approached. Melanin, if present, is in nevus cells in the upper dermis and epidermis.

The clinical appearance varies according to the microscopic pattern, and thus it is possible to predict the histological type from the clinical appearance (Table 3).

Intradermal Nevus.   In contrast to junctional and compound nevi, this entity is believed to have little or no malignant potential. Clusters of nevus cells are confined to the dermis; multinucleated cells indicate a mature nevus (Fig. 12). Melanin, if present, is in the most superficial cells. Clinically, the presence of hairs on an elevated pigmented nodule usually indicates an intradermal nevus. Rupture of a hair follicle can occur occasionally and is associated with inflammation and an increase in the size of the nevus. These findings may cause clinical concern that malignant change has taken place.

Table 2   Tumors and Related Lesions of Melanocytes of Eyelid and Their Cells of
Origin

Nevus cell	Epidermal melanocyte	Dermal melanocyte
Intradermal nevus	Freckle (ephelis)	Blue nevus
Junctional nevus	Lentigo simplex	Nevus of Ota
Compound nevus	Lentigo senilis	Mongolian spot
Variants of nevocellular nevi		
Balloon cell nevus		
Halo nevus		
Benign juvenile melanoma		
Congenital giant pigmented nevus		

A neural nevus is a variant in which the nevus cells are spindle shaped and embedded in the loose collagenous tissue of the lower dermis. There is no malignant potential.

Junctional Nevus.   In contrast to the intradermal nevus, this lesion can become malignant. Circumscribed nests of cuboidal cells occupy the lower epidermis. A few clusters appear to "drop off" into the dermis but retain their connection to the epidermis. The upper dermis may contain a few scattered nevus cells with various amounts of pigment.

Compound Nevus.   The compound nevus has features of both junctional and intradermal nevi, and a malignant potential is inherent. Melanin may or may not be present in the nevus cells.

Variants of Nevocellular Nevi.   Four variants of nevocellular nevi exist: the balloon cell nevus, the halo nevus, the benign juvenile melanoma, and the congenital giant pigmented nevus. To date, the halo nevus and giant pigmented nevus have not involved the eyelids.

Balloon cell nevus.   This is a small, elevated, soft, lightly pigmented lesion that is indistinguishable clinically from other nevocellular nevi. Microscopically, however, characteristic cells constitute part or all of the tumor mass. These cells, designated "balloon cells," are 20–40 μm in diameter and usually have a central nucleus with abundant clear or finely granular cytoplasm. Electron microscopy has disclosed that the cytoplasmic distension is caused by vacuolar degeneration and subsequent coalescence of melanosomes.

Benign juvenile melanoma.   The benign juvenile melanoma is a form of compound nevus occurring predominantly in children and young adults as a tiny, dome-shaped pinkish nodule on the face and extremities. The active junctional zone, together with cellular pleomorphism and inflammation, creates a disturbing histological picture, but circulating antibodies to malignant melanoma are absent. Melanin is present in only small amounts because of the partial lysosomal degradation of melanosomes and incomplete melanization.

Blue Nevus.   In contrast to the nevocellular nevi described earlier, the blue nevus arises from dermal melanocytes. It is a benign tumor that may occur anywhere on the skin, including the eyelids, but also on mucosal surfaces, such as the conjunctiva. Within the skin there are two types, the common blue nevus and the cellular variety. The former is small, blue, and dome shaped. The blue color results from the scattering

Table 3   Expected Histological Findings of Nevocellular Nevi on Basis
of Clinical Appearance

Color	Shape	Type of nevus
Pigmented	Flat	Junctional
	Slightly elevated	Compound
	Papillomatous	Compound
Minimally pigmented or amelanotic	Papillomatous	Intradermal
	Dome shaped	Intradermal
	Pedunculated	Intradermal

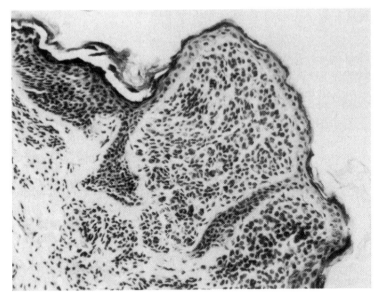

Figure 12 Intradermal nevus. Clusters of nevus cells are confined to the dermis. (Hematoxylin and eosin, ×200)

of light as it strikes melanin particles within spindle-shaped melanocytes in the deep dermis after passing through the superficial layer of skin (Fig. 13). A compound nevus occasionally is present over the lesion; the term "combined nevus" is then applied.

The cellular blue nevus has deeply pigmented, plump, and delicate spindle-shaped cells (melanocytes). Rarely, cellular blue nevi metastasize to regional lymph nodes, but death from metastasis has not been reported.

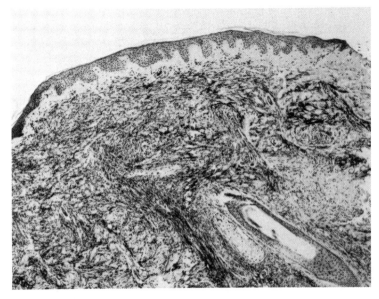

Figure 13 Blue nevus. Spindle-shaped melanocytes with pigment lie within the dermis, separated from the epidermis by a zone of connective tissue. (Hematoxylin and eosin, ×64)

Nevus of Ota.   This malformation, which arises from dermal melanocytes, is discussed in Chapter 48.

Benign Pigmented Lesions of Epidermal Melanocytes

Freckle (Ephelis).   This pigmented macule is commonly found on the eyelid, and pigmentation increases with exposure to sunlight, in contrast to lentigo simplex (discussed next). The basal layer of the epidermis contains large, strongly dihydroxyphenylalanine (dopa)-positive melanocytes, but the actual number of melanocytes is not increased. Unlike lentigo simplex, there is no elongation of the rete ridges.

Lentigo Simplex.   Clinically, lentigo simplex is indistinguishable from a junctional nevus. It may occur on the skin anywhere on the body, including the eyelids, and is not affected by exposure to sunlight. It appears as a flat brown or black lesion only a few millimeters in diameter. Microscopically, there are increased numbers of basal melanocytes, elongation of rete ridges, and melanophages in the upper dermis. The congenital "split nevus," which involves both eyelids and arises in utero when these structures are still fused, may have a histological appearance similar to that of lentigo simplex or of a junctional nevus.

Lentigo Senilis.   This closely resembles seborrheic keratosis and, as its name implies, is a flat, pigmented macule of variable size that occurs in the exposed skin of elderly people. Histologically it differs from lentigo simplex in that rete ridges are longer and tortuous; occasionally, nevus cells are present at the epidermal-dermal junction.

Malignant Melanomas

These tumors comprise only 1% of all malignant neoplasms of the eyelids and can be divided into two main groups: those that occur in situ and those that invade [37,83,94,139,153].

Lentigo Maligna (Freckle of Hutchinson, Circumscribed Precancerous Melanosis of Dubreuilh).   This lesion occurs as an uneven macule with various degrees of pigmentation, is usually several centimeters in diameter, and most commonly occurs on the face of elderly people. Peripheral extension is extremely slow (over many years), and depigmentation occurs at sites of regression. This relatively benign behavior contrasts sharply with that of in situ pagetoid melanoma. Microscopically, pleomorphic melanocytes in the epidermis are increased in number, contain more pigment, and are irregularly arranged.

Pagetoid Malignant Melanoma.   This invasive growth develops in an undetermined number of cases of in situ pagetoid melanoma and often within 1 year, contrasting sharply with the slow progression of lentigo maligna to lentigo maligna melanoma. Invasive growth is indicated by induration, ulceration, and increased pigmentation. Superficial spreading melanoma represents 70% of all cutaneous melanomas. A cure rate of 78% has been obtained during an average posttreatment follow-up period of 7.4 years [83].

Nodular Malignant Melanoma.   This lesion appears as a small, blue-black or gray smooth nodule in the age group from 40 to 50 years and is twice as common in men as in women. Growth involves the epidermis and the dermis simultaneously. Large anaplastic neoplastic cells predominate and show a tendency to lie in alveolar groups, but spindle and pleomorphic cells are also present. Although inflammatory cells are present in the early stages, they tend to decrease in number as the tumor invades. Growth is more rapid and the depth of invasion is more extensive than in other types of melanoma. As a result, the nodular variety has the worst prognosis; the death rate after 5 years is 60% [153]. Nodular lesions in the eyelid margin have a worse prognosis than those elsewhere on the eyelid skin [37,83].

In 1969, Clark and colleagues [33] introduced a classification of cutaneous melanomas based on the depth of invasion of the skin by the neoplastic cells:

    I.   Confined to epidermis
   II.   Invasion of the papillary dermis
  III.   Filling of papillary dermis, with abutment on reticular dermis
  IV.   Invasion of reticular dermis
   V.   Invasion of subcutaneous tissues

Breslow [24] also contributed to the further understanding and estimation of prognosis by considering the thickness, cross-sectional area, and depth of invasion. The methods of Clark and Breslow do not correspond exactly, and on occasion, Clark's level III or IV tumors are less than 1 mm in thickness [10]. Studies have indicated that thickness is the most reliable prognostic factor [43].

A more recent proposal for estimating expected survival takes account of the patient's sex and the thickness of the primary lesion [116]. This method is based on a study of 371 patients with stage I malignant melanoma. In female patients with a 1 mm tumor, the estimated 5 year survival rate was 94%; for each 1 mm increment in thickness, the survival rate declined by approximately 3% up to the 6 mm level. Beyond this level and up to 15 mm thickness, the survival rate declined by approximately 8% for each additional millimeter. For the male patient, the prognosis was slightly worse. Currently, however, the staging of melanoma of the eyelid is based on Clark's levels [7]. Thus, level for level, lentigo maligna melanoma appears to have a better prognosis than other types of melanoma; the 5 year survival rate is 89% (compared with 68.5% of the superficial spreading melanomas). Differentiation among the three types of invasive melanoma is thus of prognostic significance. Lentigo melanoma rarely metastasizes, but superficial spreading melanoma frequently gives rise to metastases.

When invasive melanoma of the eyelid extends to the conjunctiva, the characteristic pathological features of the various types are maintained.

D. Miscellaneous

Merkel Tactile Cell Tumor

Merkel, in 1875 [159], described the so-called Merkel tactile cell in the snout of the mole. The cell is oval and dendritic, with a round to oval nucleus that contains finely dispersed chromatin and one to three small nucleoli. The cytoplasm is scanty.

Tumors of these cells are rare but are increasingly recognized and so reported in the literature [125]. The Merkel tactile cell tumor has several synonyms, including primary small cell cutaneous carcinoma, trabecular carcinoma, small cell neuroepithelial tumor, cutaneous APUDoma, and neuroendocrine tumor. These names reflect the appearance and the function of the cell, which is derived from the neural crest. It migrates to the deep layers of the epidermis, where it forms complexes with nerve endings to function as mechanoreceptors for the sensation of touch (*Tastzellen*).

This tumor is malignant, most commonly occurs in the elderly, and is found most frequently on the head and neck. It may also occur on the trunk and limbs. The first Merkel tactile cell tumor of the eyelid was described in 1983 [14]. Since then, approximately 20 cases have been reported. In the series of Searl and colleagues [197], of 69 such patients, 7 (9%) had eyelid involvement. Six of the seven tumors affected the upper eyelid, and one was on the eyebrow. Predilection for the upper eyelid has been observed by others [125]. Most of these tumors have occurred in women.

Clinically, the tumor appears as a nontender, reddish blue nodule with telangiectatic vessels on its surface. Thus, it appears angiomatous. One case manifested as a recurrent chalazion [144]. The median age of patients is 71 years [197], but a Merkel tactile cell tumor of the eyelid has been described in a 15-year-old girl with ectodermal dysplasia [84].

Microscopically, the cells may be confused with other small cell neoplasms, such as oat cell carcinoma of the lung and lymphoma. Immunohistochemical and ultrastructural studies help to characterize the cell [201]. The cell stains positively for neuron-specific enolase, keratin, and epithelial membrane antigen [49,60] and *met*-enkephalin [60]. Peptides, such as calcitonin, somatostatin, and adrenocorticotropic hormone, have also been demonstrated in the tumor cells [89].

Rapid growth and local and distant metastases may occur. Fine-needle biopsy with immuno-histochemical studies has established the nature of such metastases to the parotid gland [84]. In the series of Searl and colleagues [197], death due to metastasis occurred in approximately 20% of patients.

Because the number of reported cases of Merkel cell tumors of the eyelid is still small, the best form of management cannot be determined; currently, wide local excision is recommended.

Fibrous Histiocytoma

The eyelids [4,105,114,115,189], conjunctiva [4,55,171], and corneoscleral limbus [58,100] are rare locations for fibrous histiocytoma. It is more commonly found in the orbit (see Chap. 50). As a single entity, it is usually solid, and those in the eyelid are usually deeply situated. Its average diameter is 1.5 cm. One patient with multiple bilateral eyelid tumors has been reported [189]. Most of these lesions are benign.

As the name implies, the tumor is composed of spindle cells and large foamy histiocytes. The fibroblasts are arranged in interlacing fascicles and may exhibit a storiform pattern. Scattered throughout the tumor are giant cells of the Touton or foreign body type, lymphocytes, and other inflammatory cells.

Myxoma

Myxomas of the eyelid or conjunctiva are rare tumors [28,175]. As an entity, the myxoma is the most common primary tumor of the heart. Approximately 90% are found in the atria; the left-right ratio is 4:1. Recently recognized is Carney's syndrome, in which a myxoma of the heart coexists with a myxoma of the skin, that may include the eyelid or conjunctiva [29,42,119,120,174,176]. In addition, there is spotty pigmentation of the skin and overactivity of various endocrine glands. Recognition of the association is important because a patient with a myxoma of the eyelid or conjunctiva requires examination by a cardiologist to exclude a cardiac myxoma. Sudden death may occur from blockage of the atrial valves during diastole, chronic wearing of the leaflets may occur, or the tumor may fragment and embolize.

Intravascular Endothelial Papillary Hyperplasia

This entity is interesting because, although benign, it may be confused histologically with angiosarcoma. Essentially the lesion is an organizing thrombus within a vessel, most commonly a vein, and consists of papillary fibrous fronds covered by proliferating pleomorphic endothelium and surrounded by the muscle coat and adventitia of the vessel. The lesion has been described in the eyelid and eyebrow as well as the orbit [73,206].

Complex Choristoma

Ectopic tissue within the eyelid is uncommon. A complex choristoma that consists of various displaced elements is extremely rare. Gordon and coworkers [87] reported such a case: in a 2-year-old child, a nodule composed of cilia and lacrimal gland was present in the outer aspect of the upper eyelid. Tears drained intermittently from the base of the cilia.

Juvenile Xanthogranuloma

As its name implies, this tumor is a histiocytic lesion of children, and giant cells are of the Touton type. It is found in the skin but rarely in the eyelid. On rare occasions, it is also found within the eye. A large macronodular juvenile xanthogranuloma was reported in the upper eyelid of a 2-day-old infant by Schwartz and coworkers [196]. Clinically the lesion was thought to be a capillary hemangioma because of its violaceous color. Histologically, the differential diagnosis included dermatofibrosarcoma protuberans, which attests to the solid spindle cells that were present. The profile with immunohistochemical studies confirmed the nature of the lesion as juvenile xanthogranuloma and showed positive staining for histiocytes (G3D3) but negative staining for CD1 (T6) and S-100 protein. Treatment with intralesional cortisone led to a complete regression of the lesion.

Lymphoma

Non-Hodgkin's lymphoma may be of B or T cell lineage. It is the former type that more commonly involves the ocular adnexa. Non-Hodgkin's lymphoma of the T cell type is composed of two categories: one gives rise to lymphoblastic lymphoma or leukemia (prethymic and thymic lymphocytes) and the second gives rise to peripheral T cell lymphoma (postthymic lymphocytes). Of the latter, mycosis fungoides is the most common type to involve the ocular adnexa [110]. A 59-year-old patient who presented with immunoblastic T cell lymphoma of the eyelid was described by Kirsch et al. [124]. Because of the histology, both local radiation and chemotherapy were given, but 3 months later multiple skin nodules developed and the second eyelid also became involved. After further radiation and chemotherapy, 2 years later the patient had no recurrence of the eyelid tumor.

III. TUMORS, CYSTS, AND RELATED LESIONS OF THE CONJUNCTIVA: EPITHELIUM

Benign

Cysts.   Epithelial cysts of the conjunctiva are usually acquired as a result of epithelial implantation or obstructed ducts. Implantation cysts are lined by regular conjunctival epithelium and contain clear fluid.

Papilloma. Recent advances in immunohistochemical methods have allowed identification of papillomavirus common antigen within the epithelial cell nuclei of most conjunctival papillomas; this supports the causal role of papillomaviruses in these benign tumors [135,150,219]. In situ hybridization studies have demonstrated several types of papillomavirus in association with the lesion [62,134, 145,152,178]. Human papillomavirus type 6 is apparently responsible for most of the conjunctival papillomas of children and young adults [152]. The presence of genital tract human papillomavirus type 6 in the lesion suggests that some of the infections are acquired during passage through an infected birth canal. Human papillomavirus type 6a has also been demonstrated in a caruncular papilloma of a patient who suffered from genital warts [62] and in the conjunctiva of a child born of a mother with genital warts [162].

The papilloma of the conjunctiva occurs most commonly in children and young adults at the limbus, eyelid margins, and lacrimal caruncle. The surface is cauliflowerlike, the consistency is soft, and there is frequently a peduncle. In dark-skinned individuals, the presence of melanin within the lesion may lead the clinician to suspect a melanoma. Microscopically, a connective tissue stalk is covered by epithelium containing goblet cells, and numerous mucous glands are frequently present.

The verrucal type of conjunctival papilloma tends to be multiple and recurrent, but despite the common recurrence there is no apparent malignant potential. Human papillomavirus type 16 has been demonstrated in bilateral lesions [168]. On occasion, recurrent conjunctival papilloma can cause nasal lacrimal duct obstruction [136,161].

An unusual benign conjunctival neoplasm is the inverted papilloma [107,211]. The juxtalimbal area, the plica semilunaris, the caruncle, or the tarsal conjunctiva may be involved. The squamous epithelium undergoes acanthosis and invaginates the underlying connective tissue without evidence of keratinization or inflammation. Initially the invaginations appear cystic, but solid lobules develop secondarily and mucus-producing goblet cells are scattered throughout. The lesion appears benign, does not exhibit local aggressive growth, and does not involve extensive segments of the conjunctival epithelium. Thus, it is distinct from its counterpart in the nasal cavity and sinuses, where it frequently recurs and, on rare occasions, becomes carcinomatous.

Oncocytoma of the Caruncle. The Greek term *onco* means increase in size. The oncocytoma may develop in the lacrimal gland, lacrimal sac, or the caruncle and canthal conjunctiva. It grows slowly, and caruncular tumors are usually benign. Malignant forms may arise in the lacrimal gland or its sac. It occurs in middle-aged and elderly persons and is more common in women [17].

The tumor may be solid or cystic or a combination of the two patterns. The cells are characteristically large, the nuclei are small, and the cytoplasm is deeply eosinophilic. It is believed that the tumor arises from oncocytic metaplasia of ductal and acinar cells in the ocular adnexa.

An ultrastructural study by Freddo and Leibowitz [75] showed that two types of mitochondria fill the cytoplasm. Most of the mitochondria are very large, and the cristae show a wide variation in pattern. Granular inclusions, presumed to be α- and β-glycogen deposits, are present in a few of the large mitochondria. Smaller slender mitochondria are less numerous and have more typical cristae. The cells show apical surface villi and poorly defined desmosomes at the lateral borders. An interesting finding is the attachment of occasional mitochondria to the cytoplasmic surface. This feature has not previously been described in oncocytomas at this location. Such desmosomal-mitochondrial complexes are present in various normal secretory epithelium in other glandular tissues.

Hereditary Benign Intraepithelial Dyskeratosis. Dyskeratosis refers to individual cell keratinization seen as eosinophilic intracytoplasmic bodies measuring 10 μm in diameter, and it may occur in benign keratoses, precancerous lesions, and squamous cell carcinoma [139]. It is also the predominant abnormality in a rare inherited disease (autosomal dominant) known as hereditary benign intraepithelial dyskeratosis. This disorder, with lesions of the bulbar and oral mucosa, was first recognized in North Carolina and affects descendants of a triracial isolate called the Haliwa [183]. Bilateral horseshoe-shaped plaques at the nasal and temporal aspects of the limbus are conspicuous abnormalities in hereditary benign intraepithelial dyskeratosis. The plaques, which are typified morphologically by a dyskeratotic hyperplastic epithelium, become apparent from birth or early infancy and persist throughout life, with fluctuations in thickness. These perfectly benign lesions recur after excision and may give the clinician a false impression of malignancy [183].

Precancerous

Dysplasia.   Dysplasia is a disturbance in the differentiation of the epithelium, characterized by variation in size, shape, and organization of hyperplastic cells. Although the degree of cellular abnormality can vary from mild to severe, the superficial layers of the conjunctiva are usually spared. Conjunctival dysplasia is analogous to the epithelial component of actinic (senile) keratosis of the eyelid and, like the latter, is usually associated with an actinic elastosis of the underlying connective tissue (pinguecula) and sometimes also a pterygium. The term "conjunctival intraepithelial neoplasia" is commonly used for various degrees of dysplasia [179]. Studies with the polymerase chain reaction assay have detected the presence of human papillomavirus type 16 in some of these intraepithelial neoplasms [137,149].

Treatment requires local excision with adequate margins. The cell type, clinical appearance, and degree of dysplasia do not necessarily correlate with the recurrence; involvement of the margins of the initial excision is an important prognostic sign for recurrence [57], as is the demonstration of human papillomavirus type 16.

Studies have shown that involucrin (see Chap. 32), which is a precursor of the cross-linked envelope protein of the human corneal stromal cells, is present in the upper layers of the epidermis and reflects normal differentiation of keratinocytes. With the use of immunoperoxidase techniques for localization of involucrin, it has been found in normal conjunctiva, conjunctival dysplasia, carcinoma in situ, and invasive carcinoma [97]. The distribution patterns for involucrin have been found to differ in precancerous and cancerous conjunctival lesions. Normal conjunctiva shows involucrin only in the three superficial cell layers; it is absent from the epithelium of the fornix. In contrast, involucrin involves the deeper layers of the epithelium, sparing the basal layers, in cases of conjunctival dysplasia. All epithelial layers are involved in carcinoma in situ and invasive squamous cell carcinoma. This characteristic suggests that the immunohistochemical demonstration of involucrin may help in differentiating the various degrees of epithelial neoplasia.

Malignant

Despite the histological similarity of malignant cutaneous and conjunctival epithelial neoplasms, their biological behavior is often different. Local recurrence is common, but metastasis is rare. The histological picture of the recurrent tumor may differ from the initial growth pattern. Not only may a lesion that is initially benign appear malignant on recurrence but also an initially malignant lesion may appear more quiescent on recurrence. This histological variability makes prognostic predictions difficult.

Epibulbar epithelial tumors tend to lie in a horizontal position in the palpebral fissure, the area relatively unprotected by the eyelids. They occur in the form of either a single plaque of acanthotic epithelium or, more commonly, a papillary growth with a broad base at the corneoscleral limbus. The tendency is toward exophytic growth, and even when the basal lamina is disrupted the tumor remains superficial, in contrast to cutaneous lesions. Usually, an abrupt transition from abnormal to normal epithelium is seen (Fig. 14), but occasionally multicentric growth occurs, and the transition is then not as distinct.

Any lesion with a hydrated keratin covering of appreciable thickness appears white (leukoplakia), whether it is benign or malignant; therefore, the term "leukoplakia" is without clinicopathological correlation.

An epidemiological survey imputes exposure to ultraviolet radiation as the main influence in the development of squamous cell carcinoma of the conjunctiva [34].

In Situ Squamous Cell Carcinoma.   In situ squamous cell carcinoma of the conjunctiva occurs at the corneoscleral limbus as a firm white plaque or fleshy mass. Atypical pleomorphic cells replace the entire thickness of the epithelium, and the atypical area may be sharply demarcated from the adjacent normal epithelium (Fig. 14).

Squamous Cell Carcinoma.   Conjunctival squamous cell carcinoma commonly appears papillomatous, with a tendency to spread superficially onto the cornea (Fig. 15). It is often preceded by a known in situ carcinoma, but despite malignant cells breaking through the basement membrane, growth remains superficial. The sclera and Bowman's layer of the cornea are excellent barriers to invasion, and only rarely are these structures directly penetrated [45,129]. This is a tumor of the later decades of life, and growth is slow and indolent; it is one of the least malignant forms of squamous cell carcinoma, particularly if treated early. In Saudi Arabia, it appears that squamous cell carcinoma of the conjunctiva follows a more

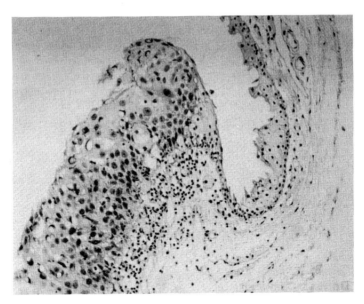

Figure 14 In situ carcinoma of conjunctival epithelium. Note the sharp line of demarcation between normal and abnormal epithelium. (Hematoxylin and eosin, ×160)

aggressive course and metastasizes widely [213]. Rarely the tumor may masquerade as orbital cellulitis [190] or necrotizing scleritis [123,141].

Pigmentation may be a feature and cause confusion with malignant melanoma, both clinically and histologically. Such cases have been reported in blacks, who normally have conjunctival melanocytes, but dark-skinned whites can be affected. Ultrastructural studies have demonstrated the presence of melanin granules within squamous cells as well as Langerhans cells, melanocytes, and macrophages [193]. There is a need to distinguish this pigmented squamous cell tumor from nodular melanoma, which has a more ominous prognosis.

Spindle cell carcinoma. Spindle cell carcinoma, a variant of squamous cell carcinoma, is a well-known tumor in many tissues but has seldom been diagnosed in the conjunctiva [36,99,165]. It may appear as a single nodule or a diffuse growth; six cases have presented in phthisical or atrophic eyes [99,165].

The tumor is characterized by spindle-shaped cells in continuity with an overlying dysplastic epithelium. Ultrastructural studies confirm the epithelial origin of the tumor, and immunohistochemistry shows that polyclonal and antikeratin antibody give the most consistent results compared with other monoclonal antikeratin antibodies [99,165].

The number of these tumors in the conjunctiva is insufficient to permit conclusions about their biological behavior; however, some of them have been locally aggressive.

Mucoepidermoid Carcinoma. As an entity, this tumor is most common in the salivary glands of both children and adults. Its occurrence in the conjunctiva is rare. It was first described at this site in a review of five patients by Rao and Font [180]. An additional nine cases have since been recorded [25, 48,81,146,147,198].

Clinically, mucoepidermoid carcinoma may be indistinguishable from squamous cell carcinoma. It is noteworthy that invasion of the conjunctiva and skin may not be clinically appreciated [81]. The tumor usually occurs in elderly persons in the seventh decade of life, but it may present as early as the fourth decade [48,147]. The most common presenting signs and symptoms are a conjunctival mass arising at the corneoscleral limbus accompanied by redness and irritation, but tumor may also occur in the lower fornix [180] and caruncle [147]. In addition, it may present as a diffuse limbal thickening or as a quiescent corneoscleral ulcer [48]. Histologically, the appearance is distinctive and the mucus-secreting cells can be demonstrated with the appropriate stains. The mucin is resistant to hyaluronidase digestion. Mucin

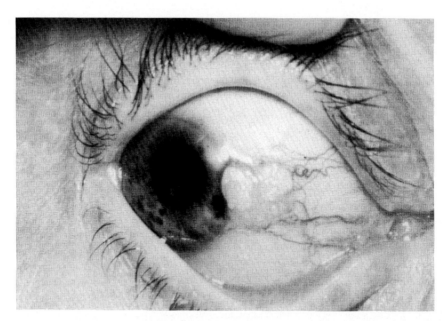

Figure 15   Squamous cell carcinoma of the nasal limbus of the right eye in line of palpebral fissure in a 62-year-old man. The surface is irregular and white because of the keratin coat. Several feeder vessels are evident.

production may be confined to a small portion of the tumor, and in one patient it was seen for the first time in the recurrent lesion [198].

Tumor growth is aggressive, and recurrence following excision is common. Wide local excision and frequent follow-up are advised. Distinction from squamous cell carcinoma is of practical importance because of the marked difference in behavior between these two tumors; squamous cell carcinoma is indolent, and mucoepidermoid carcinoma is rapid and aggressive.

Kaposi's Sarcoma.   Kaposi's sarcoma is a multicentric malignant process of endothelial cell derivation. Dorfman [50,51] was the first to suggest that the tumor cells were of lymphatic endothelial cell origin. Subsequent immunohistochemical studies with the vascular endothelial markers lectin, *Ulex europaeus* I, and monoclonal antibodies PAL E and EN4 also suggested that the tumor cells were of lymphatic origin [12].

The classic lesions consist of red to purple-brown nodules up to 1.0 cm in diameter on the skin of the lower extremities of older men, particularly those of Italian and Jewish descent. This variant of the disease is not necessarily associated with the acquired immunodeficiency syndrome (AIDS). Isolated lesions may also occur on the eyelid, conjunctiva, and episcleral tissue with or without AIDS. The tumor, unassociated with AIDS, has been reported in a patient with myasthenia gravis [13]. Multicentric conjunctival lesions have also been reported [143].

Particles resembling a retrovirus have been described in a case of conjunctival Kaposi's sarcoma [55]. Human immunodeficiency virus (HIV, HTLV-III) has been isolated in both asymptomatic and symptomatic patients with HIV antibody [80]. Patients with Kaposi's sarcoma lacking antibodies to HIV (HTLV-III) have a normal T4/T8 lymphocytic ratio [92]. The occurrence of Kaposi's sarcoma in HIV-negative homosexuals has led to a search for another virus [77]. Cytomegalovirus has been considered a possible causative agent because cytomegalovirus DNA has been found in cell lines from Kaposi's sarcoma [18]. Genetic predisposition may play a major role in determining which persons with AIDS develop Kaposi's sarcoma. Those with the HLA-DR5 phenotype seem to be susceptible [76].

The epidemic of AIDS continues and increases in incidence, as does the number of patients with immunosuppressed disorders, such as those with organ transplants. As the life of these patients lengthens as the result of new methods of management and new medicines, ophthalmic manifestations of the disease will be increasingly recognized.

In one study of 100 male homosexuals with the AIDS-related Kaposi's sarcoma, 16 had eyelid tumors, and in 7 patients the tumor was located on the conjunctiva. In 4 patients the tumor was the initial manifestation of this systemic disease [200]. Lebughe and colleagues [138], in a study of 290 patients with AIDS, found that Kaposi's sarcoma of the conjunctiva was present in 14 (23%) HIV-positive patients and in 1 HIV-negative patient.

Dugel and colleagues [54] classified adnexal Kaposi's sarcoma into three types based on the histological appearance in 18 patients with AIDS. Type 1 is composed of dilated vascular channels containing erythrocytes and lined by flat endothelial cells. Type 2 consists of plump endothelial cells and foci of immature spindle cells; vascular slits are infrequent. The features of type 3 include densely packed aggregates of spindle cells with hyperchromatic nuclei, occasional mitotic figures, and multiple vascular slits with erythrocytes between the slits. Type 1 and 2 tumors are less than 3.0 mm thick, and type 3 tumors are more than 3.0 mm thick.

In patients with AIDS, Kaposi's sarcoma has been considered relatively benign, and local treatment by excision, irradiation, application of strontium, and cryotherapy has proved successful. The tumor also responds to systemic drug therapy [200].

Lymphocytic Infiltrates of the Conjunctiva.   Small cell lymphocytic infiltrates of the conjunctiva may be part of a local benign reactive process or a manifestation of non-Hodgkin's lymphoma, B cell type. In both types, patients may present with unilateral or bilateral adnexal infiltrates (Fig. 16), and they are similar with respect to age, sex, and duration of symptoms [155]. However, lymphoid infiltrates that are confined to the conjunctiva are associated with a lower incidence of systemic lymphoma than are those of the orbit and eyelid [56,108,127,217]. Thus, the anatomical localization of the infiltrate is an important factor because the clinical behavior cannot always be determined from the histopathological findings or from the immunohistochemical studies. Lymphoid infiltrates of the conjunctiva have been extensively studied with immunohistochemical methods [56,108,109,126,158,217], and these studies gave some insight into the pathogenesis of the disease.

Genetic probe studies show that monoclonal populations exist in immunotypical polyclonal lesions and suggest that the disease evolves in situ [109]. There is a reasonably close correlation between polyclonal and well-differentiated tumors with regard to prognosis, and this may suggest that most are hyperplasias or primary lymphomas [126,155]. Less than half of all monotypic infiltrates disseminate [158], and the term "benign monoclonal lesion" has been suggested for these entities [108]. The well-differentiated subtypes predominate, and monoclonal B cells predominate over polyclonal lesions [109].

Dissemination of the cells occurs when the proliferation rate is 20% or more [158]. Thus, it is possible that determination of the fraction of proliferating cells must be assessed and so the risk of dissemination determined. Many aspects of these lymphoid infiltrates remain a challenge.

Melanocytes.   Within the ophthalmic literature, there has been a redefining of conjunctival pigmented lesions in the past decades. Nevocellular nevi remain the most common tumors of the conjunctiva and are of subepithelial, junctional, or compound type. Rarer entities, such as the blue nevus, spindle cell nevus, Spitz nevus, and epithelioid nevus, have also found their way into the literature [26,67].

The various forms of melanosis as precursors of conjunctival melanoma have been redefined because many benign conjunctival melanocytic lesions may mimic malignancy both clinically and histologically [68,69,106].

The ophthalmic pathologist recognizes that the conjunctival epithelium is not truly analogous with the epidermis and that the biological behavior of conjunctival pigmented lesions does not necessarily correlate with a counterpart of the skin. The dermatopathologist may question this nosology, but it has proved of practical importance in the management of such entities and is understood by the ophthalmologist who is caring for the patient.

The melanocytes of the eyelid epidermis and the conjunctiva arise from the neural crest. These cells contain tyrosine and therefore can replenish melanin stores and transfer melanin to neighboring epithelial cells by their dendritic processes. Melanocytes in the connective tissue, also derived from the neural crest, have low levels of tyrosine and neither replenish their stores nor transfer melanin to neighboring cells. From the epithelial melanocytes arise the conjunctival compound, junctional, and subepithelial nevi. The connective tissue gives rise to ocular dermal melanosis, blue nevi, and melanocytoma.

Conjunctival Nevi.   Most nevi develop during the first two decades of life and occur on the upper epibulbar surface, plica semilunaris, caruncle, and eyelid margin [26,67]. Usually there is no risk for the

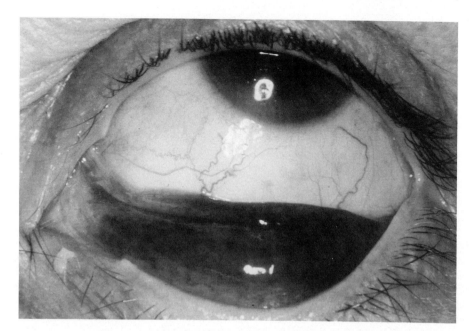

Figure 16   "Salmon pink" patch of conjunctival lymphoma.

development of melanoma, but rarely malignancy can occur in childhood and has a variable prognosis [41,148]. Nevi adjacent to the corneoscleral limbus tend to be flat, whereas those elsewhere tend to be elevated. The morphology of conjunctival nevi is similar to that of cutaneous nevi, except that the common addition of proliferating goblet cells can create cysts within the lesion; enlargement of the lesions may result from an accumulation of mucus within the cyst to produce a false clinical impression of malignancy.

Congenital Conjunctival Melanosis (in Conjunction with Melanosis Oculi). Congenital melanosis oculi, including oculodermal melanosis (nevus of Ota), is discussed in Chapter 48.

Acquired Conjunctival Melanosis. Acquired melanosis oculi can be subdivided into primary (idiopathic) and secondary types (Table 4). Because primary acquired melanosis is rare, the individual clinician and pathologist see only a small number of affected patients. Studies of large series of patients have helped to elucidate the natural history, course, and prognosis of this entity [68,106].

Reese [184] recognized that there were two forms of the disease: one form remained benign (83%), and the second form (17%) progressed to melanoma. Zimmerman [228] later introduced a staging classification based on the presence or absence of junctional activity and the degree of invasion:

Stage I
    a.   Minimal or no junctional activity
    b.   Marked junctional activity
Stage II
    a.   Superficial invasion
    b.   Deep invasion

Subsequently, Folberg and colleagues [68,69] defined two groups of lesions based on the presence or absence of atypical cells. Primary acquired melanosis without atypia carries a low risk for the development of melanoma and consists of increased numbers of melanocytes that populate the epithelium. Primary acquired melanosis with atypia is a precursor of melanoma and is characterized by polyhedral cells, spindle cells, large dendritic melanocytes, or epithelioid cells. These cells remain localized as nests in the basilar region, may proliferate to involve the epithelium, or may show pagetoid extension. Malignant melanoma occurs in 90% of lesions with pagetoid spread and 75% of lesions with epithelioid cells [70]. If malignancy

Table 4 Secondary Acquired Melanosis

Endogenous pigment
    Metabolic disease (e.g., Addison's disease)
    Chemically induced (e.g., thorazine)
    Radiation induced
    Chronic disorders (e.g., trachoma, vernal conjunctivitis)
Exogenous pigment (pseudomelanin)
    Epinephrine
    Silver
    Mascara
    Foreign bodies

supervenes, it does so at many sites and at irregular intervals, and this relatively benign course is in strong contrast to that observed in the skin.

Primary acquired melanosis usually occurs in persons aged 40–50 years and is slightly more common in women than in men. It appears as a unilateral diffuse pigmentation of variable extent, and the significant features are the diffuseness of the lesion, the distinct variability of its pattern of behavior, and its prolonged course. It is not possible to distinguish clinically primary acquired melanosis with atypia from primary acquired melanosis without atypia. The pigmented area may remain stationary, it may grow while remaining histologically benign, or it may regress. Waxing and waning of size may be associated with inflammation or may be the result of a hormonal influence.

Conjunctival Malignant Melanoma. A conjunctival melanoma is usually a flat, pigmented lesion of variable size, most commonly located at the corneoscleral limbus (Fig. 17). Tumor located in the

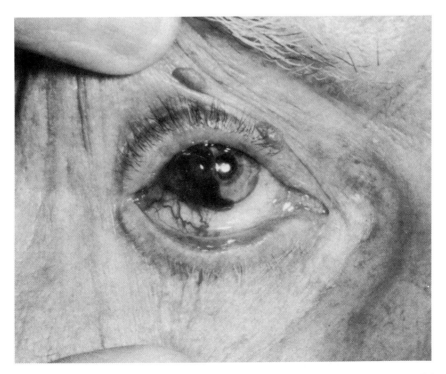

Figure 17 Nodular malignant melanoma. Conjunctiva of the right eye has a black, smooth nodule with an irregular advancing edge. Feeder vessels are present. The tumor arose de novo. Note two elevated intradermal nevi on the upper eyelid.

palpebrum has the poorest prognosis [47,113]. The tumor may arise from primary acquired melanoma with atypia, junctional or compound nevi, or de novo. Estimates of the frequency of melanomas arising from different sources have varied [102,140,184,228]. Prognosis is affected by the site and size of the lesion [78,113]. The depth of invasion is also an important prognostic factor [113,202,208,218]. However, the critical depth is in dispute. Patients with local intralymphatic spread are at risk for metastases [104].

Leiomyosarcoma of the Conjunctiva. Light microscopy, immunohistochemistry, and electron microscopy studies supported the diagnosis of this rare conjunctival tumor in the case reported by White and coworkers [221]. The patient, a 66-year-old man, had a 26 year history of a limbal lesion for which he had multiple operations; ultimately subtotal exenteration was performed. The spindle cell neoplasm showed positive staining with vimentin and muscle-specific actin and moderate staining for smooth muscle α-actin. Staining was weak for desmin and negative for S-100 protein, keratins, and α_1-antichymotrypsin. The authors attributed the protracted course in this patient to the superficial site of the tumor.

IV. TUMORS OF THE CORNEA AND ITS ADJACENT STRUCTURES

Acquired tumors of the cornea are most commonly found at the corneoscleral limbus and were discussed in Section III.

Congenital tumors include the various types of choristoma. The choristoma is a nodule of normal tissue that is ectopic. Such entities include the dermoid, dermolipoma, complex choristoma of lacrimal tissue, and the osseous choristoma.

A. Dermoid

The designation "dermoid" refers to a congenital lesion occurring at the temporal aspect of the corneoscleral limbus as an elevated, white, rounded, solid mass with a smooth surface, partly over the cornea and partly over the sclera (Fig. 18). Hairs may or may not extrude from the keratinized surface. It is a choristoma containing cutaneous appendages that are foreign to the anatomical site at which it is found. Rarely, multiple or bilateral dermoids occur, and even more rarely, intraocular extension is evident. The association of ocular dermoids with auricular appendages (Goldenhar's syndrome) [86] is a recognized entity that may be inherited. Other associated anomalies include defects of the first branchial arch and of the vertebral column.

Dermoids may enlarge at puberty and recur after incomplete surgical removal; vision may be impaired as a consequence of astigmatism or involvement of the pupillary margin. In the adjacent cornea, lipid infiltration of an arcus may be evident. It is the experience of the Mayo Clinic that most of these lesions are best left untreated because removal may lead to extensive corneal scarring. Conjunctival irritation by cilia, however, may necessitate surgical removal.

B. Dermolipoma

The dermolipoma, a common congenital anomaly of the bulbar conjunctiva with a smooth, rounded surface, occurs at the upper temporal quadrant near the lateral canthus. This variant of a dermoid consists of epithelium, appendages of the skin, and fatty tissue, the last of which predominates.

C. Complex Choristoma

The complex choristoma contains a variable admixture of cartilage, fat, smooth muscle, skin appendages, and lacrimal tissue. The lacrimal tissue almost always predominates. Usually the lesion is a single mass on the superior temporal quadrant. It has been reported in association with other ocular abnormalities in connection with the facial nevus of Jadassohn [222].

D. Episcleral-Osseous Choristoma

This solitary nodule of compact bone 0.5–2.5 mm in diameter is found in the superior temporal quadrant 5.0–10.0 mm posterior to the limbus. It may be adherent to the underlying tissue or freely movable.

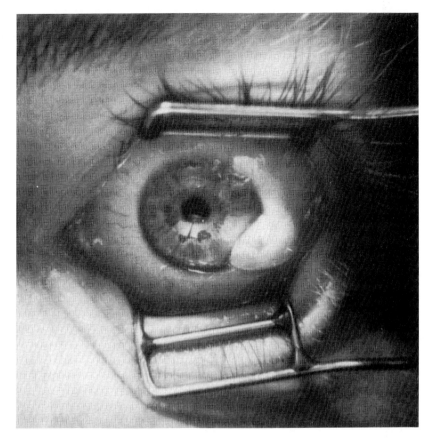

Figure 18 Corneal limbal dermoid in typical temporal position.

E. Fibroma and Fibromatosis

Fibrous lesions occurring as enlarging nodules at the limbus or in the episcleral tissues and consisting of bundles of fibroblasts with a variable variant of intracellular myxoid ground substance have been described. They may be up to 1.5 cm in diameter and are rounded but nonencapsulated. Usually there is no history of trauma or preceding inflammation, and the lesion is managed by simple excision. As entities, these lesions are more commonly located in the eyelids [61].

REFERENCES

1. Abe, M., Ohnishi, Y., Hara, Y., Shinoda, Y., and Jingu, K. Malignant tumor of the eyelid—clinical survey during 22-year period. *Jpn. J. Ophthalmol. 27*:175–184, 1983.
2. Ahluwalia, B.K., Khurana, A.K., Chugh, A.D., and Mehtani, V.G. Eccrine spiradenoma of eyelid: Case report. *Br. J. Ophthalmol. 70*:580–583, 1986.
3. Albert, D.M., McGhee, C.N.J., Seddon, J.M., and Weichselbaum, R.R. Development of additional primary tumors after 62 years in the first patient with retinoblastoma cured by radiation therapy. *Am. J. Ophthalmol. 97*:189–196, 1984.
4. Albert, D.M., and Smith, R.S. Fibrous xanthomas of the conjunctiva. *Arch. Ophthalmol. 80*:474–479, 1968.
5. Aldred, W.V., Ramirez, V.G., and Nicholson, G.H. Intraocular invasion by basal cell carcinoma of the lid. *Arch. Ophthalmol. 98*:1821–1822, 1980.
6. Ambrojo, P., Requena Caballero, L., Aguilar Martínez, A., Sánchez Yus, E., and Furió, V. Clear-cell syringoma: Immunohistochemistry and electron microscopy study. *Dermatologica 178*:164–166, 1989.

7. American Joint Committee on Cancer. Staging of cancer at specific anatomic sites: Ophthalmic tumors. In *Manual for Staging of Cancer*, 3rd ed., O.H. Beahrs, D.E. Henson, R.V.P. Hutter, and M.H. Myers (Eds.), J.B. Lippincott, Philadelphia, pp. 213–248, 1988.

8. Ashton, N. Benign calcified epithelioma of eyelid. *Trans. Ophthalmol. Soc. UK 71*:301–307, 1951.

9. Aurora, A.L., and Blodi, F.C. Lesions of the eyelids: A clinicopathological study. *Surv. Ophthalmol. 15*:94–104, 1970.

10. Balch, C.M., Soong, S.-J., Milton, G.W., Shaw, H.M., McGovern, V.J., Murad, T.M., McCarthy, W.H., and Maddox, W.A. A comparison of prognostic factors and surgical results in 1,786 patients with localized (stage I) melanoma treated in Alabama, USA, and New South Wales, Australia, *Ann. Surg. 196*:677–684, 1982.

11. Bardenstein, D.S., McLean, I.W., Nerney, J., and Boatwright, R.S. Cowden's disease. *Ophthalmology 95*:1038–1041, 1988.

12. Beckstead, J.H., Wood, G.S., and Fletcher, V. Evidence for the origin of Kaposi's sarcoma from lymphatic endothelium. *Am. J. Pathol. 119*:294–300, 1985.

13. Bedrick J.J., Savino, P.J., and Schatz, N.J. Conjunctival Kaposi's sarcoma in a patient with myasthenia gravis. *Arch. Ophthalmol. 99*:1607–1609, 1981.

14. Beyer, C.K., Goodman, M., Dickersin, G.R., and Dougherty, M. Merkel cell tumor of the eyelid: A clinico-pathologic case report. *Arch. Ophthalmol. 101*:1098–1101, 1983.

15. Beyer, T.L., and Dryden, R.M. Basal cell carcinoma masquerading as ectropion (case report). *Arch. Ophthalmol. 106*:170–171, 1988.

16. Bhalla, J.S., Vashisht, S., Gupta, V.K., and Sen, A.K. Meibomian gland carcinoma in a 20-year-old patient (letter). *Am. J. Ophthalmol. 111*:114–115, 1991.

17. Biggs, S.L., and Font, R.L. Oncocytic lesions of the caruncle and other ocular adnexae. *Arch. Ophthalmol. 95*:474–478, 1977.

18. Boldogh, I., Beth, E., Huang, E.-S., Kyalwazi, S.K., and Giraldo, G. Kaposi's sarcoma. IV. Detection of CMV DNA, CMV RNA, and CMNA in tumor biopsies. *Int. J. Cancer 28*:469–474, 1981.

19. Boniuk, M., and Zimmerman, L.E. Eyelid tumors with reference to lesions confused with squamous cell carcinoma. II. Inverted follicular keratosis. *Arch. Ophthalmol. 69*:698–707, 1963.

20. Boniuk, M., and Zimmerman, L.E. Eyelid tumors with reference to lesions confused with squamous cell carcinoma. III. Keratoacanthoma. *Arch. Ophthalmol. 77*:29–40, 1967.

21. Boniuk, M., and Zimmerman, L.E. Sebaceous carcinoma of the eyelid, eyebrow, caruncle, and orbit. *Trans. Am. Acad. Ophthalmol. Otolaryngol. 72*:619–642, 1968.

22. Bowen, J.T. Precancerous dermatoses: A study of two cases of chronic atypical epithelial proliferation. *J. Cutan. Dis. 30*:251–255, 1912.

23. Brash, D.E., Rudolph, J.A., Simon, J.A., Lin, A., McKenna, G.J., Baden, H.P., Halperin, A.J., and Pontén, J. A role for sunlight in skin cancer: UV-induced p53 mutations in squamous cell carcinoma. *Proc. Natl. Acad. Sci. USA 88*:10124–10128, 1991.

24. Breslow, A. Thickness, cross-sectional areas and depth of invasion in the prognosis of cutaneous melanoma. *Ann. Surg. 172*:902–908, 1970.

25. Brownstein, S. Mucoepidermoid carcinoma of the conjunctiva with intraocular invasion. *Ophthalmology 88*:1226–1230, 1981.

26. Buckman, G., Jakobiec, F.A., Folberg, R., and McNally, L.M. Melanocytic nevi of the palpebral conjunctiva: An extremely rare location usually signifying melanoma. *Ophthalmology 95*:1053–1057, 1988.

27. Burkhart, C.G. Looking at eyelid lesions—a clinical roundup. *Geriatrics 36*:91–95, August, 1981.

28. Campbell, R.J. Multiple endocrine neoplasia syndrome. In *The Eye in Systemic Disease*, D.H. Gold and T.A. Weingeist (Eds.), J.B. Lippincott, Philadelphia, pp. 91–93, 1990.

29. Carney, J.A., Gordon, H., Carpenter, P.C., Shenoy, B.V., and Go, V.L.W. The complex of myxomas, spotty pigmentation, and endocrine overactivity. *Medicine (Baltimore) 64*:270–282, 1985.

30. Carreras, B., Jr., Lopez-Marin, I., Jr., Mellado, V.G., and Gutierrez, M.T. Trichofolliculoma of the eyelid. *Br. J. Ophthalmol. 65*:214–215, 1981.

31. Caya, J.G., Hidayat, A.A., and Weiner, J.M., A clinicopathologic study of 21 cases of adenoid squamous cell carcinoma of the eyelid and periorbital region. *Am. J. Ophthalmol. 99*:291–297, 1985.

32. Charpentier, P., Bloch-Michel, E., Caillou, B., Soussaline, M., Boudier, V., and Offret, H. A propos d'un cas de syndrome de Torre: Association d'un adénocarcinome meibomien et d'une tumeur caecale. *J. Fr. Ophtalmol. 8*:479–485, 1985.

33. Clark, W.H., Jr., From, L., Bernardino, E.A., and Mihm, M.C. The histogenesis and biologic behavior of primary human malignant melanomas of the skin. *Cancer Res. 29*:705–727, 1969.

34. Clear, A.S., Chirambo, M.C., and Hutt, M.S.R. Solar keratosis, pterygium, and squamous cell carcinoma in Malawi. *Br. J. Ophthalmol. 63*:102–109, 1979.

35. Cleaver, J.E., and Bootsma, D. Xeroderma pigmentosum: Biochemical and genetic characteristics. *Annu. Rev. Genet. 9*:19–38, 1975.

36. Cohen, B.H., Green, W.R., Iliff, N.T., Taxy, J.B., Schwab, L.T., and de la Cruz, Z. Spindle cell carcinoma of the conjunctiva. *Arch. Ophthalmol. 98*:1809–1813, 1980.

37. Collin, J.R.O., Allen, L.H., Garner, A., and Hungerford, J.L. Malignant melanoma of the eyelid and conjunctiva. *Aust. NZ J. Ophthalmol. 14*:29–34, 1986.
38. Cooper, P.H. Carcinomas of sweat glands. *Pathol. Annu. 22*:83–124, 1987.
39. Costanza, M.E., Dayal, Y., Binder, S., and Nathanson, L. Metastatic basal cell carcinoma: Review, report of a case, and chemotherapy. *Cancer 34*:230–235, 1974.
40. Cramer, S.F. The origin of epidermal melanocytes: implications for the histogenesis of nevi and melanomas. *Arch. Pathol. Lab. Med. 115*:115–119, 1991.
41. Croxatto, J.O., Iribarren, G., Ugrin, C., Ebner, R., Żarate, J.O., and Sampaolesi, R. Malignant melanoma of the conjunctiva: Report of a case. *Ophthalmology 94*:1281–1285, 1987.
42. Daicker, B.C. Multiple myxome der Lider. *Ophthalmologica 179*:125–128, 1979.
43. Day, C.L., Jr., Mihm, M.C., Jr., Lew, R.A., Kopf, A.W., Sober, A.J., and Fitzpatrick, T.B. Cutaneous malignant melanoma: Prognostic guidelines for physicians and patients. *CA 32*:113–122, 1982.
44. de Azevedo, M.L., Milani, J.A.A., de Souza, E.C., and Nemer, R.S. Pilomatrixoma: An unusual case with secondary corneal ulcer. *Arch. Ophthalmol. 103*:553–554, 1985.
45. De Felice, G.P., Viale, G., and Caroli, R. Deeply invasive squamous cell carcinoma of the conjunctiva: Case report. *Int. Ophthalmol. 14*:241–244, 1990.
46. de Weerd-Kastelein, E.A., Keijzer, W., and Bootsma, D. Genetic heterogeneity of xeroderma pigmentosum demonstrated by somatic cell hybridization. *Nature New Biol. 238*:80–81, 1972.
47. de Wolff-Rouendaal, D., and Oosterhuis, J.A. Conjunctival melanomas in the Netherlands: A follow-up study. *Doc. Ophthalmol. 56*:49–54, 1983.
48. Dhermy, P., Pouliquen, Y., Haye, C., and Parent, A. Carcinome muco-épidermoïde de la conjunctive: Étude clinique, histologique et ultrastructurale. *J. Fr. Ophtalmol. 6*:553–563, 1983.
49. Dhermy, P., Sterkers, M., Morax, S., Charlot, J.C., and Savoldelli, M. Localisation palpébrale de la tumeur à cellules de Merkel (carcinome trabéculaire). *J. Fr. Ophtalmol. 10*:155–164, 1987.
50. Dorfman, R.F. Kaposi's sarcoma: The contribution of enzyme histochemistry to the identification of cell types. *Acta Unio. Int. Contra Cancrum 18*:464–476, 1962.
51. Dorfman, R.F. Kaposi's sarcoma revisited. *Hum. Pathol. 15*:1013–1017, 1984.
52. Doxanas, M.T., and Green, W.R. Sebaceous gland carcinoma: Review of 40 cases. *Arch. Ophthalmol. 102*: 245–249, 1984.
53. Doxanas, M.T., Iliff, W.J., Iliff, N.T., and Green, W.R. Squamous cell carcinoma of the eyelids. *Ophthalmology 94*:538–541, 1987.
54. Dugel, P.U., Gill, P.S., Frangieh, G.T., and Rao, N.A. Ocular adnexal Kaposi's sarcoma in acquired immunodeficiency syndrome. *Am. J. Ophthalmol. 110*:500–503, 1990.
55. Dugel, P.U., Gill, P.S., Frangieh, G.T., Rasheed, S., and Rao, N.A. Particles resembling retrovirus and conjunctival Kaposi's sarcoma. *Am. J. Ophthalmol. 110*:86–87, 1990.
56. Ellis, J.H., Banks, P.M., Campbell, R.J., and Liesegang, T.J. Lymphoid tumors of the ocular adnexa: Clinical correlation with the Working Formulation classification and immunoperoxidase staining of paraffin sections. *Ophthalmology 92*:1311–1324, 1985.
57. Erie, J.C., Campbell, R.J., and Leisegang, T.J. Conjunctival and corneal intraepithelial and invasive neoplasia. *Ophthalmology 93*:176–183, 1986.
58. Faludi, J.E., Kenyon, K., and Green, W.R. Fibrous histiocytoma of the corneoscleral limbus. *Am. J. Ophthalmol. 80*:619–624, 1975.
59. Farmer, E.R., and Helwig, E.B. Metastatic basal cell carcinoma: A clinicopathologic study of seventeen cases. *Cancer 46*:748–757, 1980.
60. Fawcett, I.M., and Lee, W.R. Merkel cell carcinoma of the eyelid. *Graefes Arch. Clin. Exp. Ophthalmol. 224*:330–335, 1986.
61. Ferry, A.P., and Sherman, S.E. Nodular fasciitis of the conjunctiva apparently originating in the fascia bulbi (Tenon's capsule). *Am. J. Ophthalmol. 78*:516–517, 1974.
62. Fierlbeck, G., Rassner, G., Thiel, H.J., and Pfister, H. Virusinduziertes Papillom der Bindehaut. Nachweis von HPA 6a DNA. *Z. Hautkr. 65*:497–499, 1990.
63. Finan, M.C., and Connolly, S.M. Sebaceous gland tumors and systemic disease: A clinicopathologic analysis. *Medicine (Baltimore) 63*:232–242, 1984,
64. Fischer, E., Keijzer, W., Thielmann, H.W., Popanda, O., Bohnert, E., Edler, L., Jung, E.G., and Bootsma, D. A ninth complementation group in xeroderma pigmentosum, XPI. *Mutat. Res. 145*:217–225, 1985.
65. Fitzpatrick, P.J., and Harwood, A.A. Acute epithelioma—an aggressive squamous cell carcinoma of the skin. *Am. J. Clin. Oncol. 8*:468–471, 1985.
66. Flament, J., Kouhil, M., Amiar, M.K., Boukoffa, O. S., and Forest, M. Giant keratoacanthoma of the palpebral region (diagnostic and therapeutic problems). *Bull Soc. Ophtalmol. Fr. 81*:611–615, 1981.
67. Folberg, R., Jakobiec, F.A., Bernardino, V.B., and Iwamoto, T. Benign conjunctival melanocytic lesions: Clinicopathologic features. *Ophthalmology 96*:436–461, 1989.
68. Folberg, R., McLean, I.W., and Zimmerman, L.E. Conjunctival melanosis and melanoma. *Ophthalmology 91*:673–678, 1984.

69. Folberg, R., McLean, I.W., and Zimmerman, L.E. Malignant melanoma of the conjunctiva. *Hum. Pathol.* *16*:136–143, 1985.

70. Folberg, R., McLean, I.W., and Zimmerman, L.E. Primary acquired melanosis of the conjunctiva. *Hum. Pathol.* *16*:129–135, 1985.

71. Font, R.L. Eyelids and lacrimal drainage system: Nevoid basal cell carcinoma syndrome. In *Ophthalmic Pathology: An Atlas and Textbook*, Vol. 3, W.J. Spencer (Ed.), W.B. Saunders, Philadelphia, pp. 2177–2178, 1986.

72. Font, R.L., Stone, M.S., Schanzer, M.C., and Lewis, R.A. Apocrine hidrocystomas of the lids, hypodontia, palmar-plantar hyperkeratosis, and onychodystrophy: A new variant of ectodermal dysplasia. *Arch. Ophthalmol.* *104*:1811–1813, 1986.

73. Font, R.L., Wheeler, T.M., and Boniuk, M. Intravascular papillary endothelial hyperplasia of the orbit and ocular adnexa: A report of five cases. *Arch. Ophthalmol.* *101*:1731–1736, 1983.

74. Ford, H.C., Delahunt, J.W., and Teague, C.A. Squamous cell carcinoma of the eyelid masquerading as "malignant" ophthalmopathy of Graves's disease. *Br. J. Ophthalmol.* *67*:596–599, 1983.

75. Freddo, T.F., and Leibowitz, H.M. Oncocytoma of the caruncle: A case report and ultrastructural study. *Cornea* *10*:175–182, 1991.

76. Friedman-Kien, A.E., Laubenstein, L.J., Rubinstein, P., Buimovici-Klein, E., Marmor, M., Stahl, R., Spigland, I., Kim, K.S., and Zolla-Pazner, S. Disseminated Kaposi's sarcoma in homosexual men. *Ann. Intern. Med.* *96*:693–700, 1982.

77. Freidman-Kien, A.E., Saltzman, B.R., Cao, Y., Nestor, M.S., Mirabile, M., Li, J.J., and Peterman, T.A. Kaposi's sarcoma in HIV-negative homosexual men (letter). *Lancet 335*:168–169, 1990.

78. Fuchs, U., Kivelä, T., Liesto, K., and Tarkkanen, A. Prognosis of conjunctival melanomas in relation to histopathological features. *Br. J. Cancer 59*:261–267, 1989.

79. Galimova, R.Z., and Bastimieva, B.E. Malherbe's necrotizing epithelioma of the eyelid without malignant degeneration. (in Russian) *Vestn. Oftalmol.* *106*:62–64, 1990.

80. Gallo, D., Kimpton, J.S., and Dailey, P.J. Comparative studies on use of fresh and frozen peripheral blood lymphocyte specimens for isolation of human immunodeficiency virus and effects of cell lysis on isolation efficiency. *J. Clin. Microbiol.* *25*:1291–1294, 1987.

81. Gamel, J.W., Eiferman, R.A., and Guibor, P. Mucoepidermoid carcinoma of the conjunctiva. *Arch. Ophthalmol.* *102*:730–731, 1984.

82. Gardner, E.J. Follow-up study of a family group exhibiting dominant inheritance for a syndrome including intestinal polyps, osteomas, fibromas and epidermal cysts. *Am. J. Hum. Genet.* *14*:376–390, 1962.

83. Garner, A., Koornneef, L., Levene, A., and Collin, J.R.O. Malignant melanoma of the eyelid skin: Histopathology and behaviour. *Br. J. Ophthalmol.* *69*:180–186, 1985.

84. Gherardi, G., Marveggio, C., and Stiglich, F. Parotid metastasis of Merkel cell carcinoma in a young patient with ectodermal dysplasia: Diagnosis by fine needle aspiration cytology and immunocytochemistry. *Acta Cytol.* *34*:831–836, 1990.

85. Glatt, H.J., Proia, A.D., Tsoy, E.A., Fetter, B.F., Klintworth, G.K., Neuhaus, R., and Font, R.L. Malignant syringoma of the eyelid. *Ophthalmology 91*:987–990, 1984.

86. Goldenhar, M. Associations malformatives de l'oeil et de l'oreille, en particuliar le syndrome dermoïde épibulbaire—appendices auriculaires—fistula auris congénita et ses relations avec la dysostose mandibulofaciale. *J. Genet. Hum.* *1*:243–282, 1952.

87. Gordon, A.J., Patrinely, J.R., Knupp, J.A., and Font, R.L. Complex choristoma of the eyelid containing ectopic cilia and lacrimal gland. *Ophthalmology 98*:1547–1550, 1991.

88. Gorlin, R.J., and Goltz, R.W. Multiple nevoid basal-cell epithelioma, jaw cysts and bifid rib: A syndrome. *N. Engl. J. Med.* *262*:908–912, 1960.

89. Gould, V.E., Dardi, L.E., Memoli, V.A., and Johannessen, J.V. Neuroendocrine carcinoma of the skin: Light microscopic, ultrastructural and immunohistochemical analysis. *Ultrastruct. Pathol.* *1*:499–509, 1980.

90. Graham, J.H., and Helwig, E.B. Premalignant cutaneous and mucocutaneous diseases. In *Dermal Pathology*, J.H. Graham, W.C. Johnson, and E.B. Helwig (Eds.), Harper and Row, Hagerstown, MD, pp. 561–624, 1972.

91. Grossniklaus, H.E., and Knight, S.H. Eccrine acrospiroma (clear cell hidradenoma) of the eyelid: Immunohistochemical and ultrastructural features. *Ophthalmology 98*:347–352, 1991.

92. Harper, M.E., Kaplan, M.H., Marselle, L.M., Pahwa, S.G., Chayt, K.J., Sarngadharan, M.G., Wong-Staal, F., and Gallo, R.C. Concomitant infection with HTLV-I and HTLV-III in a patient with T8 lymphoproliferative disease. *N. Engl. J. Med.* *315*:1073–1078, 1986.

93. Hashimoto, K., Blum, D., Fukaya, T., and Eto, H. Familial syringoma: Case history and application of monoclonal anti-eccrine gland antibodies. *Arch. Dermatol.* *121*:756–760, 1985.

94. Haye, C., Saragoussi, J.J., Asselain, B., Schlienger, P., and Calle, R. Le pronostic des mélanomes malins de la conjonctivite et des paupières: Étude statistique sur 56 patients. *J. Fr. Ophtalmol.* *5*:159–166, 1982.

95. Helwig, E.B. Inverted follicular keratosis. In *Seminar on the Skin: Neoplasms and Dermatoses*, Proceedings of 20th Seminar, American Society of Clinical Pathology, Washington, D.C., Indianapolis, IN, American Society of Clinical Pathology, p. 38, 1955.

96. Hidayat, A.A., and Font, R.L. Trichilemmoma of eyelid and eyebrow: A clinicopathologic study of 31 cases. *Arch. Ophthalmol. 98*:844–847, 1980.
97. Holbach, L., Hofmann, C., Völcker, H.E., and Naumann, G.O.H. Immunzytochemischer Nachweis von involucrin im präkarzinomatösen und karzinomatösen nicht-pigmentierten Bindehauttumoren. *Klin. Monatsbl. Augenheilkd. 189*:128–132, 1986.
98. Hornblass, A., and Stefano, J.A. Pigmented basal cell carcinoma of the eyelids. *Am. J. Ophthalmol. 92*:193–197, 1981.
99. Huntington, A.C., Langloss, J.M., and Hidayat, A.A. Spindle cell carcinoma of the conjunctiva: An immunohistochemical and ultrastructural study of six cases. *Ophthalmology 97*:711–717, 1990.
100. Iwamoto, T., Jakobiec, F.A., and Darrell, R.W. Fibrous histiocytoma of the corneoscleral limbus: The ultrastructure of a distinctive inclusion. *Ophthalmology 88*:1260–1268, 1981.
101. Jakobiec, F.A. Sebaceous adenoma of the eyelid and visceral malignancy. *Am. J. Ophthalmol. 78*:952–960, 1974.
102. Jakobiec, F.A. Conjunctival melanoma: Unfinished business. *Arch. Ophthalmol. 98*:1378–1384, 1980.
103. Jakobiec, F.A., Austin, P., Iwamoto, T., Trokel, S.L., Marquardt, M.D., and Harrison, W. Primary infiltrating signet ring carcinoma of the eyelids. *Ophthalmology 90*:291–299, 1983.
104. Jakobiec, F.A., Buckman, G., Zimmerman, L.E., Le Piana, F.G., Levine, M.R., Ferry, A.P., and Crawford, J.B. Metastatic melanoma within and to the conjunctiva. *Ophthalmology 96*:999–1005, 1989.
105. Jakobiec, F.A., Devoe, A.G., and Boyd, J. Fibrous histiocytoma of the tarsus. *Am. J. Ophthalmol. 84*:794–797, 1977.
106. Jakobiec, F.A., Folberg, R., and Iwamoto, T. Clinicopathologic characteristics of premalignant and malignant melanocytic lesions of the conjunctiva. *Ophthalmology 96*:147–166, 1989.
107. Jakobiec, F.A., Harrison, W., and Aronian, D. Inverted mucoepidermoid papillomas of the epibulbar conjunctiva. *Ophthalmology 94*:283–287, 1987.
108. Jakobiec, F.A., Iwamoto, T., Patell, M., and Knowles, D.M., II. Ocular adnexal monoclonal lymphoid tumors with a favorable prognosis. *Ophthalmology 93*:1547–1557, 1986.
109. Jakobiec, F.A., and Knowles, D.M. An overview of ocular adnexal lymphoid tumors. *Trans. Am. Ophthalmol. Soc. 87*:420–442, 1990.
110. Jakobiec, F.A., Lefkowitch, J., and Knowles, D.M., II. B- and T-lymphocytes in ocular disease. *Ophthalmology 91*:635–654, 1984.
111. Jakobiec, F.A., Streeten, B.W., Iwamoto, T., Harrison, W., and Smith, B. Syringocystadenoma papilliferum of the eyelid. *Ophthalmology 88*:1175–1181, 1981.
112. Jakobiec, F.A., Zimmerman, L.E., La Piana, F., Hornblass, A., Breffeilh, R.A., and Lackey, J.K. Unusual eyelid tumors with sebaceous differentiation in the Muir-Torre syndrome: Rapid clinical regrowth and frank squamous transformation after biopsy. *Ophthalmology 95*:1543–1548, 1988.
113. Jeffrey, I.J.M., Lucas, D.R., McEwan, C., and Lee, W.R. Malignant melanoma of the conjunctiva. *Histopathology 10*:363–378, 1986.
114. John, T., Yanoff, M., and Scheie, H.G. Eyelid fibrous histiocytoma. *Ophthalmology 88*:1193–1195, 1981.
115. Jordan, D.R., Addison, D.J., and Anderson, R.L. Fibrous histiocytoma: An uncommon eyelid lesion. *Arch. Ophthalmol. 107*:1530–1531, 1989.
116. Karakousis, C.P., Emrich, L.J., and Rao, U. Tumor thickness and prognosis in clinical stage I malignant melanoma. *Cancer 64*:1432–1436, 1989.
117. Kass, L.G., and Hornblass, A. Sebaceous carcinoma of the ocular adnexa. *Surv. Ophthalmol. 33*:477–490, 1989.
118. Keijzer, W., Stefanini, M., Westerveld, A., and Bootsma, D. Mapping of the XPAC gene involved in complementation of the defect in xeroderma pigmentosum group A cells (abstract). *Birth Defects 20*:508, 1984.
119. Kennedy, R.H., Flanagan, J.C., Eagle, R.C., Jr., and Carney, J.A. The Carney complex with ocular signs suggestive of cardiac myxoma. *Am. J. Ophthalmol. 111*:699–702, 1991.
120. Kennedy, R.H., Waller, R.R., and Carney, J.A. Ocular pigmented spots and eyelid myxomas. *Am. J. Ophthalmol. 104*:533–538, 1987.
121. Keramidas, D.C., and Anagnostou, D. Basal-cell carcinoma of the lower lid in a 27-month-old child. *Z. Kinderchir. 42*:250–251, 1987.
122. Khalil, M., Brownstein, S., Codère, F., and Nicolle, D. Eccrine sweat gland carcinoma of the eyelid with orbital involvement. *Arch. Ophthalmol. 98*:2210–2214, 1980.
123. Kim, R.Y., Seiff, S.R., Howes, E.L., Jr., and O'Donnell, J.J. Necrotizing scleritis secondary to conjunctival squamous cell carcinoma in acquired immunodeficiency syndrome. *Am. J. Ophthalmol. 109*:231–233, 1990.
124. Kirsch, L.S., Brownstein, S., and Codère, F. Immunoblastic T-cell lymphoma presenting as an eyelid tumor. *Ophthalmology 97*:1352–1357, 1990.
125. Kivelä, T., and Tarkkanen, A. The Merkel cell and associated neoplasms in the eyelids and periocular region. *Surv. Ophthalmol. 35*:171–187, 1990.
126. Knowles, D.M., II, and Jakobiec, F.A. Ocular adnexal lymphoid neoplasms: Clinical, histopathologic, electron microscopic, and immunologic characteristics. *Hum. Pathol. 13*:148–162, 1982.

127. Knowles, D.M., Jakobiec, F.A., McNally, L., and Burke, J.S. Lymphoid hyperplasia and malignant lymphoma occurring in the ocular adnexa (orbit, conjunctiva and eyelids): A prospective multiparametric analysis of 108 cases during 1977 to 1987. *Hum. Pathol. 21*:959–973, 1990.

128. Kraemer, K.H., Myung, M.L., and Scotto, J. Xeroderma pigmentosum: Cutaneous, ocular, and neurologic abnormalities in 830 published cases. *Arch. Dermatol. 123*:241–250, 1987.

129. Ku, E., and Avendano, J. Intraocular extension of a squamous cell carcinoma of the conjunctiva. *Rev. Oftalmol. 7*:35–39, 1986.

130. Kunnert, C., Boukoffa, W., Forest, M., Rebel, J.M., Flament, J., Bronner, A., and Brini, A. Xeroderma pigmentosum: A propos des localisations conjonctivales et palpébrales dans 2 cas. *Bull. Soc. Ophtalmol. Fr. 88*:1145–1146, 1988.

131. Kwitko, M.L., Boniuk, M., and Zimmerman, L.E. Eyelid tumors with reference to lesions confused with squamous cell carcinoma. I. Incidence and errors in diagnosis. *Arch. Ophthalmol. 69*:693–697, 1963.

132. Lahav, M., Albert, D.M., Bahr, R., and Craft, J. Eyelid tumors of sweat gland origin. *Graefes Arch. Clin. Exp. Ophthalmol. 216*:301–311, 1981.

133. Langer, K., Konrad, K., and Smolle, J. Multiple apocrine hidrocystomas on the eyelids. *Am. J. Dermatopathol. 11*:570–573, 1989.

134. Lass, J.H., Grove, A.S., Papale, J.J., and Albert, D.M. Detection of human papillomavirus DNA sequences in conjunctival papilloma. *Am. J. Ophthalmol. 96*:670–674, 1983.

135. Lass, J.H., Jenson, A.B., Papale, J.J., and Albert, D.M. Papillomavirus in human conjunctival papillomas. *Am. J. Ophthalmol. 95*:364–368, 1983.

136. Lauer, S.A. Recurrent conjunctival papilloma causing nasolacrimal duct obstruction (letter). *Am. J. Ophthalmol. 110*:580–581, 1990.

137. Lauer, S.A., Malter, J.S., and Meier, J.R. Human papillomavirus type 18 in conjunctival intraepithelial neoplasia. *Am. J. Ophthalmol. 110*:23–27, 1990.

138. Lebughe, I., Colebunders, R., Kapita, B., Francis, H., Nelson, A., Ndangi, K., et al. Clinical manifestations of Kaposi sarcoma (KS) in central Africa (meeting abstract). Second International Symposium on AIDS and Associated Cancers in Africa. October 7–9, 1987, Naples, Italy, p. 135, 1987.

139. Lever, W.F., and Schaumburg-Lever, G. *Histopathology of the Skin*, 7th ed., J.B. Lippincott, Philadelphia, 1990.

140. Liesegang, T.J., and Campbell, R.J. Mayo Clinic experience with conjunctival melanomas. *Arch. Ophthalmol. 98*:1385–1389, 1980.

141. Lindenmuth, K.A., Sugar, A., Kincaid, M.C., Nelson, C.C., and Comstock, C.P. Invasive squamous cell carcinoma of the conjunctiva presenting as necrotizing scleritis with scleral perforation and uveal prolapse. *Surv. Ophthalmol. 33*:50–54, 1988.

142. Liszauer, A.D., Brownstein, S., and Codère, F. Mucinous eccrine sweat gland adenocarcinoma of the eyelid. *Can. J. Ophthalmol. 23*:17–21, 1988.

143. Macher, A.M., Palestine, A., Masur, H., Bryant, G., Chan, C.-C., Nussenblatt, R.B., and Rodrigues, M.M. Multicentric Kaposi's sarcoma of the conjunctiva in a male homosexual with the acquired immunodeficiency syndrome. *Ophthalmology 90*:879–884, 1983.

144. Mamalis, N., Medlock, R.D., Holds, J.B., Anderson, R.L., and Crandall, A.S. Merkel cell tumor of the eyelid: A review and report of an unusual case. *Ophthalmic Surg. 20*:410–414, 1989.

145. Mäntyjärvi, J., Syrjänen, S., Kaipiainen, S., Mäntyjärvi, R., Kahlos, T., and Syrjänen, K. Detection of human papillomavirus type 11 DNA in a conjunctival squamous cell papilloma by in situ hybridization with biotinylated probes. *Acta Ophthalmol. (Copenh.) 67*:425–429, 1989.

146. Margo, C.E., and Groden, L.R. Intraepithelial neoplasia of the conjunctiva with mucoepidermoid differentiation. *Am. J. Ophthalmol. 108*:600–601, 1989.

147. Margo, C.E., and Weitzenkorn, D.E. Mucoepidermoid carcinoma of the conjunctiva: Report of a case in a 36-year-old with paranasal sinus invasion. *Ophthalmic Surg. 17*:151–154, 1986.

148. McDonnell, J.M., Carpenter, J.D., Jacobs, P., Wan, W.L., and Gilmore, J.E. Conjunctival melanocytic lesions in children. *Ophthalmology 96*:986–993, 1989.

149. McDonnell, J.M., Mayr, A.J., and Martin, W.J. DNA of human papillomavirus type 16 in dysplastic and malignant lesions of the conjunctiva and cornea. *N. Engl. J. Med. 320*:1442–1446, 1989.

150. McDonnell, J.M., McDonnell, P.J., Mounts, P., Wu, T.-C., and Green, W.R. Demonstration of papillomavirus capsid antigen in human conjunctival neoplasia. *Arch. Ophthalmol. 104*:1801–1805, 1986.

151. McDonnell, J.M., McDonnell, P.J., Stout, W.C., and Martin, W.J. Human papillomavirus DNA in a recurrent squamous carcinoma of the eyelid. *Arch. Ophthalmol. 107*:1631–1634, 1989.

152. McDonnell, P.J., McDonnell, J.M., Kessis, T., Green, W.R., and Shah, K.V. Detection of human papillomavirus type 6/11 DNA in conjunctival papillomas by in situ hybridization with radioactive probes. *Hum. Pathol. 18*:1115–1119, 1987.

153. McGovern, V.J., Mihm, M.C., Jr., Bailly, C., Booth, J.C., Clark, W.H., Jr., Cochran, A.J., Hardy, E.G., Hicks, J.D., Levene, A., Lewis, M.G., Little, J.H., and Milton, G.W. The classification of malignant melanoma and its histologic reporting. *Cancer 32*:1446–1457, 1973.

154. McKusick, V.A. *Mendelian Inheritance in Man: Catalogs of Autosomal Dominant, Autosomal Recessive, and X-Linked Phenotypes*, 9th ed., Johns Hopkins University Press, Baltimore, 1990.

155. McNally, L., Jakobiec, F.A., and Knowles, D.M., II. Clinical, morphologic, immunophenotypic, and molecular genetic analysis of bilateral ocular adnexal lymphoid neoplasms in 17 patients. *Am. J. Ophthalmol. 103*:555–568, 1987.

156. McNutt, N.S., Shea, C.R., Volkenandt, M., Lugo, J., Prioleau, P.G., and Albino, A.P. p53 protein expression is frequent in basal cell carcinomas (abstract). *Lab. Invest. 66*(1):33A, 1992.

157. McNutt, N.S., Volkenandt, M., Shea, C.R., Lugo, J., Prioleau, P.G., and Albino, A.P. Expression of p53 protein and statin in normal skin, actinic keratoses, and basal cell carcinomas (abstract). *J. Cutan. Pathol. 18*:380, 1991.

158. Medeiros, L.J., and Harris, N.L. Immunohistologic analysis of small lymphocytic infiltrates of the orbit and conjunctiva. *Hum. Pathol. 21*:1126–1131, 1990.

159. Merkel, F. Tastzellen und Taskorperchen bei den Hausthieren und beim Menschen. *Arch. Mikrost. Anat. 11*:636, 1875.

160. Mert, M., and Wozniewicz, B. Keratoacanthoma. *Klin. Oczna 81*:537–538, 1979.

161. Migliori, M.E., and Putterman, A.M. Recurrent conjunctival papilloma causing nasolacrimal duct obstruction. *Am. J. Ophthalmol. 110*:17–22, 1990.

162. Naghashfar, Z., McDonnell, P.J., McDonnell, J.M., Green, W.R., and Shah, K.V. Genital tract papillomavirus type 6 in recurrent conjunctival papilloma. *Arch. Ophthalmol. 104*:1814–1815, 1986.

163. Nerad, J.A., and Whitaker, D.C. Periocular basal cell carcinoma in adults 35 years of age and younger. *Am. J. Ophthalmol. 106*:723–729, 1988.

164. Netland, P.A., Townsend, D.J., Albert, D.M., and Jakobiec, F.A. Hidradenoma papilliferum of the upper eyelid arising from the apocrine gland of Moll. *Ophthalmology 97*:1593–1598, 1990.

165. Ni, C., and Guo, B.-K. Histological types of spindle cell carcinoma of the cornea and conjunctiva: A clinicopathologic report of 8 patients with ultrastructural and immunohistochemical findings in three tumors. *Chin. Med. J. 103*:915–920, 1990.

166. Ni, C., Wagoner, M., Kieval, S., and Albert, D.M. Tumours of the Moll's glands. *Br. J. Ophthalmol. 68*:502–506, 1984.

167. Nicolau, S.G., Bădănoiu, A., and Băluş, L. Untersuchungen über spezifische antitumorale Reaktionen bei an Keratoakanthom leidenden Kranken mit einigen Betrachtungen bezüglich des Eingreifens von Immunitätsprozessen bei der spontanen Heilung dieser Geschwulst. *Arch. Klin. Exp. Dermatol. 217*:308–320, 1963.

168. Odrich, M.G., Jakobiec, F.A., Lancaster, W.D., Kenyon, K.R., Kelly, L.D., Kornmehl, E.W., Steinert, R.F., Grove, A.S., Jr., Shore, J.W., Gregoire, L., and Albert, D.M. A spectrum of bilateral squamous conjunctival tumors associated with human papillomavirus type 16. *Ophthalmology 98*:628–635, 1991.

169. Oldfield, M.C. The association of familial polyposis of the colon with multiple sebaceous cysts. *Br. J. Surg. 41*:534–541, 1954.

170. Orlando, R.G., Rogers, G.L., and Bremer, D.L. Pilomatricoma in a pediatric hospital. *Arch. Ophthalmol. 101*:1209–1210, 1983.

171. Paglen, P.G., Karcher, D.S., and McMahon, R.T. Fibrous histiocytoma of the conjunctiva. *Ann. Ophthalmol. 12*:522–525, 1980.

172. Parsa, F.D. Sebaceous gland carcinoma of the eyelids in Hawaii. *Hawaii Med. J. 48*:165–166, 1989.

173. Parshad, R., Sanford, K.K., Kraemer, K.H., Jones, G.M., and Taronen, R.E. Carrier detection in xeroderma pigmentosum. *J. Clin. Invest. 8*:135–138, 1990.

174. Patrinely, J.R., and Green, W.R. Conjunctival myxoma: A clinicopathologic study of four cases and a review of the literature. *Arch. Ophthalmol. 101*:1416–1420, 1983.

175. Pe'er, J., and Hidayat, A.A. Myxomas of the conjunctiva. *Am. J. Ophthalmol. 102*:80–86, 1986.

176. Pe'er, J., Levinger, S., Ilsar, M., Climenhaga, H., and Okon, E. Malignant fibrous histiocytoma of the conjunctiva. *Br. J. Ophthalmol. 74*:624–628, 1990.

177. Peterka, E.S., Lynch, F.W., and Goltz, R.W. An association between Bowen's disease and internal cancer. *Arch. Dermatol. 84*:623–629, 1961.

178. Pfister, H., Fuchs, P.G., and Völcker, H.E. Human papillomavirus DNA in conjunctival papilloma. *Graefes Arch. Clin. Exp. Ophthalmol. 223*:164–167, 1985.

179. Pizzarello, L.D., and Jakobiec, F.A. Bowen's disease of the conjunctiva: A misnomer. In *Ocular and Adnexal Tumors*, F.A. Jakobiec (Ed.), Aesculapius Publishing, Birmingham, AL, pp. 553–571, 1978.

180. Rao, N.A., and Font, R.L. Mucoepidermoid carcinoma of the conjunctiva: A clinicopathologic study of five cases. *Cancer 38*:1699–1709, 1976.

181. Rao, N.A., Hidayat, A.A., McLean, I.W., and Zimmerman, L.E. Sebaceous carcinomas of the ocular adnexa: A clinicopathologic study of 104 cases, with five-year follow-up data. *Hum. Pathol. 13*:113–122, 1982.

182. Rao, N.A., McLean, I.W., and Zimmerman, L.E. Sebaceous carcinoma of eyelids and caruncle: Correlation of clinicopathologic features with prognosis. In *Ocular and Adnexal Tumors*, F.A. Jakobiec (Ed.), Aesculapius Publishing, Birmingham, AL, pp. 461–476, 1978.

183. Reed, J.W., Cashwell, L.F., and Klintworth, G.K. Corneal manifestations of hereditary benign intraepithelial dyskeratosis. *Arch. Ophthalmol. 97*:297–300, 1979.

184. Reese, A.B. Precancerous and cancerous melanosis. In *Ocular and Adnexal Tumors: New and Controversial Aspects*, M. Boniuk (Ed.), C.V. Mosby, St. Louis, pp. 19–23, 1964.

185. Reifler, D.M., and Hornblass, A. Squamous cell carcinoma of the eyelid. *Surv. Ophthalmol. 30*:349–365, 1986 (published erratum appears in *Surv. Ophthalmol. 31*:77, 1986).

186. Robbins, H.H., Kraemer, K.H., and Andrews, A.D. Inherited DNA repair defects in *H. sapiens*: Their relation to UV-associated processes in xeroderma pigmentosum. In *Biology of Radiation Carcinogenesis*, J.M. Yuhas, R.W. Tennani, and J.D. Regan (Eds.), Raven Press, New York, p. 115, 1976.

187. Rodriguez-Sains, R.S., Robins, P., Smith, B., and Bosniak, S.L. Radiotherapy of periocular basal cell carcinomas: Recurrence rates and treatment with special attention to the medial canthus. *Br. J. Ophthalmol. 72*: 134–138, 1988.

188. Rogers, P.A. The ophthalmological significance of the basal cell naevus syndrome. *Aust. NZ J. Ophthalmol. 11*:275–279, 1983.

189. Ronan, S.G., and Tso, M.O.M. Multiple periorbital fibrous histiocytomas: A light and electron microscopic study. *Arch. Dermatol. 114*:1345–1347, 1978.

190. Rootman, J., Roth, A.M., Crawford, J.B., Fox, L.P., and Patel, S. Extensive squamous cell carcinoma of the conjunctiva presenting as orbital cellulitis: The hermit syndrome. *Can. J. Ophthalmol. 22*:40–44, 1987.

191. Russell, W.G., Page, D.L., Hough, A.J., and Rogers, L.W. Sebaceous carcinoma of meibomian gland origin: The diagnostic importance of pagetoid spread of neoplastic cells. *Am. J. Clin. Pathol. 73*:504–511, 1980.

192. Sacks, E., Jakobiec, F.A., McMillan, R., Fraunfelder, F., and Iwamoto, T. Multiple bilateral apocrine cyst-adenomas of the lower eyelids: Light and electron microscopic studies. *Ophthalmology 94*:65–71, 1987.

193. Salisbury, J.A., Szpak, C.A., and Klintworth, G.K. Pigmented squamous cell carcinoma of the conjunctiva: A clinicopathologic ultrastructural study. *Ophthalmology 90*:1477–1481, 1983.

194. Sanderson, K.V. Precancerous conditions of the skin. In *Precancerous States*, R.L. Carter (Ed.), Oxford University Press, London, pp. 74–92, 1984.

195. Santa Cruz, D.J., Prioleau, P.G., and Smith, M.E. Hidradenoma papilliferum of the eyelid. *Arch. Dermatol. 117*:55–56, 1981.

196. Schwartz, T.L., Carter, K.D., Judisch, G.F., Nerad, J.A., and Folber, S.R. Congenital macronodular juvenile xanthogranuloma of the eyelid. *Ophthalmology 98*:1230–1233, 1991.

197. Searl, S.S., Boynton, J.R., Markowitch, W., and diSant'Agnese, P. A. Malignant Merkel cell neoplasm of the eyelid. *Arch. Ophthalmol. 102*:907–911, 1984.

198. Searl, S.S., Krigstein, H.J., Albert, D.M., and Grove, A.S., Jr. Invasive squamous cell carcinoma with intraocular mucoepidermoid features: Conjunctival carcinoma with intraocular invasion and diphasic morphology. *Arch. Ophthalmol. 100*:109–111, 1982.

199. Shea, C.R., McNutt, N.S., Volkenandt, M., Lugo, J., Prioleau, P.G., and Albino, A.P. Overexpression of p53 protein in basal cell carcinomas of human skin. *Am. J. Pathol. 141*:25–29, 1992.

200. Shuler, J.D., Holland, G.N., Miles, S.A., Miller, B.J., and Grossman, I. Kaposi sarcoma of the conjunctiva and eyelids associated with the acquired immunodeficiency syndrome. *Arch. Ophthalmol. 107*:858–862, 1989.

201. Sidhu, G.S., Feiner, H., Flotte, T.J., Mullins, J.D., Schaefler, K., and Schultenover, S.J. Merkel cell neoplasms: Histology, electron microscopy, biology, and histogenesis. *Am. J. Dermatopathol. 2*:101–119, 1980.

202. Silvers, D.N., Jakobiec, F.A., Freeman, T.R., Lefkowitch, J.H., and Elie, R.C. Melanoma of the conjunctiva: A clinicopathologic study. In *Ocular and Adnexal Tumors*, F.A. Jakobiec (Ed.), Aesculapius Publishing, Birmingham, AL, pp. 583–599, 1978.

203. Simpson, W., Garner, A., and Collin, J.R.O. Benign hair-follicle derived tumours in the differential diagnosis of basal-cell carcinoma of the eyelids: A clinicopathological comparison. *Br. J. Ophthalmol. 73*:347–353, 1989.

204. Soffer, D., Kaplan, H., and Weshler, Z. Meningeal carcinomatosis due to basal cell carcinoma. *Hum. Pathol. 16*:530–532, 1985.

205. Sommerville, J., and Milne, J.A. Familial primary self-healing squamous epithelioma of the skin (Ferguson Smith type). *Br. J. Dermatol. 62*:485–490, 1950.

206. Sorenson, R.L., Spencer, W.H., Stewart, W.B., Miller, W.W., and Kleinhenz, R.J. Intravascular papillary endothelial hyperplasia of the eyelid. *Arch. Ophthalmol. 101*:1728–1730, 1983.

207. Southwick, G.J., and Schwartz, R.A. The basal cell nevus syndrome: Disasters occurring among a series of 36 patients. *Cancer 44*:2294–2305, 1979.

208. Stefani, F.H. A prognostic index for patients with malignant melanoma of the conjunctiva. *Graefes Arch. Clin. Exp. Ophthalmol. 224*:580–582, 1986.

209. Stewart, W.B., Nicholson, D.H., Hamilton, G., Tenzel, R.R., and Spencer, W.H. Eyelid tumors and renal transplantation. *Arch. Ophthalmol. 98*:1771–1772, 1980.

210. Stoll, H.L., Jr. Squamous cell carcinoma. In *Dermatology in General Medicine*, T.B. Fitzpatrick, K.A. Arndt, W.H. Clark, A.Z. Eisen, E.J. VanScott, and J.H. Vaughan (Eds.), McGraw-Hill, New York, pp. 407–425, 1971.

211. Streeten, B.W., Carrillo, R., Jamison, R., Brownstein, S., Font, R.L., and Zimmerman, L.E. Inverted papilloma of the conjunctiva. *Am. J. Ophthalmol. 88*:1062–1066, 1979.

212. Sun, W., Yao, Y., and Yi, G. Clinicopathological analysis of 30 cases of meibomian gland carcinoma. *Chung Hua Yen Ko Tsa Chih 18*:363–365, 1982.

213. Tabbara, K.F., Kersten, R., Daouk, N., and Blodi, F.C. Metastatic squamous cell carcinoma of the conjunctiva. *Ophthalmology 95*:318–321, 1988.

214. Takabe, H. Personal communication.

215. Tillawi, I., Katz, R., and Pellettiere, E.V. Solitary tumors of meibomian gland origin and Torre's syndrome. *Am. J. Ophthalmol. 104*:179–182, 1987.
216. Torre, D. Multiple sebaceous tumors. *Arch. Dermatol. 98*:549–551, 1968.
217. Turner, R.R., Egbert, P., and Warnke, R.A. Lymphocytic infiltrates of the conjunctiva and orbit: Immuno-histochemical staining of 16 cases. *Am. J. Clin. Pathol. 81*:447–452, 1984.
218. Uffer, S. Mélanomes malins de la conjonctive: Étude histopathologique. *Klin. Monatsbl. Augenheilkd. 196*:290–294, 1990.
219. Vadot, E., and Merignargues, G. Papillomes conjonctivaux et papillomavirus. *Bull. Soc. Ophtalmol. Fr. 90*:789–790, 1990.
220. Wesley, R.E., and Collins, J.W. Basal cell carcinoma of the eyelid as an indicator of multifocal malignancy. *Am. J. Ophthalmol. 94*:591–593, 1982.
221. White, V.A., Damji, K.F., Richards, J.S.F., and Rootman, J. Leiomyosarcoma of the conjunctiva. *Ophthalmology 98*:1560–1564, 1991.
222. Wilkes, S.R., Campbell, R.J., and Waller, R.R. Ocular malformation in association with ipsilateral facial nevus of Jadassohn. *Am. J. Ophthalmol. 92*:344–352, 1981.
223. Wolfe, J.T., III, Yeatts, R.P., Wick, M.R., Campbell, R.J., and Waller, R.R. Sebaceous carcinoma of the eyelid: Errors in clinical and pathologic diagnosis. *Am. J. Surg. Pathol. 8*:597–606, 1984.
224. Wright, J.D., and Font, R.L. Mucinous sweat gland adenocarcinoma of eyelid: A clinicopathologic study of 21 cases with histochemical and electron microscopic observations. *Cancer 44*:1757–1768, 1979.
225. Wright, P., Collin, R.J.O., and Garner, A. The masquerade syndrome. *Trans. Ophthalmol. Soc. UK 101*(Part 2):244–250, 1981.
226. Yaun, N.F. Meibomian gland adenocarcinoma with regional lymph node metastasis. *Chung Hua Yen Ko Tsa Chih 25*:144–145, 1989.
227. Zelickson, A.S., and Lynch, F.W. Electron microscopy of virus-like particles in a keratoacanthoma. *Invest. Dermatol. 37*:79–83, 1961.
228. Zimmerman, L.E. Criteria for management of melanosis (letter to the editor). *Arch. Ophthalmol. 76*:307–308, 1966.
229. Zimmerman, L.E., and Sobin, L. (Eds.). Histological typing of tumours of the central nervous system. In *International Histological Classification of Tumours*. No. 21, World Health Organization, Geneva, 1979.

47

Intraocular Epithelial Tumors and Cysts

Alison C. E. McCartney

United Medical and Dental Schools of Guy's and St. Thomas's Hospitals, London, England

I. EPITHELIAL TUMORS OF THE IRIS

A. Spontaneous Congenital and Posttraumatic Nonpigmented Cysts of the Iris Stroma

Spontaneously occurring cysts are uncommon lesions usually present in the first few months of life, appearing as thin-walled vesicles that project into the anterior chamber [97,105]. Clinically and histologically they can be difficult to distinguish from acquired posttraumatic cysts, which may also be lined by epithelium resembling that of the conjunctiva. Spontaneous iris stromal cysts [85] are lined by stratified squamous epithelium or cuboidal epithelium (occasionally mucus-secreting [58]), with subjacent melanocytes and occasionally other structures, such as accessory lacrimal gland. Immunohistochemical staining for cytokeratins within the epithelium suggests that the cysts arise from ectopic surface ectoderm rather than neuroectoderm [77]. They should be removed in toto [73,74]. Acquired cysts arise after epithelium is implanted as a result of trauma or surgery and usually give rise to more complications, such as secondary glaucoma, corneal edema, and iridocyclitis [101], than congenital cysts. Cysts arising from the iris pigment epithelium are considered in Section III.

II. TUMORS OF THE NONPIGMENTED CILIARY EPITHELIUM (PARS CILIARIS RETINAE)

A. Embryonal Tumors (Medulloepitheliomas)

The first description of a medulloepithelioma of the ciliary body was by Badal and Lagrange in 1892 [4], using the name *carcinome primitif*. In 1904, Verhoeff [107] introduced the name "teratoneuroma." A few years later, Fuchs, adding a new case of his own, suggested *diktyoma* (Greek *diktyon*, a net) [28]. The term "diktyoma" is still occasionally used today, but the designation "medulloepithelioma," first used by Grinker [36], was preferred by the World Health Organization ocular tumor panel [124].

Clinical Features

In the 56 cases described by Broughton and Zimmerman [10], the median age at the time of surgery was 5 years. In Andersen's series of 23 cases reported in 1962 [1], the mean ages of the benign and malignant cases were 4.5 and 7 years, respectively; subsequent series [16,101] have shown the same pattern, although late presentations [17] may give rise to diagnostic confusion with malignant melanoma [23], and the tumor may recur after surgery [51]. There is equal involvement of right and left eyes, and of males and females, with no apparent racial predilection. All cases described are unilateral, the other eye being normal in all but a very few cases. Klein [52] reported cases associated with bilateral megalocornea and bilateral congenital glaucoma, and another case was thought to be bilaterally anophthalmic but later developed a unilateral orbital mass [10]. In the series reported from the Armed Forces Institute of Pathology in the United States [10] iris neovascularization was not common, being seen in only 20% of cases, but in the series of Canning and colleagues [16], 13 of 16 cases were noted to have this clinical sign. No relationship with neoplasms or malformations of other tissues or organs is usually demonstrated, but Kivelä and colleagues described a glioneuromatous lesion that resembled a medulloepithelioma clinically when it arose in conjunction with a coloboma [50].

Pain and poor vision are the predominant symptoms, especially when the tumors become necrotic [108,109,117], and leukocoria and a discrete gray-white mass in the ciliary body [41], iris [69], or anterior chamber are also frequent presenting signs. The tumor may present with hemorrhage or scleral perforation [10]. Glaucoma and cataract are frequently associated. Irregularity and dilatation of the pupil are recorded in some cases, but colobomas of the iris have never been documented in a true medulloepithelioma [51]. The differential diagnosis includes persistent hyperplastic primary vitreous [48] and juvenile nevoxantho-granuloma [3]. This tumor can also be found in goldfish, cockatiels, dogs [88], and horses [20,98] and in some breeds of dogs [57] has been described as the most common primary intraocular tumor.

Histopathology

Medulloepitheliomas are believes to arise during embryonic development of the immature nonpigmented ciliary epithelium [121]. In a very few cases they arise from remaining embryonic retina in the posterior part of the sensory retina or in the optic nerve (Fig. 1) [2,35,38,80,90]. Mullaney [71] published a case apparently arising in a persistent Bergmeister's papilla, and persistent hyperplastic primary vitreous is reported as concomitant in 20% of cases.

Nonteratoid Medulloepithelioma

Multilayered sheets of poorly differentiated neuroepithelial cells resembling the primary medullary epithelium of the optic cup are the most noticeable component of the nonteratoid form, presenting in two-thirds of cases [13,39]. Tubular and papillary structures composed of a single layer of cuboidal cells resembling more differentiated ciliary epithelium are also formed, often with gradual transitions between these two components (Fig. 2). The sheets of medullary epithelium are polarized, forming along one

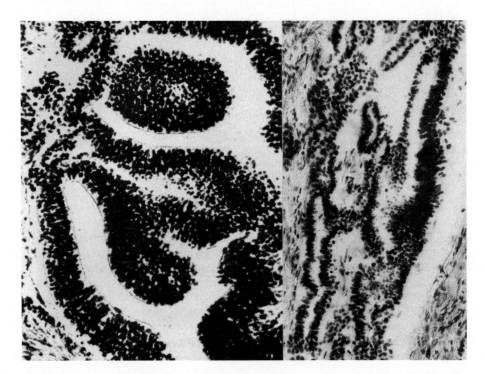

Figure 1   Nonteratoid medulloepithelioma from posterior retina and optic nerve. Multilayered membranes on left, single-layered on the right. (Hematoxylin and eosin, ×140)

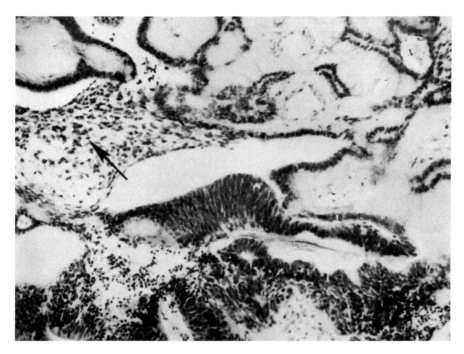

Figure 2 Nonteratoid medulloepithelioma; multilayered epithelium cut transversely in parts, forming rosettes and tubules. Single-layered areas are also present. The arrow shows glial elements. (Hematoxylin and eosin, ×140)

surface tissue that resembles the myxoid connective tissue of the primary vitreous and along the opposite surface a structure analogous to the external limiting membrane of the retina. When the multilayered tubular structures are cut transversely, they may appear as rosettes resembling to a certain extent Flexner-Wintersteiner rosettes of retinoblastoma and, in some cases, are similar to retinal anlage and primitive neuroectodermal tumors elsewhere.

Electron microscopically, cilia remnants and three types of rosettes have been described [41,42,111], and in another case the lumina of the rosettes were shown to contain microvilli [75]. The multilayered tubular structures, which have been described as neuroepithelial sheaths, stain positively for neuron-specific enolase and vimentin but not with markers of the more mature retina, such as S100 protein, glial fibrillary acid protein (GFAP), or neurofilaments [51]. This observation does not preclude other better differentiated glial elements being demonstrable, separate from the tubules, as they can be demonstrated by GFAP immunohistochemistry.

When the single-layered tubules are cut transversely, they may resemble the adenoid structures of the adult-type tumors of the differentiated ciliary epithelium. The proliferating medullary epithelium may form anastomosing cords and sheets separated by loose tissue, giving these tumors a netlike appearance—hence the old term "diktyoma." These structures are S100 positive, as is the adult ciliary epithelium [51].

Rarely, Homer-Wright rosettes (without lumen or limiting membrane) are observed [1]. Usually, the folding of the medullary epithelium occurs in such a way that the lumen of the resulting rosette or tubule is empty, lined by a surface with zonulae adherentes corresponding to the external limiting membrane, and it is here that the mitotic activity is most marked. This mitotic activity may be entirely appropriate, since in the developing retina, which this tumor mimics, mitosis of all cells of the neuroblastic retina occurs adjacent to the external (outer) limiting membrane. Confusion with the smaller [10] rosettes of retinoblastoma is usually avoidable since in medulloepithelioma a stromal component is almost always found, whereas in retinoblastoma there is no true stroma, the connective tissue being confined to the perivascular supporting tissues. The loose tissue surrounding the rosettes and tubules resembles primitive vitreous and stains intensely for glycosaminoglycans (GAG) sensitive to bovine testicular and streptococcal hyaluronidase [122].

In a few cases, free-floating cysts filled with hyaluronic acid occur in the anterior or posterior chambers. Differentiation into astrocytes (Fig. 2) and some formation of pigment epithelium is commonly observed.

Teratoid Medulloepithelioma

The teratoid medulloepithelioma is a tumor with all the foregoing characteristics but in addition containing heteroplastic tissues [121] not normally found during either embryonic or postnatal development of the eye: mature hyaline cartilage or chondroblasts, rhabdomyoblasts, with or without cross-striations [18,112,122], and cerebral tissue, including specialized CNS structures, such as ependyma or choroid plexus [120,121,123,124]. Ganglion cells are normal constituents of the retina, however, and as such probably should not be regarded as unusual within a medulloepithelioma. The heteroplastic elements may be inconspicuous, with only tiny islands of hyaline cartilage or occasional rhabdomyoblasts, sometimes in the form of strap cells with cross-striations [118]. In other cases the tumors are composed largely of mesenchymal tissue elements, such as chondroblastic (Fig. 3) or rhabdomyosarcomatous tissue (Figs. 4 through 6). Dendritic melanocytes may be another feature [9], as described in Barron and Saunders' case of "chondrosarcoma" in the eye of a cat [6].

Histopathological Criteria for Malignancy

Distinction between benign and malignant medulloepitheliomas is difficult. Malignancy may be inferred by the presence of overtly sarcomatous or carcinomatous tissues [35], but in some reports the designation malignant has been used for tumors that are aggressive and invade adjacent tissues. This is not normally taken as an absolute criterion for malignancy, and most "malignant" medulloepitheliomas have not metastasized, the "gold standard" for malignancy. In the extensive literature review performed by Kivelä

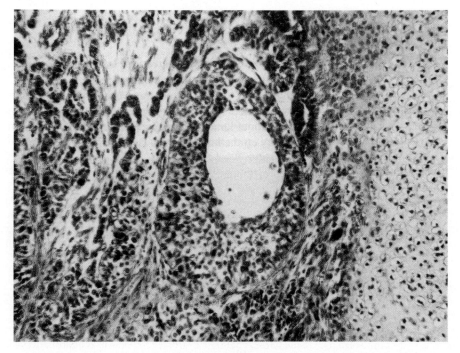

Figure 3   Teratoid medulloepithelioma with areas of hyaline cartilage on the right. (Hematoxylin and eosin, ×140)

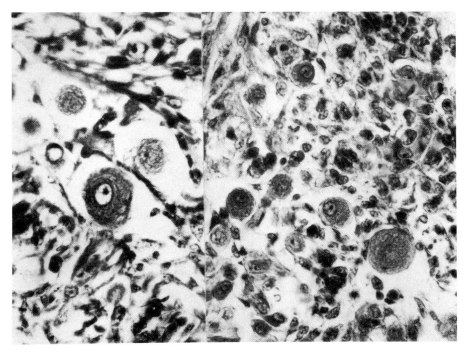

Figure 4 Ganglion cells within medulloepithelioma. (Hematoxylin and eosin, ×140)

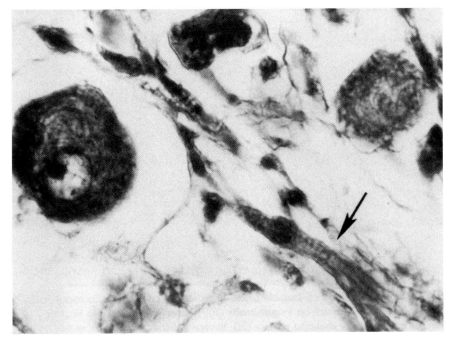

Figure 5 Malignant teratoid medulloepithelioma. Arrow points to rhabdomyoblast with cross-striations. (Wilder's reticulin stain, ×1090)

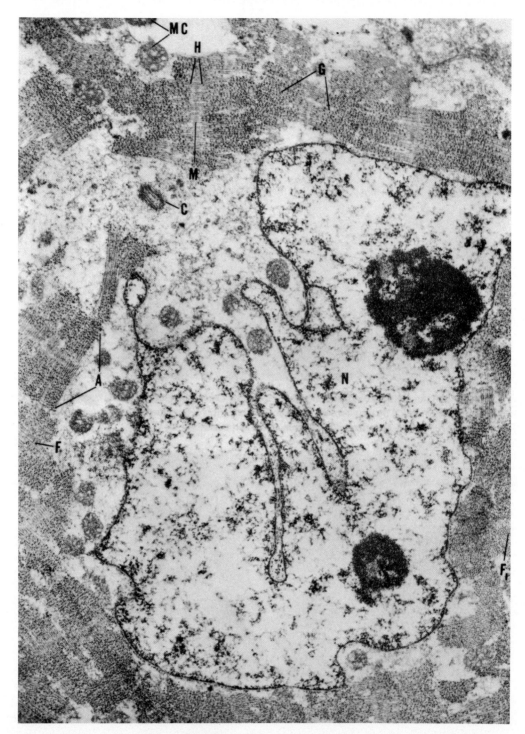

Figure 6 Ganglion cells in medulloepithelioma. Ganglion cells with numerous bundles of myofilaments, some of which are cut longitudinally (F), whereas others are seen in cross section (F₁) arranged concentrically about the nucleus (N). Several A bands (A) containing light H bands (H) with their dark central M lines (M) are present. Mitochondria (MC) are also present. (Electron micrograph, ×19,000) (Reproduced with permission from L.E. Zimmerman, R.L. Font, and S.R. Andersen. Rhabdomyosarcomatous differentiation in malignant intraocular medulloepitheliomas. *Cancer 30*:817–835, 1972.)

and Tarkkanen [51], only four cases of lymph node metastasis, two of parotid gland metastasis, and a single case of lung metastasis were found.

In most malignant tumors, the tubules and rosettes are retained, but they may be only an inconspicuous component of a largely undifferentiated neuroblastic tumor with some resemblance to a retinoblastoma. In Andersen's report of 1962 [1], his criteria for malignancy were numerous mitotic figures, pronounced pleomorphism, and extraocular extension, and although only one-quarter of the cases satisfied these requirements, he believed that all medulloepitheliomas should be considered potentially malignant. Broughton and Zimmerman [10] classified two-thirds of their cases as malignant, and in addition to the criteria for malignancy just listed, they included areas of poorly differentiated neuroblastic, chondroblastic and rhabdomyoblastic cells, and invasion of the uvea, cornea, sclera, and or optic nerve. In their malignant group 46% of tumors were teratoid, compared to 21% in the benign group. It is noteworthy that in both these series and in a later series [16] the mortality, which was due to invasion of the brain or to distant metastases, was very low. Deaths were recorded in less than 10% of the combined groups, when they were usually due to local aggressive growth, including growth into the orbit and brain; some patients were lost to follow-up, however.

Early recognition and surgical intervention was important. Enucleation may be the method of choice, although a few cases seem to have been treated successfully by iridocyclectomy, indicating that local excision might be appropriate when the tumor is small and well circumscribed; intractable iris neovascularization, however, may prejudice the eye [16], or the tumor may recur [51]. Tumors invading the optic nerve are usually treated by exenteration. The tumors appear to be radioresistant.

Histogenesis

At about week 7 of human embryonic development (20 mm stage), the iridic, ciliary, and sensory part of the inner wall of the optic cup are similar in appearance, although the development of the central retina is slightly advanced compared to the periphery. The cells are arranged in ranks or rows, with an overall appearance that might be called the embryonal retina stage [1] (Fig. 7), which still resembles the medullary epithelium (Fig. 8) of the brain of which it is an outgrowth with a direct connection. In the embryo the outer layer of the optic cup at 20 mm is still partly multilayered, but melanin granules have become visible in the pigment epithelial portions of the iridic and ciliary parts as well as in the retinal pigment epithelium (RPE). The cells of the retina form a structure that was previously called the transient layer of Chievitz (see Chap. 42), and later, the cells differentiate, forming specialized tissues. The "embryonal retina" stage disappears completely after the third embryonal month (about 60 mm) [113].

Morphologically, all ocular medulloepitheliomas seem to reflect to some extent this early embryonal retina. Even when the rosettes and tubules in these tumors have ostensibly neoplastic features, they resemble the mitotic and developmental stages of the medullary tube. Folding and displacement of premature retinal tissue may give rise to structures that are analogous to the rosettes in other types of "dysplastic" retinal tissue [2], which might perhaps be more accurately described as dystrophic or distorted. In the rare cases of medulloepitheliomas presenting in adults, it is unclear whether they have been present since birth, have arisen from residual embryonic retina, or have emerged as a result of dedifferentiation. The single-layered tubules, which are almost ubiquitous in medulloepitheliomas, resemble more differentiated ciliary epithelium rather than the mature ependymal layer.

In the teratoid medulloepitheliomas the mature mesenchymal heteroplastic tissues, such as hyaline cartilage and well-differentiated cross-striated rhabdomyoblasts, may be explained as metaplasia of the stromal elements of these tumors. Hyaline cartilage is often present in trisomy 13 and other chromosomal disorders and has been described in microphthalmic eyes with persistent hyperplastic primary vitreous [117]. The chondroblastic and rhabdomyoblastic elements [17] with features of malignancy in some of the teratoid forms are more difficult to explain but may reflect malignant change within mesenchymal components, ostensibly derived from neuroectoderm [120]. (Striated muscle in avian eyes is derived from the neuroectoderm [93].) Since the neural crest is capable of evolving mesenchymal components, other parts of the developing neuroectoderm may retain this potential pathway of development, or alternatively the neural crest itself may contribute. Neural crest mesenchymal differentiation is postulated to give rise to other tumors, including smooth muscle tumors of the orbit [45,47], and such disorders as the neurocristopathies [9].

The medullary neuroectodermal epithelium of the optic vesicle gives rise to a remarkable variety of tissues, including photoreceptors, neurons, neuroglia, pigmented and nonpigmented epithelia, the vitreous

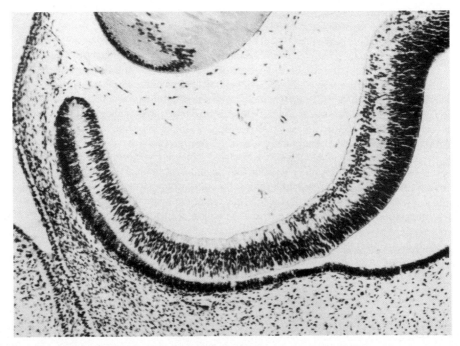

Figure 7 Anterior part of the optic cup in human fetus of 22 mm in week 7, showing multilayered undifferenti-ated epithelium resembling the medullary epithelium of the brain as the inner layer of the cup and pigment formation in the outer layer. (Hematoxylin and eosin, ×140)

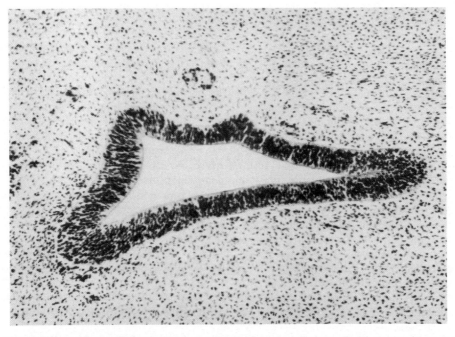

Figure 8 Undifferentiated medullary epithelium within the lateral verticular wall of the brain of the same fetus. (Hematoxylin and eosin, ×140)

body, and the involuntary smooth muscles of the iris and ciliary body. The medulloepitheliomas of the eye are further evidence of the pluripotentiality of this epithelium [24].

The neural crest does not participate in the development of normal peripheral retina derived from the neuroectoderm, however, although it contributes to the mesenchyme (mesectoderm) of the ciliary body. To postulate that the neural crest is responsible for the formation of mesectodermal elements in medullo-epitheliomas means that tissue derived from two different areas of neuroectoderm must first be separated and then grow normally in space and time before becoming inextricably entwined in the resulting tumor. If this is the case, then this pattern of growth is more akin to the development of a choristoma, with localized failure to control growth, and less like a neoplasm, which usually involves a single tissue or cell of origin, although biphasic tumors, such as pulmonary blastoma, uterine carcinosarcoma, and synovial sarcoma, are recognized [54].

Comparison with Medulloepitheliomas of the Brain

Medulloepitheliomas are even more rare in the brain than in the eye and have been regarded as embryonic ependymomas, with a rapid clinical course, usually causing death within 6 months. Karch and Urich [49], in a critical review of reported cases, accepted the diagnosis in only 11 instances. Histologically, both cerebral and intraocular medulloepitheliomas seem to mimic the primitive neural tube, and although blepharoplasts, primitive cilial remnants reported in intracerebral tumors, do not appear to have been reported in ocular tumors, cilia have been [41]. The apparently greater morbidity in the intracerebral tumors may reflect their mass effect within the cranial cavity and their propensity to seed along the spinal canal in the manner of other ependymomas.

Rhabdomyosarcomatous and chondroblastic elements associated with neuroepithelial elements have sometimes been described in brain tumors [87], and Rubinstein [86] interpreted this as evidence of a teratomatous nature.

B.   Adult-Type Tumors

Tumors, either neoplastic or hyperplastic, may arise from the mature nonpigmented ciliary epithelium after it has completed its differentiation. Usually they show some evidence of differentiation toward pigmented as well as nonpigmented epithelium, and it may be difficult to ascertain from which layer the tumor has originated. Intraocular choristomas of lacrimal gland type may also lead to confusion [33].

Hyperplasias

Fuchs' "Adenoma."   First described by Fuchs [27,28], this is a small, discrete, hyperplastic nodule: it is observed almost exclusively as an incidental finding in eyes enucleated for other reasons or examined postmortem, where it is very common, increasing in incidence with age, although often inconspicuous. They are thought to represent degenerative change within the ciliary body [83].

Reactive Hyperplasia.   Reactive hyperplasia of nonpigmented (and pigmented) ciliary epithelium occurs typically in eyes that previously suffered injury or long-standing inflammation. Clinically and histologically, it is easily confused with neoplasia, but evidence of active inflammation, scarring, and excessive production of basement membrane material by the hyperplastic ciliary epithelium helps to differentiate the lesion from a benign adenoma. When present in eyes with retinal detachment it may be described as a *Ringschwiele* (see Chap. 21).

Adenoma and Adenocarcinoma

Clinical Features.   Analysis of 30 adenomas, which are rare tumors [2], gives a mean age at the time of enucleation of 43 years, with a range of 1.5–82 years. Of the 7 posttraumatic cases 6 involved male patients. Among the spontaneous cases (about three-quarters of the material) there is no difference in incidence between the sexes. All tumors are single and unilateral. There are no associated tumors or malformations involving other tissues and no apparent racial or other genetic predisposition.

The most frequent presenting manifestations are recognition of a mass arising from the iris or ciliary body and decreased visual acuity. Less frequent causes of presentation are complications, such as glaucoma and cataract, or congenital coloboma of the iris. The posttraumatic tumors most often develop in eyes that have been blind for many years as a result of the initial injury.

Histopathology.   On gross examination an adenoma most often presents as a variably pigmented, circumscribed, round or oval solid tumor of the ciliary body and iris root, often encroaching on the lens, which might reveal a localized cataract. The upper and temporal quadrants are the preferred regions. Histopathologically, a rather uniform proliferation of cuboidal and columnar epithelial cells, similar cytologically to those of the nonpigmented ciliary epithelium, is seen. Often papillary structures or adenoidlike tubules dominate. Adenomas do not imitate embryonal retina or show spongioblastic or neuroblastic differentiation. The pigmentation varies considerably, but the melanin granules (melanosomes) are larger than those derived from the neural crest, being of the size seen in the neuroectodermally derived iris, ciliary body, and retinal pigment epithelia [66]. In very heavily pigmented lesions, an origin from the pigmented ciliary epithelium is sometimes impossible to rule out, and these tumors are probably able to differentiate toward pigmented as well as nonpigmented epithelium.

As a rule the stroma is loosely organized, with many reticulin fibers in a netlike pattern and a rich content of GAG mostly sensitive to bovine testicular hyaluronidase (in contrast to most metastatic tumors, in which the GAG are resistant) [90]. The tumor cells may show some pleomorphism and most often some mitoses and/or invasion of adjacent structures. The pleomorphism and the delicate stroma help to distinguish the adenomas from localized hyperplasias. Invasion of the iris root, ciliary muscle, or anterior chamber-angle structures is not necessarily an indication of malignancy [96], because such invasion is noticed sometimes in such nonneoplastic lesions as unequivocal hyperplasias, melanocytomas, and juvenile nevoxanthogranulomas.

Histopathological Criteria for Malignancy.   Differentiation between a benign adenoma and a malignant adenocarcinoma is difficult. In Andersen's own material [2] he classified only 3 of 23 tumors as malignant, using stricter criteria of malignancy than most other investigators, including many mitoses, pronounced pleomorphism and marked invasion of the choroid, optic nerve, orbit, or facial bones (Figs. 9 and 10). One of Andersen's cases [2] metastasized to the mandible (Fig. 10). The good prognosis in almost all published cases seems to justify the use of these strict criteria. They follow a very slow course over many years but may in extremely rare instances become malignant and run a lethal course, especially in phthisical eyes, in which symptoms are late and adequate examination of the eye may be impossible [93].

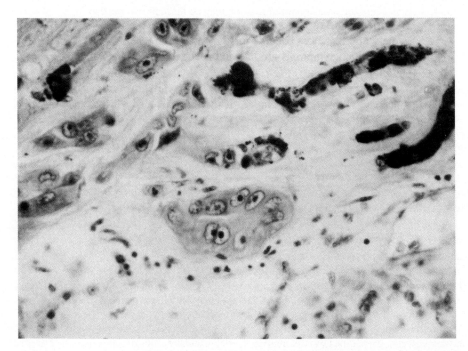

Figure 9   Pigment epithelial carcinoma showing variably pigmented tubular structures. (Hematoxylin and eosin, ×355)

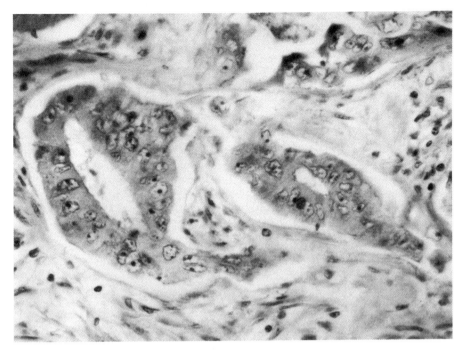

Figure 10   Metastasis in the mandible from the tumor illustrated in Figure 9. (Hematoxylin and eosin, ×355)

Treatment.   In most cases enucleation has been performed, but in early tumors iridocyclectomy is the treatment of choice and the prognosis is excellent if the surgical margins of resections contain healthy tissue on all sides. The tumors seem to be radioresistant.

Tumors Arising in a Congenital Malformation

Glioneuroma is an extremely rare benign tumor resembling brain tissue and containing ganglion cells and axons as well as neuroglia arising in a malformed sector of the optic cup [50,55]. Adenoid nonpigmented tubules seem to imitate the single-layered adult ependymal lining of the cerebral ventricles. Nothing resembling the embryonic retina or ciliary epithelium is observed in ganglioneuroma.

III.   HYPERTROPHY, TUMORS, AND CYSTS OF THE PIGMENT EPITHELIA OF THE IRIS, CILIARY BODY, AND RETINA

A.   Congenital Anomalies of Pigment Epithelium

Gass [31] in an extensive review of congenital lesions of the RPE defined and classified them into four major categories primarily on their clinical and fluorescein angiographic appearances. Two categories included RPE hamartomas [30], which could also involve the retina; the other categories were regarded as melanotic or amelanotic nevi of the RPE. Within this group of nevi he included the solitary congenital hypertrophy of the RPE (CHRPE) [14,18]. CHRPE lesions occur typically in otherwise normal individuals and in association with Gardner's syndrome [7,18,34,40,59,63,64,84,95,102,103,104], an autosomal dominant form of familial adenomatous polyposis of the intestine, with heightened potential for colonic adenocarcinoma, associated with skeletal and soft tissue hamartomas. CHRPE does not arise in other forms of familial polyposis coli, including those with hepatoblastoma [60], or in hereditary non–polyposis-associated colorectal neoplasia [103] or Peutz-Jeghers syndrome (intestinal polyposis with excessive melanin pigmentation of the skin and mucous membranes) [67]. However, CHRPE-like anomalies have been recorded in microcephalic children [89] without mental retardation or Gardner's syndrome.

Histologically few cases have been examined, but these show tall epithelial cells, tightly packed with large spheroidal mature somes, obscuring nuclear detail [14]. The bilateral diffuse uveal melanocytic hyperplasia associated with occult malignancy, especially intraabdominal [82], may also be confused with these lesions.

Black lesions of the RPE are capable of being misdiagnosed as melanocytomas or uveal melanomas [8,19], and carcinomas of the RPE may simulate melanoma (see later) [81].

Hyperplasia

The pigment epithelia of the eye are highly reactive and are prone to exhibit an exuberant hyperplasia [110] in response to a variety of insults, including old injury, chronic inflammation in adjacent structures, or long-standing retinal detachment with traction. The pigment epithelium rarely produces spontaneous neoplasms [25], and metastases from such tumors have never been documented.

Reactive hyperplasia of the pigment epithelium is often accompanied by abundant basement membrane material. Migration and invasion of the uvea and retina and even the sclera can be invaded [94] and is common but pleomorphism and mitoses are absent or inconspicuous. Differentiation from a neoplasm may be difficult [29,56,106]. Proliferation and migration can be accompanied by a metaplastic response, both fibrous and osseous and with or without calcification [26].

B. Adenoma

It is probable that most if not all tumors of the pigment epithelial of the iris, ciliary body, and retina [28,29,106] are adenomas rather than adenocarcinomas. In one series [105] the most common presenting symptom of adenomas of the pigment epithelium was a decrease in visual acuity, and the average duration of symptoms was 2.5 years before enucleation, the latter taking place at a mean age of 45.8 years. Some arise in children, however [65,76]. In some instances there is a history of inflammation, which raises the possibility of a preceding hyperplastic proliferation. Most neoplasms arise in otherwise normal eyes with clear media. Invasion of the retina and choroid is common [68,105], but not extraocular extension or metastasis. Local invasiveness and some pleomorphism and mitotic activity may not necessarily justify a diagnosis of adenocarcinoma.

Ciliary body [12,62,78,99] and RPE neoplasms often contain abundant nonsulfated GAG within intracytoplasmic vacuoles, which compress the melanosomes of the pigment epithelial cells [12,25]. The enlarging vacuoles displace the melanosomes to the periphery, which may account in part for their dark appearance. Five histological types of these tumors have been described [105]. Three of them have regular mosaic or tubular or papillary patterns, and in addition patternless variants containing vacuolated and anaplastic cells may occur. Although reactive hyperplasia of the RPE may simulate malignancy [100], neoplastic RPE lesions lose their cellular polarity, manifest greater atypia, and usually form less basement membrane.

Metastatic [5,46,79] and astrocytic [21] lesions must also be excluded in the differential diagnosis of tumors of the pigment epithelium of the iris, ciliary body, and retina.

Primary neoplasms of the pigment epithelia of the iris are extremely rare, and origin from the ciliary body epithelium cannot always be excluded [70]. They may invade the iris stroma and from there the anterior chamber [94].

C. Adenocarcinoma

As with nonpigmented ciliary epithelium, the existence of true adenocarcinomas of the RPE is doubted by some authors [94], and no metastatic deaths have been reported from these lesions, which are usually described as carcinomas [29,37,76] on the basis of local invasiveness [68]. Melanocytomas (see Chap. 50) may also be locally aggressive and are also heavily pigmented, causing diagnostic confusion [8].

D. Cysts

Separation of the anterior and posterior layers of iridic or ciliary epithelium may produce a black cyst that fills the posterior chamber or becomes prolapsed through the pupil. Pieces of proliferated epithelium may become detached and be carried into the anterior chamber, where they may give rise to cysts [32,91] that may be mistaken clinically for melanomas.

IV. MUSCLE TUMORS OF NEUROECTODERMAL ORIGIN

Rarely, leiomyomas arising from neuroectodermally derived sphincter and dilator muscles of the iris have been described [61], and leiomyomas of the ciliary body thought to be of mesectodermal origin have also been reported [15,43,44,92,114,119], which may need to be differentiated from other spindle cell tumors, including unusual tumors of the ciliary body, such as hemangiopericytoma [11] and hemangioblastoma [47], as well as from melanomas. Rhabdomyosarcomas of the iris and ciliary body have been documented [72,116], and although their origin is uncertain, some investigators have considered a neuroepithelial origin. They are described more fully in Chapter 48.

ACKNOWLEDGMENTS

Portions of the material included in this chapter were originally presented in the first edition authored by S. Ry Andersen.

REFERENCES

1. Andersen, S.R. Medulloepithelioma of the retina. *Int. Ophthalmol. Clin.* 2:483–506, 1962.
2. Andersen, S.R. Differentiation features in some retinal tumors and in dysplastic retinal conditions. *Am. J. Ophthalmol.* 71:231–241, 1971.
3. Andersen, S.R. Medulloepithelioma (diktyoma). In *Current Ocular Therapy*, F.T. Fraunfelder and F.T. Roy (Eds.), W.B. Saunders, Philadelphia, p. 240, 1980.
4. Badal, J., and Lagrange, F. Carcinome primitif des procés et du corps ciliare. *Arch. Ophtalmol. (Paris) 12*:143–148, 1892.
5. Bardenstein, D.S., Char, D.H., Jones, C., Crawford, J.B., Miller, T.R., and Riehof, F.T. Metastatic ciliary body carcinoid tumor. *Arch. Ophthalmol. 108*:1590–1594, 1990.
6. Barron, C.N., and Saunders, L.Z. Intraocular tumors in animals. II. Primary nonpigmented intraocular tumors. *Cancer Res. 19*:1171–1174, 1959.
7. Berk, T. Cohen, Z., McLeod, R.S., and Parker, J.A. Congenital hypertrophy of the retinal pigment epithelium as a marker for familial adenomatous polyposis. *Dis. Colon Rectum 31*:252–257, 1988.
8. Blodi, F.C., Reuling, F.H., and Sornson, E.T. Pseudomelanocytoma at the optic nerve head: An adenoma of the retinal pigment epithelium. *Arch. Ophthalmol. 73*:353–355, 1965.
9. Bolande, R.P. The neurocristopathies: A unifying concept of disease arising in neural crest maldevelopment. *Hum. Pathol. 5*:409–429, 1974.
10. Broughton, W.L., and Zimmerman, L.E. A clinicopathologic study of 56 cases of intraocular medulloepitheliomas. *Am. J. Ophthalmol. 85*:407–418, 1978.
11. Brown, H.H., Brodsky, M.C., Hembree, K., and Mrak, R.E. Supraciliary hemangiopericytoma. *Ophthalmology 98*:378–379, 1991.
12. Brown, H.H., Glasgow, B.J., and Foos, R.Y. Ultrastructural and immunohistochemical features of coronal adenomas. *Am. J. Ophthalmol. 112*:34–40, 1991.
13. Brownstein, S., Barsoum-Homsy, M., Conway, V.H., Sales, C., and Condon, G. Non-teratoid medullepithelioma of the ciliary body. *Ophthalmology 91*:1118–1122, 1984.
14. Buettner, H. Congenital hypertrophy of the retinal pigment epithelium. *Am. J. Ophthalmol. 79*:177–189, 1975.
15. Burk, R.O., Volcker, H.E, Daus, W., and Born, I.A. Mesectodermal leiomyoma of the ciliary body—clinical aspects, surgery and immunohistochemistry. *Fortschr. Ophthalmol. 86*:631–635, 1989.
16. Canning, C.R., McCartney, A.C.E., and Hungerford, J.L. Medullo-epithelioma (Diktyoma). *Br. J. Ophthalmol. 72*:764–767, 1988.
17. Carillo, R., and Streeten, B.W. Malignant teratoid medulloepithelioma in an adult. *Arch. Ophthalmol. 97*:695–699, 1979.
18. Champion, R., and Daicker, B.C. Congenital hypertrophy of the pigment epithelium: Light microscopic and ultrastructural findings in young children. *Retina 9*:44–48, 1989.
19. Char, D.H., Miller, T.R., and Crawford, J.B. Cytopathologic diagnosis of benign lesions simulating choroidal melanoma. *Am. J. Ophthalmol. 112*:70–75, 1991.
20. Eagle, R.C., Jr., Font, R.L., and Swerczek, T.W. Malignant medulloepithelioma of the optic nerve in a horse. *Vet. Pathol. 15*:488–494, 1978.

21. Farber, M.G., Smith, M.E., and Gans, L.A. Astrocytoma of the ciliary body. *Arch. Ophthalmol. 105*:536–537, 1987.
22. Fiar, J.R. Tumors of the retinal pigment epithelium. *Am. J. Ophthalmol. 45*:495–505, 1958.
23. Floyd, B.B., Minckler, D.S., and Valentin, L. Intraocular medulloepithelioma in a 79 year old man. *Ophthalmology 89*:1088–1094, 1982.
24. Font, R.L., Keener, M.J., Quiambo, A.B., Baehr, W., and Al-Ubaidi, M.R. An animal model of trilateral primitive neuroectodermal tumor (PNET) in transgenic mice. An immunohistochemical study. *Invest. Ophthalmol. Vis. Sci. (Suppl.) 33*:875, 1992.
25. Font, R.L., Zimmerman, L.E., and Fine, B.S. Adenoma of the retinal pigment epithelium: Histochemical and electron microscopic observations. *Am. J. Ophthalmol. 73*:544–554, 1972.
26. Frayer, W.C. Reactivity of the retinal pigment epithelium: An experimental and histopathologic study. *Trans. Am. Ophthalmol. Soc. 64*:587–643, 1966.
27. Fuchs, E. Anatomische Mischellen. *Graefes Arch. Clin. Exp. Ophthalmol. 29*:209–219, 1983.
28. Fuchs, E. Wucherungen and Geschwülste des Ciliarepithels. *Graefes Arch. Clin. Exp. Ophthalmol. 68*:534–587, 1908.
29. Garner, A. Tumours of the retinal pigment epithelium. *Br. J. Ophthalmol. 54*:715–723, 1970.
30. Gass, J.D.M. An unusual hamartoma of the retinal pigment epithelium and retina simulating choroidal melanoma and retinoblastoma. *Trans. Am. Ophthalmol. Soc. 71*:171–185, 1973.
31. Gass, J.D.M. Focal congenital abnormalities of the retinal pigment epithelium. *Eye 3*:1–18, 1989.
32. Ghabrial, R., Francis, I.C., and McClellan, K.A. Free-floating iris cyst in the anterior chamber. *Aust. NZ J. Ophthalmol. 19*:79–80, 1991.
33. Ghadially, F.N., Chisholm, I.A., and Lalonde, J.M. Ultrastructure of an intraocular lacrimal gland choristoma. *J. Submicrosc. Cytol. 18*:189–198, 1986.
34. Giardello, F.M., Offerhaus, G.J., Traboulsi, E.I., Graybeal, J.C., Maumenee, I.R., Krush, A.J., Levin, L.S., Booker, S.V., and Hamilton, S.R. Value of combined phenotypic markers in identifying inheritance of familial adenomatous polyposis. *Gut 32*:1170–1174, 1991.
35. Green, W.R., Iliff, W.J., and Trotter, R.R. Malignant teratoid medulloepithelioma of the optic nerve. *Arch. Ophthalmol. 91*:451–456, 1974.
36. Grinker, R.R. Gliomas of the retina including results of studies with silver impregnations. *Arch. Ophthalmol. 5*:920–935, 1931.
37. Grossniklaus, H.E., Zimmerman, L.E., and Krachmer, M.L. Pleomorphic adenocarcinoma of the ciliary body. Immunohistochemical and electron microscopic features. *Ophthalmology 97*:763–768, 1990.
38. Hamburg, A. Medullepithelioma arising from the posterior pole. *Ophthalmologica 181*:152–159, 1980.
39. Hausmann, N., and Stefani, F. Medulloepithelioma of the ciliary body. *Acta Ophthalmol. (Copenh.) 69*:398–401, 1991.
40. Heyen, F., Jagelman, D.G., Romania, A., Zakov, Z.N., Lavery, I.C,. Fazio, V.W., and McGannon, E. Predictive value of congenital hypertrophy of the retinal pigment epithelium as a clinical marker for familial denomatous polyposis. *Dis. Colon Rectum 33*:1003–1008, 1990.
41. Iwamoto, T., Witmer, R., and Landolt, E. Diktyoma, a clinical, histological and electron microscopical observation. *Graefes Arch. Clin. Exp. Ophthalmol. 172*:293–316, 1967.
42. Jakobiec, F.A., Howard, G.M., Ellsworth, R.M., and Rosen, M. Electron microscopic diagnosis of medulloepithelioma. *Am. J. Ophthalmol. 79*:321–329, 1975.
43. Jakobiec, F.A., and Tannenbaum, M. Embryological perspectives on the fine structure of orbital tumors. *Int. Ophthalmol. Clin. 15*:85–110, 1974.
44. Jakobiec, F.A., Font, R.L., Tso, M.O.M., and Zimmerman, L.E. Mesectodermal leiomyoma of the ciliary body: A tumor of presumed neural crest origin. *Cancer 39*:2102–2113, 1977.
45. Jakobiec, F.A., Mitchell, J.P., Chauhan, P.M., and Iwamoto, R. Mesectodermal leiomyosarcoma of the antrum and orbit. *Am. J. Ophthalmol. 85*:51–57, 1978.
46. Jakobiec, F.A., Zimmerman, L.E., Spencer, W.H., Slatker, J.S., and Krebs, W. Metastatic colloid carcinoma versus primary carcinoma of the ciliary epithelium. *Ophthalmology 94*:1469–1480, 1987.
47. Jefferies, P., and Clemett, R. An unusual ciliary body tumour: A haemangioblastoma. *Aust. NZ Ophthalmol. 19*:183–186, 1991.
48. Jensen, O.A. Persistent hyperplastic primary vitreous. Cases in Denmark 1942–1966: A mainly histopathological study. *Acta Ophthalmol. (Copenh.) 46*:418–429, 1968.
49. Karch, S.B., and Urich, H. Medulloepithelioma: Definition of an entity. *J. Neuropathol. Exp. Neurol. 31*:27–53, 1972.
50. Kivelä, T., Kauniskangas, L., Miettinen, P., and Tarkanen, A. Glioneuroma associated with colobomatous dysplasia of the anterior uvea and retina: A case simulating medullepithelioma. *Ophthalmology 96*:1799–808, 1989.
51. Kivelä, T., and Tarkkanen, A. Recurrent medulloepithelioma of the ciliary body: Immunohistochemical characteristics. *Ophthalmology 95*:1565–1575, 1988.
52. Klein, B.A. Diktyoma retinae. *Arch. Ophthalmol. 22*:432–438, 1939.
53. Konstantinov, G.S., and Ledovskii, V.G. Teratoid diktyoma of the eye (Russian). *Arkh. Patol. 49*:67–69, 1987.

54. Koss, M.N., Hochholzer, L., and O'Leary, T. Pulmonary blastomas. *Cancer 6*:2368–2381, 1991.
55. Kuhlenbeck, H., and Haymaker, W. Neuroectodermal tumors containing neoplastic neuronal elements: Gan-glioneuroma, spongioneuroblastoma and glioneuroma, with a clinicopathologic report of eleven cases, and a discussion of their origin and classification. *Milit. Surg. 99*:273–304, 1946.
56. Kurz, G.H., and Zimmerman, L.E. Vagaries of the retinal pigment epithelium. *Int. Ophthalmol. Clin. 2*:441–464, 1962.
57. Langloss, J.M., Ziommerman, L.E., and Krehbiel, J.D. Malignant intraocular teratoid medulloepithelioma in three dogs. *Vet. Pathol. 13*:343–352, 1976.
58. Layden, W.E., Toriynski, E., and Font, R.L. Mucogenic glaucoma and goblet cell cyst of the anterior chamber. *Arch. Ophthalmol. 96*:2259–2263, 1978.
59. Lewis, R.A., Crowder, W.E., Eierman, L.A., Nussbaum, R.L., and Ferrell, R.E. The Gardner syndrome. Significance of ocular features. *Ophthalmology 91*:916–925, 1984.
60. Li, F.P., Thurber, W.A., Seddon, J., and Holmes, G.E. Hepatoblastoma in families with polyposis coli. *J. Am. Med. Acad. 257*:2475–2477, 1987.
61. Li, Z.Y., Tso, M.O., and Sugar, J. Leiomyoepithelioma of iris pigment epithelium. *Arch. Ophthalmol. 105*: 819–824, 1987.
62. Lieb, W.E., Shields, J.A., Eagle, R.C., Jr., Kwa, D., and Shields, C. Cystic adenoma of the pigmented ciliary epithelium: Clinical, pathologic and immuno-histopathologic findings. *Ophthalmology 97*:1489–1493, 1990.
63. Lynch, H.T., Priluck, I., and Fitzsimmons, M.L. Congenital hypertrophy of retinal pigment epithelium in non-Gardner's polyposis kindreds. *Lancet 2*:333, 1987.
64. Lyons, L.A., Lewis, R.A., Strong, L.C., Zuckerbrod, S., and Ferrell, R.E. A genetic study of Gardner syndrome and congenital hypertrophy of the retinal pigment epithelium. *Am. J. Hum. Genet. 42*:290–296, 1988.
65. Margo, C.E., and Brooks, H.L., Jr. Adenocarcinoma of the ciliary epithelium in a 12-year-old black child. *J. Pediatr. Ophthalmol. Strabismus 28*:232–235, 1991.
66. McCartney, A.C.E., Bull, T.B., and Spalton, D.J. Fuchs' heterochromic cyclitis: An electron microscopic study. *Trans. Ophthalmol. Soc. UK 105*:324–329, 1986.
67. McKusick, V.A. *Mendelian inheritance in Man. Catalogs of Autosomal Dominant, Autosomal Recessive, and X-Linked Phenotypes*, Johns Hopkins University Press, Baltimore, p. 612, 1988.
68. Minckler, D., and Allen, A.W. Adenocarcinoma of the retinal pigment epithelium. *Arch. Ophthalmol. 96*:2252–2254, 1978.
69. Morris, A.T., and Garner, A. Medulloepithelioma involving the iris. *Br. J. Ophthalmol. 59*:276–278, 1975.
70. Morris, D.A., and Henkind, P. Neoplasms of the iris epithelium. *Am. J. Ophthalmol. 66*:31–41, 1968.
71. Mullaney, J. Primary malignant medulloepithelioma of the retinal stalk. *Am. J. Ophthalmol. 77*:499–504, 1974.
72. Naumann, G., Font, R.L., and Zimmerman, L.E. Electron microscopic verification of primary rhabdomyosar-coma of the iris. *Am. J. Ophthalmol. 74*:110–117, 1972.
73. Naumann, G.O., and Rummelt, V. Congenital nonpigmented epithelial iris cyst removed by block-excision. *Graefes Arch. Clin. Exp. Ophthalmol. 228*:392–397, 1990.
74. Naumann, G., Völcker, H.E., and Lerche, W. Adenom des pigmentierten Ciliarepithels. Klinische, histo-chemische und elektronemnikroskopische Befunde und Literatur-Übersicht. *Graefes Arch. Ophthalmol. 198*:245–258, 1976.
75. Orellana, J., Moura, R.A., Font, R.L., Moura, M., and Murphy, D. Medulloepithelioma diagnosed by ultrasound and vitreous aspiration: Electron microscopic observations. *Ophthalmology 90*:1531–1539, 1983.
76. Papale, J.J., Akiwama, K., Hilrose, T., Tsubota, K., Hanaoka, K., and Albert, D.M. Adenocarcinoma of the ciliary body pigment epithelium in a child. *Arch. Ophthalmol. 102*:100–103, 1984.
77. Paridaens, A.D.A., Deuble, K., and McCartney, A.C.E. Spontaneous non-pigmented cysts of the iris stroma. *Br. J. Ophthalmol. 76*:39–42, 1992.
78. Pe'er, J., and Hidyat, A.A. Malignant teratoid medulloepithelioma manifesting as a black epibulbar mass with expulsive hemorrhage. *Arch. Ophthalmol. 102*:1523–1527, 1984.
79. Purgason, P.A., Hornblass, A., and Harrison, W. Metastatic Merkel cell carcinoma to the eye. *Ophthalmology 98*:1432–1434, 1991.
80. Reese, A.B. Medulloepithelioma (diktyoma) of the optic nerve. *Am. J. Ophthalmol. 44*:4–6, 1957.
81. Rodrigues, M., Hidyat, A., and Karesh, J. Pleomorphic adenocarcinoma of ciliary epithelium simulating an epibulbar tumor. *Am. J. Ophthalmol. 106*:595–600, 1988.
82. Rohrbach, J.M., Roggendorf, W., Thanos, S., Steul, K.P., and Thiel, H.J. Simultaneous bilateral diffuse melanocytic uveal hyperplasia. *Am. J. Ophthalmol. 110*:49–56, 1990.
83. Rohrbach, J.M., Steul, K.P., and Theil, H.J. Zysten und Fuchssche Adenome der Pars plicata corporis ciliaris. Degenerationsprodukte als Ausdruck verschiedene Ziliarkorperleistungen? *Klin. Monatsbl. Augenheilkd 198*:195–200, 1991.
84. Romania, A., Zakov, Z.N., McGannon, E., Schroeder, T., Heyen, F., and Jagelman, D.G. Congenital hypertro-phy of the retinal pigment epithelium in familial adenomatous polyposis. *Ophthalmology 96*:879–884, 1989.
85. Roy, R.H., and Hanna, C. Spontaneous congenital iris cysts. *Am. J. Ophthalmol. 72*:97–108, 1971.
86. Rubinstein, L.J. Tumors of the central nervous system. In *Atlas of Tumor Pathology*, Series 2. Fasc. 6. Armed Forces Institute of Pathology, Washington, DC, pp. 127–129, 1972.

87. Rubenstein, L.J. Embryonal central neuroepithelial tumors and their differentiating potential. A cytogenetic view of a complex neuro-oncological problem. *J. Neurosurg.* *62*:795–805, 1985.
88. Saunders, L.Z., Geib, L.W., and Barron, C.N. Intraocular ganglioneuroma in a dog. *Pathol. Vet.* *6*:525–533, 1969.
89. Sheriff, S.M., and Hegab, S. A syndrome of multiple fundus anomalies in siblings with microcephaly but without mental retardation. *Ophthalmic Surg.* *19*:353–355, 1988.
90. Shields, J.A. *Diagnosis and Management of Intraocular Tumors*, C.V. Mosby, St. Louis, pp. 329–358, 1983.
91. Shields, J.A., Kline, M.W., and Ausberger, J.J. Primary iris cysts: A review of the literature and report of 62 cases. *Br. J. Ophthalmol.* *68*:152–166, 1984.
92. Shields, J.A., and Shields, C.L. Observations on intraocular leiomyomas. *Trans. Am. Acad. Ophthalmol. Otolaryngol.* *42*:945–950, 1990.
93. Shields, J.A., and Shields, C.L. Tumors of the non-pigmented ciliary epithelium. In *Intraocular Tumors. A Text and Atlas*, W.B. Saunders, Philadelphia, pp. 461–487, 1992.
94. Shields, J.A., and Shields, C.L. Tumors and related lesions of the pigment epithelium. In *Intraocular Tumors. A Text and Atlas*, W.B. Saunders, Philadelphia, pp. 437–459, 1992.
95. Stein, E.A., and Brady, K.D. Ophthalmologic and electro-oculographic findings in Gardner's syndrome. *Am. J. Ophthalmol.* *106*:326–331, 1988.
96. Streeten, B.W., and McGraw, J.L. Tumor of the ciliary pigment epithelium. *Am. J. Ophthalmol.* *74*:420–429, 1972.
97. Sugar, H.S., and Nathan, L.E. Congenital epithelial cysts of the iris stroma. *Ann. Ophthalmol.* *14*:483–485, 1982.
98. Szymanski, C.M. Malignant teratoid medulloepithelioma in a horse. *J. Am. Vet. Med. Assoc.* *190*:301–302, 1987.
99. Takagi, T., Tsuda, N., Wanatabe, F., and Takaku, I. An epithelioma of the ciliary body. *Ophthalmologica* *195*:13–20, 1987.
100. Theobald, G.D., Floyd, G., and Kirk, H.Q. Hyperplasia of the retinal pigment epithelium simulating a neoplasm: Report of two cases. *Am. J. Ophthalmol.* *45*:235–240, 1958.
101. Torczynski, E., Jakobiec, F.A., Johnston, M.A., Font, R.L., and Madwell, J.A. Synophthalmia and cyclopia: A histopathologic, radiographic and organogenetic analysis. *Doc. Ophthalmol.* *44*:311–378, 1977.
102. Traboulsi, E.I., Krush, A.J., Gardner, E.J., Booker, S.V., Offerhaus, G.J.A., Yardley, J.H., Hamilton, S.R., Luk, G.D., Giardello, F.M., Welsh, S.B., Hughes, J.P., and Maumenee, I.R. Prevalence and importance of pigmented ocular fundus lesions in Gardner's syndrome. *N. Engl. J. Med.* *316*:661–667, 1987.
103. Traboulsi, E.I., Maumenee, I.R., Krush, A.J., Giardello, F.M., Levin, L.S., and Hamilton, S.R. Pigmented ocular fundus lesions in the inherited nonpolyposis colorectal cancer. *Ophthalmology* *95*:964–969, 1988.
104. Traboulsi, E.I., Murphy, S.F., de la Cruz, Z.C., Maumenee, I.H., and Green, W.R. A clinicopathologic study of the eyes in familial adenomatous polyposis: Extracolonic manifestations (Gardner's syndrome). *Am. J. Ophthalmol.* *110*:550–561, 1990.
105. Tso, M.O.M., and Albert, D.M. Pathological condition of the retinal pigment epithelium: Neoplasms and nodular nonneoplastic lesions. *Arch. Ophthalmol.* *88*:27–38, 1972.
106. Turut, P., and Madelain, J. Les adénomes de l'epithélium pigmentaire rétinien. *J. Fr. Ophtalmol.* *11*:17–23, 1988.
107. Verhoeff, F.H. A rare tumor arising from the pars ciliaris retinae (terato-neuroma), of a nature hitherto unrecognized and its relation to the so-called glioma retinae. *Trans. Am. Ophthalmol. Soc.* *10*:351–377, 1904.
108. Virji, M.A. Medullepithelioma (diktyoma) presenting with a perforated, infected eye. *Br. J. Ophthalmol.* *61*:229–232, 1977.
109. Vit, V.V. Necrotic medulloepithelioma of the eye (Russian). *Arkh. Patol.* *53*:65–68, 1991.
110. Vogel, M.H., Zimmerman, L.E., and Gass, J.D.M. Proliferation of the juxtapapillary retinal pigment epithelium simulating malignant melanoma. *Doc. Ophthalmol.* *26*:461–481, 1969.
111. Wakakura, M., and Lee, W.R. Ultrastructural pleomorphism in medulloepithelioma of the ciliary body: A comparative study of tumour cells and fetal ciliary epithelium. *Jpn. J. Ophthalmol.* *34*:364–380, 1990.
112. Watts, M.T., and Rennie, I.G. Detached iris cyst presenting as an intraocular foreign body. *J. R. Soc. Med.* *84*:172–173, 1991.
113. Weston, J.A. The migration and differentiation of neural crest cells. *Adv. Morphol.* *8*:41–114, 1970.
114. White, V., Stevenson, K., Garner, A., and Hungerford, J. Mesectodermal leiomyoma of the ciliary body: A case report. *Br. J. Ophthalmol.* *73*:12–18, 1989.
115. Wilson, M.E., McClatchey, S.K., and Zimmerman, L.E. Rhabdomyosarcoma of the ciliary body. *Ophthalmology* *97*:1484–1488, 1990.
116. Woyke, S., and Chwirot, R. Rhabdomyosarcoma of the iris: Report of the first recorded case. *Br. J. Ophthalmol.* *56*:60–64, 1972.
117. Yanoff, M., and Font, R.L. Intraocular cartilage in a microphthalmic eye of an otherwise healthy girl. *Arch. Ophthalmol.* *81*:238–240, 1969.
118. Yanko, L., and Behar, A. Teratoid intraocular medullo-epithelioma. *Am. J. Ophthalmol.* *85*:850–853, 1978.

119. Yu, D.H., Cohen, S.B., Peyman, G., and Tso, M.O. Mesectodermal leiomyoma of the ciliary body: New evidence for neural crest origin. *J. Pediatr. Ophthalmol. Strabismus 27*:317–321, 1990.
120. Zimmerman, L.E. The remarkable polymorphism of tumors of the ciliary epithelium. *Trans. Cong. Aust. Coll. Ophthalmol.*, pp. 114–125, 1970.
121. Zimmerman, L.E. Verhoeff's "terato-neuroma," a critical reappraisal in light of new observations and current concepts of embryonic tumors: The fourth Frederick H. Verhoeff lecture. *Am. J. Ophthalmol. 72*:1039–1057, 1971.
122. Zimmerman, L.E., and Fine, B.S. Production of hyaluronic acid by cysts and tumors of the ciliary body. *Arch. Ophthalmol. 72*:365–379, 1964.
123. Zimmerman, L.E., Font, R.L., and Andersen, S.R. Rhabdomyosarcomatous differentiation in malignant intraocular medulloepitheliomas. *Cancer 30*:817–835, 1972.
124. Zimmerman, L.E., and Sobin, L. (Eds.) Histological typing of tumors of the eye and its adnexa. In *International Histological Classification of Tumors*, No. 21. World Health Organization, Geneva, 1981.

48
Uveal Tumors

Hans E. Grossniklaus
Emory University School of Medicine, Atlanta, Georgia

W. Richard Green
The Johns Hopkins University School of Medicine, Baltimore, Maryland

I. MELANOTIC TUMORS

A. Nevi

Nevi of Iris

Aggregates of variably pigmented melanocytic cells arranged in a mass or nodule with distortion or replacement of normal iris architecture constitute a nevus [343]. The classification of melanocytic tumors of the iris, including nevi, is presented elsewhere (pp. 1439–1440). As in the choroid, melanocytic cells of variable shape and size make up an iris nevus. Iris nevi are visible in approximately 50% of adults [299]. The incidence of iris nevi has been reported increased in eyes with choroidal melanomas [341,459], but more recent studies have not shown this to be true [299]. A melanocytoma of the iris undergoing necrosis and producing secondary glaucoma may be clinically suspected of being a melanoma [402].

Iris Nevus Syndrome

The iris nevus syndrome is a curious condition with a predilection for middle-aged women, characterized by iris whorls and/or nodules of nevi, atrophy of the iris stroma, heterochromia iridis, ectropion uveae, and peripheral anterior synechiae [90]. Histopathological studies have shown a diffuse nevus of the anterior surface of the iris and overgrowth of endothelium, with descemetization of the anterior chamber angle and the anterior iris surface [125,228,381,466]. Eagle and colleagues [125] postulate that some cases lack nevi and that the apparent nevi are due to defects in the corneal endothelium and basement membrane that extends over the anterior iris surface. The condition has features in common with Chandler's syndrome and essential iris atrophy, which may represent part of a spectrum of the same condition (see Chap. 17) now known as the iridocorneal endothelial syndrome.

Ciliary Body Nevi

A 2% incidence of ciliary body nevi was noted in a postmortem histopathological study of 400 eyes [201]. Nevi of the ciliary body do not ordinarily reach sufficient size to be clinically evident. A study of 23 melanocytomas of the ciliary body disclosed that they are unilateral, extend into contiguous structures, and slowly enlarge [157]. On rare occasions ciliary body melanocytomas undergo partial necrosis with liberation of pigment [157]. This situation can lead to secondary open-angle glaucoma as a result of blockage of the trabecular meshwork by melanin-laden macrophages. A melanocytoma of the ciliary body may extend anteriorly to involve the base of the iris and lead to a clinical misdiagnosis of a primary iris melanoma [54].

Choroidal Nevi

Usual Nevi.   Choroidal nevi are common, and an indication of their frequency has been obtained in a Maryland county, where they were found clinically in 3.1% of eyes [175]. In postmortem studies they have been found in approximately 10% of eyes by transillumination [201,312]. Most nevi are less than 4.5 mm in diameter, are slightly thicker than the adjacent normal choroid, and occur predominantly in the posterior region of the eye [315]. Their degree of pigmentation ranges from homogeneous black to yellow-white, with only scattered pigmentation.

The types of cells comprising a choroidal nevus vary and are generally classified as plump polyhedral, slender spindle, plump spindle or fusiform, dendritic, or balloon cells [317] (Figs. 1 through 3). Large round cells with abundant densely pigmented cytoplasm (melanocytoma nevus cells; magnacellular nevus cells) may be present. However, the entire spectrum of cells may be present in a single nevus.

Subretinal fluid associated with a pigmented choroidal lesion strongly suggests a melanoma rather than a nevus [266,346,363]. In a study of 933 choroidal nevi examined by fluorescein angiography, however, approximately 2% had subretinal fluid in the foveal area [335]. The ophthalmoscopic appearance and the clinical course over a 10 year period of all nevi, except one, suggested that they were benign nevi. One nevus enlarged after remaining stable for 4 years and, following enucleation, was found to be a melanoma. Serous retinal detachment associated with subretinal pigment epithelial neovascularization over a choroidal nevus has also been observed [418].

Since it has been estimated that only 1 in 5000 choroidal nevi in whites transforms into a malignant melanoma each year [175], there is a need to identify high-risk nevi. In this regard, four features of nevi have been evaluated by Mims and Shields as incurring special risk [302]: (1) nevi with dimensions of two to five disk diameters, (2) nevi with an apparent elevation on clinical examination or stereoscopic fundus photographs of at least 3 mm, (3) nevi with significant disruption of the retinal pigment epithelium, and (4) nevi associated with subretinal fluid. Mims and Shields [302] followed 50 suspicious choroidal nevi with these criteria and 194 nonsuspicious nevi over a 4 year period: 5 (10%) of the suspicious nevi manifested photographic evidence of enlargement over a 4–30 month period. The eyes containing these lesions were enucleated, and all were found to contain melanomas. None of the apparently innocuous nevi demonstrated growth. However, at least one histopathologically confirmed choroidal nevus has been documented to enlarge [271].

B. Melanocytoma

A melanocytoma is a densely pigmented tumor composed of relatively uniform, plump, round or polyhedral cells with abundant deeply pigmented cytoplasm and small round or oval nuclei without a conspicuous nucleolus (Fig. 4). This distinctive nevus [400,483,485], which was originally described in the optic nerve head, is deeply and usually uniformly pigmented. It may be located anywhere in the uveal tract [157,215,483], where it may be difficult to distinguish clinically from a melanoma [54,382,405]. These nevi are prone to necrosis, and in some instances, the pigment becomes dispersed [157]. Hemorrhage under the retinal pigment epithelium adjacent to a melanocytoma may simulate its growth [215], but they very rarely affect vision or undergo malignant transformation [30,130,370,442].

A melanocytoma of the optic nerve head appears as an elevated jet black epipapillary mass located eccentrically over the edge of the optic disk. In this location the melanocytoma may involve the nerve fiber layer of the peripapillary retina, producing a fibrillated, filigree, or feathery pattern at its margin. There may be a predilection for melanocytomas to occur in persons with dark pigmentary characteristics [483].

C. Congenital Ocular Melanocytosis

Congenital ocular melanocytosis (melanosis oculi) is due to increased pigmentation of the uveal tract or a portion of it. Clinical features include heterochromia iridis, grayish episcleral pigmentation (Figs. 5 and 6), and a dark fundus appearance. The episcleral pigmentation has a gray appearance because the pigmentation is viewed through the conjunctiva. The prevalence of ocular melanocytosis is 0.038% [183]. The melanocytes present in ocular melanocytosis are morphologically unremarkable and identical to those normally found in the uveal tract. Melanosis oculi may be associated with ipsilateral dermal melanocytosis in variable distributions of the ophthalmic division of the trigeminal nerve (nevus of Ota). The prevalence of this condition is 0.014% [185].

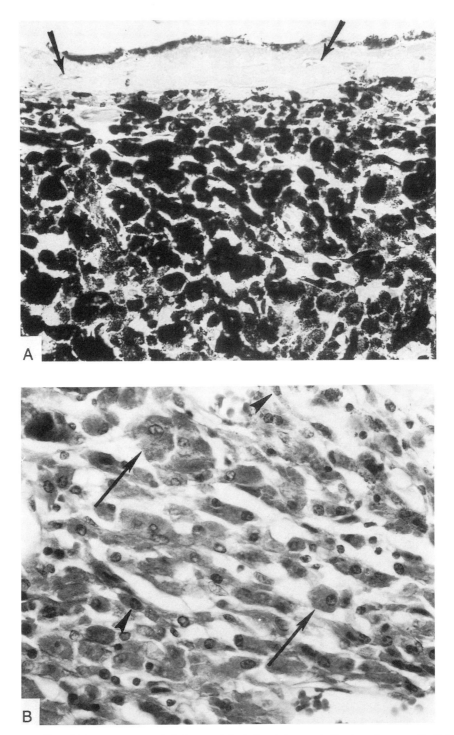

Figure 1 (A) Choroidal nevus composed of plump polyhedral and plump spindle-shaped nevus cells. Subretinal pigment epithelium neovascularization (arrows) is present over the lesion. (Hematoxylin and eosin, ×300) (B) Bleaching of pigment with potassium permanganate shows the plump polyhedral (arrows) and plump spindle-shaped nevus cells (arrowheads) more clearly. (Hematoxylin and eosin, ×480)

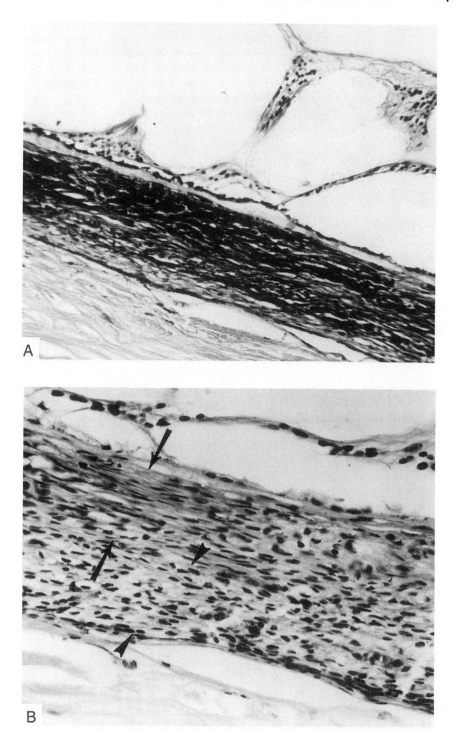

Figure 2 (A) Unbleached section of a nevus involving the peripheral choroid and pars plana. (Hematoxylin and eosin, ×170) (B) Bleached section, showing slender spindle-shaped (between arrows) and slightly plump spindle-shaped (between arrowheads) nevus cells. (Hematoxylin and eosin, ×410)

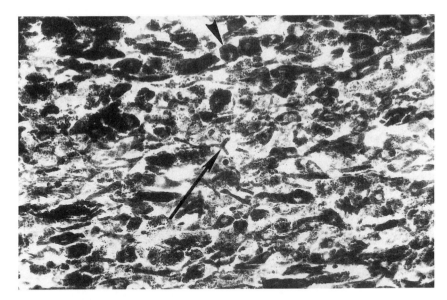

Figure 3 Unbleached section of choroidal nevus composed of dendritic (arrows) and plump polyhedral (arrowhead) nevus cells. (Hematoxylin and eosin, ×300)

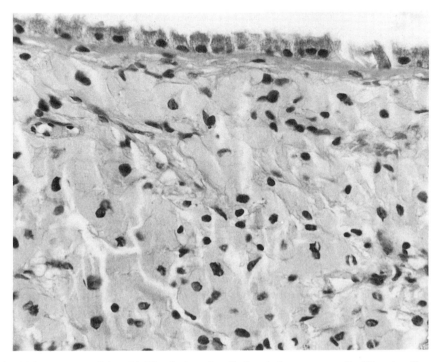

Figure 4 Melanocytoma of choroid. Bleached section disclosed plump nevus cells. (Hematoxylin and eosin, ×520)

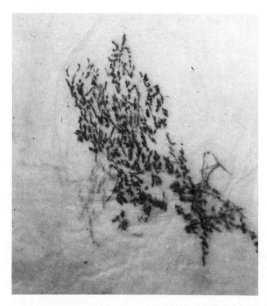

Figure 5   Gross appearance of episcleral pigmentation in eye with melanosis oculi (ocular melanocytosis). (×13)

According to Reese, eyes with melanocytosis have a propensity for the development of melanoma [340]. Others [45,334,375] have also reported an increased incidence of uveal melanoma in patients with ocular melanocytosis, and multiple independent choroidal melanomas have been observed in eyes with this condition.

The hypothesis that ocular melanocytosis is a precancerous condition that may lead to a choroidal melanoma has been questioned [45] because the incidence of malignant change in melanosis oculi is not known, because bilateral melanomas have not been reported with bilateral melanosis oculi, and because melanomas have been observed in the normally pigmented fellow eye of a patient with ocular melanocytosis.

D. Primary Melanomas of Uvea

Choroidal Melanomas

Clinical Features.   Melanoma is the most common primary malignant intraocular tumor in adults [482].

The average age of patients with choroidal melanomas is about 50 years, although less than 4% of all patients are younger than 30 years. A choroidal melanoma has been reported in a 2½-year-old girl [82]. The incidence of choroidal melanomas at specific ages increases steeply from the age of 30 to the age of 70, after which the tumor decreases in frequency.

Choroidal melanomas are slightly more common in women than in men [233]. Although heredity is not thought significantly to predispose individuals to uveal melanomas, several reports document familial examples of uveal melanomas [53,268,438]. There may be some relationship between the dysplastic nevus syndrome and the development of uveal melanoma [32,361,451].

Uveal melanomas mainly occur in whites, and in a series of 2535 eyes enucleated for uveal melanomas in the United States, only 11 were black patients [329]. Black patients with choroidal melanoma are more likely to have tumor necrosis and more darkly pigmented tumors than white patients [280]. These tumors are extremely rare in non-whites living in Asia [100,436] and Africa [440]. Persons of Northern European ancestry and greater than 5 years residence below latitude N-40° are at increased risk for development of uveal melanoma [388]. Patients with ocular melanocytosis [45,185,340], oculodermal melanocytosis [184,185], and neurofibromatosis [475] may have an increased risk of developing uveal melanoma.

Bilateral choroidal melanomas are rare [37,64,94,393,434,447,449]. It has been estimated that in a population of 50 million whites, 1 person will develop bilateral choroidal melanomas. A bilateral case is therefore expected to occur about once every 18 years in the United States [393].

The usual initial symptom with which patients with posterior-pole choroidal melanomas present is increasing hyperopia. At first this may be correctable by lenses but is usually followed by blurred vision that is uncorrectable. Of all patients with choroidal melanomas, 65% give a history of visual symptoms of 6 months duration or less [233]. If the tumor is located some distance from the macular area, however, the patient may be asymptomatic.

Certain clinical signs found on examination of the anterior segment of the globe are helpful in diagnosing choroidal melanomas [340,344,346]. Dilated episcleral vessels corresponding to the site of the tumor are seen in about one-third of all cases. These are interpreted as nutrient vessels of the tumor [344] or reflections of poor venous drainage [51]. On rare occasions hemorrhage into the vitreous is the initial sign of a necrotic melanoma [176].

Origin.   For many years, primary uveal melanomas were considered of mesodermal origin and were classified as sarcomas. In 1937, Dvorak-Theobald suggested that uveal melanomas arose from Schwann cells [124]. It is widely believed that many melanomas originate from preexisting nevi: histopathological studies [151,317,475,476] have shown that about 70% of uveal melanomas appear to develop from nevi. However, the conclusion reached by these studies depends on the interpretation of the so-called nevus cells at the base and periphery of choroidal melanomas. These "nevoid" cells may represent a local, mechanical, compressive tumor effect on the cells of the choroid [2] rather than constituting a true nevus. That these cells may not be nevi is supported by studies of Albert and colleagues [3], who showed that cells at the base of experimentally induced ocular melanomas in hamsters are morphologically similar to the nevus-like cells that have been described beneath and adjacent to primary choroidal melanomas [475].

In clinical studies of choroidal nevi, evidence of malignant transformation to melanomas is rarely seen [346]. Hogan [210] reported that he followed only one choroidal nevus that later became a melanoma. Smolin [417] reported one case of malignant transformation of a choroidal nevus occurring more than 5 years after the lesion was first seen. Two case histories in which apparent choroidal nevi suddenly changed into malignant melanomas have also been reported [346]. Unfortunately, in all these cases the diagnosis of the nevus was based solely on the clinical appearance of the lesion, and the possibility that the original lesion was a low-grade malignant melanoma, not a nevus, cannot be ruled out. In one large clinical study of choroidal nevi, no malignant transformation of nevi was noted during follow-up periods of 6 months to 16 years [302]. Since in clinical [210] and postmortem studies [201,312] the incidence of choroidal nevi varies from 6.5 to 11.0% in the general population, the incidence of malignant transformation, should it occur, must be rare.

Several reports describe uveal melanomas associated with ocular trauma [129,267,454]. Trauma may be a "promoter" of neoplasia after initiation of neoplastic transformation. Virus particles have been found in isolated cases of uveal melanoma [1], although there is little chance that there is a casual relationship. Chemicals, such as methylcholanthrene, N-Z-fluorenylacetamide, ethiorine, radium, nickel subsulfide, and polychorinated biphenyls, have been linked to the pathogenesis of uveal melanoma in some instances [4,5,47,128].

Abnormalities of the Iris.   Choroidal melanomas rarely spread to the iris, causing implantation growth as reported in one case by Reese [346]. Reese [341], however, noted the presence of increased numbers of iris nevi in histopathological examination of eyes containing choroidal melanomas. This finding was later confirmed by Wilder [459]. Although Reese [344] initially believed that this would be a clinically useful sign, it did not prove to be so, because these nevi lie so deep in the iris that they are not appreciated clinically. In a clinical study to test Reese's original observation, Michelson and Shields [299] performed slit lamp examination on 50 patients with unilateral choroidal or ciliary body melanomas and did not find a significant increase in iris nevi in eyes with posterior uveal melanomas compared to age-matched controls without melanomas.

Iris neovascularization (rubeosis iridis) may be seen in eyes with choroidal melanomas, and in one series [73] it was present in 46 of 308 eyes enucleated for melanoma. Neovascular glaucoma was the reason for the enucleation of 18 eyes in 59 patients (31%) following plaque radiotherapy for posterior uveal melanoma [397].

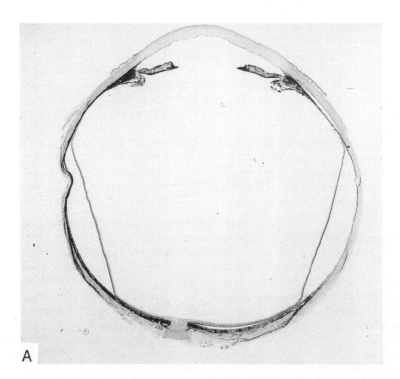

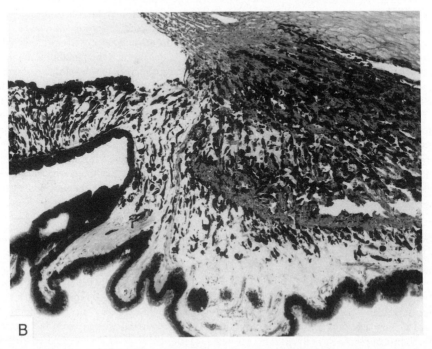

Figure 6   (A) Melanosis oculi with diffuse hyperpigmentation of iris, ciliary body, choroid, and scleral canals. (Hematoxylin and eosin, ×3) (B) Higher power, showing hyperpigmentation of iris and ciliary body due to increased number of melanocytes. (Hematoxylin and eosin, ×165) (C) Higher power of choroid posteriorly and scleral canal with ciliary nerve (asterisk) due to an increased number of melanocytes (Hematoxylin and eosin, ×165)

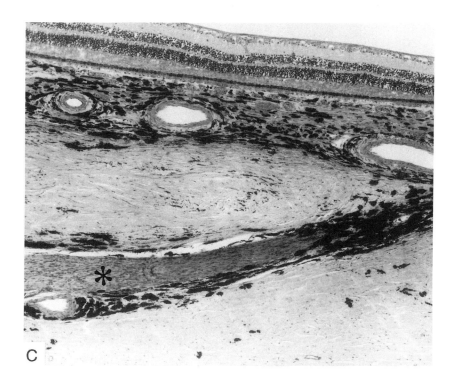

Glaucoma. Unilateral elevation of intraocular pressure may be a sign of a choroidal melanoma [410]. Reese [346] reported that about one-third of eyes enucleated for melanoma of the choroid were glaucomatous. Dunnington [122] stressed that secondary glaucoma usually develops in eyes harboring large melanomas and that the intraocular pressure is decreased in a high percentage of eyes with melanomas. In one series 19 (20%) of 96 eyes with uveal melanomas presented clinically with secondary glaucoma [473], and in many of these cases the melanoma was missed clinically, especially in eyes with opaque media and no diagnostic ultrasonography. The two major mechanisms producing glaucoma are (1) formation of peripheral anterior synechiae with angle closure or (2) cellular obstruction of the trabecular meshwork in the presence of an open angle. With a partially necrotic choroidal melanoma the glaucoma may be associated with macrophages with phagocytosed melanin pigment (melanomalytic cells) in the trabecular meshwork of an eye [130].

Pigmentation. Choroidal melanomas appear as gray, light tan, brown, or black lesions with slight to marked elevation. An abnormal vascular pattern is visible on the tumor surface in 20% of cases [344] and a yellow-orange pigment lies on the surface of some choroidal melanomas. On fluorescein angiography, this pigment blocks the background fluorescence within the tumor. It has been shown by histochemical and electron microscopic studies [30,152] that the yellow-orange pigment is lipofuscin contained in both proliferated retinal pigment epithelial cell over the tumor and in macrophages present in clusters within and beneath the sensory retina overlying the tumor. The presence of this pigment has some diagnostic significance, because although often observed over choroidal melanomas, it is rarely seen over nevi, metastatic carcinomas, or hemangiomas of the choroid [413]. Lipofuscin granules are normally found in retinal pigment epithelial cells and increase with age [429]. However, the numbers of these granules in retinal pigment epithelial cells and macrophages overlying choroidal melanomas is markedly increased, although the clinical absence of this pigment does not rule out melanoma.

Retinal Detachment. A serous retinal detachment often overlies a choroidal melanoma (Fig. 7). Occasionally, a flat melanoma of the choroid may be associated with a total retinal detachment [247]. Boniuk and Zimmerman [50] reported clinicopathological features of 57 eyes with choroidal melanomas from patients who were operated on for retinal detachment. These authors estimated that 2% of the cases of

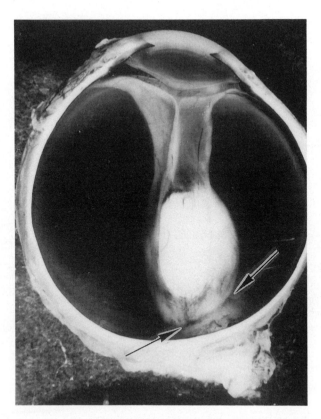

Figure 7   Melanoma of choroid with an elongated, mushroom configuration and total retinal detachment. The narrowed area (between the arrows) of the tumor is the point at which the tumor has broken through Bruch's membrane.

choroidal melanomas on file in the Registry of Ophthalmic Pathology in the United States at the Armed Forces Institute of Pathology had one or more operations for retinal detachment before enucleation. It should therefore be stressed that the presence of retinal tears does not exclude a choroidal tumor [51]. At least 13 cases of retinal detachment with retinal breaks and a melanoma of the choroid or ciliary body have been documented [35,36,50,275,276,287,307]. A retinal tear may overlie the tumor [275] or may occur far from the location of the tumor [35]. An overlying detachment may follow the development of a hole in an area of cystic degeneration in the retina overlying the tumor.

Retinal exudates are not usually a feature of choroidal melanomas, although their presence does not eliminate such a diagnosis [44]. Subretinal exudates are common at the edges of choroidal melanomas and are frequent in the inferior hemisphere in relation to superior tumors. Subretinal exudation may occur in eyes with choroidal melanoma treated with irradiation [279].

Visual Fields.   A dense visual field defect may be present [386] if the function of the retinal photoreceptors overlying the melanomas is compromised, and if the tumor is surrounded by an area of serous retinal detachment, there is a surrounding area of partial visual field defect. Visual field examination can also disclose scotomas in eyes with choroidal nevi.

Cystoid Macular Edema.   Symptoms and signs related to cystoid macular edema without serous detachment of the macula may be the initial findings in a patient with a peripherally located choroidal melanoma [57]. Although the occurrence of unilateral cystoid macular edema and choroidal melanoma may be coincidental, some authors [57] consider the association causally related.

Shape.   Although most choroidal melanomas present as localized mushroom-shaped (Fig. 7) or globular (Fig. 8) masses with growth toward the interior of the eye, 5% have a flat or diffuse type of growth

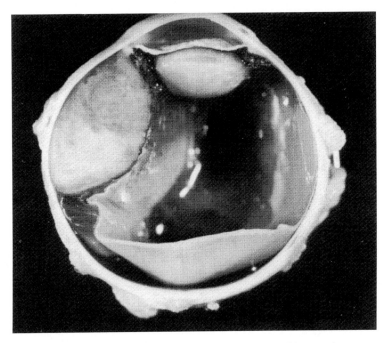

Figure 8 Melanoma of ciliary body and anterior choroid of a 56-year-old man who presented with visual complaints that were attributed to pressure on the lens. Two family members had also had choroidal melanomas.

and remain external to Bruch's membrane [206,294,349,367]. On fundoscopic examination a diffuse choroidal melanoma may resemble chorioretinitis [74] or choroidal sclerosis [27]. A conspicuous feature of diffuse uveal melanomas is the long duration of visual symptoms and sometimes pain, ranging from 7 months to 10 years, before the diagnosis becomes established [233]. Delayed diagnoses are frequent in cases of diffuse melanomas, and thus the tendency to extraocular extension is greater and the prognosis is worse than in the usual type of choroidal melanoma [151]. A unique, diffuse melanoma of the uvea with extrascleral extension presented clinically as a ring-shaped amelanotic limbal tumor [420], suggestive of a diffuse squamous cell carcinoma.

Inflammation. Necrotic melanomas can cause considerable inflammation and result in a florid uveitis, and rarely severe panophthalmitis with exophthalmos develops. Granulomatous inflammation has been reported in an eye treated with proton beam irradiation for a choroidal melanoma [279].

Hemorrhage. Most uveal melanomas slowly grow and the clinical observation of rapidly expanding, relatively flat, pigmented lesion at the posterior pole should suggest a hemorrhagic rather than a neoplastic lesion [350].

Hemorrhage into the vitreous may prevent visualization of the fundus and contain varying amounts of hemosiderin, which may impart a brownish discoloration to the hemorrhage and lead to the clinical impression of melanoma. In Ferry's series [138], 5% of eyes that were mistakenly enucleated for choroidal melanomas had vitreous hemorrhage.

Occasionally, vitreous hemorrhages occur from the dilated vascular channels in eyes with choroidal melanomas that have ruptured through Bruch's membrane to produce a mushroom-shaped lesion. Necrosis of the tumor may contribute to vitreous hemorrhage [344].

Histopathology. Callender [67] originally classified uveal melanomas as consisting of three basic types of tumor cells: (1) spindle A cells with small hyperchromatic, spindle-shaped nuclei without distinct nucleoli but often with a central dark stripe produced by a nuclear fold (Fig. 9). The cytoplasm is indistinct without well-defined borders, and mitotic figures are almost never seen. The tumor cells are cohesive, and pure spindle A melanomas account for 5% of all choroidal and ciliary body melanomas and 90% of iris melanomas. (2) Spindle B cells are also cohesive with prominent spindle-shaped nuclei, but they have

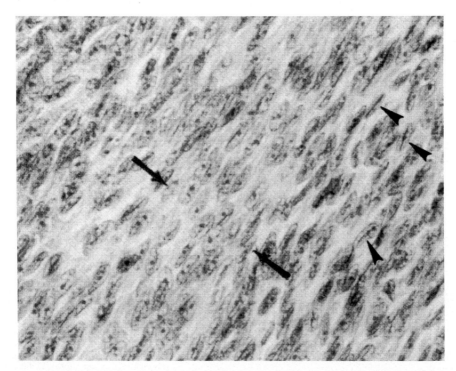

Figure 9   Choroidal melanoma with spindle A (arrowheads) and spindle B (between arrows) cells. (Hematoxylin and eosin, ×550)

distinct nucleoli (Fig. 9). Like spindle A cells, their cell borders are indistinct and mitoses are rarely seen. About 39% of choroidal and ciliary body melanomas are spindle B melanomas. In about 6% of spindle B melanomas, the cells have a palisaded arrangement that creates a fascicular pattern [329]. (3) Epithelioid melanoma cells (not to be confused with the epithelioid cells of granulomatous inflammation) are noncohesive cells with large, round nuclei, prominent nucleoli, abundant eosinophilic cytoplasm with distinct cell borders, and frequent mitotic figures (Fig. 10). A fourth cell type is now recognized by the members of the Pathology Committee of the Collaborative Ocular Melanoma Study in the United States and is referred to as intermediate epithelioid cells. These cells are similar to epithelioid cells but may be smaller and have indistinct cell borders (Fig. 11). Pure epithelioid cell tumors are the rarest of uveal melanomas, accounting for only 3% of choroidal and ciliary body melanomas.

Melanomas may be composed almost entirely of one of the foregoing cell types, or they may consist of mixtures of these cell types. According to Callender's original classification, a melanoma of the mixed cell type consists of a significant component of spindle cells (usually, spindle B cells) and epithelioid cells. This type of tumor is the most common type of uveal melanoma and accounts for 45% of these tumors. The designation "necrotic melanoma" refers to those in which the cell type cannot usually be identified because of necrosis. About 7% of choroidal melanomas are of this variety [329]. The cause of necrosis in melanomas is unknown, but ischemia and autoimmunity may play roles [346,347].

Electron Microscopy.   Electron microscopic examination of uveal melanomas [33,37,218,250] reveals the following characteristics: the size and reticulation of nucleoli and the number of free ribosomes and mitochondria increases from spindle A to spindle B and epithelioid cells. Nuclear membrane infolding is seen in spindle A cells. Rough-surfaced endoplasmic reticulum is most prominent in the spindle B cell type. Cytoplasmic filaments (see Chap. 1) are most numerous in the spindle A cells and least common in epithelioid cells. Melanomas of the mixed cell type contain features of both spindle cells and epithelioid cells [31,218]. Viruslike particles have been identified by electron microscopy in the metastases of human malignant melanoma (origin not stated) [39], but it is uncertain whether these particles are viruses.

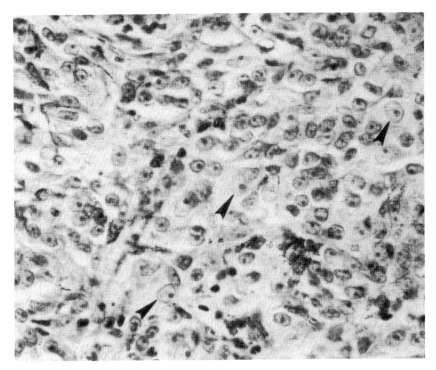

Figure 10   Choroidal melanoma with epithelioid cells (arrowheads). (Hematoxylin and eosin, ×550)

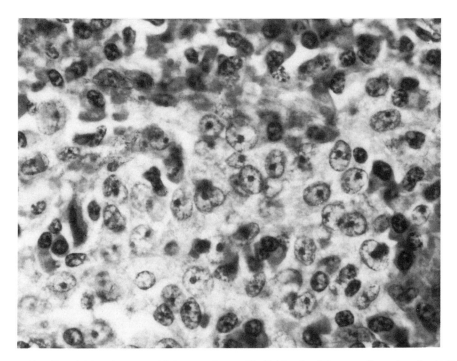

Figure 11   Choroidal melanoma with intermediate epithelioid cells. (Hematoxylin and eosin, ×900)

Morphometry. Traditionally, the histological cell type of uveal melanoma, as first proposed by Callender [67], has been useful in predicting death after enucleation [329]. Statistical analysis has shown cell type to be a prognostic indicator superior to other factors, including tumor size, mitotic activity, pigmentation, and extrascleral extension [291,482,486]. The subjective nature of the Callender and the modified Callender classifications [292] is demonstrated by 12–17% interobserver variability regarding classification [79,291]. A quantitative analysis of the Callender classification showed that six morphological factors were useful in classifying melanoma cells, although even then some melanoma cells could not be precisely classified [167]. These findings led to the development of computerized histological assessment of malignant potential analysis of uveal melanomas [168–173,387,444]. Computerized histological assessment has thus far shown that the mean size of the 10 largest nucleoli [217] is the most useful morphometric criteria with regard to long-term patient survival.

DNA Studies. Recent advances have taken morphometric analysis of tissue one step further, to that of actually measuring the DNA content of cells via flow cytometric analysis [60,93,158,165,294,371]. This technique of flow cytometric analysis has been applied to human uveal melanoma [166,293]. Results have shown 35–60% of uveal melanoma cells to have a diploid (normal) amount of DNA; 40–61% of cells to have more than diploid DNA content, and approximately 4% to have less than diploid DNA content [293]. Also, RNA content in uveal melanoma as determined by cell flow cytometry correlates with patient prognosis [83]. To date morphometric analyses have not been compared, however, either prospectively or retrospectively, with flow cytometry studies regarding prognosis in patients with uveal melanoma.

Another way to measure DNA content uses the Feulgen stain [200,301]. The prognostic value of morphometric determination of nucleolar size has been compared with that of DNA content as determined by Feulgen staining in uveal melanoma, and it appears that morphometric analysis is the better predictor of survival [288,289].

A corollary of studies regarding morphometric analysis and DNA content is that of DNA activity. The cell cycle can be divided into four sequential cycles: mitosis (M), gap 1 ($G1$), DNA synthesis (S), and gap 2($G2$) [193]. Cell cycle analysis for mitosis, gap 1, DNA synthesis, and gap 2 has been determined for human uveal melanoma utilizing flow cytometry [77], showing that there are relatively few tumor cells in the phase of DNA synthesis (S phase) at a given time [77]. The correlation of cell cycle studies and prognosis has not been determined to date regarding uveal melanoma. Another measure of DNA activity is that of nucleolar activity. Nucleolar organizing regions (NOR) are genes that code for ribosomal RNA, and it has already been shown that the RNA content correlates with prognosis in patients with uveal melanoma [83]. NOR are demonstrated by staining the associated rDNA nonhistone acid phosphoproteins [63,95,461]. Previous studies have examined Hodgkin's lymphoma, small cell tumors of childhood, and skin tumors for NOR [126,127]. Other studies have shown an increased number of NOR in cutaneous malignant melanoma versus nevus [260] and increased NOR in the vertical versus radial growth phase of cutaneous melanoma [8]. A recent study showed higher mean NOR in uveal melanomas than benign uveal nevi [277], as well as demonstrated a significant correlation between the number of NOR in uveal melanoma and computerized cytomorphometric analyses [277].

Immunophenotype. Specific antigenic determinants have been demonstrated in uveal melanoma cells by immunohistochemistry. Previous studies have shown uveal melanoma cells to be S-100 protein-positive [212], although the monoclonal antibody 079 epitope of S-100 stains cutaneous but not uveal melanomas [238,239]. Other studies have shown uveal melanoma cells to be ME 491 [146], NR MI 05, and 9.2.27/HB50 positive [146]. Additionally, the monoclonal antibody Ki67 recognizes a proliferation-associated nuclear antigen and stains nuclei in uveal melanomas [306].

There appear to be immunophenotypic differences between normal uveal melanocytes and uveal melanoma cells [146]. There also is evidence of immunophenotypic heterogeneity among uveal melanoma cells [103]. The prognostic implications of the various immunophenotypic expressions in uveal melanoma are not known.

DNA in situ hybridization [188,189,450] provides distinct advantages over immunohistochemistry, but to date in situ DNA hybridization studies have not been reported in uveal melanoma.

Immunological Studies. Reports of spontaneous regression of uveal melanoma [235,256,347], the presence of circulating tumor-associated antibodies in patients with uveal melanoma [58,134,135,338, 467], cutaneous delayed hypersensitivity to uveal melanoma antigen [80], and in vitro studies [472] suggest an immune response to uveal melanoma. The frequency of lymphocytic infiltration in uveal

Chapter 39

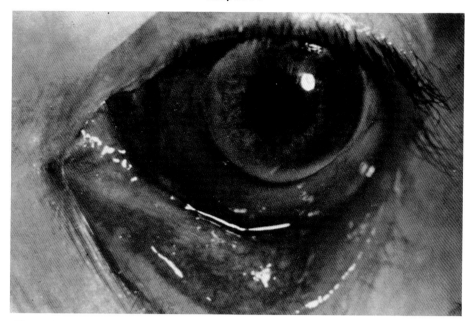

Figure 4 Argyrosis of the conjunctiva. (Courtesy of Drs. C. Hanna and F. T. Fraunfelder.)

Chapter 52

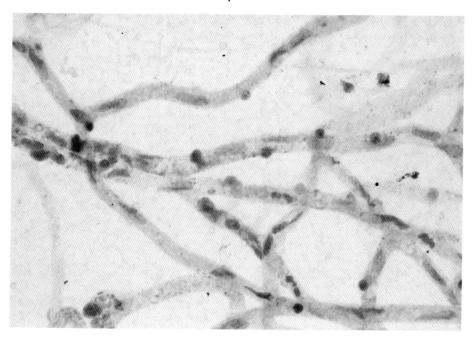

Figure 31 Enzyme digest preparation of a retina from a patient with diabetic retinopathy. The nuclei of the endothelial cells are elongated, whereas the pericyte nuclei are rounded and appear to be located on the outside of the vessel. Some of the pericyte nuclei are normal and stain intensely with hematoxylin, but many are degenerate and show marked eosinophilia. (Hematoxylin and eosin, ×145)

melanoma is variously reported as 18.6–50% [106,233,243]. There is morphological evidence of cellular interaction between uveal melanoma cells and lymphocytes [106]. The inflammatory response to uveal melanoma has been shown to be composed primarily of T cells [336] and macrophages [414]. Although one study showed no apparent associated between tumor cell type and the presence of T cells [336], a more recent report noted an increased presence of T cells in tumors of the epithelioid cell type [414]. Another recent study confirmed the presence of T cells in uveal melanoma and, further, found a higher percentage of T suppressor cells than T helper cells [123]. It is also noteworthy that tumor necrosis may be associated with a prominent lymphocytic infiltrate [347] and natural killer-lymphocytes (discussed in Chap. 53) have been found in necrotic uveal melanomas [414]. Moreover, T cells have been shown to be involved in preventing metastasis of intraocular melanoma in mice [320], and a strain of swine with a syndrome like Vogt-Koyanagi-Harada has been shown to undergo spontaneous regression of melanoma and atrophy of uveal melanocytes in the presence of large granular lymphocytes [355].

The precise relationship between lymphocytes and the prognosis of patients with uveal melanoma is unclear [106,110]. The temporal relationship regarding the type of tumor-associated lymphocytes present at a given time has yet to be determined. It is possible that antitumor lymphocytes are present at some point, portending a favorable prognosis; absence of antitumor lymphocytes may be associated with a worse prognosis.

Spread.   Choroidal melanoma primarily spreads via blood vessels. Extrascleral extension has been noted in 13% [427] and 10.4% [390] of enucleated eyes with choroidal melanomas and is almost invariably through emissary canals. Unlike retinoblastoma, optic nerve extension of these tumors is uncommon, occurring in only 5% of choroidal melanomas in one series [233]. Nevertheless, it is important to recognize that peripapillary choroidal melanomas are associated with a high incidence of tumor extension along the optic nerve and its sheaths [391]. Approximately 80% of such tumors are noted to extend into the optic nerve or its meningeal sheaths [248]. Most melanomas that extend into the optic nerve are necrotic or of mixed or epithelioid cell type and almost invariably occur in eyes with secondary glaucoma. Therefore, the presence of a necrotic melanoma in a blind painful eye with glaucoma should always lead to the suspicion the optic nerve extension may have occurred [422]. Choroidal melanomas may break through the retina and seed within the vitreous [121].

Biological Behavior.   It has long been suspected that the development and dissemination of a malignant lesion may depend largely on the immune competence of the host, although uveal melanomas rarely undergo spontaneous regression [235,256,346,347]. It is possible that the long delays in the clinical appearance of orbital or distant metastases after enucleation for a primary choroidal melanoma in some patients indicates that immunological host resistance to tumor cells plays a role [319]. These studies are interesting, but the evidence that immunological factors bear on the prognosis of melanoma is yet to be firmly substantiated.

Since the natural history of uveal melanomas is not known, attempts have been made to relate the behavior of these tumors to numerous histopathological features, including the cell type according to Callender's classification [67,69,234,272,329,392], pigmentation [291,392], reticulin fiber content [69,291], mitotic activity [291], rupture of Bruch's membrane [145,392,471], transscleral extension [234, 291,392], optic nerve extension [291], tumor shape [471], location [291], size [107,152,234,272,291,392, 443,471,482], and morphometric analysis [173,174].

Tumor size has been a confusing issue in the past regarding uveal melanomas [482]. Clinicians now generally classify melanomas in the following way based on size [482]:

1. Small melanomas are less than 10 mm in maximum diameter and less than 3 mm in maximum elevation.
2. Medium-sized melanomas are between 10 and 15 mm in maximum diameter and 3 and 5 mm in maximum thickness.
3. Large melanomas are greater than 15 mm in maximum diameter and greater than 5 mm in maximum thickness.

One should classify the tumor according to its greatest measurement (i.e., a tumor that is 9 mm maximum diameter and 6 mm maximum height is classified as large).

Analysis of these various parameters has disclosed morphometric analysis to be distinctly superior to the others in judging prognosis (see Morphometry in Section I.D.) [173,174]. However, among the features of a choroidal melanoma that can be determined clinically, the size of the tumor is thought to be the most important prognostic indicator [392,440]. That small choroidal melanomas carry a favorable prognosis is clinically significant, because it is the small choroidal melanoma that is often difficult to differentiate from other lesions, such as nevi, hemangiomas, hematomas, granulomas, proliferated pigment epithelium, and metastatic carcinoma.

Callender's classification of uveal melanomas has been useful in predicting prognosis of groups of cases after enucleation for choroidal and ciliary body melanomas [67,69,145,329,456] but is of almost no value in predicting the biological behavior of an individual case.

The 15 year actuarial survival rates based on a study of 2652 cases by Paul and colleagues [329] using the Callender classification are 81.2% for patients with spindle A tumors, 73.6% for patients with spindle B and fascicular tumors, 40.6% for patients with mixed cell and necrotic melanomas, and 28% for patients with purely epithelioid tumors.

Subsequent reappraisal of 105 melanomas of the choroid and ciliary body that were originally classified as Callender's spindle A type has raised a question of the malignancy of a tumor composed purely of this cell [292]. Only 15 of the 105 cases were of pure spindle A cell type, and there were no tumor deaths in this group. The remaining 90 cases had variable percentages of spindle B and/or epithelioid cells. It is now widely believed that spindle A cells are nevus cells. A new classification (modified Callender classification) [290] recognizes spindle cell nevi, spindle cell malignant melanomas, mixed cell melanomas, and epithelioid melanomas.

Diagnosis and Differential Diagnosis. Numerous lesions are known to simulate choroidal melanomas clinically (Table 1), and a variety of benign lesions may lead to enucleation [244,303,344], accounting for 10–50% of eyes enucleated for suspected melanomas. Benign lesions accounted for about 20% of enucleations for suspected melanoma in eyes with clear media and ophthalmoscopically visible lesions reported in 1964 [138] and 1973 [409]. Lower rates of clinical misdiagnosis of choroidal or ciliary body melanomas have been noted in series reported from teaching institutions to which large numbers of patients are referred for clinical evaluation. Blodi and Roy [46] found that the rate of misdiagnosis was 10.2% for 82 enucleated eyes sent from outside sources to their pathology laboratory, but only 5.6% among the eyes enucleated at their hospital. A recent report from the Collaborative Ocular Melanoma Study has shown a very low misdiagnosis rate (0.48%) for choroidal melanoma [92]. Lower rates of misdiagnosis in patients with intraocular tumors have been attributed to a greater clinical awareness of lesions that simulate melanomas, use of indirect ophthalmoscopy, serial fundus photography, fluorescein angiography, transillumination (Fig. 12) of the globe, and multiple ophthalmological consultations. Computed tomography, ultrasonography, and most recently magnetic resonance imaging [75,270] aid in the diagnosis in the choroidal melanoma and help to differentiate simulating lesions. Fine-needle aspiration has been utilized to identify malignant cells in choroidal melanoma [23,182]. Examiner experience is likely to be the single most important factor in the low rate of misdiagnosis.

Benign Lesions Simulated by Melanomas. Although a number of benign lesions may clinically simulate choroidal melanomas, some choroidal melanomas mimic benign lesions on rare occasions, leading to delays in diagnosis. For example, a multinodular uveal melanoma has appeared to be a postoperative choroidal detachment [374], and choroidal melanoma with an overlying neovascular membrane has been clinically misdiagnosed as diskiform macular degeneration [72].

The possibility that testing for certain immune responses of the host may prove useful in diagnosing uveal melanomas has been investigated. Rahi [338] tested the sera of 21 melanoma patients for antibodies against living cultures of their own melanoma cells. In the presence of specific autoantibodies and complement, some melanoma cells undergo necrosis. The synthesis of ribonucleic acid is interrupted in other melanoma cells. Immunofluorescence microscopy discloses that the patient's antibodies attach to antigens on the surface of the malignant cells as well as within the cells. Rahi's results contrast markedly with the earlier study of Howard and Spalter [216], which failed to detect antibodies to melanoma antigens in patients with ocular melanomas using less sensitive immunological tests.

The intradermal injection of a soluble extract of melanoma cells can elicit a delayed hypersensitivity reaction in the skin of persons with melanomas [80].

Association of Uveal Melanomas with Other Tumors. Multiple primary malignant neoplasms sometimes occur in the same patient, and at least 39 patients with nonocular malignant tumors have had

Table 1 Differential Diagnosis of Choroidal Melanoma

Condition	References
Retinal lesions	
Retinal detachment (rhegmatogenous, serous, or hemorrhagic)	97,236,409
Diskiform macular degeneration	344
Senile retinoschisis	138,409
Chorioretinitis	138,409
Hyperplasia or hypertrophy of retinal pigment epithelium	452
Hemorrhage from macroaneurysm of retinal arteries	331
Solitary retinal cyst with hemorrhage	386
Subretinal pigment epithelial hematoma	34,445
Congenital pits of optic nerve head with serous macular degeneration	139
Choroidal lesions	
Detachment	27,55,246,323,374
Nevi (including melanocytoma)	138, 409
Hemorrhage	24,108,233,243,366
Hemangioma	138,409
Metastatic carcinoma	140
Lymphoid hyperplasia	372,373
Osteoma	181,373
Scleral lesions	
Cellular blue nevus	416
Orbital mass	488

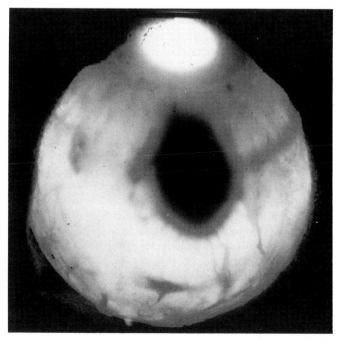

Figure 12 Melanoma of choroid and ciliary body demonstrated by transillumination.

independent primary intraocular neoplasms [10,19,208,309,322], especially choroidal melanomas. Therefore, from a clinical standpoint an intraocular mass in a patient with a history of known cancer should not be dismissed simply as a metastatic lesion.

Bilateral Diffuse Uveal Melanocytic Proliferation

Bilateral diffuse uveal melanocytic proliferation (supernevus syndrome) is associated with visceral malignancies, in particular ovarian carcinoma [29,180,281]. Multiple patchy uveal tumors giving a "giraffe skin" appearance, diffuse uveal thickening, cataract, and exudative retinal detachment are present in this paraneoplastic syndrome [180].

Multicentric Melanomas

At least 8 patients with unilateral multicentric malignant melanomas of the choroid and 11 bilateral multicentric malignant melanomas of the uvea have been identified [38,300,393,449,453].

Treatment of Choroidal Melanomas

The traditional method of treating choroidal melanomas has been enucleation of the eye, and this is still the most common form of treatment for large melanomas. There is considerable controversy, however, concerning the management of small choroidal melanomas. Some believe that eyes with small melanomas should be enucleated as soon as the diagnosis is suspected to give the patient the best chance of survival [392]; others believe that since the clinical diagnosis of melanoma is never completely free of error; despite the use of ancillary diagnostic tests, a period of observation to document tumor growth is essential [101]. The conservative management of small pigmented lesions in the fundus is now considered the standard practice [138,178,339], particularly since there is no apparent difference in the mortality rate among patients having prompt enucleations for melanoma after diagnosis compared to those whose tumor-containing eyes were observed for some time before enucleation [339].

Since enlargement of the tumor under observation is probably the most reliable indicator of malignancy, the role of observation in management of small tumors has been stressed [178], and serial photographs showing the crossing of retinal blood vessels in relation to the tumor have been recommended to help determine whether growth has occurred. Although observation for evidence of growth is reasonable, an extremely rare but potential danger of observation is the finding that a choroidal melanoma may remain clinically stationary in appearance for as long as 3 years yet develop significant extrascleral extension [72]. Conversely, apparent spontaneous regression of a choroidal melanoma has been reported [256].

Since many patients with medium-sized choroidal melanomas are asymptomatic and have normal vision, alternative forms of treatment rather than enucleation are being investigated. These include photocoagulation [15], transscleral diathermy, cryosurgery, various forms of radiation [22,191], and tumor resection.

Enucleation has traditionally been thought to provide the best prognosis for life, and animal studies [62] suggest that early enucleation may prevent metastases and prolong life. Ocular massage of experimentally produced intraocular tumors decreased the longevity of animals [159].

Zimmerman and colleagues [487] have drawn attention to an observation, yet to be statistically proven, that may influence treatment of uveal melanomas. They postulate that the tumor-related mortality rate in patients who have undergone enucleation for ocular melanomas is higher than in patients in whom the tumors were left untreated. They implicate conventional methods of enucleation in the dissemination of tumor emboli and believe that enucleation may have an adverse rather than beneficial effect regarding metastasis from the eye. Currently, the Collaborative Ocular Melanoma Study in the United States is addressing this issue in a prospective manner [359]. In this study, eyes with small melanoma are observed, whereas those with medium-sized melanomas are enucleated with or without preoperative irradiation and eyes with large melanomas are enucleated.

It is thought that malignant melanomas continuously shed cells into the bloodstream but that these cells usually do not cause metastases. If showers of cells occur during surgical intervention, however, as in a study of colonic carcinoma [448], patient survival is decreased because of increased rates of metastatic disease. Clumps of malignant cells are present in the peripheral bloodstream during or immediately after enucleation in patients with choroidal melanomas [425]. The number of tumor cells in the blood is critical and is directly proportional to the incidence of metastases [143].

The survival rate after enucleation for melanomas in patients more than 60 years of age is as good as their expected lifetime expectancy [143].

Although circulating antibodies may in theory prevent the metastasis of choroidal melanomas, it appears likely that cell-mediated defense reactions are of greater significance in causing the regression or local destruction of tumors [324,441]. Relevant evidence is still awaited, however.

The incidence of orbital extension of choroidal melanomas ranges from 10 to 23% [65,330,427] and reflects the cell type and the size of the intraocular melanoma. When there is histological evidence of extrascleral extension at the time of enucleation and this is not treated by early exenteration, orbital recurrence can be expected in about 22% of cases. The 5 year survival rate of patients without orbital extension of the uveal melanoma is 78% [390] compared with 27% with orbital extension.

Some experts [240,352] believe that exenteration is not indicated in cases of orbital extension of choroidal melanomas, and instead they recommend local excision of the orbital extension. There is anecdotal evidence that minimal surgery in patients with massive orbital extension may result in survival similar to or better than that in patients in whom extensive surgery is undertaken [358].

E. Ciliary Body Melanomas

Clinical Features

Circumscribed ciliary body melanomas constitute 2–9% of all uveal melanomas (Fig. 13) [119] and usually occur in the sixth decade of life, with an equal incidence in males and females. Like other uveal melanomas, they predominate in whites [213].

The earliest and most consistent symptom in patients with melanomas of the ciliary body is an unexplained progressive decrease in vision not correctable with lenses and without apparent clinical cause [153,395]. Reduction in vision, usually in the range 20/40–20/70 [213], is usually due to encroachment by tumor on the lens (Figs. 8 and 13). The mechanisms thought to be responsible for these optical effects principally involve displacement and changes in lens shape. Melanomas of the ciliary body and the choroid have at times been discovered only after cataract extraction [43] and sometimes after cataract extraction and intraocular lens implantation. Preoperative ultrasonography is essential on eyes in which dense cataracts preclude internal examination [84,403].

Episcleral and bulbar conjunctival vascular engorgement is common over a ciliary body melanoma, and the overlying sclera may manifest an increased local resistance to identation.

If the tumor extends into the periphery of the iris and toward the pupil, the pupil may become irregular in shape and may react sluggishly to light. The iris adjacent to the tumor is often displaced anteriorly, causing the anterior chamber to be shallow in that area. Occasionally, however, the tumor deepens the chamber and displaces the pars plicata and iris root posteriorly.

Transillumination through the pupil usually discloses a shadow on the sclera, except when cysts of the nonpigmented epithelium of the ciliary body coexist [395]. Slit lamp examination and gonioscopy with a maximally dilated pupil is necessary to detect small ciliary body melanomas.

An early but subtle sign of a ciliary body melanoma is a slightly lower (2–3 mm Hg) intraocular pressure in the involved eye compared with its fellow eye [153]. Although the exact mechanism of this relative hypotony is not known, it may reflect diminished aqueous secretion because of tumor in the ciliary body.

Spread

Ciliary body melanomas may spread to distant sites via the bloodstream or they may spread to surrounding structures by one of four routes [213]. (1) The tumor may spread anteriorly to the iris root, sometimes giving the appearance of an iridodialysis (tear at base of iris). As with melanomas of the iris, those in the ciliary body may extend circumferentially along the major arterial circle to produce a "ring melanoma" [482]. A ring melanoma may also arise from the coalescence of tumors arising at multiple sites, as is suggested by a melanoma of the ciliary body and iris that was manifested in two locations in the same eye [252]. (2) The tumor may extend centrally into the posterior chamber and vitreous. This may result in

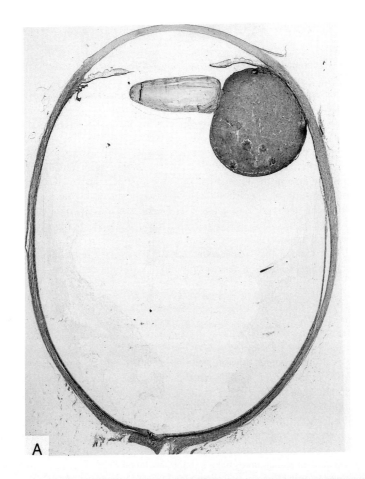

A

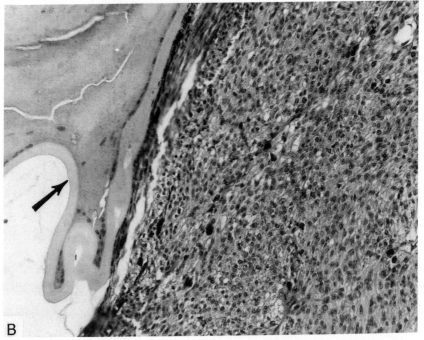

B

1442

lenticular astigmatism, subluxation, and cataract formation. Initially, the resultant opacity is restricted to that portion of the lens that is contiguous with the tumor, but eventually the entire lens becomes opaque. (3) Posterior extension of the tumor tends to be relatively late, and when the melanoma arises in the posterior portion of the pars plana, choroidal invasion may suggest a primary choroidal melanoma. A visual field defect accompanies a choroidal extension, which produces a secondary retinal detachment. (4) An extrabulbar extension to an episcleral location may occur along the scleral emissaries of the ciliary nerves and vessels, producing an episcleral pigmented lesion, but it is unusual for this to be the presenting sign [284].

Glaucoma

Pain is an infrequent symptom with ciliary body melanomas but occurs when the tumor causes glaucoma. Glaucoma may occur by one or more of three methods [213]: (1) most commonly, the tumor infiltrates the iris root against the trabecular meshwork and Schlemm's canal; (2) the tumor may displace the iris root against the trabecular meshwork and mechanically obstruct aqueous outflow; or (3) less commonly, tumor cells exfoliate and are carried by the aqueous circulation into the anterior chamber, where they may block the trabecular outflow channels.

Secondary glaucoma is usually one of the earliest findings in diffuse melanomas of the anterior uvea and is usually due to a circumferential infiltration of the chamber angle. Before or after the secondary glaucoma becomes evident, the clinical picture may resemble iridocyclitis with pigmented keratic precipitates.

If a ciliary body melanoma becomes necrotic, unilateral acute open-angle glaucoma may result from an obstruction to the trabecular meshwork by macrophages containing phagocytozed melanin pigment and other cellular debris liberated from necrotic tumor cells (melanomalytic glaucoma) [474].

Diagnosis and Differential Diagnosis

Benign solid tumors may be difficult to differentiate from malignant ciliary body melanomas by clinical appearance. Ultrasonography, although helpful in some cases, cannot help differentiate small tumors of the ciliary body [91].

When flare and cells are seen in the anterior chamber of an eye with a suspected ciliary body melanoma, aqueous aspiration and a cytological study may differentiate between inflammatory and neoplastic cells [211].

A variety of benign lesions arising in the ciliary body can simulate malignant melanomas clinically (Table 2).

Histopathology

The morphological features of ciliary body melanomas and choroidal melanomas are similar (see Choroidal Melanomas in Section I.D.).

Treatment

In the past, enucleation was the treatment of choice for any malignant melanoma of the ciliary body. The general view today, however, is that these tumors should be treated conservatively [273]. If the lesion is small and is discovered incidentally during a routine examination, it may safely be observed for signs of growth [211], but once symptoms are present, there is little time for observation.

Among eyes that have undergone local resection of iris-ciliary body or ciliary body melanomas, 10–20% have eventually required enucleation because of lack of total tumor resection, extensive hemorrhage at time of operation, secondary glaucoma, retinal detachment, or inflammation [154,273]. Even if a ring melanoma of the ciliary body is present or if widespread epibulbar extension is noted, patients may survive for long periods of time after enucleation [246].

Figure 13   (A) Melanoma of ciliary body with compression of lens from a 27-year-old woman who presented because of visual complaints and the appearance of a pigmented area in the periphery of the iris. (Partially bleached; hematoxylin and eosin, ×4) (B) Higher power, showing distortion of the lens (arrow) by ciliary body malignant melanoma. (Partially bleached; hematoxylin and eosin, ×195)

Table 2 Differential Diagnosis of Ciliary Body Melanoma

Condition	References
Cysts	
Ciliary body cyst	274,342,477
Inflammatory lesions	
Juvenile xanthogranuloma	415
Inflammatory pseudotumor	372,373
Granulomatous inflammation	278,279
Nevi	
Ciliary body nevus	201
Melanocytoma of ciliary body with extrascleral extension	381
Neoplasms	
Medulloepithelioma	273
Leiomyoma	273
Metastatic carcinoma	141,273
Hyperplastic lesions	
Hyperplasia of pigmented ciliary epithelium	273

F. Iris Melanomas

Clinical Features

The first description of an iris melanoma was by Tay in 1866 [439]. Iris melanomas are uncommon, occurring in only 0.9–1.3% of enucleated eyes before the conservative treatment of these lesions [20,61,251], but they account for between 0.5 and 8% of all uveal tract melanomas in adults and are thought clinically to arise from iris nevi [298,459]. Rarely, iris melanomas may be bilateral [112].

Since the iris is an easily observed part of the eye, changes in iris color, distortion of the pupil, or other abnormalities related to neoplastic growth can be noted early. Thus, these tumors are usually detected in patients earlier than melanomas of the posterior uveal tract. The average age of patients with iris melanomas is in the fifth decade of life [18,20,61,251], which is 10–20 years younger than pertains for ciliary body or choroidal melanomas [164].

Iris melanomas are uncommon in young patients, however. Lerner [261] reported 16 cases in patients under the age of 10 years and 25 cases between the ages of 10 and 19 years; Apt [16] described 19 juvenile iris melanomas and noted an increased incidence after puberty. In Apt's series, 14 of the patients were older than 11 years. Arentsen and Green [18], in a series of 72 iris melanomas, found that 10% of the patients were under the age of 20 years. Nevertheless, an iris melanoma has been reported in a 7½-month-old infant [61], and even a unique congenital melanoma of the iris has been documented [195]. Although these iris tumors are much less common in children than in adults, they represent 41% of all uveal melanomas in childhood [16]. Some studies have reported a slightly higher incidence in females [18,61,113,468], whereas others have described an excess of males [91,366]. Probably there is no significant difference in the incidence of iris melanomas between the sexes [20].

Like other uveal melanomas, those in the iris are rare in non-whites, and of 125 patients with iris melanomas in one series, only 2 were black [366].

Although visual symptoms are frequently denied, on close questioning the patient may have noted a pigmented spot on the iris that recently enlarged or became darker (Fig. 14). In the presence of a diffuse iris melanoma (Fig. 15), the patient may comment on the gradual development of heterochromia iridis, the involved eye having the darker iris. The hyperpigmentation in a diffuse iris melanoma is often irregular and blotchy, and tumor growth obscures the iris architecture and causes stromal thickening.

Iris melanomas are usually present in the stroma and anterior border layer of the iris but may break through the surface or extend out from the iris crypts to grow on the surface. They may have a nodular appearance and bulge into the anterior chamber or may spread as a relatively flat mass on the iris surface to infiltrate the anterior chamber angle and be inapparent for some time. Iris melanomas are usually densely pigmented, but when the tumor lacks pigment, prominent, dilated blood vessels occur on the fleshy tumor

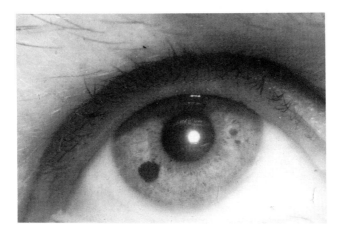

Figure 14 Melanocytic lesions of iris of a 43-year-old woman who noted enlargement during the preceding 4–5 months. Histopathological examination disclosed a compact spindle cell tumor containing spindle B cells.

surface. These superficial newly formed vessels are a feature of from 7% [18] to 20% [365] of cases, and sometimes the vessels may be sufficiently prominent to cause confusion with hemangiomas [25,202,273].

Other associated preoperative clinical features of iris melanomas include spontaneous hyphema (7–13% of cases) [365], secondary glaucoma (14% of cases) [18], and cataractous lens changes (10% of patients) [18]. Hyphema may also be a first indication of iris melanoma recurrence after previous excision [253]. Since heterochromia iridis occurs infrequently with iris melanomas [164,298,346], a low index of clinical suspicion in eyes with this finding sometimes delays diagnosis.

Most iris melanomas are located inferiorly, and the majority involve the midzone and periphery of the iris [18,87,365]. A melanoma of the superior iris is most unusual [399]. These tumors grow more slowly than choroidal melanomas but may suddenly enlarge. An increase in pigmentation alone should not be

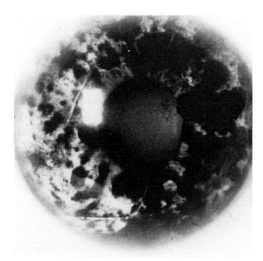

Figure 15 Diffuse, multinodular iris melanoma of a 66-year-old woman who noted darkening of the iris over a 3 year period. The eye was enucleated because of blindness and pain from secondary glaucoma. Histopathological study disclosed a diffuse, nodular, and cohesive spindle cell melanoma containing spindle B cells, with invasion of the chamber angle and anterior aspect of ciliary body. (Courtesy of Dr. Roy Scholz.)

considered definite evidence of tumor growth, since it may occur at puberty or during pregnancy. Indicators of tumor growth include increase in size of the lesion and new vessel formation, and incomplete dilation of the pupil in the area of the tumor signifies stromal invasion. The pupil is often distorted, being elongated toward the lesion, and this appearance may be accentuated by ectropion uveae.

Conjunctival hyperpigmentation in the vicinity of the iris tumor has been noted in one study [348], but it was not observed in one large series [18].

A melanoma in the extreme periphery of the iris may not be detected during a routine examination. Dilated episcleral vessels corresponding to the location of the iris tumor are generally indicative of ciliary body involvement [153].

Iris melanomas may extend around the anterior chamber angle and block enough trabecular meshwork to cause a secondary glaucoma, which can be the initial cause of symptoms [273,286]. The combination of increased pigmentation of one iris (heterochromia iridis) and ipsilateral glaucoma should arouse suspicion of a diffuse malignant melanoma of the iris [364]. The glaucoma in diffuse cases is relentless, does not respond to treatment, and eventually leads to visual loss. Occasionally, an iris melanoma extends circumferentially in the anterior chamber angle and anterior aspect of ciliary body and produces a so-called ring melanoma [213].

Fine granular pigment over the trabecular meshwork in the dependent part of the filtration angle is an almost constant finding during gonioscopy of an eye with an iris melanoma. This pigment differs from implantations of tumor cells, which are larger and tend to grow over the iris surface. Seeding of tumor cells is an important mode of intraocular spread to the angle structures and eventual extrabulbar extension.

If the iris melanoma becomes necrotic, cells and a flare appear in the anterior chamber. Rarely, an iris melanoma clinically simulates granulomatous uveitis, with iris nodules, aqueous flare, and glaucoma [231]. Tumor cells of an iris melanoma are reported to have implanted on the surface of the optic nerve head and inner surface of the retina [377]. Extraocular spread in iris melanomas presents clinically as an extrabulbar pigmented mass and, as with those of the ciliary body, is usually via scleral vascular and neural channels. One iris melanoma without choroidal involvement has been noted with extrascleral extension into the optic nerve head [424].

An unusual clinical variant of iris melanoma (tapioca melanoma) is characterized by lightly pigmented and translucent nodules, resembling tapioca pudding [231,351]. Reese and colleagues [351] documented this entity in nine patients and noted that the tapioca melanoma of the iris presents as a large irregular segmental nodule or as multifocal nodules, and the individual masses are sometimes pedunculated. Even when the nodules are multifocal, they are thought to represent separate primary growths rather than secondary implantations, because they have been shown histopathologically to lie within the iris stroma rather than on the iris surface. The average age of onset of presentation of tapioca melanomas is about 30 years (younger than with the usual type of iris melanoma) [18]. They have histopathological features [219] and prognosis similar to those of other iris melanomas.

Diagnosis and Differential Diagnosis

In one review [137] of 69 eyes enucleated with a clinical diagnosis of iris melanoma, the clinical impression was not confirmed in 24 eyes (35%). This surprising high rate of misdiagnosis was partly because one-fourth of the patients in this series were not white (iris melanomas being very uncommon in non-whites). In another series of 48 cases examined at a single university-based teaching center, incorrect clinical diagnoses were made in only 2% of the cases [214]. A large study performed on 200 patients referred to a major center with a clinical diagnosis of melanoma found that only 42 patients (24%) had melanoma [406].

Although transillumination, which is often useful in evaluating lesions of the posterior uveal tract, is of limited value in differentiating melanomas from other lesions of the iris [119], it remains a useful procedure in clinically suspected iris melanomas because it helps exclude certain lesions, such as an anterior staphyloma.

Ultrasonography is generally not useful in the evaluation of possible iris melanomas, since small tumors of the iris cannot with certainty be differentiated from each other because they reflect insufficient internal acoustic information [91].

Iris fluorescein angiography is helpful in distinguishing benign from malignant melanocytic tumors [220]. In clinically obvious melanomas of the iris, which are nonpigmented or lightly pigmented, fluorescein angiograms of the anterior segment consistently disclose an abnormal pattern of disorderly interconnected vascular channels. These always leak fluorescein to permit dye pools in or around the tumor

[111], but in heavily pigmented lesions the vascular pattern of the tumor may be obscured. Disorganized vasculature and gross leakage are more apt to be associated with melanomas and tumors of intermediate cytology than with nevi [104]. Iris angiography may be normal in histopathologically proven malignant melanomas [248].

Fine-needle aspiration biopsy may provide an adequate specimen for cytological diagnosis, although the experience of the pathologist examining the specimen is imperative [78].

Many lesions need to be considered in the differential diagnosis of iris melanomas (Table 3) [273]. An anterior staphyloma and sudden prolapse of hemorrhagic intraocular contents through the site of a corneal or scleral perforation may simulate extrabulbar extension of an iris melanoma [348].

Histopathology

The histopathological classification of melanocytic iris tumors proposed by Jakobiec and Silbert [226] has merit and is based on the study of the large series of iris lesions on file in the Harkness Institute in New York. This classification is as follows:

Group 1. Melanocytosis. Increased number of densely pigmented fusiform, multipolar, or polyhedral melanocytes resembling normal stromal melanocytes with small orthochromatic nuclei generallydevoid of nucleoli; pigment accumulation in trabecular meshwork; ectropion uveae may be present; no surface plaque growth; no mitotic figures.

Group 2. Melanocytoma. Densely pigmented lesion composed of large, uniform, plump round or oval cells with abundant, densely pigmented cytoplasm and small, centrally placed nuclei; interspersed spindle-shaped cells and macrophages; no surface plaque extension; no mitoses.

Table 3 Differential Diagnosis of Iris Melanoma

Conditions	References
Conditions with diffuse pigmentation of iris	
Congenital ocular melanosis	45,137
Herpes zoster ophthalmicus	244
Cysts	
Cysts of the iris pigment epithelium	45,477
Neoplasms	
Leiomyoma	273
Metastatic carcinoma	141,273
Inflammatory lesions	385
Syphilis	385
Inflammatory pseudotumor	404,479
Sarcoidosis	273
Tuberculosis	273
Juvenile xanthogranuloma	137
Abscess	177
Vascular lesions	
Organized thrombus of iris	376
Pigmented iris and retrocorneal membrane secondary to old central retinal vein occulsion	394
Ectropion uveae associated with iris neovascularization	348
Hemangioma	25,202,273
Nevi	
Iris nevus (Cogan-Reese) syndrome	90,228,466
Necrotic melanocytoma of iris, producing secondary glaucoma	402
Melanocytoma of the ciliary body with anterior extension into the base of the iris	54
Miscellaneous	
Stromal atrophy of the iris with baring of iris pigment epithelium	137
Metallic foreign bodies embedded in the iris	137
Anterior staphyloma	137,348

Group 3. Epithelioid cell nevus. Nests of small, round, or polyhedral nevoid cells with one or more nuclei that have a vesicular or finely stippled chromatin pattern; small basophilic nucleolus near nuclear membrane; low nuclear-cytoplasmic ratio; no mitoses; no surface plaque growth; cells separated by abundant reticulin.

Group 4. Intrastromal spindle cell nevus. Variably pigmented ovoid or spindle-shaped cells arranged in short fascicles or nests; may be nonpigmented or lightly pigmented; densely pigmented in about 20% of cases; no surface plaque formation; nuclei are small, oval or spindle-shaped, and have fine, stippled chromatin with occasional intranuclear vacuoles and an occasional central chromatin strip; low nuclear-cytoplasmic ratio; no mitoses; occasional individual cells with larger nuclei that frequently have intranuclear vacuoles; stromal sclerosis; abundant reticulin.

Group 5. Spindle cell nevus with surface plaque. Spindle-shaped cells with low nuclear-cytoplasmic ratio located intrastromally and on the iris surface; stroma component is hypocellular with abundant reticulin; plaque lesions are hypercellular with no reticulin; nuclei of both components are oval or spindle shaped with small or absent nucleoli and frequent vacuoles; no mitoses; may have stromal nests of nonpigmented or lightly pigmented larger polygonal nevoid cells; multifocal or satellite lesions demonstrate features of predominant components of tumor; may extend over angle and onto back of cornea; both components may involve entire iris; may be arranged in individual discontinuous stromal and plaque lesions ("tapioca").

Group 6. Borderline spindle cell nevus. Features of lesions in this group are essentially the same as in group 5, but in addition there are a few cells with small nucleoli.

Group 7. Spindle cell melanoma. This may have both stromal and plaque components; spindle-shaped cells (equivalent to Callender's spindle B type cells) with high nuclear-cytoplasm ratios; clumping and peripheral margination and prominent nucleoli; mitotic figures (one to three per 10 high-power fields); low reticulin content; half of the tumors have areas of nevoid cells with heavy reticulin; plaques when present consist of malignant cells.

Group 8. Spindle and epithelioid cell melanoma. These lesions have malignant spindle-shaped cells with plump nuclei, prominent nucleoli (spindle B cells), and larger polyhedral cells (epithelioid cells); abundant glassy cytoplasm, and large nuclei containing prominent eosinophilic nuclei; coarse chromatin pattern in both cell types; mitotic figures are present; may have nevoid areas; reticulin in sparse.

Group 9. Epithelioid cell melanoma. Composed of large and smaller epithelioid cells with plump nuclei and prominent eosinophilic nucleoli, abundant glassy cytoplasm and high nuclear-cytoplasm ratio; grow in sheets and nests in stroma and surface plaques; plaques are nests in stroma and surface plaques; plaques are discohesive, with shedding of tumor cells to the anterior chamber angle and back of cornea; no nevoid component; minimal reticulin in stromal component; scattered pigmented macrophages in stroma and plaque components and in the anterior chamber angle.

Prognosis

Even mixed and epithelioid cell types of iris melanomas are relatively benign compared with posterior uveal tumors of similar types. Of approximately 800 iris melanomas, only 37 deaths have been attributed to metastases, but in only 7 of the patients who died was the nature of the metastases confirmed histologically [16,18,45,61,87,197,226,233,348,365,399,430]. The length of time that an iris melanoma is present does not seem to affect longevity [365]. In a series of 22 cases observed for 1–20 years, no tumor-related metastatic deaths were reported [348]. Morphological features of iris melanomas that relate to benign behavior include the predominance of spindle-shaped cells and the cohesiveness of these cells. In one series histopathological studies were interpreted as showing 92% of the tumors to be compact and cohesive [18]. It is also possible that many tumors previously classified as melanomas were nevi. The favorable outcome of patients with iris melanomas may also reflect their early diagnosis and small size even when the anterior chamber is filled with tumor.

Treatment

Pigmented lesions of the iris should be managed conservatively by observation and, if treatment is required, local resection because (1) the eye is usually otherwise normal, (2) iris melanomas behave in a benign fashion and rarely metastasize, and (3) the lesion may not be a melanoma [61,69,87]. After iridectomy, correct handling of the excised specimen allows accurate histopathological examination and determination of the extent of the tumor.

Despite the potential risk of dissemination associated with surgery, iridectomy for an iris melanoma does not seem to increase the incidence of metastases [365]. The cohesiveness of cells constituting these tumors probably prevents their shedding during the procedure [486]. Epibulbar seeding of tumor in an eye treated by iridectomy [18] and trabeculectomy [197] has been documented. Follow-up studies of patients with iris melanomas treated by excisional iridectomy have disclosed no metastatic deaths [273,425], some patients being followed for over 20 years [348].

Glaucoma surgery may have an adverse effect on the outcome of patients with iris melanoma. In two series [18,365] 4 of the 11 deaths occurred among patients younger than 30 years, and 3 had undergone a glaucoma filtering procedure. Resection is recommended for suspected small iris melanomas. If the suspected iris melanoma is large and/or if there is diffuse pigmentation of the trabecular meshwork, a fine-needle aspiration of cells from the surface or from within the tumor is recommended. If spindle B cells or epithelioid cells are present, more aggressive therapy is warranted depending on other clinical features, such as patient age, status of the fellow eye, and the presence of glaucoma. Some large tumors with angle involvement of 30° or less may be resected by an inner lamellar, corneoscleral iridocyclectomy.

II. NONMELANOTIC TUMORS

A. Benign Tumors

Hemangioma

Hemangiomas of the uveal tract, which can be considered hamartomas rather than neoplasms, are most frequently located in the choroid. It is useful to subdivide choroidal hemangiomas into two categories: solitary and diffuse, each having fairly characteristic clinical and pathological features [463].

Solitary choroidal hemangiomas occur in young and middle-aged adults and are not related to systemic disease. They grow slowly and often remain stationary in size, but because of a predilection for the temporal side of the disk, the macular area may be affected, with reduction in central vision at an early stage.

On funduscopic examination, solitary hemangiomas are only slightly elevated, with pale yellow or gray surfaces. A lack of pigmentation makes their clinical distinction from metastatic carcinoma more difficult than their differentiation from malignant melanomas. Occasionally, the nature of the lesion can be suspected clinically because of large tortuous choroidal vessels behind the retina. Transillumination is helpful in distinguishing a hemangioma from a melanoma, because the hemangioma appears somewhat translucent when viewed against the light of a transilluminator. When external pressure is applied to the globe, a choroidal hemangioma may become paler, and if the jugular veins are compressed, the lesion may enlarge.

Ancillary techniques useful in diagnosing hemangiomas are fluorescein angiography [321] and ultrasonography [91]. On fluorescein angiography choroidal hemangiomas fill quickly before the retinal vessels and often show a characteristic lacy pattern with late staining. It is said that the quantitative A scan obtained with ultrasound allows an easy and reliable differentiation from a choroidal melanoma [91].

Histopathologically, solitary choroidal hemangiomas are noncapsulated but are more sharply delineated from surrounding choroidal tissue than are the diffuse choroidal hemangiomas of Sturge-Weber syndrome. Hemangiomas are composed of endothelium-lined blood-filled channels. In a study of 45 cases of solitary choroidal hemangiomas, 3 were classified as capillary, 20 as cavernous, and 22 as mixed [463]. The retinal pigment epithelium overlying the hemangioma may undergo metaplasia and form a fibrous membrane that may hyalinize, calcify, and even ossify. The retina overlying the lesion may become edematous and undergo cystic degeneration and atrophy, causing a visual field defect. Retinal detachment and glaucoma are important complications of such eyes.

Diffuse choroidal hemangiomas occur in up to 40% of patients with Sturge-Weber syndrome [148], an entity that accounts for one-half of all choroidal hemangiomas (Figs. 16 and 17). Diffuse choroidal hemangiomas contain a mixture of capillary and cavernous patterns [463]. When the upper eyelid is the site of a hemangioma, ipsilateral intraocular involvement is common [11]. The median age of onset of ocular symptoms is 7.6 years [463]. In whites, there is a dramatic color difference between the two fundi, the involved eye having a bright red fundus and the normal eye showing a light blonde tessellated fundus. This type of choroidal hemangioma is flat and involves the posterior pole and peripapillary region. The term "tomato catsup fundus" has been given to this characteristic ophthalmoscopic appearance [431].

Glaucoma is an important complication of a choroidal hemangioma [332]. In the adult type of solitary hemangioma, extensive detachment of the retina may lead to iris neovascularization, peripheral anterior synechiae, and intractable secondary glaucoma. In the diffuse choroidal hemangioma of Sturge-Weber syndrome, several mechanisms have been proposed to explain the development of glaucoma. The two most popular theories are (1) a malformation of the anterior chamber angle with an anterior insertion of the longitudinal ciliary muscle and uveal tissue in the angle (i.e., an angle similar to that of some patients with congenital glaucoma not associated with a systemic disease) and (2) the presence of a limbal and episcleral vasculature, which increases the episcleral venous pressure and thus impedes aqueous outflow from the eye [155,332].

Photocoagulation of a choroidal hemangioma does not significantly reduce its size, but it changes the permeability of the surface vessels so that they are no longer a source of subretinal fluid. In most cases there is prompt absorption of subretinal fluid [321,411], but complications, such as intraretinal hemorrhage, traction folds of the retina, and vitreous hemorrhage [175], may follow photocoagulation treatment.

Hemangiomas of the ciliary body are extremely rare, and only five cases have been reported [326]. A review of these cases has indicated that in four [102,196,205], the original histopathological diagnosis was in error, the lesions now being considered to represent juvenile xanthogranuloma in one instance and zones of hyperemia [136] in the other three cases. The histological features of the one remaining case [326] are more those of a capillary hemangioma than of a cavernous or mixed hemangioma, as is found in the choroid.

Hemangiomas of the iris are rare, with an incidence of 2% in a series of 145 primary tumors of the iris [20]. Hence the probability that a prominently vascularized tumor of the iris is a true hemangioma is low [136]. Some cases reported to be iris hemangiomas [354,431] have proved on reexamination and further sectioning to be juvenile xanthogranulomas [362,484], malignant melanomas [25], or a fibrovascular proliferative response following inflammation or hemorrhage [136]. Ferry [136] has questioned the validity of the diagnosis of some reported iris hemangiomas and has provided evidence that diagnoses of hemangioma of the iris and ciliary body reported between 1963 and 1972 were equivocal at best.

Histologically, iris hemangiomas vary from the capillary type to the cavernous type with delicate

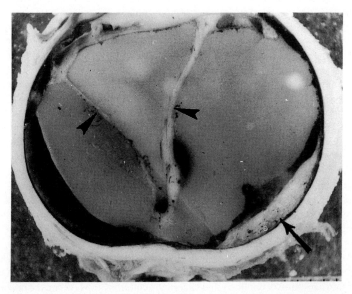

Figure 16 Surgically enucleated left eye of a 27-year-old woman with Sturge-Weber syndrome. The eye had become glaucomatous, blind, and painful. A partially ossified choroidal hemangioma (arrow) is present temporally, and the retina (arrowheads) is detached in a funnel-shaped configuration.

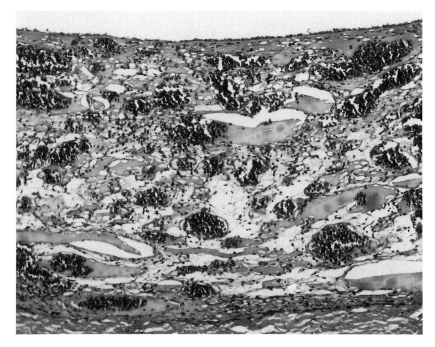

Figure 17   Small and medium-sized, thin-walled blood vessels of choroidal hemangioma of enucleated right eye of a 28-year-old man with Sturge-Weber syndrome. The patient had congenital glaucoma in both eyes and a retinitis pigmentosa–like picture in the right eye. (Hematoxylin and eosin, ×70)

fibrous stroma and varying amounts of hemorrhage [423]. A cavernous hemangioma of the iris has been reported in a neonate with diffuse congenital hemangiomatosis (Fig. 18) [310].

There has been one report of a varix of the iris [13].

Hemangiopericytoma

There has been one reported case of a choroidal hemangiopericytoma occurring in a 40-year-old woman with secondary retinal detachment [328].

Leiomyoma

A leiomyoma of the iris is rare and appears as a slowly growing, grayish white, vascularized nodule in or on the iris surface. It is usually located in the inferior portion of the iris, closer to the pupillary border than to the ciliary body. To date, there have been 45 reported cases of leiomyoma of the iris [20,109,116], but the diagnosis in these cases is equivocal because none of them were documented by electron microscopic examination and specific marker studies [190]. Leiomyomas of the ciliary body are also rare. There is one report of a tumor arising in the anterior iris pigment epithelium in a 4-year-old boy with ultrastructural features of both pigment epithelium and smooth muscle [265]. This tumor was classified as a "leiomyoepithelioma" [265]. Blodi reviewed 10 alleged cases in the literature, all of which he found equivocal [42], and added one acceptable case [42]. Since then several additional cases have been reported [48,66,70,120,297], including 2 with ultrastructural confirmation. A recent report also documents a locally resected transscleral leiomyoma that was thought to have arisen in the supraciliary area [398].

A leiomyoma examined solely by light microscopy may be confused with an amelanotic spindle A melanoma, neurofibroma, or a schwannoma (neurilemmoma; Fig. 19). Electron microscopic examination is helpful in confirming the diagnosis, because the smooth muscle cells have distinctive ultrastructural features [297], which include cytoplasmic filaments (myofibrils), rod- or cigar-shaped nuclei, basement membrane production, surface-connected vesicles (caveoli), and plasmalemmal and cytoplasmic densities. Masson's trichrome or phosphotungstic acid and hematoxylin stains may disclose intracytoplasmic fila-

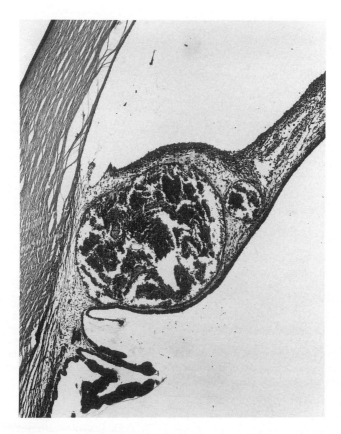

Figure 18 Iris hemangioma in an infant who died from complications of diffuse congenital hemangiomatosis. (Hematoxylin and eosin, ×36)

ments of smooth muscle cells. Immunohistochemical techniques for desmin, muscle-specific actin, and myoglobin stain smooth muscle.

Some authors have pointed out that ocular leiomyomas are of mesectodermal (neural crest) origin [224]. These mesectodermal leiomyomas are benign tumors composed of cells with both myogenic and neurogenic features [221,222]. The neurogenic features of axis cylinders, cystic degeneration, and palisading are presumably related to the embryonic neural crest origin of smooth muscle of the ciliary body [236]. Evidence of the smooth muscle nature of this tumor is the ultrastructural features of cytoplasmic filaments (4–8 nm in diameter) with fusiform densities and basement membrane [221]. Immuno-histochemical analysis of the mesectodermal leiomyoma indicates positive reactivity of tumor cells with antibodies for desmin and muscle-specific actin but negative staining for cytokeratins, glial fibrillary acid protein, neuron-specific enolase, and S-100 protein [408,458]. A mesectodermal leiomyoma can be removed successfully by partial lamellar iridocyclochoroidectomy [408]. Uveal leiomyomas presumably arise from either smooth muscle cells of pericytes [223,224,354]. There have been two documented cases to date of choroidal leiomyoma with ultrastructural confirmation [227,311].

Peripheral Nerve Sheath Tumors

Neurogenic tumors of the uveal tract are rare and include schwannomas (neurilemmomas) and neuro-fibromas. Schwannomas are very slowly growing benign tumors originating from Schwann cells, which sheath the axons of peripheral nerves. When present in the choroid, these tumors may be confused clinically and histopathologically with melanomas. By light microscopy they are composed of long, narrow, spindle-shaped cells, often with a palisade arrangement. Neurofibromas are also probably derived from Schwann

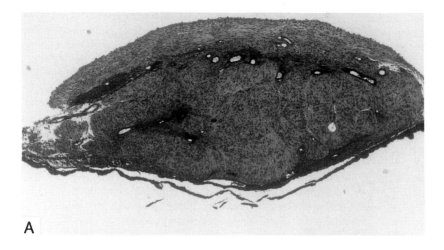

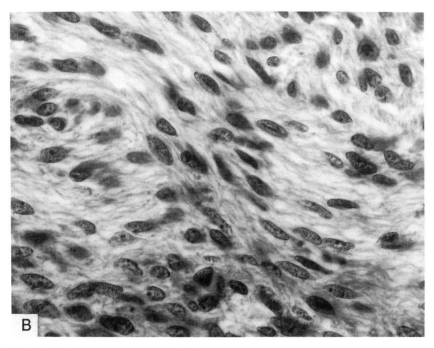

Figure 19 (A) Small iris leiomyoma in a surgically enucleated eye of a 16-year-old girl who was considered to have malignant ocular melanoma. (Hematoxylin and eosin, ×50) (B) The tumor cells have spindle-shaped nuclei with blunted ends and small nucleoli. The cells are separated by an abundant fibrillary material and contain no melanin pigment. (Hematoxylin and eosin, ×750)

cells, although perineural fibroblasts and endoneural cells are thought to be the source of some of these tumors. Schwannomas are composed of abundant bipolar or tripolar spindle-shaped cells, and they occasionally cause marked thickening of the uveal tract. Greatly thickened nonmyelinated nerve fibers and ganglion cells are occasionally associated and are suggestive of a ganglioneuroma, but the neurons are probably not neoplastic. Both schwannomas and neurofibromas may occur as solitary tumors in the eye or as part of von Recklinghausen's neurofibromatosis [119]. There is one report of a neurofibroma occurring in the iris of a patient with neurofibromatosis [464]; it is difficult, if not impossible to distinguish unequivocally between a melanocytic proliferation (Lisch nodule), neurofibroma, neurilemmoma, or leiomyoma without ultrastructural confirmation [194]. Neurofibromas of the ciliary body occur most often in association with iris and choroidal neurofibromas in patients with neurofibromatosis [68,194]. There is one report of a solitary neurofibroma of the ciliary body [114] and a solitary neurilemmoma of the ciliary body without ultrastructural confirmation [194], although a mesectodermal leiomyoma must be considered in the later case. Craig [96] presented a patient with a solitary choroidal neurofibroma, and Freedman and coworkers [163] reported a patient with neurofibromatosis and an intraocular neurilemmoma arising from a long posterior ciliary nerve. In a report describing 20 patients with solitary nerve sheath tumors of the eye (1 new case and 19 previously reported cases), Shields and colleagues [407] described 11 patients with choroidal, 3 with ciliary body, and 1 with choroidal and ciliary body tumors. One patient with neurofibromatosis and a choroidal ganglioneuroma has been reported [469].

Iris Cyst

Iris cysts can be classified into primary and secondary [401]. Primary stroma cysts are lined by surface epithelium, contain a clear fluid and are congenital and dysembryogenic [88,314]. Primary cysts of the iris pigment epithelium may involve any portion of the iris and may occasionally dislodge in the posterior and anterior [142] chambers and the vitreous [327].

Secondary iris cysts following surgery or trauma are lined by surface epithelium and are apparently due to implantation of epithelium [52,133]. Secondary surface epithelial cysts usually contain a clear fluid but rarely may contain keratin (pearl cyst) when keratinized squamous epithelium lines the cyst. Secondary cysts of the iris pigment epithelium are induced by drugs, such as phospholine iodide (echothiophate iodide).

Osteoma

Aside from occurring on the epibulbar surface [49], an intraocular osseous tumor can arise in the choroid [181,460] of otherwise normal eyes. This benign lesion represents a primary osseous choristoma or an ossified cavernous hemangioma of the choroid (Fig. 20) [183,463]. Most patients reported have usually been healthy young white women in their second or third decades with no previous history of eye disease and whose symptoms included blurred vision and central or paracentral scotomas [181,396]. The lesions are usually peripapillary in location and yellowish white in color, with mild irregular elevation and well-defined borders. Of all cases 25% are bilateral. On scleral depression choroidal osteomas behave as rigid bodies. The overlying retinal pigment epithelium has a mottled depigmented appearance and may have overlying pigmentation, and multiple small vascular networks are seen on the tumor surface. Although the ophthalmoscopic appearance of this tumor is characteristic, it may be confused with a metastatic carcinoma or amelanotic melanoma.

B. Malignant Tumors

Leiomyosarcoma

Leiomyosarcomas of the iris are extremely rare neoplasms [20,115] differentiated from leiomyomas solely on the basis of invasive properties rather than histological features. Of four cases treated by iridectomy, no deaths from metastases occurred within 3–5 years of surgery [20]. However, the diagnosis in none of the reported leiomyosarcomas of the iris was confirmed by electron microscopic or immunohistological examination [194].

Rhabdomyosarcoma

Rhabdomyosarcomas arise from primitive mesenchymal cells and can be present in structures devoid of striated muscle, such as the uterus, urinary bladder, and prostate; rhabdomyosarcomas may develop in the

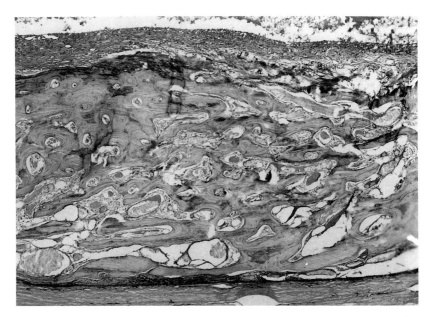

Figure 20 Choroidal osteoma or totally ossified choroidal hemangioma in a blind painful eye of a 27-year-old woman with no nevus flammeus. (Hematoxylin and eosin, ×140)

iris, but only three such cases have been documented [132,313,470]. Primitive, undifferentiated cells of the iris stroma have been postulated to give rise to this tumor [313]. An additional origin might be from iris pigment epithelium: Tso (personal communication) has shown differentiation of striated muscle from iris pigment epithelium in a sequential ultrastructural study of the developing chick.

The first reported rhabdomyosarcoma of the iris [470] occurred in a 4-year-old girl as a profusely vascularized grayish pink tumor initially suspected of being a juvenile xanthogranuloma. Neither irradiation nor corticosteroid therapy produced regression of the lesion, which was excised with a sector iridectomy. A 4 year follow-up revealed no local recurrence or metastasis. In the second case [313], the tumor recurred after sector iridectomy and extended into the ciliary body to produce a secondary glaucoma requiring enucleation. The patient was in good health 1 year later. The third case [132] was a 4-year-old girl in whom the diagnosis was established by biopsy; the child was free of tumor 7 months after enucleation. The diagnosis of rhabdomyosarcoma in these three cases was made on the basis of the pleomorphism, high nuclear-cytoplasmic ratio, the local invasiveness of the tumor cells, and, in addition, by electron microscopic features in the second and third cases.

Wilson et al. [462] described a rhabdomyosarcoma arising in the ciliary body of a 12-year-old boy. Diagnosis was based on the demonstration of cells with cross-striations, positive immunohistochemical staining for muscle-specific actin, and myosin in the neoplastic rhabdomyoblasts.

C. Miscellaneous Tumors

Several rare miscellaneous primary tumors of the iris have been reported: granular cell tumor [99], xanthoma [316], adenoma [194,335], nodular adenomatosis [446]. A case of what was interpreted as bilateral primary choroidal neonatal neuroblastomas has also been demonstrated [85].

III. METASTATIC TUMORS

A. Carcinoma and Sarcoma

Metastatic carcinoma is more frequent than primary intraocular tumors in autopsy material [6,7,40, 198,318]. The frequency of ocular involvement by metastatic carcinomas has been determined by clinical

[6,7] and postmortem studies [40,198,318]. In one series [6] ocular examinations were performed on 213 adult patients with proven metastatic carcinoma in other sites but without symptomatic evidence of ocular metastasis; 2.35% of these patients were found to have tumors metastatic to the choroid. Guthert and colleagues [198], in a histopathological study of the posterior segments of the eyes of 853 patients who had died of carcinoma, found that the incidence of ocular metastasis was 0.5%. Bloch and Gartner [40], in a postmortem investigation of the eyes and adjacent orbital structures of 230 patients with cancer, found an incidence of intraocular metastasis of 11%. Nelson and coworkers [318] found ocular metastases in 9.3% of all cancer-related fatalities. These percentages based on histological findings are higher than clinically recognized ocular metastases, which range from 0.06% [187] to 2.3% [6], probably because some metastases are not clinically apparent and individuals with terminal cancer usually do not undergo comprehensive eye examinations. Multiple foci of ocular metastasis occur in 13.2% [140] to 21.4% [428] of cases. Metastatic cancer to the eye portends a poor prognosis. The approximate average survival after ocular diagnosis is 13 and 5.2 months for breast and lung carcinoma, respectively [428]. Metastatic carcinoid tumors have a much more favorable prognosis (see later).

The most frequent presenting ocular symptom of metastatic carcinoma in the eye is decreased vision. Typically, the ocular lesion appears as a nonpigmented flat thickening of the posterior choroid (Fig. 21). The surface of the tumor may appear mottled, its edges are usually ill defined, and frequently there is an associated overlying shallow serous retinal detachment. The early occurrence of pain, the relatively acute onset of the lesion, its rapid increase in size, and the presence of additional tumors in the same eye aid in the clinical differentiation of metastatic carcinoma from malignant melanoma.

Most ocular metastases occur in the choroid, followed in frequency by the iris and ciliary body. Spontaneous hyphema [117,285], iridocyclitis [117,263,285,308], and glaucoma [140] may accompany involvement of the anterior uvea.

For a long time it was widely believed that metastatic carcinoma affected the left eye more often than the right eye, because of the anatomical arrangement of the carotid arterial system [203,345,455], but more recent studies have shown no significant predilection for left-sided involvement [6,40,140]. Metastatic tumors effect the posterior uvea more often than the anterior uvea [140], and multiple sites may be involved. Ferry and Font [140] found that 26 of 227 (11.4%) cases of metastatic carcinoma to the eye involved only the anterior segment. The iris alone was involved in 6, and the iris and ciliary body were involved in 20 cases. Metastases to the iris can mimic anterior uveitis, including inflammation due to tuberculosis [437], and sarcoidosis [383] and syphilis [386]. Metastatic carcinoma in the iris most frequently arises in the lung followed by the breast [194]. Paracentesis utilizing a 24 gauge needle with the bevel toward the tumor can be utilized in the diagnosis of metastatic carcinoma to the iris [162,383] and ciliary body [308].

The most common primary sites of carcinomas that metastasize to the choroid are the breast and lung [428], followed by the genitourinary and gastrointestinal systems. Numerous reports describe clinical and histopathological features of metastatic uveal carcinomas from the breast [229,296,333,353] and lung [97,192,232,245,249,263,264,478,480]. Fine-needle aspiration biopsy can provide useful information regarding metastatic cancers in the choroid [21].

Ocular metastases from the breast generally appear after detection of the primary tumor, but when the primary site is the lung or kidney, ocular metastases may appear before the primary tumor is known [140,156]. Numerous other malignant neoplasms may metastasize to the choroid, including neuroblastoma [6], Ewing's sarcoma [230], fibrosarcoma [369], and osteogenic sarcoma [258,421].

Radiotherapy is the usual form of treatment of ocular metastatic carcinoma, and sometimes it results in a dramatic regression of lesions [333]. One study demonstrated that chemotherapy is as useful as radiotherapy in treatment of metastatic breast carcinoma of the choroid [262].

B. Carcinoid

Several reports describe metastatic carcinoid tumors to the uvea [17,26,28,31,71,149,186,190,254, 283,356,357,360,368,419]. These tumors arise from amine precursor uptake decarboxylase (APUD) cells derived from the primitive foregut, midgut, and hindgut. Although gastrointestinal carcinoid tumors are more common than bronchial carcinoid tumors, most carcinoid tumors in the uvea metastasize from the bronchus [71]. Carcinoid tumors are composed of uniform cells arranged in chords and nests with granular cytoplasm and bland nuclei. Carcinoid tumors of foregut origin (lung, pancreas, stomach, and medi-

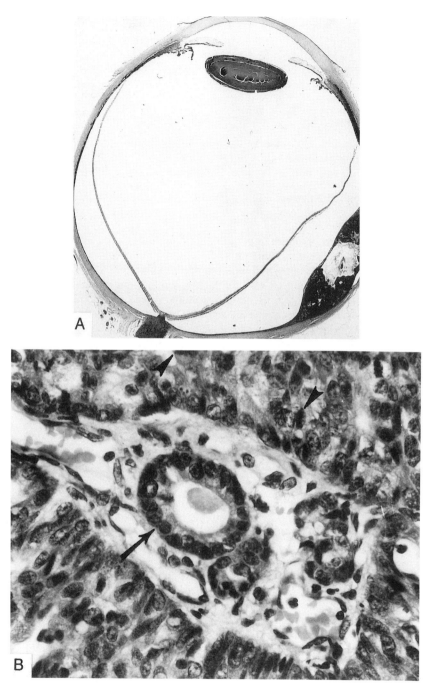

Figure 21 (A) Metastatic breast carcinoma in choroid. (Hematoxylin and eosin, ×33) (B) Higher magnification, showing acinus (arrow) and mitotic figures (arrowheads). (Hematoxylin and eosin, ×850)

astinum) react with argyrophilic stains (i.e., reduce silver) but usually not with argentaffinophilic stains (i.e., take up reduced silver), whereas those of midgut origin (small intestine and ascending colon) are both argyrophilic and argentaffinophilic; those of hindgut origin (descending colon and rectum) are negative by both reactions. These stains are of practical importance since in some instances the metastasis appears before the primary tumor is recognized. Ultrastructural examination of carcinoid tumors discloses intracytoplasmic dense-core granules. Immunohistochemical stains are positive for neuron-specific enolase, chromogranin and synaptophysin in tumor cells. Unlike metastatic carcinoma to the uvea, patients with metastatic carcinoid often have long-term survival [71].

C. Metastatic Melanoma of the Eye

Metastatic intraocular melanomas, usually from cutaneous sites, are uncommon. Font and colleagues [150] found 17 cases in the literature and reported 10 additional examples. The average age of the patients when the ocular metastases were detected was 40 years, and the average period of survival following diagnosis was 5 months. In a histopathological study of the eyes of 15 consecutive patients who died from metastatic malignant melanoma arising in the skin, asymptomatic microscopic intraocular metastases were detected in 5 patients [144]. The microscopic metastases were in multiple sites in both the choroid and retina, were of "epithelioid cell" type, and were minimally pigmented. Large or symptomatic ocular metastases from cutaneous melanoma are rare, but the frequency of microscopic uveal metastases from cutaneous melanomas is similar to that reported for metastatic breast carcinoma [40].

A large clinical study of 654 patients with cutaneous melanoma [105] found only 1 patient with ocular metastases. This clinical incidence may be underestimated since a histopathological investigation found 33% of patients with cutaneous melanoma to have intraocular metastases [147]. Microscopic metastatic foci tend to be intravascular clusters of epithelioid cells, which together with the lack of adjacent nevi helps distinguish metastatic melanoma from primary uveal melanoma. Ciliary body metastasis of cutaneous melanoma has been observed [337,426,432]. There is one report of a solitary metastases to the iris without ciliary body involvement [209]. Fine-needle aspiration cytology may be helpful in establishing a diagnosis [81,426].

D. Leukemia

It is estimated that 50–90% of patients with leukemia have ocular involvement [9,118,242,259], leukemic infiltrations occurring in the conjunctiva, corneoscleral limbus, vitreous, retina, uveal tract, optic nerve, and orbit. Ocular lesions are present more often in acute than in chronic leukemia.

Clinically the retina is the most affected ocular structure, but histopathological studies have shown the choroid to be most often involved [9,241,259,318], with an incidence ranging from 28 to 81.8% [241] of cases.

Retinal lesions include hemorrhages, cotton-wool spots, and white-centered hemorrhages. In a prospective clinical study of the ocular manifestations of 120 patients at the time of diagnosis of leukemia, Schachat et al. [380] observed changes in 66% of the patients, including retinal hemorrhages in 42 (35%), of which 13 (11%) had white centers; cotton-wool spots in 19 (16%) of patients; conjunctival hemorrhage in 10 (8%); central retinal vein occlusion in 5 (4%) patients; vitreous hemorrhage in 3 (2%); and localized choroid hemorrhage in 1 (1%) of the patients. Guyer et al. [199], in a study of 117 consecutive patients with acute leukemia, found an association between the presence of retinal hemorrhages and thrombocytopenia. The presence of anemia was related to white-centered hemorrhages in patients with acute nonlymphocytic leukemia. Cotton-wool spots were not associated with hematological parameters. Leukemic infiltrates in the choroid are more common in chronic leukemia [241] and can cause drusen, retinal pigment epithelial defects and foci of hyperplasia [86,242], and serous retinal pigment epithelial detachments. When choroidal leukemic infiltrates precede the diagnosis of chronic leukemia, the features may be mistaken for a choroidal melanoma.

Leukemic infiltrates in the iris may be either nodular or diffuse and may or may not be associated with involvement elsewhere in the eye [282,379,433]. The nodules have ill-defined borders and extend up to the pupillary margin, but if the infiltration is diffuse, iris discoloration and heterochromia may occur. Secondary glaucoma may result from blockage of aqueous outflow channels by leukemic cells. Other findings include hyphema and the presence of numerous leukemic cells in the anterior chamber (pseudo-hypopyon). In reported cases with involvement of the iris [237,379], there was little difficulty in establishing the diagnosis clinically because the presence of systemic disease was already known; however, anterior chamber paracentesis can be utilized to establish a diagnosis [379].

E. Lymphoma

Unlike leukemia, intraocular involvement in patients with lymphoma is relatively uncommon [194]. Isolated reports document uveal involvement in Burkitt's lymphoma [194], lymphoblastic lymphoma [41,76], malignant histiocytosis [89], Hodgkin's disease [194,223], mycosis fungoides [194,465], and multiple myeloma [389]. Uveal involvement is usually widespread, but the iris is rarely affected [9]. Perhaps the most common type of lymphoma to involve the uvea is large cell lymphoma (reticulum cell sarcoma), although fewer than 100 cases have been reported [161]. In a review of 32 histopathologically proven examples of ocular large cell lymphoma, Freeman and colleagues [161] found central nervous system (CNS) involvement in 56% of patients, isolated ocular involvement in 22%, visceral involvement in 16%, and CNS as well as visceral involvement in 6%. When there is visceral involvement the uvea is usually involved [160,194]. Isolated ocular or combined ocular and CNS involvement is usually associated with subretinal pigment epithelial infiltration, clinically causing a mottled appearance [257]. Cytological examination of vitreous aspiration specimens can provide a diagnosis. Large cell lymphoma cells have a large nucleus with one or more nucleoli, nuclear membrane abnormalities, and scant cytoplasm [194].

Angiotropic large cell lymphoma is a rare, generally fatal disease characterized by intravascular proliferation of neoplastic B lymphocytes with only minor extravascular lesions [305]. Ocular manifestations include choroidal distension, retinal pigment epithelial defects and foci of hyperplasia, and serous detachments of the retinal pigment epithelium and retina [131].

A diffuse infiltrate of lymphocytes in the uveal tract in a condition that has been called reactive lymphoid hyperplasia [372,373] may be a low-grade B cell lymphoma [481].

Another related malignant condition that can involve the uvea is Langerhans cell histiocytosis [12,14,204,255,269,304,484].

IV. INFLAMMATORY MASS LESIONS

A. Juvenile Xanthogranuloma

Juvenile xanthogranuloma is a benign, self-limited cutaneous disease characterized by infiltrates of chronic granulomatous inflammatory cells affecting infants and children [98], although occasional cases have been reported in adults [415]. Clinical features include a bimodal age distribution, including adults, a male-female ratio of 4:1, multiple lesions in 20% of cases, and common involvement of the head region [435].

The two most common sites involved by juvenile xanthogranulomas are the skin and the eye [207]. The iris is the most common part of the uvea affected [194], but the ciliary body [484], choroid, retina, and optic nerve can also be involved [457]. Of patients with ocular lesions, 65% are less than 7 months of age and 85% are younger than 1 year of age.

The ocular lesions of juvenile xanthogranuloma are usually unilateral and may precede the onset of yellowish orange cutaneous nodules. The eyelids, conjunctiva, cornea, sclera, and orbit are involved less often than the anterior uvea.

Patients with iris involvement may present with a localized or diffuse tumor, congenital or acquired heterochromia, spontaneous hyphema, and features of inflammatory disease and/or glaucoma that may mask the underlying tumor [484]. In one series of 20 patients, hyphema was a presenting manifestation in 17 cases [378].

Histopathologically, the lesions consist of varying proportions of lymphocytes, histiocytes, and Touton giant cells (Fig. 22). Most lesions also have eosinophils, and a few have neutrophils. Tahan et al. [435] observed that S-100+ cells accounted for 1–10% of cells, lysosome-positive mononuclear cells were scattered throughout all lesions, and Touton giant cells were positive for lysozyme and negative for S-100. Numerous thin-walled blood vessels (Fig. 22) are associated, and the vascularity may be so pronounced that the lesion may be confused with a hemangioma on microscopic examination [484].

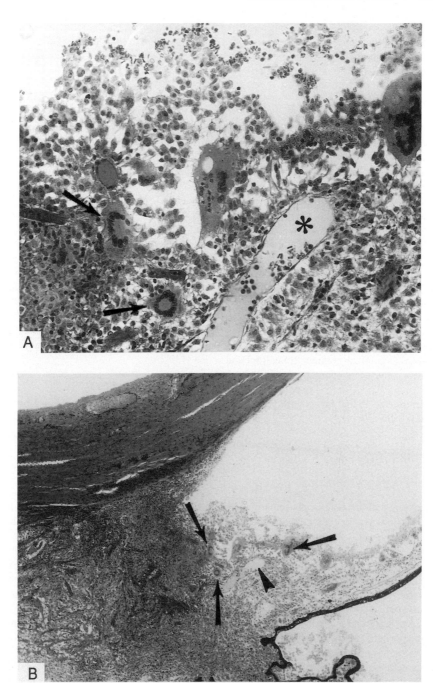

Figure 22   Juvenile xanthogranuloma with involvement of iris and ciliary body. (A) The infiltrate consists mainly of macrophages and some Touton giant cells (arrows); a thin-walled blood vessel (asterisk) extends near the anterior surface of the infiltrate. (Hematoxylin and eosin, ×230) (B) Lower power, showing Touton giant cells (arrows) and thin-walled blood vessel (arrowhead) present. (Hematoxylin and eosin, ×55)

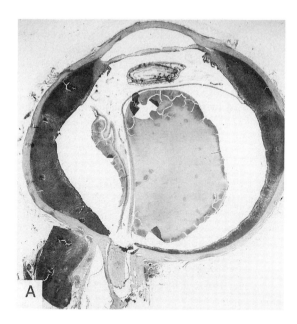

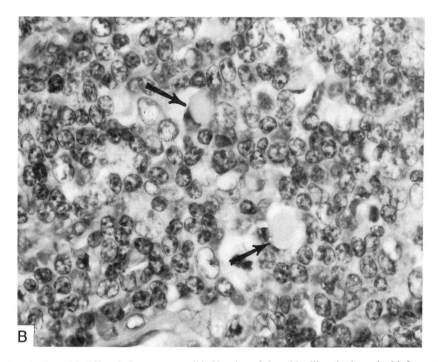

Figure 23   (A) Eye with diffuse inflammatory cell infiltration of choroid, ciliary body, and orbit from a 44-year-old man who was thought to have a malignant melanoma. There is total serous detachment of the retina. (Hematoxylin and eosin, ×3) (B) The infiltrate consists of lymphocyte, plasma cells, and some plasmacytoid cells with Russell bodies (arrows). (Hematoxylin and eosin, ×800) (Courtesy of Dr. Richard B. O'Grady.)

The diagnosis of juvenile xanthogranuloma can be confirmed by a biopsy of lesions in accessible tissues, such as the skin, conjunctiva, or cornea. Since macrophages may collect on the anterior border of the iris, they may enter the aqueous, and in two reported cases [59,384] paracentesis was helpful in establishing the diagnosis, although in another patient [412] paracentesis was followed by loss of the eye. In this disease the iris should not be biopsied unless the diagnosis is seriously in doubt, because excising this friable vascular lesion may cause extensive bleeding [484].

Although cutaneous juvenile xanthogranulomas resolve spontaneously, the intraocular lesions may seriously damage the eye by repeated hemorrhage and secondary glaucoma.

B. Inflammatory Pseudotumor

Inflammatory pseudotumors of the eye may occur as a localized or diffuse process (Fig. 23). Local iris involvement [403], iris and ciliary body [479], and the choroid [225] have been observed. Cytological examination of cells obtained from the surface of the iris may be helpful with the diagnosis [479].

Diffuse uveal inflammatory pseudotumors may be clinically indistinguishable from melanomas of the choroid [373] and should be considered in the clinical differential diagnosis of conditions that lead to thickening of the choroid and ciliary body, progressive nonrhegmatogenous retinal detachment, and unilateral narrow-angle glaucoma [179,372,373].

Histopathologically, the lesion is a nonspecific inflammatory process consisting of numerous lymphocytes, plasma cells, eosinophils, and macrophages. In some instances the finding of germinal centers with mantle zone formation helps in the histopathological diagnosis.

Entities including melanoma, metastatic carcinoma, and lymphoma are considered in the clinical differential diagnosis. Ryan and coworkers [373] reported 13 of 19 eyes (68.4%) with pseudotumor that were enucleated with a clinical diagnosis of melanoma.

Both the cause and pathogenesis of uveal tract inflammatory pseudotumors are unknown, although it has been interpreted as a lymphoid hyperplasia, analogous perhaps to the inflammatory lymphoid pseudotumors of the orbit, lacrimal gland, and conjunctiva. Propranolol was incriminated in the pathogenesis of a localized uveal inflammatory pseudotumor in one patient [486]. Some of the diffuse cases of uveal inflammatory pseudotumors are apparently low-grade, B cell lymphomas [481]. As with pseudotumors in these locations, those in the uvea usually respond well to systemic corticosteroids.

REFERENCES

1. Albert, D.M. The association of viruses with uveal melanomas. *Trans. Am. Ophthalmol. Soc. 77*:367–421, 1979.
2. Albert, D.M., Gaasterland, D.E., Caldwell, J.B., Howard, R.D., and Zimmerman, L.E. Bilateral metastatic choroidal melanoma, nevi and cavernous degeneration. *Arch. Ophthalmol. 87*:39–47, 1972.
3. Albert, D.M., Lahav, M., and Packer, S. Histogenesis of malignant melanomas of the uvea: Occurrence of nevus-like structures in experimental choroidal tumors. *Arch. Ophthalmol. 92*:318–323, 1974.
4. Albert, D.M., and Puliafito, C.A. Choroidal melanoma. Possible exposure to industrial toxins. *N. Engl. J. Med. 294*:634–635, 1977.
5. Albert, D.M., Puliafito, C.A., Fulton, A.B., Robinson, N.L., Zakov, Z.N., Dryja, T.P., Smith, A.B., Egan, E., and Leffingwell, S.S. Increased incidence of choroidal malignant melanoma occurring in a single population of chemical workers. *Am. J. Ophthalmol. 89*:323–337, 1980.
6. Albert, D.M., Rubenstein, R.A., and Scheie, H.G. Tumor metastasis to the eye. Part I. Incidence in 213 adult patients with generalized malignancy. *Am. J. Ophthalmol. 63*:723–726, 1967.
7. Albert, D.M., Rubenstein, R.A., and Scheie, H.G. Tumor metastasis to the eye. Part II. Clinical study of infants and children. *Am. J. Ophthalmol. 63*:727–732, 1967.
8. Albrecht, S., Jambrosic, J.A., and Kahn, H. Nucleolar organizer regions in superficial spreading melanoma with nodule. *Mod. Pathol. 2*:666–671, 1989.
9. Allen, R.A., and Straatsma, B.R. Ocular involvement in leukemia and allied disorders. *Arch. Ophthalmol. 66*:490–508, 1961.
10. Algan, B., Peyresblanques, J., and Reny, A. Les tumeurs primitives multiples à localisation ophtalmologique. *Arch Ophthalmol. (Paris) 25*:705–722, 1965.
11. Anderson, J.R. *Hydrophthalmia or Congenital Glaucoma, Its Causes, Treatment and Outlook.* Cambridge University Press, Cambridge, pp. 180–210, 1939.

12. Anderson, K.B., Margolis, G., and Lynn, W.S. Ocular lesions related to disturbances in fat metabolism. *Am. J. Ophthalmol. 45*:23–41, 1958.

13. Andersen, S.R., and Other, A. Varix of the iris. *Arch. Ophthalmol. 93*:32–33, 1975.

14. Angell, L.K., and Burton, T.C. Posterior choroidal involvement in Letter-Siwe disease. *J. Pediatr. Ophthalmol. Strabismus 15*:79–81, 1978.

15. Apple, D.J., Goldberg, M.F., Wybinny, G., and Levi, S. Argon laser photocoagulation of choroidal malignant melanoma. Tissue effects after a single treatment. *Arch. Ophthalmol. 90*:97–101, 1973.

16. Apt, L. Uveal melanomas in children and adolescents. *Int. Ophthalmol. Clin. 2*:403–410, 1962.

17. Archer, D.B., and Gardiner, T.A. An ultrastructural study of carcinoid tumor of the iris. *Am. J. Ophthalmol. 94*:357–368, 1982.

18. Arensten, J.J., and Green, W.R. Melanoma of the iris: Report of 72 cases treated surgically. *Ophthalmol. Surg. 6*:23–37, 1975.

19. Ashbury, M.K., and Vail, D. Multiple primary malignant neoplasms: Report of a case of malignant melanoma of the choroid and glioblastoma multiforme of the right cerebral hemisphere. *Am. J. Ophthalmol. 26*:688–693, 1943.

20. Ashton, N. Primary tumours of the iris. *Br. J. Ophthalmol. 48*:650–668, 1964.

21. Augsburger, J.J. Fine needle aspiration biopsy of suspected metastatic cancers to the posterior uvea. *Trans. Am. Ophthalmol. Soc. 86*:499–560, 1988.

22. Augsburger, J.J., Gamel, J.W., Sardi, V.F., Greenberg, R.A., Shields, J.A., and Brady, L.W. Enucleation vs cobalt plaque radiotherapy for malignant melanomas of the choroidal and ciliary body. *Arch. Ophthalmol. 104*:655–661, 1986.

23. Augsberger, J.J., Shields, J.A., Folberg, R., Lang, W., O'Hara, B.J., and Claricca, B.A. Fine needle aspiration biopsy in the diagnosis of intraocular cancer: Cytologic-histologic correlations. *Ophthalmology 92*:39–49, 1985.

24. Auw-Yange, S. Case of choroidal apoplexy diagnosed as sarcoma of choroid. *Ophthalmologica 115*:1–10, 1948.

25. Baghdassarian, S.A., and Spencer, W.H. Pseudoangioma of the iris: Its association with melanoma. *Arch. Ophthalmol. 82*:69–71, 1969.

26. Balestrazzi, E., di Tondo, U., delle Noci, N., and Blasi, M.A. Metastasis of bronchial carcinoid tumor to choroid. *Ophthalmologica 198*:104–109, 1989.

27. Bard, L.A. Eyes with choroidal detachments removed for suspected melanoma. *Arch. Ophthalmol. 73*:320–323, 1965.

28. Bardenstein, D.S., Char, D.H., Jones, C., Crawford, J.B., Miller, T.R., and Rickhof, T. Metastatic ciliary body carcinoid tumor. *Arch. Ophthalmol. 108*:1590–1594, 1990.

29. Barr, C.C., Zimmerman, L.E., Curtin, V.T., and Font, R.L. Bilateral diffuse melanocytic uveal tumors associated with systemic malignant neoplasms: A recently recognized syndrome. *Arch. Ophthalmol. 100*:249–255, 1982.

30. Barker-Griffith, A.E., McDonald, P.R., and Green, W.R. Malignant melanoma arising in a choroidal magnacellular nevus (melanocytoma). *Can. J. Ophthalmol. 11*:140–146, 1976.

31. Bell, R.M., Bullock, J.D., and Albert, D.M. Solitary choroidal metastasis from bronchial carcinoid. *Br. J. Ophthalmol. 59*:155–163, 1975.

32. Bellet, R., Shields, J., Soll, D., and Bernardino, E.A. Primary choroidal and cutaneous melanomas occurring in a patient with the B-K mole syndrome phenotype. *Am. J. Ophthalmol. 89*:567–570, 1980.

33. Berard-Badier, M., and Cesarini, J.P. Melanomas malius de l'uvee: Etude anatomopatholique et ultrastructurale. *Ann. Ocul. 204*:1244–1245, 1971.

34. Berkow, J.W., and Font, R.L. Disciform macular degeneration with subpigmentepithelial hematoma. *Arch. Ophthalmol. 82*:51–56, 1969.

35. Berson, E., Bigger, J.F., and Smith, M.E. Malignant melanoma, retinal hole and retinal detachment. *Arch. Ophthalmol. 77*:223–225, 1967.

36. Bierman, E.O. Retinal tears associated with tumors. *Am. J. Ophthalmol. 46*:74–75, 1958.

37. Bierring, F., and Jensen, O.A. Electron microscopy of melanosomes of the human uveal tract: The ultrastructure of four malignant melanomas of the mixed cell type. *Acta Ophthalmol. (Cophenh.) 42*:665–671, 1964.

38. Bietti, G., and Vozza, R. Melanoblastoma bilaterale della coroide. *Clin. Ocul. 12*:52–61, 1968.

39. Birkmayer, G.D., Blada, B.R., and Miller, F. Virus-like particles in metastases of human malignant melanomas. *Naturwissenschaften 59*:369–370, 1972.

40. Bloch, R.S., and Gartner, S. The incidence of ocular metastatic carcinoma. *Arch. Ophthalmol. 85*:673–675, 1971.

41. Blodi, F.C. Intraocular and orbital lymphoma. Verhoeff Society, Washington, D.C., April 24–25, 1980.

42. Blodi, F.C. Leiomyoma of the ciliary body. *Am. J. Ophthalmol. 33*:939–942, 1950.

43. Blodi, F.C. Ursache und Haufigkeit der Enukleation nach Starausziehung. *Klin. Monatsbl. Augenheilkd. 140*:504–510, 1962.

44. Blodi, F.C. The difficult diagnosis of choroidal melanoma. *Arch. Ophthalmol. 69*:253–256, 1963.

45. Blodi, F.C. Ocular melanocytosis and melanoma. *Am. J. Ophthalmol. 80*:389–395, 1975.

46. Blodi, F.C., and Roy, P.E. The misdiagnosed choroidal melanoma. *Can. J. Ophthalmol. 2*:209–211, 1967.

47. Boffey, P.M. Cancer from chemicals. *Science 194*:1252–1256, 1976.
48. Bonamour, M.M., Bonnet, J.C., and Jambon, M. Leiomyome du corps ciliaire; quelques considerations a propos du diagnostic et du traitement des tumeur benignes de l'iris et du corps ciliaire. *Bull. Soc. Ophtalmol. Fr. 7–8*:482–485, 1957.
49. Boniuk, M., and Zimmerman, L.E. Epibulbar osteoma (episcleral osseous choristoma). *Am. J. Ophthalmol. 53*:290–296, 1962.
50. Boniuk, M., and Zimmerman, L.E. Occurrence and behavior of choroidal melanomas in eyes subjected to operations for retinal detachment. *Trans. Am. Acad. Ophthalmol. Otolaryngol. 66*:642–658, 1962.
51. Boniuk, M., and Zimmerman, L.E. Problems in differentiating idiopathic serous detachments from solid retinal detachments. *Int. Ophthalmol. Clin. 2*:411–430, 1962.
52. Boruchoffs, S.A., Kenyon, K.R., Foulks, G.N., and Green, W.R. Epithelial cyst of the iris following penetrating keratoplasty. *Br. J. Ophthalmol. 64*:440–445, 1980.
53. Bowen, S.F., Jr., Brady, H., and Jones, V.L. Malignant melanoma of eye occurring in two successive generations. *Arch. Ophthalmol. 71*:805–806, 1964.
54. Bowers, J.F. Melanocytoma of the ciliary body. *Arch. Ophthalmol. 71*:649–652, 1964.
55. Brav, S.S. Serous choroidal detachment. *Surv. Ophthalmol. 6*:395–415, 1961.
56. Brown, D., Boniuk, M., and Font, R.L. Diffuse malignant melanoma of iris with metastases. *Surv. Ophthalmol. 34*:357–364, 1990.
57. Brownstein, S., Orton, R., and Jackson, W.B. Cystoid macular edema with equatorial choroidal melanoma. *Arch. Ophthalmol. 96*:2105–2107, 1978.
58. Brownstein, S., Sheikh, N.M., and Lewis, M.G. Immunological studies in patients with malignant melanoma of the uvea. *Can. J. Ophthalmol. 12*:16–23, 1977.
59. Bruner, W.E., Stark, W.J., and Green, W.R. Presumed juvenile xanthogranuloma of the iris and ciliary body in an adult. *Arch. Ophthalmol. 100*:457–459, 1982.
60. Büchner, T., Hiddemann, W., Wörmann, B., Kleinemeier, B., Schumann, J., Gohde, W., Ritter, J., Müller, K.M., von Bassewitz, D.B., and Roessner, A. Differential patterns of DNA aneuploidy in human malignancies. *Pathol. Res. Pract. 179*:310, 1985.
61. Burki, E. Über ein Sarkom der Iris im Sauglingsalter. *Ophthalmologica 142*:487–499, 1961.
62. Burns, R.P., Fraunfelder, F.T., and Klass, A.M. A laboratory evaluation of enucleation in treatment of intraocular malignant melanoma. *Arch. Ophthalmol. 67*:490–500, 1962.
63. Busch, H., Lischwe, M.A., Michalik, J., Chan, P.K., and Busch, R.K. Nucleolar proteins of special interest: Silver staining proteins B23 and C23 and antigens of human tumor nucleoli. In *The Nucleolus*, E.G. Jordan and C.A. Cullis (Eds.), Cambridge University Press, Cambridge, p. 43, 1982.
64. Buschmann, W., and Goder, G. Das doppelseitige maligne Melanoblastom der Aderhaut. *Graefes Arch. Ophthalmol. 167*:225–238, 1964.
65. Byers, W.G.M., and MacMillan, J.A. Treatment of sarcoma of the uveal tract. *Arch. Ophthalmol. 14*:967–973, 1935.
66. Calhoun, F.P., Jr. Leiomyoma of the ciliary body. Verhoeff Society, Washington, D.C., April 26–29, 1976.
67. Callender, G.R. Malignant melanotic tumors of the eye: A study of histologic types in 111 cases. *Trans. Am. Acad. Ophthalmol. 167*:225–238, 1964.
68. Callender, G.R., and Thigpen, C.A. Two neurofibromas in one eye. *Am. J. Ophthalmol. 13*:121–124, 1930.
69. Callender, G.R., Wilder, H.C., and Ash, J.E. Five hundred melanomas of the choroid and ciliary body, followed five years or longer. *Am. J. Ophthalmol. 25*:962–967, 1942.
70. Calmettes, L., Deodati, F., and Bec, P. Leiomyome du corps ciliaire. *Bull. Soc. Ophtalmol. Fr. 74*:158–168, 1961.
71. Campbell, R.J. Carcinoid tumor metastatic to the uvea. Verhoeff Society, Houston, Texas, April 5–8, 1990.
72. Canny, C.L.B., Shields, J.A., and Kay, M.L. Clinically stationary choroidal melanoma with extraocular extension. *Arch. Ophthalmol. 96*:436–439, 1978.
73. Cappin, J.M. Malignant melanoma and rubeosis iridis: Histopathological and statistical study. *Br. J. Ophthalmol. 57*:815–824, 1973.
74. Cargill, L.V., and Mayou, S. A case of flat sarcoma of the choroid. *Trans. Ophthalmol. Soc. UK 27*:149–155, 1907.
75. Chambers, R.B., Davidorf, F.H,. McAdoo, J.F., and Chakeres, D.W. Magnetic resonance imaging of uveal melanomas. *Arch. Ophthalmol. 105*:917–921, 1987.
76. Chambers, J.D., and Mosher, M.L., Jr. Intraocular involvement in systemic lymphoma. *Surv. Ophthalmol. 11*:562–564, 1966.
77. Char, D. DNA cell cycle studies in uveal melanoma. *Trans. Am. Ophthalmol. Soc. 87*:561–580, 1988.
78. Char, D.H., Crawford, J.B., Gonzales, J., and Miller, T. Iris melanoma with increased intraocular pressure. Differentiation of focal solitary tumors from diffuse or multiple tumors. *Arch. Ophthalmol. 107*:548–551, 1989.
79. Char, D.H., Crawford, J.B., Irvine, A.R., Hogan, M.J., and Howes, E.L., Jr. Correlation between degree of malignancy and the radioactive phosphorus uptake test in melanomas. *Am. J. Ophthalmol. 81*:71–75, 1976.
80. Char, D.H., Hollinshead, A., Cogan, D.G., Ballintine, E.J., Hogan, M.J., and Haberman, R.B. Cutaneous

delayed hypersensitivity to soluble melanoma antigen in patients with ocular malignant melanoma. *N. Engl. J. Med.* 291:274–277, 1974.

81. Char, D.H., Schwartz, A., Millter, T.R., and Abele, J.S. Ocular metastases from systemic melanoma. *Am. J. Ophthalmol.* 90:702–707, 1980.

82. Chaves, E., and Granville, R. Choroidal malignant melanoma in a two-and-one-half year-old girl. *Am. J. Ophthalmol.* 74:20–23, 1972.

83. Chen, T.C., Char, D.H., and Waldman, E. Differentiation of uveal melanoma cell type by flow cytometry. *Invest. Ophthalmol. Vis. Sci. (Suppl.)* 28:26, 1987.

84. Ches, J., Henkind, P., Albert, D.M., Gragoudas, E.S., Reidel, K., Weiss, J., McMahon, M., and Abramson, D. Uveal melanoma presenting after cataract extraction with intraocular lens implantation. *Ophthalmology* 92:827–830, 1985.

85. Cibis, G.W., Freeman, A.I., Pang, V., Roloson, G.J., Case, W.F., Ost, M., Huntrakoon, M., and Rothberg, P.G. Bilateral choroidal neonatal neuroblastoma. *Am. J. Ophthalmol.* 109:445–449, 1990.

86. Clayman, H.M., Flynn, J.T., Koch, K., and Israel, C. Retinal pigment epithelium abnormalities in leukemic disease. *Am. J. Ophthalmol.* 74:416–419, 1973.

87. Cleasby, G.W. Malignant melanoma of the iris. *Arch. Ophthalmol.* 60:403–417, 1958.

88. Coburn, A., Messmer, E.P., Boniuk, M., and Font, R.L. Spontaneous intrastromal iris cyst. A case report with immunohistochemical and ultrastructural observations. *Ophthalmology* 92:1661–1695, 1985.

89. Cogan, D.G. Choroidal histiocytes in histiocytic medullary reticulosis. Verhoeff Society, Washington, D.C., April 22–23, 1974.

90. Cogan, D.G., and Reese, A.B. A syndrome of iris nodules, ectopic Descemet's membrane, and unilateral glaucoma. *Doc. Ophthalmol.* 26:424–433, 1969.

91. Coleman, D.J., and Abramson, D.H. Ocular ultrasonography. In *Clinical Ophthalmology*, Vol., 2, T.D. Duane (Ed.), Harper & Row, New York, pp. 1–16, 1976.

92. Collaborative Ocular Melanoma Study Group. Accuracy of diagnosis of choroidal melanomas in the Collaborative Ocular Melanoma Study. COMS Report No. 1. *Arch. Ophthalmol.* 108:1268–1273, 1990.

93. Coon, J.S., Landay, A.L., and Weinstein, R.S. Advances in flow cytometry for diagnostic pathology. *Lab. Invest.* 57:453, 1987.

94. Cordes, F.C., and Cook, R.D. Simultaneous bilateral primary ocular malignant melanoma. Report of a case. *Trans. Am. Ophthalmol. Soc.* 47:80–92, 1949.

95. Courvalin, J.C., Hernandey-Verdun, D., Gosti-Testu, F., Marty, M.C., Maunaury, R., and Bornens, M. A protein of Mr 80,000 is associated with the nucleolus organizer human cell lines. *Chromosoma* 94:353–361, 1986.

96. Craig, E.L. Intraocular neurofibroma. Verhoeff Society, Washington, D.C., April 1973.

97. Crawford, J.B., and Reese, G.A. Rapid loss of vision: Initial manifestation of bronchogenic carcinoma (a clinicopathologic case report). *Trans. Am. Acad. Ophthalmol. Otolaryngol.* 73:964–968, 1969.

98. Crocker, A. The histiocytosis syndromes. In *Dermatology in General Medicine*, T. Fitzpatrick, K. Arndt, W. Clark, A. Eisen, E. Van Scott, and J. Vaughan (Eds.), McGraw-Hill, New York, pp. 1328–1338, 1971.

99. Cunha, S.L., and Lobo, F.G. Granular cell myoblastoma of the anterior uvea. *Br. J. Ophthalmol.* 50:99–101, 1966.

100. Cunningham, E.R. Ocular tumors of west China, a statistical and clinical study. *Trans. Can. Ophthalmol. Soc.* 5:102–121, 1952.

101. Curtin, V.T. Malignant melanoma management. In *Controversy in Ophthalmology*, R.J. Brockhurst, S.A. Boruchoff, B.T. Hutchinson, and S. Lessell (Eds.), W.B. Saunders, Philadelphia, pp. 635–640, 1977.

102. Daily, R.K. Hemangioma of the ciliary body. *Am. J. Ophthalmol.* 14:653–654, 1931.

103. Damato, B.E., Campbell, A.M., McGuire, B.J., Lee, W.R., and Foulds, W.S. Monoclonal antibodies to human primary uveal melanomas demonstrate tumor heterogeneity. *Invest. Ophthalmol. Vis. Sci.* 27:1362–1367, 1986.

104. Dart, J.K., Marsh, R.J., Garner, A., and Cooling, R.J. Fluorescein angiography of anterior uveal melanocytic tumors. *Br. J. Ophthalmol.* 72:326–377, 1988.

105. Das Gupta, T., and Brasfield, R. Metastatic melanoma. A clinicopathologic study. *Cancer* 17:1323–1339, 1964.

106. Davidorf, F.H., and Lang, J.R. Immunologic and immunotherapy of malignant uveal melanomas. In *Intraocular Tumors*, G. Peyman (Ed.), Appleton-Century-Crofts, New York, 1977.

107. Davidorf, F.H., and Lang, J.R. The natural history of malignant melanoma of the choroid: Small vs. large tumors. *Trans. Am. Acad. Ophthalmol. Otolaryngol.* 79:310–320, 1975.

108. Davies, W.S. Malignant melanomas of the choroid and ciliary body: A clinicopathological study. *Am. J. Ophthalmol.* 55:541–546, 1963.

109. De Buen, S., Olivares, M.L., and Charlin, V. Leiomyoma of the iris. Report of a case. *Br. J. Ophthalmol.* 55:353–356, 1971.

110. De La Cruz, P.O., Specht, C.S., and McLean, I.W. Lymphocytic infiltration of uveal melanoma. *Invest. Ophthalmol. Vis. Sci.* 29 (Suppl.):365, 1988.

111. Demeler, U., and Domarus, D.V. Klinik, Fluoreszenzangiographie und Histologie eines Ringmelanoms der Iris. *Klin. Monatsbl. Augenheilkd.* 168:387–395, 1976.

112. Diamond, S., Borley, W.E., and Miller, W.W. Partial iridocyclectomy for chamber angle tumors. *Am. J. Ophthalmol.* 57:88–94, 1964.

113. Doherty, W.B. Melanosarcoma of the iris. *Am. J. Ophthalmol.* 22:239–249, 1939.

114. Donovan, B.F. Neurilemoma of the ciliary body. *Arch. Ophthalmol.* 55:672–675, 1956.

115. Dugmore, W.N. 11 Year follow-up of a case of iris leiomyosarcoma. *Br. J. Ophthalmol.* 56:366–367, 1972.

116. Duke, J.R., and Dunn, S.N. Primary tumor of the iris. *Arch. Ophthalmol.* 59:204–214, 1958.

117. Duke, J.R., and Kennedy, J.J. Metastatic carcinoma of the iris and ciliary body. *Arch. Ophthalmol.* 60:1092–1103, 1958.

118. Duke-Elder, S. and Dobree, J.H. The leukemias. In *System of Ophthalmology*, Vol. 10, S. Duke-Elder (Ed.), C.V. Mosby, St. Louis, MO, pp. 387–393, 1966.

119. Duke-Elder, S., and Perkins, E.S. Malignant melanoma. In *System of Ophthalmology*, Vol. 9, S. Duke-Elder (Ed.), C.V. Mosby, St. Louis, MO, pp. 841–911, 1967.

120. Dunbar, J.C. Leiomyoma of the ciliary body. Report of a case exhibiting a significant uptake of radioactive phosphorus. *Am. J. Ophthalmol.* 42:204–207, 1956.

121. Dunn, W.J., Lambert, H.M., Kincaid, M.C., Dieckert, J.P., and Shore, J.W. Choroidal malignant melanoma with early vitreous seeding. *Retina* 8:188–192, 1988.

122. Dunnington, J.H. Intraocular tension in cases of sarcoma of the choroid and ciliary body. *Arch. Ophthalmol.* 20:359–363, 1938.

123. Durie, F.H., Campbell, A.M., Lee, W.R., and Damato, B.E. Analysis of lymphocytic infiltration in uveal melanoma. *Invest. Ophthalmol. Vis. Sci.* 31:2106–2110, 1990.

124. Dvorak-Theobald, G. Neurogenic origin of choroidal sarcoma. *Arch. Ophthalmol.* 18:971–997, 1937.

125. Eagle, R.C., Font, R.L., Yanoff, M., and Fine, B.S. Proliferative endotheliopathy with iris abnormalities: The iridocorneal endothelial syndrome. *Arch. Ophthalmol.* 97:2104–2111, 1979.

126. Egan, M.J., and Crocker, J. Nucleolar organizer regions in cutaneous tumours. *J. Pathol.* 154:247–253, 1988.

127. Egan, M.J., Raafat, F., Crocker, J., and Smith, K. Nucleolar organizers regions in small cell tumours of childhood. *J. Pathol.* 153:275–280, 1987.

128. Egan, K.M., Sedden, J.M., Glynn, R.J., Gradoudas, E.S., and Albert, D.M. Epidemiologic aspects of uveal melanoma. *Surv. Ophthalmol.* 32:239–251, 1988.

129. El-Baba, F., and Blumenkranz, M. Malignant melanoma at the site of penetrating ocular trauma. *Arch. Ophthalmol.* 104:405–409, 1986.

130. El-Baba, F., Hagler, W.S., De La Cruz, A., and Green, W.R. Choroidal melanoma with pigment dispersion in vitreous and melanomalytic glaucoma. *Ophthalmology* 95:370–377, 1988.

131. Elner, V., Hidayat, A.A., Charles, N.C., Davity, M.A., Smith, M.E., Burgess, D., and Dawson, N. Neoplastic angioendotheliomatosis. A variant of malignant lymphoma. Immunohistochemical and ultrastructural observations of three cases. *Ophthalmology* 93:1237–1243, 1986.

132. Elsas, F.J., Mroczek, E.C., Kelly, D.R., and Specht, C.S. Primary rhabdomyosarcoma of the iris. *Arch. Ophthalmol.* 109:982–984, 1991.

133. Farmer, S.G., and Kalina, R.E. Epithelial implantation cyst of the iris. *Ophthalmology* 88:1286–1289, 1981.

134. Federman, J.L., Lewis, M.G., and Clark, W.H. Tumor-associated antibodies to ocular and cutaneous melanomas: negative interaction with normal choroidal melanocytes. *J. Natl. Cancer Inst.* 52:587–589, 1974.

135. Federman, J.L., Lewis, M.G., Clark, W.H., Egerer, I., and Sarin, L.K. Tumor-associated antibodies in the serum of ocular melanoma patients. *Trans. Am. Acad. Ophthalmol. Otolaryngol.* 78:784–794, 1974.

136. Ferry, A.P. Hemangioma of the iris and ciliary body. Do they exist? A search for a histologically proved case. *Int. Ophthalmol. Clin* 12:177–194, 1972.

137. Ferry, A.P. Lesions mistaken for malignant melanoma of the iris. *Arch. Ophthalmol.* 18:9–18, 1965.

138. Ferry, A.P. Lesions mistaken for malignant melanoma of the posterior uvea: A clinicopathologic analysis of 100 cases with ophthalmoscopically visible lesions. *Arch. Ophthalmol.* 72:463–469, 1964.

139. Ferry, A.P. Macular detachment associated with congenital pit of the optic nerve head: Pathologic finding in two cases simulating malignant melanoma of the choroid. *Arch. Ophthalmol.* 70:346–357, 1963.

140. Ferry, A.P., and Font, R.L. Carcinoma metastatic to the eye and orbit. I. Clinicopathologic study of 227 cases. *Arch. Ophthalmol.* 92:276–286, 1974.

141. Ferry, A.P., and Font, R.L. Carcinoma metastatic to the eye and orbit. II. A clinicopathologic study of 26 patients with carcinoma metastatic to the anterior segment of the eye. *Arch. Ophthalmol.* 93:472–582, 1975.

142. Fine, B.S. Free-floating pigmented cyst in the anterior chamber. A clinicohistopathologic report. *Am. J. Ophthalmol.* 67:493–500, 1969.

143. Fisher, E.R., and Fisher, B. Experimental studies of factors influencing hepatic metastases. Part I. *Cancer* 12:926–928, 1959.

144. Fishman, M.L., Tomaszewski, M.M., and Kuwabara, T. Malignant melanoma of the skin metastatic to the eye: Frequency in autopsy series. *Arch. Ophthalmol.* 94:1309–1311, 1976.

145. Flocks, M., Gerende, J.H., and Zimmerman, L.E. The size and shape of malignant melanomas of the choroid and ciliary body in relation to prognosis and histologic characteristics: A statistical study of 210 tumors. *Trans. Am. Acad. Ophthalmol. Otolaryngol.* 59:740–758, 1955.

146. Folberg, R., Donoso, L.A. Monoclonal antibodies and ocular melanoma. Part II. Applications to pathology. *Invest. Ophthalmol. Vis. Sci. (Suppl.) 25*:82, 1984.

147. Fishman, M.L., Tomaszewski, M.M., and Kuwabara, T. Malignant melanoma of the skin metastatic to the eye. Frequency in autopsy series. *Arch. Ophthalmol. 94*:1309–1311, 1976.

148. Font, R.L., and Ferry, A.P. The phakomatoses. *Int. Ophthalmol. Clin. 12*:1–50, 1972.

149. Font, R.L., Kaufer, G., and Winstanley, R.A. Metastasis of bronchial carcinoid tumor to the eye. *Am. J. Ophthalmol. 62*:723–727, 1966.

150. Font, R.L., Naumann, G., and Zimmerman, L.E. Primary malignant melanoma of the skin metastatic to the eye and orbit: Report of ten cases and review of the literature. *Am. J. Ophthalmol. 63*:738–754, 1967.

151. Font, R.L., Spaulding, A.G., and Zimmerman, L.E. Diffuse malignant melanoma of the uveal tract: A clinicopathologic report of 54 cases. *Trans. Am. Acad. Ophthalmol. Otolaryngol. 72*:877–895, 1968.

152. Font, R.L., Zimmerman, L.E., and Armaly, M.F. The nature of the orange pigment over a choroidal melanoma: Histochemical and electron microscopic observations. *Arch. Ophthalmol. 91*:359–362, 1974.

153. Foos, R.Y., Hull, S.N., and Straatsma, B.R. Early diagnosis of ciliary body melanomas. *Arch. Ophthalmol. 81*:336–344, 1969.

154. Forrest, A.W., Keyser, R.B., and Spencer, W.H. Iridocyclectomy for melanomas of the ciliary body: A follow-up study of pathology and surgical morbidity. *Ophthalmology 85*:1235–1249, 1978.

155. Francois, J. Ocular aspects of the phakomatoses. In *Handbook of Clinical Neurology*, Vol. 15, *The Phakomatoses*, P.J. Vinken and G.W. Bruyn (Eds.), American Elsevier, New York, pp. 643–644, 1972.

156. Francois, J., Hanssens, H., and Verbraeken, H. Intraocular metastasis at first sign of generalized carcinomatosis. *Ann. Ophthalmol. 8*:405–419, 1976.

157. Frangieh, G.T., El-Baba, F., Traboulsi, E.I., and Green, W.R. Melanocytoma of the ciliary body: Presentation of four cases and review of nineteen reports. *Surv. Ophthalmol. 29*:328–334, 1985.

158. Frankfurt, O.S., Arbuck, S.G., Chin, J.L., Greco, W.R., Pavelic, Z.P., Slocum, H.K., Mittelman, A., Piver, S.M., Pontes, E.J., and Rustum, Y.M. Prognostic application of DNA flow cytometry for human solid tumors. *Ann. NY Acad. Sci. 468*:276–290, 1986.

159. Fraundfelder, F.T., Boozman, F.W., Wilson, R.S., and Thomas, A.H. No-touch technique for intraocular malignant melanomas. *Arch. Ophthalmol. 95*:1616–1620, 1977.

160. Frederick, D.R., Char, D.H., Ljung, B.M., and Brinton, D.A. Solitary intraocular lymphoma as an initial presentation of a widespread disease. *Arch. Ophthalmol. 107*:395–397, 1989.

161. Freeman, L.N., Schachat, A.P., Knox, D., Michels, R.G., and Green, W.R. Clinical features, laboratory investigations and survival in ocular reticulum cell sarcoma. *Ophthalmology 94*:1631–1639, 1987.

162. Freeman, T.R., and Friedman, A.H. Metastatic carcinoma of the iris. *Am. J. Ophthalmol. 80*:557–558, 1975.

163. Freedman, S.F., Elner, V.M., Donev, I., Gunta, R., and Albert, D.M. Intraocular neurilemmoma arising from the posterior ciliary nerve in neurofibromatosis: Pathologic findings. *Ophthalmology 95*:1559–1564, 1988.

164. Friedenwald, J.S., Wilder, H.C., Maumanee, A.E., Sanders, T.E., Keyes, J.E.L., Hogan, M.H., Owens, W.C., and Owens, E.U. *Ophthalmic Pathology: An Atlas and Textbook*, W.B. Saunders, Philadelphia, p. 398, 1952.

165. Friedlander, M.L., Hedley, D.W., Taylor, I.W. Clinical and biological significance of aneuploidy in human tumors. *J. Clin. Pathol. 37*:961–974, 1984.

166. Fuglestad, S.J., Campbell, R.J., Tsushima, K., Ilstrup, D.M., and Lieber, M.M. Malignant melanoma of the choroid nuclear DNA ploidy pattern studied by flow cytometry. *Invest. Ophthalmol. Vis. Sci. (Suppl.) 28*:5° 1987.

167. Gamel, J.W., and McLean, I.W. Quantitative analysis of the Callender classification of uveal melanoma cells. *Arch. Ophthalmol. 95*:686–691, 1977.

168. Gamel, J.W., and McLean, I.W. Computerized histopathologic assessment of malignant potential. II. A practical method for predicting survival following enucleation for uveal melanoma. *Cancer 52*:1032–1038, 1983.

169. Gamel, J.W., and McLean, I.W. Computerized histopathologic assessment of malignant potential. *Invest. Ophthalmol. Vis. Sci. (Suppl.) 24*:50, 1983.

170. Gamel, J.W., and McLean, I.W. Computerized histopathologic assessment of malignant potential. III. Refinements of measurement and data analysis. *Analy. Quant. Cytol. 6*:37–44, 1984.

171. Gamel, J.W., and McLean, I.W. Modern developments in histopathologic assessment of uveal melanomas. *Ophthalmology 91*:679–684, 1984.

172. Gamel, J.W., and McLean, I.W. Corrected lifetime risk of death for ciliochoroidal melanoma as a function of largest tumor dimension measured on a microslide. *Invest. Ophthalmol. Vis. Sci. (Suppl.) 29*:210, 1988.

173. Gamel, J.W., McLean, I.W., Greenberg, R.A., Zimmerman, L.E., and Lichtenstein, S.J. Computerized histologic assessment of malignant potential. I. A method for determining the prognosis of uveal melanomas. *Hum. Pathol. 13*: 893–897, 1982.

174. Gamel, J.W., McLean, I.W., Foster, W.D., and Zimmerman, L.E. Uveal melanomas: Correlation of cytologic features with prognosis. *Cancer 41*:1897–1901, 1978.

175. Ganley, J.P., and Comstock, G.W. Benign nevi and malignant melanomas of the choroid. *Am. J. Ophthalmol. 76*:19–25, 1973.

176. Gass, J.D.M. Hemorrhage into vitreous, a presenting manifestation of malignant melanoma of choroid. *Arch. Ophthalmol. 69*:778–779, 1963.
177. Gass, J.D.M. Iris abscess simulating malignant melanoma. *Arch. Ophthalmol. 90*:300–302, 1973.
178. Gass, J.D.M. Problems in the differential diagnosis of choroidal nevi and malignant melanomas. *Trans. Am. Acad. Ophthalmol. Otolaryngol. 83*:19–48, 1977.
179. Gass, J.D.M. Retinal detachment and narrow angle glaucoma secondary to inflammatory pseudotumor of the uveal tract. *Am. J. Ophthalmol. 64*:612–621, 1967.
180. Gass, J.D.M., Gieser, R.G. Wilkinson, C.P., Beahm, D.E. and Pautler, S.E. Bilateral diffuse uveal melanocytic proliferation in patients with occult carcinoma. *Arch. Ophthalmol. 108*:527–533, 1990.
181. Gass, J.D.M., Guerry, R.K., Jack, R.L., and Harris, G. Choroidal osteoma. *Arch. Ophthalmol. 96*:428–435, 1978.
182. Glasgow, B.J., Brown, H.H., Zargoza, A.M., and Foos, R.Y. Quantitation of tumor seeding from fine needle aspiration of ocular melanomas. *Am. J. Ophthalmol. 105*:538–546, 1988.
183. Gonder, J.R., Ezell, P.C., Shields, J.A., and Augsberger, J.J. Ocular melanocytosis. A study to determine the prevalence rate of ocular melanocytosis. *Ophthalmology 89*:950–952, 1982.
184. Gonder, J.R., Shields, J.A., and Albert, D.M. Malignant melanoma of the choroid associated with oculodermal melanocytosis. *Ophthalmology 88*:372–376, 1981.
185. Gonder, J.R., Shields, J.A., Albert, D.M., Augsburger, J.J., and Lavin, P.T. Uveal malignant melanoma associated with ocular and oculodermal melanocytosis. *Ophthalmology 89*:953–960, 1982.
186. Gonzales, R., and Cubillos, T.M.E. Metastasis coroidea de un adenoma bronzuial lip carcinoide. *Arch. Chil. Oftalmol. 30*:101, 1973.
187. Gotfredsen, E. On the frequency of secondary carcinomas in the choroid. *Acta Ophthalmol. (Copenh.) 22*:394–400, 1944.
188. Grady, W.W., Cheng, L., and Lewin, K.J. Application of in situ DNA hybridization to diagnostic surgical pathology. *Pathol. Annu. 22*:151–175, 1987.
189. Grady, W.W., Cheng, L., and Lewin, K.J. In situ viral DNA hybridization in diagnostic surgical pathology. *Hum. Pathol. 18*:535, 1987.
190. Gragoudas, E.S., and Carroll, J.M. Multiple choroidal metastasis from bronchial carcinoid and proton beam irradiation. *Am. J. Ophthalmol. 87*:299–304, 1979.
191. Gragoudas, E.S., Seddon, J., Egan, K., Glynn, R., Munzenrider, J., Austin-Seymour, M., Goiten, M., Verhey, L., Urie, M., and Kochler, A. Long term results of proton beam irradiated uveal melanomas. *Ophthalmology 94*:349–353, 1987.
192. Graveto, M.A., De Abreu, F., Campas, J.R., and Rasteiro, A. Metastase coroideia de carcinoma do pulmao. *Exp. Ophthalmol. (Coimbra) 6*:43–45, 1980.
193. Gray, J.W., and Coffino, P. Cell cycle analysis by flow cytometry. *Methods Enzymol. 58*:233–248, 1979.
194. Green, W.R. The uveal tract. In *Ophthalmic Pathology, An Atlas and Textbook*, W.H. Spencer (Ed.), W.B. Saunders, Philadelphia, pp. 1352–2072, 1986.
195. Greer, C.H. Congenital melanoma of the anterior uvea. *Arch. Ophthalmol. 76*:77–78, 1966.
196. Griffith, A.H. The diagnosis of intraocular growths. *Med. Chron. Manchester 16*:1–86, 1892.
197. Grossniklaus, H.E., Brown, R.H., Stulting, R.D., and Blasberg, R.D. Iris melanoma seeding through a trabeculectomy site. *Arch. Ophthalmol. 108*:1287–1290, 1990.
198. Guthert, H., Janisch, W., and Rossbach, K. Über die Haufigkeit der Augenmetastasen. *Muench. Med. Wochenschr. 107*:939–941, 1965.
199. Guyer, D.R., Schachat, A.P., Vitale, S., Markowitz, J.A., Braine, H., Burke, P.J., Karp, J.E., and Graham, M. Leukemic retinopathy. Relationship between fundus lesions and hematologic parameters at diagnosis. *Ophthalmology 96*:860–864, 1989.
200. Hale, A.J. Feulgen microspectrophotometry and its correlation with other cytochemical methods. In *Introduction to Quantitative Chemistry*, G.L. Wied (Ed.), Academic Press, New York, pp. 183–199, 1966.
201. Hale, P.N., Allen, R.A., and Straatsma, B.R. Benign melanomas (nevi) of the choroid and ciliary body. *Arch. Ophthalmol. 74*:532–538, 1965.
202. Hamburg, A. Iris melanoma with vascular proliferation simulating a hemangioma. *Arch. Ophthalmol. 82*:72–76, 1969.
203. Hart, W.M. Metastatic carcinoma to the eye and orbit. *Int. Ophthalmol. Clin. 2(2)*:465–482.
204. Heath, P. The ocular features of a case of acute reticuloendotheliosis (Letterer-Siwe type). *Trans. Am. Ophthalmol. Soc. 57*:290–302, 1959.
205. Heine, L. Hamangiome des Ziliarkorpers mit Bemerkungen über Hypertrophie der Ziliarfortsatze. *Z. Augenheilkd. 58*:191–193, 1926.
206. Heitmann, K.F., Kincaid, M.C., and Stehly, L. Diffuse malignant change in a ciliochoroidal melanocytoma in a patient of mixed racial background. *Retina 8*:67–72, 1988.
207. Helwig, E.B. Histiocytic and fibrocytic disorder. In *Dermal Pathology*, J.G. Graham, W. Johnson, and E. Helwig (Eds.), Harper & Row, New York, pp. 715–730, 1972.
208. Henkind, P., and Roth, M.S. Breast carcinoma and concurrent uveal melanoma. *Am. J. Ophthalmol. 71*:198–203, 1971.

209. Hirst, L.W., Reich, J., and Galbraith, J.E.K. Primary cutaneous malignant melanoma metastatic to the iris. *Br. J. Ophthalmol.* 63:165–168, 1979.

210. Hogan, M. Melanomas of the uvea and optic nerve: Clinical aspects, management and prognosis. *Highlights of Ophthalmology*, Vol. 6, No. 2, Pan American Institute of Ophthalmology, pp. 146–166, 1963.

211. Hogan, M.J. Pigmented intraocular tumors: Clinical aspects, management and prognosis of melanomas of the uvea and optic nerve. In *Ocular and Adnexal Tumors: New and Controversial Aspects*, M. Boniuk (Ed.), C.V. Mosby, St. Louis, MO, pp. 203–302, 1964.

212. Holland, G.N., Cochran, A.J., Duan-Ren, W., Herschman, H.R., Lee, W.R., Foos, R.Y., and Straatsma, B.R. Detection of S-100 protein in intraocular melanomas. *Invest. Ophthalmol. Vis. Sci. (Suppl.)* 24:50, 1983.

213. Hopkins, R.E., and Carriker, F.R. Malignant melanomas of the ciliary body. *Am. J. Ophthalmol.* 45:835–843, 1958.

214. Howard, G.M. Erroneous clinical diagnoses of retinoblastoma and uveal melanoma. *Trans. Am. Acad. Ophthalmol. Otolaryngol.* 73:199–203, 1969.

215. Howard, G.M., and Forrest, A.W. Incidence and location of melanocytomas. *Arch. Ophthalmol.* 77:61–66, 1967.

216. Howard, G.M., and Spalter, H.F. Study of autoimmune serologic reactions to ocular melanoma. *Arch. Ophthalmol.* 76:399–402, 1966.

217. Huntington, A.C., Haugan, P., McLean, I.W., and Gamel, J.W. The mean of the ten largest nucleoli as a measure of malignant potential in ciliochoroidal melanoma. *Invest. Ophthalmol. Vis. Sci. (Suppl.)* 29:210, 1988.

218. Iwamoto, T., Jones, I.S., and Howard, G.M. Ultrastructural comparison of spindle-A, spindle-B, and epithelioid cells in uveal malignant melanoma. *Invest. Ophthalmol.* 11:873–889, 1972.

219. Iwamato, T., Reese, A.B., and Mund, M.L. Tapioca melanoma of the iris. Part 2. Electron microscopy of the melanoma cells compared with normal iris melanocytes. *Am. J. Ophthalmol.* 74:851–861, 1972.

220. Jakobiec, F.A., Depot, M.J., Henkind, P., and Spencer, W.H. Fluorescein angiographic patterns of iris melanocytic tumors. *Arch. Ophthalmol.* 100:1288–1299, 1982.

221. Jakobiec, F.A., Font, R.L., Tso, M.O.M., and Zimmerman, L.E. Mesectodermal leiomyoma of the ciliary body: A tumor of presumed neural crest origin. *Cancer* 39:2102–2113, 1977.

222. Jakobiec, F.A., and Iwamoto, T. Mesectodermal leiomyoma of the ciliary body associated with a nevus. *Arch. Ophthalmol.* 96:692–695, 1978.

223. Jakobiec, F.A., Jones, I.S., and Tannenbaum, M. Leiomyoma: An unusual tumour of the orbit. *Br. J. Ophthalmol.* 57:825–831, 1973.

224. Jakobiec, F.A., Mitchell, J.P., Chauhan, P.M., and Iwamato, T. Mesectodermal leiomyosarcoma of the antrum and orbit. *Am. J. Ophthalmol.* 57:825–831, 1973.

225. Jakobiec, F.A., Sacks, E., Kronish, J.W., Weiss, T., and Smith, M. Multifocal static creamy choroidal infiltrates: An early sign of lymphoid neoplasia. *Ophthalmology* 94:397–406, 1987.

226. Jakobiec, F.A., and Silbert, G. Are most iris "melanomas" really nevi? A clinicopathologic study of 189 lesions. *Arch. Ophthalmol.* 99:2117–2132, 1981.

227. Jakobiec, F.A., Witschel, H., and Zimmerman, L.E. Choroidal leiomyoma of vascular origin. *Am. J. Ophthalmol.* 82:205–212, 1976.

228. Jakobiec, F.A., Yanoff, M., Mottow, L., Anker, P., and Jones, I.S. Solitary iris nevus associated with peripheral anterior synechiae and iris endothelialization. *Am. J. Ophthalmol.* 83:884–891, 1977.

229. Jakobiec, F.A., Zimmerman, L.E., Spencer, W.H., Slakter, J.S., and Krebs, W. Metastatic colloid carcinoma versus primary carcinoma of the ciliary epithelium. *Ophthalmology* 94:1469–1480, 1987.

230. Jampol, L.M., Cottle, E., Fischer, D.S., and Albert, D.M. Metastasis of Ewing's sarcoma to the choroid. *Arch. Ophthalmol.* 89:207–209, 1973.

231. Jarrett, W.H., Goldberg, M.F., and Schulze, R.R. An unusual iris melanoma. *Arch. Ophthalmol.* 75:469–474, 1966.

232. Jarrett, W.H., II, Green, W.R., Berlin, A.J., Jr., and Brawner, J.N., III. Retinal detachment as the initial manifestation of carcinoma of the lung. *Trans. Am. Acad. Ophthalmol. Otolaryngol.* 74:52–58, 1970.

233. Jensen, O.A. Malignant melanomas of the uvea in Denmark, 1943–1952: A clinical histopathological and prognostic study. *Acta Ophthalmol. Suppl. (Copenh.)* 75:1–220, 1963.

234. Jensen, O.A. Malignant melanomas of the human uvea: Recent follow-up of cases in Denmark, 1943–1952. *Acta Ophthalmol. (Copenh.)* 48:1113–1128, 1970.

235. Jensen, O.A., and Anderson, S.R. Spontaneous regression of a malignant melanoma of the choroid. *Acta Ophthalmol. (Copenh.)* 52:173–182, 1974.

236. Johnston, M.C., Noden, D.M., Hazelton, R.D., Coulombe, J.L., and Coulombe, A.J. Origins of avian ocular and periocular tissues. *Exp. Eye Res.* 29:27–43, 1979.

237. Johnston, S.S., and Ware, C.F. Iris involvement in leukemia. *Br. J. Ophthalmol.* 57:320–324, 1973.

238. Kan-Mitchell, J., Albert, D.M., Rao, N., and Taylor, C.R. Immunophenotype of uveal melanoma: A comparison with cutaneous melanoma. *Invest. Ophthalmol. Vis. Sci. (Suppl.)* 30:58, 1989.

239. Kan-Mitchell, J., Rao, N., Albert, D.M., Van Eldik, L.J., and Taylor, C.R. S100 immunophenotypes of uveal melanomas. *Invest. Ophthalmol. Vis. Sci.* 31:1492–1496, 1990.

240. Kersten, R.C., Tse, D.T., Anderson, R.L., and Blodi, F.D. The role of orbital exenteration in choroidal melanoma with extrascleral extension. *Ophthalmology 92*:436–443, 1985.

241. Kincaid, M.C., and Green, W.R. Ocular and orbital involvement in leukemia. *Surv. Ophthalmol. 27*:211–232, 1983.

242. Kincaid, M.C., Green, W.R., and Kelley, J.S. Acute ocular leukemia. *Am. J. Ophthalmol. 87*:698–702, 1979.

243. Kirk, H.Q., and Petty, R.W. Malignant melanoma of the choroid: A correlation of clinical and histological findings. *Arch. Ophthalmol. 56*:843–860, 1956.

244. Klein, B.A., and Farkas, T.G. Pseudomelanoma of the iris after herpes zoster ophthalmicus. *Am. J. Ophthalmol. 57*:392–397, 1964.

245. Klein, R., Nicholson, D.H., and Luxenberg, M.N. Retinal metastasis from squamous cell carcinoma of the lung. *Am. J. Ophthalmol. 83*:358–361, 1977.

246. Knapp, H. Cited by W.S. Duke-Elder in *Textbook of Ophthalmology*, Vol. 3, C.V. Mosby, St. Louis, MO, pp. 2538–2543, 1941.

247. Kolb, H., and Vollmar, F. Beitrag zum flachenhaften malignen Melanom der Choroidea. *Graefes Arch. Ophthalmol. 191*:45–52, 1974.

248. Kottow, M. Fluorescein angiographic behaviour of iris masses. *Ophthalmologica 174*:217–223, 1977.

249. Kreiger, A.E., Meyer, D., Smith, T.R., and Riemer, K. Metastatic carcinoma to the choroid with choroidal detachment. A case presenting as uveal effusion. *Arch. Ophthalmol. 82*:209–213, 1969.

250. Kroll, A.J., and Kuwabara, T. Electron microscopy of uveal melanoma: A comparison of spindle and epithelioid cells. *Arch. Ophthalmol. 73*:378–386, 1965.

251. Kronenberg, B. Topography and frequency of complications of uveal sarcoma. *Arch. Ophthalmol. 20*:290–298, 1938.

252. Kurz, G.H. Malignant melanoma of ciliary body and iris manifested in two locations. *Am. J. Ophthalmol. 59*:917–921, 1965.

253. Kurz, G.H., and Zimmerman, L.E. Spontaneous hyphema and acute glaucoma as initial signs of recurrent iris melanoma. *Arch. Ophthalmol. 59*:917–921, 1965.

254. Lack, E.E., Harris, G.B.C., Eraklis, A.J., and Vawter, G.F. Primary bronchial tumors in childhood: A clinicopathologic study of six cases. *Cancer 51*:492–497, 1983.

255. Lahav, M., and Albert, D.M. Unusual ocular involvement in acute disseminated histiocytosis X. *Arch. Ophthalmol. 92*:455–458, 1974.

256. Lambert, S.R., Char, D.H., Howes, E., Crawford, J.B., and Wells, J. Spontaneous regression of a choroidal melanoma. *Arch. Ophthalmol. 104*:732–734, 1986.

257. Lang, G.K., Surer, J.L., Green, W.R., Finkelstein, D., Michels, R.G., and Maumenee, A.E. Ocular reticulum cell sarcoma. Clinicopathologic correlation of a case with multifocal lesions. *Retina 5*:79–86, 1985.

258. Lees, V.T. A case of metastatic osteosarcoma in the choroid. *Br. J. Ophthalmol. 31*:713–716, 1947.

259. Leonardy, N.J., Rupani, M., Dent, G., and Klintworth, G.K. Analysis of 135 autopsy eyes for ocular involvement in leukemia. *Am. J. Ophthalmol. 109*:436–444, 1990.

260. Leong, A.S., and Gilham, P. Silver staining of nucleolar organizer regions in malignant melanoma and melanotic nevi. *Hum. Pathol. 20*:257–262, 1989.

261. Lerner, H.A. Malignant melanoma of the iris in children. *Arch. Ophthalmol. 84*:754–757, 1970.

262. Letson A.D., Davidorf, F.H., and Bruce, R.A., Jr. Chemotherapy for treatment of choroidal metastases from breast carcinoma. *Am. J. Ophthalmol. 93*:102–106, 1982.

263. Levine, R.A., and Williamson, D.E. Metastatic carcinoma simulating a postoperative endophthalmitis. *Arch. Ophthalmol. 83*:59–60, 1970.

264. Levy, R.M., and De Venecia, G. Trypsin digest study of retinal metastasis and tumor cell emboli. *Am. J. Ophthalmol. 70*:778–782, 1970.

265. Li, Z., Tso, M.O.M., and Sugar, J. Leiomyoepithelioma of iris pigment epithelium. *Arch. Ophthalmol. 105*:819–824, 1987.

266. Lincoff, H,. and Kreissig, I. Patterns of non-rhegmatogenous elevation of the retina. *Br. J. Ophthalmol. 58*: 899–906, 1974.

267. Litricin, O. Unsuspected uveal melanomas. *Am. J. Ophthalmol. 76*:734–738, 1973.

268. Lynch, H.T., Anderson, D.E., and Krush, A.J. Heredity and intraocular malignant melanoma. *Cancer 21*: 119–125, 1968.

269. MacCumber, M.W., Hoffman, P.N., Wand, G.S., Epstein, J.I., Beschorner, W.E., and Green, W.R. Ophthalmic involvement in aggressive histiocytosis X. *Ophthalmology 97*:22–27, 1990.

270. Macfee, M.F., Peyman, G.A., Peace, J.H., Cohen, S.B., and Mitchell, M.W. Magnetic resonance imaging in the evaluation and differentiation of uveal melanoma. *Ophthalmology 94*:341–348, 1987.

271. MacIlwaine, IV, W.A., Anderson, B., Jr., and Klintworth, G.K. Enlargement of a histologically documented nevus. *Am. J. Ophthalmol. 87*:480–486, 1979.

272. MacRae, A. Prognosis in malignant melanoma of choroid and ciliary body. *Trans. Ophthalmol. Soc. UK 73*: 3–30, 1953.

273. Makley, T.A. Management of melanomas of the anterior segment. *Surv. Ophthalmol. 19*:135–153, 1974.

274. Makley, T.A., and King, G.L. Multiple cysts of the iris and ciliary body simulating a malignant melanoma. *Trans. Am. Acad. Ophthalmol. Otolaryngol.* 62:441–443, 1958.
275. Manschot, W.A. Retinal hole in a case of choroidal melanoma. *Arch. Ophthalmol.* 73:666–668, 1965.
276. Manschot, W.A. Ring melanoma. *Arch. Ophthalmol.* 71:625–632, 1964.
277. Marcus, D.M., Minkovitz, J.B., Wardwell, S.D., and Albert D.M. The value of nucleolar organizer regions in uveal melanoma. *Am. J. Ophthalmol.* 110:527–534, 1990.
278. Margo, C.E., Hidayat, A.A., and Polack, F. Ciliary body granuloma. Simulating malignant melanoma after herpes zoster ophthalmicus. *Cornea* 1:147–153, 1982.
279. Margo, C.E., and Pautler, S.E. Granulomatous uveitis after treatment of a choroidal melanoma with proton-beam irradiation. *Retina* 10:141–143, 1990.
280. Margo, C.E., and McLean, I.W. Malignant melanoma of the choroid and ciliary body in black patients. *Arch. Ophthalmol.* 102:77–79, 1984.
281. Margo, C.E., Pavan, P.R., Gendelman, D., and Gragoudas, E. Bilateral melanocytic uveal tumors associated with systemic non-ocular malignancy. Malignant melanomas or benign paraneoplastic syndrome? *Retina* 7:137–141, 1987.
282. Martin, B. Infiltration of the iris in chronic lymphatic leukemia. *Br. J. Ophthalmol.* 52:781–785, 1968.
283. Masek, P., Janula, J., and Rejthar, A. Ocular metastasis of bronchial carcinoid. *Czech. Oftalmol.* 37:60–63, 1981.
284. Matas, B.R. Unusual course of a ciliary body melanoma. *Am. J. Ophthalmol.* 72:592–594, 1971.
285. Mayer, W., and Ray, E.S. Metastatic carcinoma of the iris and ciliary body. *Am. J. Ophthalmol.* 39:37–43, 1955.
286. Mayou, M.S. Sarcoma of the iris. *Br. J. Ophthalmol.* 14:152–157, 1930.
287. McGraw, J.L. Malignant melanoma associated with retinal hole. *Arch. Ophthalmol.* 46:666–667, 1951.
288. McLean, I.W., and Gamel, J.W., Comparison of morphometric determination nucleolar size and spectrophotometric determination of DNA in prediction of metastasis of uveal melanoma. *Invest. Ophthalmol. Vis. Sci. (Suppl.)* 28:59, 1987.
289. McLean, I.W., and Gamel, J.W. Prediction of metastasis of uveal melanoma: Comparison of morphometric determinations of nucleolar size and spectrophotometric determination of DNA. *Invest. Ophthalmol. Vis. Sci.* 29:507–511, 1988.
290. McLean, I.W., Foster, W.D., and Zimmerman, L.E. Modifications of Callender's classification of uveal melanoma·at the Armed Forces Institute of Pathology. *Am. J. Ophthalmol.* 96:502–509, 1983.
291. McLean, I.W., Foster, W.D., and Zimmerman, L.E. Prognostic factors in small malignant melanomas of choroid and ciliary body. *Arch. Ophthalmol.* 95:48–58, 1977.
292. McLean, I.W., Zimmerman, L.E., and Evans, R.M. Reappraisal of Callender's spindle A type of melanoma of choroid and ciliary body. *Am. J. Ophthalmol.* 86:557–564, 1978.
293. Meecham, W.J., Char, D.H., Huhta, K., and Juster, R. Correlation of DNA content abnormality in uveal melanoma prognosis. *Invest. Ophthalmol. Vis. Sci. (Suppl.)* 27:259, 1986.
294. Merkel, D.E., Dressler, L.G., and McGuire, W.L. Cellular DNA content in human malignancy. *J. Clin Oncol.* 5:1690, 1987.
295. Merrill, R.H. Ueber seltenere ophthalmoskopische Befunde bei Sarkom der Aderhaut. *Klin. Monatsbl. Augenheilkd.* 91:598–609, 1933.
296. Mewis, L., and Young, S.R. Breast carcinoma metastatic to the choroid: Analysis of 67 patients. *Ophthalmology* 89:147–151, 1982.
297. Meyer, S.L., Fine, B.S., Font, R.L., and Zimmerman, L.E. Leiomyoma of the ciliary body: Electron microscopic verification. *Am. J. Ophthalmol.* 66:1061–1068, 1968.
298. Meyer-Schwickerath, G. The preservation of vision by treatment of intraocular tumors with light coagulation. *Arch. Ophthalmol.* 66:458–466, 1961.
299. Michelson, J.B., and Shields, J.A. Relationship of iris nevi to malignant melanoma of the uvea. *Am. J. Ophthalmol.* 83:694–696, 1977.
300. Migdal, C., and Macfarlane, A. Bilateral primary choroidal melanoma. *Br. J. Ophthalmol.* 68:268–271, 1984.
301. Mikel, U.V., Fishbein, W.N., and Bahr, G.F. Some practical considerations in quantitative absorbance microspectrophotometry: Preparation techniques in DNA cytomorphometry. *Anal. Quant. Cytol.* 7:107, 1985.
302. Mims, J.L., and Shields, J.A. Follow-up studies of suspicious choroidal nevi. *Trans. Am. Acad. Ophthalmol. Otolaryngol.* 85:929–943, 1978.
303. Minckler, D., Font, R.L., and Shields, J.A. Non-melanoma ocular lesions with positive P[32] tests. In *Ocular and Adnexal Tumors*, F. Jakobiec (Ed.), Aesculapius, Birmingham, AL, pp. 245–256, 1978.
304. Mittleman, D., Apple, D.J., and Goldberg, M.F. Ocular involvement in Letter-Siwe disease. *Am. J. Ophthalmol.* 75:261–265, 1973.
305. Molina, A. Immunohistochemical and cytogenetic studies indicate that angiotrophic large cell lymphoma is a primary intravascular (angiotropic) lymphoma. *Cancer* 66:470–474, 1990.
306. Mooy, C.M., de Jong, P.T.V.M., Van der Kwast, T.H., Mulder, P.G.H., Jager, M.J., and Ruiter, D.J. Ki-67 immunostaining in uveal melanoma. The effect of pre-enucleation radiotherapy. *Ophthalmology* 97:1275–1280, 1990.

307. Morgan, O.G. Some problems arising in a case of malignant melanoma of the choroid. *Trans. Ophthalmol. Soc. UK* 76:649–657, 1956.
308. Morgan, W.E., Malmgren, R.A., and Albert, D.M. Metastatic carcinoma of the ciliary body simulating uveitis: Diagnosis by cytologic examination of aqueous tumor. *Arch. Ophthalmol.* 83:54–58, 1970.
309. Nadbath, R.P., and Bullwinkel, H.G. Coexistence of intraocular melanoma and lymphatic leukemia. *Arch. Ophthalmol.* 48:349–351, 1952.
310. Naidoff, M.A., Kenyon, K.R., and Green, W.R. Iris hemangioma and abnormal retinal vasculature in a case of diffuse congenital hemangiomatosis. *Am. J. Ophthalmol.* 72:633–644, 1971.
311. Naumann, G.O.H. Leiomyoma of the choroid. Seventh Biennial Meeting of the Association of Ophthalmology. Alumni, Armed Forces Institute of Pathology, Washington, D.C., June 3–4, 1977.
312. Naumann, G. Pigmenfierte naevi der Aderhaut und des Ciliakorpers. *Fortschr. Augenheilkd.* 23:187–272, 1970.
313. Naumann, G., Font, R.L., and Zimmerman, L.E. Electron microscopic verification of primary rhabdomyosarcoma of the iris. *Am. J. Ophthalmol.* 74:110–117, 1972.
314. Naumann, G., and Green, W.R. Spontaneous nonpigmented iris cysts. *Arch. Ophthalmol.* 78:496–500, 1967.
315. Naumann, G.O.H., Hellner, K., and Namann, L.R. Pigmented nevi of the choroid. Clinical study of secondary changes in the overlying tissues. *Trans. Am. Acad. Ophthalmol. Otolaryngol.* 75:110–123, 1971.
316. Naumann, G.O.H., and Ruprecht, K.W. Xanthom der iris. Ein klinisch-pathologischer Befundbericht. *Ophthalmologica* 164:293–305, 1972.
317. Naumann, G., Yanoff, M., and Zimmerman, L.E. Histogenesis of malignant melanomas of the uvea. I. Histopathologic characteristics of nevi of choroid and ciliary body. *Arch. Ophthalmol.* 76:784–796, 1966.
318. Nelson, C.C., Hertzberg, B.S., and Klintworth, G.K. A histopathologic study of 716 unselected eyes in patients with cancer at the time of death. *Am. J. Ophthalmol.* 95:788–793, 1983.
319. Newton, F.H. Malignant melanoma of choroid: Report of a case with clinical history of 36 years and follow-up of 32 years. *Arch. Ophthalmol.* 73:198–199, 1965.
320. Niederkorn, J.Y. T cell subsets involved in the rejection of metastases arising from intraocular melanomas in mice. *Invest. Ophthalmol. Vis. Sci.* 28:1397–1403, 1987.
321. Norton, E.W.H., and Gutman, H. Fluorescein angiography and hemangiomas of the choroid. *Arch. Ophthalmol.* 78:121–125, 1967.
322. Nover, A. Über das workommen multipler maligner Primartumoren. *Graefes Arch. Ophthalmol.* 157:237–251, 1956.
323. O'Brien, C.S. Detachment of the choroid after cataract extraction: Clinical and experimental studies with a report of 75 cases. *Arch. Ophthalmol.* 14:527–540, 1935.
324. O'Connor, G.R. The uveal annual review. *Arch. Ophthalmol.* 89:505–518, 1973.
325. Offret, H., and Saraux, H. Adenoma of the iris pigment epithelium. *Arch. Ophthalmol.* 98:875–883, 1980.
326. Oksala, A., Lingren, I., and Ahlas, A. Haemangioma of the ciliary body. *Br. J. Ophthalmol.* 48:669–672, 1964.
327. Orellana, J., O'Malley, R.E., McPherson, A.R., and Font, R.L. Pigmented free-floating vitreous cysts in two young adults. Electron microscopic observations. *Ophthalmology* 92:297–302, 1985.
328. Papale, J.J., Frederick, A.R., Albert, D.M. Intraocular hemangiopericytoma. *Arch. Ophthalmol.* 101:1409–1411, 1983.
329. Paul, E.V., Parnell, B.L., and Fraker, M. Prognosis of malignant melanomas of the choroid and ciliary body. *Int. Ophthalmol. Clin.* 2:387–402, 1962.
330. Pawel, E. Beitrag zur Lehre von dein Choriodealsarkom. *Graefes Arch. Ophthalmol.* 49:71–124, 1900.
331. Perry, H.D., Zimmerman, L.E., and Benson, W.E. Hemorrhage from isolated aneurysm of a retinal artery: Report of two cases simulating malignant melanoma. *Arch. Ophthalmol.* 95:281–283, 1977.
332. Phelps, C.D. The pathogenesis of glaucoma in Sturge-Weber syndrome. *Tr. Am. Acad. Ophthalmol. Otolaryngol.* 85:276–286, 1978.
333. Piro, P., Pappas, H.R., Erozan, Y.S., Michels, R.G., Sherman, S.H., and Green, W.R. Diagnostic vitrectomy in metastatic breast carcinoma to the vitreous. *Retina* 2:182–188, 1982.
334. Pomeranz, G.A., Bunt, A.H., and Kalina, R.E. Multifocal choroidal melanoma in ocular melanocytosis. *Arch. Ophthalmol.* 99:857–863, 1981.
335. Pro, M., Shields, J.A., and Tomer, T.L. Serous detachment of the macula associated with presumed choroidal nevi. *Arch. Ophthalmol.* 96:1374–1377, 1978.
336. Puliafito, C.A., Wilkes, B.M., and Albert, D.M. Direct identification of T cells in malignant melanoma of the choroid. *Int. Ophthalmol. Clin.* 20:93–102, 1980.
337. Radnot, M. Metastatisches Melanosarkom des Strahlenkorpers. *Klin. Monatsbl. Augenheilk.* 121:352–354, 1952.
338. Rahi, A.H.S. Autoimmune reactions in uveal melanoma. *Br. J. Ophthalmol.* 55:793–807, 1971.
339. Raivio, I. Uveal melanoma in Finland. *Acta Ophthalmol. Suppl. (Copenh.)* 133:1–64, 1977.
340. Reese, A.B. Melanosis oculi: A case with microscopic findings. *Am. J. Ophthalmol.* 8:865–870, 1925.
341. Reese, A.B. Pigment freckles of the iris (benign melanomas): Their significance in relation to malignant melanoma of the uvea. *Am. J. Ophthalmol.* 27:217–226, 1944.
342. Reese, A.B. Spontaneous cysts of the ciliary body simulating neoplasms. *Am. J. Ophthalmol.* 33:1738–1746, 1950.

343. Reese, A.B. The association of uveal nevi with skin nevi. *Trans. Am. Ophthalmol. Soc. 49*:47–57, 1951.
344. Reese, A.B. The differential diagnosis of malignant melanoma of the choroid. *Arch. Ophthalmol. 58*:477–482, 1957.
345. Reese, A.B. *Tumors of the Eye*, 2nd ed. P.B. Hoeber, New York, pp. 519–523, 1963.
346. Reese, A.B. *Tumors of the Eye*, 3rd ed. Harper & Row, New York, pp. 174–262, 1976.
347. Reese, A.B., Archila, E.A., Jones, I.S., and Cooper, W.C. Necrosis of malignant melanoma of the choroid. *Am. J. Ophthalmol. 69*:91–104, 1970.
348. Reese, A.B., and Cleasby, G.W. The treatment of iris melanomas. *Am. J. Ophthalmol. 47*:118–125, 1959.
349. Reese, A.B., and Howard, G.M. Flat uveal melanomas. *Am. J. Ophthalmol. 64*:1021–1028, 1967.
350. Reese, A.B., and Jones, I.S. Hematomas under the retinal pigment epithelium. *Trans. Am. Ophthalmol. Soc. 59*:43–79, 1961.
351. Reese, A.B., Mund, M.L., and Iwamoto, T. Tapioca melanoma of the iris. Part I. Clinical and light microscopy studies. *Am. J. Ophthalmol. 74*:840–850, 1972.
352. Rendahl, I. Does execteratio orbitae improve the prognosis in orbital tumours? *Acta Ophthalmol. (Copenh.) 32*:431–449, 1954.
353. Reynard, M., and Font, R.L. Two cases of uveal metastasis from breast carcinoma in men. *Am. J. Ophthalmol. 95*:208–215, 1983.
354. Rhodin, J.A.G. Ultrastructure of mammalian venous capillaries, venules, and small collecting veins. *J. Ultrastruct. Res. 25*:452–500, 1968.
355. Richerson, J.T., Burns, R.P., and Misfeldt, M.L. Association of uveal melanocyte destruction in melanoma-bearing swine with large granular lymphocytes. *Invest. Ophthalmol. Vis. Sci. 30*:2455–2460, 1989.
356. Ricketts, M.M., Price, K.T., and Thomas, M. Choroidal metastasis of bronchial adenoma: Adenoid-cystic carcinoma type. *Am. J. Ophthalmol. 39*:33–36, 1955.
357. Riddle, P.J., Font, R.L., and Zimmerman, L.E. Carcinoid tumors of the eye and orbit: A clinicopathologic study of 15 cases, with histochemical and electron microscopic observations. *Hum. Pathol. 13*:459–469, 1982.
358. Rini, F.J., Jakobiec, F.A., Hornblass, A., Beckerman, B.L., and Anderson, R.L. The treatment of advanced choroidal melanoma with massive orbital extension. *Am. J. Ophthalmol. 104*:634–640, 1987.
359. Robertson, D.M. A rationale for comparing radiation to enucleation in the management of choroidal melanoma. *Am. J. Ophthalmol. 108*:448–451, 1989.
360. Rodriques, M.M., and Shields, J.A. Iris metastasis from a bronchial carcinoid tumor. *Arch. Ophthalmol. 96*:77–83, 1978.
361. Rodriquez-Sains, R.S., Abramson, D.H., and Rubman, R.H. B-K mole syndrome: Cutaneous and ocular malignant melanoma. *Invest. Ophthalmol. Vis. Sci. (Suppl.) 19*:108, 1980.
362. Rodin, F.H. Angioma of the iris: First case to be reported with histologic examination. *Arch. Ophthalmol. 2*:679–690, 1929.
363. Rones, B., and Linger, H.T. Early malignant melanoma of the choroid. *Am. J. Ophthalmol. 38*:163–170, 1954.
364. Rones, B., and Zimmerman, L.E. The production of heterochromia and glaucoma by diffuse malignant melanoma of the iris. *Trans. Am. Acad. Ophthalmol. Otolaryngol. 61*:447–463, 1957.
365. Rones, B., and Zimmerman, L.E. The prognosis of primary tumors of the iris treated by iridectomy. *Arch. Ophthalmol. 60*:193–205, 1958.
366. Rones, B., and Zimmerman, L.E. An unusual choroidal hemorrhage simulating malignant melanoma. *Arch. Ophthalmol. 70*:30–32, 1963.
367. Rosenbaum, P.S., Boniuk, M., and Font, R.L. Diffuse uveal melanoma in a 5-year old child. *Am. J. Ophthalmol. 106*:601–606, 1988.
368. Rosenbluth, J., Laval, J., and Weil, J.V. Metastasis of bronchial adenoma to the eyes. *Arch. Ophthalmol. 63*:47–50, 1960.
369. Rootman, J., Carvounis, E.P., Dolman, E.P., and Dimmick, J.E. Congenital fibrosarcoma metastatic to the choroid. *Am. J. Ophthalmol. 87*:632–638, 1979.
370. Roth, A.M. Malignant change in melanocytomas of the uveal tract. *Surv. Ophthalmol. 22*:402–412, 1976.
371. Ryan, D.H., Falon, M.A., and Horan, P.K. Flow cytometry in the clinical laboratory. *Clin. Chim. Acta 171*:125–173, 1988.
372. Ryan, S.J., Frank, R.N., and Green, W.R. Bilateral inflammatory pseudotumor of the ciliary body. *Am. J. Ophthalmol. 72*:586–591, 1971.
373. Ryan, S.J., Zimmerman, L.E., and King, F.M. Reactive lymphoid hyperplasia: An unusual form of intraocular pseudotumor. *Trans. Am. Acad. Ophthalmol. Otolaryngol. 76*:652–671, 1972.
374. Rycroft, B.W. Choroidal detachment. *Br. J. Ophthalmol. 27*:283–291, 1943.
375. Sabates, F.N., and Yamashita, T. Congenital melanosis oculi: Complicated by two independent malignant melanomas of the choroid. *Arch. Ophthalmol. 77*:801–803, 1967.
376. Safar, K. Pseudo-melanoblastom der Iris durch groben Thrombus vorgetauscht. *Klin. Monatsbl. Augenheilkd. 139*:835–840, 1961.
377. Samuels, S.L., and Payne, B.F. Malignant melanoma of the iris: Mode of extension and dissemination. *Am. J. Ophthalmol. 55*:629–631, 1963.
378. Sanders, T. Intraocular juvenile xanthogranuloma. *Am. J. Ophthalmol. 53*:455–562, 1962.

379. Schachat, A.P., Jabs, D.A., Graham, M.L., Ambinder, R.F., Green, W.R., and Saral, R. Leukemic iris infiltration. *J. Pediatr. Ophthalmol. Strabismus* 25:135–138, 1988.

380. Schachat, A.P., Markowitz, J.A., Guyer, D.R., Burke, P.J., Karp, J.E., and Graham, M.L. Ophthalmic manifestations of leukemia. *Arch. Ophthalmol.* 107:697–700, 1989.

381. Scheie, H.G., and Yanoff, M. Iris nevus (Cogan-Reese) syndrome: A cause of unilateral glaucoma. *Arch. Ophthalmol.* 93:963–970, 1975.

382. Scheie, H.G., and Yanoff, M. Pseudomelanoma of the ciliary body. *Arch. Ophthalmol.* 77:81–83, 1967.

383. Scholz, R.T., Green, W.R., Baranano, E.C., Erozan, Y.S., and Montgomery, B.J. Metastatic carcinoma to the iris: Diagnosis by aqueous paracentesis and response to irradiation and chemotherapy. *Ophthalmology* 90:1524–1527, 1983.

384. Schwartz, L., Rodiques, M.M., and Hallett, J. Juvenile xanthogranuloma diagnosed by paracentesis. *Am. J. Ophthalmol.* 77:243–246, 1974.

385. Schwartz, L.K., and O'Connor, R. Secondary syphilis with iris papules. *Am. J. Ophthalmol.* 90:380–384, 1980.

386. Scruggs, J.H. Malignant melanoma of the uvea. *Am. J. Ophthalmol.* 49:594–605, 1960.

387. Seddon, J.M., Friedenberg, G.R., Albert, D.M., and Gamel, J.W. Cell type of uveal melanoma assessed by number of epithelioid cells per HPF and ISDNA: Correlation and prognostic value. *Invest. Ophthalmol. Vis. Sci. (Suppl.)* 25:83, 1984.

388. Seddon, J.M., Gragoudas, E.S., Glynn, R.J., Egan, K.M., Albert, D.M., and Blitzer, P.H. Host factors, UV radiation, and risk of uveal melanoma. A case-control study. *Arch. Ophthalmol.* 108:1274–1280, 1990.

389. Shakin, E.P., Augsburger, J.J., Eagle, R.C., Ehya, H., Shields, J.A., Fischer, D., and Koepsell, D.G. Multiple myeloma involving the iris. *Arch. Ophthalmol.* 106:524–526, 1988.

390. Shammas, H.F., and Blodi, F.C. Orbital extension of choroidal and ciliary body melanomas. *Arch. Ophthalmol.* 95:2002–2005, 1977.

391. Shammas, H.F., and Blodi, F.C. Peripapillary choroidal melanomas: Extension along the optic nerve and its sheaths. *Arch. Ophthalmol.* 96:440–445, 1978.

392. Shammas, H.F., and Blodi, F.C. Prognostic factors in choroidal and ciliary body melanomas. *Arch. Ophthalmol.* 95:63–69, 1977.

393. Shammas, H.F., and Watzke, R.C. Bilateral choroidal melanomas: Case report and incidence. *Arch. Ophthalmol.* 95:617–623, 1977.

394. Shaver, R.P. Pigmented iris and retrocorneal membrane simulating an iris melanoma. *Arch. Ophthalmol.* 78:55–57, 1967.

395. Shaw, H. Melanoma of ciliary body. *Am. J. Ophthalmol.* 38:104–105, 1954.

396. Shields, C.L., Shields, J.A., and Augsburger, J.J. Choroidal osteoma. *Surv. Ophthalmol.* 33:17–27, 1988.

397. Shield, C.L., Shields, J.A., Karlson, U., Menduke, H., and Brady, L.W. Enucleation after plaque radiotherapy for posterior uveal melanoma. *Ophthalmology* 97:1665–1670, 1990.

398. Shields, C.L., Shields, J.A., and Varenhorst, M.P. Transscleral leiomyoma. *Ophthalmology* 98:84–87, 1991.

399. Shields, J.A. *Diagnosis and Management of Intraocular Tumors.* C.V. Mosby, St. Louis, MO, 1983.

400. Shields, J.A. Melanocytoma of optic nerve head: A review. *Int. Ophthalmol.* 1:31–37, 1978.

401. Shields, J.A. Primary cysts of the iris. *Trans. Am. Ophthalmol. Soc.* 79:771–809, 1981.

402. Shields, J.A., Annesley, W.H., and Spaeth, G.L. Necrotic melanocytoma of iris with secondary glaucoma. *Am. J. Ophthalmol.* 84:826–829, 1977.

403. Shields, J.A., and Augsburger, J.J. Cataract surgery and intra-ocular lenses in patients with unsuspected malignant melanoma of the ciliary body and choroid. *Ophthalmology* 92:823–826, 1985.

404. Shields, J.A., Augsburger, J.J., Gonder, J.R., and MacLeod, D. Localized benign lymphoid tumor of the iris. *Arch. Ophthalmol.* 99:2147–2148, 1981.

405. Shields, J.A., and Font, R.L. Melanocytoma of the choroid clinically simulating a malignant melanoma. *Arch. Ophthalmol.* 87:396–400, 1972.

406. Shields, J.A., Sanborn, G.E., and Augsberger, J.J. The differential diagnosis of malignant melanoma of the iris: A clinical study of 200 patients. *Ophthalmology* 90:716–720, 1983.

407. Shields, J.A., Sanborn, G.E., Kurz, G.H., and Augsburger, J.J. Benign peripheral nerve tumor of the choroid: A clinicopathologic correlation and review of the literature. *Ophthalmology* 88:1322–1329, 1981.

408. Shields, J.A., Shields, C.L., and Eagle, R.C. Mesectodermal leiomyoma of the ciliary body managed by partial lamellar iridocyclochoroidectomy. *Ophthalmology* 96:1369–1376, 1989.

409. Shields, J.A., and Zimmerman, L.E. Lesions simulating malignant melanoma of the posterior uvea. *Arch. Ophthalmol.* 89:466–471, 1973.

410. Shields, M.B., and Klintworth, G.K. Anterior uveal melanomas and intraocular pressure. *Ophthalmology* 87:503–517, 1980.

411. Smith, J.L., David, N.J., Hart, L.M., Levenson, D.S., and Tillet, C.W. Hemangioma of the choroid: Fluorescein angiography and photocoagulation. *Arch. Ophthalmol.* 69:51–54, 1963.

412. Smith, J.L.S., and Ingram, R.M. Juvenile oculodermal xanthogranuloma. *Br. J. Ophthalmol.* 52:696–763, 1968.

413. Smith, L.T., and Irvine, A.R. Diagnostic significance of orange pigment accumulation over choroidal tumors. *Am. J. Ophthalmol.* 76:212–216, 1973.

414. Smith, M.D., Liggett, P.E., and Rao, N.A. Immunohistochemical characterization of lymphoid infiltration in human choroidal melanomas. *Invest. Ophthalmol. Vis. Sci. (Suppl.)* 29:365, 1988.

415. Smith, M.R., Sanders, T.W., and Bresnick, G.H. Juvenile xanthogranuloma of the ciliary body in an adult. *Arch. Ophthalmol.* 81:813–814, 1969.

416. Smith, T.R., and Brockhurst, R.J. Cellular blue nevus of the sclera. *Arch. Ophthalmol.* 94:618–620, 1976.

417. Smolin, G. Malignant change of a benign melanoma. *Am. J. Ophthalmol.* 61:174–177, 1966.

418. Snip, R.C., Green, W.R., and Jaegers, K.R. Choroidal nevus with subretinal pigment epithelial neovascular membrane and a positive P^{32} test. *Ophthalmol. Surg.* 9:35–42, 1978.

419. Southren, A.L. Functioning metastatic bronchial carcinoid with elevated levels of serum and cerebrospinal fluid serotonin and pituitary adenoma. *J. Clin. Endocrinol.* 20:298–305, 1960.

420. Spaulding, A.G., Green, W.R., and Font, R.L. Ring-shaped limbal tumor, secondary to unrecognized diffuse malignant melanoma of the uvea. *Arch. Ophthalmol.* 77:76–80, 1967.

421. Spaulding, A.G., and Woodfin, M.C., Jr. Osteogenic sarcoma metastatic to the choroid. *Arch. Ophthalmol.* 80:84–86, 1968.

422. Spencer, W.H. Optic nerve extension of intraocular neoplasms. *Am. J. Ophthalmol.* 80:465–471, 1975.

423. Spencer, W., and Ferguson, W. Hemangioma of the iris. *Arch. Ophthalmol.* 69:51–54, 1963.

424. Spencer, W.H., and Iverson, H.A. Diffuse melanoma of the iris, with extrabulbar extension via the optic nerve. *Surv. Ophthalmol.* 10:365–371, 1965.

425. Stanford, G.B., and Reese, A.B. Malignant cells in the blood of eye patients. *Trans. Am. Acad. Ophthalmol. Otolaryngol.* 75:102–109, 1971.

426. Stark, W.J., Rosenthal, A.R., Mullins, G.M., and Green, W.R. Simultaneous bilateral uveal melanomas responding to BCNU therapy. *Trans. Am. Acad. Ophthalmol. Otolaryngol.* 75:70–83, 1971.

427. Starr, H.J., and Zimmerman, L.E. Extrascleral extension and orbital recurrence of malignant melanomas of the choroid and ciliary body. *Int. Ophthalmol. Clin* 2:369–384, 1962.

428. Stephens, R.F., and Shields, J.A. Diagnosis and management of cancer metastatic to the uvea: A study of 70 cases. *Ophthalmology* 86:1336–1349, 1979.

429. Streeten, B.W. The sudanophilic granules of the human retinal pigment epithelium. *Arch. Ophthalmol.* 66:391–398, 1961.

430. Sunba, M.S.N., Rahi, A.H.S., and Morgan, G. Tumours of the anterior uvea. I. Metastasizing malignant melanoma to the iris. *Arch. Ophthalmol.* 98:82–85, 1980.

431. Susac, J.O., Smith, J.L., and Scelfo, R.J. The "tomato-catsup" fundus in Sturge-Weber syndrome. *Arch. Ophthalmol.* 92:69–70, 1974.

432. Szeps, J., and Patterson, T.D. Metastatic malignant melanoma of ciliary body and choroid from a primary melanoma of the skin. *Can. J. Ophthalmol.* 4:394–399, 1969.

433. Tabbara, K.F., and Beckstead, J.H. Acute promonocytic leukemia with ocular involvement. *Arch. Ophthalmol.* 98:1055–1058, 1980.

434. Tade, A.A. Bilateral primary melanoblastoma of the choroid (Russian). *Vestn. Oftalmol.* 4:30–35, 1960.

435. Tahan, S.R., Pastel-Levy, C., Bhan, A.K., and Mihm, M.C., Jr. Juvenile xanthogranuloma. Clinical and pathologic characterization. *Arch. Pathol. Lab. Med.* 113:1057–1061, 1989.

436. Takahashi, K., Hattori, Ho., Ieb, Q.S., Nagayama, R., and Kato, T. Statistical observation on ocular tumors (Japanese). *Rinsho Ganka* 23:295–300, 1969.

437. Talegaonkar, S.K. Anterior uveal tract metastasis as the presenting feature of bronchial carcinoma. *Br. J. Ophthalmol.* 53:123–126, 1969.

438. Tasman, W. Familial intraocular melanoma. *Trans. Am. Acad. Ophthalmol. Otolaryngol.* 74:955–958, 1970.

439. Tay, W. Primary cancer of the iris. *R. Lond. Ophthalmol. Hosp. Rep.* 5:230, 1866.

440. Templeton, A.C. Tumors of the eye and adnexa in Africans of Uganda. *Cancer* 20:1689–1698, 1967.

441. The, T.H., Eibergen, R., and Lamberts, H.B. Immune phagocytosis in vivo of human malignant melanoma cells. *Acta Med. Scand.* 192:141–144, 1972.

442. Thomas, C.I., and Purnell, E.W. Ocular melanocytoma. *Am. J. Ophthalmol.* 67:79–86, 1969.

443. Thomas, J.V., Green, W.R., and Maumenee, A.E. Small choroidal melanomas: A long-term follow-up study. *Arch. Ophthalmol.* 97:861–864, 1979.

444. Thomas, R.A., Jacobs, P.M., Liggett, P.E., Azan, S.P., Barlow, W.E., Affelt, J.C., and Rao, N.A. Comprehensive examination of histopathologic factors that determine prognosis of ciliochoroidal melanoma with extrascleral extension. *Invest. Ophthalmol. Vis. Sci. (Suppl.)* 28:26, 1987.

445. Tredici, T.J., and Fenton, R.H. Hematoma beneath the retinal pigment epithelium: Report of a case mistaken clinically for a malignant melanoma of the choroid. *Arch. Ophthalmol.* 72:796–799, 1964.

446. Tso, M.O.M., Goldberg, M.F., and Sugar, J. Nodular adenomatosis of iris pigment epithelium. *Am. J. Ophthalmol.* 100:87–95, 1985.

447. Tsukahara, S., Wakui, K., and Ohzeki, S. Simultaneous bilateral primary diffuse malignant uveal melanoma: Case report with pathologic examination. *Br. J. Ophthalmol.* 70:33–38, 1986.

448. Turnbull, R.B., Kyle, K., Watson, F.R., and Spratt, J. Cancer of the colon: The influence of the no-touch isolation technique on survival rates. *Ann. Surg.* 166:420–427, 1967.

449. Uliesinger, H., Phipps, G.W., and Guerry, D. Bilateral melanoma of the choroid associated with leukemia and meningioma. *Arch. Ophthalmol.* 62:889–893, 1959.

450. Unger, E.R., Budgeon, L.R., Myerson, D., and Brigati, D.J. Viral diagnosis by in situ hybridization: Description of a rapid simplified colorimetric method. *Am. J. Surg. Pathol.* 10:1–8, 1986.

451. Vink, J., Grijns, M.B., Mooy, C.M., Bergman, W., Oosterhuis, J.A., and Went, L.N. Ocular melanoma in families with dysplastic nevus syndrome. *J. Am. Acad. Dermatol.* 23:858–862, 1990.

452. Vogel, M.H., Zimmerman, L.E., and Gass, J.D.M. Proliferation of the juxtapapillary retinal pigment epithelium simulating malignant melanoma. *Doc. Ophthalmol.* 26:461–481, 1969.

453. Volcker, H.E., and Naumann, G.O.H. Multicentric primary malignant melanomas of the choroid: Two separate malignant melanomas of the choroid and two uveal naevi in one eye. *Br. J. Ophthalmol.* 62:408–413, 1978.

454. Volcker, H.E., and Naumann, G.O.H. Klinisch underwartete maligne Melanoma der hinteren Uvea. *Klin. Monatsbl. Augenheilkd.* 168:311–317, 1976.

455. Walsh, F.B., and Hoyt, W.F. *Clinical Neuro-ophthalmology*, Vol. 3, 3rd ed. Williams and Wilkins, Baltimore, pp. 2044–2058, 1969.

456. Warren, R.M. Prognosis of malignant melanomas of the choroid and ciliary body. In *Current Concepts in Ophthalmology*, Vol. 4, F.C. Blodi (Ed.), C.V. Mosby, St. Louis, MO, pp. 158–166, 1974.

457. Wertz, F.D., Zimmerman, L.E., McKeown, C.A., Croxatto, J.O., Whitmore, P.V., and La Piana, F.G. Juvenile xanthogranuloma of the optic nerve, disc, retina and choroid. *Ophthalmology* 89:1331–1335, 1982.

458. White, V., Stevenson, K., Garner, A., and Hungerford, J. Mesectodermal leiomyoma of the ciliary body: Case report. *Br. J. Ophthalmol.* 73:12–18, 1989.

459. Wilder, H.C. Relationship of pigment cell clusters in the iris to malignant melanoma of the uveal tract. In *The Biology of Melanomas*, Vol. 4, New York Academy of Sciences, New York, pp. 137–143, 1948.

460. Williams, A.T., Font, R.L., Van Kyk, H.J.L., and Riekof, F.T. Osseous choristoma of the choroid simulating a choroidal melanoma. *Arch. Ophthalmol.* 96:1874–1877, 1978.

461. Williams, M.A., Kleinschmidt, J.A., Krohne, G., and Franke, W.W. Argyrophilic nuclear and nucleolar proteins of *Xenopus laevis* oocytes identified by gel electrophoresis. *Exp. Cell Res.* 137:341–351, 1982.

462. Wilson, M.E., McClatchey, S.K., and Zimmerman, L.E. Rhabdomyosarcoma of the ciliary body. *Ophthalmology* 97:1484–1488, 1990.

463. Witschel, H., and Font, R.L. Hemangioma of the choroid: A clinicopathologic study of 71 cases and a review of the literature. *Surv. Ophthalmol.* 20:415–431, 1976.

464. Wolter, J.R. Solitary neurofibroma of the iris: Report of a case. *J. Pediatr. Ophthalmol.* 6:84–87, 1969.

465. Wolter, J.R., Leenhouts, T.M., and Hendrix, R.C. Corneal involvement in mycosis fungoides. *Am. J. Ophthalmol.* 55:317–322, 1963.

466. Wolter, J.R., and Makley, T.A., Jr. Cogan-Reese syndrome: Formation of a glass membrane on an iris nevus clinically simulating tumor growth. *J. Pediatr. Ophthalmol.* 9:102–105, 1972.

467. Wong, L.D., and Oskvig, R.M. Immunofluorescent detection of antibodies to ocular melanoma. *Arch. Ophthalmol.* 92:98–102, 1974.

468. Wood, C.A., and Pusey, B. Primary sarcoma of the iris. *Arch. Ophthalmol.* 31:323–383, 1902.

469. Woog, J.J., Albert, D.M., Craft, J., Siberman, N., and Horns, D. Choroidal ganglioneuroma in neurofibromatosis. *Graefes Arch. Clin. Exp. Ophthalmol.* 220:25–31, 1983.

470. Woyke, S., and Chwirot, R. Rhabdomyosarcoma of the iris. Report of the first recorded case. *Br. J. Ophthalmol.* 56:60–64, 1972.

471. Wright, C.J.E. Prognosis in cutaneous and ocular malignant melanoma: A study of 222 cases. *J. Pathol. Bacteriol.* 61:507–525, 1949.

472. Wybran, J., Hellstrom, I., Hellsgrom, K.E., and Fundenberg, H. Cytotoxicity of human rosette-forming blood lymphocytes on cultivated human tumor cells. *Int. J. Cancer* 13:515–521, 1974.

473. Yanoff, M. Glaucoma mechanisms in ocular malignant melanomas. *Am. J. Ophthalmol.* 70:898–904, 1970.

474. Yanoff, M., and Scheie, H.G. Melanomalytic glaucoma: Report of a case. *Arch. Ophthalmol.* 84:471–473, 1970.

475. Yanoff, M., and Zimmerman, L.E. Histogenesis of malignant melanomas of the uvea. II. Relationship of uveal nevi to malignant melanomas. *Cancer* 20:493–507, 1967.

476. Yanoff, M., and Zimmerman, L.E. Histogenesis of malignant melanomas of the uvea. III. The relationship of congenital ocular melanocytosis and neurofibromatosis to uveal melanomas. *Arch. Ophthalmol.* 77:331–336, 1967.

477. Yanoff, M., and Zimmerman, L.E. Pseudomelanoma of anterior chamber caused by implantation of iris pigment epithelium. *Arch. Ophthalmol.* 74:302–305, 1965.

478. Yeo, J.H., Jakobiec, F.A., Iwamoto, T., Brown, R., and Harrison, W. Metastatic carcinoma masquerading as scleritis. *Ophthalmology* 90:184–194, 1983.

479. Yeomans, S., Knox, D.L., Green, W.R., and Murgatroyd, G.W. Ocular inflammatory pseudotumor associated with propranolol therapy. *Ophthalmology* 90:1422–1425, 1983.

480. Young, S.E., Cruciger, M., and Lukeman, J. Metastatic carcinoma to the retina: Case report. *Trans. Am. Acad. Ophthalmol. Otolaryngol.* 86:1350–1354, 1979.

481. Zimmerman, L.E. Discussion of Freeman, L.N., Schachat, A.P., Knox, D.L., Michels, R.G., and Green, W.R.

Clinical features, laboratory investigations and survival in ocular reticulum cell sarcoma. *Ophthalmology* *94*:1631–1639, 1987.

482. Zimmerman, L.E. Malignant melanoma of the uveal tract. In *Ophthalmic Pathology: An Atlas and Textbook*, W.H. Spencer (Ed.), W.B. Saunders, Philadelphia, pp. 2072–2139, 1986.

483. Zimmerman, L.E. Melanocytes, melanocytic nevi and melanocytomas. *Invest. Ophthalmol. 4*:11–41, 1965.

484. Zimmerman, L.E. Ocular lesions of juvenile xanthogranuloma (nevoxanthoendothelioma). *Trans. Am. Acad. Ophthalmol. Otolaryngol. 69*:412–442, 1965.

485. Zimmerman, L.E., and Garron, L.K. Melanocytoma of the optic disc. *Int. Ophthalmol. Clin. 2*:431–440, 1962.

486. Zimmerman, L.E., and McLean, I.W. Changing concepts of the prognosis and management of small malignant melanomas of the choroid. *Trans. Ophthalmol. Soc. UK 95*:487–494, 1975.

487. Zimmerman, L.E., McLean, I.W., and Foster, W.D. Does enucleation of the eye containing a malignant melanoma prevent or accelerate the dissemination of tumour cells? *Br. J. Ophthalmol. 62*:420–425, 1978.

49

Tumors of the Retina

José A. Sahel
Clinique Ophtalmologique, Hôpitaux Universitaires, Strasbourg, France

Daniel M. Albert
University of Wisconsin—Madison, Madison, Wisconsin

I. RETINOBLASTOMA

Retinoblastoma is the most common malignant eye tumor of childhood, and after malignant melanoma, it is the most common primary intraocular malignancy of the eye. The tumor, although accounting for only approximately 1% of all deaths from cancer under 15 years of age [100], is attracting interest from various disciplines, such as epidemiology, genetics, and molecular biology, as a consequence of the recent isolation and cloning of the gene altered in this disease [138,242,279]. In recent years retinoblastoma has emerged as a model of oncogenesis and the literature on the tumor has grown dramatically. Moreover, recent advances in cell culture studies and immunohistochemistry have provided useful clues to a better understanding of the histogenesis, growth, and differentiation of the tumor. With recent significant progress in achieving early and accurate diagnosis, the improved prognosis for survival and vision is leading to new concepts in the management of early cases [259,324,371,372].

A. Epidemiology

Incidence

An accurate determination of the incidence of retinoblastoma is difficult to achieve. Even in industrialized countries differences in methods of study, sample size, and stage at diagnosis may account for the variations in reported data [100,190]. Nevertheless, useful estimates have been derived from population-based studies. Since 1970 the incidence is evaluated at 11 cases per 1 million children under 5 years of age or 1 per 18,000 live births [100] and 3.58 cases per 1 million children under the age of 15 [9,100,309]. Recent data from the Surveillance, Epidemiology, and End Results (SEER) Study from 1974 through 1984 have established an average incidence of 10.9 per 1 million for children under 5 years of age and 5.8 per 1 million children younger than 10 years [388]. A British study (1969–1980) provides a registration rate of 1 per 23,000 births [352]. Most studies from Australia, Sweden, and New Zealand report similar rates [176,225,304,381].

An increased incidence in Finland and Holland between 1915 and 1965 has been reported [36,164,359,393]. It seems likely that improvement in methods of diagnosis may account for this apparent increase [452]. Schipper, after a thorough analysis of the Dutch registry, demonstrated stabilization at around 1 per 15,560 births since 1950 [361].

Although retinoblastoma affects all ethnic groups and is encountered throughout the world [45], based on studies from Nigeria [226] and Jamaica [57], it does not appear as evenly distributed in view of evidence for a higher incidence in black populations. In addition, Macklin [261] described a higher mutation rate for retinoblastomas in blacks than in whites in Ohio. Yet, several authors are of the opinion that these variations may result from differences in referral pattern and methods of case ascertainment. In the last SEER report blacks were found to have a higher incidence than whites, although not greater than about 75% [388]. No sex predilection has been demonstrated [100,352,388].

Age at Diagnosis

The average age at the time of diagnosis is about 18 months of age. Most reports [7,215] have found that the mean age at diagnosis for the hereditary type, which is characteristically bilateral, is earlier (between 12 and 14 months of age) than pertains in the sporadic (usually unilateral) variety. In the latter the diagnosis is made at about 24–30 months of age [214,215]. A few retinoblastomas have been observed at birth or in premature babies [316]. In a recent study of 220 cases, 95% were diagnosed before 5 years of age and 40% before 1 year. Exceptional cases have occurred after 10 years, and Takahashi and colleagues studied 11 retinoblastomas in patients older than 20 years [385].

Epidemiological studies of age at diagnosis have provided crucial information relevant to understanding the pathogenesis of retinoblastoma. Knudson, in 1971, designed a semilogarithmic plot of the age in months versus the fraction of unilateral and bilateral types of retinoblastoma not yet diagnosed. He showed that for bilateral cases the curve fits a simple exponential pattern; for unilateral cases the curve fits a second-order regression pattern [216,219].

Since a strong association exists between bilaterality and the hereditary type of retinoblastoma and, conversely, between unilateral involvement and the sporadic variety, Knudson concluded that in heritable retinoblastoma, only one event is required after birth for tumor induction. In contrast in nonheritable retinoblastoma, two events are necessary for tumorigenesis. From these data, Knudson and Strong postulated that two mutations were necessary for oncogenesis in retinoblastoma, as well as other childhood tumors, such as Wilms' tumor [221]. Knudson and colleagues estimated a mutation frequency of 2×10^{-7} per year. If one of the mutations is inherited, the tumors develop at an earlier age [214–216].

Age at diagnosis is also providing information relevant to prognosis and course [1,2]. Since laterality is correlated with age at diagnosis, this can confound the analysis. Actually, no definitive and clear association has emerged from recent studies. The most recent data from the SEER study are in agreement with previous findings [2] showing worsening survival with increasing age at diagnosis. Yet, beyond 2 years of age, this relationship becomes less clear. In the British findings children older than 2 years at the time of diagnosis had a worse prognosis [352]. Abramson and colleagues showed also that the best survival was in children older than 7 years at the time of diagnosis [1,2]. These conflicting data could be accounted for by (1) a smaller size of tumors when diagnosed in children under the age of 2 years or (2) a different biological behavior of tumors in younger and older children [1]. These findings may be related to the increased mortality in blacks ($>2.5 \times$ whites) [192,301]. As shown by Newell and colleagues [301], more than half of whites with retinoblastoma were diagnosed before 2 years of age, whereas in blacks the diagnosis was established in less than one-fourth of the group studied by this time. This suggests that the higher mortality in blacks is at least in part due to a delay in both diagnosis and treatment.

B. Genetics

Despite its infrequency, retinoblastoma has become a paradigm in the understanding of a major category of oncogenesis.

Historical Background

Familial transmission of a retinoblastoma from an enucleated survivor to its offspring was apparently first reported in 1886 by DeGouveia [9], although we have been unable to confirm this. Despite a few reports of families with tumors in sibships, it was not until the beginning of the twentieth century that the role of heredity was really appreciated, when survivors and their offspring became more numerous [9].

Between 60 and 70% of retinoblasmas appear sporadically and are not transmitted to offspring, and 30–40% of cases [9,136,151,261,327,452] appear clinically to be transmitted as an "irregular" autosomal dominant trait with "incomplete" penetrance (hereditary retinoblastomas) [9,151,327]. Sporadic cases develop unilateral and unifocal tumors at a later age than the inherited retinoblastomas. Hereditary retinoblastomas appear in about 85% of cases as multifocal or bilateral lesions [9,354,421].

Knudson's Hypothesis

The original theory of retinoblastoma as inherited as an irregular autosomal dominant trait was widely recognized as unsatisfactory until Knudson proposed an alternative model in 1971 [214]. From an epidemiological and statistical study of the ages at diagnosis and the laterality of tumors, Knudson and colleagues derived a "two-hit" model involving a double mutational event [214–221]. Patients with nonhereditary retinoblastoma develop two mutations in the same postzygotic somatic cell, giving rise to a single unilateral tumor. Since both mutations occur in the same cell, multifocality of tumors should not be expected.

In contrast, in hereditary retinoblastoma the first mutation occurs in germinal cells either as a result of inheritance of a predisposing mutation from a carrier parent (accounting for one-third of cases, according to Vogel) [418] or through a new germ-line mutation, which although not present in either parent can be transmitted to their offspring [295]. The second mutation occurs in a postzygotic retinal cell (or cells). Consequently, every retinal cell contains the first mutation. Should the second mutational event occur, which is likely in the millions of developing retinal cells, tumors then appear. Comings, suggesting a general model of oncogenesis, proposed that inactivation of the two alleles of a single regulatory locus could release the cell from normal growth control [81].

Chromosomal Studies

The well-recognized hereditary aspect of retinoblastoma, together with the occasional occurrence of congenital malformations in some of these patients [94,280,387], stimulated a search for chromosomal abnormalities [136,354]. In 1962, Stallard reported investigations in a female infant with retinoblastoma and deletion in the D group of chromosomes [9,189]. Subsequently additional similar findings were reported, and improvement in cytogenetic techniques in the 1970s allowed assignment of the chromosome abnormality to chromosome 13 [182]. Retinoblastoma came to be included with the 13q$^-$ syndromes [220,292,426]. A site for skin fibroblast radiosensitivity was also postulated on that chromosome [22,425]. Yunis and Ramsay and others observed that all deletions in the long arm of chromosome 13 in patients with retinoblastomas involved the 13q14 band [182,448]. Moreover, if the 13q14 was not deleted, retinoblastoma was not encountered; consequently this became the possible locus for the candidate gene [219,448]. In 1980 Sparkes and colleagues demonstrated that the polymorphic marker enzyme esterase D locus also maps to chromosome band 13q14 [87,374]. In patients with no cytogenetic abnormality of 13q14 esterase D levels were normal, but in all patients with retinoblastoma and 13q14 deletion low esterase D levels were found. Despite the finding of such a 13q14 deletion in only 5% of patients with retinoblastoma, these data directed attention of this locus site of the "retinoblastoma gene" [72,109,289,374,376].

Molecular Genetics: Identifying the Rb Gene

By comparing constitutional and tumor genotypes through the use of restriction fragment-length polymorphisms, the Benedict [43], Cavenee [70,71], and Dryja groups [108,109,112] provided evidence that in some retinoblastomas the tumor cells had become homozygous for loci on the chromosome 13. In inherited retinoblastoma it was shown that the chromosome 13 homolog present in tumors was derived from the affected parent. Using a DNA probe (H3-8) previously assigned to the region 13q14-1, analysis of 37 retinoblastomas showed that these tumors displayed hybridization patterns consistent with homologous deletions [70,108]. These data, taken together with various studies using restriction fragment-length polymorphisms, confirmed that loss of heterozygosity for chromosome 13 in tumors was a key factor for a recessive mechanism at the molecular level [42–44,109,112]. The mutations of the Rb locus responsible for cancer appear as loss of function (whether or not the loss can be detected at the cytogenetic level). One copy of the normal allele is able to prevent malignant transformation. In nonheritable retinoblastoma, both alleles of the Rb locus are normal in the germinal cells. A mutation at both loci (equating the two hits of Knudson) is therefore necessary to induce tumorigenesis in a retinal cell. In contrast, in heritable retinoblastoma, one copy of the gene is altered in all cells. A second mutational event in a retinal cell is sufficient to produce the retinoblastoma [9,88]. This event appears more commonly to be a conspicuous abnormality of chromosome 13 rather than a point mutation.

Starting from the H3-8 probe, chromosome walking techniques allowed identification of a cDNA sequence coding for a 4.7 kb mRNA representing the Rb transcript [138]. Friend and colleagues detected this RNA transcript in adenovirus 12-immortalized retinal cells, normal human adult retina, and many tumor types, but no transcript was found in retinoblastomas or osteosarcomas [138]. These investigators found partial and internal deletions of the gene in the tumor. Others have demonstrated structural changes within 16 of 40 retinoblastomas, but among the other tumors the Rb transcript was absent or truncated [139,242]. Methods of amplification and sequencing of the Rb gene, as well as techniques using ribonuclease production, allowed identification of point mutations within the Rb gene [174,443]. Shortly after identification of the Rb transcript, the sequence of the cDNA was established. The Rb gene is now known to have a complex organization spanning over 200 kb DNA that includes 27 exons [55,170,242,258]. The isolation of the Rb gene, the first recessive cancer suppressive gene to be described, provided the basis for advances in both basic and clinical sciences:

1. Understanding the causes of Rb gene inactivation [68,86,167,174,240,241,243,429]
2. Investigation of the role of Rb and other "recessive oncogenes" [143,160,272,293,441,445]
3. Developing animal models of retinoblastoma [434]
4. Attempts at reversing malignant properties by genetic manipulation [262].
5. Establishing probes and techniques for genetic counseling [85,86,155,295]

The Rb gene product has been characterized as a 110 kD nuclear phosphoprotein with DNA binding properties, as shown by immunocytochemistry [245]. This protein, p105-Rb, may be a regulatory protein inhibiting cellular proliferation. p105-Rb is underphosphorylated in nonproliferating cells and phosphorylated in proliferating cells [28,60,76,97]. Maximal phosphorylation is associated with the S phase of the cell cycle [60,76,83,140,256,277]. Rb dephosphorylation precedes the arrest of cell growth during differentiation [60,76].

Rb gene loss has been demonstrated in osteosarcomas [111,132,161], small cell lung cancer [162], bladder carcinoma, and breast cancer [389], and its loss is widely seen as a factor in the initiation of several tumor types [173].

Attempts have been made to reintroduce the Rb gene into cultured retinoblastoma cell lines (the WERI-27 line) using a retrovirus containing the full-length cDNA with normal chromosome 13 by microcell fusion [262]. The treated cells produced p105-Rb with an associated decrease in the growth rate and reduced tumorigenicity in nude mice [262].

Although this avenue of research has clinical implications, a more immediate application of the Rb gene discovery is likely to be in determining whether a given retinoblastoma is heritable [61,85,100, 155,431,432]. Wiggs and colleagues identified restriction fragment-length polymorphisms within the Rb gene and tested their usefulness in predicting the risk of retinoblastoma in families with a positive story of familial retinoblastoma [431]. They were successful in 19 of 20 kindreds. The use of enzymatic amplification and DNA sequence analysis has allowed Yandell and colleagues to identify oncogenic point mutations in seven retinoblastoma patients with a negative family history [443]. Using this technique they showed that four of these were sporadic cases and three others had new germ cell mutations. Such studies have made possible a major improvement in genetic counseling accuracy [62,155]. Also of interest in these studies was the demonstration that new germline mutations occur primarily during spermatogenesis [110, 443,449].

C. Histopathology

Despite tremendous advances in the understanding of the molecular biology of retinoblastoma, the controversy over the cell of origin is not yet resolved. Data from tissue culture studies, immunohistochemistry, and animal models have provided new insights and complemented the earlier histopathological and ultrastructural findings.

Historical Aspects

Retinoblastoma was first recognized as a discrete tumor, distinct from "fungus haematodes," or soft cancers that arose from the breast and limbs, by the Scottish surgeon Wardrop in 1809 [9,115,424]. Wardrop's astute observations, based on dissections made without benefit of the microscope, convinced him that the tumor arose from the retina. His observations were subsequently confirmed by various pathologists of the nineteenth century, including Robin and Langenbeck [115]. Virchow concluded that the tumor arose from the glial cells and named it a glioma of the retina [416]. Flexner and later Wintersteiner described the characteristic rosettes named after them. Both suggested the use of the term "neuro-epithelioma," believing that the tumor was of neuroepithelial origin, and regarded rosettes as an attempt to form photoreceptors [132,402,435]. This led to the use of the term "retinoblastoma," suggested by Verhoeff, who concluded that the tumor was derived from undifferentiated embryonic retinal cells called retinoblasts, comparable to the neuroblasts originating from the medullary epithelium [165,412,433]. Between 1922 and 1924, Mawas [271a] in France proposed the terms "retinoblastoma" for undifferentiated tumors and "retinocytoma" for differentiated tumors. The name was adopted in 1926 by the American Ophthalmological Society. Zimmerman [452] has proposed that the designation *retinocytoma* be restricted to differentiated retinal tumors that display benign features after thorough histological sampling [452].

The most popular concept regarding retinoblastoma histogenesis holds that the tumor generally arises from a multipotential precursor cell that can develop into almost any type of inner or outer retinal cell. This view can account for the heterogeneity of the histopathological, ultrastructural, and immunohistochemical features described in retinoblastoma. [26,452]

Light Microscopic Appearance

Undifferentiated areas of retinoblastoma are composed of small round cells with large variably shaped, hyperchromatic nuclei and scanty cytoplasm (Fig. 1). Differentiated areas are present within many retinoblastomas, the most characteristic of these being the rosettes first described by Flexner and Winter-steiner in the 1890s [132,435]. These structures consist of clusters of cuboidal or short columnar cells arranged around a central lumen (Fig. 2). The nuclei are displaced away from the lumen, which by light microscopy appears to have a limiting membrane, resembling the external limiting membrane, of the retina. Photoreceptor-like elements protrude through the membrane, and some taper into fine filaments [402,452]. The lumen of these rosettes contains hyaluronidase-resistant glycosaminoglycans similiar to those found between normal photoreceptors and the retinal pigment epithelium (RPE). They are similar to the material that normally surrounds photoreceptors [450]. Less common are the rosettes of the Homer Wright type composed of radial arrangements of cells around a central tangle of fibrils [440]. These are identical to the rosettes found in neuroblastomas and medulloblastomas. Electron microscopic studies, as described later, confirm that the cells around rosettes share many characteristics of photoreceptors.

An additional differentiated structure is the fleurette, first described by Tso and colleagues, which represents a higher degree of photoreceptor differentiation [405]. Fleurettes are seen by light microscopy in areas having larger cells with abundant eosinophilic cytoplasm and fewer hyperchromatic nuclei than the surrounding areas. The term "fleurette" was applied to denote the arrangement like a "fleur-de-lis" of the apparently abortive photoreceptor structures. Whereas fleurettes were initially described in 18 of 200 consecutive cases of retinoblastoma, serial sectioning in our laboratory indicated that these may be found in about one-fourth of retinoblastomas. Tso and colleagues suggested that tumors containing such differentiated components are less radioresponsive [403]. A few tumors are exclusively composed of cells exhibiting photoreceptor differentiation with almost no mitoses. As noted, it has been suggested that these tumors be called retinomas or retinocytomas [269]. These could represent a benign example of the retinal tumor possibilities induced by abnormal retinoblastoma gene function. Interestingly, malignant transformation of this variant has been reported [118].

Growth Pattern

Two patterns of macroscopically observed growth are classically described. Demonstration of both types of growth pattern in the same tumor is often demonstrable on histological examination, but this distinction is still clinically relevant.

An *exophytic pattern* denotes growth primarily in the subretinal space, giving rise to a retinal detachment. Tumor cells may then infiltrate through Bruch's membrane into the choroid [439] and subsequently invade either blood vessels or ciliary nerves or vessels (Fig. 3).

An *endophytic pattern* describes growth into the vitreous space. The tumor is seen ophthalmo-scopically as one or more masses on the surface of the retina (Fig. 4). In contrast to the exophytic pattern, retinal vessels are not visible above the tumor. Neoplastic cells may also be seen as round masses floating in the vitreous and anterior chamber. Such an appearance may render the clinical diagnosis difficult

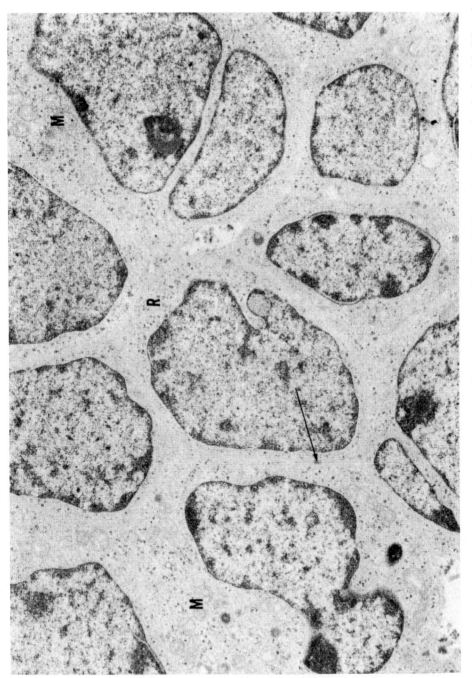

Figure 1 Undifferentiated retinoblastoma by transmission electron microscopy, showing cellular attachment (arrow), mitochondria (M), and aggregates of ribosomes (R) throughout the cytoplasm. Note the infoldings of some nuclear membranes. (×4000)

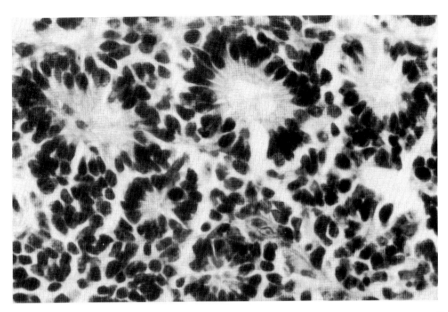

Figure 2 High-power light microscope view of Flexner-Wintersteiner rosette in a retinoblastoma. (Hematoxylin and eosin, ×700)

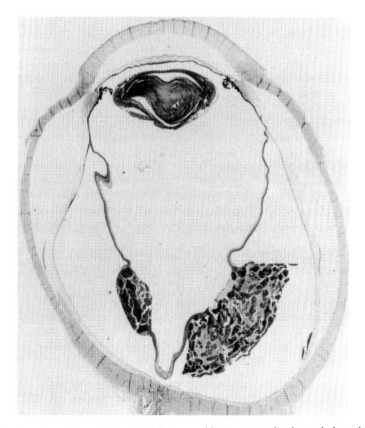

Figure 3 Exophytic pattern of growth in retinoblastoma with tumor growing beneath the retina. The retina is entirely detached. (Hematoxylin and eosin, ×5.2)

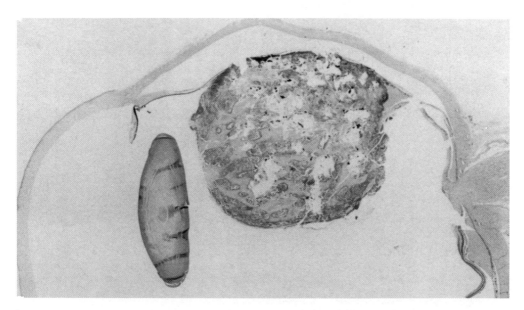

Figure 4   Endophytic retinoblastoma arising from the surface of the retina. (Hematoxylin and eosin, ×6.5)

since the appearance may simulate endophthalmitis or iridocyclitis. Secondary deposits or seeding of tumor cells into other areas of the retina may be confused with multicentric tumors.

Another presentation, which may pose diagnostic difficulties clinically, is an extensive retinoblastoma with necrosis, especially if it evokes much inflammation. Areas of necrosis are common, particularly in large retinoblastomas. Examination of these areas shows several prominent features: collars of viable tumor cells of uniform thickness surround the remaining blood vessels, often designated inappropriately as pseudorosettes; beyond these collars, areas of infarction are prominent. Frequently associated with the necrosis are areas of intra- and extracellular calcification (Figs. 5 and 6). In other areas of necrosis, numerous lymphocytes are observed, and the vascular endothelium is hyperplastic, which may occlude the vascular lumen in some areas [20,228,411]. Precipitated DNA originating from tumor cells occasionally surrounds and involves the wall of vessels and other structures at a distance from the tumor [290]. Areas of photoreceptor cell differentiation are characteristically devoid of necrosis. As a result of inflammation, probably related to necrosis, numerous inflammatory cells may be present, and in some cases, secondary endophthalmitis or panophthalmitis may occur [73,366,452]. Iris neovascularization accompanied by peripheral anterior synechiae or ectropion uveae may develop, with resultant glaucoma and/or hyphema [145].

Ultrastructure

Transmission Electron Microscopy.   Retinoblastoma cells have been examined by transmission electron microscopy (TEM) in some detail [26,46,110,135,184,271,318,319,320,397,402–405], and the ultrastructure of this tumor can be summarized as follows. (1) Photoreceptor cell elements occur within Flexner-Wintersteiner rosettes, and fleurettes represent photoreceptor cell differentiation. (2) Triple-membrane structures involving both the nuclear and cytoplasmic membranes are extremely common in retinoblastoma and fetal retina (Fig. 7). (3) Annulate lamellae, cytomembranes that structurally resemble a nuclear envelope, occur in a high percentage of the cells (Fig. 8). (4) Cilia are plentiful and appear in longitudinal, oblique, and transverse planes (Fig. 9). In transverse views, nine double tubules with no central pairs are seen. Most cilia in the body contain the central pair of tubules; the "9 + 0" type of cilia seen in retinoblastoma are also characteristic of the photoreceptor cell (Fig. 9). (5) Microtubules can be identified in most retinoblastoma cells, most commonly in the Golgi area, but may be diffusely distributed throughout the cytoplasm. These cytoplasmic components, of wide distribution, have an outside diameter of 15–27 nm, a wall thickness of approximately 5 nm, and an indefinite length. The microtubules are often

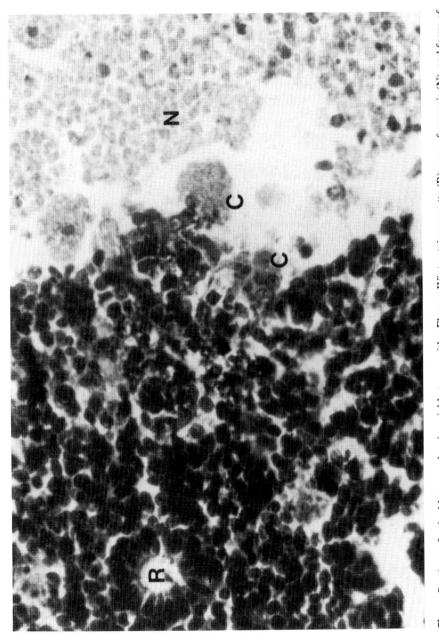

Figure 5 Area of retinoblastoma showing viable tumor with a Flexner-Wintersteiner rosette (R), area of necrosis (N), and focus of calcium deposition (C). (Hematoxylin and eosin, ×24)

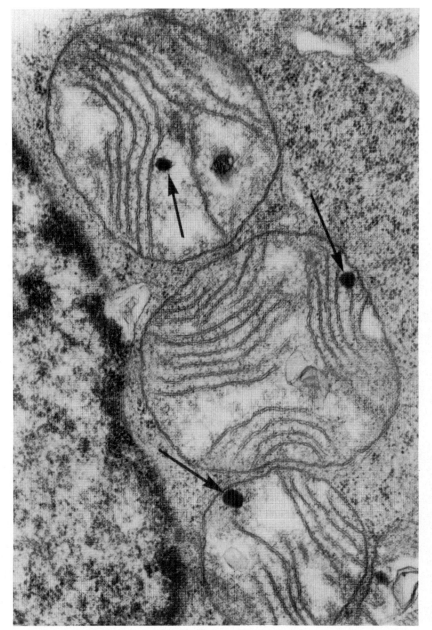

Figure 6 Giant mitochondria within a retinoblastoma cell. The dark material within the mitochondria (arrows) is calcium. This appears to be one of the earliest stages in the calcification of retinoblastoma cells. (×33,750)

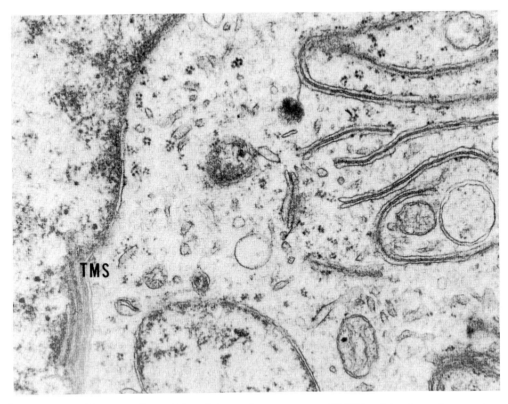

Figure 7 Retinoblastoma cell containing triple-membrane structures (TMS) involving the nuclear membrane. Note that triple-membrane infoldings are also present in the cytoplasm. (×32,000)

clumped together (Fig. 10) and on occasion may appear in the nucleus. The tubular structures observed by Fine [128] and by Sheffield [365] in rod fibers behave in a similar manner. In contrast, microtubules were not observed in chrome-osmium–fixed preparations of the nerve fiber layer or in Müller cells. (6) Bristle-coated vesicles are found free in cytoplasm, budding from the cell membrane, and in the intercellular spaces (Fig. 10). The coated vesicles are believed to form at the cell surface by a pinocytic invagination of the apical membrane and subsequently to move toward and fuse with multivesicular bodies, which serve to transport protein. (7) In addition, occasional retinoblastoma cells contain numerous dense-core granules structurally similar to those in cells of sympathetic innervation (Fig. 11). (8) Zonula adherens-like cell attachments occur that are similar to the junctions between normal photoreceptor cells (Fig. 12). Giant cells have occasionally been demonstrated in retinoblastoma, but their significance is not clearly understood [178].

Scanning Electron Microscopy. Scanning electron microscopy (SEM) has been applied in the study of the surface morphology of retinoblastoma [10,89]. This mode of investigation has disclosed two distinct populations of retinoblastoma cells. The first type of cell has abundant distinctive surface features, in contrast to the relatively featureless surface morphology of the second cell type (Fig. 13). The first type of cell exhibits surface projections (microvilli) that are continuous with the plasma membrane, have a diameter of 0.1 µm, and are of varying lengths (Fig. 14). Spherical extensions of the cell surface represent transient extrusions of cytoplasm (zeiotic blebs; Fig. 15). Rufflelike structures having a thickness of 1 µm, a height of 6–8 µm, and a length of 8 µm (lamellipodia) form on the free margin of the cell. Long, slender projections with a variable diameter ranging from 50 to 100 µm and a length of 18 µm (filopodia) also develop (Fig. 16). The second population of cells are spherical and smooth (Fig. 13) and are thought to represent cells in mitosis. The rosette pattern of a well-differentiated retinoblastoma is strikingly demonstrated by scanning electron microscopy.

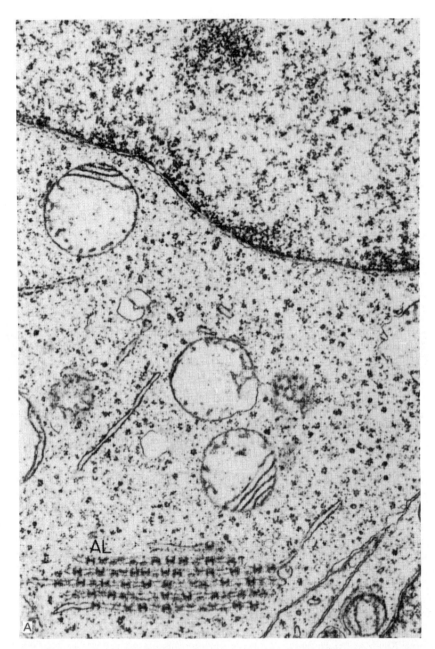

Figure 8 Annulate lamellae. (A) Longitudinal view of an annular lamella (AL). (×46,800) (B) Cross section. These structures have on occasion been mistaken for virus particles. (×52,000)

Immunocytochemistry

Neuron-Specific Enolase. "Neuron-specific" enolase (NSE) is a glycolytic isoenzyme of 2-phospho-glycerate and phosphoenolpyruvate [267,332]. This dimeric protein, composed of two γ subunits, is present in most neurons of the retina and central nervous system (CNS), and in neuroendocrine cells but also in neuroectodermal malignant tumors and in some reactive glia [54,101,150,157,270,305,343, 344,347,348,362,390,413–415,430]. In the retina NSE is detected in neuronal perikarya and in proteins, but not in the glia [206,207]. Many reports have demonstrated NSE in retinoblastoma and in tumor cell

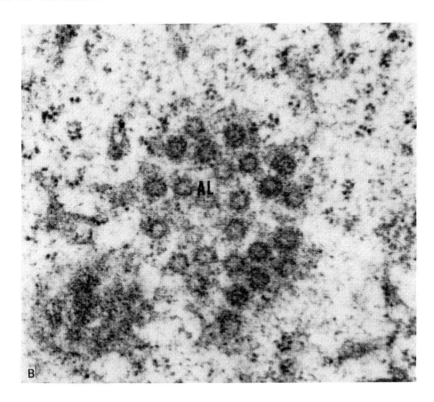

lines [4,206,207,224]. NSE has been detected both in undifferentiated areas and in well-differentiated Flexner-Wintersteiner rosettes and fleurettes [206,207,386].

Synaptophysin. Synaptophysin, a neural membrane glycoprotein of presynaptic vesicles, was detected immunohistochemically in 45 of 54 formalin-fixed and paraffin-embedded retinoblastoma specimens [417]. Western blotting of a major polypeptide conjugating with human brain synaptophysin was detected in retinoblastomas [211].

Neurofilaments. Neurofilaments (NF) are intermediate filaments composed of three triplet polypeptides of 68, 145, and 200 kD respectively, which may be phosphorylated [400]. Since malignant transformation is seldom reputed to alter cell intermediate filaments, these are seen as good markers of tumor cell origin and differentiation [307,356,401]. Kivela and colleagues have demonstrated neurofilaments (200 kD) in rare processes in the nerve fiber and inner plexiform layers in normal retinas; on the other hand, retinoblastoma cells were not stained [207,210,417]. Perentes and colleagues, however, detected NF (200 kD) in three of seven retinoblastomas [310]. Tarlton and Easty, using two different neurofilament antigens (155 and 210 kD) against retinoblastoma cells, found mild and no reactivity, respectively [394]. Further studies using phosphorylated and nonphosphorylated epitopes of the 68 and 145 kD neurofilament polypeptides are certainly needed [148].

Miscellaneous Biologically Active Peptides. Various markers of biologically active peptide synthesis, such as substance P and proenkephalon A, have been shown in a few retinoblastoma cells. These markers are usually attributed to amacrine cells [391,392]. Similarly, somatostatin-like and insulin-like immunoreactivity has been detected in both retinoblastoma specimens and cultured Y-79 retinoblastoma cells [107,207]. Tetanus toxin receptor, as well as dopamine β-hydroxylase, has been demonstrated in tumor cell lines [107,207]. The latter could be linked to the occasional ultrastructural finding of dense-core neurosecretory granules and of small amounts of catecholamines within retinoblastoma cells demonstrated by fluorescent and histochemical techniques [237,355]. Nevertheless, neurotransmitters and their receptors are not good markers of retinoblastoma.

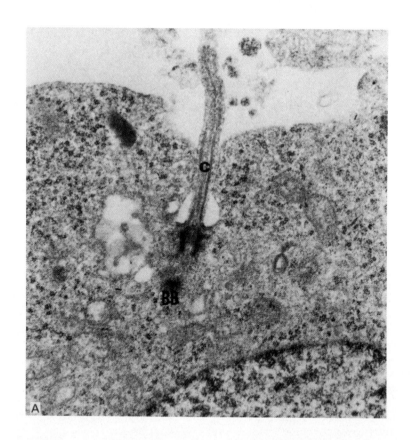

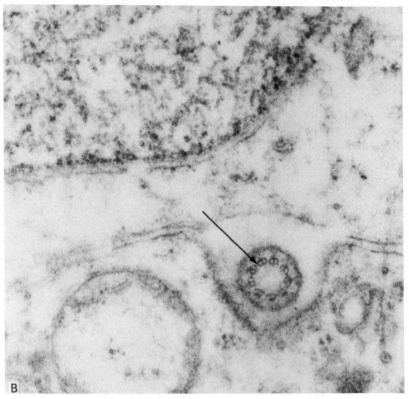

Photoreceptor Cell-Associated Antigens.   Strong evidence exists for the presence of photoreceptor cell elements in retinoblastoma. After preliminary studies by Felberg and Donoso [125], many antigens attributed to retinal photoreceptor cells have been scrutinized [420]. Rhodopsin has been demonstrated in fleurettes and Flexner-Wintersteiner rosettes using monoclonal antibodies [105]. S-antigen (arrestin) was detected by the use of both monoclonal and polyclonal antibodies [103,104,106,283,410] in the same differentiated structures, in diffuse areas of differentiated retinoblastoma, in trilateral retinoblastoma, and in cell lines, but not in nondifferentiated retinoblastomas. Donoso and colleagues further demonstrated that monoclonal antibodies to rhodopsin and S-antigen bound to the same areas [105]. Donoso and colleagues [107] mention a personal observation of retinoblastoma staining positively for α-transducin. This can be related to the finding of transcripts for the L-transducin, as well as for the red or green cone cell photo-pigment in all of seven low-passage retinoblastoma cell lines [49]. No marker genes to rod cells were expressed, and it is conceivable that retinoblastoma has a cone lineage.

Interphotoreceptor Cell Binding Protein.   Interphotoreceptor cell binding protein (IRBP), which is secreted by the rod photoreceptor cells into the extracellular matrix, has been detected in the lumen of Flexner-Wintersteiner rosettes [339–341], the amount of IRPB in tumor samples correlating with the degree of tumor differentiation [339].

Using Western and Northern blots and radiolabeled ligand binding techniques, Fong and colleagues investigated retinoid binding proteins in fresh tumors and cell lines [58,133]. They concluded that (1) the expression of retinoid binding proteins is variable in tumor cells; (2) the only retinoid binding protein consistently expressed by both types of cells is IRPB at a level similar to that in the normal retina at 22 weeks gestation; and (3) these findings are consistent with an embryonic origin for the cells. Fong and colleagues further speculated that the tumor does not arise earlier than the 22 week stage.

Tarlton and Easty tested a panel of 18 monoclonal antibodies against six retinoblastomas and compared the reactivity of the tumors with adult and fetal retina. They concluded that the closest normal cell type is a 13–16 week outer retinal cell. The antigens expressed in the tumor could be detected in both the inner and outer nuclear layers of the retina [394]. Because of the potential of the precursor cell to differentiate into photoreceptor cells as well as "inner" retinal cells, Tarlton and Easty propose that the tumor arises from a primitive multipotential cell type that predominates before week 8 of gestation and declines in parallel with later retinal development.

Glia-Associated Antigens.   A few studies have provided support for glial differentiation in retino-blastomas. Shuangshoti and colleagues [373] detected glial markers in 23 of 39 retinoblastomas, whereas 18 contained neuronal markers. These findings are consistent with those of Molnar and colleagues [285] and of Messmer and colleagues [274], who observed glial fibrillary acidic protein (GFAP), an intermediate filament typical of astrocytes, in 1 of 7 and 2 of 50 tumors, respectively. Most reports, however, interpret GFAP as well as S-100 staining as markers of reactive astrocytes in retinoblastoma since positive cells are located around blood vessels and in reactive areas of the tumor or radiating into the tumor from the bordering retina and optic nerve [209,210,238,349,396,452]. Most cell culture experiments demonstrated exclusive neuronal differentiation, but a few independent studies document coexpression of neuronal and glial markers in tumor cell lines and fresh tumor tissue [65,66,207,234]. In tissue studies a glial component has been demonstrated in Flexner-Wintersteiner rosettes and is suspected of being neoplastic [90]. As emphasized by several authors, the hypothesis that a multipotential neuroectodermal precursor of both neurons and glia exists is not ruled out [99,234].

HNK-1 Epitope.   HNK-1 monoclonal antibody raised against HSB-2 human T lymphoblastoid cell lines recognizes a carbohydrate epitope shared by various molecules (myelin-associated glycoproteins, neuroendocrine secretory granules [207,311], and neural cell adhesion molecules) [206,207,311]. The HNK-1 epitope is expressed in the embryonic retina on putative precursor cells of both neuronal and glial cells [205]. This epitope is detected in ganglion cell bodies near the inner limiting membrane and neuronal

Figure 9   (A) Longitudinal section of a cilium (C) and a basal body (BB) in a retinoblastoma cell. ($\times 21{,}600$) (B) Transverse section of a cilium in a retinoblastoma, illustrating a ring of nine double tubules: the central pair is absent. ($\times 45{,}000$)

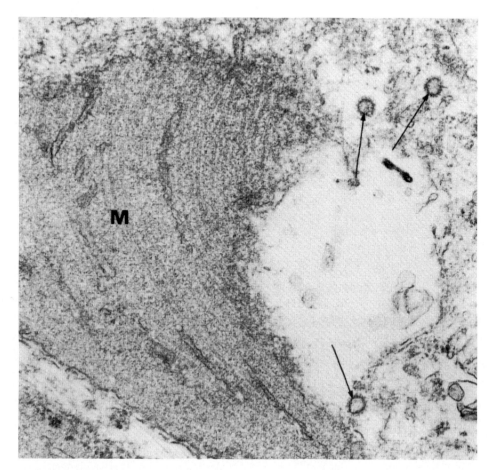

Figure 10　TEM of microtubules. A cluster of microtubules (M) is seen within a retinoblastoma; coated vesicles are also present (arrows). (×43,000)

processes in both plexiform layers [205]. Myelin-associated glycoprotein is present in Müller cells [205,207].

Leu-7 Antigen.　The Leu-7 antigen, a glycoprotein of natural killer lymphocytes sharing epitopes with myelin-associated glycoprotein and detectable in cell processes of all retinal layers, has not been detected in retinoblastoma cells [205,310,311]. Carcinoembryonic antigen, which is elevated in the plasma of some patients with retinoblastoma, was not detected by immunohistochemistry in the tumors [208]. Kivela demonstrated in 10 retinoblastomas lectin binding properties similar to those of photoreceptor cells (concanavalin A conjugates) [205,207]. Kivela's findings, as well as those of others [34,125], in cell lines demonstrate similarities between photoreceptors and both differentiated and undifferentiated retinoblastoma cells. However, the specificity of most lectin bindings must be interpreted with caution.

It is difficult to draw conclusions from such contradictory data. Tissue culture studies were first attempted to determine the cell of origin and differentiation patterns of retinoblastoma [166,234,246]. Both plasticity and multipotentiality were demonstrated, which contradicts many studies providing evidence for a neuronal nature and differentiation. Therefore, the data from animal studies, such as transgenic mouse models, concerning the origin of the tumor should be of great interest.

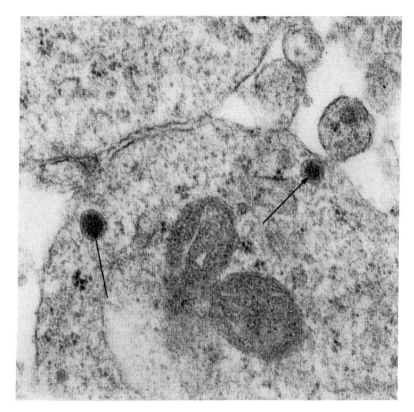

Figure 11   TEM of dense-core granules within a retinoblastoma cell (arrows). ($\times 43,000$)

D. Natural History

Spontaneous Regression

Complete spontaneous regression of retinoblastoma is an unusual but well-documented entity. It is usually characterized by a severe inflammatory reaction followed by phthisis bulbi, and 22 histopathological reports of 39 such tumors have been published [20,52,53,197,253,287,298,327,380]. Most authors have incriminated infarction of the tumor consecutive to a central vessel obstruction [20,356]. Histopathological reports of these cases demonstrate dense calcification , necrotic tissue, fossilized tumor cells, massive proliferation of the RPE, inflammatory reaction, and variable degrees of ossification. Marcus and colleagues emphasize that a reliable distinction between such spontaneous necrosis and retinomas-retinocytomas in nonphthisical eyes has not been made [268]. These authors concur with Zimmerman in viewing such tumors as benign variants of retinoblastoma [452]. Reports of a malignant transformation of a retinoma-retinocytoma variant support this concept [118]. Both completely regressed retinoblastomas and retinocytomas differ from regression patterns observed after irradiation (i.e., formation of a glial scar with complete destruction of the tumor and associated atrophy of surrounding choroid and vessels following treatment) [268].

Intraocular Spread

The pattern of retinoblastoma spread both within and outside the eye is well recognized and documented [169,327,444,452]. Retinoblastoma is generally a poorly cohesive neoplasm that may grow in all directions. This poor cohesion may be related to the apparently defective or absent zonula adherens and/or filopodia, which normally contribute to cell-cell attachment. Tumor cells commonly seed anteriorly, in the vitreous and aqueous. Cells may be deposited on the surface of the iris and in the anterior chamber angle,

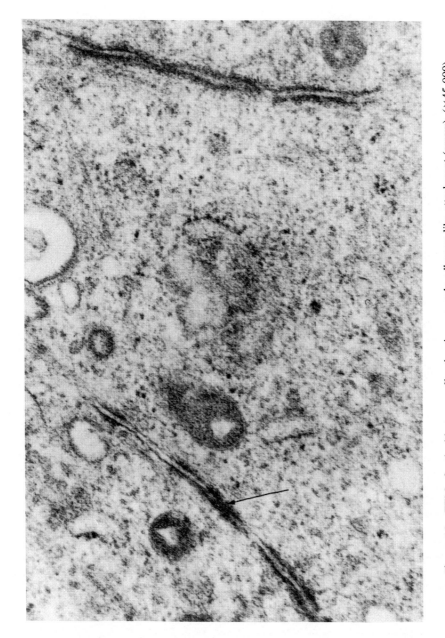

Figure 12   TEM of retinoblastoma cells, showing a zonula adherens-like attachment (arrow). (×45,000)

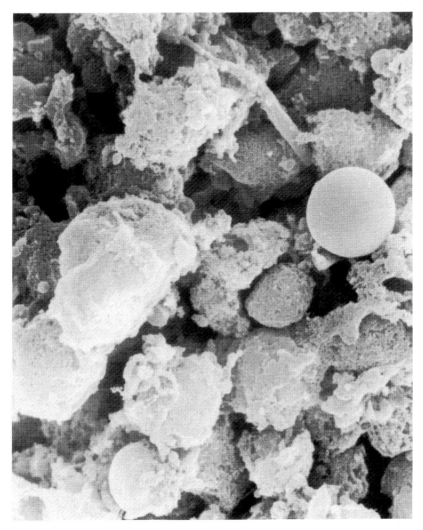

Figure 13 SEM of retinoblastoma cells, showing two general types: the smooth, spherelike cell and the more numerous cells with profuse surface features. (×2500)

giving rise to a secondary glaucoma and/or pseudohypopyon [159]. Clusters of tumor cells may collect on the inner surface of the retina and grow as separate foci, particularly in the peripheral retina and at the ora serrata. These secondary lesions may be mistaken for additional primary sites of retinoblastoma development. The presence of intravitreal clusters of cells and of the major portion of the tumor at the inner retinal surface is helpful in distinguishing secondary deposits from additional primary foci [452]. Another common pattern of spread is posteriorly into the subretinal space. The significance of minimal choroidal invasion is still disputed. Massive choroidal invasion, however, usually correlates with a high risk of scleral, orbital, and hematogenous spread. Invasion of the optic nerve may occur at the base of the optic cup, in the area of the central vessels, or into the subarachnoid space adjacent of optic nerve (Fig. 17).

Extraocular Spread

Tumor cells may disseminate hematogenously through choroidal or other vessels in proximity to the subarachnoid space [444,452]. Infiltrative spread through the optic nerve [264] or subarachnoid space gives access to orbital tissues and brain [423a]. Retinoblastoma may also reach the orbit through the

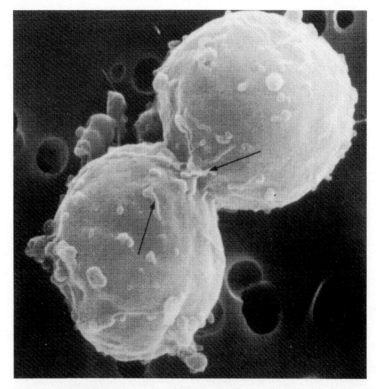

Figure 14 SEM of two retinoblastoma cells with microvilli on a Nucleopore filter (arrows). (×5000)

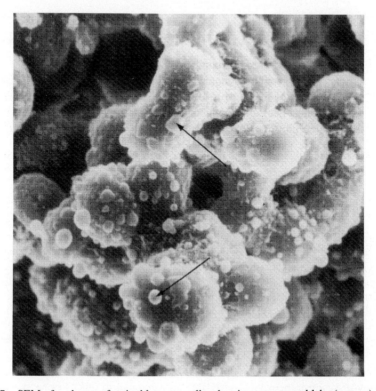

Figure 15 SEM of a cluster of retinoblastoma cells, showing numerous blebs (arrows). (×2000)

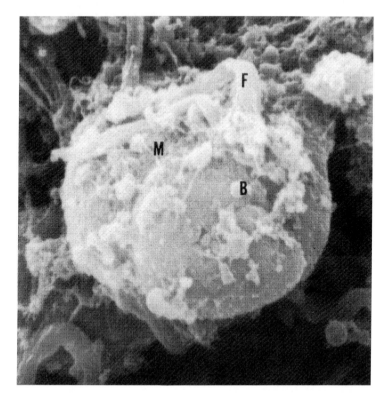

Figure 16   Retinoblastoma cells by SEM showing zeiotic blebs (B), microvilli (M), and thick filopodia (F). ($\times 5000$)

emissarium. In a similar manner, tumor may grow through paracentesis sites and spread subconjunctivally [379]. In advanced cases, retinoblastoma may massively penetrate through the sclera and grow extensively into the orbit [122]. Metastases to the preauricular and cervical lymph nodes usually follow such massive extraocular metastases [69]. Recurrence of retinoblastoma in the orbit following enucleation is suspected of being the consequence of subclinical orbital involvement escaping recognition or from residual tumor in the remaining optic nerve.

Metastases

The most common sites of distant metastasis of retinoblastoma are the CNS, skull, distal bones, lymph nodes, and spinal cord [273] with spread to bones beyond the skull noted in about 50% of patients dying from the neoplasm. Although most metastases are detected within the first 2 years after diagnosis, some may become apparent many years after the last evidence of tumor activity in the retina is noted [185,447]. In such cases, a new primary tumor should be considered. Usually metastases to bone and brain from retinoblastoma do not show evidence of rosette and fleurette formation and may resemble Ewing's sarcoma, neuroblastoma, or other small round cell tumors of childhood. In such cases, immunohistochemistry and tissue culture, as well as electron microscopy, may be of diagnostic value [12,82,452]. This lack of differentiation is helpful to distinguish such lesions from midbrain tumors in trilateral retinoblastoma.

E. Tumor Cell Biology: Cell Culture

Biology of the tumor cells has been best studied in tissue culture since the early 1970s, particularly after the establishment of the Y-79 cell line [244] and the WERI-Rb1 line [17,142]. These cell lines, as well as other systems, have been used for studies on cell growth, differentiation, attachment, and tumorigenicity, as well as experimental evaluation of new therapeutic approaches [65,66].

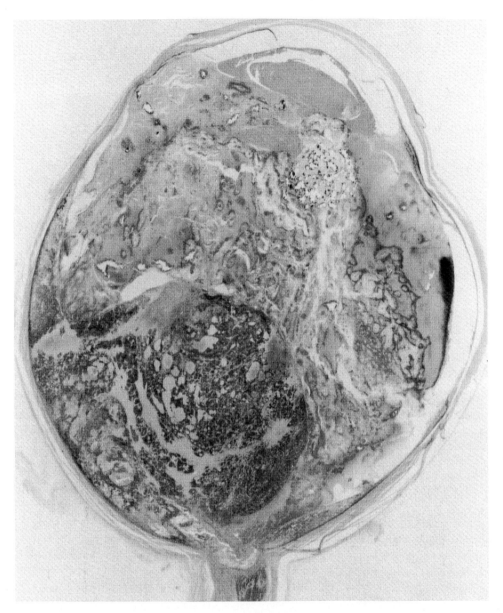

Figure 17   Low-power view of a section of an eye with a retinoblastoma extending to fill vitreous cavity. Also note the presence of tumor in the optic nerve. (Hematoxylin and eosin, ×7)

The Y-79 cell line was first established in 1974 [330] from an undifferentiated tumor. Electron microscopy shows close similarities between cultured cells and the original tumor [66]. Another cell line, WERI-Rb1, was established in 1977 [260]. The two cell lines are similar except for their doubling times: 33 h for the Y-79 compared with 96 h for the WERI-Rb1 cells. Short-term cultures of tumor-derived cells are also feasible. Tumor cells usually retain their differentiation potential in this model. Both established cell lines grow as monolayers on special layers, such as poly-D-lysine or laminin. They attach directly to feeder cell layers (iris pigment epithelium, RPE, rat smooth muscle, human embryonic fibroblasts, and conjunctival fibroblasts).

Tumorigenicity was analyzed principally by injecting Y-79 or WERI-Rb1 into the anterior chambers of athymic "nude" mice [141,262,428,436]. These cells rapidly filled the eyes and invaded the optic nerve, orbit, subarachnoid space, and brain, and a characteristic fibrovascular stroma became prominent. Although tumor cells from fresh retinoblastomas can grow inside the eyes, no invasion beyond the eye was observed in this model. This difference may be related to the more aggressive behavior of Y-79 cells. In parallel with these tumorigenicity assays, growth control parameters, such as oncogenes and growth factors, have been investigated. As oncogenes, the increased expression of N-myc in tumor cells may simply reflect the rapidly proliferating state of these cells and may not be a factor in their malignant transformation [28,244,377]. A growth factor called RDGF (retinoblastoma-derived growth factor) was extracted in 1981 from the media of Y-79 cells [346]. Its action may be mediated through protein tyrosine kinase activities in a manner similar to that of epidermal growth factor or platelet-derived growth factor. Phosphorylation of tyrosine as a consequence of RDGF elaboration may contribute to tumor growth.

Other substances produced by tumor cells, such as basic fibroblast growth factor, may account for the angiogenic activity of Rb cells [64,67,230–233,364]. The effects on tumor growth of differentiating agents, such as retinoids (retinol and retinoic acid), butyrate, cAMP, or vitamin D, have been assayed on cultured cells [254–258]. Retinol, butyrate, retinoic acid, and vitamin D inhibit cell growth in both cultures and nude mouse eyes. Butyrate appears to block the cells in the G phase of the cell cycle. Experiments from Kyritsis and colleagues argue for an action of butyrate at the nuclear level on a regulatory subunit of the type I cAMP-dependent protein kinase [230,232]. Abnormalities of this enzyme system in the Y79 cells have been demonstrated [231,232,235]. Studies on retinol and retinoic acid argue for an irreversible effect through the cytoplasm, causing cell death by the former and a reversible, nuclear hormone-like effect by the latter [65,230]. Studies of the effects of vitamin D on retinoblastoma cells both in culture systems and in the nude mouse model indicate inhibition of tumor growth [80].

The numerous immunohistochemical studies of cultured retinoblastomas and of cells derived from them suggest that retinoblastomas have a multipotential nature and amazing plasticity [48,149,166,234, 246,398,406,417]. Interestingly, Turner and Cepko showed an in vivo conservation of multipotential differentiation patterns in the normal retina [408]. In cell culture, differentiation of tumor cells toward almost any particular cell type, including RPE, can be induced by appropriately adding culture substrate (laminin, fibronectin, and integrin) and differentiating agents (butyrate and laminin) [67,236]. For example, laminin, an extracellular matrix attachment molecule, promoted the axonal outgrowth of retinal ganglion cells and attachment and neurite outgrowth of Y-79 cells [67]. However, the susceptibility of these tissue culture models to microenvironmental factors must arouse caution in the interpretation of such findings as the multipotentiality of retinoblastoma cells [303]. Studies of animal models are needed to evaluate the in vitro studies.

F. Animal Models

Beside the nude mouse model of retinoblastoma [41], which represents an extrapolation of the culture systems model, two types of retinal tumors have been induced by viruses [15,45,144,302,384,434,451].

Human Adenovirus 12 Model

A retinal tumor develops in the eyes of newborn rats after an intraocular injection of human adenovirus [12,222,223,224,288]. However, despite ultrastructural and immunohistochemical [224] similarities to retinoblastoma, the search for human adenovirus markers in human tumors has been negative [265]. Yet the enzyme RNA-directed DNA polymerase (reverse transcriptase) was detected in a human retinoblastoma by Albert and colleagues [11,15,16,19,328,329] as well as in various animal tumors [33,144].

Simian Virus 40 Large T Antigen Transgenic Models

In 1990 a new model of retinoblastoma was described in transgenic mice [302,434]. This heritable tumor was created by the retinal expression of simian virus 40 (SV40) large T-antigen (T-Ag), and the resultant T-Ag oncoprotein. The construct used (luteininizing hormone β subunit gene/SV large T antigen) was designed to cause pituitary tumors. However, one transgenic male developed bilateral ocular tumors. This founder subsequently gave rise to a colony of transgenic mice inheriting retinal tumors with SV40 T-Ag. Morphological and immunohistochemical characterization of these tumors indicates that they mimic human retinoblastoma. Moreover, a similar progression pattern and a primary midbrain tumor ("trilateral" retinoblastoma) were observed [434].

In this model, immunoprecipitation and western blot analysis showed that SV40 T-Ag and p105-Rb were found together within tumor cells.

The inactivation of the retinoblastoma protein (p105Rb) by a viral oncoprotein (SV40 T-Ag) has now led to a renewed investigation of the role of viruses in oncogenesis [29,116,117,302,434]. Other studies of this model with regards to tumor ontogeny, proliferation, and treatment are also in progress.

A second transgenic model of retinoblastoma expressing the SV40 large T antigen contains the phenylethanolamine methyltransferase promoter [32a]. A third transgenic model of an ocular tumor occurs in mice expressing the SV40 large T antigen controlled by the promoter of the gene for human inter-photoreceptor cell-binding protein (IRBP) [133a]. The tumors in these mice have similarities to retino-blastomas.

G. Clinical Diagnosis

The presenting signs and symptoms in over 65% of retinoblastomas are in order of decreasing frequency: leukocoria or "cat's eye" reflex [37,38,148,180], strabismus, and a red and painful eye with or without glaucoma and poor vision [59,73,293,327,366,367]. Less frequent modes of presentation include ocular inflammation (granulomatous iridocyclitis), hyphema, and glaucoma or, in neglected cases, suspected trauma to the eye, fundus observed by hazy media, or metastatic disease [163,375,427]. Ocular inflammation, is often a misdiagnosed presentation and is a poor prognostic sign [159,378].

A child under 3 years of age with any of these signs and symptoms should be suspected of retinoblastoma. The finding of multiple tumors arising from the retina of variable color and appearance is almost diagnostic, as well as a large unilateral calcified tumor [181]. Retinoblastoma is diagnosed occasionally in the first weeks of life. This occurs particularly when there is a family history of the disease and ocular examination is carried out under general anesthesia and indentation of the peripheral globe [181]. Multiple tumor nodules can reflect either a true multifocality in origin or vitreous seeding of the tumor.

Computed tomography (CT) is sometimes a useful ancillary test in the diagnosis of retinoblastoma, since more than 90% of these tumors contain calcium as detected by light microscopy; x-ray examination is far less sensitive [213,278,314,422]. High-resolution computed tomography can also detect retroorbital and intracranial tumor growth [278]. Spread past the lamina cribrosa is sometimes less reliably demonstrated [278].

Ultrasonography is also able to detect calcifications [369] within the tumor and orbit. Optic nerve invasion is less accurately visualized with this diagnostic procedure, and intracranial metastases or pinealomas are beyond the scope of this technique. Measurement of the axial length of the globe can be helpful since eyes with retinoblastoma are almost never microophthalmic, except for regressed tumors with phthisis bulbi [114].

Magnetic resonance imaging (MRI) has proven inferior to CT scan with regards to diagnostic specificity and sensitivity in detecting calcifications and small tumors [263,313,363]. Yet, the pattern observed may prove useful in the differential diagnosis with Coats' disease, toxocariasis, or persistent hyperplastic primary vitreous [263,313,453] and in the determination of tumor differentiation. The use of [123I]*meta*-iodobenzylguanidine scintigraphy may also become helpful in imaging occult metastatic disease [50,51].

Assays of aqueous lactic dehydrogenase [102,193,296,342,383] or neuron-specific enolase [39,45] and serum levels of αfetoprotein, carcinoembryonic antigen, and catecholamines [156,276,282,290, 325,329,331,354] have been inconsistent and unreliable in the diagnosis of retinoblastoma.

Despite the availability of fine-needle aspiration biopsy to diagnose retinoblastoma [30,73,75], this technique has not been generally accepted as a safe by the ophthalmic community. The usefulness of bone marrow aspirations and lumbar punctures in the initial metastatic work-up of patients with retinoblastoma [24,351] was recently called into question in view of the very infrequent positivity of those tests in children without clinical or histological evidence of extraocular tumor dissemination [322].

II. NONOCULAR TUMORS AND TRILATERAL RETINOBLASTOMA

A. Trilateral Retinoblastoma

The association of bilateral retinoblastoma with a midline intracranial malignancy located in the pineal or parasellar region has become appreciated during the past decade and termed trilateral retinoblastoma [31,32,188,312,370]. Although such intracranial tumors were reported previously, they were considered either metastases or unrelated to retinoblastoma. Jakobiec and colleagues [188] recorded two indisputable cases, and this entity was characterized by Bader and colleagues in 1980 [31,32]. These intracranial tumors are most often suprasellar or parasellar neuroblastomas and undifferentiated neuroblastic pineal tumors (pinealoblastomas). About 50 such cases have now been reported [312,370]. A unilateral retinoblastoma is only exceptionally associated with midline intracranial neoplasms [188,452].

These case reports on all trilateral retinoblastomas and histological data, together with the description of retinoblastoma-like differentiation in pineal tumors associated with retinoblastoma and the report of a suprasellar tumor in the sister of a child affected with trilateral retinoblastoma, all suggest that such midbrain tumors represent a third site of expression of the Rb genetic predisposition. This is similar to the transgenic mouse model [434]. Since midline intracranial neoplasms are the most frequent cause of death in patients with bilateral retinoblastomas before the age of 10 years, the use of high-resolution imaging techniques to allow their early detection is mandatory.

B. Nonintracranial Second Tumors

As demonstrated by Abramson and colleagues [3], the genetic predisposition to heritable retinoblastoma may also result in nonocular tumors (such as osteosarcomas) [161] or soft tissue sarcomas in retinoblastoma survivors or in their relatives [14,78,79,98,257,284,323,437]. The development of such tumors is related to the existence of structural deletions or mutations of the retinoblastoma gene in osteosarcomas [161], small cell lung cancers, breast carcinomas, and other tumors [162,247,257]. The risk of nonocular cancer in survivors of bilateral retinoblastoma was recently calculated [5,98,272,335]. The 30 year cumulative index was 35.1% for patients subjected to radiation therapy, and the rate within the field of radiation was 29.3%. This is in comparison with an incidence of 5.8% during the same period for patients who had not received radiotherapy and with a rate of 8.1% for tumors outside the field of radiation. The use of cyclophosphamide is also incriminated. Tumors reported in the field of radiation include osteosarcomas, chondrosarcomas, malignant melanomas, and sebaceous and other carcinomas [14,78,79,98,257,284, 323,437]. The relative risk of such nonocular cancer in carriers of the retinoblastoma predisposition was evaluated by Sanders and colleagues in a large population sample and found to be 9.9 greater than in noncarriers [353]. The risk for death from lung cancer was 15 times higher for carriers of the abnormal Rb gene than in the general population [272,381].

C. Staging and Prognosis

The overall 92% 5 year survival rate commonly quoted for patients treated for retinoblastoma is misleading since many different clinical situations are lumped together [279].

Two clinical staging systems are now available to predict the local outcome of eye-saving conservative treatment. It should be emphasized that both are intended to provide information within the context of treatment regimens only. The Reese-Ellsworth classification (Table 1) was developed to predict the chance of survival of the eye after external beam radiotherapy. It has been widely used for more than 30 years, but many ocular oncologists, including Ellsworth himself, believe it requires significant changes [120,121, 123], and an alternative working classification proposed by De Sutter and colleagues is at present employed in several oncology centers [96,171].

The following clinical considerations are important in terms of prognosis [227]: (1) professional competence, (2) age at diagnosis, (3) time at which diagnosis is made, (4) staging, and (5) bilaterality.

A multivariate statistical analysis of tumors in Ellsworth group V tumors [345] showed that all prognostic factors are related to "histological" features, namely optic nerve length < 5 mm removed at enucleation (p = 0.001), optic nerve involvement (p = 0.004), and large tumor size (p = 0.01). It seems that histological features are the best survival predictors [96]. The degree of optic nerve involvement is

Table 1   Classification of Retinoblastomas Based in Prognostic Indicators

Group 1: very favorable
   Solitary tumor smaller than 4 disk diameters, at or behind the equator
   Multiple tumors, none larger than 4 disk diameters, all at or behind the equator
Group 2: favorable
   Solitary tumor 4–10 disk diameters in size, at or behind the equator
   Multiple tumors 4–10 disk diameters in size, all behind the equator
Group 3: doubtful
   Any lesion anterior to the equator
   Solitary tumor larger than 10 disk diameters, behind the equator
Group 4: unfavorable
   Multiple tumors, some larger than 10 disk diameters
   Any lesion extending anterior to the ora serrata
Group 5: very unfavorable
   Massive tumors involving over half the retina
   Vitreous seeding

generally considered the most reliable single prognostic indicator (Fig. 18) [444,452]. The mortality rate varies with the extent of the optic nerve involvement, and it is essential that the surgeon excise a length section of the optic nerve of at least 10 mm at enucleation. Some authors advocate the use of frozen sections at the time of surgery to check the adequacy of optic nerve section [195]. Magramm and colleagues [264], in a review of 814 patients, found 240 cases of optic nerve invasion (29.5%). These were classified as follows:

Grade I. Superficial invasion of the optic nerve head only; mortality rate 10%
Grade II. Involvement up to and including the lamina cribrosa; mortality rate 29%
Grade III. Involvement beyond the lamina cribrosa; mortality rate 42%
Grade IV. Involvement up to and including the surgical margin; mortality rate 78%

These investigators did not find choroidal involvement, scleral extension, or laterality to be significant covariants. The only other significant association was age at diagnosis. Other authors have found massive choroidal extension and iris neovascularization (rubeosis iridis) to be associated with poor prognosis [45,326]. Many conflicting data exist on retinoblastoma prognosis; we emphasize the following:

1. The lack of an incontrovertible correlation between the degree of differentiation and prognosis, except for retinocytomas, is in contrast to the initial studies, which assigned a sixfold better prognosis to differentiated tumors [404,407,452].
2. The impact on prognosis of the occurrence of nonocular cancers [69,165].

D. Management

A detailed discussion of treatment modalities exceeds the scope of this text [121,163,172,324]. We believe that it is important to stress the importance of referral to oncology centers able to combine such various techniques as cryotherapy, external beam radiotherapy, rotating ^{125}I plaque therapy, chemotherapy, and bone marrow replacement [8,26,27,56,138,177,179,198,286,333,350,368,438]. With the increasing use of improved therapeutic modalities, a gradual but definite decrease in the frequency of enucleation as the primary treatment for both unilateral and bilateral tumors was recently reported [371,372]. The experience, which has been gained principally in large referral centers, is a significant prognostic factor [73,121,123,294,366].

III. RETINAL INVOLVEMENT IN LEUKEMIA

Ocular manifestations of leukemia are common, although they may not be detected clinically [203] for want of careful fundus examination. Prevalence figures vary from 28% [299] through 50% [25] to

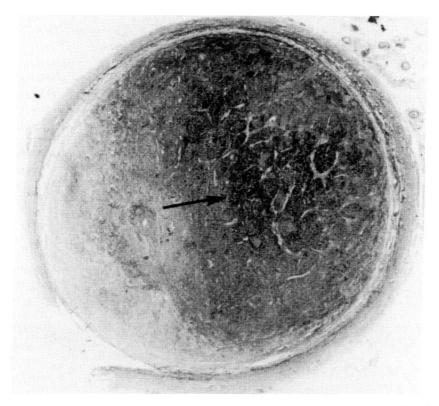

Figure 18   Massive invasion of the optic nerve by retinoblastoma (arrow). (Hematoxylin and eosin, ×18)

approximately 80% [203]. The study by Kincaid and Green [203] showed no variation in this percentage between 1923 and 1980 and little difference between acute (82%) and chronic (75%) leukemia. Duke-Elder asserted that at some stage of the disease 90% of patients display fundus abnormalities [113].

These high rates are the reflection of various mechanisms of dysfunction involving the eye in leukemia: (1) direct invasion by neoplastic cells whether definite (leukemic infiltrates) or putative (white-centered ocular hemorrhages); (2) hematological abnormalities associated with leukemia (anemia and thrombocytopenia); (3) complications of hyperviscosity (microaneurysms, closure of capillaries, ischemia, and neovascularization); and (4) opportunistic infections.

More prospective studies of patients examined at the time of diagnosis are needed to determine accurately the prevalence of ocular changes: Guyer and colleagues found ocular abnormalities in 42% of 117 consecutive patients with acute leukemia (51 acute lymphocytic and 66 acute myelogenous). They found an association between thrombocytopenia and retinal hemorrhages for all patients, and a lower hematocrit level was counted in patients with acute lymphocytic leukemia and retinal hemorrhages. Anemia was correlated with the finding of a white-centered hemorrhage in patients with nonlymphocytic leukemia [158].

Retinal infiltrates appear as gray-white nodules of varying size or streaks alongside the vessels [25,204,229,336] and are reportedly associated with an elevated leukocyte count, a high proportion of blast cells, and a poor prognosis. Some authors emphasize that ocular leukemic infiltration detected in autopsy series could be related to the peripheral leukocyte count during the final hours of life [248]. Choroidal infiltrates are more common than retinal infiltrates but are often undetectable clinically except when indicated by the occurrence of RPE alterations (atrophy, hypertrophy, or hyperplasia) or serous detachment of the RPE or the sensory retina [25,63,77,147,186]. Vitreous infiltration is less usual than in large-cell lymphoma ("reticulum cell sarcoma").

IV. LYMPHOMAS OF RETINA

A. General

Except for the so-called reticulum cell sarcoma vitreoretinal involvement by tumor cells in Hodgkin's or non-Hodgkin's lymphoma has rarely been documented pathologically [146,196,199,299,357]. Diffuse large cell lymphomas have often referred to as reticulum cell sarcomas or histiocytic lymphomas and microgliomatosis. [129,130,266,304,360]. However, the large cells composing the tumors are transformed B and T lymphocytes, according to immunocytochemical and in vitro lymphocyte function studies [321]. Unfortunately, the lack of a fully accepted definitive classification of non-Hodgkin's lymphomas and the relative paucity of information on intraocular involvement by lymphomas has unfortunately led to the continued use of the misnomer "reticulum cell sarcoma" instead of large cell lymphoma. This tumor occurs most frequently between 37 and 82 years, with a mean age of diagnosis at 61 years. More than 120 cases have now been reported, making this disease far less novel than it was a decade ago [25,35,82, 82,137,152,156,212,275,281,300,303,304,308,327,382,419]. There is no clear sexual or ethnic predisposition, and 80% of reported cases have appeared bilaterally, although they were frequently asymmetrical. The mean interval between diagnosis and death according to one report was 39 months [137].

Two forms of clinical presentation are recognized: (1) a systemic form and (2) a primary CNS form [200,297]. Ocular involvement is detected more usually in association with CNS participation (56% in one series) [137]; visceral involvement is less often associated with ocular involvement, being present in 22% of cases in another report [137]. Isolated ocular involvement is rare [35,212,382]. In the CNS form the tumor probably develops multicentrically in the eye and brain [137,201,202,297]. Nevertheless, it should be emphasized that large cell lymphoma is likely to be seen first by the ophthalmologist. A delay of more than 1 year between the onset of symptoms and definitive diagnosis is usual. Prompt diagnosis and radiotherapy can lead to prolonged survival, however, and it is important to suspect this diagnosis in older patients with torpid, idiopathic uveitis.

Indeed, the most common initial manifestation of intraocular large cell lymphomas mimics uveitis, especially choroiditis [29]. The symptoms, usually floaters or loss of vision, commonly precede the onset of neurological symptoms. Clinical findings at the posterior pole may include an "inflammatory" vitreous haze and subretinal cellular infiltrations, characteristically appearing as large yellowish multifocal subpigment epithelial plaques with sharp margins and progressive confluence [137,212,239,275]. Various other signs have been reported, including retinal or vitreous hemorrhages, optic neuropathy, papilledema, exudative retinal detachment, and punched-out lesions of the RPE [137,212].

The clinically apparent "inflammatory cells" are found on histopathological examination to be tumor cells in combination with a reactive inflammatory leukocyte reactive compound. Alternatively, it is possible that the inflammatory process precedes neoplasia [200].

B. Diagnosis

A systemic and neurological workup is mandatory both to help establish the diagnosis and to determine the necessary therapeutic approach. The workup should include hematological studies, CT scan, MRI, lumbar puncture, and possibly visceral biopsies.

Lumbar puncture and cerebrospinal fluid cytological examination may obviate the need for diagnostic vitrectomy, yet, in many cases the tissue diagnosis requires a vitreous examination. This vitreous surgery is often aimed at both establishing an earlier diagnosis and also eventually helping to improve vision [156,275].

C. Histopathology

Vitreous samples from suspected cases are passed through a Millipore filter and stained with Papanicolaou stain [154,275]. Typically the tumor cells are large pleomorphic cells with scant cytoplasm and have round, oval, or indented nuclei with prominent, eccentrically located nucleoli [91,266,317,419]. Characteristic fingerlike outpouchings are seen in some nuclei.

On cytopathological examination the presence of an intense inflammatory element may be confusing. Some authors emphasize that the finding of apparently normal lymphocytes only in an aspirate does not eliminate the diagnosis [73,154]. Immunocytochemical identification of monoclonal B cells is indicative of neoplasia [84,194]. Transmission electron microscopy may demonstrate intranuclear inclusions, cytoplasmic crystalloids, and occasional pseudopodial extensions and cytosomes, as well as autophagic vacuoles [175]. When a high level of clinical suspicion exists, some authors advocate a retinochoroidal biopsy, arguing that the uvea is more densely infiltrated than the vitreous [73]. Studies of enucleated eyes have disclosed that the tumor cells in the retina, like those in brain, have a perivascular pattern, whereas the uvea usually contains diffuse infiltrations of closely packed cells arranged in closely packed plaques. Characteristically the cells tend to accumulate between the RPE and Bruch's membrane [266]. This uveal infiltration differs from uveal infiltration by low-grade small lymphoplasmacytic lymphomas that do not involve the retina and vitreous and were formerly termed reactive lymphoid hyperplasia [40,187].

Since the tumors are highly radiosensitive, bilateral palliative ocular radiation is usually recommended. The efficiency of chemotherapy still needs to be clearly established.

V. RETINAL METASTATIC CARCINOMA AND MELANOMA

A. General

In contrast to the uvea, metastases to the retina are rare. In a recent report of two additional cases and a survey of the literature, Leys and colleagues found that 11 examples of retinal metastasis from carcinoma and 11 instances from skin melanoma had been documented [250]. Nevertheless, the use of diagnostic vitreous aspiration or vitrectomy [74,124,338] should demonstrate foci of clinically silent metastatic cells. In a prospective study Fishman and colleagues [131] found retinal metastases in 2 of 15 consecutive autopsies in fatal skin melanomas. Because this rate is far higher than expected from the total case reports, one anticipates that the actual incidence is higher. Moreover, patients with carcinomas are surviving longer, and this is likely to be reflected in a similarly rising incidence of retinal metastases.

The primary tumor is usually a carcinoma of the lung, breast, stomach, rectosigmoid colon, or uterus or a skin melanoma [6,13,18,23,47,74,93,95,126,131,153,249,251,306,334,338,358,395,409,423, 446]. The tumor cells gain access to the retina by the internal carotid artery [23], and this may account for the frequent association of retinal and brain metastases [18]. The vitreous may be involved in eyes with retinal metastases following infiltration of the superficial retina and retinal vessels [74,134,251,315, 338,358,446].

B. Clinical Findings

Patients with retinal metastases usually complain of blurred or decreased vision or of floaters; a few asymptomatic cases have been detected during systematic ocular examination or at autopsy [131,249]. Metastatic carcinomas may present as papilledema [127,446], white intraretinal patches, or perivascular infiltrates, and vitreous or aqueous cells sometimes occur with secondary glaucoma. Metastatic melanomas to the retina are often associated with brown spherules and retinal plaques [74,119,338]. Hemorrhages and exudates are also common. Metastatic carcinoma of the retina may masquerade as a panuveitis. In immunosuppressed patients the differential diagnosis includes opportunistic infection. In some patients with a known primary malignancy and metastases, tissue diagnosis may not be necessary. In other instances vitreous surgery or aspiration [119,124,250,315,338,358] is necessary and facilitates the planning of treatment. A modified Papanicolaou stain and cytological analysis by an experienced pathologist using immunocytochemistry or electron microscopy may be required. However, metastatic tumors have been totally eliminated by palliative therapeutic, such as external beam radiation, or systemic and local cytostatic drug administration in very few eyes [252,446]. In these cases involvement of the retinal vessels by tumor cells has generally been reported [250,315]. Ocular metastases signify a poor prognosis for life, the average survival being 11.5 months and the median 6 months.

REFERENCES

1. Abramson, D.H., Ellsworth, R., Grumbach, N., Sturgis-Buckhout, L., and Haik, B.G. Retinoblastoma: Correlation between age at diagnosis and survival. *J. Pediatr. Ophthalmol. Strabismus* 23:174–177, 1986.
2. Abramson, D.H., Ellsworth, R.M., Grumbach, N., and Kitchin, F.D. Retinoblastoma: Survival, age at detection and comparison 1914–1958, 1958–1983. *J. Pediatr. Ophthalmol. Strabismus* 22:246–250, 1985.

3. Abramson, D.H., Ellsworth, R.M., Kitchin, F.D., and Tung G. Second nonocular tumors in retinoblastoma survivors. Are they radiation induced? *Ophthalmology 91*:1351–1355, 1984.
4. Abramson, D.H., Greenfield, D.S., Ellsworth, R.M., Fleischer, M., Weiss, R., Haik, B., Schwartz, M.K., and Bhalla, R. Neuron-specific enolase and retinoblastoma: Clinicopathologic correlations. *Retina 9*:148–152, 1989.
5. Abramson, D.H., Piro, P.A., Ellsworth, R.M., Kitchin, F.D., and McDonald, M. Lactate dehydrogenase levels and isoenzyme patterns: Measurements in the aqueous humor of retinoblastoma patients. *Arch. Ophthalmol. 97*:870–871, 1979.
6. Adamuk, V. Ein Fall von metastatischem Melanosarcom der Uvea. *Z. Augenh. 21*:505, 1909.
7. Aherne, G., and Roberts, D.F. Retinoblastoma. A clinical survey and its genetic implications. *Clin. Genet. 8*:275–290, 1975.
8. Akiyama, K., Iwasaki, M., Amemiya, T., and Yanai, M. Chemotherapy for retinoblastoma. *Ophthalmic Paediatr. Genet. 10*:111–116, 1989.
9. Albert, D.M. Historic review of retinoblastoma. *Ophthalmology 94*:654–662, 1987.
10. Albert, D.M., Craft, J.L., and Sang, D.N. Ultrastructure of retinoblastoma: Transmission and scanning electron microscopy. In: *Ocular and Adnexal Tumors*, F.A. Jakobiec (Ed.), Aesculapius Press, Birmingham, AL, 1978, pp. 157–171.
11. Albert, D.M., Lahav, M., Colby, E.D., Shadduck, J.A., and Sang, D.N. Retinal neoplasia and dysplasia. I. Induction by feline leukemia virus. *Invest. Ophthalmol. Vis. Sci. 16*:325–337, 1977.
12. Albert, D.M., Lahav, M., Lesser, R., and Craft, J.L. Recent observations regarding retinoblastoma. I. Ultrastructure, tissue culture growth, incidence and animal models. *Trans. Ophthalmol. Soc. UK 94*:909–928, 1974.
13. Albert, D.M., Lahav, M., Torczynski, E., and Bahr, R. Black hypopion: Report of two cases. *Graefes Arch. Clin. Exp. Ophthalmol. 193*:81–94, 1975.
14. Albert, D.M., McGee, C.N.J., Seddon, J.M., and Weichselbaum, R.R. Development of additional primary tumors after 62 years in the first patient with retinoblastoma cured by radiation therapy. *Am. J. Ophthalmol. 97*:189–196, 1984.
15. Albert, D.M., and Rabson, A.S. The role of viruses in the pathogenesis of ocular tumors. *Int. Ophthalmol. Clin. 12*:195–224, 1972.
16. Albert, D.M., Rabson, A.S., and Dalton, A.J. In vitro neoplastic transformation of uveal and retinal tissue by oncogenic DNA viruses. *Invest. Ophthalmol. 7*:357–365, 1968.
17. Albert, D.M., Rabson, A.S., and Dalton, A.J. Tissue culture study of human retinoblastoma. *Invest. Ophthalmol. Vis. Sci. 9*:64–72, 1970.
18. Albert, D.M., Rubenstein, R.A., and Scheie, H.G. Tumor metastasis to the eye. I. Incidence in 213 adult patients with generalized malignancy. *Am. J. Ophthalmol. 63*:723–726, 1967.
19. Albert, D.M., and Reid, T.W. RNA-directed DNA polymerase activity in retinoblastoma: Report of its presence and possible significance. *Trans. Am. Acad. Ophthalmol. Otolaryngol. 77*:630–640, 1973.
20. Albert, D.M., Sang, D.N., and Craft, J.L. Clinical and histopathologic observations regarding cell death and tumor necrosis in retinoblastoma. *Jap. J. Ophthalmol. 22*:358–374, 1978.
21. Albert, D.M., Tapper, D., Robinson, N.L., and Felman, R. Retinoblastoma and angiogenesis activity. *Retina 4*:189–194, 1984.
22. Albert, D.M., Walton, D.S., Weichselbaum, R.R., Cassady, J.R., Little, J.B., Leombruno, D., Trantravahi, R., and Puliafito, C.A. Fibroblast radiosensitivity and intraocular fibrovascular proliferation. *Br. J. Ophthalmol. 70*:336–342, 1986.
23. Albert, D.M., Zimmerman, A.W., Jr., and Zeidman, I. Tumor metastasis to the eye. II. The fate of circulating tumor cells to the eye. *Am. J. Ophthalmol. 63*:733–738, 1967.
24. Alexander, R.F., and Spriggs, A.I. The differential diagnosis of tumor cells in circulating blood. *J. Clin. Pathol. 13*:414–424, 1960.
25. Allen, R.A., and Straatsma, B.R. Ocular involvement in leukemia and allied disorders. *Arch. Ophthalmol. 66*:490–508, 1961.
26. Allen, R.A., Latta, H., and Straatsma, B.R. Retinoblastoma. *Invest. Ophthalmol. 1*:728–744, 1962.
27. Amendola, B.E., Markoe, A.M, Augsburger, J.J., Karlsson, U.L., Giblin, M., Shields, J.A., Brady, L.W., and Woodleigh, R. Analysis of treatment results in 36 children with retinoblastoma treated by scleral plaque irradiation. *Int. J. Radiat. Oncol. Biol. Phys. 17*:63–70, 1989.
28. Amy, C.M., and Bartholomew, J.C. Regulation of the N-myc transcript stability in human neuroblastoma and retinoblastoma cells. *Cancer Res. 47*:6310–6314, 1987.
29. Appen, R.E. Posterior uveitis and primary cerebral reticulum cell sarcoma. *Arch. Ophthalmol. 93*:123–124, 1975.
30. Augsburger, J.J., Shields, J.A., and Goldberg, R.E. Classification and management of hereditary retinal angiomas. *Int. Ophthalmol. 30*:173–181, 1985.
31. Bader, J.L., Meadows, A.T., Zimmerman, L.E., Rorke, L.B., Voute, P.A., Champion, I.A.A., Miller, R.W. Bilateral retinoblastoma with ectopic intracranial retinoblastoma: Trilateral retinoblastoma. *Cancer Genet. Cytogenet. 5*:203–213, 1982.

32. Bader, J.L., Miller, R.W., Meadows, A.T., Zimmerman, L.E., Champion, I.A.A., and Voute, P.A. Trilateral retinoblastoma. *Lancet* 2:582–583, 1980.

32a. Baetge, E.E., Behringer, R.R., Messing, A., Brimster, R.L., and Palmiter, R.D. Transgenic mice express the human phenylethanolamine-methyl-transferase gene in adrenal medulla and retina. *Proc. Natl. Acad. Sci. USA* 85:3648–3652, 1988.

33. Balda, B.R., Hehlman, R., Cho, J.R., and Spiegelman, G. Oncornavirus-like particles in human skin cancers. *Proc. Natl. Acad. Sci. USA* 72:3697–3700, 1975.

34. Bardenstein, D.S., Rodrigues, M.M., Alroy, J., and Brownstein, S. Lectin binding in retinoblastoma. *Curr. Eye Res.* 6:1141–1150, 1987.

35. Barr, C.C., Green, W.R., Payne, J.W., Knox, J.W., Jensen, A.D, and Thompson, R.L. Intraocular reticulum cell sarcoma: Clinicopathologic study of four cases and review of the literature. *Surv. Ophthalmol.* 19:224–239, 1975.

36. Barry, G., and Mullaney, J. Retinoblastoma in the Republic of Ireland. *Trans. Ophthalmol. Soc. UK* 91:839–855, 1971.

37. Bedford, M.A. Treatment of retinoblastoma. *Adv. Ophthalmol.* 31:2–32, 1975.

38. Bedford, M.A., Bedotto, C., and MacFaul, P.A. Retinoblastoma: A study of 139 cases. *Br. J. Ophthalmol.* 55:19–27, 1971.

39. Beemer, F.A., Vlug, A.M.C., van Veelen, C.W.M., Rijksen, G., and Staal, G.E.J. Isozyme pattern of enolase of childhood tumors. *Cancer* 54:293–296, 1984.

40. Ben Ezra, D., Sahel, J.A., Harris, N.L., Hemo, I., and Albert, D.M., Uveal lymphoid infiltrates: Immuno-histochemical evidence for a lymphoid neoplasia. *Br. J. Ophthalmol.* 73:846–851, 1989.

41. Benedict, W.F., Dawson, J.A., Banerjee, A., and Murphree, A.L. The nude mouse model for human retino-blastoma: A system for evaluation of retinoblastoma therapy. *Med. Pediatr. Oncol.* 8:391–395, 1980.

42. Benedict, W.F., Fung, Y.K.T., and Murphree, A.L. The gene responsible for the development of retinoblastoma and osteosarcoma. *Cancer (Suppl.)* 62:1691–1694, 1988.

43. Benedict, W.F., Murphree, A.L., Banerjee, A., Spina, C.A., Sparkes, M.C., and Sparkes, R.S. Patient with 13 chromosome deletion: Evidence that the retinoblastoma gene is a recessive cancer gene. *Science* 219:973–975, 1983.

44. Benedict, W.F., Xu, H.J., Hu, S.X., and Takahashi, R. Role of the retinoblastoma gene in the initiation and progression of human cancer. *J. Clin. Invest.* 85:988–993, 1990.

45. Berkow, R.L., and Fleshman, J.K. Retinoblastoma in Navajo Indian Children. *Am. J. Dis. Child.* 137:137–138, 1983.

46. Bierring, F., Egeberg, J., and Jensen, O.A. A contribution to the ultrastructural study of retinoblastoma. *Acta Ophthalmol. (Copenh.)* 45:424–428, 1967.

47. Boente, R. Metastatische Melanoblastome in der Retina. *Klin. Montasbl. Augenheilkd.* 82:732–740, 1929.

48. Bogenmann, E. Retinoblastoma cell differentiation in culture. *Int. J. Cancer* 38:883–887, 1986.

49. Bogenmann, E., Lochrie, M.A., and Simon, M.I. Cone cell specific genes expressed in retinoblastoma. *Science* 240:76–78, 1988.

50. Bomanji, J., Hungerford, J.L., Kingstone, J.E., Levison, D.A., and Britton, K.E. I-123 metalodobenzyl-guanidine (MIBG) scintigraphy of retinoblastoma—preliminary experience. *Br. J. Ophthalmol.* 73:146–150, 1989.

51. Bomanji, J., Hungerford, J.L., and Britton, K.E. I-123 metalodobenzylguanidine scintigraphy of ectopic intracranial retinoblastoma. *Med. Pediatr. Oncol.* 17:66–68, 1989.

52. Boniuk, M., and Girard, L.J. Spontaneous regression of bilateral retinoblastoma. *Trans. Am. Acad. Ophthalmol. Otolaryngol.* 73:194–198, 1969.

53. Boniuk, M., and Zimmerman, L.E. Spontaneous regression of retinoblastoma. *Int. Ophthalmol. Clin.* 2:525–542, 1962.

54. Bonnin, J.M., and Rubenstein, L.J. Immunohistochemistry of central nervous system tumors: Its contributions to neurosurgical diagnosis. *J. Neurosurg.* 60:1121–1133, 1984.

55. Bookstein, R., Lee, E.Y., To, H., Young, L.J., Sery, T.W., Hayes, R.C., Friedmann, T., and Lee, W.H. Human retinoblastoma susceptibility gene: Genomic organization and analysis of heterozygous intragenic deletion mutants. *Proc. Natl. Acad. Sci. USA* 85:2210–2214, 1988.

56. Brady, L.W., Markoe, A.M., Amendola, B.E., Karrisson, U.L., Micaily, B., Shields, J.A., and Augsburger, J.J. The treatment of primary intraocular malignancy. *Int. J. Radiat. Oncol. Biol. Phys.* 15:1355–1361, 1988.

57. Bras, G., Cole, H., Ashemeade-Dyer, A., and Walter, D.C. Report on 151 childhood malignancies observed in Jamaica. *J. Natl. Cancer Inst.* 43:417–421, 1969.

58. Bridges, C.D.B., Fong, S.L., Landers, R.A., Liou, G.I., and Font, R.L. Interstitial retino-binding protein (IRBP) in retinoblastoma. *Neurochem. Int.* 7:875–881, 1985.

59. Brini, A., Dhermy, P., and Sahel, J.A. *Oncology of the Eye and Adnexa.* Kluwer, Dordrecht, 1990.

60. Buchkovich, K., Duffy, L.A., and Harlow, E. The retinoblastoma protein is phosphorylated during specific phases of the cell cycle. *Cell* 58:1097–1105, 1989.

61. Bunin, G.R., Emanuel, B.S., Meadows, A.T., Buckley, J.D., Woods, W.G., and Hammond, G.D. Frequency of 13q abnormalities among 203 patients with retinoblastoma. *J. Natl. Cancer Inst.* 81:370–374, 1989.

62. Bunin, G.R., Emanuel, B.S., Meadows, A.T., Buckley, J.D., Woods, W.G., and Hammond, G.D. Pre- and postconception factors associated with sporadic heritable and nonheritable retinoblastoma. *Cancer Res. 49*: 5730–5735, 1989.
63. Burns, C.A., Blodi, F.C., and Williamson, B.K. Acute lymphocytic leukemia and central serous retinopathy. *Trans. Am. Acad. Ophthalmol. Otolaryngol. 69*:307–309, 1965.
64. Byrd, P., Brown, K.W., and Gallimore, P.H. Malignant transformation of human embryo retinoblasts by cloned adenovirus 12 DNA. *Nature 298*:69–71, 1982.
65. Campbell, M., and Chader, G. Retinoblastoma cells in tissue culture. *Ophthalmic Pediatr. Genet. 9*:171–199, 1988.
66. Campbell, M., Karras, P., and Chader, G.J. Y-79 retinoblastoma cells—isolation and characterization of clonal lineages. *Exp. Eye Res. 48*:75–85, 1989.
67. Campbell, M.A., and Chader, G.J. Effects of laminin on attachment, growth and differentiation of cultured Y-70 retinoblastoma cells. *Invest. Ophthalmol. Vis. Sci. 29*:1517–1522, 1988
68. Canning, S., and Dryja, T.P. Short direct repeats at the breakpoints of deletions of the retinoblastoma gene. *Proc. Natl. Acad. Sci. USA 86*:5044–5048, 1989.
69. Carbajal, U.M. Metastasis in retinoblastoma. *Am. J. Ophthalmol. 48*:47–69, 1959.
70. Cavenee, W.K., Dryja, T.P., Phillips, R.A., Benedict, W.F., Godbout, R., Gallie, B.L., Murphree, A.L., Strong, L.C., and White, R.L. Expression of recessive alleles by chromosomal mechanisms in retinoblastoma. *Nature 305*:779–784, 1983.
71. Cavenee, W.K., Koufos, A., and Hansen, M.F. Recessive mutant genes predisposing to human cancer. *Mutat. Res. 168*:3–14, 1986.
72. Cavenee, W.K., Murphree, A.L., Shull, M.M., Benedict, W.F., Sparkes, R.S., Kock, E., and Nordenskjold, M. Prediction of familial predisposition to retinoblastoma. *N. Engl. J. Med. 314*:1201–1207, 1986.
73. Char, D.H. *Clinical Ocular Oncology.* Churchill-Livingstone, New York, 1989.
74. Char, D.H., Schwartz, A., Miller, T.R., and Abele, J.S. Ocular metastases from systemic melanoma. *Am. J. Ophthalmol. 90*:702–707, 1980.
75. Char, D.H., and Miller, T.R. Fine needle biopsy in retinoblastoma. *Am. J. Ophthalmol. 97*:686–690, 1984.
76. Chen, P.L., Scully, P., Shew, J.Y., Wang, J.Y., Lee, W.H. Phosphorylation of the retinoblastoma gene product is modulated during the cell cycle and cellular differentiation. *Cell 58*:1193–1198, 1989.
77. Clayman, H.M., Flynn, J.T., Koch, K., and Israel, C. Retinal pigment epithelial abnormalities in leukemic disease. *Am. J. Ophthalmol. 74*:416–419, 1972.
78. Cohen, M.S., Augsburger, J.J., Shields, J.A., Amsel, J., and Felberg, N.T. Cancer in relatives of retinoblastoma patients. *Jpn. J. Ophthalmol. 33*:173–176, 1989.
79. Cohen, R. Metachronous sarcomas in a patient with bilateral retinoblastomas—a case report. *S. Afr. Med. J. 76*:117–118, 1989.
80. Cohen, S.M., Saulenas, A.M., Sullivan, C.R., and Albert, D.M. Further studies on the effect of vitamin D on retinoblastoma with 1,25-dihydroxycholecalciferol. *Arch. Ophthalmol. 106*:541–543, 1988.
81. Comings, D.E. A general theory of carcinogenesis. *Proc. Natl. Acad. Sci. USA 70*:3324–3328, 1973.
82. Cooper, E.L., and Riker, J.L. Malignant lymphoma of the uveal tract. *Am. J. Ophthalmol. 34*:1153–1158, 1951.
83. Cooper, J.A., and Whyte, P. RB and the cell cycle: Entrance or exit? *Cell 58*:1009–1011, 1989.
84. Corriveau, C., Easterbrook, M., and Payne, D. Lymphoma simulating uveitis (masquerade syndrome). *Can. J. Ophthalmol. 21*:144–149, 1986.
85. Cowell, J.K. Should all patients with retinoblastoma be screened for chromosome deletions? *Lancet 2*:544–545, 1987.
86. Cowell, J.K. One hundred years of retinoblastoma research from clinic to the gene and back again. *Ophthalmic Pediatr. Genet. 10*:75–88, 1989.
87. Cowell, J.K., Hungerford, J., Rutland, P., and Jay M. Genetic and cytogenetic analysis of patients showing reduced esterase D levels and mental retardation from a survey of 500 individuals with retinoblastoma. *Ophthalmic Pediatr. Genet. 10*:117–128, 1989.
88. Cowell, J.K, Rutland, P., Hungerford, J., and Jay M. Deletion of chromosome 13q14 is transmissible and does not always predispose to retinoblastoma. *Hum. Genet. 80*:43–45, 1988.
89. Craft, J.L., Robinson, N.L., Roth, N.A., and Albert, D.M. Scanning electron microscopy of retinoblastoma. *Exp. Eye Res. 27*:519–531, 1978.
90. Craft, J.L., Sang, D.N., Dryja, T.P., Brockhurst, R.J., Robinson, N.L., and Albert, D.M. Glial cell component in retinoblastoma. *Exp. Eye Res. 40*:647–659, 1985.
91. Cravioto, H. Human and experimental reticulum cell sarcoma (Microglia of the nervous system). *Acta Neuropathol. Suppl. (Berl.) 4*:135–140, 1975.
92. Currey, T.A., and Deutsch, A.R. Reticulum cell sarcoma of the uvea. *South. Med. J. 58*:919–922, 1965.
93. Das Gupta, T., and Brasfield, R. Metastatic melanoma. *Cancer 17*:1323–1339, 1964.
94. Day, R.W., Wright, S.W., Koons, A., and Quigley, M. XXX 21-trisomy and retinoblastoma. *Lancet 2*:154–155, 1963.
95. De Bustros, S., Augsburger, J.J., Shields, J.A., Shakin, E.P., and Pryor, C.C. 2nd Intraocular metastases from cutaneous melanoma. *Arch. Ophthalmol. 103*:937–940, 1985.

96. De Sutter, E., Havers, W., Hopping, W., Zeller, G., and Alberti, W. The prognosis of retinoblastoma in terms of globe saving treatment. *Ophthalmic Pediatr. Genet. 8*:77–84, 1987.
97. Decaprio, J.A., Ludlow, J.W., Lynch, D., Furukawa, Y., Griffin, J., Piwnica-Worms, H., Huang, C.M., and Livingston, D.M. The product of the retinoblastoma susceptibility gene has properties of a cell cycle regulatory element. *Cell 58*:1085–1095, 1989.
98. DerKinderen, D.J., Koten, J.W, Nagelkerke, N.J., Tan, K.E., Beemer, F.A., and DenOtter, W. Non-ocular cancer in patients with hereditary retinoblastoma and their relatives. *Int. J. Cancer 41*:499–504, 1988.
99. Detrick, B., Chader, G.J., Rodrigues, M., Kyritsis, A.P., Chan, C.C., and Hooks, J.J. Coexpression of neuronal, glial, and major histocompatibility complex class II antigens on retinoblastoma cells. *Cancer Res. 48*:1633–1641, 1988.
100. Devesa, S.S. The incidence of retinoblastoma. *Am. J. Ophthalmol. 80*:263–265, 1975.
101. Dhillon, A.P., and Rode, J. Patterns of staining for neuron specific enolase in benign and malignant melanocytic lesions of the skin. *Diagn. Histopathol. 5*:169–174, 1982.
102. Dias, P.L.R., Shanmuganathan, S.S., and Rajartham, M. Lactic dehydrogenase activity of aqueous humor in retinoblastoma. *Am. J. Ophthalmol. 79*:697–698, 1975.
103. Donoso, L.A., Folberg, N.T., Augsburger, J.J., and Shields, J.A. Retinal S-antigen and retinoblastoma: A monoclonal antibody and flow cytometric study. *Invest. Ophthalmol. Vis. Sci. 26*:568–571, 1985.
104. Donoso, L.A., Folberg, N.T., and Arbizo, V. Retinal S. antigen and retinoblastoma. A monoclonal antibody histopathologic study. *Arch. Ophthalmol. 103*:855–857, 1985.
105. Donoso, L.A., Hamm, H., Dietzschold, B., Augsburger, J.J, Shields, J.A., and Arbizo, V. Rhodopsin and retinoblastoma. *Arch. Ophthalmol. 104*:111–113, 1986.
106. Donoso, L.A., Rorke, L.B., Shields, J.A., Augsburger, J.J., Browstein, S., and Lahoud, S. S-antigen immunoreactivity in trilateral retinoblastoma. *Am. J. Ophthalmol. 103*:57–62, 1987.
107. Donoso, L.A., Shields, C.L., and Lee, E. Immunohistochemistry of retinoblastoma. *Ophthalmic Pediatr. Genet. 10*:3–32, 1989.
108. Dryja, T.P., Cavenee, W., White, R., Rapaport, J.M., Petersen, R., Albert, D.M., and Bruns, G.A.P. Homozygosity of chromosome 13 in retinoblastoma. *N. Engl. J. Med. 310*:550–553, 1984.
109. Dryja, T.P., Friend, S., and Weinberg, R.A. Genetic sequence that predisposes to retinoblastoma and osteosarcoma. *Symp. Fund. Cancer Res. 39*:115–119, 1986.
110. Dryja, T.P., Mukai, S., Petersen, R., Rapaport, J.M., Walton, D., and Yandell, D.W. Parental origin of mutations of the retinoblastoma gene (letter). *Nature 339*:556–557, 1989.
111. Dryja, T.P., Rapaport, J.M., Epstein, J., Goorin, A.M., Weichselbaum, R., Koufos, A., and Cavenee, W.K. Chromosome homozygosity in osteosarcoma without retinoblastoma. *Am. J. Hum. Genet. 38*:59–66, 1986.
112. Dryja, T.P., Rapaport, J.M., Joyce, J.M., and Petersen, R.A. Molecular detection of deletions involving band q14 of chromosome 13 in retinoblastoma. *Proc. Natl. Acad. Sci. USA 83*:7391–7394, 1986.
113. Duke-Elder, S. *System of Ophthalmology*, Vol. IX, *Diseases of the Uveal Tract*. C.V. Mosby, St. Louis, pp. 775–937, 1966.
114. Duke-Elder, S. *System of Ophthalmology*, Vol. XII, *Diseases of the Lens and Vitreous; Glaucoma and Hypotony*. C.V. Mosby, St. Louis, pp. 637–640, 1969.
115. Dunphy, E.B. The story of retinoblastoma. *Trans. Am. Acad. Ophthalmol. Otolaryngol. 68*:249–264, 1964.
116. Dyson, N., Buchovich, K., Whyte, P., and Harlow, E. The cellular 107K protein that binds to adenovirus E1A also associates with the large T antigen of SV40 and JC virus. *Cell 58*:249–255, 1989.
117. Dyson, N., Howley, P.M., Munger, K., and Harlow, E. The human papilloma virus cells E7 oncoprotein is able to bind to the retinoblastoma gene product. *Science 243*:934–937, 1989.
118. Eagle, R.C., Shields, J.A., Donoso, L., and Milner, R. Malignant transformation of spontaneously regressed retinoblastoma, retinoma/retinocytoma variant. *Ophthalmology 96*:1389–1395, 1989.
119. Eide, N., and Syrdalen, P. Intraocular metastases from cutaneous malignant melanoma. *Acta Ophthalmol. (Copenh). 68*:102–106, 1990.
120. Ellsworth, R.M. Treatment of retinoblastoma. *Am. J. Ophthalmol. 66*:49–51, 1968.
121. Ellsworth, R.M. The practical management of retinoblastoma. *Trans. Am. Ophthalmol. Soc. 67*:462–534, 1969.
122. Ellsworth, R.M. Orbital retinoblastoma. *Trans. Am. Ophthalmol. Soc. 72*:79–88, 1974.
123. Ellsworth, R.M. Current concepts in the treatment of retinoblastoma. In *Intraocular Tumors*, G.A. Peyman, D.J. Apple, and D.R. Sanders (Eds.), Appleton-Century-Crofts, New York, pp. 335–355, 1977.
124. Engel, H.M., Green, W.R., Michels, R.G., Rice, T.A., and Erozan, Y.S. Diagnostic vitrectomy. *Retina 1*:121–149, 1981.
125. Felberg, N.T., and Donoso, L.A. Surface cytoplasmic antigens in retinoblastoma. *Invest. Ophthalmol. Vis. Sci. 19*:1242–1245, 1980.
126. Ferry, A.P. Primary malignant melanoma of the skin metastatic to the eye. *Am. J. Ophthalmol. 74*:12–19, 1979.
127. Ferry, A.P., and Font, R.L. Carcinoma metastatic to the eye and orbit. I. A clinicopathologic study of 227 cases. *Arch. Ophthalmol. 92*:276–286, 1974.
128. Fine, B.S. Observations on the axoplasm of neural elements in the human retina. In *Proceedings of the Third European Regional Conference on Electron Microscopy*, Vol. B. Czechoslovak Academy of Science, Prague, p. 319, 1964.

129. Fisher, D., Mantell, B.S., and Urich, H. The clinical diagnosis and treatment of microgliomatosis: Report of a case. *J. Neurol. Psychiatry 32*:474–478, 1969.
130. Fisher, E.R., Davis, E.R., and Lemmen, L.J. Reticulum cell sarcoma of the brain (microglioma). *Arch. Neurol. Psychiatry 81*:591–598, 1959.
131. Fishman, M.L., Tomaszewski, M.M., and Kuwabara, T. Malignant melanoma of the skin metastatic to the eye. Frequency in autopsy series. *Arch. Ophthalmol. 94*:1309–1311, 1976.
132. Flexner, S. A peculiar glioma (neuroepithelioma) of the retina. *Bull. Johns Hopkins. Hosp. 2*:115–119, 1891.
133. Fong, S.L., Balakier, H., Canton, M., Bridges, C.D., Gallie, B. Retinoid binding proteins in retinoblastoma tumors. *Cancer Res. 48*:1124–1128, 1988.
133a. Font, R.L., Keener, M.J., Quimbao, A.B., Baehr, W., and Al-Ubaidi, A. An animal model of trilateral primitive neuroectodermal tumors (PNET) in transgenic mice: An immunohistochemical study. *Invest. Ophthalmol. Vis. Sci. (Suppl.) 33*:875, 1992.
134. Font, R.L., Naumann, G., and Zimmerman, L.E. Primary malignant melanoma of the skin metastatic to the eye and orbit: Report of ten cases and review of the literature. *Am. J. Ophthalmol. 63*:738–754, 1967.
135. Francois, J.M., Hanssens, M., and Lagasse, A. The ultrastructure of retinoblastoma. *Ophthalmologica 149*:53–67, 1965.
136. Francois, J.M., Matton, M.T., Debie, S., Tanaka, Y., and Van den Bulke, D. Genesis and genetics of retinoblastoma. *Ophthalmologica 170*:405–425, 1975.
137. Freeman, L.N., Schachat, A.P., Knox, D.L., Michels, R.G., and Green, W.R. Clinical features, laboratory investigation, and survival in ocular reticulum cell sarcoma. *Ophthalmology 94*:1631–1639, 1987.
138. Friend, S.H., Bernards, R., Rogelj, S., Weinberg, R.A., Rapaport, J.M., Albert, D.M., and Dryja, T.P. A human DNA segment with properties of the gene that predisposes to retinoblastoma and osteosarcoma. *Nature 323*:643–646, 1986.
139. Fung, Y.K., Murphree, A.L., Tang, A., Qian, J., Hinrichs, S.H., and Benedict, W.F. Structural evidence for the authenticity of the human retinoblastoma gene. *Science 236*:1657–1661, 1987.
140. Furukawa, Y., Decaprio, J.A., Freedman, A., Kanakura, Y., Nakamura, M., Ernst, T.J., Livingston, D.M., and Griffin, J.D. Expression and state of phosphorylation of the retinoblastoma susceptibility gene product in cycling and noncycling human hematopoeitic cells. *Proc. Natl. Acad. Sci. USA 87*:2770–2774, 1990.
141. Gallie, B.L., Albert, D.M., Wong, J.J., Buyukmihci, N., and Puliafito, C.A. Heterotransplantation of retinoblastoma into the athymic "nude" mouse. *Invest. Ophthalmol. Visual Sci. 16*:256–259, 1977.
142. Gallie, B.L., Holmes, W., and Phillips, R.A. Reproducible growth in tissue culture of retinoblastoma tumor specimens. *Cancer Res. 42*:301–305, 1982.
143. Gallie, B.L., Squire, J.A., Goddard, J., Dunn, J.M., Canton, M., Hinton, D., Zhu, X., and Phillips, R.A. Mechanisms of oncogenesis in retinoblastoma. *Lab. Invest. 62*:394–408, 1990.
144. Gallo, R.C. *Recent Advances in Tumor Research: Cell Biology, Molecular Biology and Tumor Virology*, Vol. 1. CRC Press, Cleveland, OH, 1977.
145. Garrido, C.M., and Arra, A. Studies of ocular retinoblastoma with immunoperoxidase techniques. *Ophthalmologica 193*:242–247, 1986.
146. Gartner, J. Mycosis fungoides mit Beteiligung der Aderhaut. *Klin. Monatsbl. Augenheilkd. 131*:61–69, 1957.
147. Gass, J.D.M. *Differential Diagnosis of Intraocular Tumors*, C.V. Mosby, St. Louis, 1977.
148. Gass, J.D.M. *Stereoscopic Atlas of Macular Disease*, 3rd ed. C.V. Mosby, St. Louis, pp. 654–657, 1987.
149. Gass, P., Frankfurter, A., Katsetos, C.D., Herman, M.M., Donoso, L.A., and Rubenstein, L.J. Antigenic expression of neuron associated class III beta tubulin isotype (hB4) and microtubule associated protein 2 (MAP2) by the human retinoblastoma cell line WERI-Rb1. *Ophthalmic Res. 22*:57–66, 1990.
150. Ghandour, M.S., Langley, O.K., and Keller, A. A comparative immunohistological study of cerebellar enolases. Double labelling technique and immunoelectronmicroscopy. *Exp. Brain Res. 41*:271–279, 1981.
151. Gifford, A.M., and Sorsby, A. The genetics of retinoblastoma. *Br. J. Ophthalmol. 28*:279–293, 1944.
152. Givner, I. Malignant lymphoma with ocular involvement. *Am. J. Ophthalmol. 39*:29–32, 1955.
153. Graham, J.H., Johnson, W.C., and Helwig, E.B. (Eds.). *Dermal Pathology*. Harper & Row, New York, 1972.
154. Green, W.R. The retina. In *Ophthalmic Pathology: An Atlas and Textbook*, 3rd ed., W.H. Spencer (Ed.), W.B. Saunders, Philadelphia, pp. 589–1271, 1986.
155. Greger, V., Kerst, S., Messmer, E., Hopping, W., Passarge, E., and Horsthemke, B. Application of linkage analysis to genetic counselling in families with hereditary retinoblastoma. *J. Med. Genet. 25*:217–221, 1988.
156. Groover, J.R., and Rogers, A.I. Immunologic tests for the detection of gastrointestinal cancers: Status report on carcinoembryonic antigen (CEA) and alpha-fetoprotein (AFP). *South. Med. J. 66*:1218–1221, 1973.
157. Gu, J., Polak, J.M., Noorden V., Pearse, A., Marangos, P.J., and Azzopardi, J.G. Immunostaining of neuron specific enolase as a diagnostic tool for Merckel cell tumors. *Cancer 52*:1039–1043, 1983.
158. Guyer, D.R., Schachat, A.P., Vitale, S., Markowitz, J.A., Braine, H., Burke, P.J., Karp, J.E., and Graham, M. Leukemic retinopathy. Relationship between fundus lesions and hematologic parameters at diagnosis. *Ophthalmology 96*:860–864, 1989.
159. Haik, B.G., Dunleavy, S.A., Cooke, C., Ellsworth, R.M., Abramson, D.H., Smith, M.E., and Karcioglu, Z.A. Retinoblastoma with anterior chamber extension. *Ophthalmology 94*:367–370, 1987.

160. Hansen, M.F., and Cavenee, W.K. Retinoblastoma and the progression of tumor genetics. *Reviews 4*:123–129, 1988.
161. Hansen, M.F., Koufos, A., Gallie, B.L., Phillips, R.A., Fodstad, O., Brogger, A., Gedde-Dahl, T., and Cavanee, W.K. Osteosarcoma and retinoblastoma: A shared chromosomal mechanism recessive predisposition. *Proc. Natl. Acad. Sci. USA 82*:6216–6220, 1985.
162. Harbour, J.W., Lai, S.L., Whang-Peng, J., Gazdar, A.F., Minna, J.D., and Kaye, F.J. Abnormalities in the structure and expression of human retinoblastoma gene in SCLC. *Science 241*:353–357, 1988.
163. Helveston, E.M., Knuth, K.R., Ellis, F.D. Retinoblastoma. *J. Pediatr. Ophthalmol. Strabismus 24*:296–300, 1987.
164. Hemmes, G.D. Untersuchung nach dem Vorkommen von Glioma retinae bei Verwandten von mit dieser Krankheit Behafteten. *Klin. Montasbl. Augenheilkd. 86*:331–335, 1931.
165. Herm, R.L., and Heath, P. A study of retinoblastoma. *Am. J. Ophthalmol. 41*:22–30, 1956.
166. Herman, M.M., Perentes, E., Katsetos, C.D., Darcel, F., Frankfurter A., Collins, P., Donoso, L.A., Eng, L.F., Manganos, P.J., Weichmann, A.F., May, E.M., Thomas, C.B., and Rubenstein, L.J. Neuroblastic differentiation potential of the human retinoblastoma cell line Y-79 and WERI-Rb1 maintained in an organ culture system. *Am. J. Pathol. 134*:115–132, 1989.
167. Higgins, M.J., Hansen, M.F., Cavenee, W.K., and Lalande, M. Molecular detection of chromosomal translocations that disrupt the putative retinoblastoma susceptibility locus. *Mol. Cell. Biol. 9*:1–5, 1989.
168. Hogan, M.J., and Zimmerman, L.E. *Ophthalmic Pathology: An Atlas and Textbook*, 2nd ed. W.B. Saunders, Philadelphia, pp. 433–607, 1962.
169. Hogan, M.J., and Zimmerman, L.E. *Ophthalmic Pathology: An Atlas and Textbook*, 2nd ed. W.B. Saunders, Philadelphia, pp. 516–534, 1962.
170. Hong, F.D., Huang, H.J.S., To, H., Young, L.-J.S., Oro, A., Bookstein, R., Lee, E.Y.-H.P., and Lee, W.H. Structure of the retinoblastoma gene. *Proc. Natl. Acad. Sci. USA 86*:5502–5506, 1989.
171. Hopping, W. The new Essen prognosis classification for conservation of sight saving treatment of retinoblastoma. In *Intraocular Tumors*, Akademieverlag, Berlin, 1983.
172. Hopping, W., and Renelt, P. The treatment of retinoblastoma. *Mod. Probl. Ophthalmol. 12*:580–587, 1974.
173. Horowitz, J.M., Park, S.H., Bogenmann, E., Cheng, J.C., Yandell, D.W., Kaye, F.J., Minna, J.D., Dryja, T.P., and Weinberg, R.A. Frequent inactivation of the retinoblastoma anti-oncogene is restricted to a subset of human tumor cells. *Proc. Natl. Acad. Sci. USA 87*:2775–2779, 1990.
174. Horowitz, J.M., Yandell, D.W., Park, S.H., Canning, S., Whyte, P., Buchkovich, K., Harlow, E., Weinberg, R.A., and Dryja, T.P. Point mutational inactivation of the retinoblastoma anti-oncogene. *Science 243*:937–940, 1989.
175. Horvat, B., Pena, C., and Fisher, E.R. Primary reticulum cell sarcoma (microgliosis) of the brain. An electron microscopy study. *Arch. Pathol. 87*:609–616, 1969.
176. Horven, I. Retinoblastoma in Norway. *Acta Ophthalmol. (Copenh.) 6*:103–109, 1973.
177. Horwarth, C., Meyer, D., Husto, H.O., Johnson, W.W., Shanks, E., and Pratt, C. Stage-related combined modality treatment of retinoblastoma: Results of a prospective study. *Cancer 45*:851–858, 1980.
178. Howard, M.A., Dryja, T.P., Walton, D.S., and Albert, D.M. Identification and significance of multinucleate tumor cells in retinoblastoma. *Arch. Ophthalmol. 107*:1025–1030, 1989.
179. Howard, G.M. Ocular effects of radiation and photocoagulation. *Arch. Ophthalmol. 76*:7–10, 1966.
180. Howard, G.M., and Ellsworth, R.M. Differential diagnosis of retinoblastoma: A statistical survey of 500 children. II. Factors relating to the diagnosis of retinoblastoma. *Am. J. Ophthalmol. 60*:618–621, 1965.
181. Howard, G.M., and Ellsworth, R.M. Findings in the peripheral fundi of patients with retinoblastoma. *Am. J. Ophthalmol. 62*:243–251, 1966.
182. Howard, R.O., Warburton, D., Breg, W.R., Miller, O.J., McKeeown, J., and Rubin, S.P. Retinoblastoma and partial deletion of the long arm of chromosome 13. *Trans. Am. Ophthalmol. Soc. 76*:172–183, 1978.
183. Hu, Q.J., Dyson, N., and Harlow, E. The regions of the retinoblastoma protein needed for binding to adenovirus E1A or SV40 large T antigen are common sites for mutations. *EMBO J. 9*:1147–1155, 1990.
184. Ikui, H., Tominaya, Y., Konomi, I., and Ueno, K. Electron microscopic studies on the histogenesis of retinoblastoma. *Jpn. J. Ophthalmol. 10*:282–290, 1966.
185. Jafek, B.W., Lindford, R., and Foos, R.Y. Late recurrent retinoblastoma in the nasal vestibule. *Arch. Otolaryngol. 94*:264–267, 1971.
186. Jakobiec, F.A., Brodie, S.E., Haik, B., Iwamoto, T. Giant cell astrocytoma. A tumor of possible Mueller cell origin. *Ophthalmology 90*:1565–1575, 1983.
187. Jakobiec, F.A., Sacks, E., Kronish, J.W., Weiss, T., and Smith, M. Multifocal static creamy choroidal infiltrates: An early sign of lymphoid neoplasia. *Ophthalmology 94*:397–406, 1987.
188. Jakobiec, F.A., Tso, M.O.M., Zimmerman, L.E., and Danis, P. Retinoblastoma and intracranial malignancy. *Cancer 39*:2048–2058, 1977.
189. Jay, M. Deficiencies of group D chromosome. In *The Eye in Chromosomal Duplications and Deficiencies*, Marcel Dekker, New York, pp. 77–100, 1977.
190. Jay, M., Cowell, J.K., Kingston, J.E., Hungerford, J. Demonstration of bias in an early series of retinoblastoma. *Ophthalmic Pediatr. Genet. 10*:89–92, 1989.

191. Jensen, O.A. Choroidal metastasis from a malignant melanoma of the skin. *Arch. Ophthalmol. 38*:91, 1947.
192. Jensen, R.D., and Miller, R.W. Retinoblastoma: Epidemiologic characteristics. *N. Engl. J. Med. 285*:307–311, 1971.
193. Kabak, J., and Romano, P.E. Aqueous humor lactic dehydrogenase isoenzyme in retinoblastoma. *Br. J. Ophthalmol. 59*:268–269, 1975.
194. Kaplan, H.J., Meridith, T.A., Aaberg, T.M., and Keller, R.H. Reclassification of intraocular reticulum cell sarcoma (histiocytic lymphoma): Immunologic characterization of vitreous cells. *Arch. Ophthalmol. 98*:707–710, 1980.
195. Karcioglu, Z.A., Haik, B.G., and Gordon, R.A. Frozen section of the optic nerve in retinoblastoma surgery. *Ophthalmology 95*:674–676, 1988.
196. Karp, L.A., Zimmerman, L.E., and Payne, T. Intraocular involvement in Burkitt's lymphoma. *Arch. Ophthalmol. 85*:295–298, 1971.
197. Karsgaard, A.T. Spontaneous regression of retinoblastoma: A report of two cases. *Can. J. Ophthalmol. 6*:218–222, 1971.
198. Keith, C.G. Chemotherapy in retinoblastoma management. *Ophthalmic Pediatr. Genet. 10*:93–98, 1989.
199. Keltner, J.L., Fritsch, E., Ciekert, R.C., and Albert, D.M. Mycosis fungoides: Intraocular and central nervous system involvement. *Arch. Ophthalmol. 95*:645–650, 1977.
200. Kennerdell, J.S., Johnson, B.L., and Wisotzkey, H.M. Vitreous cellular reaction: Association with reticulum cell sarcoma of the brain. *Arch. Ophthalmol. 93*:1341–1345, 1975.
201. Kernohan, J.W., and Uihlein, A. Sarcoma of the reticuloendothelial system. In *Sarcomas of the Brain* Charles. C. Thomas, Springfield, IL, 1962, pp. 54–54.
202. Kincaid, M.C. Ocular and orbital tumors. *Ophthalmology 95*:1588–1595, 1988.
203. Kincaid, M.C., and Green, W.R. Ocular and orbital involvement in leukemia. *Surv. Ophthalmol. 27*:211–232, 1983.
204. Kincaid, M.C., Green, W.R., and Kelley, J.S. Acute ocular leukemia. *Am. J. Ophthalmol. 87*:698–702, 1979.
205. Kivela, T. Expression of the HNK-1 carbohydrate epitope in human retina and retinoblastoma: An immuno-histochemical study with the anti-leu-7 monoclonal antibody. *Virchows Arch. [A] 510*:139–146, 1986.
206. Kivela, T. Neuron-specific enolase in retinoblastoma. An immunohistochemical study. *Acta Ophthalmol. (Copenh.)-64*:19–25, 1986.
207. Kivela, T. Antigenic properties of retinoblastoma tissue. Thesis, University of Helsinki, Finland, 1987.
208. Kivela, T., and Tarkkanen, A. Carcinoembryonic antigen in retinoblastoma. An immunohistochemical study. *Graefes Arch. Clin. Exp. Ophthalmol. 221*:8–11, 1983.
209. Kivela, T., and Tarkkanen, A. S-100 protein in retinoblastoma revisited. *Acta Ophthalmol. (Copenh.) 64*:664–673, 1986.
210. Kivela, T., Tarkkanen, A., and Virtanen, I. Intermediate filaments in the human retina and retinocytoma: An immunohistochemical study of vimentin, glial fibrillary acidic protein, and neurofilaments. *Invest. Ophthalmol. Vis. Sci. 27*:1075–1084, 1986.
211. Kivela, T., Tarkkanen, A., and Virtanen, I. Synaptophysin in the human retina and retinoblastoma: An immunohistochemical and western blotting study. *Invest. Ophthalmol. Vis. Sci. 30*:212–219, 1989.
212. Klingele, T.G., and Hogan, M.J. Ocular reticulum cell sarcoma. *Am. J. Ophthalmol. 79*:39–47, 1975.
213. Klintworth, G.K. Radiographic abnormalities in eyes with retinoblastoma and other disorders. *Br. J. Ophthalmol. 62*:365–372, 1978.
214. Knudson, A.G., Jr. Mutation and cancer: Statistical study of retinoblastoma. *Proc. Natl. Acad. Sci. USA 68*:820–823, 1971.
215. Knudson, A.G., Jr. The genetics of childhood cancer. *Cancer 35*:1022–1026, 1975.
216. Knudson, A.G., Jr. Genetics and the etiology of childhood cancer. *Pediatr. Res. 10*:513–517, 1976.
217. Knudson, A.G., Jr. Persons at high risk of cancer. *N. Engl. J. Med. 301*:606–607, 1979.
218. Knudson, A.G., Jr. Hereditary cancer, oncogenes, and antioncogenes. *Cancer Res. 45*:1437–1443, 1985.
219. Knudson, A.G., Jr., Hethcote, H.W., and Brown, B.W. Mutation and childhood cancer. A probabilistic model for the incidence of retinoblastoma. *Proc. Natl. Acad. Sci. USA 72*:5116–5120, 1975.
220. Knudson, A.G., Jr., Meadows, A.T., Nichols, W.W., and Hill, R. Chromosomal deletion and retinoblastoma. *N. Engl. J. Med. 295*:1120–1123, 1976.
221. Knudson, A.G., Jr., and Strong, L.C. Mutation and cancer: A model for Wilms' tumor of the kidney. *J. Natl. Cancer Inst. 48*:313–324, 1973.
222. Kobayashi, S., and Mukai, N. Retinoblastoma-like tumors induced by human adenovirus type 12 in rats. *Cancer Res. 34*:1646–1651, 1974.
223. Kobayashi, S., and Mukai, N. Retinoblastoma-like tumors induced by human adenovirus. *Invest. Ophthalmol. Vis. Sci. 12*:853–858, 1973.
224. Kobayashi, S., Sawada, T., and Mukai, N. Immunohistochemical evidence of neuron specific enolase (NSE) in human adenovirus 12 induced retinoblastoma-like tumor cells in vitro. *Acta Histochem. Cytol. 18*:551–556, 1985.
225. Kock, E., and Naeser, P. Retinoblastoma in Sweden 1958–1971—a clinical and histopathological study. *Acta Ophthalmol. (Copenh.) 57*:344–350, 1979.

226. Kodilinye, H.C. Retinoblastoma in Nigeria: Problems of treatment. *Am. J. Ophthalmol. 63*:469–483, 1967.
227. Kopelman, J.E., McLean, I.W., and Rosenberg, S.H. Multivariate analysis of risk factors for metastasis in retinoblastoma treated by enucleation. *Ophthalmology 94*:371–377, 1987.
228. Kremer, I., Hartmann, B., Haviv, D., Krakovsky, D., and Bar Ishak, R. Immunohistochemical diagnosis of a totally necrotic retinoblastoma: A clinicopathologic case. *J. Pediatr. Ophthalmol. Strabismus 25*:90–92, 1988.
229. Kuwabara, T., and Aiello, L. Leukemic ciliary nodules in the retina. *Arch. Ophthalmol. 72*:494–497, 1964.
230. Kyritsis, A.P., Joseph, G., and Chader, G.J. Effects of butyrate, retinol and retinoic acid on human Y-79 retinoblastoma cells growing in monolayer culture. *J. Natl. Cancer Inst. 73*:649–654, 1984.
231. Kyritsis, A.P., Kapoor, C.L., and Chader, G.J. Distribution of the regulatory subunit of type II cAMP dependent protein kinase in Y-79 retinoblastoma cells. *Invest. Ophthalmol. Vis. Sci. 27*:1420–1423, 1986.
232. Kyritsis, A.P., Koh, S.W., and Chader, G.J. Modulators of cyclic AMP in monolayer cultures of Y-79 retinoblastoma cells: Partial characterization of the response with VIP and glucagon. *Curr. Eye Res. 3*:339–343, 1984.
233. Kyritsis, A.P., Tsokos, M., and Chader, G.J. Control of retinoblastoma cell growth by differentiating agents: Current work and future directions. *Anticancer Res. 6*:465–474, 1986.
234. Kyritsis, A.P., Tsokos, M., Triche, T.J., and Chader, G.J. Retinoblastoma—origin from an primitive neuroectodermal cell? *Nature 307*:471–473, 1984.
235. Kyritsis, A.P., Tsokos, M., and Chader, G.J. Attachment culture of human retinoblastoma cells. Long term culture conditions and effects of dibutyrl cyclic AMP. *Exp. Eye Res. 38*:411–421, 1984.
236. Kyritsis, A.P., Tsokos, M., Triche, T.J., and Chader, G.J. Retinoblastoma: Primitive tumor with multipotential characteristics. *Invest. Ophthalmol. Vis. Sci. 27*:1760–1764, 1986.
237. Kyritsis, A.P., Weichman, A.F., Bok, D., and Chader, G.J. Hydroxyindole-O-methyltransferase in Y-79 human retinoblastoma cells: Effect of cell attachment. *J. Neurochem. 48*:1612–1616, 1987.
238. Lane, J.C., and Klintworth, G.K. A study of astrocytes in retinoblastomas using the immunoperoxidase technique and antibodies to glial fibrillary acidic protein. *Am. J. Ophthalmol. 95*:197–207, 1982.
239. Lang, G.K., Surer, J.L., Green, W.R., Finkelstein, D., Michels, R.G., and Maumenee, A.E. Ocular reticulum cell sarcoma: Clinicopathologic correlation of a case with multifocal lesions. *Retina 5*:79–86, 1985.
240. Lee, E.Y., Bookstein, R., Young, L.H., Lin, C.J., Rosenfeld, M.G., and Lee, W.H. Molecular mechanisms of retinoblastoma gene inactivation in retinoblastoma cell line Y-79. *Proc. Natl. Acad. Sci. USA 85*:6017–6021, 1988.
241. Lee, E.Y., To, H., Shew, J.Y., Bookstein, R., Scully, P., and Lee, W.H. Inactivation of the retinoblastoma susceptibility gene. *Science 241*:218–222, 1988.
242. Lee, W.H., Bookstein, R., Hong, F., Young, L.J., Shew, J.Y., and Lee, E. Human retinoblastoma susceptibility gene: Cloning, identification, and sequence. *Science 235*:1395–1397, 1987.
243. Lee, W.H., Bookstein, R., and Lee, E.Y. Studies of the human retinoblastoma susceptibility gene. *J. Cell. Biochem. 38*:213–227, 1988.
244. Lee, W.H., Murphree, A.L., and Benedict, W.F. Expression and amplification of the N-myc gene in primary retinoblastoma. *Nature 309*:458–462, 1984.
245. Lee, W.H., Shew, J.Y., Hong, F.D., Sery, T.W., Donoso, L.A., Young, L.J., Bookstein, R., and Lee, E.Y. The retinoblastoma susceptibility gene encodes a nuclear phosphoprotein associated with DNA binding activity. *Nature 329*:642–645, 1987.
246. Lemieux, N., Leung, T., Michaud, J., Milot, J., and Richer, C.L. Neuronal and photoreceptor differentiation of retinoblastoma cells in culture. *Ophthalmic Pediatr. Genet. 11*:109–120, 1990.
247. Leonard, R.C., MacKay, T., Brown, A., Gregor, A., Crompton, G.L., and Smyth, J.F. Small-cell lung cancer after retinoblastoma. *Lancet 2*:1503, 1988.
248. Leonardy, N.J., Rupani, M., Dent, G., and Klintworth, G.K. Analysis of 135 autopsy eyes for ocular involvement in leukemia. *Am. J. Ophthalmol. 109*:436–444, 1990.
249. Letson, A.D., and Davidorf, F.H. Bilateral retinal metastases from cutaneous malignant melanoma. *Arch. Ophthalmol. 100*:605–607, 1982.
250. Leys, A.M., Van Eyck, L.M., Nuttin, B.J., Pauwels, P.A., Delabie, J.M., and Libert, J.A. Metastatic carcinoma to the retina: Clinicopathologic findings in two cases. *Arch. Ophthalmol. 108*:1448–1452, 1990.
251. Liddicoat, J.A., Wolter, J.R., and Wilkinson, W.C. Retinal metastasis of malignant melanoblastoma: A case report. *Am. J. Ophthalmol. 48*:172–177, 1959.
252. Liu, H.S., Refojo, M.F., Perry, H.D., Albert, D.M. Direct delivery of anticancer agents: Experimental treatment of intraocular malignancy. *Invest. Ophthalmol. Vis. Sci. 17*:993–1004, 1978.
253. Lindley-Smith, J.S. Histology and spontaneous regression of retinoblastoma. *Trans. Ophthalmol. Soc. UK 94*:953–967, 1974.
254. Little, J.B., Weichselbaum, R.R., Nove, J., and Albert, D.M. X-ray sensitivity of fibroblasts from patients with retinoblastoma and with abnormalities of chromosome 13. In *DNA Repair Mechanics*, E.L. Friedberg and P.C. Hanawalt (Eds.), Academic Press, New York, pp. 685–690, 1978.
255. Ludlow, J.W., Decaprio, J.A., Huang, C.M., Lee, W.H., Paucha, E., Livingston, D.M. SV40 large T antigen initially to an underphophorylated member of the retinoblastoma susceptibility gene product family. *Cell 56*:57–65, 1989.

256. Ludlow, J.W., Shon, J., Pipas, J.M., Livingston, D.M., Decaprio, J.A. The retinoblastoma susceptibility gene product undergoes cell cycle-dependent dephosphorylation in binding to and release from SV40 large T. *Cell* 60:387–396, 1990.

257. Lueder, G.T., Judisch, F., and O'Gorman, T.W. Second nonocular tumors in survivors of heritable retinoblastoma. *Arch. Ophthalmol.* 104:372–373, 1986.

258. McGee, T.L., Yandell, D.W., and Dryja, T.P. Structure and partial genomic sequence of the human retinoblastoma susceptibility gene. *Gene 80*:119–128, 1989.

259. McCartney, A.C.E., Olver, J.M., Kingston, J.E., and Hungerford, J.L. Forty years of retinoblastoma: Into the fifth age. *Eye (Suppl.)* 2:513–518, 1988.

260. McFall, R.C., Sery, T.W., and Makadon, M. Characterization of a new continous cell line derived from human retinoblastoma. *Cancer Res.* 37:1003–1010, 1977.

261. Macklin, M.T. A study of retinoblastoma in Ohio. *Am. J. Hum. Genet.* 12:1–43, 1960.

262. Madreperla, S.A., Whittum-Hudson, J. Prendergast, R.A., Chen, R.L., and Lee, W-H. Suppression of intraocular retinoblastoma xenograft growth by the retinoblastoma gene. *Invest. Ophthalmol. Vis. Sci. (Suppl.)* 32:981, 1991.

263. Mafee, M.F., Goldberg, M.F., Cohen, S.B., Gotsis, E.D., Safran, M. Chekuri, L., Raofi, B., and Haik, B.G. Magnetic resonance imaging versus computed tomography of leukocoric eyes and use of in vitro proton magnetic resonance spectroscopy of retinoblastoma. *Ophthalmology* 96:965–976, 1989.

264. Magramm, I., Abramson, D.H., and Ellsworth, R.M. Optic nerve involvement in retinoblastoma. *Ophthalmology* 96:217–222, 1989.

265. Mak, S., Mak, I., Gallie, B.L., Godbout, R., and Phillips, R.A. Adenovirus 12 genes undetectable in human retinoblastoma. *Int. J. Cancer 30*:607–700, 1982.

266. Mann, R.B., Jaffee, E.S., and Berard, C.W. Malignant lymphoma a conceptual understanding of morphologic diversity. *Am. J. Pathol.* 94:105–197, 1979.

267. Marangos, P.J. Schmechel, D., Zis, A.P., and Goodwin, F.K. The existence and neurobiological significance of neuronal and glial forms of the glycolytic enzyme enolase. *Biol. Psychiatry 14*:563–579, 1979.

268. Marcus, D.M., Craft, J.L., and Albert, D.M. Histopathologic verification of Verhoeff's 1918 irradiation cure of retinoblastoma. *Ophthalmology* 97:221–224, 1990.

269. Margo, C., Hidayat, A., Kopelman, J., and Zimmerman, L.E. Retinocytoma. A benign variant of retinoblastoma. *Arch. Ophthalmol.* 101:1519–1531, 1983.

270. Margo, C.E., and Lavellee, M. Gamma-enolase activity in choroidal melanoma. *Graefes Arch Clin Exp. Ophthalmol.* 224:374–376, 1986.

271. Matsuo, N., and Takayama, T. Electron microscopic observations of visual cells in a case of retinoblastoma. *Folia Ophthalmol. Jpn.* 16:574–580, 1965.

271a. Mawas, J. Les cancers de la rétine optique. *Bull. Mem. Soc. Fr. Ophtalmol.* 37:512–515, 1924.

272. Meadows, A.T. Risk factors for second malignant neoplasms: Report from the late effects study group. *Bull Cancer 75*:125–130, 1988. Molecular mechanisms in familial and sporadic cancers (editorial). *Lancet 1*(8577):92, 1988.

273. Merriam, G.R. Retinoblastoma, analysis of 17 autopsies. *Arch. Ophthalmol.* 44:71–108, 1950.

274. Messmer, E.P., Font, R.L., Kirkpatrick, J.B., and Hopping, W. Immunohistochemical demonstration of neuronal and astrocytic differentiation in retinoblastoma. *Ophthalmology* 92:167–173, 1985.

275. Michels, R.G., Knox, D.L., Erozan, Y.S., and Green, W.E. Intra-ocular reticulum cell sarcoma: Diagnosis by pars plana vitrectomy. *Arch. Ophthalmol.* 93:1331–1335, 1975.

276. Michelson, J.B., Felberg, N.T., and Shields, J.A. Fetal antigens in retinoblastoma. *Cancer 37*:719–723, 1976.

277. Mihara, K., Cao, X.R., Yen, A., Chandler, S., Driscoll, B., and Murphree, A.L. Cell cycle-dependent regulation of phosphorylation of the human retinoblastoma gene product. *Science 246*:1300–1303, 1989.

278. Mikolajewski, V.J., Messmer, E., Sauerwain, W., Freundlieb, O. Orbital computed tomography. Does it help in diagnosing the infiltration of choroid, sclera, and/or optic nerve in retinoblastoma. *Ophthalmic Pediat. Genet.* 8:101–104, 1987.

279. Miller, R.W. Fifty-two forms of childhood cancer: United States mortality experience 1960–1966. *J. Pediatr.* 75:685–689, 1969.

280. Miller, R.W. Neoplasia and Down's syndrome. *Ann. NY Acad. Sci.* 171:637–645, 1970.

281. Minckler, D.S., Font, R.L., and Zimmerman, L.E. Uveitis and retinoblastoma cell sarcoma of the brain with bilateral neoplastic seeding of vitreous without retinal or uveal involvement. *Am. J. Ophthalmol.* 80:433–439, 1975.

282. Minei, M., Yamana, Y., and Ohnishi, Y. Carcinoembryonic antigena and alpha foeto-protein levels in retinoblastoma. *Jpn. J. Ophthalmol.* 27:185–192, 1983.

283. Misrhahi, M., Boucheix, C., Dhermy, P., Haye, C., and Faure, J.P. Expression of photoreceptor-specific S-antigen in human retinoblastoma. *Cancer 57*:1497–1500, 1986.

284. Mitchell, C. Second malignant neoplasms in retinoblastoma. *Ophthalmic Pediatr. Genet.* 9:161–165, 1988.

285. Molnar, M.L., Stefansson, K., Marton, L.S., Tripathi, R.S., and Molnar, G.K. Immuno-histochemistry of retinoblastoma in humans. *Am. J. Ophthalmol.* 97:301–307, 1984.

286. Moro, F., Secchi, A.G., Moschini, G.B., Pinello, L., Sotti, G., and Zanesco, L. Retinoblastoma. Combined treatment of 21 cases. Critical review of the results. *Ophthalmic Paediat. Genet.* *10*:107–110, 1989.
287. Morris, W.E., and LaPiana, F.G. Spontaneous regression of bilateral retinoblastoma with preservation of normal visual acuity. *Ann. Ophthalmol.* *6*:1192–1194, 1974.
288. Mukai, N., and Murao, T. Retinal tumor induction by ocular inoculation of human adenovirus in 3-days-old rats. *J. Neuropathol. Exp. Neurol.* *34*:28–35, 1975.
289. Mukai, S., Rapaport, J.M., Shields, J.A., Augsburger, J.J., and Dryja, T.P. Linkage of genes for human esterase D and hereditary retinoblastoma. *Am. J. Ophthalmol.* *97*:681–685, 1984.
290. Mullaney, J. DNA in retinoblastoma. *Lancet* *2*:918, 1968.
291. Munger, K., Werness, B.A., Dyson, N., Phelps, W.C., Harlow, E., and Howley, P.M. Complex formation of human papillomavirus E7 proteins with the retinoblastoma tumor suppressor gene product. *EMBO J.* *8*:4099–5015, 1989.
292. Munier, F., Pescia, G., Jotterand-Bellomo, M., Balmer, A., Gailloud, C., and Thonney, F. Constitutional karyotype in retinoblastoma. Case report and review of literature. *Ophthalmic Pediatr. Genet.* *10*:129, 1989.
293. Murphree, A.L., and Benedict, W.F. Retinoblastoma: Clues to human oncogenesis. *Science* *223*:1028–1033, 1984.
294. Murphree, A.L., and Rother, C. Retinoblastoma. In *Retina*, Vol. 1, J. Ryan (Ed.), C.V. Mosby, St. Louis, pp. 517–556, 1989.
295. Musarella, M.A., and Gallie, B.L. A simplified scheme for genetic counseling in retinoblastoma. *J. Pediatr. Ophthalmol.* *24*:124–125, 1987.
296. Nakajima, T., Kato, K., Kaneko, A., Tsumuraya, M., Morinaga, S., and Shimosato, Y. High concentration of enolase, alpha and y-subinits in the aqueous humor in cases of retinoblastoma. *Am. J. Ophthalmol.* *101*:102–106, 1986.
297. Neault, R.W., Van Scoy, R.E., Okazaki, H., and MacCarty, C.S. Uveitis associated with isolated reticulum cell sarcoma of the brain. *Am. J. Ophthalmol.* *73*:431–436, 1972.
298. Nehen, J.H. Spontaneous regression of retinoblastoma. *Acta Ophthalmol. (Copenh.)* *53*:647–651, 1975.
299. Nelson, C.C., Hertzberg, B.S., and Klintworth, G.K. A histopathologic study of 716 unselected eyes in patients with cancer at the time of death. *Am. J. Ophthalmol.* *95*:788–793, 1983.
300. Nevins, R.C., Jr., Frey, W.W., and Elliott, J.H., Primary solitary intraocular reticulum cell sarcoma (microgliomatosis): A clinicopathologic case report. *Trans. Am. Acad. Ophthalmol. Otolaryngol.* *72*:867–876, 1968.
301. Newell, G.R., Robert, J.D., and Baranovsky, A. Retinoblastoma: Presentation and survival in Negro children compared with whites. *J. Natl. Cancer Inst.* *49*:989–992, 1972.
302. O'Brien, J., Marcus, D.M., Niffeneger, A.S., Bernards, R., Carpenter, J.L., Windle, J.J., Mellon, P., and Albert, D. Trilateral retinoblastoma in transgenic mice. *Trans. Amer. Ophthalmol. Soc.* *87*:301–326, 1989.
303. O'Connor, G.R. The uvea (annual review). *Arch. Ophthalmol.* *89*:505–518, 1973.
304. O'Day, J., Billson, F.A., and Hoyt, C.S. Retinoblastoma in Victoria. *Med. J. Aust.* *2*:428–432, 1977.
305. Odelstad, L., Pahlman, S., Bilsson, K., Larsson, E., Lackgren, G., Johansson, K.E., Hjerten, S., and Grotte, G. Neuron-specific enolase in relation to differentiation in human neuroblastoma. *Brain Res.* *224*:69–82, 1981.
306. Oosterhuis, J.A, de Keizer, R.J., de Wolff-Rouendaal, D., Kakebeeke-Kemme, H.M., and de Graaff, M.L. Ocular and orbital metastases of cutaneous melanomas. *Int. Ophthalmol.* *10*:175–184, 1987.
307. Osborn, M., and Weber, K. Tumor diagnosis by intermediate filament typing: A novel tool for surgical pathology. *Lab. Invest.* *48*:372–394, 1983.
308. Owens, G., and Babel, J. Sarcome réticulaire intra-oculaire et cérébral. *Arch. Ophtalmol. (Paris)* *35*:409–416, 1975.
309. Pendergrass, T.N., and Davis, S. Incidence of retinoblastoma in the United States. *Arch. Ophthalmol.* *98*:1204–1210, 1980.
310. Perentes, E., Herbort, C.P., Rubinstein, L.J., Hermann, M.M., Uffer, S., Donoso, L.A., and Collins, V.P. Immunohistochemical characterization of human retinoblastoma in situ with multiple markers. *Am. J. Ophthalmol.* *103*:647–658, 1987.
311. Perentes, E., and Rubinstein, L.J. Immunohistochemical recognition of human neuroepithelial tumors by anti-leu 7 (HNK-1) monoclonal antibody. *Acta Neuropathol. (Berl.)* *69*:227–233, 1986.
312. Pesin, S.R., and Shields, J.A. Seven cases of trilateral retinoblastoma. *Am. J. Ophthalmol.* *107*:121–126, 1989.
313. Peyster, R.G., Augsburger, J.J., Shields, J.A., Hershey, B.L., Eagle, R., and Haskin, M.E. Intraocular tumors: Evaluation with MR imaging. *Radiology* *168*:773–779, 1988.
314. Pfeiffer, R.L. Roentgenographic diagnosis of retinoblastoma. *Arch. Ophthalmol.* *15*:811–821, 1936.
315. Piro, P., Pappas, H.R., Erozan, Y.S., Michels, R.G., Sherman, S.H., and Green, W.R. Diagnostic vitrectomy in metastatic breast carcinoma in the vitreous. *Retina* *2*:182–188, 1982.
316. Plotsky, D., Quinn, G., Eagle, R., Shields, J., and Granowetter, L. Congenital retinoblastoma: A case report. *J. Pediatr. Ophthalmol. Strabismus.* *24*:120–123, 1987.
317. Polak, M. Microglioma and/or reticulosarcoma of the nervous system. *Acta Neuropathol. Suppl. (Berl.)* *6*: 115–118, 1975.

318. Popoff, N. Filamentous alteration in photoreceptors from human eyes with retinoblastoma. *J. Ultrastruct. Res.* *42*:244–254, 1973.

319. Popoff, N., and Ellsworth, R.M. The fine structure of retinoblastoma: In vivo and in vitro observations. *Lab. Invest. 25*:389–402, 1971.

320. Popoff, N., and Ellsworth, R.M. The fine structure of nuclear alterations in retinoblastoma and the developing human retina: In vivo and in vitro observations. *J. Ultrastruct. Res. 29*:535–549, 1969.

321. Portlock, C.S. The non-Hodgkin's lymphomas. In *Cecil Textbook of Medicine*, J.B. Wyngaarden and L.H. Mith (Eds.), W.B. Saunders, Philadelphia, pp. 994–999, 1988.

322. Pratt, C.B., Meyer, D., Chenaille, P., and Crom, D.B. The use of bone marrow aspirations and lumbar punctures at the time of diagnosis of retinoblastoma. *J. Clin. Oncol. 7*:140–143, 1989.

323. Pratt, C.B., and George, S.L. Second malignant neoplasms among children and adolescents treated for cancer. *Proc. Am. Assoc. Cancer Res. 22*:151, 1981.

324. Raab, E.L., Shields, J.A., Augsburger, J.J., and Donoso L.A. Pediatric update. Recent developments—related to retinoblastoma. *J. Pediatr. Ophthalmol. Strabismus 23*:148–152, 1986.

325. Rapin, A.M.C., and Burger, M.M. Tumor cell surfaces. *Adv. Cancer Res. 20*:1–91, 1974.

326. Redler, L.D., and Ellsworth, R.M. Prognostic importance of choroidal invasion in retinoblastoma. *Arch. Ophthalmol. 90*:294–296, 1973.

327. Reese, A.B. *Tumors of the Eye*, 3rd ed. Harper & Row, New York, pp. 89–132, 1976.

328. Reid, T.W., and Albert, D.M. RNA-dependent DNA polymerase activity in human tumors. *Biochem. Biophys. Res. Commun. 46*:383–390, 1972.

329. Reid, T.W., and Russell, P. Recent observations regarding retinoblastoma. II. An enzyme study of retinoblastoma. *Trans. Ophthalmol. Soc. UK 94*:929–937, 1974.

330. Reid, T.W., Albert, D.M., Rabson, A.S., Russell, P., Craft, J., Chu, E.W., Tralka, T.S., and Wilcox, J.L. Characteristics of an established cell line of retinoblastoma. *J. Natl. Cancer Inst. 53*:347–352, 1974.

331. Renelt, P., and Trieschmann, W. Vanilmandelic acid urinary excretion in the diagnostic of retinoblastoma. *Graefes Arch. Clin. Exp. Ophthalmol. 188*:281–283, 1973.

332. Rider, C.C., and Taylor, C.B. Enolase isoenzymes in rat tissues. Electrophoretic, chromatographic, immunological and kinetic properties. *Biochim. Biophys. Acta 365*:285–300, 1974.

333. Riedel, K.G. Hypertherme Therapieverfahren in Ergänzung zur Strahlenbehandlung maligner intraokularer Tumoren. *Klin. Monatsbl. Augenheilkd. 193*:131–137, 1988.

334. Riffenburgh, R.S. Metastatic malignant melanoma to the retina. *Arch. Ophthalmol. 66*:447–449, 1961.

335. Roarty, J.D., McLean, I.W., and Zimmermann, L.E. Incidence of second neoplasms in patients with bilateral retinoblastoma. *Ophthalmology 95*:1583–1587, 1988.

336. Robb, R.M., Ervin, L.D., and Sallan, S.E. A pathological study of eye involvement in acute leukemia of childhood. *Trans. Am. Ophthalmol. Soc. 76*:90–101, 1978.

337. Roberts, D.F., Duggan-Keen, M., Aherne, G.E.S., Long, D.R. Immunogenetic studies in retinoblastoma. *Br. J. Ophthalmol. 70*:686–691, 1986.

338. Robertson, D.M., Wilkinson, C.P., Murray, J.L., and Gordy, D.D. Metastatic tumor to the retina and vitreous cavity from primary melanoma of the skin: Treatment with systemic and subconjunctival chemotherapy. *Ophthalmology 88*:1296–1301, 1981.

339. Rodrigues, M.M., Wiggert, B., Shields, J., Donoso, L., Bardenstein, D., Katz, N., Friendly, D., and Chader, G. Retinoblastoma. Immunohistochemistry and cell differentiation. *Ophthalmology 94*:378–387, 1987.

340. Rodrigues, M.M., Wilson, M.E., Wiggert, B., Krishna, G., and Chader, G.J. Retinoblastoma. A clinical immunohistochemical, and electron microscopic case report. *Ophthalmology 93*:1010–1015, 1986.

341. Rodriguez, M.N., Bardenstein, D.S., Donoso, L.A., Rajagopalan, S., and Brownstein, S. An immunohistopathologic study of trilateral retinoblastoma. *Am. J. Ophthalmol. 103*:776–781, 1987.

342. Romano, P.E., and Kabok, J. Aqueous humor lactic acid dehydrogenase in retinoblastoma. *Am. J. Ophthalmol. 79*:697–698, 1975.

343. Royds, J.A., Parsons, M.A., Rennie, I.G., Timperley, W.R., and Taylor, C.B. Enolase isoenzymes in benign and malignant melanocytic lesions. *Diagn. Histopathol. 5*:175–181, 1982.

344. Royds, J.A., Parsons, M.A., Taylor, C.B., and Timperley, W.R. Enolase isoenzyme distribution in the human brain and its tumors. *J. Pathol. 137*:37–49, 1982.

345. Rubin, C.M., Robinson, L., Cameron, J.D., Woods, W.G., Nesbit, M.E., Krivit, W., Jr., Kim, T.H., Letson, R.D., and Ramsay, N.K.C. Intraocular retinoblastoma group V: An analysis of prognostic factors. *J. Clin. Oncol. 3*:680–685, 1985.

346. Rubin, N.A., Tarsio, J.F., Borthwick, A.C., Gregerson, D.S., and Reid, T.W. Identification and characterization of a growth factor secreted by an established cell line of human retinoblastoma maintained in serum-free medium. *Vision Res. 21*:105–112, 1981.

347. Rubinstein, L.J. Embryonal central neuroepithelial tumors and their differentiating potential: A cytogenetic view of a complex neuro-oncological problem. *J. Neurosurg. 62*:795–805, 1985.

348. Russell, D.S., and Rubinstein, L.J. *Pathology of the Nervous System*, 4th ed. Williams and Wilkins, Baltimore, pp. 299–330, 1977.

349. Sahel, J.A., Frederick, A.R., Pesavento, R., and Albert, D.M. Idiopathic retinal gliosis mimicking a choroidal melanoma. *Retina* 8:282–287, 1988.

350. Sahel, R.A., Gross, S., Cassano, W., and Gee, A. Metastatic retinoblastoma successfully treated with immunomagnetically purged autologous bone marrow transplantation. *Cancer* 62:2301–2303, 1988.

351. Salsbury, A.J., Bedford, M.A., and Dobree, J.H. Bone marrow appearances in children suffering from retinoblastoma. *Br. J. Ophthalmol.* 52:388–395, 1968.

352. Sanders, B.M., Draper, G.J., and Kingston. J.E. Retinoblastoma in Great Britian 1969–80: Incidence, treatment, and survival. *Br. J. Ophthalmol.* 72:576–583, 1988.

353. Sanders, B.M., Jay, M., Draper, G.J., and Roberts, E.M. Non-ocular cancer in relatives of retinoblastoma patients. *Br. J. Cancer* 60:358–365, 1989.

354. Sang, D.N., and Albert, D.M. Recent advances in the study of retinoblastoma. In *Intraocular Tumors*, G.A. Peyman, D.J. Apple, and D.R. Sanders (Eds.), Appleton-Century-Crofts, New York, pp. 285–329, 1977.

355. Sang, D. N., and Albert, D.M. Catecholamine levels in retinoblastoma. In *Ocular and Adnexal Tumors*, F.A. Jakobiec (Ed.), Aesculapius, Birmingham, AL, pp. 172–180, 1978.

356. Sasaki, A., Ogawa, A., Nakazato, Y., and Ishida, Y. Distribution of neuro-filament protein and neuron-specific enolase in peripheral neuronal tumors. *Virchows Arch. [A] 407*:33–41, 1985.

357. Schachat, A.P. Leukemias and lymphomas. In *Retina*, Vol. 1, Ryan, S.J. (Ed.), C.V. Mosby St. Louis, pp. 775–793, 1989.

358. Schachat, A.P. Tumor involvement of the vitreous cavity. In *Retina*, Vol. 1, Ryan S.J. (Ed.), C.V. Mosby, St. Louis, pp. 805–818, 1989.

359. Schappert-Kimmijser, J., Hemmes, G.D., and Nijland, R. The heredity of retinoblastoma. *Ophthalmologica 151*:197–213, 1966.

360. Schaumburg, H.H., Plank, C.R., and Adams, R.D. The reticulum cell sarcoma microglioma group of brain tumors: A consideration of their clinical features and therapy. *Brain 95*:199–212, 1972.

361. Schipper, J. *Retinoblastoma: A Medical and Experimental study*. Ph.D. Thesis, University Utrecht, 1980.

362. Schmechel, D., Marangos, P.J., Zis, A.P., Brightman, M., and Goodwin, F.K. Brain enolases as specific markers of neuronal and glial cells. *Science 199*:313–315, 1978.

363. Schulman, J.A., Peyman, G.A., Mafee, M.F., Lawrence, L., Bauman, A.E., Goldman, A., and Kurwa, B. The use of magnetic resonance imaging in the evaluation of retinoblastoma. *J. Pediatr. Ophthalmol. Strabismus 23*:144–147, 1986.

364. Schweigerer, L., Neufeld, G., and Gospodarowicz, D. Basic fibroblast growth factor in present in cultured human retinoblastoma cells. *Invest. Ophthalmol. Vis. Sci.* 28:1838–1843, 1987.

365. Sheffield, J.B. Microtubules in the outer nuclear layer of rabbit retina. *J. Microsc.* 5:173–180, 1966.

366. Shields, J.A. *Diagnosis and Management of Intraocular Tumors*. C.V. Mosby, St. Louis, 1983.

367. Shields, J.A., and Augsburger, J.J. Current approaches to the diagnosis and management of retinoblastoma. *Surv. Ophthalmol.* 25:347–371, 1981.

368. Shields, J.A., Giblin, M.E., Shields, C.L., Maroke, A.M., Karlsson, U., Brady, L.W., Amendola, B.E., and Woodleigh, R. Episclera plaque radiotherapy for retinoblastoma. *Ophthalmology* 96:530–537, 1989.

369. Shields, J.A., Leonard, B.C., Michelson, J.B., and Sarin, L.K. B-scan ultrasonography in the diagnosis of atypical retinoblastoma. *Can. J. Ophthalmol. 11*:42–51, 1976.

370. Shields, J.A., Pesin, S.R., and Shields, C.L. Trilateral retinoblastoma—feature photo. *J. Clin. Neuro Ophthalmol. 9*:222–223, 1989.

371. Shields, J.A., Shields, C.L., Donoso, L.A., and Lieb, W.E. Changing concepts in the management of retinoblastoma. *Ophthalmic Surg. 21*:72–76, 1990.

372. Shields, J.A., Shields, C.L., and Sivalingam, V. Decreasing frequency of enucleation in patients with retinoblastoma. *Am. J. Ophthalmol. 108*:185–188, 1989.

373. Shuangshoti, S., Chaiwun, B., and Kasantikul, V. A study of 39 retinoblastomas with particular reference to morphology, cellular differentiation, and tumor origin. *Histopathology 15*:113–124, 1989.

374. Sparkes, R.S., Murphree, A.L., Lingua, R.W., Sparkes, M.C., Field, I.L., Funderburk, S.J., and Benedict, W.F. Gene for hereditary retinoblastoma assigned to human chromosome 13 by linkage to esterase D. *Science 219*:971–973, 1983.

375. Spaulding, A.G., and Naumann, G. Unsuspected retinoblastoma. *Arch. Ophthalmol.* 76:575–579, 1966.

376. Squire, J., Dryja, T.P., Dunn, J., Goddard, A., Hofmann, T., Musarella, M., Willard, H.F., Becker, A.J., Gallie, B.L., and Philips, R.A. Cloning of the esterase D gene. A polymorphic gene probe closely linked to the retinoblastoma locus on chromosome 13. *Proc. Natl. Acad. Sci. USA 83*:6573–6577, 1986.

377. Squire, J., Goddard, A.D., Canton, M., Becker, A., Phillips, R.A., and Gallie, B.L. Tumor induction by the retinoblastoma mutation is independent of N-myc expression. *Nature 322*:555–557, 1986.

378. Stafford, W.R., Yanoff, M., and Parnell, B.L. Retinoblastoma initially misdiagnosed as primary ocular inflammation. *Arch. Ophthalmol. 82*:771–773, 1969.

379. Stevenson, K.E., Hungerford, J., and Garner, A. Local extraocular extension of retinoblastoma following intraocular surgery. *Br. J. Ophthalmol.* 73:739–742, 1989.

380. Stewart, J.K., Smith, J.L.S., and Arnold, E.L. Spontaneous regression of retinoblastoma. *Br. J. Ophthalmol. 40*:449–461, 1956.

381. Suckling, R.D., Fitzgerald, P.H., and Wells, E. The incidence and epidemiology of retinoblastoma in New Zealand: A 30 year survey. *Br. J. Cancer 46*:729–736, 1982.

382. Sullivan, S.F., and Dallow, R.L. Intraocular reticulum cell sarcoma: Its dramatic response to systemic chemotherapy and its angiogenic potential. *Ann. Ophthalmol. 9*:401–406, 1977.

383. Swartz, M. Aqueous humor lactic acid dehydrogenase in retinoblastoma. In *Intraocular Tumors*, G.A. Peyman, D.J. Apple, and D.R. Sanders (Eds.), Appleton-Century-Crofts, New York, pp. 331–335, 1977.

384. Symington, T., and Carter, R.L. *Scientific Foundations of Oncology*. William Heinemann, London, 1976.

385. Takahashi, T., Tamura, S., Inoue, M., Isayama, Y., and Sashikata, T. Retinoblastoma in a 26 year old adult. *Ophthalmology 90*:179–183, 1983.

386. Takayama, S., Yamomoto, M., and Ito, H. 27 Cases of retinoblastoma-pathological and immunohistological studies. *Nippon Ganka Gakkai Zasshi 89*:797–803, 1985.

387. Taktikos, A. Association of retinoblastoma with mental defect and other pathological manifestations. *Br. J. Ophthalmol. 48*:495–498, 1964.

388. Tamboli, A., Podgor, M.J., and Horm. J.W. The incidence of retinoblastoma in the United States: 1974–1985. *Arch. Ophthalmol. 108*:128–132, 1990.

389. Tang, A., Varley, J.M., Chakraborty, S., Murphree, A.L., and Fung, Y.K. Structural rearrangement of the retinoblastoma gene in human breast carcinoma. *Science 242*:263–266, 1988.

390. Tapia, F.J., Polak, J.M., Barbosa, A.J.A., Bloom, S.R., Marangos, P.J., Dermody, C., and Pearse, A.G.E. Neuro-specific enolase is produced by neuroendocrine tumors. *Lancet 1*:808–811, 1981.

391. Tarkkanen, A., Tervo, K., Eranko, L, Eranko, O., and Cuello, A.C. Substance P immunoreactivity in normal human retina and in retinoblastoma. *Ophthalmic Res. 15*:300–306, 1983.

392. Tarkkanen, A., Tervo, T., Tervo, K., and Panula, P. Immunohistochemical evidence for preproenkephalin. A synthesis in human retinoblastoma. *Invest. Ophthalmol. Vis. Sci. 25*:1210–1212, 1984.

393. Tarkkanen, A., and Tuovinen, E. Retinoblastoma in Finland 1912–1964. *Acta Ophthalmol. (Copenh.) 49*:293–300, 1971.

394. Tarlton, J.F., and Easty, D.L. Immunohistological characterization of retinoblastoma and related ocular tissue. *Br. J. Ophthalmol. 74*:144–149, 1990.

395. Ten Doesschate, G. Ueber metastatisches Sarkom des Auges. *Klin. Monatsbl. Augenheilkd. 66*:766, 1921.

396. Terenghi, G., Polak, J.M., Ballesta, J., Cocchia, D., Michetti, F., Dahl, D., Marangos, P.J., and Garner, A. Immunocytochemistry of neuronal and glial markers in retinoblastoma. *Virchows Arch. [A] 404*:61–73, 1984.

397. Tokunaya, T., and Nakamura, S. Electron microscopic figure of retinoblastoma. *Acta Soc. Ophthalmol. Jpn. 67*:1358–1368, 1963.

398. Tombran-Tink, J., and Johnson, L.V. Neuronal differentiation of retinoblastoma cells induced by medium conditioned by human RPE cells. *Science 30*:1700–1707, 1989.

399. Totsuka, S., Akazawa, K., and Minoda, K. Transplantation of retinoblastoma into the nude mouse-tumor doubling time of retinoblastoma. *Acta Soc. Ophthalmol. Jpn. 86*:418–425, 1982.

400. Trojanowski, J.Q., Obrocka, M.A., and Lee, V.M.-Y. Distribution of neurofilament subunits in neurons and neuronal processes: Immunohistochemical studies of bovine cerebellum with subunit-specific monoclonal antibodies. *J. Histochem. Cytochem. 33*:557–563, 1985.

401. Trojanowski, J.Q., Walkenstein, N., and Lee, V.M.Y. Expression of neurofilament subunits in neurons of the central and peripheral nervous system: An immunohistochemical study with monoclonal antibodies. *J. Neurosci. 6*:650–660, 1986.

402. Tso, M.O.M., Fine, B.S., and Zimmerman, L.E. The Flexner-Wintersteiner rosette in retinoblastoma. *Arch. Pathol. 88*:664–671, 1969.

403. Tso, M.O.M., Zimmerman, L.E., and Fine, B.S. The nature of retinoblastoma: Photoreceptor differentiation. *Trans. Am. Acad. Ophthalmol. Otolaryngol. 74*:959–989, 1970.

404. Tso, M.O.M., Zimmerman, L.E., and Fine, B.S. The nature of retinoblastoma. II. Photoreceptor differentiation an electronic microscopic study. *Am. J. Ophthalmol. 89*:350–359, 1970.

405. Tso, M.O.M., Zimmerman, L.E., and Fine, B.S. The nature of retinoblastoma. I. Photoreceptor differentiation: A clinical and histopathologic study. *Am. J. Ophthalmol. 89*:339–348, 1970.

406. Tsokos, M., Kyritsis, A.P., Chader, G.J., and Triche, T.J. Differentiation of human retinoblastoma in vitro into cell types with characteristics observed in embryonal or mature retina. *Am. J. Pathol. 123*:542–552, 1986.

407. Tsukahara, I. A histopathological study on the prognosis and radiosensitivity of retinoblastoma. *Arch. Ophthalmol. 63*:1005–1008, 1960.

408. Turner, D.L., and Cepko, C.L. A common progenitor for neurons and glia persists in rat retina late in development. *Nature 328*:131–136, 1987.

409. Uhler, E.M. Metastatic malignant melanoma of the retina. *Am. J. Ophthalmol. 23*:158–162, 1940.

410. Uusitalo, H., Lehtosalo, J.I., Gregerson, D.S., Uusitalo, R., and Palkama, A. Ultra-structural localization of retinal S-antigen in the rat. *Graefes Arch. Clin. Exp. Ophthalmol. 222*:118–122, 1985.

411. Verhoeff, F.H. Retinoblastoma undergoing spontaneous regression: Calcifying agent suggested in treatment of retinoblastoma. *Am. J. Ophthalmol. 62*:573–575, 1966.

412. Verhoeff, F.H., and Jackson, E. Minutes of the proceedings. Sixty-second Annual Meeting. *Trans. Am. Ophthalmol. Soc. 24*:38–39, 1926.

413. Vinores, S.A., Bonnin, J.M., Rubinstein, L.J., and Marangos, P.J. Immunohistochemical demonstration of neuron-specific enonase in neoplasms of the CNS and other tissues. *Arch. Pathol. Lab. Med. 108*:536–540, 1984.

414. Vinores, S.A., Herman, M.M., Rubinstein, L.J., and Marangos, P.J. Electron microscopic localization of neuron-specific enolase in rat and mouse brain. *J. Histochem. Cytochem. 32*:1295–1302, 1984.

415. Vinores, S.A., and Rubinstein, L.J. Simultaneous expression of glial fibrillary acidic (GFA) protein and neuron-specific enolase (NSE) by the same reactive or neoplastic astrocytes. *Neuropathol. Appl. Neurobiol. 11*:349–359, 1985.

416. Virchow, R. *Die kranklaften Gesschwuelste*, Vol. 2, August Hirschwald, Berlin, 1864.

417. Virtanen, I., Kivela, T., Bugnoli, M., Mencarelli, C., Pallini, V., Albert, D.M, and Tarkkanen, A. Expression of intermediate filaments and synaptophysin show neuronal properties and lack of glial characteristics in Y79 retinoblastoma cells. *Lab. Invest. 59*:649–655, 1988.

418. Vogel, F. Genetics of retinoblastoma. *Hum. Genet. 52*:1–54, 1979.

419. Vogl, M.H., Font, R.L., Zimmerman, L.E., and Levine, R.A. Reticulum cell sarcoma of the retina and uvea: Report of six cases and review of the literature. *Am. J. Ophthalmol. 66*:205–215, 1968.

420. Vrabec, T., Arbizo, V., Adamus, G., McDowell, J.H., Hargrave, P.A., and Donoso, L.A. Rod cell-specific antigens in retinoblastoma. *Arch. Ophthalmol. 107*:1061–1063, 1989.

421. Waardenburg, P.J., Franceschetti, A., and Klein, D. *Genetics and Ophthalmology*, Vol. 2. Charles C. Thomas, Springfield, IL, 1963.

422. Wackenheim, A., van Damme, W., Kosmann, P., and Bittighoffer, B. Computed tomography in ophthalmology. *Neuroradiology 13*:135–138, 1977.

423. Wagenmann, D. Ein Fall von multipler Melanosarkomen mit eigenartigen Komplikationen beider Augen. *Deutsch. Med. Wochenschr. 25*:262–263, 1900.

423a. Walsh, F.B., Hoyt, W.F., and Miller, N. *Clinical Neuro-Ophthalmology*, 4th ed. Williams and Wilkins, Baltimore, 1989.

424. Wardrop, J. *Observations on the Fungus Haematodes*. Constable, Edinburgh, 1809.

425. Weichselbaum, R.R., Nove, J., and Little, J.B. Skin fibroblasts from D-deletion type retinoblastoma patients are abnormally radiosensitive. *Nature 266*:726–727, 1977.

426. Weichselbaum, R.R., Zakov, Z.N., Albert, D.M., Friedman, A.H., Nove, J., and Little, J.B. New findings in the chromosome 13 long are deletion syndrome and retinoblastoma. *Ophthalmology 86*:1191–1198, 1979.

427. Weizenblatt, S. Differential diagnostic difficulties in atypical retinoblastoma. *Arch. Ophthalmol. 58*:699–709, 1957.

428. White. L., Reed, C., and Tobias, V. Comparison of cyclophosphamide and diaziquone in a retinoblastoma xenograft model. *Ophthalmic Pediatr. Genet. 10*:99–106, 1989.

429. Whyte, P., Buchkovich, K.J., Horowitz, J.M., Friend, S.H., Raybuck, M., Weinberg, R.A., and Harlow, E. Association between an oncogene and an anti-oncogene: The adenovirus E1A proteins bind to the retinoblastoma gene product. *Nature 334*:124–129, 1988.

430. Wick, M.R., Scheithauer, B.W., and Kovacs, K. Neuron-specific enolase in neuroendocrine tumors of the thymus, bronchus, and skin. *Am. J. Clin. Pathol. 79*:703–707, 1988.

431. Wiggs, J., Nordenskjold, M., Yandell, D., Rapaport, J., Grondin, V., et al. Prediction of the risk of hereditary retinoblastoma using DNA polymorphisms within the retinoblastoma gene. *N. Engl. J. Med. 318*:151–157, 1988.

432. Wiggs, J.L., and Dryja, T.P. Predicting the risk of hereditary retinoblastoma. *Am. J. Ophthalmol. 106*:346–351, 1988.

433. Willis, R.A. Pathology of tumors, 3rd ed. Butterworths, Washington, D.C., 1960.

434. Windle, J.J., Albert, D.M., O'Brien, J.M, Marcus, D.M., Disteche, C.M., Bernards, R., and Mellon, P.L. Retinoblastoma in transgenic mice. *Nature 343*:665–669, 1990.

435. Wintersteiner, H. *Die Neuroepithelioma retinae. Eine anatomische und klinische Studie*. Leipzig, Dentisae, p. 14, 1897.

436. Winther, J. Photodynamic therapy effect in an intraocular retinoblastoma-like tumor assessed by an in vivo to in vitro colony forming assay. *Br. J. Cancer 59*:869–872, 1989.

437. Winther, J., Olsen, J.H., and De Nully Brown, P. Risk of non-ocular cancer among retinoblastoma patients and their parents: A population based study in Denmark, 1943–1984. *Cancer 62*:1458–1462, 1988.

438. Winther, J., and Overgaard, J. Photodynamic therapy of experimental intraocular retinoblastomas—dose response relationships to light energy and photofrin II. *Acta Ophthalmol. (Copenh.) 67*:44–50, 1989.

439. Wolter, J.R. Retinoblastoma extension into the choroid. Pathological study of the neoplastic process and thoughts about its prognostic significance. *Ophthalmic Pediatr. Genet. 8*:151–157, 1987.

440. Wright, J.H. Neurocytoma or neuroblastoma, a kind of tumor not generally recognized. *J. Exp. Med. 12*:556–561, 1910.

441. Xu, H.J., Hu, S.X., Hashimoto, T, Takahashi, R., and Benedict, W.F. The retinoblastoma susceptibility gene product: A characteristic pattern in normal cells and abnormal expression in malignant cells. *Oncogene 4*:807–812, 1989.

442. Yandell, D.W. Parental origin of mutations of the retinoblastoma gene. *Nature 339*:556–558, 1989.
443. Yandell, D.W., Campbell, T.A., Dayton, S.H., Petersen, R., Walton, D., Little, J.B., McConkie-Ravell, A., Buckley, E.G., and Dryja, T.P. Oncogenic point mutations in the human retinoblastoma gene: Their application to genetic counseling. *N. Engl. J. Med. 321*:1689–1695, 1989.
444. Yanoff, M., and Fine, B.S. *Ocular Pathology: A Text and Atlas*. Harper and Row, New York, pp. 686–698, 1989.
445. Yokoyama, T., Tsukahara, T., Nakagawa, C., Kikuchi, T., Minoda, K., and Shimatake, H. The N-myc gene product in primary retinoblastomas. *Cancer 63*:2134–2138, 1989.
446. Young, S.E. Retinal metastases. In Ryan S.J. (Ed.), *Retina*, Vol. 1, C.V. Mosby, St. Louis, pp. 591–596, 1989.
447. Yttebsorg, J., and Arnesen, K. Late recurrence of retinoblastoma. *Acta Ophthalmol. (Copenh.) 50*:367–374, 1972.
448. Yunis, J.J., and Ramsay, N. Retinoblastoma and subband deletion of chromosome 13. *Am. J. Dis. Child. 132*:161–163, 1978.
449. Zhu, X., Dunn, J.M., Phillips, R.A., Goddard, A.D., Paton, K.E., Becker, A., and Gallie, B.L. Preferential germline mutation of the paternal allele in retinoblastoma (letter). *Nature 340*:312–313, 1989.
450. Zimmerman, L.E. Application of histochemical methods for the demonstration of acid mucopolysaccharides to ophthalmic pathology. *Trans. Am. Acad. Ophthalmol. Otolaryngol. 62*:697–703, 1958.
451. Zimmerman, L.E. Changing concepts concerning the pathogenesis of infectious disease. *Am. J. Ophthalmol. 69*:947–964, 1970.
452. Zimmerman, L.E. Retinoblastoma and retinocytoma. In *Ophthalmic Pathology: An Atlas and Textbook*, W.H. Spencer (Ed.), W.B. Saunders, Philadelphia, pp. 1292–1351, 1985.
453. Zimmerman, R.A., and Bilaniuk, L.T. Ocular MR imaging (editorial). *Radiology 168*:875–876, 1988.

50

Tumors of the Orbit, Optic Nerve, and Lacrimal Sac

Alec Garner
Institute of Ophthalmology, University of London, London, England

Gordon K. Klintworth
Duke University Medical Center, Durham, North Carolina

I. INTRODUCTION

For its small size, the orbit comprises a considerable variety of tissues: apart from the eye, muscle, collagen, cartilage, bone, fat, nerves, blood vessels, and glandular tissue are all features. It can also form a focus for lymphocytic aggregation. Consequently, it should occasion little surprise that the orbit can be a target for a wide range of tumor types. In this chapter the cardinal aspects only of orbital tumor pathology are discussed: for a full account, including therapeutic considerations, recourse should be made to the several comprehensive texts on the subject [172,197,226,362,374].

The frequency of the various types of orbital tumor in the population is difficult to define. Much depends on the source of the statistics [287], the experience in general hospitals tending to reflect a relatively high incidence of secondary and metastatic tumors and exclusively ophthalmic units attracting perhaps more of the esoteric primary tumors. There seems little doubt, however, that the majority of expanding lesions in the orbit are benign [124,362,405]. A listing of biopsied or resected neoplastic and other tumors seen during a 25 year period at the Institute of Ophthalmology, London (Table 1) points to a predominance of lymphoproliferative conditions followed by vascular lesions. In childhood the proportion of hamartomatous and developmental disorders, mostly capillary hemangiomas and dermoid cysts, is, not surprisingly, relatively greater than pertains in adults (Table 2). Lesions of this type accounted for an average 40% of the total in a cumulative analysis of several published series of orbital tumors in children [46,335]. Conversely, a review from Pakistan, which is likely to typify many other countries, revealed that over half the space-occupying orbital masses in children represented extraocular spread of retinoblastoma [328].

Immunocytochemical studies with the immunoperoxidase technique using monoclonal antibodies that recognize specific cellular antigens, such as structural proteins and cytoskeletal components (desmin and vimentin), increase the diagnostic accuracy of different orbital neoplasms and may suggest a firm diagnosis or aid in differentiating between different diagnostic possibilities [62,341,433].

Orbital fine-needle aspiration biopsy, especially if guided by computed tomography, provides a simple alternative to more invasive procedures [75,89,289,343,409,439,482]. Despite its limitations the technique is simple, rapid, inexpensive, and well accepted by patients and has not produced significant complications. Fine-needle aspiration biopsies can prevent unnecessary exploratory surgery, especially in patients with metastatic orbital tumors. The method also avoids radical surgery of benign lesions and can be used when a recurrence of an orbital neoplasm is suspected, as when a new mass is detected by computed tomography. All tumors cannot be recognized by fine-needle aspiration, but many conditions can be reliably diagnosed with this method if it is applied in cooperation with an experienced pathologist [343].

Table 1 Relative Incidence of Expanding Lesions of the Orbit Examined at the Institute of Ophthalmology, London, 1966–1990

Inflammatory	183 (12.3%)
Nonspecific	169
Sarcoidosis	11
Fasciitis	3
Fibrous tissue tumors	20 (1.32%)
Fibrous histiocytoma (benign)	8
Fibrous histiocytoma (malignant)	6
Fibrosarcoma	6
Histiocytic tumors	9 (0.6%)
Xanthogranuloma	5
Histiocytosis X	4
Adipose tissue tumors	10 (0.7%)
Lipoma	3
Liposarcoma	7
Muscle tumors	78 (5.3%)
Rhabdomyosarcoma	78
Vascular tumors	231 (15.6%)
Capillary hemangioma	26
Cavernous hemangioma	101
Malformations	93
Hemangiopericytoma	7
Angiosarcoma	4
Bone and cartilage tumors	10 (0.6%)
Chondroma	1
Chondrosarcoma	2
Benign osteoblastoma	3
Aneurysmal bone cyst	2
Osteoma	2
Periopheral nerve tumors	93 (6.3%)
Neurofibroma	36
Schwannoma	45
Granular cell	7
Malignant	5
Optic nerve tumors	109 (7.3%)
Astrocytoma (juvenile)	33
Malignant astrocytoma	2
Meningioma[a]	74
Germ cell tumors	100 (6.7%)
Dermoid cyst	99
Teratoma	1
Lymphoid tumors	353 (23.8%)
Lymphoid hyperplasia	151
Lymphoma (non-Hodgkins)	142
Indeterminate	60
Lacrimal gland tumors	132 (8.9%)
Pleomorphic adenoma	76
Adenocarcinoma	16
Adenoid cystic carcinoma	39
Mucoepidermoid	1
Secondary tumors	113 (7.6%)
Local spread	56
Metastases	57
Miscellaneous	49 (3.3%)
Mucocele	7
Cholesterol granuloma	9
Others	33

[a]Number almost certainly includes several unsuspected intracranial primary tumors.

Table 2 Frequency or Orbital Tumors in Children Based on Several Series

	Number of cases	%
Dermoid cyst	134	37.4
Hemangioma	42	11.7
Rhabdomyosarcoma	31	8.7
Glioma of optic nerve	20	5.6
Neurofibroma	14	3.9
Neuroblastoma	12	3.4
Lymphangioma	10	2.8
Inflammatory pseudotumor	9	2.5
Leukemia and lymphoma	9	2.5
Lipoma	7	2.0
Meningioma (orbit/sphenoid ridge)	8	2.2
Schwannoma	6	1.7
Microphthalmos with cyst	5	1.4
Teratoma	4	1.1
Prominent palpebral lobe of lacrimal gland	4	1.1
Retinoblastoma		
Orbital recurrence	4	1.1
Orbital presentation	2	0.6
Undifferentiated sarcoma	3	0.8
Epithelial or "sebaceous" cysts	3	0.8
Noninflammatory pseudotumor	3	0.8
Arteriovenous malformation	3	0.8
Ectopic lacrimal gland	2	0.6
Epibulbar, eyelid, and obital osseous choristoma	2	0.6
Dermolipoma	2	0.6
Lacrimal gland duct cyst	2	0.6
Alveolar soft-part sarcoma	2	0.6
Fibrous dysplasia	2	0.6
Neurosarcoma	1	
Metastatic embryonal sarcoma	1	
Pleomorphic adenoma of lacrimal gland	1	
Benign adenomatous epithelial hyperplasia of sweat or lacrimal gland	1	
Osteoma	1	
Meningoencephalocele	1	
Amyloidosis	1	
Eosinophilic granuloma	1	
Malignant teratoid epithelioma of optic nerve	1	
"Metastatic" astrocytoma	1	
Posttraumatic hemorrhagic cyst	1	
Myxosarcoma	1	
Prolapsed orbital fat	1	
Total	358	100

Source: Modified from Reference 189.

Nevertheless, the technique is not without problems. Strict radiological control is necessary to ensure that the appropriate tissue is being sampled, and cell aspiration is rarely feasible for fibrotic lesions. Furthermore, caution is needed in the interpretation of the cytological preparations because benign lesions, such as meningioma and reactive lymphoid hyperplasia, may be misinterpreted as malignant and non-Hodgkin's lymphoma may be regarded as benign [439].

The value of clinical staging of soft tissue sarcomas in general for the purposes of management and prognostication has been gaining acceptance in recent years and might well be applied in the context of the orbit with advantage. Staging is based on tumor size, involvement of regional lymph nodes, evidence of distant metastasis, and the histological grade of malignancy [383]. Apart from the last, the parameters are objective and can be summed to give a grading within the range I–IV. An analysis along these lines of 1215 soft tissue tumors representing 13 histological types of sarcoma has shown good correlation with survival and indicates that staging creates a sound base from which to determine therapeutic modalities [383,432].

II. TUMORS OF THE LACRIMAL GLAND

A. Benign

Pleomorphic Adenoma

Accounting for slightly more than half of all lacrimal gland tumors [22,116,147,403], pleomorphic adenoma most often presents during the fourth decade with proptosis or displacement of the eye. A common but less appropriate name for pleomorphic adenoma is benign mixed tumor, since according to evidence originally drawn from its counterpart in the parotid salivary gland, there is reason to regard the stromal components as, like the acinar and ductal tissue, of epithelial origin. This view was initially based on the character of the mucinous elements of the tumors but was more recently supported by immunohistochemical evidence that suggests that the more obviously glandular elements derive from ductal epithelium and the "stromal" components are of myoepithelial origin [322,419]. Moreover, it is possible that the tumor represents neoplastic transformation of a single stem cell of myoepithelial type [419]. Direct evidence derived from an immunohistochemical study of lacrimal gland tumors points similarly to a pure epithelial histogenesis [158]. Theoretically, it is conceivable that, as in the salivary glands, there should be a range of adenomatous tumors ranging from those with a pure ductal element to those composed exclusively of myoepithelium. As yet instances of such monomorphic adenomas in the lacrimal gland are

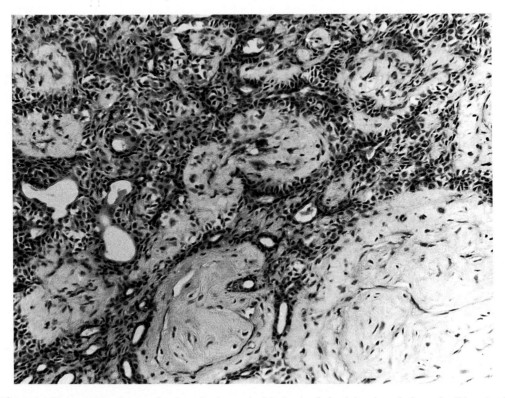

Figure 1 Pleomorphic adenoma (benign mixed tumor) of the lacrimal gland showing tubules and solid cords of epithelium together with islands of hyalinized stroma formed by myoepithelial cells. (Hematoxylin and eosin, ×180)

limited to rare cases of myoepithelioma [117,171], but it seems sensible to consider the pleomorphic adenoma as occupying an intermediate position in a continuous spectrum of neoplastic development.

Histologically, the tumor is composed of a predominantly double cell layer of epithelium arranged in interlacing ducts and solid strands surrounded by a matrix of myxoid epithelial secretion in which islands of chondroid differentiation are common (Fig. 1). The overtly epithelial component is distinguished by a conspicuous keratin content, whereas the myoepithelial stromal cells stain for smooth muscle actin and, less consistently, glial fibrillary acid protein and vimentin [158].

Despite being encapsulated, it is not uncommon for histopathological examination of a pleomorphic adenoma to disclose small groups of tumor cells extending through the capsule. This is likely to contribute to a tendency to recur after surgical excision [22,116,125,484]. It is also to be noted that the tumor may be surrounded by a marked lymphocytic reaction, which, when biopsy specimens are taken from the edge of the lesion, may lead to a mistaken diagnosis of inflammatory pseudotumor.

B. Malignant

Pleomorphic Adenocarcinoma

Malignant types of mixed lacrimal tumors carry a moderately poor prognosis and account for between 10 and 20% of all such neoplasms [22,116,474]. They may arise de novo, but more commonly they develop within a preexisting benign adenoma, and a typical history is of removal of a pleomorphic adenoma followed by one or more recurrences and evidence of a more aggressive behavior in the form of local invasion or distant metastasis. The malignant component appears to originate within the overtly epithelial tissue, where it gives rise to an adenocarcinomatous (Fig. 2) or, less often, a squamous carcinomatous

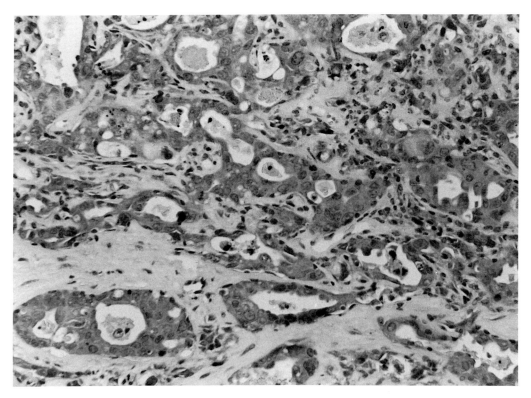

Figure 2   Pleomorphic adenocarcinoma (malignant mixed tumor) of the lacrimal gland. The epithelium forming the ductular tissue is irregular, with nuclear hyperchromatism and increased mitotic activity. (Hematoxylin and eosin, ×280)

picture. Rare involvement of the "stromal" element can result in a pseudosarcomatous spindle cell histology.

Adenoid Cystic Carcinoma

Adenoid cystic carcinoma accounted for 30% of all lacrimal gland neoplasms in the series reported by Font and Gamel [116] and is much the most common form of malignancy in this situation [22,116,126,477]. In the series reported from the Armed Forces Institute of Pathology in the United States, about one in nine adenoid cystic carcinomas developed within a pleomorphic adenoma [116].

The histology of the usual cribiform tumor is one of anastomosing cords of small cells with hyperchromatic nuclei and sparse cytoplasm within a hyalinized or hypocellular fibrous stroma (Fig. 3). The individual cords are perforated by multiple cystic spaces, which create a swiss cheese cylindromatous pattern. This tumor can be diagnosed by fine-needle aspiration [289]. Electron microscopy shows that the tumor cells contain granules normally seen in the terminal ducts, indicating that adenoid cystic carcinoma probably originates from the duct epithelium. There are a number of histological variants, however, including basaloid and sclerosing patterns. The basaloid variant (Fig. 4), which is formed by solid lobules of densely compacted cells with basophilic nuclei and scanty cytoplasm, is particularly noteworthy because it carries a decidedly worse prognosis than the other types [138,477]. Pathologists need to be aware of the basaloid variant of the adenoid cystic carcinoma because it can be confused with orbital invasion by a basal carcinoma.

A proclivity to infiltrate along nerves and blood vessels is the likely explanation for the rapidity with which adenoid cystic carcinoma invades adjacent structures, including the brain. Distant metastasis may also occur, and the overall prognosis is poor, with a 10 year survival rate between 10 and 25% [138,477].

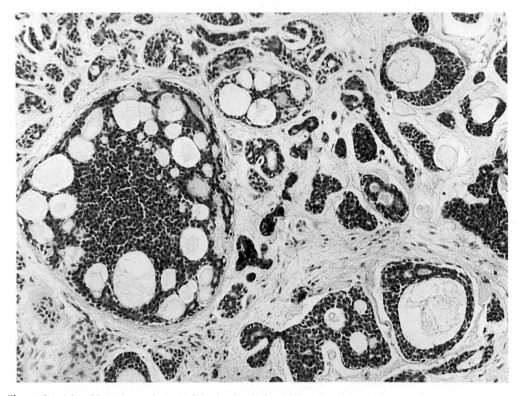

Figure 3   Adenoid cystic carcinoma of the lacrimal gland. Groups of closely packed tumor cells surround tubular spaces of varying size to create a cribiform appearance (Hematoxylin and eosin, ×180)

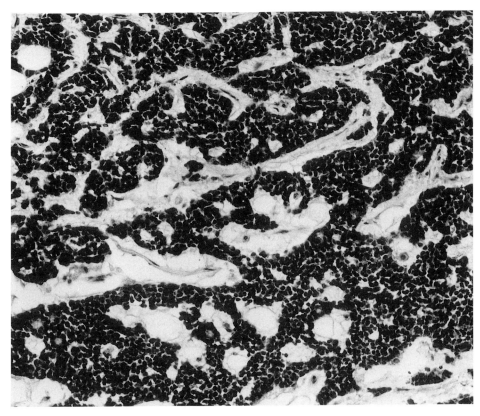

Figure 4   Adenoid cystic carcinoma of the lacrimal gland. The arrangement of the cells is characteristic of the basaloid variant. (Hematoxylin and eosin, ×180)

Monomorphic Adenocarcinoma

Lacrimal gland carcinoma arising de novo in which the malignancy is confined to a pure adenoid type of differentiation is fairly uncommon. The prognosis for carcinomas developing de novo is considerably worse than for malignant transformation within pleomorphic adenomas, with medium survival rates of 3.5 and 12.0 years, respectively [116].

Mucoepidermoid Tumors

A not uncommon type of salivary gland tumor characterized by proliferation of intimately related squamous and mucus-secreting epithelium occurs, as a rarity, in the lacrimal gland [358]. However, unless sufficient sections are examined to exclude other kinds of tissue differentiation that would establish a diagnosis of pleomorphic adenoma (or carcinoma), recognition of mucoepidermoid tumor is tenuous, and Ashton [22] found only one acceptable case in his review of the published cases. The tumor is considered to stem from the duct epithelium and can show a variable degree of malignancy, which is not always reflected in the histological appearance. Correspondingly, some workers prefer not to define mucoepidermoid tumors in terms of adenoma or carcinoma.

Other Carcinomas

Squamous cell and, rarely, sebaceous gland [252] differentiation or anaplasia may also be encountered in lacrimal gland neoplasia with a prognosis comparable to that of other carcinomas at this site.

III. TUMORS OF THE LACRIMAL SAC

Lined by pseudostratified columnar (transitional cell) epithelium with an admixture of mucus-secreting goblet cells, neoplasms originating within the lacrimal sac reflect their histogenesis from ectodermal epithelium continuous with the schneiderian membrane of the nasal passages and usually present with epiphora, swelling, and inflammation due to obstructed outflow. Pain is a feature of the malignant lesions.

A. Benign

Transitional Cell Papilloma

According to two studies covering a total of 35 epithelial neoplasms of the lacrimal sac [169,384], transitional cell papillomas composed of columnar cells, commonly with evidence of early squamous differentiation and growing toward the wall of the sac as a result of infolding, are the most common type of benign neoplasm in this situation (Fig. 5). Mitotic activity is slight, differentiation is good, and the basement membrane of the proliferating epithelium is intact. The prognosis for a well-differentiated papilloma is excellent if completely excised, but recurrences are not uncommon because of surgical difficulties in guaranteeing complete removal, and in some of these tumors malignant transformation can supervene [169,384].

Squamous Cell Papilloma

A minority of tumors consist entirely of differentiated squamous epithelium, and although it may be that such papillomas have a preference for proliferation within the cavity of the lacrimal sac, as op-

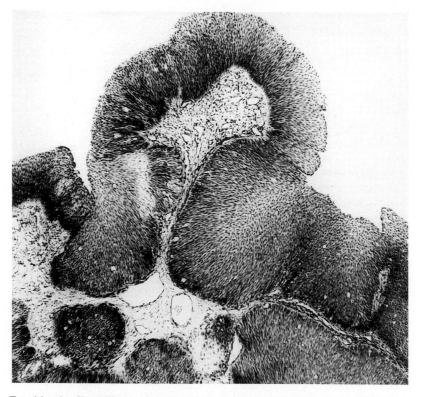

Figure 5 Transitional cell papilloma of the lacrimal sac, showing folding of the proliferated epithelium. (Hematoxylin and eosin, ×70) (Reproduced with permission from Harry, J., and Ashton, N. The pathology of tumours of the lacrimal sac. *Trans. Ophthalmol. Soc. UK* 88:19–35, 1968.)

posed to "transitional" cell papillomas, which grow mainly into the supporting stroma, there is no reason to regard them separately. It has been proposed that the designation "schneiderian papilloma" is a convenient inclusive term [232].

B. Malignant

Transitional Cell Carcinoma

Malignant tumors with recognizable stratified columnar epithelium may arise de novo or complicate a papilloma. Diagnosis is based on a conspicuous level of mitotic activity, cellular pleomorphism with nuclear irregularity, and, ultimately, evidence of extension into the wall of the sac with penetration of the epithelial basement membrane. Local recurrence after surgery with spread into the orbit has complicated about one-half of the cases in two reported series, and exceptionally, widespread carcinomatosis has been recorded [169].

In addition to frank carcinoma, Ryan and Font [384] have described instances of focal malignant change within transitional cell papillomas. Harry and Ashton [169] also recognized a state intermediate between benignity and unequivocal malignancy, and there appears to be a correlation between repeated recurrence and increasing histological evidence of malignancy.

Histological distinction between benign and malignant epithelial tumors can be very difficult and is sometimes impossible, in which case the initial surgery should aim for complete excision in all cases [113]. The prognosis for histologically malignant lesions is not encouraging [334].

Squamous Cell Carcinoma

In the experience of Ryan and Font [384], squamous cell carcinoma is the most frequent form of lacrimal sac malignancy, some arising de novo but others complicating benign transitional cell or squamous cell papillomas. As with transitional cell tumors, conservative surgery is the treatment of choice in the first instance.

Other Tumors

Isolated examples of fibrous histiocytoma [65,239], benign and malignant oncocytic tumors [24,349], lymphoma [468], angiosarcoma [169,222], schwannoma [339], malignant melanoma [93,106,169,442, 480], hemangiopericytoma [53], adenoid cystic carcinoma [240], and mucoepidermoid carcinoma [39] have also been reported in the lacrimal sac.

IV. TUMORS OF FIBROUS TISSUE

A. Benign

Fibroma

The diagnosis of fibroma is somewhat nebulous, relying for its recognition on finding a circumscribed proliferation of regular collagen-producing fibroblasts in the absence of an obvious predisposing condition, such as inflammation or a hematoma. In view of this difficulty, very few substantiated discrete fibromas have been described, and those in the orbit have been adjacent to the periosteum [54,325].

Fibromatosis

Fibromatosis describes a proliferation of fibroblasts that, although lacking the metastasizing potential of a fibrosarcoma, are prone to be locally invasive and to lack the distinct capsule of a benign fibroma [395,428]. A variety of names have been applied to lesions of this sort, reflecting their congenital or acquired nature, as the case may be, and their anatomical distribution [283]. In general, fibromatoses occurring in young subjects exhibit the most aggressive behavior [6]. Orbital involvement is uncommon but not unknown [175,330,408], most cases presenting in the first decade of life and showing a predilection for the inferior orbit and lower eyelid.

B. Malignant

Fibrosarcoma

An uncommon tumor in the orbit, most adequately documented fibrosarcomas in this location have followed irradiation of retinoblastomas; when the latter are inherited, there is a distinct possibility that both retinal and fibrous tissue tumors are linked to the same genetic defect [3,5]. Instances of spontaneous orbital fibrosarcoma are very rare in adults and children, but it is noteworthy that the juvenile form carries much the best prognosis [457].

The histological appearance is of a highly cellular proliferation of spindle cells commonly organized in a fascicular or even a "herringbone" pattern. Mitotic figures are prominent, but as a corollary, synthetic function is diminished and amounts of collagen are slight or undetectable. In the latter case the electron microscopical demonstration of a prominent rough-surfaced endoplasmic reticulum with absence of intercellular digitations but with poorly developed desmosomes may be useful in excluding other spindle cell tumors, such as meningioma and fibrous histiocytoma [211].

V. TUMORS OF HISTIOCYTIC ORIGIN

A distinction needs to be made between cells whose primary function is phagocytosis and those that acquire phagocytic properties (facultative phagocytosis) as a secondary activity. The first type describes cells that originate in the bone marrow and either become fixed histiocytes lining such structures as hepatic, splenic, and lymph node sinuses during intrauterine life or circulate as blood monocytes and migrate through the tissues, where they are recognized as macrophages. Facultative histiocytes include vascular endothelium (as well as the corneal and trabecular meshwork endothelium) and fibroblasts. Neoplasia of cells showing secondary phagocytic properties may well be the basis of fibrous histiocytomas [203]. An excellent review of the histiocytoses and of the distinctions among them was written by Malone [290a].

The ensuing descriptions relate primarily to tumors of essential phagocytes.

A. Benign

Xanthoma

Tumors referred to as xanthomas are composed of cells with small, round nuclei and abundant foamy or finely granular cytoplasm, which is rich in neutral lipid. They are rarely encountered in the orbit [315]. Whether xanthomas are true neoplasms or represent a localized phagocytic response to some undisclosed event, such as a hematoma, is arguable but of little practical significance, since they are self-limiting and utterly benign.

Juvenile Xanthogranuloma

Although the term "xanthogranuloma" has been used to describe a xanthomalike lesion associated with chronic inflammatory cell infiltration, a juvenile xanthogranuloma is a well-documented self-limiting proliferation of histiocytes presenting in infancy (Fig. 6). Compared with the iris and eyelids, involvement of the orbit is rare [391,483].

Necrobiotic Xanthogranuloma

This is an uncommon condition resembling the juvenile form in many respects but differing in involving adults, in having zones of stromal necrosis that may be slowly progressive, and in being linked in most instances with a dysproteinemia. Periocular and anterior orbital involvement is a frequent site for the lesions [370,377].

Fibrous Histiocytoma

Alternatively known as fibrous xanthoma, there is reason to believe that this tumor arises from facultative phagocytes rather than primary histiocytes since the cells have interdigitating processes and form rudimentary desmsomal junctions [203]. Such morphology is characteristic of fibroblasts rather than of true macrophages.

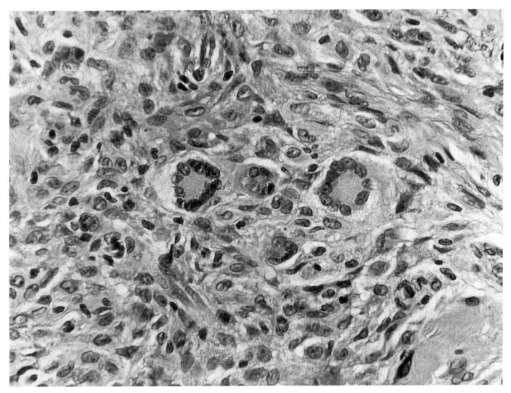

Figure 6 Juvenile xanthogranuloma of the orbit, showing proliferation of histiocytes, some of which have a rather foamy cytoplasm, with two Touton giant cells, each consisting of a ring of nuclei around a core of finely granular material. (Hematoxylin and eosin, ×450)

Fibrous histiocytomas usually present in adult life [199,303] but have been observed in infancy [207], and there is a more or less equal sex incidence. Within the orbit, the upper nasal quadrant appears to be a favored site, and the patient generally presents with proptosis and diplopia caused by infiltration of the extraocular muscles. Since the tumors tend not to have a significant capsule, they can be difficult to remove, which probably contributes to a recurrence after surgery of about 30% [118]. There is some evidence, based on DNA measurements, that the "histiocytic" cells are the more malignant component of the tumor, although both they and the spindle cell forms stem from a common precursor [144].

The histological picture is of cells that are mostly spindle shaped arranged in a characteristic storiform (matted) or cartwheel pattern (Fig. 7). Extracellular connective tissue is variable but rarely conspicuous. Cells with a histiocytic morphology complemented by appropriate enzyme properties are an inconstant feature, although multinucleated giant cells may sometimes be present. Mitotic activity is minimal and metastasis does not occur.

B. Malignant

Malignant Fibrous Histiocytoma

Tumors distinguished by hypercellularity and other histological features of malignancy, such as nuclear irregularity, hyperchromatism, and prominent mitotic activity, accounted for 17 of 150 fibrohistiocytic tumors reported by Font and Hidayat [118] (Fig. 8). Such tumors may be seen at the time of surgery to be infiltrating the surrounding tissues so that repeated local recurrences are common, death ensuing in some patients because of direct spread to vital structures or distant metastasis [372]. A ten year survival rate of about 25% has been cited [118]. Some fibrous histiocytomas are locally aggressive but have no apparent metastatic potential: they are distinguished histologically by showing definite infiltrative activity, as do the

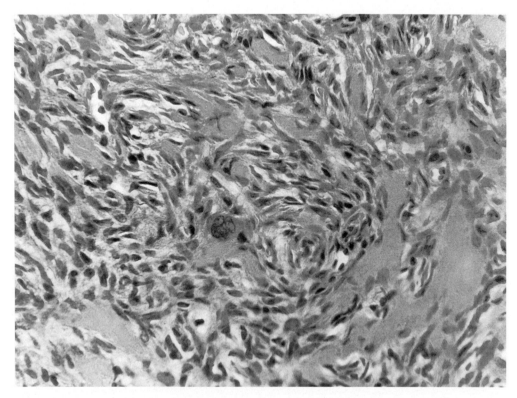

Figure 7 Fibrous histiocytoma. Spindle-shaped cells intermingled with wisps of collagenous tissue are arranged in a matted and slightly whorled pattern. A multinucleated cell is also present but has no sinister implication, and the overall cytology is regular. (Hematoxylin and eosin, ×450)

overtly malignant tumors, in the absence of the cytological features of malignancy. A macrophage origin has been postulated on the basis of immunohistochemistry [430].

C. Histiocytic Tumors of Uncertain Nature

Histiocytosis X (Langerhans Cell Histiocytosis)

"Histiocytosis X" is the term introduced by Lichtenstein [269] to describe a spectrum of arguably neoplastic proliferations of histiocytes occurring in osseous and soft tissues. The cells are now recognized as Langerhans cells, and the proliferation is generally regarded as reactive rather than neoplastic [107]. They may show varying degrees of maturation, the more primitive cells having a slightly basophilic cytoplasm and little evidence of phagocytic function, whereas those presumed to be more mature have eosinophilic cytoplasm and often contain ingested lipid.

At one end of the histiocytosis X spectrum is an acute disseminated form (Letterer-Siwe disease) that develops in infancy, with widespread bony and visceral involvement producing hepatosplenomegaly and myelophthisic anemia. The acute form of the disease is frequently fatal, and the histiocytic proliferation is predominantly of the immature cell type. Uveal involvement is well documented in Letterer-Siwe disease [313], but orbital involvement is exceptional [431], owing perhaps to a relative infrequency of destructive bone disease in this variant of histiocytosis X. Conversely, lytic lesions of bone are an integral component of the chronic disseminated form (Hand-Schüller-Christian disease), and orbital involvement occurs in about one-quarter of patients [316]. The classic triad of this variety consists of punched-out bone defects in the skull, unilateral or bilateral exophthalmos, and diabetes insipidus, with, in some patients, other manifestations of pituitary failure. Hand-Schüller-Christian disease occurs in childhood, as opposed to infancy, and is characterized by multifocal proliferation of mature histiocytes that have foamy cytoplasm

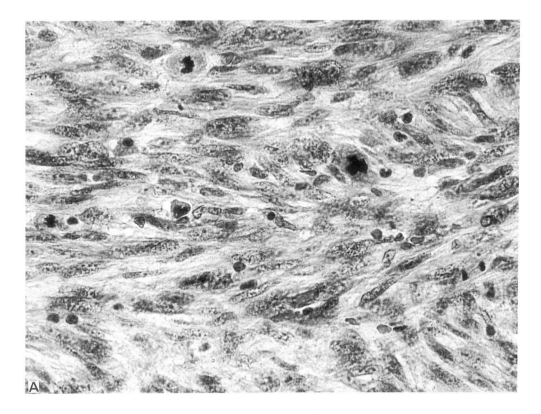

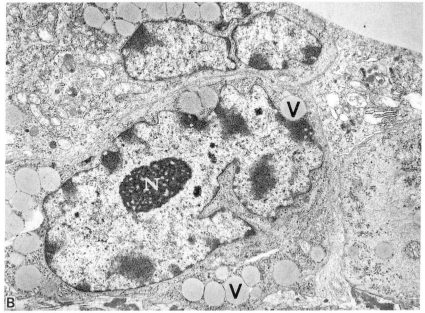

Figure 8 Malignant fibrous histiocytoma. (A) The cells remain predominantly spindle shaped but have increased nuclear-cytoplasmic ratios and conspicuous nucleoli and show prominent abnormal mitotic activity. (Hematoxylin and eosin, ×450) (B) Ultrastructure of tumor cell in malignant fibrous histiocytoma. Note the prominent nucleolus (N) and numerous cytoplasmic vacuoles (V). (×6600) (Courtesy of Dr. J. Shelburne.)

and, in frozen sections, demonstrable lipid. Eosinophils may also be present. The prognosis is a little better, with a 50% mortality, than pertains in Letterer-Siwe disease (mortality approximately 70%) [102]. A rare disseminated form occurring in an adult has also been described [282].

Whether eosinophilic granuloma of bone represents the other end of the histiocytosis X spectrum, as proposed by Lichtenstein [268], is disputed. The arguments in favor of an association rest on the presence of mature Langerhans cells, although these are less foamy than those seen in Hand-Schüller-Christian disease, and the presence of other leukocytes, including numerous eosinophils. The counterarguments are based on the nonprogressive behavior of a solitary lesion, which in contrast to accepted forms of histiocytosis X presents no threat to survival [26,63]. Orbital involvement in eosinophilic granuloma occurs between the ages of 3 and 10 years [27,212], which is earlier than often pertains in other bones.

Confirmation of the Langerhans cell presence is provided by an anti-T6 antibody response using an immunohistochemical technique, and electron microscopy reveals characteristic granules (histiocytosis X bodies, Birbeck granules, Langerhans granules, or racquet bodies) in the cytoplasm, which are formed, possibly, by fusion of contiguous surface ruffles and their subsequent ingestion [339]. The granules have a laminated rod-shaped profile (see Chap. 1, Fig. 73).

Sinus Histiocytosis with Massive Lymphadenopathy

In 1969, Rosai and Dorfman [376] described a self-limiting lesion in which there is bilateral cervical lymphadenopathy with fever, predominantly affecting children. Other sites are involved, including the orbit [64,231], where extranodal collections of large pale histiocytes surrounded by lymphoid cells are seen. A notable feature of the histiocytes is the presence of phagocytozed intact lymphocytes, plasma cells, and erythrocytes.

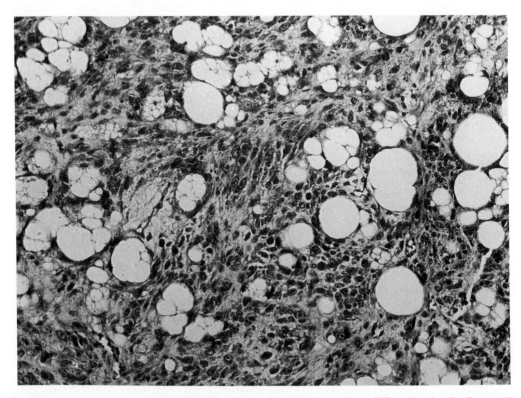

Figure 9 Liposarcoma of the orbit, showing pleomorphic and frequently undifferentiated cells. Some cells contain multiple vacuoles within the cytoplasm, however, and in places the lipid content has been liberated to create larger vacuolar spaces. Oil red O staining of frozen sections serves to confirm the lipid nature of the material within the vacuoles. (Hematoxylin and eosin, ×180)

VI. TUMORS OF ADIPOSE TISSUE

A. Benign

Lipoma

To distinguish between benign neoplasia of mature fat cells and normal adipose tissue is impossible on histological grounds. Recognition is based on clinical evidence of an increased amount of adipose tissue in the orbit sufficient to cause proptosis or displacement of the eyeball, but even then it is necessary to exclude herniation of normal orbital adipose tissue through the orbital septum [228]. A rare type of lipoma in which mature lipocytes are admixed with spindle cells has also been described in the orbit [31,220], as has a presumed hamartomatous lipoma present from birth [45].

Lipomatosis

An increase in orbital fat associated with subcutaneous lipomas involving the limbs and fatty infiltration of the myocardium is on record [323].

B. Malignant

Liposarcoma

Liposarcoma involving the orbit is a rare but highly malignant tumor, arising, it is believed, not from mature adipose tissue but from primitive mesenchymal cells located in the fascial planes [103]. If the latter contention is correct, it would go a long way toward explaining the variable histological picture seen not only between tumors but within the same tumor. Thus, although rounded cells with vaculated lipid-filled cytoplasm may be seen (Fig. 9), the predominant form is a myxoid liposarcoma composed of stellate or spindle-shaped cells within a mucoid matrix (Fig. 10) [105,258,396]. The degree of anaplasia and

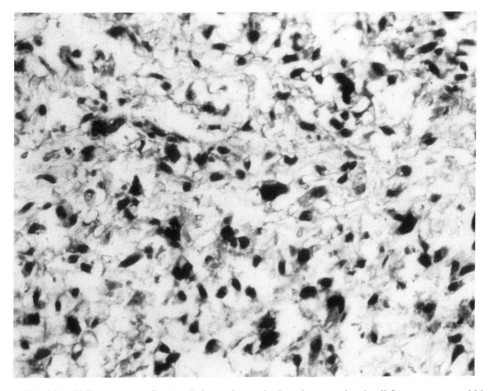

Figure 10   Myxoid liposarcoma. Scattered signet ring and otherwise vacuolated cell forms are seen within a loose stroma, and the cell nuclei show moderate pleomorphism. (Hematoxylin and eosin, ×480)

cytological evidence of malignancy in the form of nuclear atypia, hyperchromatism, and excessive mitotic activity is related to the risk of metastasis. Histological diagnosis is facilitated by the examination of frozen sections stained for fat, although it is to be emphasized that cells other than lipoblasts may contain lipid. Liposarcoma in general is an adult tumor, but an exceptional example of a pleomorphic liposarcoma supervening within an ostensibly benign lipoblastoma in a 12-year-old boy is recorded [309].

Wide local resection may be appropriate for the better differentiated myxoid variants, but in general exenteration is needed to prevent recurrence and even then there is a risk of metastases at a later date [209,258,392].

VII. TUMORS OF MUSCLE

A. Striated Muscle

Rhabdomyoma

Benign tumors of striated muscle in any situation are extremely rare, and an accepted example occurring in the orbit has yet to be presented [247].

Rhabdomyosarcoma

Neoplasia of established striated muscle is exceptional anywhere in the body and is virtually unknown in the orbit, although Kassel and colleagues [235] described a rhabdomyosarcoma intimately related to the extrinsic ocular muscles in a 78-year-old man. In general, tumors showing evidence of striated muscle differentiation, whatever their location, do not show an anatomical association with established muscle. They appear rather to stem from primitive mesenchymal elements and, as such, are usually tumors of childhood and adolescence. The majority (75%) of cases present in the first decade and exceptionally are present at birth [100], but orbital rhabdomyosarcoma after adolescence is uncommon [23,227,354]. A slight preponderance of male patients is evident in each of the studies reported. Rapidly progressive exophthalmos, with or without pain, is the dominant clinical feature [227], although ptosis and epiphora complicate some cases [168]. The tumor can develop anywhere in the orbit but is most commonly situated behind or above the globe [227].

From a histological standpoint four types of rhabdomyosarcoma can be recognized: pleomorphic, embryonal, botryoid, and alveolar. This classification is unfortunately not without fault, since by mixing histogenetic and morphological terms it obscures the embryonal or developmental character of the alveolar and botryoid variants. Furthermore, other than with respect to the alveolar variant, which has a generally worse prognosis, the subdivision has little bearing on clinical outcome, and classifications based solely on cell type have been proposed [344].

When the diagnosis of orbital rhabdomyosarcoma is problematical, immunohistochemical investigations are often valuable. Antibodies against desmin and α-sarcomeric actin are useful for the diagnostic definition of rhabdomyosarcoma [62,433,446], whereas α smooth muscle actin is absent and antibodies to myoglobin, vimentin, and enolase are unreliable [62,433]. The protein product of the muscle regulatory gene MyoD1 is highly restricted in its distribution in human tissue and has only been detected in skeletal muscle, especially fetal, and in rhabdomyosarcomas [84]: correspondingly, its demonstration, even in the absence of desmin expression, may be diagnostic in suspected rhabdomyosarcoma. Electron microscopy can also be extremely useful as a diagnostic tool in equivocal cases of embryonal rhabdomyosarcoma. Even poorly differentiated rhabdomyoblasts commonly contain bundles of 150 nm myosin filaments; the better differentiated cells show periodic transverse Z bands indicative of primitive sarcomere formation (Fig. 11).

Adult Rhabdomyosarcoma

Commonly referred to as pleomorphic rhabdomyosarcoma [426], this neoplasm is considered to arise from established voluntary muscle and, as discussed earlier, is extremely rare in the orbit [235,249]. Histologically, it consists of rhabdomyoblasts showing various degrees of differentiation, although cross-striations are unusual: most cells are round or strap or racquet shaped with eosinophilic cytoplasm, which is often granular, but vacuolation to create a "spider" cell may also be seen. The nucleus may be markedly

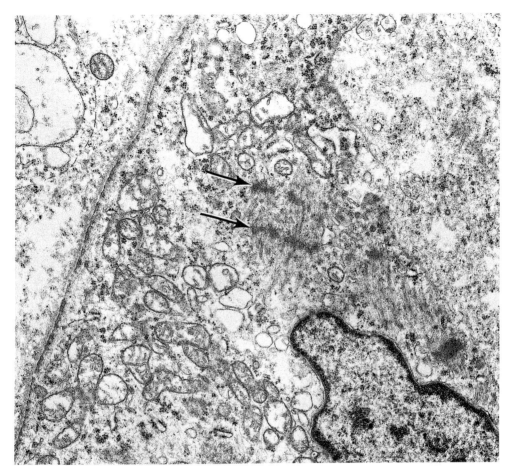

Figure 11   The diagnosis of a rhabdomyosarcoma can be established by electron microscopy when the 15 nm thick cytoplasmic filaments of myosin have a parallel arrangement and are organized into sarcomere-like units with Z lines (arrows). The cells contain both thick (myosin) and thin (actin) filaments. (×15,000)

irregular, multinucleated giant cells can occur, and mitotic activity is usually pronounced. Cell necrosis may also be noticed [80].

Embryonal Rhabdomyosarcoma

Tumors arising before adult life and differentiating toward, rather than from, striated muscle predominate in the head and neck region [425], whereas the adult rhabdomyosarcoma is essentially a tumor of the limb muscles. Several subdivisions of embryonal rhabdomyosarcoma have been described [23,227,249,354] according to the macroscopic and microscopic appearance. The degree of differentiation, taking the presence of racquet- or strap-shaped cells (Fig. 12) as evidence of myoblastic maturation, seems to be the best histological guide to behavior. Cross-striations (Fig. 13), although of inestimable value in arriving at a diagnosis, do not have much use in prognosis.

Embryonal rhabdomyosarcoma as defined in histological terms alone, and in contradistinction to the alveolar and botryoid types, covers a range of appearances. The cells may be elongated and bipolar with markedly eosinophilic cytoplasm and a darkly stained flattened nucleus, they may be racquet or strap shaped, they may exhibit cross-striations, they may be vacuolated, and they may be multinucleated. Sometimes the cells are round or spindle shaped with relatively little cytoplasm and no clear evidence of muscle differentiation (Fig. 14): such cells were termed mesenchymal cells by Ashton and Morgan [23].

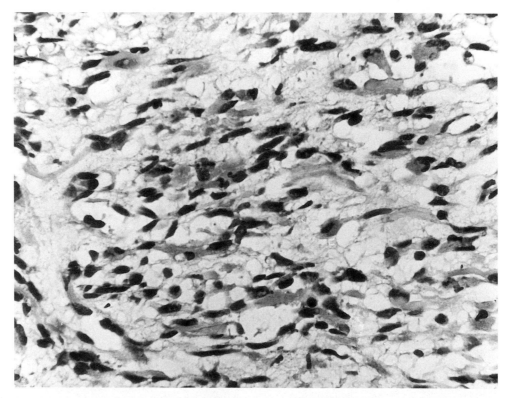

Figure 12 Well-differentiated embryonal rhabdomyosarcoma of the orbit, showing numerous strap-shaped cells, the cytoplasm of which is deeply eosinophilic. Nuclear pleomorphism is also present. (Hematoxylin and eosin, ×450)

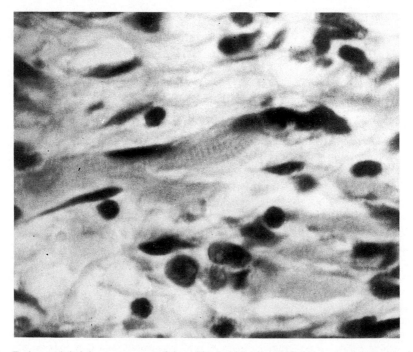

Figure 13 Embryonal rhabdomyosarcoma of the orbit. At higher magnification occasional strap-shaped cells exhibit readily recognized cross-striations. (Hematoxylin and eosin, ×980)

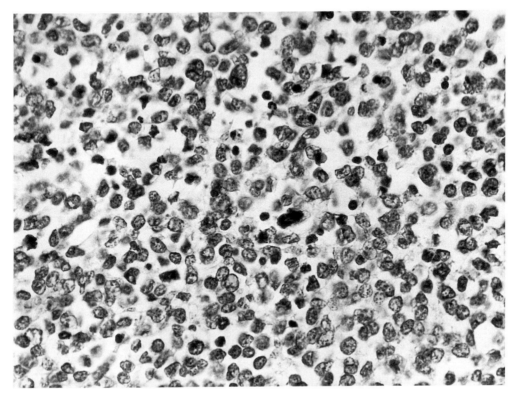

Figure 14 Undifferentiated rhabdomyosarcoma of the orbit. The cells have only scanty cytoplasm, and the nuclei are irregular and hyperchromatic. (Hematoxylin and eosin, ×450)

Botryoid Rhabdomyosarcoma

Botryoid rhabdomyosarcoma is a variant of the embryonal tumor associated with mucosa-lined hollow organs, where the capacity for unrestricted growth allows the formation of grapelike polypoid masses. The rare examples of this type of rhabdomyosarcoma in relation to the orbit have arisen beneath the conjunctiva [249]. It is comparable to the sarcoma botryoides developing in the urogenital tract of children and is distinguished histologically by nodules of neoplastic rhabdomyoblasts in varying stages of maturation surrounding a central zone of loose myxoid stroma in which there are distributed relatively smaller rhabdomyoblasts.

Alveolar Rhabdomyosarcoma

Alveolar rhabdomyosarcoma is closely related to embryonal rhabdomyosarcoma but with maximal incidence between the ages of 10 and 25 years and derives its name from a vague resemblance to lung tissue [368]. The distinctive appearance is due to interlacing bands of fibrous tissue, with intervening spaces lined and partially filled by neoplastic rhabdomyoblasts showing generally little evidence of differentiation (Fig. 15). Cross-striations are unusual. The alveolar variant behaves particularly badly [249,354] and is said to occur preferentially in the lower part of the orbit [354].

Embryonal rhabdomyosarcoma is a highly malignant neoplasm that, untreated, is rapidly fatal as a result of local extension into the brain and nasal passages or to distant metastasis. Lymphatic spread to regional lymph nodes has been reported [23,131,354], but in common with sarcomas in general, hematogenous spread to the lungs is more usual. Knowles and colleagues [249], however, comment that orbital rhabdomyosarcoma is slower to disseminate than the same tumor elsewhere in the head and neck. In a review of four reported series totaling 162 cases between 1959 and 1965 [23,131,227,354], Knowles and colleagues [249] found that only 25% of cases survived more than 3 years, but the introduction of chemo-

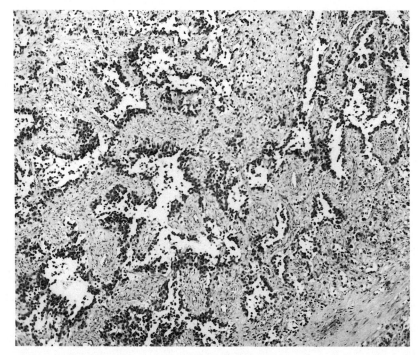

Figure 15 Alveolar rhabdomyosarcoma of the orbit. Interlacing bands of fibrous tissue are associated with irregular spaces lined by hyperchromatic tumor cells. Similar neoplastic rhabdomyoblasts are shed into the "alveoli." (Hematoxylin and eosin, ×68)

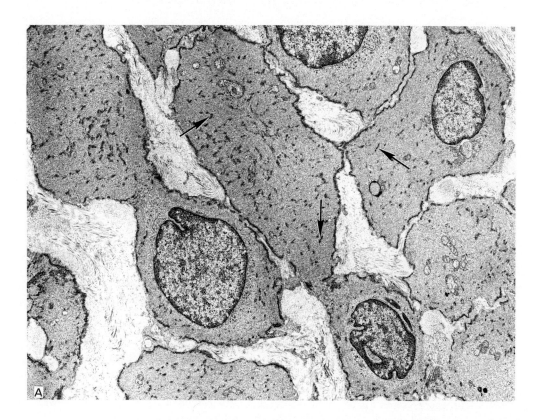

and radiotherapy [88,386] has radically improved the prognosis [193,238,298,359] to the extent that the Intergroup Rhabdomyosarcoma Study Committee, reporting on 127 patients treated between 1972 and 1983, cited a 3 year survival of 93% [461]. Others have also observed favorable results with immediate irradiation and chemotherapy for the treatment of orbital rhabdomyosarcoma [110].

B. Smooth Muscle

Leiomyoma

Benign tumors of smooth muscle origin are uncommon in the orbit and chiefly involve young adults [201,206,332,385,389]. They are encapsulated and richly vascularized, the latter finding giving support to the view that leiomyomas in this location originate from the smooth muscle or pericytes of orbital blood vessels. Histologically, the tumor consists of bundles of slender spindle cells with fine processes containing fibrils most conventionally demonstrated by trichome or phosphotungstic acid and hematoxylin staining. Alternatively, the contractile protein fibrils can be stained specifically by indirect immunofluorescence on unfixed material or demonstrated by transmission electron microscopy (Fig. 16) [206,389]. The rare association of an orbital leiomyoma with an inflammatory pseudotumor has been reported [385].

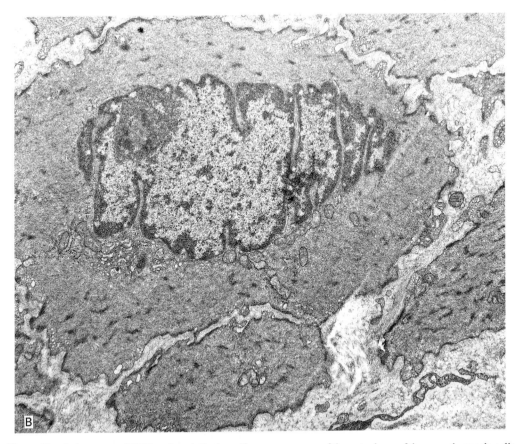

Figure 16 Leiomyoma. (A) Note the relatively uniform appearance of the cytoplasm of the smooth muscle cells caused by abundant, closely packed cytoplasmic filaments of myosin. Scattered throughout the cytoplasm are ill-defined densities (arrows), and these are particularly prominent on·the inner surface of the cell membrane. (×5000) (B) Higher magnification of smooth muscle cell. (×12,750)

Leiomyosarcoma

Spontaneously occurring malignant tumors of smooth muscle are excessively rare and occur later in adult life [201,302] than their benign counterpart, from which they are distinguished by the absence of a capsule and more numerous mitosis. They have also been observed as a sequel to radiation treatment of retinoblastoma, in which case they develop in early adult life [115,119]. Hematogenous metastasis to the lungs is prone to occur.

VIII. TUMORS OF VASCULAR ORIGIN

A. Benign

Capillary Hemangioma

Capillary hemangiomas are hamartomatous tumors that usually present at birth or shortly thereafter. A spate of proliferative activity in the next few months is frequently followed by gradual involution, so that by the age of 10 years the majority have completely regressed; alteratively, they may remain stationary. In an ophthalmic context, involvement of the skin of the eyelids is the most frequent presentation, but related or isolated involvement of the orbit is by no means unusual [34]. Exceptionally, they can originate within the frontal bone and lacrimal gland [178,410], in which case they tend to manifest in adult life.

    The tumors are not encapsulated. Histologically actively growing capillary hemangiomas consist of closely packed cords of uniform endothelial cells with few if any definitive vascular channels (Fig. 17). Such solid masses are sometimes referred to as benign hemangioendotheliomas, infantile hemangiomas, or juvenile hemangiomas. Despite a rapid growth rate, reflected in an appreciable number of mitoses, the

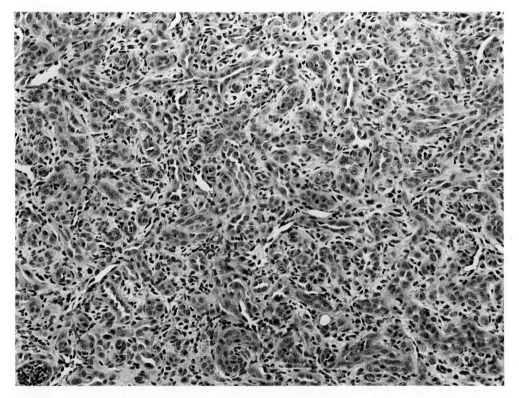

Figure 17 Benign hemangioendothelioma of the orbit. This is an actively grown capillary hemangioma composed of numerous slitlike vascular spaces lined by plump endothelial cells, which in some places form solid cords. (Hematoxylin and eosin, ×180)

cytology is entirely regular and malignancy is never a feature of these lesions, even though their histological picture may sometimes be disturbing. Mature capillary hemangiomas present an intricate network of thin-walled vascular channels the size of capillaries lined by flattened endothelial cells. Involution is associated with fibroblastic activity in the intervening stroma and the accumulation of lipid- and hemosiderin-laden macrophages.

Cavernous Hemangioma

Hemangiomas of the cavernous type are characterized by variably sized, but overall large, blood-filled spaces separated by a fibrous stroma (Figs. 18 through 20). The fibrous component can be marked, with inclusion of smooth muscle and elastic elements [192], and commonly presents foci of mucoid change. Moreover, such foci are often associated with newly formed capillary blood vessels originating from the larger cavernous spaces (Fig. 21), and it has been reasoned that this type of development may be responsible for the continued, if slow, growth of the angiomas [138,165].

Indeed, although cavernous hemangiomas have been reported in childhood the vast majority occur in adult life, chiefly in the fifth decade [138,381] and consequently cannot easily be regarded as hamartomatous. It is nevertheless conceivable that partial involution of a vascular malformation with reduced blood flow and tissue hypoxia could engender new vessel proliferation and propagation of an angiomatous process [138]. The extraocular muscle cone is the favored [288] but not exclusive site, and the tumors are circumscribed and encapsulated. In contrast to the capillary hemangioma, there is no propensity for involution and surgical intervention is usually necessary. Malignant transformation has not been recorded.

Intravascular Papillary Endothelial Hyperplasia

Generally considered an unusual form of thrombus organization characterized by a plethora of delicate fronds of fibrinous or collagenous tissue covered by a single layer of proliferated endothelium, intravascular papillary endothelial hyperplasia may occasionally be seen in the orbit [456]. It is most likely to occur

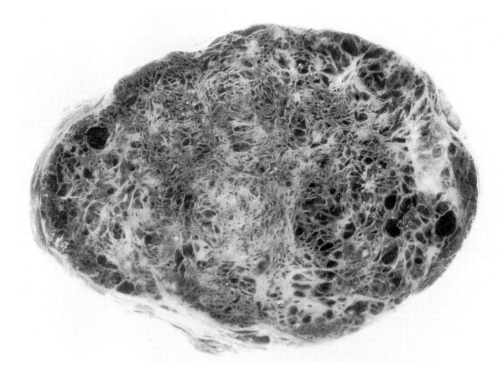

Figure 18 Cavernous hemangioma of the orbit. The cut surface of a resected specimen shows a honeycomb of large vascular spaces separated by trabeculae of fibromuscular connective tissue. (×8)

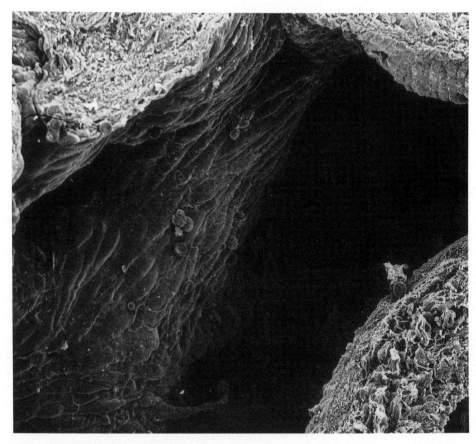

Figure 19 Cavernous hemangioma of the orbit viewed by scanning electron microscopy to show the endothelial lining of a "cavern." (×430)

as a complication of an underlying vascular malformation, and although it can be confused with an angiosarcoma the behavior is entirely benign.

Vascular Malformations

Venous. Orbital varices constitute a focal conglomeration of abnormally dilated venous channels and are associated with intermittent exophthalmos. A variable lymphocytic infiltrate may be seen in the intervening connective tissue [277]. In an analysis of 67 patients with proptosis attributable to vascular causes, Wright [472] found venous malformations to be much the most common lesion. This author considers, on the basis of venography, that many presumed lymphangiomas are really varices, but others [202] contest this statement and suggest that the demonstration of smooth muscle in the walls of true varices will help to distinguish them from the poorly supported endothelial channels of lymphangiomas. Apart from varices, venous angiomas are also described [202]: these consist of newly formed vascular channels lined by flattened endothelium with thick fibromuscular walls.

Arteriovenous. Malformations in which congeries of thick-walled vessels connect the arterial and venous sides of the orbital circulation without an intervening capillary network usually occur as part of a more widespread vascular anomaly. Most arteriovenous malformations of the orbit are linked with similar lesions in the brain [469]. The retinal and midbrain arteriovenous anomalies that constitute the Wyburn-Mason syndrome [479] may be accompanied by similar malformations in the retrobulbar region of the orbit

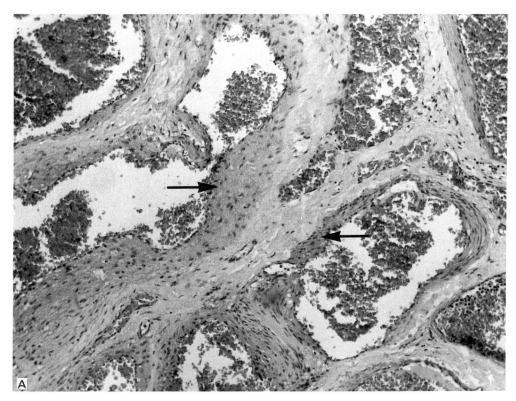

Figure 20 Cavernous hemangioma of the orbit. (A) Light microscopy shows irregular vascular spaces of considerable size lined by a single layer of endothelium. The darker areas (arrows) immediately beneath the endothelium represent smooth muscle fibers. (Hematoxylin and eosin, ×110) (B) Smooth muscle cell of connective tissue trabeculae with abundant thin filaments in peripheral cytoplasm (F). The cell membrane contains numerous flasklike invaginations (pits, P) akin to what is seen in pinocytosis and electron-dense material adjacent to the cell membrane and among the microfilaments (arrows). The cell is surrounded by a prominent basal lamina. (×19,000)

[183]. The anomalous vessels are histologically recognizable as arteries and are organized in a convoluted pulsatile mass that has been likened to a bunch of grapes (racemose angioma).

Lymphangioma

Hamartomatous and, because of the apparent absence of lymph vessels in the normal orbit, possibly choristomatous tumors, lymphangiomas usually affect children, giving rise to proptosis, which may be acute. Indeed, secondary hemorrhage is a common cause for presentation and recurrence [166]. Histologically, they consist of thin-walled vessels of varying size lined by a single layer of flattened endothelium. They are distinguished from hemangiomas by the absence of pericytes and smooth muscle and of blood, although hemorrhage may spill into a lymphangioma from poorly supported blood capillaries projecting into the lymph spaces to create a "chocolate" cyst [363]. Such hemorrhage can cause confusion with a venous malformation, as described earlier. The presence of lymphocytes, sometimes with germinal follicles, in the stroma of a lymphangioma [223,224] may account for an apparent increase in size and exacerbations of exophthalmos, which can complicate upper respiratory tract infections.

Conceptually, a case has been made for regarding orbital lymphangiomas as an abortive vascular development arising from an aberrant vascular anlage [166,197], in which case it is not illogical to consider the vascular malformations as a group. Those that are connected with the normal drainage system constitute

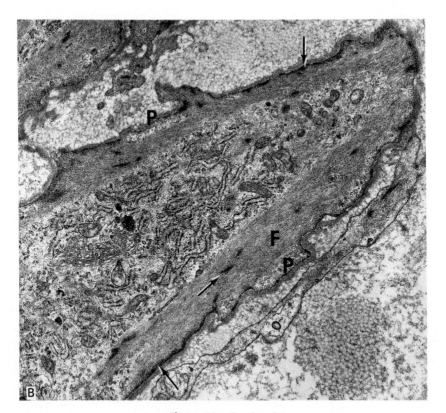

Figure 20   Continued

venous malformations, whereas those that are not and contain only clear fluid can properly be regarded as lymphangiomas.

Hemangiopericytoma

Hemangiopericytoma is essentially a tumor of adult life and can behave in either a benign or a malignant fashion. The component cells are spindle shaped, with scanty cytoplasm and centrally placed round or ovoid nuclei, and are situated between vascular spaces lined with endothelium (the latter may be difficult to discern; Fig. 22) in which case immunohistochemical staining for factor VIII–antigen may be useful [329]. The neoplastic pericytes lack the numerous organelles seen in endothelial cells, and the finding that individual cells are invested by reticulin (Figs. 22 through 24) further distinguishes them from the cells of a hemangioendothelioma in which the reticulin typically embraces clusters of proliferating endothelium.

In line with the experience of hemangiopericytomas in general, the orbital lesion is variable in behavior [432a]. Most grow slowly and rarely recur after surgical excision. Some are evidently malignant, showing nuclear pleomorphism and numerous mitoses, but between these two groups is a borderline group in which it is difficult to prognosticate on the basis of histological criteria [74]. In a consideration of hemangiopericytoma at other sites, it has been suggested that four or more mitotic figures per 10 high-power fields should be regarded as ominous [104]. Recurrence of an ostensibly benign tumor occurs not infrequently [127,174,200,427] and has been reported as late as 22 years after initial excision [345].

B. Malignant

Hemangiosarcoma

Current practice restricts the definition of hemangiosarcoma to tumors of vascular endothelium, and since capillary and lymphatic endothelium are indistinguishable, the term "angiosarcoma" is generally pre-

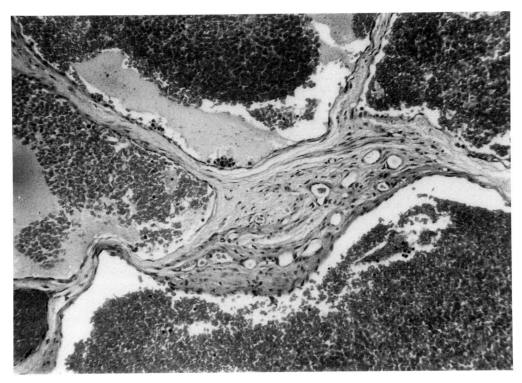

Figure 21   Cavernous hemangioma of the orbit. Clusters of capillary blood vessels within the fibrous septae are seen, and it is conjectured that these may latter dilate and provide a basis for continued growth of the tumor. (Hematoxylin and eosin, ×185)

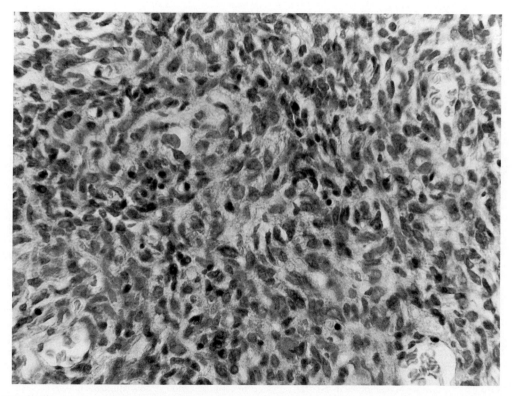

Figure 22 Benign hemangiopericytoma of the orbit. Several small endothelium-lined vascular channels are separated by densely packed spindle cells. (Hematoxylin and eosin, ×450)

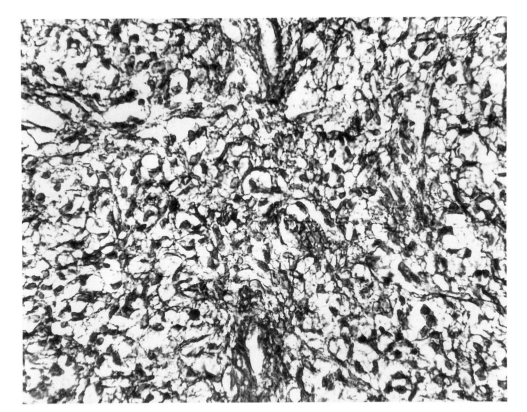

Figure 23 Benign hemangiopericytoma of the orbit, showing a dense network of "reticulin" fibers that enclose individual tumor cells, in contrast to the reticulin distribution in hemangioendotheliomas, where clusters of cells around a central blood vessel are delineated. (Gomori's reticulin stain, ×450)

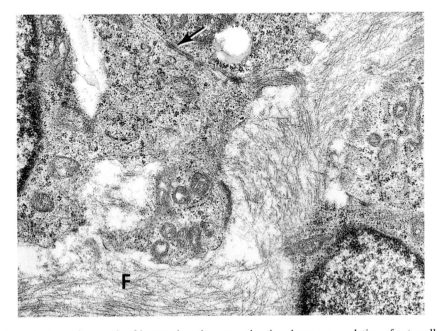

Figure 24 Electron micrograph of hemangiopericytoma, showing dense accumulation of extracellular collagenous fibrils (F), which correspond to the "reticulin" seen by light microscopy. Adjacent tumor cells are connected by macula adherens cell junctions (arrow). (×19,600) (Courtesy of Dr. J. Shelburne.)

ferred. Angiosarcomas originating in the orbit are extremely rare [52,398], a review in 1987 listing 15 cases with age at presentation ranging from 2 weeks to 66 years but with most developing in childhood [184]. Follow-up information is limited, but there appears to be a considerable risk of recurrence and metastasis following surgery. The tumor cells show a generally marked degree of pleomorphism, hyperchromatism, and mitotic activity, but histological diagnosis depends on the demonstration that the tumor cells are themselves forming the vascular channels that traverse the lesion. Immunohistochemical demonstration of factor VIII-related antigen and binding of the *Ulex europaeus* lectin can be useful in confirming the cell of origin, although the former is often negative and the latter is not wholly specific. The presence of epithelioid metaplasia as evidenced by multiple, slender microvilli, tonofilaments, and desmosomes has been observed in an orbital angiosarcoma [306].

IX. TUMORS OF BONE AND CARTILAGE

A. Benign

Chondroma

Orbital tumors composed of pure cartilage are exceedingly rare. Some develop from the adjacent bone; others are assumed to arise from the trochlea [218], the only cartilaginous structure in the normal orbit, or from pluripotential orbital mesenchyme [43]. Orbital cartilaginous hamartomas may be a manifestation of a generalized disorder characterized by multiple enchondromata (Ollier's disease) [79].

Osteoma

An osteoma is a circumscribed benign proliferation of mature lamellar bone in adults. Osteomas occurring in young adults may present signs of active growth, whereas those in older individuals tend to have thick trabeculae with fewer active osteoblasts. Orbital disturbance is due to osteomas arising in the paranasal sinuses, most commonly the maxillary sinus [136,308,440].

Osteoblastoma and Ossifying Fibroma

To what extent benign osteoblastoma and ossifying fibromas are different tumors is questionable, especially because osteoblasts are essentially modified fibroblasts. Distinction is based in part on the degree of osteoblastic differentiation of multipotential fibroblasts but also on radiological and clinical criteria [135]. It is the much greater propensity of ossifying fibroma for locally aggressive behavior and recurrence following surgery that is the principal merit of diagnostic separation. Benign osteoblastoma affects children and young adults and is characterized histologically by variably calcified osteoid trabeculae lined by plump osteoblasts and lying within a richly vascularized fibrous matrix that may contain osteoclasts [270]. Involvement of the orbital bones has been reported as a rare event [265,436] and may not be contiguous with a sinus cavity [279].

Ossifying fibroma is similar histologically, differing only in having a larger amount of fibrous tissue in which plump, active fibroblasts may assume a whorled pattern (Fig. 25). Confusion with fibrous dysplasia is also possible (see later), but authentic examples have been described in the orbit [135]. A subgroup of ossifying fibroma further defined by the presence of numerous small round psammomalike ossicles is also recognized. Known as psammomatoid ossifying fibroma [296], the tumor is largely restricted to the orbital portion of the frontal bone or ethmoid bone and, although benign, is often locally aggressive.

B. Malignant

Osteosarcoma

Osteosarcoma is a highly malignant tumor that characteristically presents between the ages of 10 and 30 years, has a male predominance, and involves the limb bone metaphyses [72]. Involvement of the skull, more particularly of the orbit, is extremely rare [362]. Although some orbital osteosarcomas may arise de novo, a considerable proportion of reported cases had received ionizing radiation for retinoblastoma some 13–20 years before [136]. Osteosarcoma originating in the skull may present in later life as a complication of Paget's disease [286], and Blodi [41] has described such a patient with orbital involvement.

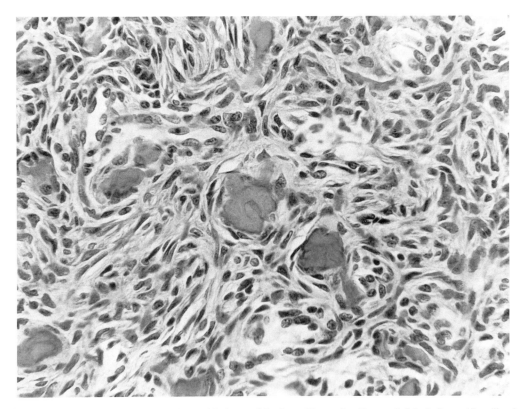

Figure 25 Ossifying fibroma of the intraorbital part of the frontal bone. Small, rounded foci of osteoid are lined by prominent osteoblasts. Similar cells and numerous blood vessels constitute the intervening stroma. (Hematoxylin and eosin, ×450)

The tumor consists of pleomorphic cells with large hyperchromatic nuclei within a connective tissue matrix that includes osteoid trabeculae of varying maturity according to the degree of osteoblastic differentiation (Fig. 26). Calcification may or may not be present. In equivocal cases in which differentiation is minimal and osteoid not discernible, the electron microscopic demonstration of collagen fibers impregnated with hydroxyapatite crystals can be a useful ploy [205].

Chondrosarcoma

Like osteosarcoma, chondrosarcoma of the orbit can develop as a complication of irradiation for retinoblastoma. It is extremely rare and usually originates within the paranasal sinuses [177]. Histological diagnosis depends on the presence of single and multinucleated cells within a variably differentiated chondroid matrix. Chondrosarcomas of low-grade malignancy alongside an adjacent area of highly malignant sarcoma of variable histogenesis, so-called dedifferentiated chondrosarcomas, are also recognized, and a case involving the orbit has been documented [355]. Irrespective of treatment, of whatever kind, the prognosis is extremely bad, only 1 of 11 cases reported by Fu and Perzin [136] surviving more than 10 years and most dying within 2 years.

Mesenchymal Chondrosarcoma

The mesenchymal chondrosarcoma is characterized by undifferentiated mesenchymal cells and islands of well-differentiated cartilage (Fig. 27) [159,387]. The first documented examples of this unusual variant of the chondrosarcoma were of bony origin, but the neoplasm can occur in soft tissues, including the orbit [51,158,400,406]. Mesenchymal chondrosarcomas tend to occur at a younger age (average age 33 years)

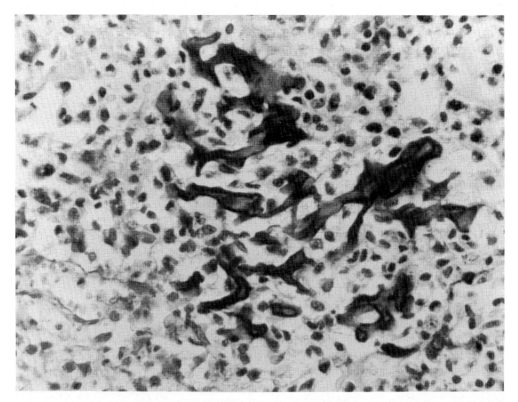

Figure 26 Osteosarcoma of the orbit. Partially calcified fragments of osteoid represent an abortive attempt at bone trabecula formation. The cells in the intervening stroma are markedly pleomorphic. (Hematoxylin and eosin, ×450)

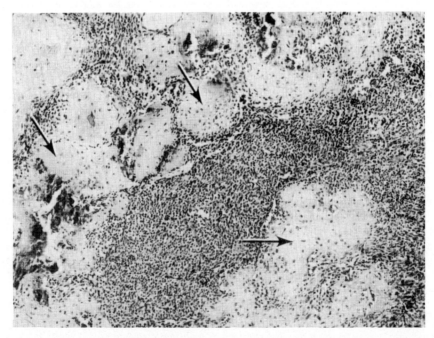

Figure 27 Mesenchymal chondrosarcoma of the orbit. Densely packed undifferentiated mesenchymal cells are associated with areas of well-differentiated cartilage (arrows). (Hematoxylin and eosin, ×100)

than chondrosarcomas in general (average age 55 years) and follow a much more aggressive course than the usual chondrosarcomas, but metastases may not occur until 23 years after treatment.

Chordoma

Chordomas arise in young adults within the remnants of the embryonic notochord and consequently may involve the vertebral column, particularly the sacrococcygeal region, and the base of the skull. Tumors in the latter situation may extend into the orbit [32,76,311] and are associated with a generally poor prognosis because of their relatively inaccessible position and advanced spread by the time diagnosis is established.

The tumor has a gelatinous consistency, is locally destructive, and presents a histological picture of scattered groups of cells with conspicuously vacuolated cytoplasm ("physaliphorous cells") within a mucoid stroma (Fig. 28). Sometimes there is a marked similarity to chondrosarcoma.

B. Tumors of Indeterminate Behavior

Giant Cell Tumor

Giant cell tumor is so designated because of the presence of large cells containing numerous centrally placed nuclei within a loose stroma composed of ovoid or spindle-shaped cells, which probably have the same histogenesis (Fig. 29). Although sometimes termed osteoclasts, the evidence provided by electron microscopy, such as a sparsity of lysosomes, does not support this view and favors a connective tissue origin [420].

Orbital involvement is uncommon [42], and the behavior of the tumor is variable. Most remain localized, but metastasis can occur, the risk is normally, but not always, being reflected in the histological evidence of malignancy.

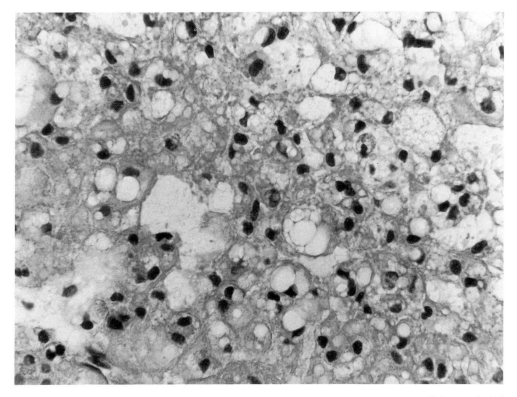

Figure 28   Chordoma invading the orbit. Lying within a mucinous matrix are so-called physaliphorous (bubble-bearing) cells, showing characteristic coarse vacuolation of the cytoplasm. (Hematoxylin and eosin, ×450)

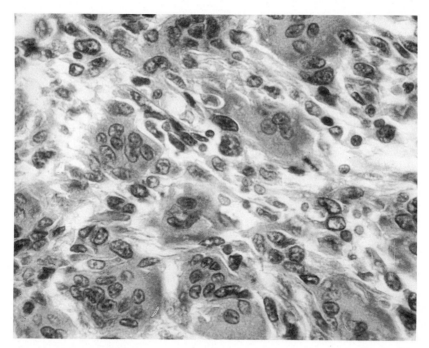

Figure 29 Giant cell tumor of the orbit. The characteristic giant cells contain large numbers of nuclei, which tend to be centrally placed and are probably of the same histogenesis as the single cells within the supporting vascularized stroma. (Hematoxylin and eosin, ×700)

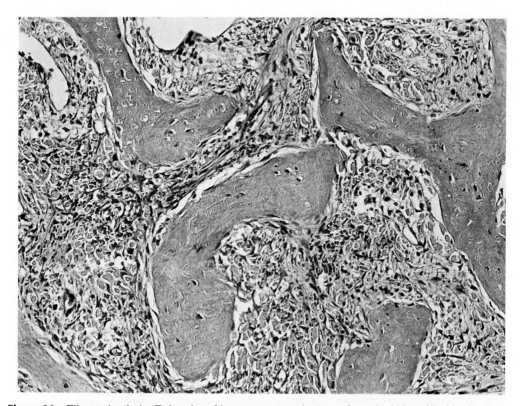

Figure 30 Fibrous dysplasia. Trabeculae of immature woven bone are formed within a fibroblastic stroma. Compared with true neoplasms of bone, there are only a few osteoblasts lining the trabeculae. (Hematoxylin and eosin, ×180)

Aneurysmal Bone Cyst

Aneurysmal bone cyst is an expanding lesion, the cavity of which is filled with reddish brown spongy material. Histology shows numerous dilated vascular channels mingled with fibrous tissue, multinucleated giant cells, foci of hemorrhage, and occasional spicules of bone. The histogenesis is uncertain, although circumstantial evidence suggests a vascular origin [382].

The skull is an unusual site and only very rarely is the orbit involved, children and young adults being the people usually at risk [185,356]. Aneurysmal bone cyst does not behave like a true neoplasm, and curettage is adequate management for most cases.

Fibrous Dysplasia

Presenting as a solitary lesion or, much less commonly, as a polyostotic disorder in conjunction with precocious puberty in girls and patchy cutaneous pigmentation (Albright's syndrome), fibrous dysplasia is a nonneoplastic osseous disorder that not infrequently affects the face and orbit [145,268]. Children and young adults are most commonly involved, the cancellous part of the affected bone being replaced by collagenous tissue, which includes numerous fibroblasts and curved spicules of nonlamellar (woven) bone resembling fragments of eggshell (Fig. 30). Although the nature of fibrous dysplasia is uncertain, it appears to be a self-limiting focal proliferation of intracameral fibrous tissue that has a restricted potential for transformation to bone. A characteristic histological feature is the absence of osteoblasts along the margins of the bony trabeculae since the transformation to bone represents metaplasia of preformed fibrous tissue; this finding can be of value in the differential diagnosis between fibrous dysplasia and benign osteoblastoma or ossifying fibroma.

X. TUMORS OF PERIPHERAL NERVE AND AUTONOMIC NERVOUS SYSTEM

The orbit contains many neurogenic derivatives that are potential sources of neoplasms. These include the ciliary ganglion and several descendants of the neural crest: (1) the Schwann cells, which wrap themselves around the axons of peripheral and cranial nerves to form the myelin sheaths; (2) meningothelial cells, which surround the optic nerve and occasionally occur in the perineurium of orbital nerves; and (3) melanocytes. In some of the tumors spawned by descendants of the neural crest, more than one cell type is a component of the tumor. The rare storiform neurofibroma and melanotic schwannomas, for example, may contain both Schwann cells and melanocytes.

A. Benign

Neurofibroma

The tumor mass of a neurofibroma is composed of a variable mix of Schwann cells, collagen fibers, and scattered nerve axons. Perineural cells may also be involved, although there is good evidence that the Schwann cells are themselves able to produce collagen. Frequently the tumor has an appreciable mucin content, making it soft and slimy. From a clinicopathological standpoint it is usual to recognize three categories of neurofibroma: localized, plexiform, and diffuse. Most localized neurofibromas in the orbit present as solitary lesions, only some 12% being associated with neurofibromatosis [129]. They are discrete with an indeterminate capsule and are composed of elongated spindle cells with a characteristic wavy nucleus in a stroma with variable mucin content. The upper part of the orbit is a preferred location, and mild discomfort as well as proptosis is common [255,378]. Plexiform neurofibroma is virtually synonymous with von Recklinghausen's disease and comprises a convoluted tangle of nerves thickened by Schwann cell proliferation [318]. In contradistinction to the solitary lesions, which occur mainly in adult life, the plexiform tumor usually presents in childhood and may be associated with bony defects of the orbit [37,50,307]. Diffuse neurofibroma is the least common form and is associated with generalized neurofibromatosis in about 10% of cases [104]. The component cells are usually less elongated than those in other neurofibromas and may include clusters of Meissner bodies, but their chief significance lies with an absence of any semblance of a capsule, such that they are intimately bound to the surrounding structures and difficult to excise [172].

Schwannoma (Neurilemmoma)

A schwannoma is a benign, slowly growing encapsulated tumor of Schwann cells that gradually enlarges the nerve in a nodular or fusiform fashion to form a mass [163,314]. Although sometimes occurring sporadically, orbital schwannomas, like those in other locations, may be a manifestation of von Recklinghausen's disease of nerves (see Chap. 45). Café-au-lait spots of the skin may be associated [324] and the only other stigma of this phakomatosis. In contrast to neurofibromas, which tend to be painless, schwannomas compress the nerve of origin so that pain is often a prominent clinical feature. The schwannoma, which does not have a predilection for any particular part of the orbit, tends to be firm and rubbery in consistency, and after sectioning cystic spaces containing mucoid material are frequently disclosed. Light microscopy presents two different patterns (Fig. 31): one is composed of closely compacted, spindle-shaped cells with eosinophilic cytoplasm, oval nuclei, and indistinct cell membranes (Antoni type A). The nuclei of the tumor cells are often palisaded, sometimes around hyalinized structures resembling tactile corpuscles ("Verocay bodies"). In other schwannomas stellate cells are haphazardly arranged in a myxomatous matrix (Antoni type B) that does not stain readily with alcian blue, in contrast to the mucoid material of neurofibromas [163].

Lymphocytes, lipid-laden macrophages, and thick-walled vessels frequently traverse schwannomas. Hyalinization and mucinous cystoid formation are particularly prone to occur in schwannomas of long standing, and so is the occasional calcification. Some schwannomas are excessively cellular, with increased

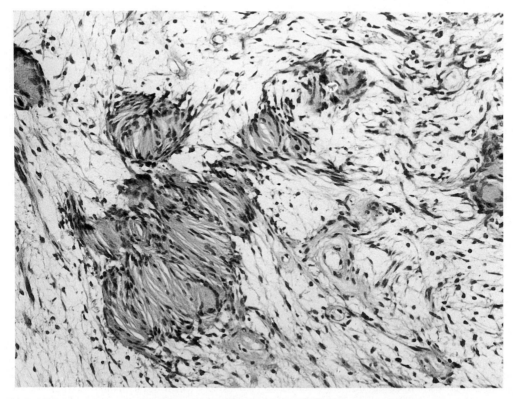

Figure 31 Schwannoma of the orbit. Cells aligned in parallel with palisading of their nuclei constitute the Antoni A component of the schwannoma, and when as well organized as in this instance resemble tactile organs and are described by Verocay bodies. The surrounding loose mucoid tissue constitutes the Antoni B component of the schwannoma. In other schwannomas, either Antoni A or B tissue may be the sole component. (Hematoxylin and eosin, ×180)

nuclear atypia but without conspicuous mitoses (cellular schwannoma). By transmission electron micro-scopy, schwannomas are characterized by cells with slender cellular processes and minimal rough-surfaced endoplasmic reticulum, a basal lamina, and long-spacing collagen with a cross-striational banding with a periodicity of 100 nm (Fig. 32). Although tumors derived from Schwann cells frequently produce conspicuous quantities of long-spacing collagen, this morphological variety of collagen also forms in some normal tissues and in many other pathological conditions, including nonschwannian tumors [28]. Endo-neurial fibroblasts without a surrounding basal lamina are scattered throughout the tumor. The tumor probably lacks a predisposition to malignancy but may recur many years after excision [57].

Granular Cell Tumor

Originally called granular cell myoblastoma because of a belief that it stems from striated muscle, this is an extremely rare orbital neoplasm [55,86,91,95,150,194,233,320,321]. This generally benign encapsulated tumor is composed of large, round, or polygonal cells with small, vesicular, or hyperchromatic nuclei (Fig. 33). The eosinophilic cytoplasm contains coarse granules that can be enhanced with the periodic acid–Schiff stain and a variety of other histological techniques. By electron microscopy most of the granules appear as amorphous, eosinophilic, lysosomelike structures, but sheaths of intracytoplasmic filaments (angulated bodies) also occur (Fig. 34) [17]. These ultrastructural features, which support its Schwann cell origin [413], are reinforced by immunohistochemical demonstration of S-100 protein, neuron-specific enolase, and various myelin proteins [104,333]. Orbital involvement is rare [86,194,321] and associated with a generally good prognosis following local excision. Malignant forms, although recognized, have not been convincingly described in the orbit.

Paraganglioma (Chemodectoma)

The term "chromaffin cells" is used to describe small clusters of epithelioid cells derived from neural crest that are innervated by preganglionic sympathetic fibers and synthesize and release catecholamines (epi-nephrine and norepinephrine). These cells develop a brown discoloration when exposed to aqueous solutions of potassium dichromate (chromaffin reaction).

Clusters of morphologically similar cells but without a positive chromaffin reaction occur as chemo-receptor cells in the carotid body at the bifurcation of the carotid artery, in the aortic arches, in the glomus jugulare, and at numerous other sites. According to ultrastructural studies, the traditional nonchromaffin paraganglia differ only in degree from the chromaffin cells of the sympathetic nervous system. These various specialized cells on occasion give rise to tumors known as chemodectomas or paragangliomas [259]. Paragangliomas are rare in the orbit, probably originating in the ciliary ganglion [12,19,83,111, 148,229,273,347,437,448,450,478], and the literature contains an exceptional report of a paraganglioma with an admix of melanin [348]. Orbital paragangliomas tend to involve the extraocular muscles, and if incompletely excised the tumor may recur and even undergo malignant change [336]. Extension to the middle cranial fossa has been reported [450]. Paragangliomas consist of variably sized cells with round to oval nuclei and finely granular eosinophilic cytoplasm arranged in nests, balls (*Zellballen*), or cords separated by septa consisting of connective tissue or sinusoids (Fig. 35). Mitotic figures are rarely seen, and the vascular component is often marked and suggestive of an angioma. Characteristic dense-core granules (50–200 nm in diameter) are disclosed in the tumor cells by electron microscopy (Fig. 36).

Traumatic Neuroma

Following the transection of peripheral nerves, the severed axons sprout from the proximal end of the cut nerve and grow in haphazard directions. These regenerating axons, together with hyperplastic fibroblasts and Schwann cells, may form a swelling of the nerve (traumatic or amputation neuroma). Despite that orbital nerves are severed during enucleations and other surgical procedures around the eye, traumatic neuromas are extremely rare in the orbit [40,114,305]. Perhaps this reflects the small size of the orbital nerves or, alternatively, a lesser capacity of cranial nerves to regenerate than nerves of the peripheral nervous system. They may be associated with slowly enlarging conjunctival inclusion cysts. Pain is rarely encountered and is probably caused by mechanical irritation of the amputation neuroma, by retracting scar tissue, or by compression from an adjacent cystic mass [305].

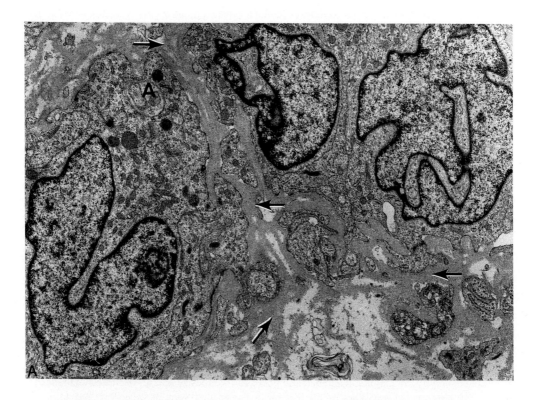

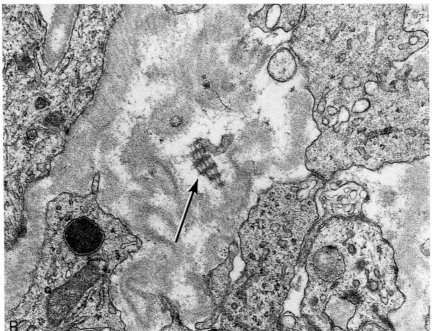

Figure 32 Electron micrographs of a Schwannoma. (A) The neoplastic Schwann cells are characteristically surrounded by a prominent basal lamina (arrows). Despite their benignity, the cells, which may encase axons (A), commonly have bizarrely shaped nuclei. (×11,800) (B) Extracellular broad-banded collagen (arrow) is frequently adjacent to the basal laminar material of Schwann cell. (×25,000) (Courtesy of Dr. J. Shelburne.)

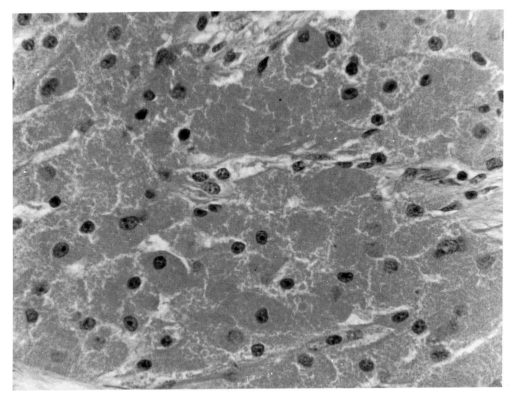

Figure 33 Granular cell tumor of the orbit. Individual tumor cells have voluminous fine granular eosinophilic cytoplasm and small regular nuclei. (Hematoxylin and eosin, ×450)

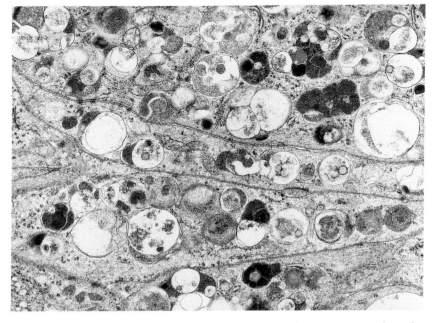

Figure 34 Ultrastructure of granular cell tumor. The cytoplasm contains numerous membrane-bound inclusions of variable size and shape. (×12,400) (Courtesy of Dr. J. Shelburne.)

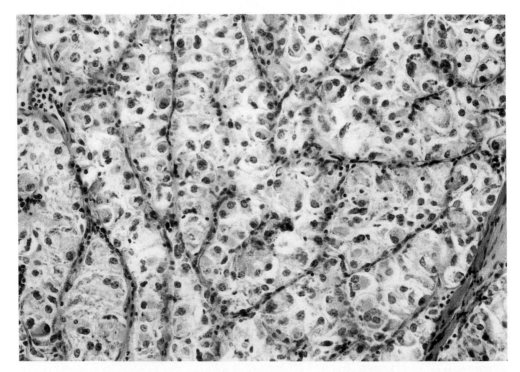

Figure 35 Paraganglioma (chemodectoma) of the orbit. The cells vary in size and have fine granular eosinophilic cytoplasm. The cells tend to form clusters separated by fibrous septa. (Hematoxylin and eosin, ×200)

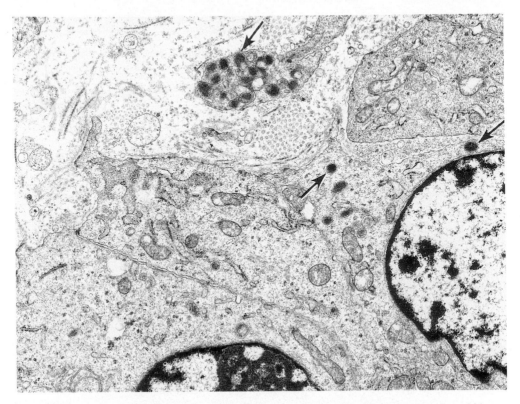

Figure 36 Electron micrograph of paraganglioma, showing characteristic dense-core granules within cytoplasm of tumor cell. (×37,500) (Courtesy of Dr. J. Shelburne.)

B. Malignant

Malignant Peripheral Nerve Sheath Tumors

Although many malignant tumors affecting peripheral nerves are reasonably attributed to a schwannian origin (Fig. 37), this is not always evident, and in consequence, there is advantage in preferring the less precise designation of malignant peripheral nerve sheath tumor. Overall about half of such tumors arise in patients with neurofibromatosis [393], but they are extremely rare in the orbit, a review in 1989 identifying 16 cases [281]. A predilection for involvement of the supraorbital nerve has been noted [157,198] and the prognosis is poor, 10 of the 16 reported cases dying within 5 years.

Alveolar Soft Part Sarcoma

The extremely rare sarcoma designated by the descriptive term "alveolar soft-part sarcoma" because of its sites of origin and the pseudoalveolar or organoid pattern of the tumor cells [59] remains a tumor of disputable origin. The sarcoma is composed of nests of large polygonal cells with abundant granular eosinophilic cytoplasm usually arranged in a distinctive alveolar pattern outlined by thin-walled capillaries. The lesion must be differentiated histologically from the alveolar rhabdomyosarcoma, nonchromaffin paraganglioma, granular cell tumor, amelanotic malignant melanoma, metastatic renal carcinoma, and certain vascular neoplasms. The cytoplasm of the alveolar soft-part sarcoma usually contains characteristic rod-shaped periodic acid–Schiff-positive, diastase-resistant crystalloids that have an 8 nm periodicity when viewed by transmission electron microscopy. The alveolar soft-part sarcoma was once believed to be the malignant counterpart of the granular cell tumor, but its granules are distinct from those of that tumor. The possibility that the alveolar soft-part sarcoma is the malignant counterpart of the paraganglioma has also been raised [459] because the two tumors may appear to differ morphologically only in the degree of nuclear atypia and the number of mitotic figures. Appealing as this may be, however,

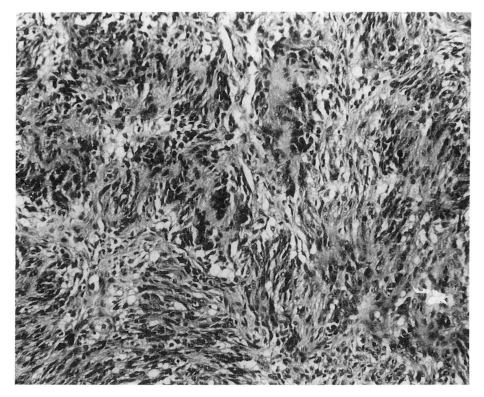

Figure 37 Malignant schwannoma. The palisade arrangement of a schwannoma is still recognizable, but the cell nuclei are unusually pleomorphic. (Hematoxylin and eosin, ×180)

the alveolar soft-part sarcoma has larger and more pleomorphic cells, and although it possesses its own characteristic crystalline granules the alveolar soft-part sarcoma lacks the dense-core granules of the paraganglioma. Other evidence that relies mainly on the immunohistochemical demonstration of muscle proteins points to a myogenic origin [176], but this too is not unequivocal. A claim has even been made that the distinctive inclusions constitute renin, such as occurs in the renal juxtaglomerular apparatus [82], but this has not been confirmed by others. The alveolar soft-part sarcoma is an extremely rare orbital tumor [2,9,123,156,449] occurring over a wide age range (1–69 years) [123]. In a review of 17 orbital cases (13 females and 4 males), Font and colleagues [120] found the median age to be 18 years. The tumor pursues a lethal course, but metastases may not develop until more than a decade after the primary tumor is discovered and treated.

XI.   TUMORS OF THE OPTIC NERVE

A.   Astrocytoma

Benign (Juvenile Pilocytic Astrocytoma)

Despite being the most common tumors of the optic nerve, astrocytomas are rare in this situation, accounting, according to one report, for 1 in 100,000 patients presenting to a general ophthalmic department [98]. Most histologically benign astrocytomas of the optic nerve develop in childhood, although up to 10% present at a later age [98], and various reports describe a moderate predominance of female patients [422,475,481]. A proportion of astrocytomas involving the optic nerve originate intracranially, and the present discussion is limited to those in which the tumor is presumed to have developed in the intraorbital portion of the nerve. An association with neurofibromatosis is well recognized [78,293,297,421], with an analysis of a total of 1412 cases reported in the literature indicating an incidence of 22% [92].

The usual histological appearance is one of compact bundles of fibrillary astrocytes with uniform round or ovoid nuclei and virtually no evidence of mitotic activity [272] (Fig. 38). Frequently the cells have elongated bipolar cytoplasmic processes (Fig. 39) that confer a piloid or hairlike pattern. Particularly in

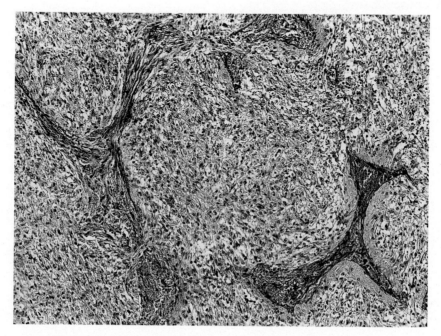

Figure 38   Juvenile pilocytic astrocytoma of the optic nerve. Cross section of optic nerve, showing enlarged bundles of tumor composed of astrocytes of uniform shape and size. (Hematoxylin and eosin, ×100)

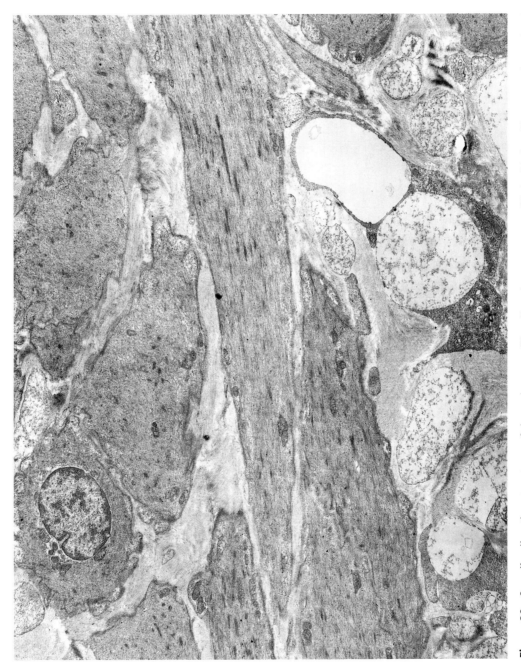

Figure 39 Juvenile pilocytic astrocytoma of the optic nerve. The pilocytic processes are filled with fine filaments and occasional mitochondria. Between the processes and the supporting collagenous stroma there is an amorphous basement membrane. (×6250)

the vicinity of blood vessels coursing through the tumor, the astrocytes may be aligned in a palisade perpendicular to the lumen, and the capillaries themselves may present a conspicuously hypertrophic endothelial lining. Homogeneous eosinophilic carrot-shaped expansions (Rosenthal fibers) are sometimes conspicuous in optic nerve astrocytomas. Transmission electron microscopy of these structures discloses condensations of microfilaments [146,160]. Rosenthal fibers stain positively for the heat-shock protein ubiquitin [280] and have been found on detailed analysis to consist of aggregates of αB-crystallin with glial fibrillary acid protein and ubiquitin [444]. Also common are areas of mucin accumulation, sometimes such as to form microcysts, and this can be a cause of tumor expansion in the absence of true proliferative activity [14].

Reduced visual acuity and moderate proptosis are the major clinical findings [61], visual disturbance being reported to occur earlier in children whose tumors are primarily intracranial [98]. Two basic behavior patterns can be recognized.

One that is slightly the more common is characterized by cessation of growth at the time of or soon after clinical presentation [11,310] and has been regarded as an essentially hamartomatous development [181]. Such lesions may nevertheless give rise to a meningeal reaction within the surrounding nerve sheath [68] that comprises a combination of arachnoidal cell hyperplasia and fibroblastic and glial cell proliferation (Figs. 40 and 41), and although it is difficult to rule out a contribution by neoplastic astrocytes, it is probable that most of the glial response is reactive [418]. It is this type of behavior that is commonly seen in patients with neurofibromatosis-associated gliomas [422,475].

The second growth pattern is more sinister since the proliferating astrocytes show a greater propensity to spread within the nerve and involve the chiasm and other intracranial structures. Conversely, invasion of the meninges is less common. Yanoff and colleagues [481] reported a 36% mortality in patients with chiasmal involvement, and whereas no treatment is required in the case of stable tumors, actively growing astrocytomas usually warrant resection of the optic nerve provided the chiasm is spared [475].

Symptoms tend to develop earlier in patients with stable tumors than in those with active lesions, with means of 5.9 and 8.3 years, respectively, in a series reported by Wright et al. [475]. This correlates to some

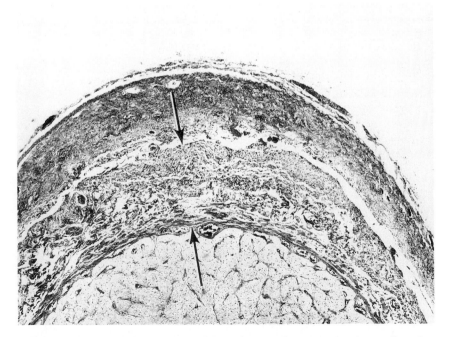

Figure 40   Thickening of subarachnoid portion of the optic nerve (between arrows) several centimeters away from juvenile pilocytic astrocytoma of optic nerve. This meningeal hyperplasia is a common response to invasion of the leptomeninges by the astrocytoma. (Masson trichome, ×40)

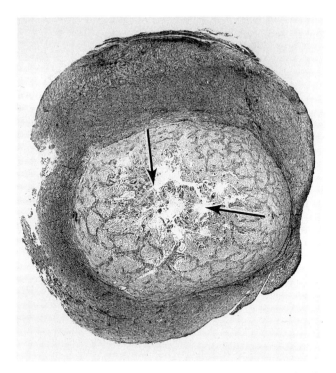

Figure 41 Cross section of juvenile pilocytic astrocytoma of the optic nerve showing enlarged nerve with mucoid-containing cystoid spaces in the center of the tumor (arrows). The dense tissue within the subarachnoid space is composed of neoplastic astrocytes, reactive fibroblasts and meningothelial cells, and collagen. (Masson's trichrome, ×5)

extent with the earlier age at diagnosis of patients in whom the tumors are linked with neurofibromatosis relative to sporadic cases (4.9 and 12.0 years, respectively) [422].

Malignant (Anaplastic Astrocytoma)

Malignant astrocytomas of the optic nerve are extremely rare, which is fortunate in view of their very poor prognosis. In contradistinction to the benign tumors of childhood, the malignant astrocytoma of middle age has a predilection for male victims [182], and although exceptionally they may develop as recurrences of childhood tumors after a prolonged period of quiescence [327], most appear to arise de novo.

The clinical history is characteristic: an episode of acute pain, impaired visual activity, and afferent pupillary defect that initially simulates retrobulbar neuritis is followed within a matter of weeks by progressive proptosis and evidence of chiasmal and contralateral ocular involvement [161,182,294]. Death usually ensues 6–9 months later as a result of extensive intracranial tumor spread.

Histology shows cellular pleomorphism, although many are still recognizable as fibrillary astrocytes, with hyperchromatic and even multilobulated nuclei (Fig. 42) [161]. The cell processes tend to be short and stubby, so that the piloid histology of the childhood gliomas is absent, and mostly it is appropriate to classify the tumors as grade 3 astrocytomas. Electron microscopy reveals a variety of abnormalities, including peculiar whorled arrangements of the endoplasmic reticulum and perinuclear swirls of cytoplasmic filaments [160]. Hyperplasia of the vascular endothelium may be conspicuous in the malignant optic nerve astrocytomas.

Immunohistochemical studies have demonstrated two antigenically different types of neoplastic astrocyte, those of a second type that expresses an A2B5 antigen behaving in the more benign fashion [38]. Also it appears that malignant gliomas are much more likely to synthesize transforming growth factor α than their benign counterparts [388]. It remains to be seen to what extent these findings are relevant in an optic nerve context.

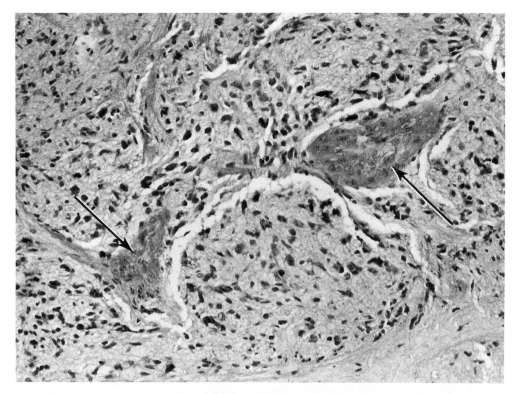

Figure 42   Malignant astrocytoma of the optic nerve. The astrocytic proliferation between the fibrous septa of the optic nerve is pleomorphic, and many of the cell nuclei are hyperchromatic. Marked endothelial cell hyperplasia is also seen in the blood vessels (arrows). (Hematoxylin and eosin, ×180)

B.   Meningioma

Meningiomas comprise less than 5% of orbital tumors (Table 1) [234,360], and the vast majority of them are direct extensions of intracranial meningiomas from along the wing of the sphenoid (sphenoidal ridge meningioma) [109,154] and the tuberculum sellae (suprasellar meningioma) or above and adjacent to the cribriform plate (olfactory groove meningioma) [423]. Patients with these tumors usually come under the initial care of neurosurgeons rather than ophthalmologists because of the associated neurological symptoms. Sphenoidal ridge meningiomas are frequently accompanied by an exuberant reactive hyperostosis of the adjacent sphenoid bone, and this is often sufficiently pronounced to produce proptosis by itself. A sphenoidal ridge meningioma occasionally spreads as far as the distal optic nerve and choroid [317]. Aside from the spread of meningiomas into the orbit from a primary intracranial focus, meningiomas may also arise anywhere along the optic nerve sheath (Fig. 43) [162,453]. Other orbital meningiomas may be unattached to the optic nerve outside the muscle cone [73,234,291,438] or rarely external to the periosteal coverings of the orbital walls [438]. Rarely orbital meningiomas are bilateral [414] or associated with multiple other meningiomas in extraorbital sites, such as the sphenoidal ridge and thoracic region [21]. Multiple meningiomas as well as meningiomas in childhood are often a manifestation of von Recklinghausen's neurofibromatosis [234,304]. Individuals may inherit a predisposition to meningioma, and a meningioma tumor suppressor gene has been identified on the long arm of chromosome 22, corresponding to the region 22q12.3-qter. The same genetic abnormality has been found with all histological variants of meningioma. Current evidence indicates that the meningioma gene is at a different point on the long arm of chromosome 22 than the gene involved in neurofibromatosis type 2 (central or bilateral acoustic neurofibromatosis) [66].

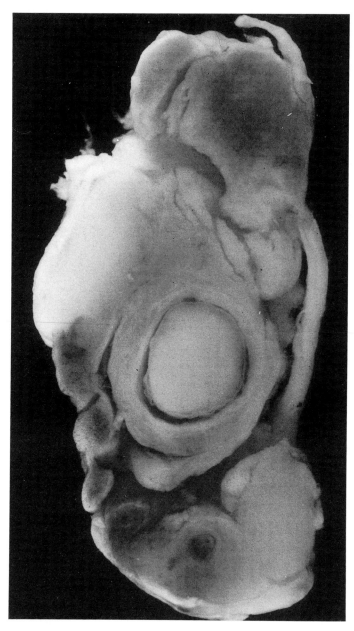

Figure 43 Meningioma of optic nerve at apex of orbit. The sheath of the nerve is greatly thickened by a primary meningioma, which has extended through the dura to spread extensively within the surrounding connective tissue of the orbit. (Resected specimen, ×10)

Nonorbital meningiomas of ophthalmological importance arise beneath the conjunctiva or caruncle [284] and within the optic canal [236,390,446], paranasal sinuses [262], and the skin around the eye [278]. The meningothelial cells of the optic nerve sheath are the source of most primary orbital meningiomas (78% in one series) [276]; other primary orbital meningiomas not connected to the optic nerve probably arise from meningothelial cells in an ectopic location. At least some of the latter cells presumably become entrapped in the perineurium of the nerves as they pass beyond the meningeal coverings of the central nervous system (CNS). The presence of meningiomas in the orbital muscle cone has led to speculation that mesenchymal elements may transform into meningothelial cells [407], but there is little evidence to support this view. As with meningiomas elsewhere in the CNS, those arising in the orbit occur more often in females than in males, although, interestingly, the less frequent tumors developing in younger subjects tend to predominate in males [476]. Conceivably, the overall preponderance of females is linked with the demonstration of receptors for progesterone and estrogen in a majority of intracranial tumors [454]. In the experience of some investigators [234], about one-fourth of the cases of primary orbital meningiomas become symptomatic before 10 years of age, in sharp contrast to intracranial meningiomas, which are rare before the age of 20 years [263,304]. However, this predilection for an early age of onset was not confirmed in other studies [172,473]. Like intracranial and intraspinal meningiomas, the majority of primary orbital meningiomas present in the fifth decade of life. As a rule the tumor spreads within the nerve sheath, causing nerve compression with relatively little expansion [8]: correspondingly, visual loss is the principal complaint, with only mild proptosis. Nerve compression may also be revealed by the emergence of prominent optociliary shunt vessels at the disk.

Because of variable morphological patterns, meningiomas are subdivided into numerous histological types, but such classifications are only of academic interest since all varieties manifest a similar biological behavior. Some meningiomas, the vast majority in the context of the optic nerve, appear as sheets of polygonal cells with indistinct cytoplasmic membranes and oval vesicular nuclei (syncytial meningioma), whereas other meningiomas are composed of densely packed interwoven bundles of spindle-shaped cells with some degree of whorl formation in a collagenous matrix that imparts toughness to the tumor (fibroblastic meningioma; Fig. 44). That these two varieties are related is underscored by meningiomas

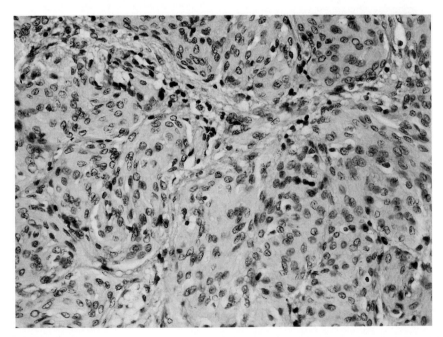

Figure 44 Meningioma of the optic nerve sheath. Clusters of syncytial cells with vesicular nuclei are surrounded by fine strands of fibrous tissue to constitute a transitional type of meningioma. (Hematoxylin and eosin, ×250)

encompassing features of both the syncytial and fibroblastic patterns (transitional meningiomas). Fibro-blastic and angioblastic meningiomas are virtually never seen in the orbit [234], and the diagnosis of those that have been documented [73,77,284] is questionable. That angioblastic meningiomas do not occur in the orbit is perhaps not surprising since the very existence of this traditional variety of meningioma is disputed [180]. As Burger and colleagues [47] have pointed out, most if not all of the so-called angioblastic meningiomas possess the attributes of a hemangiopericytoma or hemangioblastoma. Within meningiomas intranuclear invaginations of cytoplasm sometimes confer a light microscopic appearance of an intra-nuclear inclusion body, but the true nature of these pseudoinclusions (see Chap. 1) is readily discernible by electron microscopy [369]. Spherical bodies with concentric lamellae that are calcified and sometimes also impregnated with iron (psammoma bodies) are common in meningiomas (Fig. 45) and occasionally obscure most of the tumor's cellular component. Provided the degree of calcification is sufficient, many orbital meningiomas are evident radiologically (12.5%) [276]. Psammoma bodies occur in areas of high cellularity and may be of diagnostic significance since fibroblastic and Schwann cell tumors do not form them. By electron microscopy the bodies possess a substructure of radially arranged spicules of apatite crystals oriented around an amorphous mass [271]. Several theories for the genesis of psammoma bodies have been proposed, but none have received general acceptance [271,451]. Ultrastructurally, a striking feature of meningiomas is the complex interlocking of the cell processes between contiguous tumor cells, as well as the presence of desmosomes and hemidesmosomes (Fig. 46) [70,204]. Individual tumor cells often possess vast amounts of intracytoplasmic filaments, and unlike some other neoplasms, basement membrane material and microfibrils are not deposited between the tumor cells [70,278,331,352].

Metastasis is an exceedingly rare phenomenon [153,204,219,429], but the tumors can be locally infiltrative and subject to recurrence (Fig. 43) [73,234]. There is a relatively greater risk of intracranial extension, particularly in patients under 40 years of age, and although there may be little to be gained from surgery in the older age group, Wright and colleagues [476] advise total excision of the nerve in these individuals.

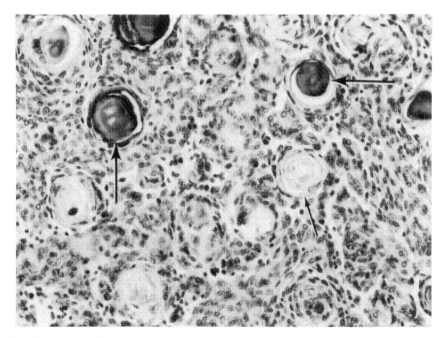

Figure 45 Meningioma of the optic nerve sheath. Within the clusters of meningothelial cells are scattered concentric calcified (psammoma) bodies (large arrows). Some of the tumor cells are arranged in concentric whorls of about the same size as the psammoma bodies (small arrow). (Hematoxylin and eosin, ×250)

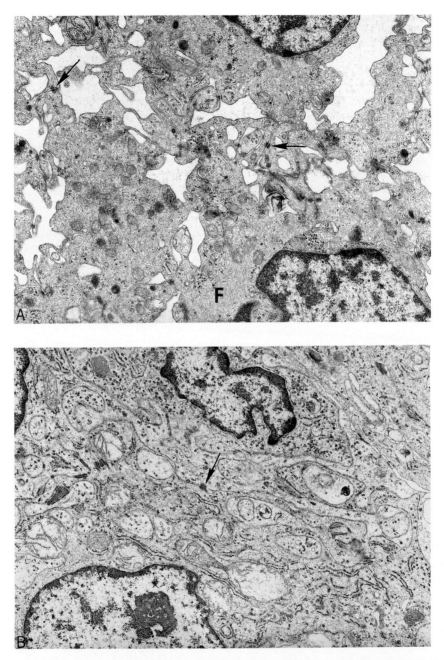

Figure 46 Electron micrographs of meningiomas. (A) The tumor cells have prominent interdigitating cytoplasmic processes, and these together with desmosomes (arrows) connect adjacent cells. These cells also have
prominent intracytoplasmic microfilaments (F). (×2500) (B) In contrast to the cells shown in A, cytoplasmic
filaments are not a feature of these meningioma cells, which are connected by desmosomes (arrow). (×7500)
(Courtesy of Dr. J. Shelburne.)

XII. TUMORS OF THE MELANOGENIC SYSTEM

A. Primary Orbital Melanoma

The vast majority of orbital malignant melanomas are secondary to intraocular melanomas of the ciliary body and choroid. Much less commonly they are blood-borne metastases from distant primary sites [340], and very rarely melanomas develop in the orbit in the absence of an intraocular tumor or evidence of a melanoma elsewhere in the body [173,361,365]. In common with many other tumors, desmosomes are evident by electron microscopy in primary orbital melanomas [71,196]. When the tumor is not pigmented, the presence of premelanosomes within the cytoplasm can be an ultrastructural diagnostic feature (Fig. 47). Primary orbital melanomas presumably arise from melanocytes in the leptomeninges or other parts of the orbit. This may occur in individuals with neurocutaneous melanosis (multiple giant hairy nevi, especially when the head is involved) or oculodermal melanosis (nevus of Ota; see Chap. 48) [160,215]. Some apparent primary orbital melanomas have developed without an apparent underlying lesion, as might occur from ectopically located melanocytes [380,470]. Although not known to predispose to orbital melanomas, other potential sites for primary orbital melanomas are melanocytic hamartomas, such as the cellular blue nevus [266,373]. Interestingly, a primary malignant melanoma of the orbit has been described in a black person despite the rarity of melanomas in blacks [90].

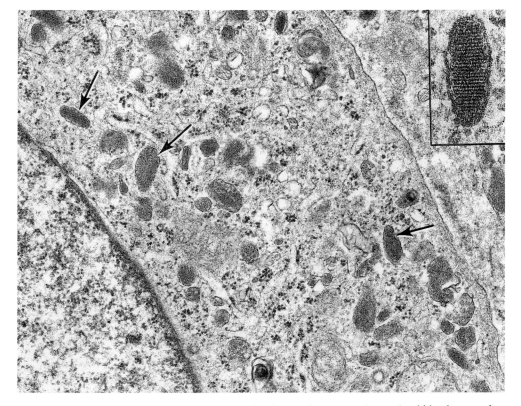

Figure 47 Electron micrograph of melanoma, showing melanosomes (arrows) within the cytoplasm. (×77,700). The inset is of a premelanosome with its characteristic 9 nm periodicity. The presence of this organelle within nonpigmented tumor cells is often helpful in establishing the diagnosis of an amelanotic melanoma. (×259,000) (Courtesy of Dr. J. Shelburne.)

B. Blue Nevus

The orbital tissues may be involved in the diffuse melanocytic proliferation that occurs in congenital ocular melanosis or oculodermal melanosis (nevus of Ota), and rarely, elongated melanin-containing cells intimately admixed with fibrous tissue form a discrete mass within the orbit [416] or adjacent to the sclera [412]. Such lesions are identical to the blue nevus of the dermis (see Chap. 46).

XIII. TUMORS OF GERM CELL (EXTRAGONADAL) AND UNCERTAIN ORIGIN

A. Benign

Dermoid Cyst

Dermoid cysts, which are among the most common orbital tumors, usually present in the superotemporal quadrant and are most often encountered in childhood. Lying in front of the orbital septum, as a rule, they rarely cause more than a painless swelling, although they may rupture and excite a chronic inflammatory reaction in which giant cells feature [257]. Radiographs may show defects in the adjacent bone and "dumbbell" extensions into the temporal fossa are common. Histological examination reveals a unilocular cyst lined by keratinizing squamous epithelium with dermal appendages in the fibrous wall (Fig. 48). Such choristomatous lesions possibly result from ectopic sequestration of skin during embryogenesis.

Teratoma

A teratoma differs from a dermoid cyst in containing tissues of ectodermal, mesodermal, and endodermal origin. Skin, colonic mucosa, bone, tooth, brain, and other tissues may be present in varying degrees of complexity [467], including, as an extreme curiosity, a partially developed fetus [94].

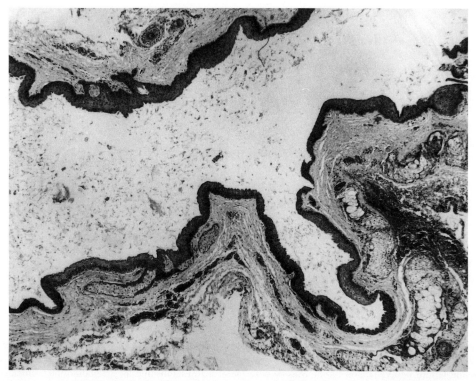

Figure 48 Dermoid cyst. The cyst cavity contains keratinous debris, and the wall includes hair follicles and sebaceous gland elements. (Hematoxylin and eosin, ×45)

This rare lesion is present at birth and is usually unilateral and of sufficient size to cause considerable enlargement of the bony orbit [30,35,187]. Secondary involvement of the orbit by a teratoma arising in a maxillary sinus is also reported [462]. A few cases with intracranial extension have been reported [35]. Rapid postnatal growth is also usual and necessitates urgent exenteration (the eye is almost always blind).

B. Malignant

Endodermal Sinus Tumor (Embryonal Carcinoma)

The endodermal sinus tumor (embryonal carcinoma) of the orbit is an exceptionally rare germ cell tumor [249,295] that corresponds to the similarly named entity found in the gonads of infants. An alternative name is yolk-sac tumor, and histologically, mantles of mucus-secreting cells are seen around blood vessels to create, in some instances, a distinctly adenocarcinomatous appearance. Orbital endodermal sinus tumors apparently occur at a younger age than comparable neoplasms in other nongonadal sites. Immuno-histochemical testing for α-fetoprotein can be helpful in distinguishing endodermal sinus tumors from rhabdomyosarcomas. The tumor is highly malignant and the prognosis is bad, but aggressive treatment can result in long-term survival [295].

Malignant Rhabdoid Tumor

The malignant rhabdoid tumor, initially portrayed as a sarcomatous variant of Wilms' tumor, is now acknowledged as a separate highly malignant neoplasm with both epithelial and mesenchymal differentia-tion. Despite a light microscopic resemblance to rhabdomyosarcoma, the polygonal neoplastic cells with eosinophilic filamentous cytoplasm, eccentric nuclei, and prominent "owl eye" nucleoli lack ultrastruc-tural and immunohistochemical evidence of rhabdomyoblastic differentiation. The tumor cells contain both mesenchyme-specific (vimentin) and epithelium-specific (epithelial membrane antigen) proteins, but they do not react with antibodies to the striated muscle proteins desmin and myoglobin. In contrast to the endodermal sinus tumor, with which it may be confused, the cells lack α-fetoprotein. Rare examples of this primary tumor in the orbit have been documented [335a,375].

XIV. TUMORS OF LYMPHOID TISSUE

Although lymphoid cells are not indigenous to the orbit, lymphoproliferative disorders rank high among the causes of proptosis. The incidence of orbital involvement in systemic lymphoma has been estimated to be in the region of 1–2.4% [112,186,261,379], but it is probable that most orbital lymphomas are primary to this site. Also seen are hyperplastic (reactive) lymphocytic lesions, frequently referred to as pseudotumors.

Following the introduction of immunological and histochemical marker techniques for the identifica-tion of the various categories of lymphocyte and monocyte and the need to correlate histological appearances with clinical behavior and prognosis, the classification of lymphocytic tumors has undergone numerous revisions within recent years [435]. Indeed, the process of reclassification is still unsettled and will remain so until the histogenesis of the various morphological cell types is completely defined. Even then it is doubtful whether the classifications, based as they are on tumors of lymph node origin, will be entirely relevant in the context of orbital and other ocular adnexal lymphoid neoplasms. Nor is ocular adnexal lymphoproliferative disease peculiar in this respect, the lung and gastrointestinal tract in particular presenting similar limitations. This has led to the emergence of a concept of mucosa-associated lymphoid tissue.

A. Mucosa-Associated Lymphoid Tissue

The concept of mucosa-associated lymphoid tissue (MALT) applies by definition to mucosal surfaces, such as the intestines and bronchi. In these locations lymphocytes are a normal component, but the concept also relates to organs, like the stomach and salivary glands, in which the lymphoid tissue is acquired as a function of aging. It is supposed that the lymphocytes constitute a protective mechanism aimed at eliminating unwanted antigens. Characteristically there is a mixed B and T cell population, most of the former being linked with IgA and IgM formation and the latter showing a CD4 helper cell predominance [191]. The lymphoid tissue seen in the conjunctiva is properly included within the MALT category.

Inclusion of orbital lymphoproliferative disorders under this heading is justifiable but open to some question since the orbit does not possess a mucosal component and there is little evidence that the presence of lymphocytes is ever a simple age-related accumulation. Nevertheless, the neoplastic lymphocytic lesions seen in the orbit resemble MALT-derived lymphomas in general in tending to remain localized for long periods and being preceded by an apparently reactive or inflammatory phase. Rarely they are also associated with lymphomas of other mucosal surfaces [167].

B. Lymphomas

Lymphoma (Non-Hodgkin's)

Medeiros and Harris [301] examined 99 lymphoid infiltrates of the orbit and conjunctiva immuno-histologically: 66 infiltrates expressed monotypic immunoglobulin; 1 case was immunoglobulin negative, B lineage; and 32 infiltrates expressed polytypic immunoglobulin. Using histological criteria, 36 cases were malignant (35 monotypic), 44 were indeterminate (31 monotypic and 13 polytypic), and 19 were benign (all polytypic). Most lymphomas (76%) were of low-grade malignancy; small lymphocytic lymphoma (45%) was the most common subtype. Cytological atypia and Dutcher bodies were peculiar to lymphomas. Bilateral involvement and dissemination at time of presentation occurred only in lymphomas. No other histological or clinical features reliably distinguished lymphomas from benign orbital lymphoid infiltrates. A total of 19 patients had a history of extraorbital malignant lymphoma, and 8 patients had a history of a reactive lesion. Patients with a history of malignant lymphoma more often presented with dissemination and less often had the small lymphocytic subtype than patients without a history of lymphoma. However, not all patients with a history of extraorbital lymphoma had monotypic orbital and conjunctival infiltrates, and the incidence of monotypic orbital and conjunctival lesions in these patients was similar to that of the patients without a history of lymphoma. The presence of either cytological atypia or Dutcher bodies is a reliable criterion of malignant lymphoma in the orbit, but for a considerable proportion of cases immunohistological studies are the only means of distinguishing malignant from benign lymphoid infiltrates [245,248,300].

Lymphoid tumors presenting in the orbit can be divided into high-grade malignant lymphoma, the more common low-grade malignant lymphoma, and indeterminate lymphocytic lesions [225]. About 15% have disseminated lymphoma at presentation [36]. The local control can be achieved with low doses of radiotherapy to the orbit, but lens opacities and dry eyes occasionally follow. The prognosis for stage I low-grade lymphoma and indeterminate lymphocytic lesions is similar to that of a normal population [36]. Most, if not all, lymphoid masses presenting in the orbit are either actually or potentially neoplastic rather than reactive in nature [36]. Any part of the orbit can be affected, including the musculature [179].

Lymphoplasmacytic lymphomas of the orbit are occasionally associated with serum paraproteinemia [44], cryoglobulinemia [261], and even amyloidosis [44].

Almost all orbital lymphomas are B cell tumors [250,292], although exceptional T cell lesions are also reported [260]. The majority are of low-grade malignancy [319] (Figs. 49 through 51), and on the basis of the Kiel classification of lymph node tumors [264] most nearly correspond to the lymphoplasmacytic and centrocytic lymphomas. As such they consist of sheets of small lymphocytes with groups of plasma cells and intermediate forms with scattered blast cells (lymphoplasmacytoid type) or a similar infiltration of lymphocytes with numerous pale-staining cells having cleared nuclei but few plasma cells (centrocytic type; Fig. 52). Some tumors have a significant addition of centroblasts. Less common, accounting for a third of the cases reported by Knowles and others [250], are rather more aggressive lesions with increased numbers of large blast cell forms. Some orbital lymphomas present an ill-defined follicular architecture, and probably a majority have evidence of previous germinal centers as revealed by the presence of reticulum cells [285]. Patients with the acquired immuno-deficiency syndrome (AIDS) are prone to non-Hodgkin's lymphomas, and on rare occasions these involve the orbit [15].

Histological diagnosis may be facilitated by the application of immunocytochemical techniques. Demonstration of antibody light-chain restriction is an irrefutable indication of neoplasia, but in cases that do not show significant plasmacytoid differentiation it may be helpful to assess the overall lymphoid population. Consonant with the observation that orbital lymphomas are usually B cell proliferations, the ratio of B to T cells is generally in excess of 4:1 [300], and only rarely do they contain more than 40% of T cells [250]. About one-fifth express the CD5 (Leu-1) antigen normally found only on the surface of T cells [250,251].

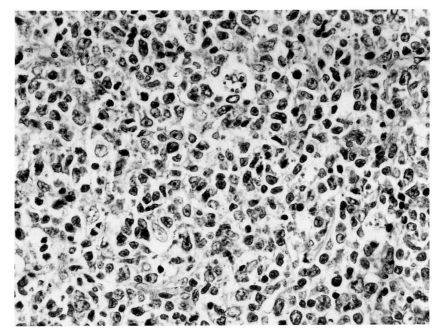

Figure 49 Diffuse histiocytic lymphoma composed of a fairly uniform population of pleomorphic cells with pale-staining cytoplasm and prominent nucleoli. (Hematoxylin and eosin, ×400)

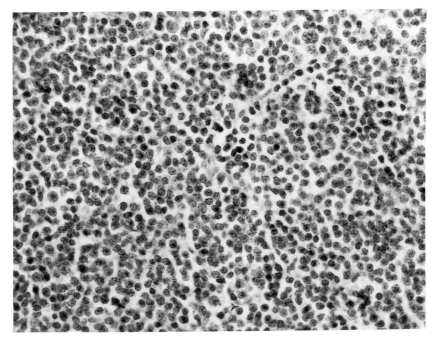

Figure 50 Well-differentiated lymphocytic lymphoma. The tumor is composed of densely packed lymphocytes of uniform size and shape. The cells have rounded nuclei and relatively little cytoplasm. (Hematoxylin and eosin, ×400)

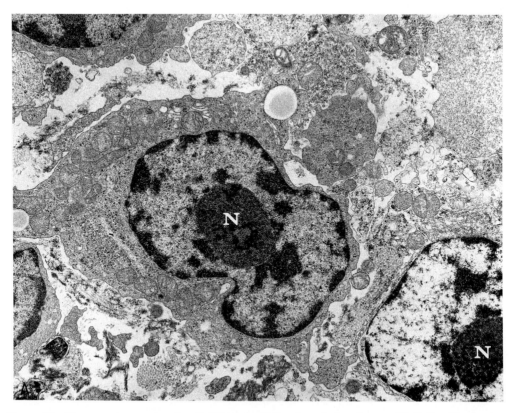

Figure 51   Electron micrographs of well-differentiated lymphocytic lymphoma. (A) Cells with prominent
nucleoli (N) and more cytoplasm than normal lymphocytes. (×11,600). (B) Cells with prominent nuclear
foldings and a prominent nuclear "pocket" (arrow). (×21,800) Although not diagnostic, these ultrastructural
features are frequently observed in lymphocytic lymphomas. (Courtesy of Dr. J. Shelburne.)

Burkitt's Lymphoma

The lymphoma described by Burkitt [48,49] primarily affects children and is most common in tropical
Africa [1], although rare cases have been observed elsewhere. The tumor involves the maxilla in about 20%
of cases, and Burkitt's lymphoma is the most common cause of proptosis among children in parts of Africa
[441]. Burkitt's lymphoma is not limited to humans and has been identified within the orbit of a cynomolgus
monkey (*Macaca fascicularis*) with a unilateral facial deformation and proptosis [216].

The histological picture is characteristic and consists of sheets of closely packed lymphoblasts that are
poorly differentiated interspersed with large macrophages (Fig. 53). Since the cytoplasm of the macrophages is essentially clear, they create an overall "starry sky" effect that is virtually pathognomonic.

The tumor grows extremely rapidly and disseminates early and widely, but in the absence of CNS or
bone marrow involvement, the response to chemotherapy or radiotherapy is good.

The serum of patients suffering from Burkitt's lymphoma is rich in antibody to the Epstein-Barr virus,
and the neoplastic lymphocytes possess a tumor-specific antigen that appears to be determined by this virus
[242]. A causal relationship is a strong possibility, at least with respect to endemic cases, the virus perhaps
being responsible for translocation of the part of chromosome 8 that carries the c-*myc* gene to the Ir region
of one of the three chromosomes concerned with immunoglobulin formation. Most Burkitt lymphomas,
murine plasmacytomas, and rat immunocytomas manifest a chromosomal translocation in which an
activated c-*myc* gene is linked to the IgH locus [164]. The pathogenic importance of this linkage has been
dramatically demonstrated in transgenic mice, in which lymphoma can be readily produced by the
introduction of foreign genes containing an immunoglobulin heavy-chain enhancer fused with the c-*myc*
oncogene [243].

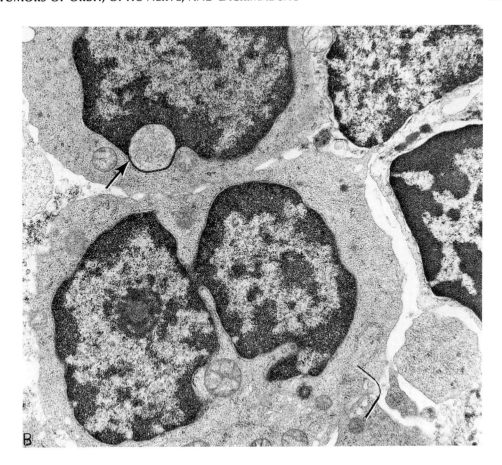

Other Lymphomas

Uncommon morphological variants of non-Hodgkin's lymphomas, such as the signet ring cell [87] and the "porcupine" lymphoma [121], involve the orbit on rare occasions. The signet ring cell lymphoma contains either vacuolated or periodic–acid Schiff-positive cytoplasmic inclusions that displace the nucleus eccentrically. The inclusions contain immunoglobulin M (IgM) trapped within distended rough endoplasmic reticulum [87]. The individual tumor cells in the porcupine lymphoma are characterized by their myriad of microvillous projections [121].

Hodgkin's Disease

Hodgkin's disease is extremely rare in the orbit [130,346,362,455], and when it does occur it is customarily part of a known systemic disease in the terminal phase. The histological picture is one of combined histiocytic and lymphocytic proliferation with an admixture of plasma cells, eosinophils, and occasional neutrophil leukocytes [342]. The diagnostic finding, however, is the Reed-Sternberg cell: a binucleate cell in which the nuclei are so arranged to suggest a mirror image and in which each nucleus has a prominent eosinophilic nucleolus surrounded by a clear halo. Recent studies strongly support a B lymphocytic origin of the Reed-Sternberg cell [394a]. Histological subdivisions of Hodgkin's disease relate very largely to the prevalence of lymphocytes and Reed-Sternberg cells, predominance of the former carrying the best prognosis and large numbers of the latter signifying a poor outcome. Tumors intersected by bands of fibrous tissue (nodular sclerosis) have an intermediate prognosis. Using the highly sensitive polymerase chain reaction, Epstein-Barr virus DNA has been detected in a relatively high percentage of cases of Hodgkin's disease [471a], but the significance of this observation awaits clarification. Recent evidence suggests that the nodular lymphocyte predominance variety of Hodgkin's disease is a distinct entity, perhaps related to

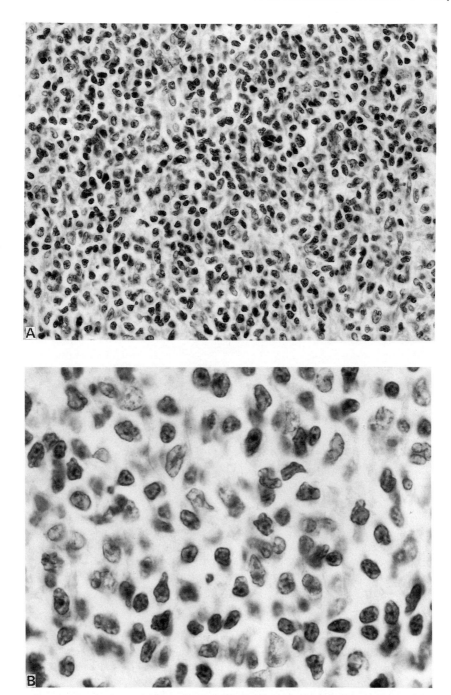

Figure 52 Moderately differentiated lymphocytic lymphomas. (A) The tumor is composed of lymphocytes in varying stages of maturation. (Hematoxylin and eosin, ×1000) (B) Higher magnification of tumor, showing lymphoblasts with clumped chromatin, recognizable nucleoli, and irregularly shaped cleft nuclei. (Hematoxylin and eosin, ×1000)

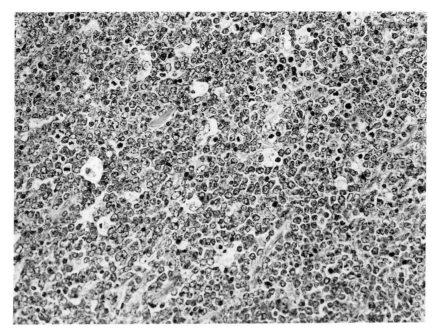

Figure 53 Burkitt's lymphoma involving the orbit. Densely packed lymphoblasts are interspersed with scattered pale-staining cells, giving a "starry sky" appearance. (Hematoxylin and eosin, ×250)

abnormal B cell proliferation, and although some reports have documented a bcl-2 gene rearrangement (present in most follicle-derived B cell lymphomas), other investigators have been unable to confirm this observation [386a,394a].

C. Reactive Lymphoid Hyperplasia

In line with the general concept of MALT, orbital lymphoproliferative disease deserves to be regarded as a continuous spectrum commencing as a nonneoplastic hyperplasia. It is presumed, although there is virtually no evidence, that the initial process is reactive. Of possible relevance is a finding that many of the patients have low serum IgA levels and an array of autoantibodies, which may point to a state of abnormal immunological function [142].

Previously referred to as inflammatory (lymphoid) pseudotumor, lymphoid hyperplasia is characterized by masses of lymphocytes with variable numbers of plasma cells and histiocytes. Germinal follicles are common (Fig. 54) but not invariable, and there may be an admixture of eosinophils (Fig. 55). The process is polyclonal, up to 60% of the lymphocytes being T cells [246], and there is no light-chain restriction. As befits their presumed inflammatory nature, perhaps, reactive lesions may be associated with pain [56] and they respond to corticosteroid therapy. Any part of the orbit can be affected, including the lacrimal gland and extraocular muscles, although inferiorly situated lesions are rare.

There is also a condition that closely resembles lymphoid hyperplasia of the orbit that develops in the region of the cavernous sinus and orbital apex, where it gives rise to intense pain and ophthalmoplegia [256,394,411]. Variously referred to as the orbital apex or Tolosa-Hunt syndrome, the lymphoid aggregation interferes with extraocular muscle function and sympathetic nerve activity in the eye. It is important to recognize, nevertheless, that the clinical features of the Tolosa-Hunt syndrome, including an initial response to corticosteroid therapy, can be mimicked by other lesions, such as vascular anomalies [128], and that some of the inflammatory processes, especially those showing sclerosis, are not pure lymphoid lesions [134].

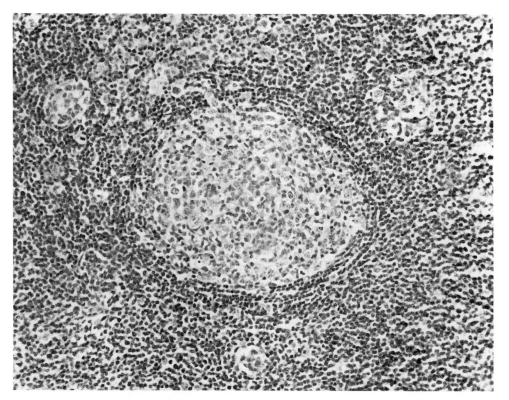

Figure 54   Lymphoid pseudotumor of the orbit, showing marked lymphocytic proliferation with, in the center of the picture, a prominent germinal follicle. (Hematoxylin and eosin, ×180)

D. Indeterminate Lymphoid Lesions

Between the established reactive and neoplastic proliferations there is a gray zone in which manifestly polyclonal lesions behave in a manner suggestive of neoplasia in that they do not respond to corticosteroid administration and sometimes disseminate. Indeed, there is good evidence that proliferations that are demonstrably polyclonal in terms of their immunoglobulin synthesis can subsequently become oligoclonal and then monoclonal with light-chain restriction [7,208]. A similar pattern of behavior has been described with respect to other MALT proliferations [29,417]. Analysis of DNA sequences has uncovered evidence of gene rearrangement in small clones of cells within ostensibly hyperplastic lesions [208], which could mean that proliferative disorders that are initially hyperplastic may spawn a neoplastic mutation. For a time the neoplastic clone coexists with the hyperplastic proliferation before gaining the upper hand to produce an exclusively lymphomatous lesion. Such an evolution could explain the unsatisfactory response to anti-inflammatory treatment despite a less than obvious neoplastic phenotype. Histologically the proliferations are characterized by sheets of mature lymphocytes with a variable admixture of diffusely disseminated blast forms in the absence of discernible follicles (Fig. 55).

From a practical standpoint it is sensible to regard any orbital lymphoproliferative process that is not unequivocally inflammatory as a potential if not actual lymphoma [142,143]. This attitude is reinforced by a comprehensive prospective study of some 69 patients followed over a 10 year period [250], which underscores the artificiality of attempting to separate presumed hyperplastic and neoplastic disorders. It was found that 27% of patients with lymphoid hyperplasia diagnosed on histopathological criteria and confirmed by immunophenotypic analysis developed lymphomas at other sites compared with 33% in those with similarly diagnosed lymphomas. This suggests that merely classifying lesions into benign and malignant categories is not useful in predicting eventual outcome, although it is recognized that identification of low and higher grades of malignancy by histopathological methods is of prognostic value [250].

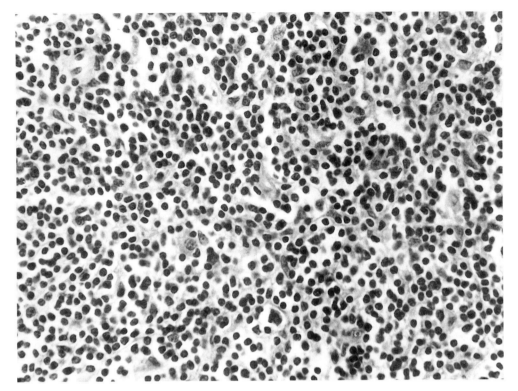

Figure 55 Lymphoid pseudotumor of the orbit, which proved resistant to corticosteroid treatment. Occasional lymphoblasts are spread diffusely through the proliferating lymphocytes, and there is an absence of germinal follicle formation. (Hematoxylin and eosin, ×450)

Even so it appears that the single most important prognostic factor is the extent of the disease at the time of presentation.

E. Plasma Cell Tumors

Plasma cell proliferation can take several forms, but the best known type and the one with most relevance to the orbit is multiple myeloma. As the name indicates, multiple myeloma is a disseminated lesion within the bone marrow characterized by masses of atypical plasma cells that are larger than normal and frequently possess multiple nuclei (binucleate forms are not diagnostic since they can occur in inflammatory processes). An uncontrolled formation of immunoglobulin is reflected in raised serum levels, most commonly expressed in the IgG but sometimes in other classes (especially IgA). Some patients have circulating antibody light chains, and about 50% pass light chains (Bence Jones protein) in their urine.

Orbital complications, which can be the presenting manifestation of multiple myeloma [33,221,397], sometimes represent involvement of the orbital bones [58], but this appears to be exceptional; more commonly they are the result of plasma cell proliferation within the soft tissues of the orbit [371]. The mean age for multiple myeloma is 64 years, but the condition can affect individuals younger than 40 years, especially in persons with AIDS, and unique bilateral orbital plasmacytomas have been documented in an otherwise apparently normal 25-year-old man [397]. It is noteworthy that although only 2% of all myelomas are of the IgD class, this variety has been conspicuous in the very few orbital myelomas that have been characterized [244]. Ostensible solitary myeloma has also been reported in the orbit [151,195,237,397], but such lesions can be regarded as substantiated only after detailed study of other potential sites and long follow-up.

Waldenström's macroglobulinemia is a rare condition that may involve the orbit, especially the lacrimal gland [274]. It is caused by the secretion of large amounts of monoclonal IgM by neoplastic B lymphocytes in a variety of lymphomas, the responsible cells often demonstrating periodic acid–Schiff-positive perinuclear (Dutcher) bodies. The hyperviscosity attributable to the macroglobulinemia can precipitate retinal vein occlusion [415].

XV. INFLAMMATORY MASSES (PSEUDOTUMORS) OF THE ORBIT

Any expanding process within the orbital confines is prone to cause proptosis and if more or less circumscribed is in danger of being confused with a neoplasm. Even so, to describe any nonneoplastic swelling as a pseudotumor is unsatisfactory because at best it merely highlights a negative property of a lesion that may or may not have a clearly defined cause, and at worst it provides a spurious diagnostic label that serves to disguise a basic lack of understanding. The issue is confused further by many workers by the arbitrary restriction of the term to idiopathic inflammatory lesions. Typically, an inflammatory swelling presents with pain, diplopia, and lid swelling as well as proptosis. As a rule, given a representative sample, histological study of a biopsy specimen allows a reliable distinction to be drawn between an inflammatory lesion and a true neoplasm. This objection apart, it is common practice to recognize three principal types of so-called orbital pseudotumor from a histopathological standpoint: lymphoid, granulomatous, and sclerosing [137].

Orbital pseudotumors rarely extend beyond the confines of the bony orbit, whether intracranially or into the ethmoid, sphenoid, or other paranasal sinuses [97,337,351]. Involvement of both orbits by the inflammatory reaction is uncommon [351]. The reason for the orbital inflammation is unknown, but there is probably more than one. Noncultivable cell wall-deficient bacteria known as mollicutes may be involved but a claim that mollicutes-like organisms are implicated [466] needs confirmation [140]. Orbital pseudotumors of childhood [326,351], in contrast to comparable lesions in adults, are often associated with peripheral blood eosinophilia and an elevated erythrocyte sedimentation rate [326], suggesting a different cause and pathogenesis.

A. Reactive Lymphoid Hyperplasia

This disorder is discussed within the context of orbital lymphoproliferative disease as a whole, as a variant of the so-called mucosa-associated lymphoid tissue (see p. 1567).

B. Nodular Fasciitis

Bearing a superficial resemblance to fibrosarcoma, nodular fasciitis is a self-limiting nonneoplastic condition that typically involves the fascial planes and subcutaneous tissue of the limbs (especially the forearm) and trunk [253]. Occasionally, the conjunctiva and anterior episclera [122,443], eyebrow [299] and the orbit [267,350] may be involved.

The lesion develops rapidly, often within a few weeks, and histological examination shows proliferating fibroblasts in a variably collagenous or myxoid matrix (Fig. 56). Capillary blood vessels are conspicuous, and there is a constant, if scanty, infiltrate of mononuclear inflammatory cells. Despite the presence of scattered mitotic figures, the cells show none of the other nuclear changes associated with malignancy, and the lesion responds well to local excision. Its true nature is elusive.

C. Lipogranuloma

"Orbital lipogranuloma" is the term given to an inflammatory reaction within the adipose tissue and has been considered to represent a response to fat necrosis [69]. Lymphocytes, macrophages, and occasional multinucleated giant cells are associated with active fibrosis, culminating in some instances in a sclerosing lipogranuloma (Fig. 57). The cause of the fat necrosis, if such really is the stimulus to the granulomatous reaction, is obscure, although trauma has been postulated in some cases [69]. In a minority there is evidence of exogenous lipid or oil such as can complicate a grease gun injury [139] or orbitography using a lipid-based contrast medium [99].

D. Multifocal Fibrosclerosis

The term "multifocal fibrosclerosis" refers to the presence in multiple sites of dense hyalinized fibrous tissue associated with a mild chronic inflammatory process (Fig. 58). Orbital involvement can occur and

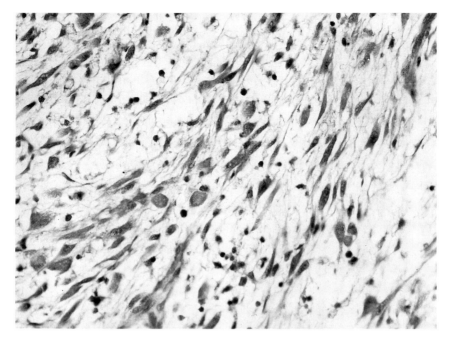

Figure 56 Nodular fasciitis causing an orbital pseudotumor. An exuberant proliferation of fibroblasts presents a superficial resemblance of fibrosarcoma. However, there the cell nuclei are small and regular and there is more collagen synthesis than is seen in most fibrosarcomas. Scattered lymphocytes suggest an inflammatory basis for the lesion. (Hematoxylin and eosin, ×250)

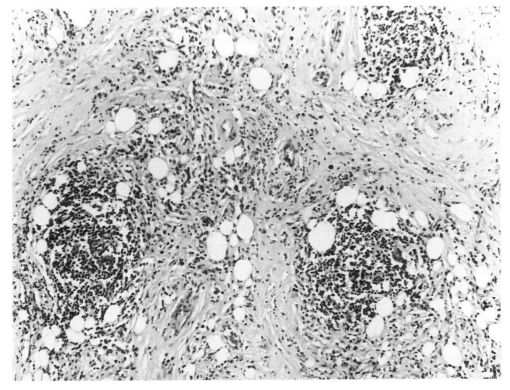

Figure 57 Lipogranuloma of the orbit. This chronic inflammatory state is associated with focal lymphocytic infiltration and reactive fibrosis around the orbital fatty tissue. (Hematoxylin and eosin, ×110)

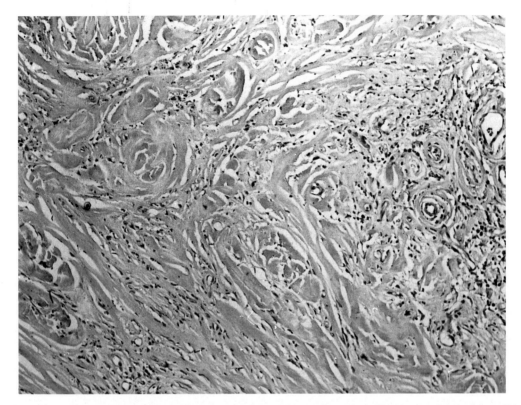

Figure 58 Multifocal fibrosclerosis. Extensive hyalinized fibrous tissue deposition in associated with a mild chronic inflammatory cell infiltration. The patient in this instance also had retroperitoneal fibrosis. (Hematoxylin and eosin, ×110)

produce proptosis. Thus, orbital fibrosclerosis has been reported as a concomitant of mediastinal fibrosis [96,366], sclerosing cholangitis [460], Riedel's thyroiditis [13,20], and retroperitoneal fibrosis [67]. In some patients there appears to be a familial aspect [67]. Occasional instances of orbital fibrosis accompanied by fibrotic nodules in the dermis of the head and neck can also be observed, the collagen bundles often showing a multiple concentric pattern.

The cause of multifocal fibrosclerosis in general as well as in an orbital context is unknown, and the significance of a report that T cell receptor gene rearrangement, with the implication that the process may be a low-grade neoplasia [81], remains to be seen.

E. Mucocele

An important cause of proptosis, more commonly seen by the rhinologist than the ophthalmologist, a mucocele is a sequel to long-standing obstruction to drainage of a paranasal sinus. The sinuses most often associated with orbital complications are those in the ethmoidal and frontal bones [188]. As a result of continued mucus secretion, the sinus expands by eroding its shell of cortical bone and enters the orbit. The excised mucocele has a lining of either pseudostratified ciliated epithelium or a thin layer of atrophic epithelium. Frequently the mucocele is infected, and rupture of its wall can result in orbital cellulitis. Exceptionally cysts of seeming respiratory epithelium derivation have been described at orbital sites remote from the sinuses [213], and it is presumed in these instances that they represent dispersion of sinus epithelium occasioned by trauma.

F. Other Causes of Orbital Inflammation

A whole host of inflammatory conditions, infective and allergic, localized and generalized, can produce proptosis and simulate an orbital neoplasm [140]. Many of these are discussed elsewhere in connection with systemic immune disorders (see Chap. 6), fungus infections (see Chap. 10), helminth infestation (see Chap. 12), and arthropod infestation (see Chap. 13). The responses associated with organizing hematomas, so-called cholesterol granulomas or hematic cysts [312,401], and occasionally with traumatic foreign body implantation are also causes of orbital inflammation and hence, on occasion, of a pseudotumor.

XVI. SECONDARY TUMORS OF THE ORBIT

Secondary tumors are a principal form of orbital neoplasia. Jakobiec and colleagues [210] quote an incidence of 10% but refer to the survey of 465 orbital tumors carried out at the Mayo Clinic, in which direct invasion from neighboring sites and metastasis accounted for just over 50% [172]. Primary ophthalmic centers, however, can expect to see a lower incidence; 7.6 and 11% being reported from the Institute of Ophthalmology, London (Table 1) and the Wills Eye Hospital, Philadelphia [405], respectively.

Diplopia, ocular motility limitation, and mass effect with displacement, proptosis, or palpable mass are common modes of presentation [149,404]. The clinical presentations can be broken down into four categories: infiltrative (53%), mass (37%), inflammatory (5%), and functional (3%) [149]. Accurate diagnosis often depends on biopsy supplemented by immunohistochemical marker examination or, less frequently, electron microscopy (Fig. 59) to determine the origin of these often poorly differentiated tumors. Proptosis is usual, and enophthalmos sometimes occurs [364] as a result of destruction of the bony orbital wall: it was present in 25% of cases in one series [149]. Goldberg and colleagues [150] found the infiltrative syndrome of presentation to be most common. The orbital metastasis is commonly detected before the realization of the primary neoplasm, accounting for 24% of cases in one series [150]. Modern therapeutic approaches often lead to long-term palliation, but the average patient survival after the diagnosis of orbital metastasis is 10.2–13 months [149,404]. Lung carcinoma carries the worst prognosis, with an average survival time of only 4 months [404].

Children

As with malignant neoplasia in general, orbital metastasis is uncommon in children. One series enumerated 4 metastatic tumors compared with 88 primary tumors (excluding retinoblastoma) [328]. Neuroblastoma appears to be the most frequently recorded [4,353], followed by Ewing's sarcoma and Wilms' tumor [18].

Neuroblastomas arise from primitive neuroblasts located within the adrenal medulla or, less commonly, in relation to the autonomic nerve chain. Most of these tumors present before the age of 5 years. Sheets of small compact cells with sparse cytoplasm and densely stained oval nuclei, which can resemble lymphocytes or retinoblastoma cells, are present on histological examination (Fig. 60). Rosettes formed by the grouping of cells around a central tangle of fibrillar cell processes are a feature of the well-differentiated primary neuroblastoma but are almost never seen in orbital metastases. Diagnosis may be facilitated by examination of the urine for catecholamines and electron microscopy of the tumor cells, which contain dark-core (bioamine) granules and microtubules [210]. The orbit appears to be a favored site for neuroblastoma metastasis [5], being located within either the soft tissues or the wall, especially the latter.

Ewing's sarcoma is a highly malignant tumor arising primarily in long bones that usually presents between the ages of 10 and 25 years. For many years the histogenesis remained elusive, the cells resembling reticular stem cells with an ill-defined cytoplasm rich in glycogen. Ewing's sarcoma cells express a specific cell surface protein (referred to as p30/32^{MIC2}, HBA71, 12E7, or O13 antigen), and the monoclonal antibody HBA71 is valuable in establishing the diagnosis immunohistochemically even in paraffin-embedded decalcified tissue [364a]. Persuasive evidence based on immunocytochemistry and cell cultures points to a neuroectodermal origin [275,338,364a]. Strong evidence that this tumor is genetically controlled finds support in the observation that a chromosomal translocation {t(11;22) (q24:q12)} (see Chap. 41 for terminology of chromosomal disorders), has been identified in 92% of patients with Ewing's sarcoma [447]. The metastases are usually located within the soft tissues, but the bones of the orbit may be involved and exceptional instances of primary orbital bone involvement by Ewing's sarcoma have been recorded [4,10,465,471].

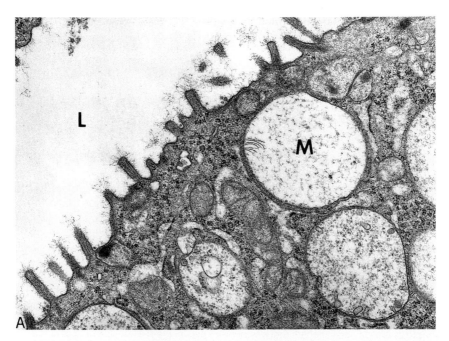

Figure 59 Ultrastructure of adenocarcinomas, showing some features that may be helpful in establishing the diagnosis. (A) Microvilli are projecting into the lumen (L) of an acinus of a mucin-secreting adenocarcinoma. Note the mucin-containing vacuoles within the cytoplasm (M). (×19,000) (B) Less differentiated adenocarcinomas commonly form a rudimentary lumen within individual tumor cells. The presence of such a "neo-lumen" (arrows) can be of diagnostic value. (×19,000) (C) This poorly differentiated adenocarcinoma has a basal lamina (BL), desmosomes (D), and a neolumen (N), which is less well developed than in B. (×19,000) (Courtesy of Dr. J. Shelburne.)

Adults

Sarcomas, such as leiomyosarcomas [230], rarely metastasize to the orbit, but carcinomatous deposits, most of them coming from the breast (Fig. 61) [108,132,404], are not infrequent. Carcinoma of the bronchus and prostate [254,404] predominates as the primary source in males. Other sources include the kidney, gastrointestinal tract, pancreas, testicle, liver [452], and urinary bladder [357], as well as cutaneous [404] or meningeal [101] melanoma (Fig. 57). Carcinoid tumors that arise in the bronchus, trachea, or ileum also occasionally metastasize to the orbit [367]. They may be associated with the carcinoid syndrome and with elevated levels of urinary 5-hydroxyindoleacetic acid. Four variants of the histological pattern are recognized: solid lobules or masses, trabecular or cordlike, tubular or rosettelike, and a mixed pattern [367]. In contrast to metastatic carcinoma, metastatic carcinoid tumors have a much more favorable prognosis. Mycosis fungoides may also involve the orbit [463].

Ferry and Font [108] make the observation that since metastases reaching the orbit necessarily pass through the lungs, it is not surprising that orbital and pulmonary metastases are often associated: accordingly, it is recommended that x-ray examination of the chest be taken in all cases in which there is a possibility of metastatic tumor.

Leukemic deposits are also known to occur in the orbits of both children and adults, particularly in the acute forms of the disease [203], and complicate the lymphoblastic disorder rather more frequently than the myelogenous. Myelogenous deposits sometimes have a greenish color attributable to myeloperoxidase activity, which in the past earned the descriptive term "chloroma." Rarely other types of acute leukemia may be involved [434].

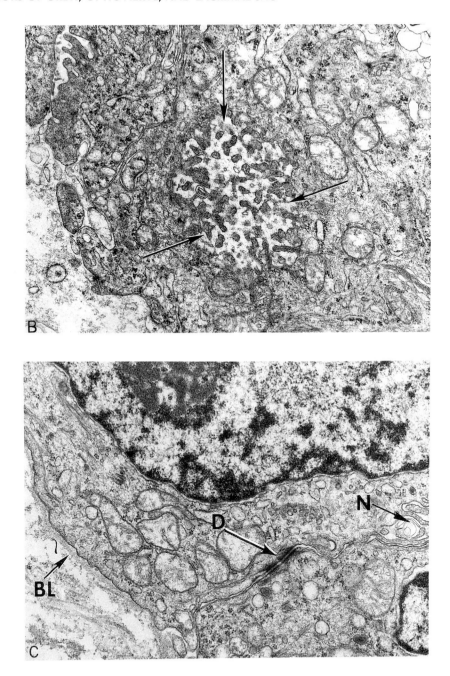

Tumors from Adjacent Structures

Neoplasia in the orbit attributable to direct invasion can originate within the eye or the periorbital tissues. Since they are the most common types of intraocular malignancy, it is not unexpected that retinoblastoma (see Chap. 49) and uveal melanoma (see Chap. 48) are the ocular tumors usually seen spreading into the orbit. The malignant cells enter the orbit by way of the scleral vascular and neural channels and, in the case

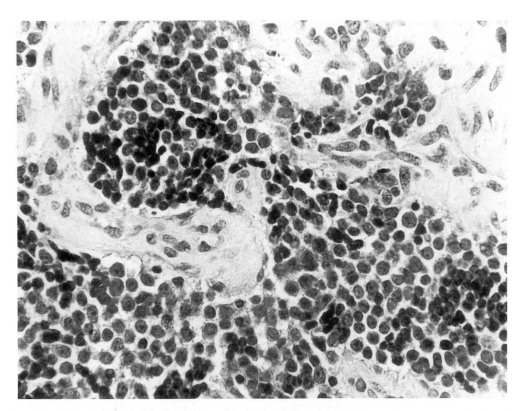

Figure 60 Metastatic neuroblastoma in the orbit of a child. The tumor cells have intensely basophilic round nuclei and little cytoplasm. Rosette formation is unusual in metastatic deposits. (Hematoxylin and eosin, ×450)

of retinoblastoma, along the optic nerve. Not all melanoma deposits in the orbit are the outcome of uveal spread, however, for apart from other tumors that are primary, metastasis from cutaneous melanoma is also seen [340].

Medulloepithelioma and malignant tumors of mature ciliary body epithelium can also extend into the orbit (see Chap. 47), but only as a very rare event in view of the low incidence of the primary tumors.

Orbital invasion from the eyelids is usually related to squamous or basal cell carcinoma [25]; squamous cell carcinoma and malignant melanoma are the usual conjunctival tumors with a propensity to involve the orbit [190,214].

There are many reports of orbital neoplasia secondary to tumors of the nasal passages and paranasal sinuses. In Henderson's series 7% of all orbital tumors originated in these sites. A rare tumor of the nasal mucosa that can invade the orbit is the esthesioneuroblastoma (olfactory neuroblastoma) [402]. Oncocytic tumors of the nose and paranasal sinuses, which tend to be low-grade malignant neoplasms, can also invade the orbit [60]. An exceptional neoplasm derived from embryonal tooth elements in the maxillary antrum (ameloblastoma) has also invaded the orbit [458]. Intracranial meningiomas are also prone to enter the orbit, and there are isolated reports of orbital invasion by a pituitary adenoma [85] and an intracranial germinoma [133], medulloblastoma [241], and a glioblastoma multiforme in the absence of previous surgical intervention [16].

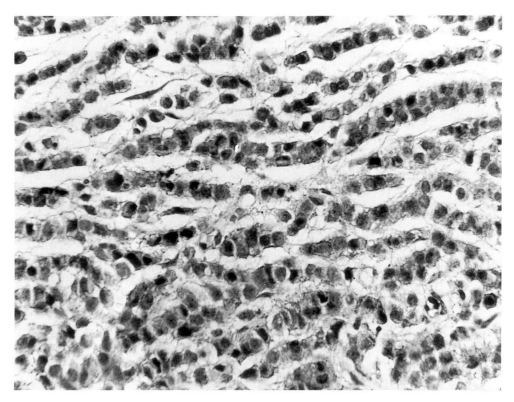

Figure 61 Metastatic breast carcinoma in the orbit. Toward the margins of secondary deposits, the cells of a breast carcinoma frequently assume a regimented arrangement where they are invading the orbital connective tissue, and this finding can be helpful in diagnosis. (Hematoxylin and eosin, ×450)

REFERENCES

1. Abiose, A., Adido, J., and Agarwal, S.C. Childhood malignancies of the eye and orbit in northern Nigeria. *Cancer 55*:2889–2893, 1985.
2. Abrahams, I.W., Fenton, R.H., and Vidone, R. Alveolar soft-part sarcoma of the orbit. *Arch. Ophthalmol. 79*:185–188, 1968.
3. Abramson, D.H., Ellsworth, R.M., and Zimmerman, L.E. Non-ocular cancer in retinoblastoma survivors. *Trans. Am. Acad. Ophthalmol. Otolaryngol. 81*:454–457, 1976.
4. Albert, D.M., Rubenstein, R.A., and Scheie, H.G. Tumor metastasis to the eye. II. Clinical study in infants and children. *Am. J. Ophthalmol. 63*:727–732, 1967.
5. Alfano, J.E. Ophthalmological aspects of neuroblastomatosis: A study of 53 verified cases. *Trans. Am. Acad. Ophthalmol. Otolaryngol. 72*:830–848, 1968.
6. Allen, P.W. The fibromatoses: A clinicopathologic classification based on 140 cases. *Am. J. Surg. Pathol. 1*:255–270, 305–321, 1977.
7. Alper, M.G., and Bray, M. Evolution of a primary lymphoma of the orbit. *Br. J. Ophthalmol. 68*:255–260, 1984.
8. Als, E. Intraorbital meningiomas encasing the optic nerve: A report of two cases. *Acta Ophthalmol. (Copenh.) 47*:900–903, 1969.
9. Altamirano-Dimas, M., and Albores-Saavedra, J. Alveolar soft part sarcoma of the orbit. *Arch. Ophthalmol. 75*:496–499, 1966.
10. Alvarez-Berdecia, A., Schut, L., and Bruce, D.A. Localized primary intracranial Ewing's sarcoma of the orbital roof: Case report. *J. Neurosurg. 50*:811–813, 1979.
11. Alvord, E.C., and Lofton, S. Gliomas of the optic nerve or chiasm: Outcome by patients' age, tumor site, and treatment. *J. Neurosurg. 68*:85–98, 1980.
12. Amemiya, T., and Kadoya, M. Paraganglioma in the orbit. *J. Cancer Res. Clin. Oncol. 96*:169–179, 1980.

13. Anderson, S.R., Seedorff, H.H., and Halberg, P. Thyroiditis with myxoedema and orbital pseudotumor. *Acta Ophthalmol. (Copenh.) 41*:120–125, 1963.

14. Anderson, D.R., and Spencer, W.H. Ultrastructural and histochemical observations of optic nerve gliomas. *Arch. Ophthalmol. 83*:324–335, 1970.

15. Antle, C.M., White, V.A., Horsman, D.E., and Rootman, J. Large cell orbital lymphoma in a patient with acquired immune deficiency syndrome. Case report and review. *Ophthalmology 97*:1494–1498, 1990.

16. Aoyama, I., Makita, Y., Nabeshima, S., Motomochi, M., and Masuda, A. Extradural nasal and orbital extension of glioblastoma multiforme without previous surgical intervention. *Surg. Neurol. 14*:343–347, 1980.

17. Aparicio, S.R., and Lumsden, C.E. Light and electron microscopic studies on the granular cell myoblastoma. *J. Pathol. 97*:339–355, 1969.

18. Apple, D.J. Wilm's tumor metastatic to the orbit. *Arch. Ophthalmol. 80*:480–483, 1968.

19. Archer, K.F., Hurwitz, J.J., Balogh, J.M., and Fernandes, B.J. Orbital nonchromaffin paraganglioma: A case report and review of the literature. *Ophthalmology 96*:1659–1666, 1989.

20. Arnott, E.J., and Greaves, D.P. Orbital involvement in Riedel's thyroiditis. *Br. J. Ophthalmol. 49*:1–5, 1965.

21. Arseni, C., Dumitrescu, I.L., and Carp, N. Orbital, sphenoidal ridge and spinal meningiomas occurring in one patient. *Neurochirurgia 27*:86–88, 1984.

22. Ashton, N. Epithelial tumours of the lacrimal gland. *Mod. Probl. Ophthalmol. 14*:306–323, 1975.

23. Ashton, N., and Morgan, G. Embryonal sarcoma and embryonal rhabdomyosarcoma of the orbit. *J. Clin. Pathol. 18*:699–714, 1965.

24. Aurora, A.L. Oncocytic metaplasia in a lacrimal sac papilloma. *Am. J. Ophthalmol. 75*:466–468, 1973.

25. Aurora, A.L., and Blodi, F.C. Lesions of the eyelids: A clinicopathologic study. *Surv. Ophthalmol. 15*:94–104, 1970.

26. Avery, M.E., McAfee, J.G., and Guild, H.G. The course and prognosis of reticuloendotheliosis (eosinophilic granuloma, Schuller-Christian disease and Letterer-Siwe disease): A study of forty cases. *Am. J. Med. 22*:636–652, 1957.

27. Baghdassarian, S.A., and Shammas, H.F. Eosinophilic granuloma of orbit. *Ann. Ophthalmol. 9*:1247–1251, 1977.

28. Banfield, W., Lee, C.K., and Lee, C.W. Myocardial collagen of the fibrous long-spacing type. *Arch. Pathol. 95*:262–266, 1973.

29. Banerjee, D., and Ahmad, D. Malignant lymphoma complicating lymphocytic interstitial pneumonia: A monoclonal B-cell neoplasm arising in a polyclonal lymphoproliferative disorder. *Hum. Pathol. 13*:780–782, 1982.

30. Barber, J.C., Barber, L.F., Guerry, D., III, and Geeraets, W.J. Congenital orbital teratoma. *Arch. Ophthalmol. 91*:45–48, 1974.

31. Bartley, G.B., Yeatts, R.P., Garrity, J.A., Farrow, G.M., and Campbell, R.J. Spindle cell lipoma of the orbit. *Am. J. Ophthalmol. 100*:605–609, 1985.

32. Bastiaensen, L.A., Leyten, A.C., Tjan, T.G., and Misere, J.F. Chondroid chordoma of the base of the skull: Orbital and other neuro-ophthalmological symptoms. *Doc. Ophthalmol. 55*:5–15, 1983.

33. Benjamin, I., Taylor, H., and Spindler, J. Orbital and conjunctival involvement in multiple myeloma. *Am. J. Clin. Pathol. 63*:811–817, 1975.

34. Bergstrom, K., Enoksson, P., Gamstrorp, I., and Naeser, P. Haemangioendothelioma of the orbit. *Ophthalmologica 177*:115–120, 1978.

35. Berlin, A.J., Rich, L.S., and Hahn, J.F. Congenital orbital teratoma. *Childs Brain 10*:208–216, 1983.

36. Bessell, E.M., Henk, J.M., Wright, J.E., and Whitelocke, R.A. Orbital and conjunctival lymphoma treatment and prognosis. *Radiother. Oncol. 13*:237–244, 1988.

37. Binet, E.F., Kieffer, S.A., Martin, S.H., and Peterson, H.O. Orbital dysplasia in neurofibromatosis. *Radiology 93*:829–833, 1969.

38. Bishop, M., and de la Monte, S.M. Dual lineage of astrocytomas. *Am. J. Pathol. 135*:517–527, 1989.

39. Blake, J., Mullaney, J., and Gillan, J. Lacrimal sac mucoepidermoid carcinoma. *Br. J. Ophthalmol. 70*:681–685, 1986.

40. Blodi, F.C. Amputation neuroma in the orbit. *Am. J. Ophthalmol. 32*:929–932, 1949.

41. Blodi, F.C. Unusual orbital neoplasms. *Am. J. Ophthalmol. 68*:407–412, 1969.

42. Blodi, F.C. Cited by F.A. Jakobiec and I.S. Jones in *Diseases of the Orbit*, I.S. Jones and F.A. Jakobiec (Eds.), Harper & Row, New York, pp. 503–569, 1979.

43. Bowen, J.H., Christensen, F.H., Klintworth, G.K., and Sydnor, C.F. A clinicopathologic study of a cartilaginous hamartoma of the orbit—a rare cause of proptosis. *Ophthalmology 88*:1356–1360, 1981.

44. Brisbane, J.U., Lessell, S., Finkel, H.E., and Neiman, R.S. Malignant lymphoma presenting in the orbit: A clinicopathologic study of a rare immunoglobulin-producing variant. *Cancer 47*:548–553, 1981.

45. Brown, H.H., Kersten, R.C., and Kulwin, D.R. Lipomatous hamartoma of the orbit. *Arch. Ophthalmol. 109*:240–243, 1991.

46. Bullock, J.D., Goldberg, S.H., and Rakes, S.M. Orbital tumors in children. *Ophthalmic Plast. Reconstr. Surg. 5*:13–16, 1989.

47. Burger, P.C., Scheithauer, B.W., and Vogel, F.S. *Surgical Pathology of the Nervous System and Its Coverings*, 3rd ed. Churchill Livingstone, New York, 1991.
48. Burkitt, D. A sarcoma involving jaws in African children. *Br. J. Surg. 46*:218–223, 1958.
49. Burkitt, D.P. Etiology of Burkitt's lymphoma—an alternative hypothesis to vectored virus. *J. Natl. Cancer Inst. 42*:19–28, 1969.
50. Burrows, E.H. Bone changes in orbital neurofibromatosis. *Br. J. Radiol. 36*:549–561, 1963.
51. Cardenas-Ramirez, L., Albores-Savedra, J., and de Buen, J. Mesenchymal chondrosarcoma of the orbit: Report of the first case in orbital location. *Arch. Ophthalmol. 86*:410–413, 1971.
52. Carelli, P., and Cangelosi, J. Angiosarcoma of the orbit. *Am. J. Ophthalmol. 31*:453–456, 1948.
53. Carnevali, L., Trimarchi, F., Rosso, R., and Stringa, M. Haemangiopericytoma of the lacrimal sac: A case report. *Br. J. Ophthalmol. 72*:782–785, 1988.
54. Case, T., and LaPiana, F. Benign fibrous tumor of the orbit. *Ann. Ophthalmol. 7*:813–815, 1975.
55. Chaves, E., Oliveira, A., and Armaud, A. Retrobulbar granular cell myoblastoma. *Br. J. Ophthalmol. 56*:854–856, 1972.
56. Chavis, R.M., Garner, A., and Wright, J.E. Inflammatory orbital pseudotumor: A clinicopathologic study. *Arch. Ophthalmol. 96*:1817–1822, 1978.
57. Chisholm, I.A., and Polyzoidis, K. Recurrence of benign orbital neurilemmoma (schwannoma) after 22 years. *Can. J. Ophthalmol. 17*:271–273, 1982.
58. Chohan, B.S., Parmar, I.P.S., Chugh, T.D., and Jain, A.L. Bilateral orbital involvement in multiple myelomatosis. *All India Ophthalmol. Soc. 18*:25–28, 1970.
59. Christopherson, W.M., Foote, F.W., and Stewart, F.W. Alveolar soft-part sarcomas: Structurally characteristic tumors of uncertain histogenesis. *Cancer 5*:100–111, 1952.
60. Chui, R.T., Liao, S.Y., and Bosworth, H. Recurrent oncocytoma of the ethmoid sinus with orbital invasion. *Otolaryngol. Head Neck Surg. 93*:267–270, 1985.
61. Chutorian, A.M., Schwartz, J.F., Evans, R.A., and Carter, S. Optic gliomas in children. *Neurology (Minneap.) 14*:83–96, 1964.
62. Cintorino, M., Vindigni, C., Del Vecchio, M.T., Tosi, P., Frezzotti, R., Hadjistilianou, T., Leoncini, P., Silvestri, S., Skalli, O., and Gabbiani, G. Expression of actin isoforms and intermediate filament proteins in childhood orbital rhabdomyosarcomas. *J. Submicrosc. Cytol. Pathol. 21*:409–419, 1989.
63. Cline, M.J., and Golde, D.W. A review and re-evaluation of the histiocytic disorders. *Am. J. Med. 55*:49–60, 1973.
64. Codling, B.W., Soni, K.C., Barry, D.R., and Martin-Walker, W. Histiocytosis presenting as swelling of orbit and eyelid. *Br. J. Ophthalmol. 56*:517–530, 1972.
65. Cole, S.H., and Ferry, A.P. Fibrous histiocytoma (fibrous xanthoma) of the lacrimal sac. *Arch. Ophthalmol. 96*:1647–1649, 1978.
66. Collins, V.P., Nordenskjold, M., and Dumanski, J.P. The molecular genetics of meningiomas. *Brain Pathol. 1*:19–24, 1990.
67. Comings, D.E., Skubi, K.B., Van Eyes, J., and Motulsky, A.G. Familial multifocal fibrosclerosis: Findings suggesting that retroperitoneal fibrosis, mediastinal fibrosis, sclerosing cholangitis, Riedel's thyroiditis, and pseudotumor of the orbit may be different manifestations of a single disease. *Ann. Intern. Med. 66*:884–892, 1967.
68. Cooling, R.J., and Wright, J.E. Arachnoid hyperplasia in optic nerve glioma: Confusion with orbital meningioma. *Br. J. Ophthalmol. 63*:596–599, 1979.
69. Coop, M.E. Pseudotumor of the orbit: A clinical and pathological study of 47 cases. *Br. J. Ophthalmol. 45*:513–542, 1961.
70. Copeland, D.D., Bell, S.W., and Shelburne, J.D. Hemidesmosome-like intercellular specializations in human meningiomas. *Cancer 41*:2242–2249, 1957.
71. Coppeto, J.R., Jaffe, R., and Gillies, C.G. Primary orbital melanoma. *Arch. Ophthalmol. 96*:2255–2258, 1978.
72. Coventry, M.B., and Dahlin, D.C. Osteogenic sarcoma: A critical analysis of 430 cases. *J. Bone Joint Surg. [Am.] 39*:741–758, 1957.
73. Craig, W., and Gogela, L. Intraorbital meningiomas: A clinicopathologic study. *Am. J. Ophthalmol. 32*:1663–1680, 1949.
74. Croxatto, J.O., and Font, R.L. Hemangiopericytoma of the orbit: A clinicopathologic study of 30 cases. *Hum. Pathol. 13*:210–218, 1982.
75. Czerniak, B., Woyke, S., Daniel, B., Krzysztolik, Z., and Koss, L.G. Diagnosis of orbital tumors by aspiration biopsy guided by computerized tomography. *Cancer 54*:2385–2389, 1984.
76. Daicker, B.C. Orbital chordoma. *Ophthalmologica 136*:236–239, 1978.
77. D'Alena, P.R. Primary orbital meningioma. *Arch. Ophthalmol. 71*:832–833, 1964.
78. Davis, F.A. Primary tumors of the optic nerve (a phenomenon of von Recklinghausen's disease): A clinical and pathological study with a report of five cases and a review of the literature. *Arch. Ophthalmol. 23*:735–821, 957–1022, 1940.
79. De Laey, J.J., De Schryver, A., Kluyskens, P., and Kunnen, M. Orbital involvement in Ollier's disease (multiple enchondromatosis). *Int. Ophthalmol. 5*:149–154, 1982.

80. Dempster, A.G., Lee, W.R., Bahnasawi, S., and Downie, T. Cell necrosis and endocytosis (apoptosis) in an embryonal rhabdomyosarcoma of the orbit. *Graefes Arch. Clin. Exp. Ophthalmol. 221*:89–95, 1983.
81. Dent, G.A., Baird, B., and Ross, D.W. Systemic idiopathic fibrosis with T-cell receptor gene rearrangement. *Arch. Pathol. Lab. Med. 115*:80–83, 1991.
82. De Schryver-Kecskemeti, K., Kraus, F.T., Engelmann, W., and Lacey, P.E. Alveolar soft part sarcoma: A malignant angioretinoma. *Am. J. Surg. Pathol. 6*:5–18, 1982.
83. Deutsch, A.R., and Duckworth, J.K. Nonchromaffin paraganglioma of the orbit. *Am. J. Ophthalmol 68*:659–663, 1969.
84. Dias, P., Parham, D.M., Shapiro, D.N., Webber, B.L., and Houghton, P.J. Myogenic regulatory protein (MyoD1) expression in childhood solid tumors: Diagnostic utility in rhabdomyosarcoma. *Am. J. Pathol. 137*:1283–1291, 1990.
85. de Divitis, E., and Cerillo, A. Pituitary adenoma with intraorbital extension: Apropos of a case. *Neurochirurgie 19*:561–566, 1973.
86. Dolman, P.J., Rootman, J., and Dolman, C.I. Infiltrating orbital granular cell tumour: A case report and literature review. *Br. J. Ophthalmol. 71*:47–53, 1987.
87. Dolman, P.J., Rootman, J., and Quenville, N.F. Signet-ring cell lymphoma in the orbit: A case report and review. *Can. J. Ophthalmol. 21*:242–245, 1986.
88. Donaldson, S.S. The value of adjuvant chemotherapy in the management of sarcomas in children. *Cancer 55*:2184–2197, 1985.
89. Dresner, S.C., Kennerdell, J.S., and Dekker, A. Fine needle aspiration biopsy of metastatic orbital tumors. *Surv. Ophthalmol. 27*:397–398, 1983.
90. Drews, R. Primary malignant melanoma of the orbit in a Negro. *Arch. Ophthalmol. 93*:335–336, 1975.
91. Drummond, J.W., Hall, D.L., Steen, W.H., Jr., and Maxey, S.A. Granular cell tumor (myoblastoma) of the orbit. *Arch. Ophthalmol. 97*:1492–1507, 1979.
92. Duffner, P.K., and Cohen, M.E. Isolated optic nerve gliomas in children with and without neurofibromatosis. *Neurofibromatosis 1*:201–211, 1988.
93. Duguid, I.M. Malignant melanoma of the lacrimal sac. *Br. J. Ophthalmol. 48*:394–398, 1964.
94. Duke-Elder, S. *Normal and Abnormal Development*, Part 2, *System of Ophthalmology*, Vol. 3, Kimpton, London, 1964.
95. Dunnington, J.H. Granular cell myoblastoma of the orbit. *Arch. Ophthalmol. 40*:14–22, 1948.
96. DuPont, H.L., Varco, R.L., and Winchell, C.P. Chronic fibrous mediastinitis simulating pulmonic stenosis, associated with inflammatory pseudotumor of the orbit. *Am. J. Med. 44*:447–452, 1968.
97. Edwards, M.K., Zauel, D.W., Gilmor, R.L., and Muller, J. Invasive orbital pseudotumor-CT demonstration of extension beyond orbit. *Neuroradiology 23*:215–217, 1982.
98. Eggers, H., Jakobiec, F.A., and Jones, I.S. Optic nerve gliomas. In *Diseases of the Orbit*, I.S. Jones and F.A. Jakobiec (Eds.), Harper & Row, New York, pp. 417–433, 1979.
99. Eifrig, D.E. Lipid granuloma of the orbit. *Arch. Ophthalmol. 79*:163–165, 1968.
100. Ellenbogen, E., and Lasky, M.A. Rhabdomyosarcoma of the orbit in the newborn. *Am. J. Ophthalmol. 80*:1024–1027, 1975.
101. Ellis, D.S., Spencer, W.H., and Stephenson, C.M. Congenital neurocutaneous melanosis with metastatic orbital malignant melanoma. *Ophthalmology 93*:1639–1642, 1986.
102. Enriquez, P., Dahlin, D.C., Hayles, A.B., and Henderson, E.D. Histiocytosis X: A clinical study. *Mayo Clin. Proc. 42*:88–99, 1967.
103. Enterline, H.T., Culberson, J.D., Rochlin, D.B., and Brady, L.W. Liposarcoma: A clinical and pathological study of 53 cases. *Cancer 13*:932–950, 1960.
104. Enzinger, F.M., and Weiss, S.W. *Soft Tissue Tumors*, 2nd ed., C.V. Mosby, St. Louis, pp. 596–613, 1988.
105. Enzinger, F.M., and Winslow, D.J. Liposarcoma: A study of 103 cases. *Virchows Arch. [A.] 335*:367–388, 1962.
106. Farkas, T.G., and Lamberson, R.E. Malignant melanoma of the lacrimal sac. *Am. J. Ophthalmol. 66*:45–48, 1968.
107. Favara, B.E., McCarthy, R.C., and Mierau, G.W. Histiocytosis X. *Hum. Pathol. 14*:663–676, 1983.
108. Ferry, A.P., and Font, R.L. Carcinoma metastatic to the eye and orbit. I. A clinicopathologic study of 227 cases. *Arch. Ophthalmol. 91*:276–286, 1974.
109. Finn, J.E., and Mount, L.A. Meningiomas of the tuberculum sellae and planum sphenoidale: A review of 83 cases. *Arch. Ophthalmol. 92*:23–27, 1974.
110. Fiorillo, A., Migliorati, R., Grimaldi, M., Vassallo, P., Canale, G., Tranfa, F., Uccello, G., Fiore, M., Muto, P., Menna, G., Parasole, R., and Bonavolont, G. Multidisciplinary treatment of primary orbital rhabdomyosarcoma. A single-institution experience. *Cancer 67*:560–563, 1991.
111. Fisher, E.R., and Hazard, J.B. Nonchromaffin paraganglioma of the orbit. *Cancer 5*:521–524, 1952.
112. Fitzpatrick, P.J., and Macko, S. Lymphoreticular tumors of the orbit. *Int. J. Radiat. Oncol. Biol. Phys. 10*:333–340, 1984.

113. Flanagan, J.C., Mauriello, J.A., Jr., and Stefanyszyn, J. Lacrimal sac tumors and inflammations. In *Management of Orbital and Ocular Adnexal Tumors and Inflammations*, J.A. Mauriello, Jr., and J.C. Flanagan (Eds.), Springer-Verlag, Berlin, pp. 187–196, 1990.

114. Folberg, R., Bernardino, V.B., Jr., Aquilar, G.L., and Shannon, G.M. Amputation neuroma mistaken for recurrent melanoma in the orbit. *Ophthalmic. Surg. 12*:275–278, 1981.

115. Folberg, R., Cleasby, G., Flanagan, J.A., Spencer, W.H., and Zimmerman, L.E. Orbital leiomyosarcoma after radiation therapy for bilateral retinoblastoma. *Arch. Ophthalmol. 101*:1562–1565, 1983.

116. Font, R.L., and Gamel, J.W. Epithelial tumors of the lacrimal gland: An analysis of 265 cases. In *Ocular and Adnexal Tumors*, F.A. Jakobiec (Ed.), Aesculapius, Birmingham, AL, pp. 787–805, 1978.

117. Font, R.L., and Garner, A. Myoepithelioma of the lacrimal gland: Report of a case with spindle cell morphology. *Br. J. Ophthalmol. 76*:634–636, 1992.

118. Font, R.L., and Hidayat, A.A. Fibrous histiocytoma of the orbit: A clinicopathologic study of 150 cases. *Hum. Pathol. 13*:199–209, 1982.

119. Font, R.L., Jurco, S., and Brechner, R.J. Postradiation leiomyosarcoma of the orbit complicating bilateral retinoblastoma. *Arch. Ophthalmol. 101*:1557–1561, 1983.

120. Font, R.L., Jurco, S., and Zimmerman, L.E. Alveolar soft part sarcoma of the orbit: A clinicopathologic analysis of seventeen cases and a review of the literature. *Hum. Pathol. 13*:569–579, 1982

121. Font, R.L., and Shields, J. Large cell lymphoma of the orbit with microvillous projections ("porcupine lymphoma"). *Arch. Ophthalmol. 103*:1715–1719, 1985.

122. Font, R.L., and Zimmerman, L.E. Nodular fasciitis of the eye and adnexa: A report of 10 cases. *Arch. Ophthalmol. 75*:475–481, 1966.

123. Font, R. L., and Zimmerman, L. E. Alveolar soft part sarcoma of the orbit: A clinicopathologic study of 15 cases, (abstract). *Lab. Invest. 40*:254, 1979.

124. Forrest, A.W. Intraorbital tumors. *Arch. Ophthalmol. 41*:198–232, 1949.

125. Forrest, A.W. Epithelial lacrimal gland tumors: Pathology as a guide to prognosis. *Trans. Am. Acad. Ophthalmol. Otolaryngol. 58*:848–865, 1954.

126. Forrest, A.W. Pathologic criteria for effective management of epithelial lacrimal gland tumors. *Am. J. Ophthalmol. 71*:178–192, 1971.

127. Fox, S.A. Hemangiopericytoma of the orbit. *Am. J. Ophthalmol. 40*:786–789, 1955.

128. Fowler, T.J., Earl, C.J., McAllister, V.L., and McDonald, W.I. Tolosa-Hunt syndrome: The dangers of an eponym. *Br. J. Ophthalmol. 59*:149–154, 1975.

129. Francois, J. Ocular aspects of the phakomatoses. In *Handbook of Clinical Neurology*, P.J. Vinken and G.W. Bruyn (Eds.), American Elsevier, New York, pp. 624–639, 1972.

130. Fratkin, J.D., Shammas, H.F., and Miller, S.H. Disseminated Hodgkin's disease with bilateral orbital involvement. *Arch. Ophthalmol. 96*:102–104, 1978.

131. Frayer, W.C., and Enterline, H.T. Embryonal rhabdomyosarcoma of the orbit in children and young adults. *Arch. Ophthalmol. 62*:203–210, 1959.

132. Freedman, M.I., and Folk, J.C. Metastatic tumors to the eye and orbit patient survival and clinical characteristics. *Arch. Ophthalmol. 105*:1215–1219, 1987.

133. Friedman, A.H., Cooperman, E.W., and Henkind, P. Chemosis, proptosis, and amaurosis in a 19-year-old male. *Surv. Ophthalmol. 20*:125–132, 1975.

134. Frohman, L.P., Kupersmith, M.J., Lang, J., Reede, D., Bergeron, D.T., Aleksic, S., and Trasi, S. Intracranial extension and bone destruction in orbital pseudotumor. *Arch. Ophthalmol. 104*:380–384, 1986.

135. Fu, Y.S., and Perzin, K.H. Non-epithelial tumors of the nasal cavity, paranasal sinuses, and nasopharynx: A clinicopathological study. II. Osseous and fibro-osseous lesions including osteoma, fibrous dysplasia, ossifying fibroma, osteoblastoma, giant cell tumor and osteosarcoma. *Cancer 33*:1289–1305, 1974.

136. Fu, Y.S., and Perzin, K.H. Non-epithelial tumors of the nasal cavity, paranasal sinuses, and nasopharynx: A clinicopathologic study. III. Cartilaginous tumors (chondroma, chondrosarcoma). *Cancer 34*:453–463, 1974.

137. Fujii, H., Fujisada, H., Kondo, T., Takahashi, T., and Okada, S. Orbital pseudotumour: Histopathological classification and treatment. *Ophthalmologica 190*:230–242, 1985.

138. Gamel, J.W., and Font, R.L. Adenoid cystic carcinoma of the lacrimal gland: The clinical significance of a basaloid histologic pattern. *Hum. Pathol. 13*:219–225, 1982.

139. Garner, A. Cavernous haemangioma of the orbit: A consideration of its origin and development. *Orbit 7*:149–156, 1988.

140. Garner, A. Pathology of "pseudotumours" of the orbit: A review. *J. Clin. Pathol. 26*:639–648, 1973.

141. Garner, A. Mollicutes: What are they? *Br. J. Ophthalmol. 73*:859, 1989.

142. Garner, A. Orbital lymphoproliferative disease. *Br. J. Ophthalmol. 76*:47–48, 1992.

143. Garner, A., Rahi, A.H.S., and Wright, J.E. Lymphoproliferative disorders of the orbit: An immunological approach to diagnosis and pathogenesis. *Br. J. Ophthalmol. 67*:561–567, 1983.

144. Genberg, J., Mark, J., Hakelius, L., Ericsson, J., and Nister, M. Origin and relationship between different cell types in malignant fibrous histiocytoma. *Am. J. Pathol. 135*:1185–1196, 1989.

145. Gibson, M.J., and Middlemiss, J.H. Fibrous dysplasia of bone. *Br. J. Radiol. 44*:1–13, 1971.

146. Gluszcz, A., Giernat, L., Habryka, K., Alwasiak, J., Lach, B., and Papierz, W. Rosenthal fibers birefringent gliofibrillary changes and intracellular homogenous conglomerates in tissue cultures of gliomas. *Acta Neuropathol. (Berl.) 17*:54–67, 1971.
147. Goder, G. Über sogenannte Mischgeschwulste der Tranendrusen-gegend und ihr histochemisches Verhalten. *Monatsbl. Klin. Augenheilkd. 141*:510–522, 1962.
148. Goder, G. Das nichtchromaffine Paragangliom der Orbita. *Zentralbl. Allg. Pathol. 113*:167–172, 1970.
149. Goldberg, R.A., and Rootman, J. Clinical characteristics of metastatic orbital tumors. *Ophthalmology 97*:620–624, 1990.
150. Goldberg, R.A., Rootman, J., and Cline, R.A. Tumors metastatic to the orbit: A changing picture. *Surv. Ophthalmol. 35*:1–24, 1990.
151. Gonazlez-Almarcz, G., de Buen, S., and Tsutsumi, V. Granular cell tumor (myoblastoma) of the orbit. *Am. J. Ophthalmol. 79*:606–612, 1975.
152. Gonnering, R.S. Bilateral primary extramedullary orbital plasmocytomas. *Ophthalmology 94*:267–270, 1987.
153. Gordon, A., and Maloney, A.F.J. A case of metastasizing meningioma. *J. Neurol. Neurosurg. Psychiatry 28*:159–162, 1965.
154. Gordon, E. Orbital extension of meningioma. *Can. J. Ophthalmol. 5*:381–385, 1970.
155. Graham, J.R. Cardiac and pulmonary fibrosis during methysergide therapy for headache. *Am. J. Med. Sci. 254*:1–12, 1967.
156. Grant, G.D., Shields, J.A., Flanagan, J.C., and Horowitz, P. The ultrasonographic and radiologic features of a histologically proven case of alveolar soft-part sarcoma of the orbit. *Am. J. Ophthalmol. 87*:773–777, 1979.
157. Grinberg, M.A., and Levy, N.S. Malignant neurilemoma of the supraorbital nerve. *Am. J. Ophthalmol. 78*:489–492, 1974.
158. Grossniklaus, H.E., Abbuhl, M.F., and McLean, I.W. Immunologic properties of benign and malignant mixed tumor of the lacrimal gland. *Am. J. Ophthalmol. 110*:540–549, 1990.
159. Guccion, J.G., Font, R.L., Enzinger, F.M., and Zimmerman, L.E. Extraskeletal mesenchymal chondrosarcoma. *Arch. Pathol. 95*:336–340, 1973.
160. Hagler, W., and Brown, C. Malignant melanoma of the orbit arising in a nevus of Ota. *Trans. Am. Acad. Ophthalmol. Otolaryngol. 70*:817–822, 1966.
161. Hamilton, A.M., Garner, A., Tripathi, R.C., and Sanders, M.D. Malignant optic nerve glioma: Report of a case with electron microscope study. *Br. J. Ophthalmol. 57*:253–264, 1973.
162. Hannesson, O.B. Primary meningioma of the orbit invading the choroid: Report of a case. *Acta Ophthalmol. (Copenh.) 49*:627–632, 1971.
163. Harkin, J., and Reed, R. Tumors of the peripheral nervous system. In *Atlas of Tumor Pathology*, Series 2, Fasc. 3. Armed Forces Institute of Pathology, Washington, D.C., 1969.
164. Harris, A.W., Langdon, W.Y., Alexander, W.S., et al. Transgenic mouse models for hematopoietic tumorigenesis. *Curr. Top. Microbiol. Immunol. 141*:82–93, 1988.
165. Harris, G.J., and Jakobiec, F.A. Cavernous hemangioma of the orbit. *J. Neurosurg. 51*:219–228, 1979.
166. Harris, G.J., Sakol, P.J., Bonovolonta, G., and de Conciliis, C. An analysis of thirty cases of orbital lymphangioma: Pathophysiologic considerations and management recommendations. *Ophthalmology 97*:1583–1592, 1990.
167. Harris, N.L., Pilch, B.Z., Bhan, A.K., Harmon, D.C., and Goodman, M.L. Immunohistologic diagnosis of orbital lymphoid infiltrates. *Am. J. Surg. Pathol. 8*:83–91, 1984.
168. Harry, J. Pathology of rhabdomyosarcoma. *Mod. Probl. Ophthalmol. 14*:325–329, 1975.
169. Harry, J., and Ashton, N. The pathology of tumours of the lacrimal sac. *Trans. Ophthalmol. Soc. UK 88*:19–35, 1968.
170. Heathcote, J.G., Allen, L.H., and Willis, N.R. Plasma cell granuloma of the lacrimal sac. *Can. J. Ophthalmol. 22*:387–390, 1987.
171. Heathcote, J.G., Hurwitz, J.J., and Dardick, I. A spindle-cell myoepithelioma of the lacrimal gland. *Arch. Ophthalmol. 108*:1135–1139, 1990.
172. Henderson, J.W. *Orbital Tumors*. W.B. Saunders, Philadelphia, 1973.
173. Henderson, J.W., and Farrow, G.M. Malignant melanoma primary in the orbit: Report of a case. *Trans. Am. Acad. Ophthalmol. Otolaryngol. 76*:1487–1490, 1972.
174. Henderson, J.W., and Farrow, G.M. Primary orbital hemangiopericytoma: An aggressive and potentially malignant neoplasm. *Arch. Ophthalmol. 96*:666–673, 1978.
175. Hidayat, A.A., and Font, R.L. Juvenile fibromatosis of the periorbital region and eyelid: A clinicopathologic study of six cases. *Arch. Ophthalmol. 98*:280–285, 1980.
176. Hirose, T., Kudo, E., Hasegawa, T., Jun-ichi, A., and Hizawa, K. Cytoskeletal properties of alveolar soft part sarcoma. *Hum. Pathol. 21*:204–211, 1990.
177. Holland, M., Allen, J., and Ichinose, H. Chondrosarcoma of the orbit. *Trans. Am. Acad. Ophthalmol. Otolaryngol. 65*:898–905, 1961.
178. Hook, S.R., Font, R.L., McCrary, J.A., and Harper, R.L. Intraosseous capillary hemangioma of the frontal bone. *Am. J. Ophthalmol. 103*:824–827, 1987.

179. Hornblass, A., Jakobiec, F.A., Reifler, D.M., and Mines, J. Orbital lymphoid tumors located predominantly within extraocular muscles. *Ophthalmology 94*:688–697, 1987.
180. Horten, B.C., Urich, H., Rubinstein, L.J., and Montague, S.R. The angioblastic meningioma: A reappraisal of a nosological problem. *J. Neurol. Sci. 31*: 387–410, 1977.
181. Hoyt, W.F., and Baghdassarian, S.B. Optic glioma of childhood: Natural history and rationale for conservative management. *Br. J. Ophthalmol. 53*:793–798, 1969.
182. Hoyt, W.F., Meshel, G., Lessell, S., Schatz, N.J., and Suckling, R.D. Malignant optic glioma of adulthood. *Brain 96*:121–133, 1973.
183. Huber, A. Angiography and differential diagnosis of orbital tumours. *Trans. Ophthalmol. Soc. UK 92*:35–50, 1972.
184. Hufnagel, T., Ma, L., and Kuo, T.-T. Orbital angiosarcoma with subconjunctival presentation: Report of a case and literature review. *Ophthalmology 94*:72–77, 1987.
185. Hunter, J.V., Yokoyama, C., Mosely, I.F., and Wright, J.E. Aneurysmal bone cyst of the sphenoid with orbital involvement. *Br. J. Ophthalmol. 74*:505–508, 1990.
186. Hunter, P. An unusual bilateral case of lymphosarcoma of the orbit. *Trans. Ophthalmol. Soc. UK 74*:223–228, 1954.
187. Ide, C.H., Davis, W.E., and Black, S.P.W. Orbital teratoma. *Arch. Ophthalmol. 96*:2093–2096, 1978.
188. Iliff, C.E. Mucoceles in the orbit. *Arch. Ophthalmol. 89*:392–395, 1973.
189. Iliff, W.J., and Green, W.R. Orbital tumors in children. In *Ocular and Adnexal Tumors*, F.A. Jakobiec (Ed.), Aesculapius, Birmingham, AL, pp. 669–684, 1978.
190. Iliff, W.J., Marback, R., and Green, W.R. Invasive squamous cell carcinoma of the conjunctiva. *Arch. Ophthalmol. 93*:119–122, 1975.
191. Isaacson, P.G., and Wright, D.H. Extranodal lymphoma. In *Recent Advances in Histopathology* (P.P. Anthony and R.N.M. MacSween, Eds.), Churchill Livingstone, Edinburgh, pp. 159–184, 1987.
192. Iwamoto, T., and Jakobiec, F.A. Ultrastructural comparison of capillary and cavernous hemangiomas of the orbit. *Arch. Ophthalmol. 97*:1144–1153, 1979.
193. Jaffe, N., Filler, R.M., Farber, S., Traggis, D.G., Vawter, G.F., Tefft, M., and Murray, J.E. Rhabdomyosarcoma in children: Improved outlook with a multidisciplinary approach. *Am. J. Surg. 125*:482–487, 1973.
194. Jaeger, M.J., Green, W.R., Miller, N.R., and Harris, G.J. Granular cell tumor of the orbit and ocular adnexae. *Surv. Ophthalmol. 31*:417–423, 1987.
195. Jain, B.S. Solitary myeloma of the orbit. *Am. J. Ophthalmol. 58*:855–858, 1964.
196. Jakobiec, F.A., Ellsworth, R., and Tannenbaum, M. Primary orbital melanoma. *Am. J. Ophthalmol. 78*:24–39, 1974.
197. Jakobiec, F.A., and Font, R.L. Orbit. In *Ophthalmic Pathology; an Atlas and Textbook*, 3rd ed., Vol. 3, W.H. Spencer (Ed.), W.B. Saunders, Philadelphia, pp. 2533–2538, 1986.
198. Jakobiec, F.A., Font, R.L., and Zimmerman, L.E. Malignant peripheral nerve sheath tumors of the orbit: A clinicopathologic study of eight cases. *Trans. Am. Ophthalmol. Soc. 83*:332–366, 1985.
199. Jakobiec, F.A., Howard, G.M., Jones, I.S., and Tannenbaum, M. Fibrous histiocytomata of the orbit. *Am. J. Ophthalmol. 77*:333–345, 1974.
200. Jakobiec, F.A., Howard, G.M., Jones, I.S., and Wolff, M. Hemangiopericytoma of the orbit. *Am. J. Ophthalmol. 78*:816–834, 1974.
201. Jakobiec, F.A., Howard, G.M., Rosen, M., and Wolff, M. Leiomyoma and leiomyosarcoma of the orbit. *Am. J. Ophthalmol. 80*:1028–1042, 1975.
202. Jakobiec, F.A., and Jones, I.S. Vascular tumors, malformations, and degenerations. In *Diseases of the Orbit*, I.S. Jones and F.A. Jakobiec (Eds.), Harper & Row, New York, pp. 269–308, 1979.
203. Jakobiec, F.A., and Jones, I.S. Lymphomatous, plasmacytic, histiocytic, and hematopoietic tumors. In *Diseases of the Orbit*, I.S. Jones and F.A. Jakobiec (Eds.), Harper & Row, New York, pp. 309–353, 1979.
204. Jakobiec, F.A., and Jones, I.S. Neurogenic tumors. In *Diseases of the Orbit*, I.S. Jones and F.A. Jakobiec (Eds.), Harper & Row, New York, pp. 371–415, 1979.
205. Jakobiec, F.A., and Jones, I.S. Mesenchymal and fibro-osseous tumors. In *Diseases of the Orbit*, I.S. Jones and F.A. Jakobiec (Eds.), Harper & Row, New York, pp. 461–502, 1979.
206. Jakobiec, F.A., Jones, I.S., and Tannenbaum, M. Leiomyoma: An unusual tumour of the orbit. *Br. J. Ophthalmol. 57*:825–831, 1973.
207. Jakobiec, F.A., Klapper, D., Maher, E., and Krebs, W. Infantile subconjunctival and anterior orbital fibrous histiocytoma. Ultrastructural and immunohistochemical studies. *Ophthalmology 95*:516–525, 1988.
208. Jakobiec, F.A., Neri, A., and Knowles, D.M. Genotypic monoclonality in immunophenotypically polyclonal orbital lymphoid tumors: A model of tumor progression in the lymphoid system. *Ophthalmology 94*:980–994, 1987.
209. Jakobiec, F.A., Rini, F., Char, D., Orcutt, J., Rootman, J., Baylis, H., and Flanagan, J. Primary liposarcoma of the orbit: Problems in the diagnosis and management of five cases. *Ophthalmology 96*:180–191, 1989.
210. Jakobiec, F.A., Rootman, J., and Jones, I.S. Secondary and metastatic tumors of the orbit. In *Diseases of the Orbit*, I.S. Jones and F.A. Jakobiec (Eds.), Harper & Row, New York, pp. 503–569, 1979.

211. Jakobiec, F.A., and Tannenbaum, M. The ultrastructure of orbital fibrosarcoma. *Am. J. Ophthalmol.* 77:899–917, 1974.
212. Jakobiec, F.A., Trokel, S.L., Aron-Rosa, D., Iwamoto, T., and Doyon, D. Localized eosinophilic granuloma (Langerhan's cell histiocytosis) of the orbital frontal bone. *Arch. Ophthalmol.* 98:1814–1820, 1980.
213. James, C.R.H., Lyness, R., and Wright, J.E. Respiratory epithelium lined cysts presenting in the orbit without associated mucocele formation. *Br. J. Ophthalmol.* 70:387–390, 1986.
214. Jay, B. Naevi and melanomata of the conjunctiva. *Br. J. Ophthalmol.* 49:169–204, 1965.
215. Jay, B. Malignant melanoma of the orbit in a case of oculodermal melanosis (naevus of Ota). *Br. J. Ophthalmol.* 49:359–363, 1965.
216. Jayo, M.J., Jayo, J.M., Jerome, C.P., Krugner-Higby, L., and Reynolds, G.D. Maxillo-orbital lymphoma (Burkitt's-type) in an infant *Macaca fascicularis. Lab. Anim. Sci.* 38:722–726, 1988.
217. Jensen, O.A. Mucosubstances of mixed tumours of the human lacrimal gland. *Acta Pathol. Microbiol. Scand.* 78:184–190, 1967.
218. Jepson, C.N., and Wetzig, P.C. Pure chondroma of the trochlea: A case report. *Surv. Ophthalmol.* 11:656–659, 1966.
219. Jestico, J.V., and Lantos, P.L. Malignant meningioma with liver metastases and hypoglycemia: A case report. *Acta Neuropathol. (Berl.)* 35:357–361, 1976.
220. Johnson, B.L., and Linn, J.G. Jr. Spindle cell lipoma of the orbit. *Arch. Ophthalmol.* 97:133–134, 1979.
221. Jonasson, F. Orbital plasma cell tumours. *Ophthalmologica* 177:152–157, 1978.
222. Jones, I.S. Tumors of the lacrimal sac. *Am. J. Ophthalmol.* 42:561–566, 1956.
223. Jones, I.S. Lymphangiomas of the ocular adnexa: An analysis of 62 cases. *Trans. Am. Ophthalmol. Soc.* 57:602–665, 1959.
224. Jones, I.S. Lymphangiomas of the ocular adnexa: An analysis of 62 cases. *Am. J. Ophthalmol.* 51:481–509, 1961.
225. Jones, S.E., Fuks, Z., Bull, M., Kadin, M.E., Dorfman, R.F., Kaplan, H.S., Rosenberg, S.A., and Kim, H. Non-Hodgkin's lymphomas. IV. Clinicopathologic correlation in 405 cases. *Cancer* 31:806–823, 1973.
226. Jones, I.S., and Jakobiec, F.A. (Eds.), *Diseases of the Orbit.* Harper & Row, New York, 1979.
227. Jones, I.S., Reese, A.B., and Krout, J. Orbital rhabdomyosarcoma: An analysis of 62 cases. *Trans. Am. Ophthalmol. Soc.* 63:223–255, 1965.
228. Jordan, D.R., and Tse, D.T. Herniated orbital fat. *Can. J. Ophthalmol.* 22:173–177, 1987.
229. Kadoya, M., and Amemiya, T. A case of orbital paraganglioma. *Acta Soc. Ophthalmol. Jpn.* 83:359–367, 1979.
230. Kaltreider, S.A., Destro, M., and Lemke, B.N. Leiomyosarcoma of the orbit. A case report and review of the literature. *Ophthalmol. Plast. Reconstruct. Surg.* 3:35–41, 1987.
231. Karcioglu, Z.A., Allam, B., and Insler, M.S. Ocular involvement in sinus histiocytosis with massive lymphadenopathy. *Br. J. Ophthalmol.* 72:793–795, 1988.
232. Karcioglu, Z.A., Caldwell, D.R., and Reed, H.T. Papillomas of lacrimal drainage system: A clinicopathologic study. *Ophthalmic Surg.* 15:670–676, 1984.
233. Karcioglu, Z.A., Hemphill, G.L., and Wool, B.M. Granular cell tumor of the orbit: Case report and review of the literature. *Ophthal. Surg.* 14:125–129, 1983.
234. Karp, L.A., Zimmerman, L.E., Borit, A., and Spencer, W. Primary intraorbital meningiomas. *Arch. Ophthalmol.* 91:24–28, 1974.
235. Kassel, S.H., Copenhaver, R., and Aréan, V.M. Orbital rhabdomyosarcoma. *Am. J. Ophthalmol.* 60:811–818, 1965.
236. Kennerdell, J.S., and Maroon, J.C. Intracanalicular meningioma with chronic optic disc edema. *Ann. Ophthalmol.* 7:507–512, 1975.
237. Khalil, M.K., Huang, S., Viloria, J., and Duguid, W.P. Extramedullary plasmacytoma of the orbit: Case report with results of immunocytochemical studies. *Can. J. Ophthalmol.* 92:39–42, 1981.
238. Kilman, J.W., Clatworthy, H.W., Newton, W.A., and Goosfeld, J.L. Reasonable surgery for rhabdomyosarcoma: A study of 67 cases. *Ann. Surg.* 178:346–351, 1973.
239. Kincaid, M.C., Green, R., and Iliff, W.J. Fibrous histiocytoma of the lacrimal sac. *Am. J. Ophthalmol.* 93:511–517, 1982.
240. Kincaid, M.C., Meis, J.M., and Lee, M.W. Adenoid cystic carcinoma of the lacrimal sac. *Ophthalmology* 96:1655–1658, 1989.
241. Kingsley, D.P.E., and Harwood-Nash, D.C.F. Orbito-facial extension of intracranial medulloblastoma. *Neuroradiology* 27:88–89, 1985.
242. Klein, G. Tumor immunology. *Transplant. Proc.* 5:31–41, 1973.
243. Klintworth, G.K. Pathologic states produced in transgenic mice. *Adv. Pathol.* 3:233–299, 1990.
244. Knowles, D.M., Halper, J.A., Trokel, S., and Jakobiec, F.A. Immunofluorescent and immunoperoxidase characteristics of IgD lamba myeloma involving the orbit. *Am. J. Ophthalmol.* 85:485–594, 1978.
245. Knowles, D.M., and Jakobiec, F.A. Ocular adnexal lymphoid neoplasms: Clinical, histopathologic, electron microscopic and immunologic characteristics. *Hum. Pathol.* 13:148–162, 1982.
246. Knowles, D.M., and Jakobiec, F.A. Identification of T lymphocytes in ocular adnexal neoplasms by hybridoma monoclonal antibodies. *Am. J. Ophthalmol.* 95:233–242, 1983.

247. Knowles, D.M., and Jakobiec, F.A. Rhabdomyoma of the orbit. *Am. J. Ophthalmol.* 80:1011–1018, 1975.
248. Knowles, D.M., Jakobiec, F.A., and Halper, J.P. Immunological characterization of ocular adnexal lymphoid neoplasms. *Am. J. Ophthalmol.* 87:603–619, 1979.
249. Knowles, D.M., Jakobiec, F.A., and Jones, I.S. Rhabdomyosarcoma. In *Diseases of the Orbit*, I.S. Jones and F.A. Jakobiec (Eds.), Harper & Row, New York, pp. 435–459, 1979.
250. Knowles, D.M., Jakobiec, F.A., McNally, L., and Burke, J.S. Lymphoid hyperplasia and malignant lymphoma occurring in ocular adnexa (orbit, conjunctiva, and eyelids): A prospective multiparametric analysis of 108 cases during 1977 to 1987. *Hum. Pathol.* 21:959–973, 1990.
251. Knowles, D.M., Jakobiec, F.A., and Wang, C.I. The expression of surface antigen Leu-1 by ocular adnexal lymphoid neoplasms. *Am. J. Ophthalmol.* 94:246–254, 1982.
252. Konrad, E.A., and Thiel, H.J. Adenocarcinoma of the lacrimal gland with sebaceous differentiation: A clinical study using light and electron microscopy. *Graefes Arch. Clin. Exp. Ophthalmol.* 221:81–85, 1983.
253. Konwaler, B.E., Keasbey, L., and Kaplan, L. Subcutaneous pseudosarcomatous fibromatosis (fasciitis). *Am. J. Clin. Pathol.* 25:241–252, 1955.
254. Kopelman, J.E., and Shorr, N. A case of prostatic carcinoma metastatic to the orbit diagnosed by fine needle aspiration and immunoperoxidase staining for prostatic specific antigen. *Ophthalmic Surg.* 18:599–603, 1987.
255. Krohel, G.B., Rosenberg, P.N., Wright, J.E., and Smith, R.S. Localized orbital neurofibromas. *Am. J. Ophthalmol.* 100:458–464, 1985.
256. Lakke, J.P. Superior orbital fissure syndrome: Report of a case caused by local pachymeningitis. *Arch. Neurol.* 7:289–300, 1962.
257. Lane, C.M., Ehrlich, W.W., and Wright, J.E. Orbital dermoid cyst. *Eye* 1:504–511, 1987.
258. Lane, C.M., Wright, J.E., and Garner, A. Primary myxoid liposarcoma of the orbit. *Br. J. Ophthalmol.* 72:912–917, 1988.
259. Lattes, R., McDonald, 9., and Sproul, E. Nonchromaffin paraganglioma of carotid body and orbit. *Ann. Surg.* 139:382–384, 1954.
260. Lauer, S.A., Fischer, J., Jones, J., Gartner, S., Dutcher, J., and Hoxie, J.A., Orbital T-cell lymphoma in human T-cell leukemia virus-1 infection. *Ophthalmology* 95:110–115, 1988.
261. Lazzarino, M., Morra, E., Rosso, R., Brusamolino, E., Pagnucco, G., Castello, A., Ghisolfi, A., Tafi, A., Zennaro, G., and Bernasconi, C. Clinicopathologic and immunologic characteristics of non-Hodgkin's lymphomas presenting in the orbit: A report of eight cases. *Cancer* 55:1907–1912, 1985.
262. Lehrer, H.Z. Ossifying fibroma of the orbital roof: Its distinction from "blistering" or "intra-osseous" meningioma. *Arch. Neurol.* 20:536–541, 1969.
263. Leibel, S.A., Wara, W.M., Sheline, G.E., Townsend, J.J., and Boldrey, E.B. Treatment of meningiomas in childhood. *Cancer* 37:2709–2712, 1976.
264. Lennert, K. *Histopathology of Non-Hogkin's Lymphomas.* Springer-Verlag, Berlin, 1981.
265. Leone, C.R., Jr., Lawton, A.W., and Leone, R.T. Benign osteoblastoma of the orbit. *Ophthalmology* 95:1554–1558, 1988.
266. Leopold, J.G., and Richards, D.B. Cellular blue naevi. *J. Pathol. Bacteriol.* 94:247–255, 1967.
267. Levitt, J.M., de Veer, J.A., and Oguzhan, M.C. Orbital nodular fasciitis. *Arch. Ophthalmol.* 81:235–237, 1969.
268. Liakos, G.M., Walker, C.B., and Carruth, J.S. Ocular complications in craniofacial fibrous dysplasia. *Br. J. Ophthalmol.* 63:611–616, 1979.
269. Lichtenstein, L. Histiocytosis X: Integration of eosinophilic granuloma of bone, "Letterer-Siwe disease", and "Schuller-Christian disease" as related manifestations of a single nosologic entity. *Arch. Pathol.* 56:84–102, 1953.
270. Lichtenstein, L., and Sawyer, W.R. Benign osteoblastoma: Further observations and report of 20 additional cases. *J. Bone Joint Surg. [Am]* 46:755–765, 1964.
271. Lipper, S., Dalzell, J.C., and Watkins, P.J. Ultrastructure of psammoma bodies of meningioma in tissue culture. *Arch. Pathol. Lab. Med.* 103:670–675, 1979.
272. Liss, L., and Wolter, J.R. The histology of the gliomas of the optic nerve: A study with silver carbonate. *Arch. Ophthalmol.* 58:689–694, 1957.
273. Litricin, O. Paraganglioma non-chromaffine de l'orbite. *Ann. Ocul.* 203:585–592, 1970.
274. Little, J.M. Waldenstrom's macroglobulinemia in the lacrimal gland. *Trans. Am. Acad. Ophthalmol. Otolaryngol.* 71:875–879, 1967.
275. Lizard-Nacol, S., Lizard, G., Justrabo, E., and Turc-Carel, C. Immunologic characterization of Ewing's sarcoma using mesenchymal and neuronal markers. *Am. J. Pathol.* 135:847–855, 1989.
276. Lloyd, G.A. Primary orbital meningioma: A review of 41 patients investigated radiologically. *Clin. Radiol.* 33:181–187, 1982.
277. Lloyd, G.A.S., Wright, J.E., and Morgan, G. Venous malformations in the orbit. *Br. J. Ophthalmol.* 55:505–516, 1971.
278. Lopez, D.A., Silvers, D.N., and Helwig, E.B. Cutaneous meningiomas: A clinicopathologic study. *Cancer* 34:728–744, 1974.
279. Lowder, C.Y., Berlin, A.J., Cox, W.A., and Hahn, J.F. Benign osteoblastoma of the orbit. *Ophthalmology* 93:1351–1354, 1986.

280. Lowe, J., and Mayer, R.J. Ubiquitin, cell stress and diseases of the nervous system. *Neuropathol. Appl. Neurobiol. 16*:281–291, 1990.

281. Lyons, C.J., McNab, A.A., Garner, A., and Wright, J.E. Orbital malignant peripheral nerve sheath tumours. *Br. J. Ophthalmol. 73*:731–738, 1989.

282. MacCumber, M.W., Hoffman, P.N., Wand, G.S., Epstein, J.I., Beschorner, W.E., and Green, W.R. Ophthalmic involvement in aggressive histiocytosis X. *Ophthalmology 97*:22–27, 1990.

283. MacKenzie, D.H. *The Differential Diagnosis of Fibroblastic Disorders*, Blackwell, Oxford, 1970.

284. MacMichael, I.M., and Cullen, J.F. Primary intraorbital meningioma. *Br. J. Ophthalmol. 53*:169–173, 1969.

285. McCartney, A.C.E. Personal communication, 1991.

286. McKenna, R.J., Schwinn, C.P., Soong, K.Y., and Higinbotham, N.L. Osteogenic sarcoma arising in Paget's disease. *Cancer 17*:42–66, 1964.

287. McFadzean, R.M., and Gowan, M.E. Orbital tumours. A review of 34 cases. *J.R. Coll. Surg. Edinb. 28*:361–364, 1983.

288. McNab, A.A., and Wright, J.E. Cavernous haemangiomas of the orbit. *Aust. NZ. J. Ophthalmol. 17*:337–345, 1989.

289. Malberger, E., and Gdal-On, M. Adenoid cystic carcinoma of the orbit diagnosed by means of aspirative cytology. *Ophthalmologica 190*:125–127, 1985.

290. Malhotra, G.S., Paul, S.D., and Batra, D.V. Mucoepidermoid carcinoma of the lacrimal gland. *Ophthalmologica 153*:184–190, 1967.

290a. Malone, M. The histiocytoses of childhood. *Histopathology 19*:105–119, 1991.

291. Mandelcorn, M.S., and Shea, M. Primary orbital perioptic meningioma. *Can. J. Ophthalmol. 6*:293–297, 1971.

292. Mann, R.B., Jaffe, E.S., and Berard, C.W. Malignant lymphomas—a conceptual understanding of morphologic diversity. A review. *Am. J. Ophthalmol. 94*:105–192, 1979.

293. Manschot, W.A. Primary tumours of the optic nerve in von Recklinghausen's disease. *Br. J. Ophthalmol. 38*:285–289, 1954.

294. Manor, R.S., Israeli, J., and Sandbank, U. Malignant optic glioma in a 70 year old patient. *Arch. Ophthalmol. 94*:1142–1144, 1976.

295. Margo, C.E., Folberg, R., Zimmerman, L.E., and Sesterhenn, I.A. Endodermal sinus tumor (yolk sac tumor) of the orbit. *Ophthalmology 90*:1426–1432, 1983.

296. Margo, C.E., Ragsdale, B.D., Perman, K.I., and Zimmerman, L.E. Psammomatoid (juvenile) ossifying fibroma of the orbit. *Ophthalmology 92*:150–159, 1985.

297. Marshall, D. Glioma of the optic nerve as a manifestation of von Recklinghausen's disease. *Am. J. Ophthalmol. 37*:15–36, 1954.

298. Maurer, H.M., Moon, T., Donaldson, M., Fernandez, C., Gehan, E.A., Hammond, D., Hays, D.M., Lawrence, W., Newton, W., Ragab, A., Raney, B., Soule, E.H., Sutow, W.W., and Tefft, M. The intergroup rhabdomyosarcoma study: A preliminary report. *Cancer 40*:2015–2026, 1977.

299. Meacham, C.T. Pseudosarcomatous fasciitis. *Am. J. Ophthalmol. 77*:747–749, 1974.

300. Medeiros, L.J., and Harris, N.L. Lymphoid infiltrates of the orbit and conjunctiva. A morphologic and immunophenotypic study of 99 cases. *Am. J. Surg. Pathol. 13*:459–471, 1989.

301. Medeiros, L.J., and Harris, N.L. Immunohistologic analysis of small lymphocytic infiltrates of the orbit and conjunctiva. *Hum. Pathol. 21*:1126–1131, 1990.

302. Meekins, B.B., Dutton, J.J., and Proia, A.D. Primary orbital leiomyosarcoma: A case report and review of the literature. *Arch. Ophthalmol. 106*:82–86, 1988.

303. Meister, P., Konrad, E., and Krauss, F. Fibrous histiocytoma: A histological and statistical analysis of 155 cases. *Pathol. Res. Pract. 162*:361–379, 1978.

304. Merten, D.F., Goodling, C.A., Newton, T.H., and Malamud, N. Meningiomas of childhood and adolescence. *J. Pediatr. 84*:696–700, 1974.

305. Messmer, E.P., Camara, J., Boniuk, M., and Font, R.L. Amputation neuroma of the orbit. Report of two cases and review of the literature. *Ophthalmology 91*:1420–1423, 1984.

306. Messmer, E.P., Font, R.L., McCrary, J.A., and Murphy, D. Epithelioid angiosarcoma of the orbit presenting as Tolosa-Hunt syndrome. A clinicopathologic case report with review of the literature. *Ophthalmology 90*:1414–1421, 1983.

307. Meyer, J.H., and Hackeloer, H. Pulsierender Exophthalmus als Zeichen eines angeborenen Kleilbeindefektes bei Neurofibromatose. *Klin. Monatsbl. Augenheilkd. 160*:452–456, 1972.

308. Miller, N.R., Gray, J., and Snip, R. Giant mushroom-shaped osteoma of the orbit originating from the maxillary sinus. *Am. J. Ophthalmol. 83*:587–591, 1971.

309. Miller, M.H., Yokohama, C., Wright, J.E., and Garner, A. An aggressive lipoblastic tumour in the orbit of a child. *Histopathology 17*:141–145, 1990.

310. Miller, N.R., Iliff, W.J., and Green, W.R. Evaluation and management of gliomas of the anterior visual pathways. *Brain 97*:743–754, 1974.

311. Miller, S.J.H. Ocular signs of chordoma. *Proc. R. Soc. Med. 65*:522–523, 1972.

312. Milne, H.L., Leone, C.R., Kincaid, M.C., and Brennan, W.M. Chronic hematic cyst of the orbit. *Ophthalmology 94*:271–277, 1987.

313. Mittelman, D., Apple, D.J., and Goldberg, M.F. Ocular involvement of Letterer-Siwe disease. *Am. J. Ophthalmol.* 75:261–265, 1973.
314. Mohan, H., and Sen, D.K. Orbital neurilemmoma: Presenting as retrobulbar neuritis. *Br. J. Ophthalmol.* 54:206–207, 1970.
315. Mohan, H., Sen, D.K., and Chatterjee, P. Localized xanthomatosis of orbit. *Am. J. Ophthalmol.* 69:1080–1082, 1970.
316. Moore, A.T., Pritchard, J., and Taylor, D.S.I. Histiocytosis X: An ophthalmological review. *Br. J. Ophthalmol.* 69:7–14, 1985.
317. Moore, C.E. Sphenoidal ring meningioma with optic nerve metastasis. *Br. J. Ophthalmol.* 52:636–639, 1968.
318. Moore, J.G. Neonatal neurofibromatosis. *Br. J. Ophthalmol.* 46:682–684, 1962.
319. Morgan, G. Lymphocytic tumours of the orbit. *Mod. Probl. Ophthalmol.* 14:355–360, 1975.
320. Morgan, G. Granular cell myoblastoma of the orbit. *Arch. Ophthalmol.* 94:2135–2142, 1976.
321. Moriarty, P., Garner, A., and Wright, J.E. Case report of granular cell myoblastoma arising within the medial rectus muscle. *Br. J. Ophthalmol.* 67:17–22, 1983.
322. Morinaga, S., Nakajima, T., and Shimosato, Y. Normal and neoplastic myoepithelial cells in salivary glands: An immunohistochemical study. *Hum. Pathol.* 18:1218–1226, 1987.
323. Morris, D., and Henkind, P. Fatty infiltration of orbits and heart. *Am. J. Ophthalmol.* 69:987–993, 1970.
324. Mortada, A. Orbital neurilemmoma with cafe-au-lait pigmentation of the skin. *Br. J. Ophthalmol.* 52:262–264, 1968.
325. Mortada, A. Fibroma of the orbit. *Br. J. Ophthalmol.* 55:350–352, 1971.
326. Mottow-Lippa, L., Jakobiec, F.A., and Smith, M. Idiopathic inflammatory orbital pseudotumor in childhood. II. Results of diagnostic tests and biopsies. *Ophthalmology* 88:565–574, 1981.
327. Mullaney, J., Walsh, J., Lee, W.R., and Adams, J.H. Recurrence of astrocytoma of optic nerve after 48 years. *Br. J. Ophthalmol.* 60:539–543, 1976.
328. Munirulhaq, M. Orbital tumors in children. *Orbit* 8:215–222, 1989.
329. Nadji, M., Gonzalez, M.S., Castro, A., and Morales, A.R. Factor VIII-related antigen: An endothelial cell marker. *Lab. Invest.* 42:139, 1980.
330. Nasr, A.M., Blodi, F.C., Lindahl, S., and Jinkins, J. Congenital generalized multicentric myofibromatosis with orbital involvement. *Am. J. Ophthalmol.* 102:779–787, 1986.
331. Napolitano, L., Kyle, R., and Fisher, E.R. Ultrastructure of meningiomas and the derivation and nature of their cellular constituents. *Cancer* 17:233–241, 1963.
332. Nath, K., and Shukla, B. Orbital leiomyoma and its origin. *Br. J. Ophthalmol.* 47:369–371, 1963.
333. Nathrath, W.B.J., and Remberger, K. Immunohistochemical study of granular cell tumors: Demonstration of neuron specific enolase, S-100 protein, laminin and alpha-1-chymotrypsin. *Virchows Arch.* 408:421–434, 1986.
334. Ni, C., D'Amico, D.J., Fan, C.Q., and Kuo, P.K. Tumors of the lacrimal sac: A clinicopathological analysis of 82 cases. *Int. Ophthalmol. Clin.* 22:121–140, 1982.
335. Nicole, S., Palma, L., Giuffr'e, R., and Fortuna, A. 31 primary orbital mass lesions in infancy and childhood. *Childs Brain* 6:255–261, 1980.
335a. Hiffenegger, J.H., Jakobiec, F.A., Shore, J.W., and Albert, D.A. Adult extrarenal rhabdoid tumor of the lacrimal gland. *Ophthalmology* 99:567–574, 1992.
336. Nirankari, M.S., Greer, C.H., and Chaddah, M.R. Malignant nonchromaffin paraganglioma in the orbit. *Br. J. Ophthalmol.* 46:357–363, 1963.
337. Noble, S.C., Chandler, W.F., and Lloyd, R.V. Intracranial extension of orbital pseudotumor: A case report. *Neurosurgery* 18:798–801, 1986.
338. Noguera, R., Triche, J.J., Navarro, S., Tsokos, M., and Llombart-Bosch, A. Dynamic model of differentiation in Ewing's sarcoma cells. *Lab. Invest.* 62:143–151, 1992.
339. Offret, H., and Saraux, H. Localizations ophtalmologiques de l'histiocytose X. *Arch. Ophthalmol. (Paris)* 37:329–349, 1977.
340. Orcutt, J.C., and Char, D.H. Melanoma metastatic to the orbit. *Ophthalmology* 95:1033–1037, 1988.
341. Orcutt, J.C., Reeh, M.J., Gown, A.M., and Lindquist, T.D. Diagnosis of orbit and periorbital tumors. Use of monoclonal antibodies to cytoplasmic antigens (intermediate filaments). *Ophthalmol. Plast. Reconstruct. Surg.* 3:159–178, 1987.
342. Order, S.E., and Hellman, S. Pathogenesis of Hodgkin's disease. *Lancet* 1:571–573, 1972.
343. Palma, O., Canali, N., Scaroni, P., and Torri, A.M. Fine needle aspiration biopsy: Its use in the management of orbital and intraocular tumors. *Tumori* 75:589–593, 1989.
344. Palmer, N., and Foulkes, M. Histopathology and prognosis in the second Intergroup Rhabdomyosarcoma Study (IRS-II). *Proc. Am. Soc. Clin. Oncol.* 2:229 (Abstr. 897), 1983.
345. Panda, A., Dayal, Y., Singhal, V., and Pattnaik, N.K. Haemangiopericytoma. *Br. J. Ophthalmol.* 68:124–127, 1984.
346. Patel, S., and Rootman, J. Nodular sclerosing Hodgkin's disease of the orbit. *Ophthalmology* 90:1433–1436, 1983.
347. Paufique, L., Girard, P.F., and Audibert, J. Une tumeur orbitaire exceptionelle: Le paragangliome non-chromaffine. *Ann. Ocul.* 195:131–141, 1962.

348. Paulus, W., Jellinger, K., and Brenner, H. Melanotic paraganglioma of the orbit: A case report. *Acta Neuropathol. (Berl.) 79*:340–346, 1989.
349. Peretz, W.L., Ettinghausen, S.E., and Gray, G.F. Oncocytic adenocarcinoma of the lacrimal sac. *Arch. Ophthalmol. 96*:303–304, 1978.
350. Perry, R., Ramani, P., McAllister, V., Kalbag, R.M., and Kanagasundaram, C.R. Nodular fasciitis causing unilateral proptosis. *Br. J. Ophthalmol. 59*:404–408, 1975.
351. Pillai, P., and Saini, J.S. Bilateral sino-orbital pseudotumour. *Can. J. Ophthalmol. 23*:177–180, 1988.
352. Popoff, N.A., Malinin, T.I., and Rosomoff, H.E. Fine structure of intracranial hemangiopericytoma and angiomatous meningioma. *Cancer 34*:1187–1197, 1974.
353. Porterfield, J.F. Orbital tumors in children. *Int. Ophthalmol. Clin. 2*:319–335, 1962.
354. Porterfield, J.F., and Zimmerman, L.E. Rhabdomyosarcoma of the orbit: A clinicopathologic study of 55 cases. *Virchows Arch. [A] 335*:329–344, 1962.
355. Potts, M.J., Rose, G.E., Milroy, C., and Wright, J.E. Dedifferentiated chondrosarcoma arising in orbit. *Br. J. Ophthalmol. 76*:49–51, 1992.
356. Powell, J., and Glaser, J. Aneurysmal bone cysts of the orbit. *Arch. Ophthalmol. 93*:340–342, 1975.
357. Prats, J., Bellmunt, J., Calvo, M.A., Sarrias, F., and Toran, N. Orbital metastasis, by transitional cell carcinoma of the bladder. *Int. Urol. Nephrol. 21*:389–392, 1989.
358. Pulitzer, D.R., and Eckert, E.R. Mucoepidermoid carcinoma of the lacrimal gland: An oxyphilic variant. *Arch. Ophthalmol. 105*:1406–1409, 1987.
359. Ransom, J.L., Pratt, C.B., and Shanks, E. Childhood rhabdomyosarcoma of the extremity: Results of combined modality therapy. *Cancer 40*:2810–2816, 1977.
360. Reese, A.B. Expanding lesions of the orbit. *Trans. Ophthalmol. Soc. UK 91*:85–104, 1971.
361. Reese, A.B. Congenital melanomas. *Am. J. Ophthalmol. 77*:798–808, 1974.
362. Reese, A.B. *Tumors of the Eye*, 3rd ed. Harper & Row, New York, 1976.
363. Reese, A.B., and Howard, G.M. Unusual manifestations of ocular lymphangioma and lymphangiectasis. *Surv. Ophthalmol. 18*:226–231, 1973.
364. Reifler, D.M. Orbital metastasis with enophthalmos: A review of the literature. *Henry Ford Hosp. Med. J. 33*:171–179, 1985.
364a. Rettig, W.J., Garin-Chesa, P., and Huvos, A.G. Ewing's sarcoma: New approaches to histogenesis and molecular plasticity. *Lab. Invest. 66*:133–137, 1992.
365. Rice, C.D., and Brown, H.H. Primary orbital melanoma associated with orbital melanocytosis. *Arch. Ophthalmol. 108*:1130–1134, 1990.
366. Richards, A.B., Skalka, H.W., Roberts, F.J., and Flint, A. Pseudotumor of the orbit and retroperitoneal fibrosis: A form of multifocal fibrosclerosis. *Arch. Ophthalmol. 98*:1617–1620, 1980.
367. Riddle, P.J., Font, R.L., and Zimmerman, L.E. Carcinoid tumors of the eye and orbit: A clinicopathologic study of 15 cases, with histochemical and electron microscopic observations. *Hum. Pathol. 13*:459–469, 1982.
368. Riopelle, J.L., and Theriault, J.P. Sur une forme méconnue de sarcome des parties molles le rhabdomyosarcoma alvéolaire. *Ann. Anat. Pathol. 1*:88–111, 1956.
369. Robertson, D.M. Electron microscopic studies of nuclear inclusions in meningiomas. *Am. J. Pathol. 45*:835–848, 1964.
370. Robertson, D.M., and Winkelmann, R.K. Ophthalmic features of necrobiotic xanthogranuloma with paraproteinemia. *Am. J. Ophthalmol. 97*:173–183, 1984.
371. Rodman, H.I., and Font, R.L. Orbital involvement in multiple myeloma: A review of the literature and report of 3 cases. *Arch. Ophthalmol. 87*:30–35, 1972.
372. Rodrigues, M.M., Furgiuele, F.P., and Weinreb, S. Malignant fibrous histiocytoma of the orbit. *Arch. Ophthalmol. 95*:2025–2028, 1977.
373. Rodriguez, H., and Ackerman, L. Cellular blue nevus: Clinicopathologic study of forty-five cases. *Cancer 21*:393–405, 1968.
374. Rootman, J. *Diseases of the Orbit: A Multidisciplinary Approach.* J.G. Lippincott, Philadelphia, 1988.
375. Rootman, J., Damji, K.F., and Dimmick, J.E. Malignant rhabdoid tumor of the orbit. *Ophthalmology 96*:1650–1654, 1989.
376. Rosai, J., and Dorfman, R.F. Sinus histiocytosis with massive lymphadenopathy: A newly recognized clinicopathological entity. *Arch. Pathol. 87*:63–70, 1969.
377. Rose, G.E., Patel, C., Garner, A., and Wright, J.E. Orbital xanthogranuloma in adults. *Br. J. Ophthalmol. 75*:680–684, 1991.
378. Rose, G.E., and Wright, J.E. Isolated peripheral nerve sheath tumors of the orbit. *Eye 5*:668–675, 1991.
379. Rosenberg, S.A., Diamond, H.D., Jaslowitz, B., and Craver, L.F. Lymphosarcoma: A review of 1269 cases. *Medicine (Baltimore) 40*:31–84, 1961.
380. Rottino, A., and Kelly, A. Primary orbital melanoma: Case report with review of the literature. *Arch. Ophthalmol. 27*:934–949, 1942.
381. Ruchman, M.C., and Flanagan, J. Cavernous hemangiomas of the orbit. *Ophthalmology 90*:1328–1336, 1983.
382. Ruiter, D.J., van Rijssel, T.G., and van der Velde, E.A. Aneurysmal bone cysts: A clinicopathological study of 105 cases. *Cancer 39*:2231–2239, 1977.

383. Russell, W.O., Cohen, J., Enzinger, F., Hajdu, S.I., Heise, H., Martin, R.G., Meissner, W., Miller, W.T., Schmitz, R.L., and Suit, H.D. A clinical and pathological staging system for soft tissue sarcomas. *Cancer* 40:1562–1560, 1977.

384. Ryan, S.J., and Font, R.L. Primary epithelial neoplasms of the lacrimal sac. *Am. J. Ophthalmol.* 76:73–88, 1973.

385. Saga, T., Takeuchi, T., and Tagawa, Y. Orbital leiomyoma accompanied by orbital pseudotumour. *Jpn. J. Ophthalmol.* 26:175–182, 1982.

386. Sagerman, R.H., Cassady, J.R., and Tretter, P. Radiation therapy for rhabdomyosarcoma of the orbit. *Trans. Am. Acad. Ophthalmol. Otolaryngol.* 72:849–854, 1968.

386a. Said, J.W., Sassoon, A.F., Shintaku, I.P., Kurtin, P.J., and Pinkus, G.S. Absence of bcl-2 major breakpoint region and J_H gene rearrangement in lymphocyte predominance Hodgkin's disease: Results of Southern blot analysis and polymerase chain reaction. *Am. J. Pathol.* 138:261–264, 1991.

387. Salvador, A.H., Beabout, J.W., and Dahlin, D.C. Mesenchymal chondrosarcoma: Observations on 30 new cases. *Cancer* 28:605–615, 1971.

388. Samuels, V., Barrett, J.M., Bockman, S., Pantazis, C.G., and Allen, M.B., Jr. Immunocytochemical study of transforming growth factor expression in benign and malignant gliomas. *Am. J. Pathol.* 134:895–902, 1989.

389. Sanborn, G.E., Valenzuela, R.E., and Green, W.R. Leiomyoma of the orbit. *Am. J. Ophthalmol.* 87:371–375, 1979.

390. Sanders, M., and Falconer, M.A. Optic nerve compression by an intracanalicular meningioma. *Br. J. Ophthalmol.* 48:13–18, 1964.

391. Sanders, T.E. Infantile xanthogranuloma of the orbit: A report of three cases. *Am. J. Ophthalmol.* 61:1299–1306, 1966.

392. Saunders, J.R., Jacques, D.A., Casterline, P.F., Percarpio, B., and Goodloe, S. Liposarcomas of the head and neck: A review of the literature and addition of four cases. *Cancer* 43:162–169, 1979.

393. Schatz, H. Benign orbital neurilemmoma: Sarcomatous transformation in von Recklinghausen's disease. *Arch. Ophthalmol.* 86:268–273, 1971.

394. Schatz, N.J., and Farmer, P. Tolosa-Hunt syndrome: The pathology of painful ophthalmoplegia. In *Neuro-Ophthalmology*, Vol. 6, J.L. Smith (Ed.), C.V. Mosby, St. Louis, pp. 102–112, 1972.

394a. Schmid, C., Pan, L., Diss, T., and Isaacson, P.G. Expression of B-cell antigens by Hodgkin's and Reed-Sternberg cells. *Am. J. Pathol.* 139:701–707, 1991.

395. Schutz, J.S., Rabkin, M.D., and Schutz, S. Fibromatous tumor (desmoid type) of the orbit. *Arch. Ophthalmol.* 97:703–704, 1979.

396. Schroeder, W., Kasrendieck, H., and Domarus, D. Primares myxoides Liposarkom der Orbita. *Ophthalmologica* 172:337–348, 1976.

397. Scroggs, M.W., Streeten, B.W., Coli, A.F., and Klintworth, G.K. Plasma cell tumors of the orbit. Unpublished observations.

398. Sekimoto, T., Nakaseko, H., and Kondo, K. A case of malignant hemangioendothelioma in the orbit. *Folia Ophthalmol. Jpn.* 22:535–538, 1971.

399. Sen, D.K., Mohan, H., and Chatterjee, P.K. Neurilemmoma of the lacrimal sac. *Eye Ear Nose Throat Mon.* 50:179–180, 1971.

400. Sevel, D. Mesenchymal chondrosarcoma of the orbit. *Br. J. Ophthalmol.* 58:882–887, 1974.

401. Shapiro, A., Tso, M.O.M., Putterman, A.M., and Goldberg, M.F. A clinicopathologic study of hematic cysts of the orbit. *Am. J. Ophthalmol.* 102:237–241, 1986.

402. Shehata, W.M. A rare disorder. Primary esthesionneuroblastoma of the orbit. *Ill. Med. J.* 172:427–429, 1987.

403. Shields, C.L., Shields, J.A., Eagle, R.C., and Rathmell, J.P. Clinicopathologic review of 142 cases of lacrimal gland lesions. *Ophthalmology* 96:431–435, 1989.

404. Shields, C.L., Shields, J.A., and Peggs, M. Tumors metastatic to the orbit. *Ophthalmol. Plast. Reconstr. Surg.* 4:73–80, 1988.

405. Shields, J.A., Bakewell, B., Augsburger, J.J., and Flanagan, J.C. Classification and incidence of space-occupying lesions of the orbit: A survey of 645 biopsies. *Arch. Ophthalmol.* 102:1606–1611, 1984.

406. Shimo-oku, M., Okamoto, N., Ogita, Y., and Sashikata, T. A case of mesenchymal chondrosarcoma of the orbit. *Acta Ophthalmol. (Copenh.)* 58:831–840, 1980.

407. Shuangshoti, S. Meningioma of the optic nerve. *Br. J. Ophthalmol.* 57:265–269, 1973.

408. Snitka, T., Asp, D., and Horner, R. Congenital generalized fibromatosis. *Cancer* 11:627–639, 1958.

409. Slamovits, T.L., Cahill, K.V., Sibony, P.A., Dekker, A., and Johnson, B.L. Orbital fine-needle aspiration biopsy in patients with cavernous sinus syndrome. *J. Neurosurg.* 59:1037–1042, 1983.

410. Slem, G., and Ikayto, R. Hemangioma of the lacrimal gland in the adult. *Ann. Ophthalmol.* 4:77–78, 1978.

411. Smith, J.L., and Taxdal, D.S.R. Painful ophthalmoplegia: The Tolosa-Hunt syndrome. *Am. J. Ophthalmol.* 61:1466–1472, 1966.

412. Smith, T.R., and Brockhurst, R.J. Cellular blue nevus of the sclera. *Arch. Ophthalmol.* 94:618–620, 1976.

413. Sobel, H.J., Marquet, E., and Schwarz, R. Is schwannoma related to granular cell myoblastoma? *Arch. Pathol.* 95:396–401, 1973.

414. Sood, G.C., Malik, S.K.R., Gupta, D.K., and Gupta, A.N. Bilateral meningiomas of the orbit. *Am. J. Ophthalmol.* 61:1533–1535, 1966.

415. Spalter, H.F. Abnormal serum proteins and retinal vein thrombosis. *Arch. Ophthalmol. 62*:868–881, 1959.
416. Speakman, J.S., and Phillips, M.J. Cellular and malignant blue nevus complicating oculodermal melanosis (nevus of Ota syndrome). *Can. J. Ophthalmol. 8*:539–547, 1973.
417. Spencer, J., Diss, T.C., and Isaacson, P.G. Primary B-cell gastric lymphoma. *Am. J. Pathol. 135*:557–564, 1989.
418. Spencer, W.H. Primary neoplasms of the optic nerve and its sheaths: Clinical features and current concepts of pathogenetic mechanisms. *Trans. Am. Ophthalmol. Soc. 70*:490–528, 1972.
419. Stead, R.H., Qizilbash, A.H., Kontozoglou, T., Daya, A.D., and Riddell, R.H. An immunohistochemical study of pleomorphic adenomas of the salivary gland: Glial fibrillary acidic protein-like immunoreactivity identifies a major myoepithelial component. *Hum. Pathol. 19*:32–40, 1988.
420. Steiner, G., Ghosh, L., and Dorfman, H. Ultrastructure of giant cell tumors of bone. *Hum. Pathol. 3*:569–586, 1972.
421. Stern, J., DiGiacinto, G.V., and Housepian, E.M. Neurofibromatosis and optic glioma: Clinical and morphological correlations. *Neurosurgery 4*:524–528, 1979.
422. Stern, J., Jakobiec, F.A., and Housepian, E.M. The architecture of optic nerve gliomas with and without neurofibromatosis. *Arch. Ophthalmol. 98*:505–511, 1980.
423. Stern, W.E. Meningiomas in the cranio-orbital junction. *J. Neurosurg. 38*:428–437, 1973.
424. Stewart, F.W., Foote, F.W., and Becker, W.F. Mucoepidermoid tumors of salivary glands. *Ann. Surg. 122*:820–844, 1945.
425. Stobbe, G.D., and Dargeon, H.W. Embryonal rhabdomyosarcoma of the head and neck in children and adolescents. *Cancer 3*:826–836, 1950.
426. Stout, A.P. Rhabdomyosarcoma of the skeletal muscles. *Ann. Surg. 123*:447–472, 1946.
427. Stout, A.P. Hemangiopericytoma: A study of 25 new cases. *Cancer 2*:1027–1035, 1949,
428. Stout, A.P., and Lattes, R. Tumors of soft tissues. In *Atlas of Tumor Pathology*, Series 2, Fasc. 1. Armed Forces Institute of Pathology, Washington, D.C., 1966.
429. Strang, R.R., Tovi, D., and Nordenstaim, H. Meningioma with intracerebral, cerebellar, and visceral metastases. *J. Neurosurg. 12*:1098–1102, 1964.
430. Strauchen, J.A., and Dimitriu-Bona, A. Malignant fibrous histiocytoma: Expression of monocyte/macrophage differentiation antigens detected with monoclonal antibodies. *Am. J. Pathol. 124*:303–309, 1986.
431. Stucchi, C.A., and Catti, A. Maladie de Abt-Letterer-Siwe avec localisation orbitaire précoce. *Confin. Neurol. (Basel) 28*:254–263, 1966.
432. Suit, H.D., Russell, W.O., and Martin, R.G. Sarcoma of soft tissue: Clinical and histopathological parameters and response to treatment. *Cancer 35*:1478–1483, 1975.
432a. Sullivan, T.J., Wright, J.E., Wule, A.E., Garner, A., Mosely, I., and Sathananthan, N. Haemangiopericytoma of the orbit. *Austral. N.Z. J. Ophthalmol. 20*:325–332, 1992.
433. Sun, X.L., Zheng, B.H., Li, B., Li, L.Q., Soejima, K., and Kanda, M. Orbital rhabdomyosarcoma. Immunohistochemical studies of seven cases. *Chin. Med. J. Peking 103*:485–488, 1990.
434. Suttorp, M., Polchau, H., Kuhn, B., Loffler, H., and Rister, M. Acute megakaryoblastic leukemia (FAB-M7) in an infant presenting with orbital chloroma and meningeal involvement. *Hamatol. Bluttransfus. 33*:368–372, 1990.
435. Symmers, W.St.C. The lymphoreticular system. In *Systemic Pathology*, 2nd ed., Vol. 2, W.St.C. Symmers (Ed.), Churchill Livingstone, Edinburgh, pp. 504–891, 1978.
436. Szlezak, L., Przybora, L., and Markowska, M. Osteoblastoma benignum blednika sitowego zatoki czolewej: Oczodulu. *Klin. Oczna 45*:247–251, 1975.
437. Takeshita, T., Kojima Y., and Ishimaru, S. A case of orbital paraganglioma (Japanese). *Folia Ophthalmol. Jpn. 40*:2306–2312, 1989.
438. Tan, K.K., and Lim, A.S.M. Primary extradural intra-orbital meningioma in a Chinese girl. *Br. J. Ophthalmol. 49*:377–380, 1965.
439. Tarkkanen, A., Koivuniemi, A., Liesmaa, M., and Merenmies, L. Fine-needle aspiration biopsy in the diagnosis of orbital tumours. *Graefes Arch. Clin. Exp. Ophthalmol. 219*:165–170, 1982.
440. Tarkannen, J.V., and Metsala, P. A case of orbital osteoma. *Acta Ophthalmol. (Copenh.) 42*:1074–1078, 1964.
441. Templeton, A.C. Orbital tumours in African children. *Br. J. Ophthalmol. 55*:254–261, 1971.
442. Thomas, A., Sujatha, S., Ramakrishnan, P.M., and Sudarsanam, D. Malignant melanoma of the lacrimal sac. *E. Arch. Ophthalmol. 3*:84–86, 1975.
443. Tolls, R.E., Mohr, S., and Spencer, W.H. Benign nodular fasciitis originating in Tenon's capsule. *Arch. Ophthalmol. 75*:482–483, 1966.
444. Tomokane, N., Iwaki, T., Tateishi, J., Iwaku, A., and Goldman, J.E. Rosenthal fibers share epitopes with alpha B-crystallin, glial fibrillary acidic protein, and ubiquitin, but not with vimentin: Immunoelectron microscopy with colloidal gold. *Am. J. Pathol. 138*:875–885, 1991.
445. Trobe, J.D., Glaser, J.S., Post, J.D., and Page, L.K. Bilateral optic canal meningiomas: A case report. *Neurosurgery 3*:68–74, 1978.
446. Tsokos, M., Howard, R., and Costa, J. Immunohistochemical study of alveolar and embryonal rhabdomyosarcoma. *Lab. Invest. 48*:148–155, 1983.

447. Turc-Carel, C., Aurias, A., Mugneret, F., Lizard, S., Sidaner, I., Volk, C., Thiery, J.P., Olschwang, S., Philip, I., Berger, M.P., Philip, T., Lenoir, G.M., and Mazabraud, A. 1. An evaluation of 85 cases and remarkable consistency of t(11;220(q24;q12). *Cancer Genet. Cytogenet. 32*:229–238, 1988.
448. Vara Thorbeck, R., Morales Valentin, O.I., and Ruiz Morales, M. Non-chromaffin paraganglioma of the orbit. Case report. *Zentralbl. Chir. 111*:46–29, 1986.
449. Varghese, S., Nair, B., and Joseph, T.A. Orbital malignant non-chromaffin paraganglioma: Alveolar soft tissue sarcoma. *Br. J. Ophthalmol. 52*:713–715, 1968.
450. Venkataramana, N.K., Kolluri, V.R., Kumar, D.V., Rao, T.V., and Das, B.S. Paraganglioma of the orbit with extension to the middle cranial fossa: Case report. *Neurosurgery 24*:762–764, 1989.
451. Virtanen, I., Lehtonen, E., and Worthovaara, J. Structure of psammoma bodies of a meningioma in scanning electron microscopy. *Cancer 38*:824–829, 1976.
452. Wakisaka, S., Tashiro, M., Nakano, S., Kita, T., Kisanuki, H., and Kinoshita, K. Intracranial and orbital metastasis of hepatocellular carcinoma: Report of two cases. *Neurosurgery 26*:863–866, 1990.
453. Walsh, F.B. Selected optic neuropathies. *Jpn. J. Ophthalmol. 18*:1–29, 1974.
454. Wan, W.L., Geller, J.L., Feldon, S.E., and Sadun, A.A. Visual loss caused by rapidly progressive intracranial meningiomas during pregnancy. *Ophthalmology 97*:18–21, 1990.
455. Watillon, M., Prijot, E., and Farra, M. Maladie de Hodgkin, localisation lacrymale. *Arch. Ophtalmol. (Paris) 24*:153–155, 1964.
456. Weber, F.L., and Babel, J. Intravascular papillary endothelial hyperplasia of the orbit. *Br. J. Ophthalmol. 65*:18–22, 1981.
457. Weiner, J.M., and Hidayat, A.A. Juvenile fibrosarcoma of the orbit and eyelid: A study of five cases. *Arch. Ophthalmol. 101*:253–259, 1983.
458. Weiss, J.S., Bressler, S.B., Jacobs, E.F., Jr., Shapiro, J., Weber, A., and Albert, D.M. Maxillary ameloblastoma with orbital invasion. A clinicopathologic study. *Ophthalmology 92*:710–713, 1985.
459. Welsh, R., Bray, D., Shipkey, F., and Meyer, A. Histogenesis of alveolar soft part sarcoma. *Cancer 29*:191–204, 1972.
460. Wenger, J., Gingrich, G.W., and Mendeloff, J. Sclerosing cholangitis—a manifestation of systemic disease. *Arch. Intern. Med. 116*:509–514, 1965.
461. Wharam, M., Beltangady, M., Hays, D., Heyn, R., Ragab, A., Soule, E., Tefft, M., and Maurer, H. Localised orbital rhabdomyosarcoma: An interim report of the Intergroup Rhabdomyosarcoma Study Committee. *Ophthalmology 94*:251–254, 1987.
462. Weiss, A.H., Greenwald, M., Margo, C.E., and Myers, W. Primary and secondary orbital teratomas. *J. Pediatr. Ophthalmol. Strabismus 26*:44–49, 1989.
463. Whitbeck, E.G., Spiers, A.S., and Hussain, M. Mycosis fungoides: Subcutaneous and visceral tumors, orbital involvement, and ophthalmoplegia. *J. Clin. Oncol. 1*:270–276, 1983.
464. Willis, R.A. *Pathology of Tumours*, Butterworth, London, 1953.
465. Wilson, W.B., Roloff, J., and Wilson, H.L. Primary peripheral neuroepithelioma of the orbit with intracranial extension. *Cancer 62*:2595–2601, 1988.
466. Wirostko, E., Johnson, L., and Wirostko, B. Chronic orbital inflammatory disease: Parasitisation of orbital leucocytes by mollicute-like organisms. *Br. J. Ophthalmol. 73*:865–870, 1989.
467. Wohlschlag, M. Orbital teratoma. *Ophthalmologica 172*:229–234, 1976.
468. Wolpiuk, M. Przypadek obutronnego chloniaka zloshiwego workow Izowych. *Klin. Oczna 45*:61–64, 1975.
469. Wolter, J.R. Arteriovenous fistulas involving the eye region. *J. Pediatr. Ophthalmol. 12*:22–39, 1975.
470. Wolter, J.R., Bryson, J.M., and Blackhurst, R.T. Primary orbital melanoma. *Eye Ear Nose Throat Mon. 45*:64–67, 1966.
471. Woodruff, G., Thorner, P., and Skarf, B. Primary Ewing's sarcoma of the orbit presenting with visual loss. *Br. J. Ophthalmol. 72*:786–792, 1988.
471a. Wright, C.F., Reid, A.H., Tsai, M.M., Ventre, K.M., Murari, P.J., Frizzera, G., and O'Leary, T.J. Detection of Epstein-Barr virus sequences in Hodgkin's disease by the polymerase chain reaction. *Am. J. Pathol. 139*:393–398, 1991.
472. Wright, J.E. Orbital vascular anomalies. *Trans. Am. Acad. Ophthalmol. Otolaryngol. 78*:606–616, 1974.
473. Wright, J.E. Primary optic nerve meningiomas: Clinical presentation and management. *Trans. Am. Acad. Ophthalmol. Otolaryngol. 87*:617–625, 1976.
474. Wright, J.E. Lacrimal gland tumours. *Trans. Ophthalmol. Soc. NZ. 35*:101–106, 1983.
475. Wright, J.E., McNab, A.A., and McDonald, W.I. Optic nerve glioma and the management of optic nerve tumours in the young. *Br. J. Ophthalmol. 73*:967–974, 1989.
476. Wright, J.E., McNab, A.A., and McDonald, W.I. Primary optic nerve sheath meningioma. *Br. J. Ophthalmol. 73*:960–966, 1989.
477. Wright, J.E., Rose, G.E., and Garner, A. Primary malignant neoplasms of the lacrimal gland. *Br. J. Ophthalmol. 76*:401–407, 1992.
478. Wu, B.F. Orbital chemodectoma: Clinical and pathologic analysis of 2 cases. *Chin. Med. J. Peking 94*:419–422, 1981.

479. Wyburn-Mason, R. Arteriovenous aneurysm of mid-brain and retina, facial naevi, and mental changes. *Brain* 66:163–203, 1943.
480. Yamade, S., and Kitagawa, A. Malignant melanoma of the lacrimal sac. *Ophthalmologica* 177:30–33, 1978.
481. Yanoff, M., Davis, R.L., and Zimmerman, L.E. Juvenile pilocytic astrocytoma ("glioma") of the optic nerve: Clinicopathologic study of sixty three cases. In *Ocular and Adnexal Tumors*, F.A. Jakobiec (Ed.), Aesculapius, Birmingham, AL, pp. 685–707, 1978.
482. Zajdela, A., de Maublanc, M.A., Schlienger, P., and Haye, C. Cytologic diagnosis of orbital and periorbital palpable tumors using fine-needle sampling without aspiration. *Diagn. Cytopathol.* 2:17–20, 1986.
483. Zimmerman, L.E. Ocular lesions of juvenile xanthogranuloma nevoxanthoendothelioma. *Trans. Am. Acad. Ophthalmol. Otolaryngol* 69:412–442, 1965.
484. Zimmerman, L.E., Sanders, T.E., and Ackerman, L.V. Epithelial tumors of the lacrimal gland: Prognostic and therapeutic significance of histologic types. *Int. Ophthalmol. Clin.* 2:333–367, 1962.

51

Immunology of Ocular Tumors

Alec Garner
Institute of Ophthalmology, University of London, London, England

Amjad H. S. Rahi
Ministry of Health, Dammam, Saudi Arabia

I. GENERAL ASPECTS

The failure to control cell growth, which is at the heart of the neoplastic process, reflects changes in the genetic code that can also have important ramifications concerning the nature of the proteins located at the surface of the cell. When this happens the character of the proteins encoded by the DNA may be so altered that they are no longer recognized by the immune surveillance system and a rejection process is initiated.

II. IMMUNE RESPONSE TO NEOPLASIA

A. Clinical Evidence

Before direct evidence of tumor antigenicity was forthcoming, observations of a clinical nature suggested that the behavior of a wide range of cancers is modified by host defense mechanisms that are possibly of an immune nature. Thus, the phenomenon of spontaneous regression had been recognized, albeit infrequently, for many years, and although there have been many spurious claims, Everson and Cole [31] were able to confirm 176 cases of histologically proven malignant tumors representing many different morphological types that behaved in this way. Metastases have been known to disappear after removal of the primary tumor [64], and conversely, metastases often fail to develop despite the presence of malignant cells in the peripheral bloodstream incurred by surgical resection of the primary growth [85,104]. Studies relating to uveal melanoma and retinoblastoma also indicate that the presence of tumor cells in the circulating blood does not correlate with the incidence of metastasis [41]. Other evidence pointing to an immune factor in the neoplastic process is the increased incidence of malignant disease, particularly within the lymphoid and cutaneous tissues, in patients receiving prolonged immunosuppressive treatment [106,121]. One analysis of over 6000 renal transplant recipients concluded that the risk of developing malignant lymphoma is about 35 times greater than in the average population [55]. Precisely why patients with renal transplants are more prone to develop malignant tumors is not clear. Conceivably, it is associated with antigenic mismatch between donor and recipient, particularly at locus B of the major histocompatibility complex–human leukocyte antigen (MHC–HLA) system, since this can be expected to lead to chronic stimulation of the host immune system with graft rejection as the end point. This, it is suggested, may detract from the immune surveillance function aimed at eliminating emergent neoplastic cell proliferation [102]. Additionally, the region on chromosome 6 responsible for HLA encoding also includes the genes for complement, tumor necrosis factor (TNF), and the heat-shock proteins; each of these is able to modify the immune response and contribute to a predisposition to neoplasia in immunosuppressed patients [126].

B. Laboratory Evidence

A high peripheral blood lymphocyte count is said to have a beneficial effect on prognosis in treated cancer patients [111], and there is a positive correlation between the degree of lymphocytic infiltration of the primary tumor and clinical outcome in a range of tumors [5,19]. Curiously, however, this does not always seem to be the case, one group reporting that the prognosis is worse with respect to patients with choroidal melanomas should they have prominent lymphocytic infiltration [101], particularly when T cells predominate [32].

III. TUMOR ANTIGENS

Most antigens exhibited by neoplastic cells are common to the tissues from which they originated and in consequence are ignored by the immune surveillance apparatus. The observation that an immune response is often forthcoming, however, suggests that other new components are produced that are treated as alien by the host. In part the expression of tumor antigens is due to oncogene activity, the oncogenes representing either normal cellular components of the genome concerned with cell growth (c-*onc*) or part of an oncogenic viral genome (v-*onc*). These oncogenes are released from physiological control mechanisms by the insertion of viral promoter DNA, by gene translocation or amplification, or by point mutations in the protooncogene attributable to the effects of chemical or physical agents. Conversely, the transformation of a normal cell to a neoplastic form includes the removal of suppressor gene activity, some of which serves to encourage cell differentiation. Suppressor oncogenes also appear to influence the production of inhibitory cytokines, which, as in the case of the p53 gene [75,144], are involved in programmed cell death or apoptosis.

It is with those tumor antigens that are incorporated within the surface membrane that interest principally lies, since antigens in the underlying cytoplasm are not accessible to patrolling lymphocytes and macrophages. Although this antigenic seclusion reduces the opportunity for sensitization, with time some exposure of the intracytoplasmic neoantigens to the immune surveillance system is inevitable because of normal tumor cell turnover involving apoptosis [66], and ultimately, it is the inability of the effector arm of the immune response to make contact with the antigens that is the important limiting factor. Alien tumor antigens located on the cell surface evince precisely the same response on the part of the host as would a heterograft and in consequence have attracted the designation of tumor-specific transplantation antigens (TSTA; Fig. 1).

Overall there are at least three distinct groups of cell surface antigens on cancerous cells:

1. *Individually distinct antigens* are unique to a given tumor.
2. *Shared antigens* are present on tumors of similar or sometimes different histogenesis.
3. *Common antigens*: tumor cells possess many of the surface features seen in normal cells and exhibit the corresponding antigens (e.g., HLA and blood group antigens).

A. Tumor-Specific Transplantation Antigens

It has been shown in experimental situations involving small animals that if a chemically induced tumor is surgically excised and viable cells from the same tumor are reintroduced at a later date, rejection occurs [69,70]. Such *rejection antigens*, as they are sometimes known, can be highly peculiar to a given tumor or may cross-react with other tumors of the same histogenesis.

Individual-Specific Antigens

Chemical carcinogenesis in laboratory animals is associated with the emergence of TSTA, which are not only peculiar to the host but are also restricted to the tumor concerned, such that a second tumor attributable to the same carcinogen, even though it is in the same animal, has a different set of antigens [2,98]. The antigens resulting from chemical carcinogenesis vary considerably in their immunogenicity but are generally weak [54]. On the other hand, experimental tumors induced by physical means (ultraviolet, UV, irradiation) give rise to a strong immune response when transplanted to syngeneic animals [72,132]. Cutaneous melanomas induced in C3H mice by a combination of UV irradiation and chemical carcinogenesis express antigens common to normal tissues in a given individual as well as some that are both

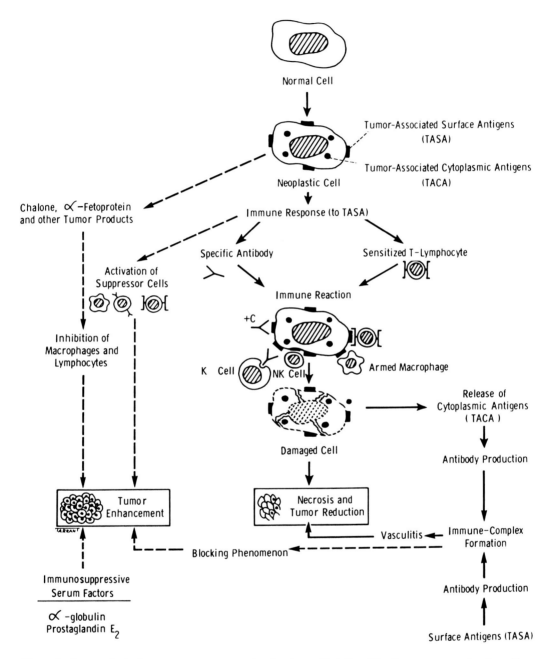

Figure 1 Immunological response to tumor-associated antigens. Both B and T cell responses can develop with a complex sequence of effects, although the latter appear to exercise the larger share of any tumoricidal effect. Moreover, antigen located at the cell surface is most susceptible to attack from the effector arm of any immune response. Antibody responses are provoked by surface or cytoplasmic antigens liberated from damaged cells and can be involved in the formation of immune complexes that may occasionally serve to interfere with cytotoxic T cell activity. These and other possible reactions are shown here (solid arrows indicate tumoricidal activity; dashed lines indicate tumor-enhancing activity).

individual and tumor specific [26]. Notwithstanding their marked antigenicity, immunologically induced tumor regression in the primary host is uncommon because of counterbalancing immunosuppression mediated to a large extent through the generation of tumor antigen-specific suppressor T cells [56]. The extent to which highly specific antigens of this sort occur in human neoplasia is not known, although it is of interest that when TSTA are demonstrable in animals with naturally occurring tumors, they are overwhelmingly individual specific [54].

Proteins that are currently attracting attention in the context of tumor immunity are the heat-shock proteins and closely related glucose-regulated proteins. These highly conserved proteins are expressed by all cells across the animal kingdom (at least all cells so far examined) under a wide range of stressful situations, including neoplasia [35,141]. Furthermore, they can behave as antigens and, should they be expressed on the surface of the tumor cell, can excite protective immunity [131]. Some of the heat-shock protein epitopes in such circumstances are specific to the host, perhaps because of point mutations affecting single amino acids or gene polymorphism. Perversely, heat-shock proteins may also potentiate tumor growth by generating suppressor T cells, which inhibit tumoricidal immunological activity [50].

Cross-Reacting Antigens

Because viral material is included in the cell genome, tumors induced by DNA viruses tend to be characterized by surface antigens that reflect the nature of the responsible virus, which means that lesions attributable to a particular virus can be expected to have at least some TSTA in common irrespective of the host or the tumor histogenesis [22,68,72]. It is much less certain that RNA virus-induced tumors express viral antigens since it is only necessary for the promoter region of the viral RNA to be encoded in the host cell DNA for neoplasia to develop. Examples of virus-induced tumors in humans are rare, although there is good reason to implicate the Epstein-Barr (EB) virus in Burkitt's lymphoma and nasopharyngeal lymphoepithelioma [130] and, possibly, Hodgkin's disease [23] and some cases of gastric adenocarcinoma [122]. The EB virus is a DNA virus that promotes such a strong TSTA response in the transformed host cells that further growth is usually prevented unless there is a degree of immunosuppression, which possibly explains the frequent association of Burkitt's lymphoma and chronic malaria [8].

B. Tumor-Associated Antigens

In addition to antigens that are apparently tumor specific, others linked with the neoplastic process are an expression of an earlier stage of development in the parent cell line. As such the antigens are the outcome of cellular dedifferentiation, with failure to suppress genes connected with embryogenesis. One of the best known instances is the carcinoembryonic antigen [43], encountered in adenocarcinomas of the human gastrointestinal tract but otherwise only in endodermal structures during early embryonic life. Another antigen of this type is α-fetoprotein, which may reemerge in patients with hepatocellular carcinoma [42]. The immune response, if any, in the autologous host is of no significance, however, and has no propensity for tumor rejection. The distinctiveness of the cytoplasmic and surface antigen profile is an indication of cellular differentiation, and the better differentiated tumors exhibit antigens peculiar to their histogenesis. Rarely these antigens can be associated with an autologous immune reaction, possibly because they are presented in a slightly modified way, but the chief significance of differentiation antigens from a clinical standpoint is that they can be used as markers in histological tumor diagnosis.

Aberrant glycosylation as a consequence of oncogenic transformation is well documented. One expression of this aberration is that some tumor-associated antigens are in the form of glycolipids or glycoproteins. These novel compounds arise either because of interference with the formation of more complex carbohydrate components of the normal cell or because there is increased synthesis of the precursor substance in response to the activation of normally silent glycosyltransferases [48].

IV. CELL-MEDIATED TUMOR IMMUNITY

It is expected that both cell- and antibody-mediated responses are provoked by tumor antigens, but in that they have any tangible effect it is the cellular defenses that are of greatest importance. They can take several forms (Figs. 1 and 2).

A. T-Cell Responses

T lymphocyte-mediated immunity, as revealed by in vitro testing, has been clearly demonstrated with respect to experimentally induced tumors in animals and to several human neoplasms (Fig. 2). Laboratory tests have shown that autologous lymphocytes undergo blastic transformation when mixed with tumor cells and are then able to initiate cell death and inhibit growth of tumor cultures [47]. Human neoplastic conditions in which cell-mediated immunity of this type has been described cover a wide spectrum, those of particular interest in an ophthalmic context including Burkitt's lymphoma [33] and cutaneous melanoma [89]. It has also been shown that lymphocytes from a cancer-bearing patient may cross-react with tumor cells from other patients with the same type of tumor [63]. In vitro blastic transformation of autologous lymphocytes and delayed hypersensitivity reactions to tumor cell extracts can be favorable prognostic signs in malignant melanoma of the skin [33,119], and improved survival prospects have been reported in patients treated for a number of cancer types in whom autologous cell-mediated cytotoxicity can be demonstrated [100,134].

It might be expected that cytotoxic lymphocytes would be the T cell subset of prime importance, but evidence is accruing that it is the helper cell that holds the key [135]. Not only does this cell regulate the overall response, but it possibly functions as an effector cell provided the tumor can be induced to express class II MHC antigens. This in turn may require the intervention of interferon-γ and other cytokines [62]. The T cells can also act indirectly through the release of cytokines, such as lymphotoxin [45] and the closely related tumor necrosis factor, both acting in concert with interferon-γ [113]. On the other hand, noncytolytic antitumor T cell responses may downregulate protective immunity and encourage tumor growth [47].

Natural Killer (NK) Cells

NK cells are lymphocytes with a cytotoxic propensity independent of specific T cell sensitization, although their activity can be augmented by T cell-derived interleukin-2 and interferon. That they can function in the absence of prior antigenic sensitization has encouraged a suggestion that they have a role in surveillance

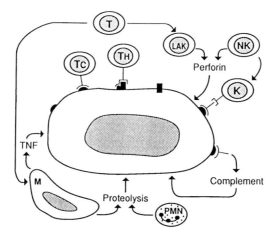

Figure 2 Tumoricidal immune mechanisms. The principal tumoricidal mechanisms are cell mediated. Antigen-specific cytotoxic T cells (Tc) act directly on the cell surface; helper T cells (Th) behave similarly if there is expression of class II MHC antigen. Sensitized T cells can also activate macrophages (M) and certain killer lymphocytes (LAK) through the release of lymphokines. LAK cells and natural killer cells (NK) damage the tumor cell nonspecifically by releasing perforin. Killer cells can also be tumoricidal through binding of receptors on the cell surface with the Fc region of antigen-bound antibody (antibody-dependent cell cytotoxicity). Complement-activating tumor-specific antibody is generally of little consequence. Proteolytic enzyme and toxic free radical release on the part of macrophages and neutrophil polymorphonuclear leukocytes (the latter entirely nonspecific) is also involved. Tumor necrosis factor is secreted by activated macrophages. [Key: ▲ tumor specific antigen; ■ class II MHC antigen].

and the elimination of incipient tumor growths. Evidence to support this idea is provided by a naturally occurring mutant in a strain of mice such that it is NK cell deficient; the mutant mice have a significantly greater risk of succumbing to spontaneous neoplasia than their normal littermates [49]. Artificially induced depletion of circulating NK cells in rats has been shown to impair the capacity for elimination of mammary carcinoma cells [4]. Low NK cell activity is often encountered clinically in patients with leukemia or lymphoma, but patients with acquired or congenital immune deficiency, such as Chédiak-Higashi syndrome, in which there is pronounced NK cell deficiency, have a high incidence of lymphoproliferative disease [139]. In view of this evidence, it is disappointing that the use of interferons to augment the therapeutic potential of NK cells appears to be limited by the transience of the effect [80].

Lymphokine-Activated Killer (LAK) Cells

There is a category of lymphocyte that, although not itself a T cell, can be made to exert tumor cytotoxicity by virtue of the cytokine interleukin-2 (IL-2) derived from T cells that have been sensitized by the tumor [88]. Normal cells are unaffected, and a beneficial response has been claimed in cancer patients following the simultaneous injection of LAK cells and interleukin-2 [115]. Most LAK cells are probably activated NK cells, although a minority may represent cytotoxic T cells [139].

Tumor-Infiltrating Lymphocytes

Solid tumors are often infiltrated by T lymphocytes which have been interpreted as representing a specific immune response [105]. It is possible to recover these tumor-infiltrating lymphocytes (TIL) by enzymatic digestion of tumor tissue followed by separation of the cells on a Ficoll gradient. The TIL are tumoricidal in cell culture, sometimes to a degree that surpasses that of LAK cells [95]. When stimulated by the preincubation with IL-2, TIL have been found to exert a beneficial effect on metastatic tumor deposits in the autologous host [47,116].

Genetically Engineered Lymphocytes

Tumor-infiltrating lymphocytes can be transfected with the gene for tumor necrosis factor and returned to the autologous host, which has the advantage of specifically targeting the cytotoxic cytokine.

B. Macrophages

The effect of macrophages on tumor behavior is complex. On the one hand, they are capable of selective tumor cytotoxicity under the influence of interferon-γ and other cytokines liberated by sensitized T lymphocytes through the release of proteolytic enzymes, oxygen radical formation, and synthesis of TNF. Experiments in rabbits have shown that TNF injected into the vitreous induces a moderate inflammatory response in the anterior segment [114]. On the other hand, macrophages can engender the suppression of both T and NK cell function and possibly encourage tumor growth [30]. Systemic administration of immunomodulator substances incorporated in liposomes has been shown to induce regression of established metastases by activating tumoricidal macrophages, which liberate TNF, IL-1, and IL-6 [29].

C. Granulocytes

Polymorphonuclear leukocytes can kill tumor cells in vitro by oxidative and nonoxidative mechanisms [77]. Their capacity for activation through IL-1, TNF, and colony-stimulating factor supplementation raises the possibility that autologous granulocytes may be provoked into tumoricidal activity in vivo.

V. TUMOR ANTIBODIES

The antibody contribution to the immune reaction to neoplastic processes was the aspect that originally attracted most attention. The epitopes with which they correspond covers the whole range of tumor-specific and tumor-associated antigens, as well as some normal tissue components, and although they belong predominantly to the IgG class, IgM tumor antibodies are also reported [87].

The contribution of the humoral response to protection against neoplasia is not now considered of great importance, although some isolated early reports commented on the beneficial effect of administering sera from patients with spontaneously regressing melanoma of the skin to other melanoma patients

[91,127]. Similar claims were made with respect to Burkitt's lymphoma patients [92]. There is also in vitro evidence of tumor cytotoxicity attributable to antibody activity, which is most effective against autologous tumor cells [76]. The relevant antibodies appear to function by fixing complement [10].

It is possible that if humoral defenses have any relevance to the prognosis in neoplasia, they are most likely to influence the viability of small tumor foci and reduce the incidence of metastasis, their effect on the larger primary tumor being minimal.

Other ways in which antibodies may affect neoplastic processes is through their interaction with cell-mediated responses. Known as antibody-dependent cell cytotoxicity, the combination of the Fc region of tumor-specific antibodies with receptor sites on certain types of killer cells serves as a homing device and thus enhances the level of cytotoxic potential at the site of the tumor [1,58]. Conversely, as previously mentioned, antibodies to tumor cells can also interfere with cell-mediated cytotoxicity.

VI. TUMOR GROWTH IN THE FACE OF AN IMMUNE RESPONSE

Given that it is the rule rather than the exception for the neoplastic process to generate tumor-specific antigens and that this is often associated with an immune response on the part of the host, it is pertinent to ask how the tumors are able to develop and progress. Even before present concepts of the immunological system had begun to be formulated, Green [46] suggested that tumors developed if there was inadequacy of a postulated immune surveillance mechanism. This hypothesis was fostered by Burnet [9] and was supported by the clinical observation that immune deficiency states, whether congenital or acquired, carry an enhanced risk of malignant disease for the patients [38,106]. Moreover, it is a common experience that cell-mediated immunity, as shown by delayed hypersensitivity to a variety of antigens, is depressed in a nonspecific manner in patients with cancer, particularly those with advanced disease [52]. If there is to be any substantial role for immunotherapy in the management of malignant disease, however, it is necessary to understand the reasons for the seeming ineffectiveness of the immune system in controlling the process in individuals who, initially at least, appear to have intact immunological function. There are several possibilities.

A. Sneaking Through

One suggestion is that there may be a delay between the emergence of the malignant cells and activation of the surveillance mechanism sufficient to allow the tumor to become established before the capacity for rejection is adequately developed [21,98]. Such "sneaking through," as it has been called, could occur because the initial small number of cells was unable to provide sufficient antigenic stimulation for the immune response to be effective. Woodruff [142] suggests that the situation may be comparable to the persistence of primary allografts in experimental animals despite the rejection of subsequent grafts from the same source, a phenomenon attributed to host immune responses being already primed at the second graft but delayed at the time of the initial transplant.

B. Blocking Antibodies

Not all the antibodies provoked by a tumor have cytotoxic potential; some may actually promote tumor growth by interfering with the T cell response [53]. Originally it was thought that antigenic sites on the surfaces of the tumor cells become coated with specific antibody, rendering the tumor inaccessible to aggressive cell-mediated reactions [59]. Now, however, it seems more likely that blocking is aimed at the T cell rather than the target cell, and it has been suggested that incomplete fragments of antigen are released into the circulation from the tumor, where they form complexes with the antibody in such a way that some antigenic sites remain free and are able to combine with specific receptors on sensitized T cells [124]. It is also conceivable that circulating fragments of antigen could themselves interfere with cell-mediated immunity by reacting directly with cytotoxic T cells before they can reach the main tumor mass [124].

C. Immune Suppression by the Tumor

The initial reaction of the immune system to neoplasia has the potential to eliminate the aberrant cells, but experiments in mice have shown that this positive response may ultimately be supplanted by predominantly suppressor T cell activity [96], which compares with the clinical observation that immunological function is often depressed in patients with advanced cancer [52]. The further finding that the tendency toward immunosuppression can be reversed in the experimental situation by excision of the tumor [96] offers a plausible explanation for the reported reemergence of antibodies after surgery [76] and the beneficial effect that removal of the primary tumor can sometimes have in promoting the regression of metastases.

The release of cytokines, such as TNF and IL-1, can sometimes have an adverse effect, serving to promote angiogenesis and contribute to the risk of metastasis by enhancing tumor cell adhesion [79]. A permissive effect on tumor growth may also occur through a loss of normal responsiveness to the regulatory effects of TGF-β and interferon [112].

VII. TUMOR IMMUNOTHERAPY

Except for a very few instances, the curative properties of naturally occurring tumor-induced immunological responses are of little consequence, and as a result there have been many attempts at artificial augmentation. The efforts have been aimed principally at boosting the activity of the cells shown to have tumoricidal potential, such as cytotoxic and helper T cells, macrophages, and natural killer cells, using a variety of bacterial adjuvants, interferons, and other cytokines [135]. Reports of the effectiveness of these measures are mildly encouraging but not overly impressive, in part because of the frequently transient nature of the suppression.

Ironically, in light of their relative ineffectiveness, it is to antibody-mediated tumor reactions that much recent attention has turned in the search for a realistic approach to cancer immunotherapy. By linking a cytotoxic agent to tumor antibodies, which target the conjugate in high concentration to a relevant tumor, it should be possible to damage the unwanted cells without harming the healthy tissues. In practice, however, this has proved a somewhat elusive goal because of problems in synthesizing stable conjugates able to penetrate capillary walls, in avoiding nonspecific binding, and in identifying surface antigens that facilitate the all-important entry of the toxin into the cytoplasm of the tumor cell [99]. Cytotoxic agents that have been used include a number of plant lectins, especially ricin, cobra venom factor, and several synthetic substances. Interferons and other immunostimulants can also be delivered in this way [137]. The antibodies are raised by the hybridoma technique and can be cloned to a high degree of specificity, although they are usually directed against tumor-associated as opposed to tumor-specific antigens and have no intrinsic cytotoxicity [3]. A patient's mononuclear cells incubated with antitumor antibodies chemically attached to anti-CD3 antigen can generate the proliferation of cytotoxic T cells, and these may induce tumor regression on reintroduction into the circulation [95]. A long-term limitation of this approach is the emergence of host antibodies to the conjugate, given that the initial immunization involves the use of xenogeneic splenocytes. Even this may be turned to advantage, however, by performing a second conjugation of antibodies resulting from the host response to the initial conjugate with the cytotoxic agent and thus achieving an even higher dosage level at the tumor site [44]. An alternative approach that minimizes the immune response to foreign antibodies is the production of genetically engineered antibodies. This involves a so-called transfectoma technique, in which the antigen binding variable region of a rodent immunoglobulin is joined to the constant region of human immunoglobulin. The genes for these regions are first isolated and cloned in a suitable vector and then transfected into a nonsecreting myeloma cell line, which then produces the desired antibody. Such chimeric humanized antibodies and lymphokines are already undergoing trial [16,86, 117,138].

VIII. TUMOR IMMUNODIAGNOSIS

Monoclonal antibodies produced by the hybridoma technique can also be used for diagnostic purposes. Clinical diagnosis can be aided by conjugating the antibodies with a radioactive label, which on injection into the circulation lodges at the site of a corresponding tumor, where it can be demonstrated by recording the scintillation profile [103]. The same method can help to detect metastatic tumor deposit.

Histological diagnosis can often be greatly facilitated using monoclonal antibodies that recognize epitopes peculiar to a specific cell type, the antibody being labeled with a marker, such as fluorescein or horseradish peroxidase, that can be detected in tissue sections.

IX. SPECIFIC OCULAR TUMOR IMMUNOLOGY

A. Malignant Melanoma

Evidence that ocular melanomas, especially those involving the uvea, are able to stimulate an immune response is slowly accumulating, and there are signs that it could have a marginal effect on clinical behavior, particularly with regard to the risk of metastasis.

Antigenicity

One of the first demonstrations that tumor-specific antigens may be expressed by ocular melanomas came from a study showing that sera from patients with choroidal lesions inhibit the growth of autologous cells salvaged from the tumors at the time of enucleation and maintained in tissue culture in up to 50% of cases [107]. As such they resemble TSTA located on the melanoma cell surface. In general, however, the frequency of individual-specific tumor antigens in melanoma patients is low, of the order of 7% [57].

Other membrane-bound antigens appear to be tumor associated rather than tumor specific, and although a considerable number have now been described, it is probable that most are, as in the similarly neural crest-derived melanomas of the skin, oncofetal or differentiation antigens. To some extent, therefore, the antigenic differences between normal and neoplastic melanocytes are quantitative rather than qualitative.

Some of these tumor-associated antigens belong to the class I and II histocompatibility system, neither class being expressed in normal melanocytes. Class II HLA antigens, particularly HLA-DR antigens, can provoke a T cell response [37] and in the context of cutaneous melanomas correlate with a high metastatic potential [7]. The less well differentiated epithelioid cell melanomas of the choroid are capable of relatively little HLA-DR antigen expression [125], but in vivo irradiation of uveal melanomas in general reduces not only the level of class II HLA expression but also the degree of lymphocytic infiltration of the tumors [60]. The cell adhesion molecule ICAM-1 [90] and expression of tumor-associated α2-macroglobulin [81] are other indices of poor prognosis.

There is evidence from studies of cutaneous melanoma that some of the differentiation antigens are stage specific. Presumed "early" markers occur on the cell surfaces of the relatively undifferentiated epithelioid and amelanotic tumors, "intermediate" markers are characteristic of spindle cells and fetal melanocytes, whereas "late" markers are associated with mature nonneoplastic melanocytes [57].

Considerable overlap is apparent in the melanoma-associated antigens on the surfaces of individual cutaneous [25] and uveal melanomas [133] as revealed by the range of monoclonal antibodies they can generate, although some seem to be more frequent than others and the overlap is far from complete [11]. In the context of skin melanomas, a monoclonal antibody R24, which recognizes a ganglioside (GD3) present in the intercellular adhesion plaques, was found to have an affinity for 58 of 60 tumors examined [25]. Similar antigenic overlap has also been observed in two smaller studies of choroidal melanoma [6,20].

At least five individual-specific cell surface antigens have been identified on cultured skin melanoma cells, one of which is a 90 kDa glycoprotein [97,110]. Moreover, more than 20 distinct monoclonal antibodies against melanoma-associated gangliosides have been produced, the most widely studied of which are AH, directed against ganglioside GD2, and R24, directed against ganglioside GD3 [97,136].

Antigens shared with normal cells, including those of different histogenesis, can also be associated with an immune response. Thus, in an examination of 120 patients with histologically proven uveal melanoma, smooth muscle antibodies were demonstrated in 32 instances [109]. The bearing of this type of reaction, if any, on prognosis is not known.

Immune Reactions

Artificial reduction in T cell activity increases the risk of metastasis of ocular melanoma after enucleation in mice [93], and reducing NK cell numbers has a comparable effect [143]. Alternatively, the infusion of T cells can reverse the risk in thymectomized and irradiated mice that have had melanoma cells inoculated into their anterior chambers [94]. Promoting NK cell and, probably, T cell activity by dosing with a quinoline 3-carboxamide immunomodulator significantly reduced the risk of metastasis of melanoma cells implanted in the anterior chambers of mice, although the primary tumors were unaffected [51].

Somewhat different findings are reported in human melanoma patients. The number of T cells, both helper and suppressor/cytotoxic subtypes, is claimed to be increased in the blood of patients with epithelioid as opposed to spindle cell melanomas [125]. There is also evidence that the total number of lymphocytes detected in histological sections of the tumors (Fig. 3) appears to be linked in an adverse way with survival prospects [101], although an earlier investigation by Rahi and Agarwal [108] failed to show any correlation. The inverse relationship between prognosis and lymphocytic infiltration appears to relate principally to the T cell component [32]. Individuals with choroidal melanomas often have increased numbers of circulating B cells and suppressor T cells [36], but a decrease in T cell activity, as measured by rosetting techniques, is common in patients with metastatic lesions [17]. Curiously, the latter study also demonstrated enhanced cell-mediated function in persons with local extrascleral spread of their tumors.

There are no reports of the use of immunological responses in the treatment of ocular melanoma. As a whole, melanoma-associated antigens are not strongly immunogenic, although there are prospects that the level may be raised using adjuvants [78]. Moreover, it is possible that some of the melanoma-associated antigens with fairly restricted affinities may be used to target cytotoxic agents.

Immunodiagnosis

Monoclonal antibodies raised against cutaneous melanoma-associated antigens and tagged with radioactive labels have been used to detect both hepatic metastases [27] and the primary tumor in patients with uveal melanomas [6,120].

Histological diagnosis is aided by immunohistochemical techniques that employ antisera to proteins in the cytoplasm of melanoma cells. The proteins demonstrated in this way have included S100 protein and neuron-specific enolase [140]. The protein gene product PGP9.5 is another antigen demonstrable in uveal melanomas, particularly in cells surrounding nerve branches [140]. Particularly valuable is the monoclonal antibody HMB 45, which not only appears to be specific but selectively identifies proliferating melanocytic lesions [44a]. Elevated levels of S100 protein have been detected by radioimmunoassay in the vitreous, but not the aqueous, of melanoma patients [18].

B.   Retinoblastoma

Spontaneous regression of retinoblastoma is a well-known, if extremely rare, occurrence [67]. Inevitably there have been attempts to explain the phenomenon in immunological terms, but as yet there is no evidence to confirm or refute the hypothesis, although there are signs that the tumor has antigenic properties and can elicit an immune response.

Antigenicity

The available information about the antigenicity of retinoblastoma cells concerns components that are either tumor associated, in the form of MHC antigens, or shared with the parent tissue.

MHC antigens belonging to both classes I and II have been described. Class I MHC antigens are uncommon, occurring in up to 10% of tumors according to the level of differentiation such that the least differentiated show virtually no activity [24]. Class II (HLA-DR) MHC antigens are much more evident and can be demonstrated in over two-thirds of differentiated tumors and up to 10% of those that are poorly differentiated [24]. Monoclonal antibody staining of cultured retinoblastoma cell lines indicates that there is some sharing of tumor-associated antigens [15].

Interest in tissue-associated antigens in retinoblastoma has been generated by the hope that it will resolve the long-standing debate about whether the tumor has a neuronal or a glial origin: the morphological evidence is overwhelmingly in favor of the former hypothesis, but some doubts have lingered. Ironically, immunohistochemical staining indicates that antigens characteristic of both neuronal and glial tissue may be present, with the inference that the tumor is derived from a primitive neurogenic cell retaining a limited capacity for glial differentiation. Evidence of a neuronal origin based on the detection of neuron-specific enolase in almost all tumors [84,129] must be treated with caution in view of the dubious specificity of this enzyme. Rather more convincing is the demonstration of an antigen shared with rod outer segments [34], which is now thought to be identical to rhodopsin [27]. Evidence of photoreceptor differentiation in the form of retinal S-antigen [83] in a proportion of cells is also supportive of this concept. Conversely, the finding of S100 protein [129] and glial fibrillary acid protein [65,123] in a minority of the retinoblastoma cells is evidence of pluripotentiality [73]. There is also a possibility that an antigen recognized by the PAL-E antibody and considered peculiar to the capillary and venous endothelium of brain tumors [74] may similarly be present in retinoblastomas.

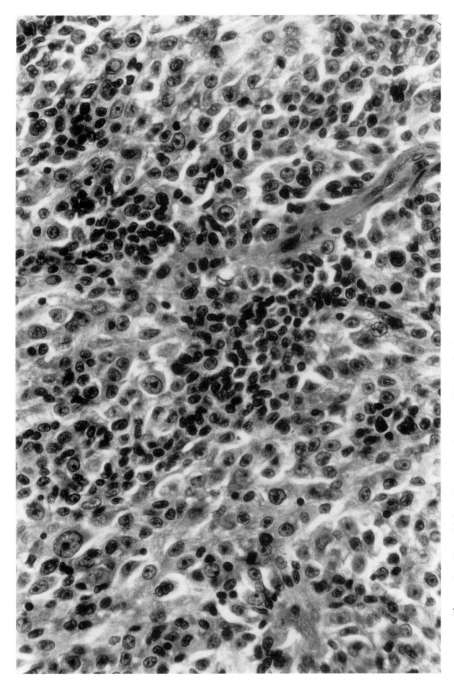

Figure 3   Choroidal malignant melanoma with patchy lymphocytic infiltration. (Hematoxylin and eosin, ×480)

Immune Reactions

Cell-mediated immunity in the form of cutaneous hypersensitivity [14] and in vitro cytotoxicity [13] has been demonstrated using crude tumor extracts. The same workers later detected increased levels of circulating immune complexes in 8 of 13 patients examined [12], but whether the complexes hinder or enhance tumor progression is not known. Reference has been made to the presence in the circulating blood of an immunosuppressive acid protein in retinoblastoma patients [128]. Raised NK cell activity that can be further enhanced by adding interferon-γ has also been described in the peripheral blood of retinoblastoma patients [118]. The relevance of these responses is obscure, and it is important to reiterate that, as Gallie and colleagues [39] remark, there is as yet no evidence that specific cytotoxicity is a feature of regressed retinoblastoma.

Immunotherapy

There have been no significant attempts to influence retinoblastoma behavior by immunological means, although Merriam and others [82] reported that a monoclonal light-chain antibody fragment conjugated with ricin was toxic in vitro to certain retinoblastoma cell lines.

C. Lymphoma

Neoplasia of the lymphoreticular system can affect the optic nerve and retina in the form of large cell lymphoma (previously known as reticulum cell sarcoma), the uvea, the conjunctiva, and the orbit. Lymphoproliferative disease of the orbit, including malignant lymphoma, is considered elsewhere (see Chap. 50), and there is not much information concerning the immunology of the other lymphoid neoplasias of the eye and its environs. It may be noted, however, that lymphomas in general are commonly associated with a degree of immunodeficiency or other systemic immunological abnormalities and that the orbit is no exception. A study in our own laboratory of patients with orbital lymphoproliferative conditions ranging from hyperplasia to neoplasia revealed abnormal levels of circulating immunoglobulins and an increased incidence of autoantibodies [40]. Also, a proportion of the lymphocytes in the undoubtedly malignant proliferations, especially the T cell component, appear to be reactive [71], and it is possible that they exert a restraining effect on the process or, conceivably, promote the tumor through a predominantly helper T cell component [61].

REFERENCES

1. Adams, D.O., Hall, T., Steplewski, Z., and Koprowski, H. Tumors undergoing rejection induced by monoclonal antibodies of the IgG_{2a} isotype contain increased numbers of macrophages activated for a distinct form of antibody dependent cytolysis. *Proc. Natl. Acad. Sci. USA 81*:3506–3510, 1984.
2. Baldwin, R.W., Barker, C.R., Embleton, M.J., Glaves, D., Moore, M., and Pimm, M.V. Demonstration of cell surface antigens on chemically induced tumors. *Ann. NY Acad. Sci. 177*:268–278, 1971.
3. Baldwin, R.W., and Byers, V.S. Monoclonal antibody targeting of cytotoxic agents for cancer therapy. In *Immunology of Malignant Diseases*, V.S. Byers and R.W. Baldwin, (Eds.), MTP Press, Lancaster, PA, pp. 44–54, 1987.
4. Barlozzari, T., Leonhardt, J., Wiltrout, R.H., Herberman, R.B., and Reynolds, C.W. Direct evidence for the role of LGL in the inhibition of experimental tumor metastasis. *J. Immunol. 134*:2783–2789, 1985.
5. Bill, J.R., Friedell, G.H., and Goldenberg, I.S. Prognostic significance of pathologic findings in human breast cancer. *Surg. Gynecol. Obstet. 129*:258–262, 1969.
6. Bomanji, J., Garner, A., Prasad, J., Albert, D.M., Hungerford, J.L., Granowska, M., and Britton, K.E. Characterisation of ocular melanoma with cutaneous melanoma antibodies. *Br. J. Ophthalmol. 71*:647–650, 1987.
7. Brocker, E.-B., Suter, L., Bruggen, J., Ruiter, D.J., Macher, E., and Sorg, C. Phenotypic dynamics of tumour progression in human malignant melanoma. *Int. J. Cancer 36*:29–35, 1985.
8. Burkitt, D.P. Etiology of Burkitt's lymphoma; an alternative hypothesis to vectored virus. *J. Natl. Cancer Inst. 42*:19–28, 1969.
9. Burnet, F.M. Immunological aspects of malignant disease. *Lancet 1*:1171–1174, 1967.
10. Capone, P.M., Papsidero, L.D., Groghan, G.A., and Chi, T.M. Experimental tumoricidal effects of monoclonal antibody against solid breast tumors. *Proc. Natl. Acad. Sci. USA 80*:7328–7332, 1983.
11. Carrel, S., Schreyer, M., Gross, N., and Zografos, L. Surface antigenic profile of uveal melanoma analysed with a panel of antibodies directed against cutaneous melanoma. *Anticancer Res. 10*:81–90, 1990.

12. Char, D.H., Christensen, M., Goldberg, L., and Stein, P. Immune complexes in retinoblastoma. *Am. J. Ophthalmol.* 86:395–399, 1978.

13. Char, D.H., Ellsworth, R., Rabson, A.S., Albert, D.M., and Herberman, R.B. Cell-mediated immunity to a retinoblastoma tissue culture line in patients with retinoblastoma. *Am. J. Ophthalmol.* 78:5–11, 1974.

14. Char, D.H., and Herberman, R.B. Cutaneous delayed hypersensitivity responses of patients with retinoblastoma to standard recall antigens and crude membrane extracts of retinoblastoma tissue culture cells. *Am. J. Ophthalmol.* 78:40–44, 1974.

15. Char, D.H., Wood, I.S., Huhta, K., Rand, N., Morita, C.T., and Howes, E.L., Jr. Retinoblastoma: Tissue culture lines and monoclonal antibody studies. *Invest. Ophthalmol. Vis. Sci.* 25:30–40, 1984.

16. Co, M.S., and Queen, C. Humanized antibodies for therapy. *Nature* 351:501–502, 1991.

17. Cochran, A.J., Foulds, W.S., Damato, B.E., Trope, G.E., Morrison, L., and Lee, W.R. Assessment of immunological techniques in the diagnosis of ocular malignant melanoma. *Br. J. Ophthalmol.* 69:171–176, 1985.

18. Cochran, A.J., Holland, G.N., Saxton, R.E., Damato, B.E., Foulds, W.S., Herschman, H.R., Foos, R.Y., Straatsma, B.R., and Lee, W.R. Detection and quantification of S100 protein in ocular tissues and fluids from patients with intraocular melanomas. *Br. J. Ophthalmol.* 72:874–879, 1988.

19. Cutler, J., Black, M.M., Mork, J., Harvei, S., and Freeman, C. Further observations on prognostic factors in cancer of the female breast. *Cancer* 24:653–667, 1969.

20. Damato, B.E., Campbell, A.M., McGuire, B.J., Lee, W.R., and Foulds, W.S. Monoclonal antibodies to human primary uveal melanomas demonstrate tumor heterogeneity. *Invest. Ophthalmol. Vis. Sci.* 27:1362–1367, 1986.

21. DeBoer, R.J., Hogeweg, P., Dullens, H.F.J., DeWeger, R.A., and DenOtter, W. Macrophage T lymphocyte interactions in the antitumor immune response: A mathematical model. *J. Immunol.* 134:2748–2758, 1985.

22. Defendi, V. Effect of SV40 virus immunization on growth of transplantable SV40 and polyoma virus tumors in hamsters. *Proc. Soc. Exp. Biol. Med.* 113:12–16, 1963.

23. Delsol, G., Brousset, P., Chittal, S., and Rigal-Huguet, F. Correlation of the expression of Epstein-Barr virus latent membrane protein and in situ hybridization with biotinylated *Bam*Hi-W probes in Hodgkin's disease. *Am. J. Pathol.* 140:247–253, 1992.

24. Detrick, B., Chader, G., Katz, N., Rodrigues, M., Suzuki, S., Percopo, C., and Hooks, J.J. Evaluation of class II antigen expression and cellular differentiation in retinoblastoma. *Invest. Ophthalmol. Vis. Sci.* 29(Suppl.):340, 1988.

25. Dippold, W.G., Lloyd, K.D., Li, L.T.C., Ikeda, H., Oettgen, H.F., and Old, L.J. Cell surface antigens of human malignant melanoma: Definition of six antigenic systems with monoclonal antibodies. *Proc. Natl. Acad. Sci. USA* 77:6114–6118, 1980.

26. Donawho, C., and Kripke, M.L. Immunogenicity and cross-reactivity of sygeneic murine melanomas. *Cancer Commun.* 2:101, 1990.

27. Donoso, L.A., Folberg, R., Naids, R., Augsberger, J.J., Shields J.A., and Atkinson, B. Metastatic uveal melanoma: Hepatic metastases identified by hybridoma secreted monoclonal antibody Mab 8-1H. *Arch. Ophthalmol.* 103:799–801, 1985.

28. Donoso, L.A., Hamm, H., Dietzschold, B., Augsberger, J.J., Shields, J.A., and Arbizo, V. Rhodopsin and retinoblastoma: A monoclonal antibody histopathologic study. *Arch. Ophthalmol.* 104:111–113, 1986.

29. Esgro, J.J., Whitworth, P., and Fidler, I.J. Macrophages as effectors of tumor immunity. *Immunol. Allerg. Clin. North Am.* 10:705–729, 1990.

30. Evans, R. Macrophage requirement for growth of a murine fibrosarcoma. *Br. J. Cancer* 37:1086–1989, 1978.

31. Everson, T.C., and Cole, W.H. *Spontaneous Regression of Cancer: A Study and Abstract of Reports in the World Medical Literature and of Personal Communications Concerning Spontaneous Regression of Malignant Disease.* W.B. Saunders, Philadelphia, 1966.

32. Farah, S., Whelchel, J.C., McLean, I.W., and Burnier, M.M. Immunohistochemistry of infiltrating lymphocytes in uveal malignant melanoma. *Invest. Ophthalmol. Vis. Sci.* (Suppl) 33:1242, 1992.

33. Fass, L., Heberman, R.B., Ziegler, J.L., and Kiryawire, J.W.M. Cutaneous hypersensitivity reactions to autologous extracts of malignant melanoma cells. *Lancet* 1:116–118, 1970.

34. Felberg, N.T., and Donoso, L.A. Surface and cytoplasmic antigens in retinoblastoma. *Invest. Ophthalmol. Vis. Sci.* 19:1242–1245, 1980.

35. Finlay, C.A., Hinds, P.W., Tan, T.-H., Eliyahu, D., Oren, M., and Levine, A.J. Activating mutations for transformation by p53 produce a gene product that forma an hsc70-p53 complex with an altered half-life. *Mol. Cell. Biol.* 8:531–539, 1988.

36. Flynn, K., Felberg, N.T., Koegel, A., Hager, R., Shields, J.A., Augsburger, J.J., and Donoso, L.A. Lymphocyte subpopulations before therapy in patients with uveal malignant melanoma. *Am. J. Ophthalmol.* 101:160–163, 1986.

37. Fossati, G., Taramelli, D., Balsari, A., Bodganovitch, S., Andreola, A., and Parmiani, G. Primary but not metastatic human melanomas expressing DR antigens stimulate autologous lymphocytes. *Int. J. Cancer* 33:591–597, 1984.

38. Fraumeni, J.F. Constitutional disorders of man leading to leukemia and lymphoma. *National Cancer Institute Monograph, Hemopoietic Neoplasms*, Vol. 32. 221–232, 1969.

39. Gallie, B., Ellsworh, R.M., Abramson, D.H., and Phillips, R.A. Retinoma: Spontaneous regression of retinoblastoma or benign manifestation of the mutation? *Br. J. Cancer. 45*:513–521, 1982.

40. Garner, A., Rahi, A.H.S., and Wright, J.E. Lymphoproliferative disorders of the orbit: An immunological approach to diagnosis and pathogenesis. *Br. J. Ophthalmol. 67*:561–569, 1983.

41. Goder, G., and Velhagen, K.H. Die Bertalanffy-Methode zum Nachweis von Tumorzellen in Blut bei Geschwulsten des Auges. *Ophthalmologica (Basel) 161*:372–384, 1970.

42. Gold, P. Antigenic reversion in human cancer. *Annu. Rev. Med. 22*:85–94, 1971.

43. Gold, P., and Freedman, S. Specific carcinoembryonic antigens of the human digestive system. *J. Exp. Med. 122*:467–481, 1965.

44. Goldenberg, D.M. Targeting of cancer with radiolabeled antibodies: Prospects for imaging and therapy. *Arch. Pathol. Lab. Med. 112*:580–587, 1988.

44a. Gown, A.M., Vogel, A.M., Hoak, D., Gough, F., and McNutt, M.A. Monoclonal antibodies specific for melanocytic tumors distinguish subpopulations of melanocytes. *Am. J. Pathol. 123*:195–203, 1986.

45. Gray, P.W., Aggarawal, B.B., Benton, C.V., Bringman, T.S., Henzel, W.J., Jarrett, J.A., Leung, D.W., Moffat, B., Ng, P., Svedvsky, L.P., Palladino, M.A., and Nadwin, G. Cloning and expression of a DNA for human lymphotoxin, a lymphokine with tumor necrosis activity. *Nature 312*:721–724, 1984.

46. Green, H.N. An immunological concept of cancer: A preliminary report. *Br. Med. J. 2*:1374–1380, 1954.

47. Hainaut, P., Weynants, P., Coulie, P.G., and Boon, T. Anti-tumor T-cell responses. *Immunol. Allergy Clin. North Am. 10*:639–662, 1990.

48. Hakamori, S. Biochemical basis of tumor-associated carbohydrate antigens. *Immunol. Allergy Clin. North Am. 10*:781–802, 1990.

49. Haliotis, T., Ball, J.K., Dexter, D., and Roder, J.C. Spontaneous and induced primary oncogenesis in natural killer (NK) cell deficient beige mutant mice. *Int. J. Cancer 35*:505–513, 1985.

50. Harboe, M., and Quayle, A.J. Heat shock proteins: Friend or foe? *Clin. Exp. Immunol. 86*:2–5, 1991.

51. Harning, R., and Szalay, J. A treatment for metastasis of murine ocular melanoma. *Invest. Ophthalmol. Vis. Sci. 29*:1505–1510, 1988.

52. Harris, J.E., and Sinkovics, J.G. *The Immunology of Malignant Disease.* C.V. Mosby, St. Louis, MO, 1970.

53. Hellstrom, I., Sjogren, H.O., Warner, G., and Hellstrom, K.E. Blocking of cell-mediated tumor immunity by sera from patients with growing neoplasms. *Int. J. Cancer 7*:226–237, 1971.

54. Hewitt, H.B. The choice of animal tumors for experimental study of cancer therapy. *Adv. Cancer Res. 27*:149–200, 1979.

55. Hoover, R., and Fraumeni, J.F., Jr. Risk of cancer in renal transplant recipients. *Lancet 2*:55–57, 1973.

56. Hostetler, L.W., Ananthaswamy, H.N., and Kripke, M.L. Generation of tumor-specific transplantation antigens by UV radiation can occur independently of neoplastic transformation. *J. Immunol. 137*:2721–2724, 1986.

57. Houghton, A.N., Cordon-Carlo, C., and Eisinger, M. Differentiation antigens of melanoma and melanocytes. *Int. Rev. Exp. Pathol. 28*:217–248, 1986.

58. Houghton, A.N., Mintzer, D., Cordon-Carlo, S., Welt, S., Fleigel, B., Vadhan, D., Carswell, E., Melamed, M.R., Oettgen, H.F., and Old, L.J. Mouse monoclonal IgG3 antibody detecting GD3 ganglioside: A phase 1 trial in patients with malignant melanoma. *Proc. Natl. Acad. Sci. USA 82*:1242–1246, 1985.

59. Hutchin, P. Mechanisms and functions of immunologic enhancement. *Surg. Gynecol. Obstet. 126*:1331–1356, 1968.

60. Jager, M.J., van der Pol, J.P., de Wolff-Rouendaal, D., de Jong, P.V.T.M., and Ruiter, D.J. Decreased expression of HLA Class II antigens on human uveal melanoma cells after in vivo x-ray irradiation. *Am. J. Ophthalmol. 105*:78–86, 1988.

61. Jakobiec, F.A., Neri, A., and Knowles, D.M., II. Genotypic monoclonality in immunophenotypically polyclonal orbital lymphoid tumors. *Ophthalmology 94*:980–994, 1987.

62. Janeway, C.A., Bottomly, K., Babich, J., Conrad, P., Conzen, S., Jones, B., Kaye, J., Katz, M., McVay, L., Murphy, D.P., and Tite, J. Quantitative variation in Ia expression plays a central role in immune regulation. *Immunol. Today 5*:99–105, 1984.

63. Jehn, M.W., Nathanson, L., and Schwartz, R. Lymphocyte sensitivity to tumor antigens in malignant melanoma (abstract). *Proc. Am. Ass. Cancer Res. 11*:40, 1970.

64. Jenkins, G.D. Regression of pulmonary metastasis following nephrectomy fot hypernephroma: Eight year follow-up. *J. Urol. 82*:37–40, 1959.

65. Jiang, Q., Lim, R., and Blodi, F.C. Dual properties of cultured retinoblastoma cells: Immunohistochemical characterization of neuronal and glial markers. *Exp. Eye Res. 39*:207–215, 1984.

66. Kerr, J.F.R., Wyllie, A.H., and Currie, A.R. Apoptosis: A basic biological phenomenon with wide ranging implications in tissue kinetics. *Br. J. Cancer 26*:239–257, 1972.

67. Khodadoust, A.A., Roozitalab, H.M., Smith, R.E., and Green, W.R. Spontaneous regression of retinoblastoma. *Surv. Ophthalmol. 21*:467–478, 1977.

68. Klein, G., and Klein, E. Evolution of tumours and the impact of molecular oncology. *Nature 315*:190–195, 1985.

69. Klein, G., and Oettgen, H.F. Immunologic factors involved in the growth of primary tumors in human or animal hosts. *Cancer Res. 29*:1741–1746, 1969.

70. Klein, G., Sjögren, H.O., Klein, E., and Hellstrom, K.E. Demonstration of resistance against methyl-cholanthrene induced sarcomas in the primary autochthonous host. *Cancer Res.* 20:1561–1572, 1960.

71. Knowles, D.M., II, and Jakobiec, F.A. Identification of T lymphocytes in ocular adnexal neoplsms by hybridoma monoclonal antibodies. *Am. J. Ophthalmol.* 95:233–242, 1983.

72. Kripke, M.L. Principles of tumor immunology: Lessons from animal models. *Immunol. Allergy Clin. North Am.* 10:595–606, 1990.

73. Kyritsis, A.P., Tsokos, M., Triche, T.J., and Chader, G.J. Retinoblastoma: Origin from a primitive neuroecto-dermal cell. *Nature 307*:471–473, 1984.

74. Leenstra, S., Das, P., Troost, D., Bosch, D., Essen, N., and Becker, A. PAL-E, monoclonal antibody with immunoreactivity for endothelium specific to brain tumours. *Lancet 335*:671, 1990.

75. Levine, A.J., Momand, J., and Finlay, C.A. The p53 tumour suppressor gene. *Nature 351*:453–456, 1991.

76. Lewis, M.G., Ikonopisor, R.L., Nairn, R.C., Philips, T.M., Fairley, G.H., Bodenham D.C., and Alexander, P. Tumour-specific antibodies in human malignant melanoma and their relationship to the extent of the disease. *Br. Med. J. 3*:547–552, 1969.

77. Lichtenstein, A. Granulocytes as possible effectors of tumor immunity. *Immunol. Allergy Clin. North Am.* 10:731–746, 1990.

78. Livingston, P., Takeyama, H., Pollack, M., Houghton, A.N., Albino, A., Oettgen, H.F., and Old, L.J. Serological responses of melanoma patients to vaccines derived from allogeneic cultured melanoma cells. *Int. J. Cancer 31*:567–575, 1983.

79. Malik, S.T.A. Tumour necrosis factor: Roles in cancer pathophysiology. *Semin. Cancer Biol. 3*:27–33, 1992.

80. Maluish, A.E., Ortaldo, J.R., Conlon, J.C., Sherwin, S.A., Leavitt, R., Strong, D.M., Wernick, P., Oldham, R.K., and Herberman, R.B. Depression of natural killer cell cytotoxicity after in vivo administration of recombinant leukocyte interferon. *J. Immunol. 131*:503–507, 1983.

81. Matoska, J., Wahlstrom, T., Vaheri, A., Bizik, J., and Grofora, M. Tumour-associated alpha-2-macroglobulin in human melanomas. *Int. J. Cancer 41*:359–363, 1988.

82. Merriam, J.C., Lyon, H.S., and Char, D.H. Toxicity of a monoclonal F(ab')2:ricin A conjugate for reti-noblastoma in vitro. *Cancer Res. 44*:3178–3183, 1984.

83. Mirshahi, M., Boucheix, C., Dhermy, P., Haye, C., and Faure, J-P. Expression of the photoreceptor-specific S antigen in human retinoblastoma. *Cancer 57*:1497–1500, 1986.

84. Molnar, M.L., Stefansson, K., Marton, L.S., Tripathi, R.S., and Molnar, G.V. Immunohistochemistry of retinoblastomas in humans. *Am. J. Ophthalmol. 97*:301–307, 1984.

85. Moore, G.E., Sandberg, A., and Silverberg, J.R. Clinical and experimental observations of the occurrence and fate of tumor cells in the blood stream. *Ann. Surg. 146*:580–587, 1957.

86. Moore, G.P. Genetically engineered antibodies. *Clin. Chem. 25*:1849–1853, 1989.

87. Morton, D.L., Malmgren, R.A., Holmes, E.C., and Ketcham, A.S. Demonstration of antibodies against human malignant melanoma by immunofluorescence. *Surgery 64*:233–240, 1968.

88. Mule, Shu S., and Rosenberg, S.A. The anti-tumour efficacy of lymphokine-activated killer cells and recombi-nant interleukin 2 in vivo. *J. Immunol. 135*:646–652, 1985.

89. Nagel, G.A., Piessens, W.F., Stilmant, M.M., and Lejeune, F. Evidence for tumor-specific immunity in human malignant melanoma. *Eur. J. Cancer 7*:1–47, 1971.

90. Natali, P., Nicotra, M.R., Cavaliere, R., Bigotto, A., Romano, G., Temponi, M., and Ferrone, S. Differential expression of intercellular adhesion molecule 1 in primary and metastatic melanoma lesions. *Cancer Res. 50*:1271–1278, 1990.

91. Nathanson, L., Hall, T.C., and Farber, S. Biological aspects of human malignant melanoma. *Cancer 20*:650–655, 1967.

92. Ngu, V.A. Host defences to Burkitt tumour. *Br. Med. J. 1*:345–347, 1967.

93. Niederkorn, J.Y. Enucleation in consort with immunologic impairment promotes metastasis of intraocular melanoma in mice. *Invest. Ophthalmol. Vis. Sci. 25*:1080–1086, 1984.

94. Niederkorn, J.Y. T cell subsets involved in the rejection of metastases arising from intraocular melanomas in mice. *Invest. Ophthalmol. Vis. Sci. 28*:1397–1403, 1987.

95. Nitta, T., Sato, K., Yagita, H., Okumura, K., and Ishi, H. Preliminary trials of specific targeting therapy against malignant glioma. *Lancet 335*:368–371, 1990.

96. North, R.J. Down-regulation of the antitumor immune response. *Adv. Cancer Res. 45*:1–43, 1985.

97. Oettgen, H.F., Retting, W.J., Lloyd, K.O., and Old, L.J. Serologic analysis of human cancers. *Immunol. Allergy Clin. North Am.* 10:607–637, 1990.

98. Old, L.J., Boyse, E.A., Clarke, D.A., and Carswell, F.A. Antigenic properties of chemically induced tumors. *Ann. NY Acad. Sci. 101*:80–106, 1962.

99. Olsnes, S., Sandvig, K., Petersen, O.W., and van Deurs, B. Immunotoxins: Entry into cells and mechanisms of action. *Immunol. Today 10*:291–295, 1989.

100. O'Toole, C., Perlmann, P., Unsgaard, B., Moberger, G., and Edsmyr, F. Cellular immunity to human urinary bladder carcinoma. *Int. J. Cancer 10*:77–98, 1972.

101. Panfilo, O., De La Cruz, P.O., Specht, C.S., and McLean, I.W. Lymphocytic infiltration of uveal melanoma. *Invest. Ophthalmol. Vis. Sci. (Suppl) 29*:365, 1988.

102. Penn, I. Why do immunosuppressed patients develop cancer? *Crit. Rev. Oncogen. 1*:27–52, 1989.
103. Pimm, M.V. Immunoscintigraphy; tumour detection with radiolabelled antitumour monoclonal antibodies. In *Immunology of Malignant Diseases*, V.S. Byers and R.W. Baldwin (Eds.) MTP Press, Lancaster, PA, pp. 21–24, 1987.
104. Pruitt, J.C., Hilberg, A.W., and Kaiser, R.F. Malignant cells in blood. *N. Engl. J. Med. 259*:1161–1164, 1958.
105. Puri, R.K., Leland, P., and Razzaque, A. Antigen specific tumor infiltrating lymphocytes from tumor induced by human herpes virus (HPV-6) DNA transfected NIH3T3 transformats. *Clin. Exp. Immunol. 83*:96–101, 1990.
106. Purtilo, D.T. Opportunistic cancers in patients with immunodeficiency syndromes. *Arch. Pathol. Lab. Med. 111*:1123–1129, 1988.
107. Rahi, A.H.S. Autoimmune reactions in malignant melanoma. *Br. J. Ophthalmol. 55*:793–807, 1971.
108. Rahi, A.H.S., and Agarwal, P.K. Prognostic parameters in choroidal melanomata. *Trans. Ophthalmol. Soc. UK 97*:368–372, 1977.
109. Rahi, A.H.S., Garner, A., and Malaty, A.H.A. Contractile protein antigen in the cells of malignant melanoma of the choroid and their diagnostic significance. *Br. J. Ophthalmol. 62*:394–401, 1978.
110. Real, F.X., Furukawa, K.S., and Mattes, M.J. Class I (unique) tumor antigens of human melanoma: Identification of unique and common epitopes on a 90KD glycoprotein. *Proc. Natl. Acad. Sci. USA 85*:3891–3895, 1988.
111. Riesco, A. Five year cancer cure: Relation to total amount of peripheral lymphocytes and neutrophils. *Cancer 25*:135–140, 1970.
112. Roberts, A.B., Kim, S., and Sporn, M.B. Is there a common pathway mediating growth inhibition by TGF-beta and the retinoblastoma gene product? *Cancer Cells 3*:19–21, 1991.
113. Robins, R. A basic tumour immunology. In *Immunology of Malignant Diseases*, V.S. Byers and R.W. Baldwin (Eds.), MTP Press, Lancaster, PA, pp. 1–28, 1987.
114. Rosenbaum, J.T., Howes, E.L., Jr., Rubin, R.M., and Samples, J.R. Ocular inflammatory effects of intravitreally-injected tumor necrosis factor. *Am. J. Pathol. 133*:47–53, 1988.
115. Rosenberg, S.A., Lotze, M.T., Muul, M., Chang, A.E., Aris, F.P., Leitman, S., Linehan, W.M., Robertson, C.M., Lee, R.E., Rubin, J.T., Seipp, C.A., Simpson, C.G., and White, D.E. A progress report on the treatment of 157 patients with advanced cancer using LAK and IL-2 or IL-2 alone. *N. Engl. J. Med. 316*:889–897, 1987.
116. Rosenberg, S., Spiess, P., and Lafrieniere, R. A new approach to adoptive immunotherapy of cancer with tumor infiltrating lymphocytes. *Science 233*:1318–1321, 1986.
117. Russell, S.J. Lymphokine gene therapy. *Immunol. Today 11*:196–200, 1990.
118. Sasabe, T., Kiritoshi, A., Ohashi, Y., and Manabe, R. Interferon enhances the natural killer cell activity of the retinoblastoma patients to autologous retinoblastoma cells. *Ophthalmic Paediatr. Genet. 8*:43–46, 1987.
119. Savel, H. Effect of autologous tumor extracts on cultured human peripheral blood lymphocytes. *Cancer 24*:56–63, 1969.
120. Schaling, D.F., van der Pol, J.P., Jager, M.J., van Kroonenburgh, M.J.P.G., Oosterhuis, J.A., and Ruiter, D.J. Radioimmunoscintigraphy and immunohistochemistry with melanoma-associated monoclonal antibodies in choroidal melanoma: A comparison of the clinical and immunohistochemical results. *Br. J. Ophthalmol. 74*:538–541, 1990.
121. Sheil, A.G.R. Cancer in organ transplant recipients: Part of an induced immune deficiency syndrome. *Br. Med. J. 288*:659–661, 1984.
122. Shibata, D., and Weiss, L.M. Epstein-Barr virus-associated gastric adenocarcinoma. *Am. J. Pathol. 140*:769–774, 1992.
123. Shuangshoti, S., Chaiwun, B., and Kasantikul, V. A study of 39 retinoblastomas with particular reference to morphology, cellular differentiation, and tumour origin. *Histopathology 15*:113–124, 1989.
124. Sjögren, H.O., Hellstrom, I., Bansal, S.C., and Hellstrom, K.E. Suggestive evidence that "blocking antibodies" of tumor-bearing individuals may be antigen-antibody complexes. *Proc. Natl. Acad. Sci. USA 68*:1372–1375, 1971.
125. Smith, M.D., Liggett, P.E., and Rao, N.A. Immunohistochemical characterization of lymphoid infiltration in human choroidal melanomas. *Invest. Ophthalmol. Vis. Sci. (Suppl) 29*:365, 1988.
126. Streilein, J.W. Immunogenetic factors in skin cancer. *N. Engl. J. Med. 325*:884–886, 1991.
127. Sumner, W.C., and Foraker, A.G. Spontaneous regression of human melanoma: Clinical and experimental studies. *Cancer 13*:79–81, 1960.
128. Takahashi, R., Yamaguchi, K., and Tamai, M. Quantitative measurement of immunosuppressive acidic protein (AP) in patients with retinoblastoma (Japanese). *Acta Soc Ophthalmol. Jpn. 94*:593–596, 1990.
129. Terenghi, G., Polak, J.M., Ballesta, J., Cocchia, D., Michetti, F., Dahl, D., Marangos, P.J., and Garner, A. Immunocytochemistry of neuronal and glial markers in retinoblastoma. *Virchows Arch. [A] 40*:61–73, 1984.
130. Thorley-Lawson, D.A. Basic virologic aspects of Epstein-Barr virus infection. *Semin. Hematol. 25*:247–260, 1988.
131. Ullrich, S.J., Robinson, E.A., Law, L.W., Willingham, M., and Appella, E. A mouse tumor-specific transplantation antigen is a heat-shock related protein. *Proc. Natl. Acad. Sci. USA 83*:3121–3125, 1986.
132. Urban, J.L., van Waes, C., and Schreiber, H. Pecking order among tumour specific antigens. *Eur. J. Immunol. 14*:181–187, 1984.

133. van der Pol, J.P., Jager, M.J., de Wolff-Rouendaal, D., Ringens, P.J., Vernegoor, C., and Ruiter, D.J. Heterogenous expression of melanoma associated antigens in uveal melanomas. *Curr. Eye Res.* 6:757–765, 1987.
134. Vanky, F., Klein, E., Williams, J., Brook, K., Ivert, T., Petterfy, A., Nilsonne, V., Kreicbergs, A., and Aparisi, T. Lysis of autologous tumor cells by blood lymphocytes tested at the time of surgery: Correlation with postsurgical course. *Cancer Immunol. Immunother.* 21:69–76, 1986.
135. Vose, B.M. Immunomodulating agents. In *Immunology of Malignant Diseases*, V.S. Byers and R.W. Baldwin (Eds.), MTP Press, Lancaster, PA, pp. 70–82, 1987.
136. Watanabe, T., Pukel, C.S., and Takeyama, H. Human melanoma antigen AH is an autoantigenic ganglioside related to GD2. *J. Exp. Med.* 156:1884–1886, 1982.
137. Wawrzynczak, E.J., and Davies, A.J.S. Strategies in antibody therapy of cancer. *Clin. Exp. Immunol.* 82:189–193, 1990.
138. Weatherall, D. Tomorrow's biotechnology. *Br. Med. J.* 303:1282–1283, 1991.
139. Whiteside, T.L., and Herberman, R.B. Characteristics of natural killer cells and lymphokine-activated killer cells. *Immunol. Allergy Clin. North Am.* 10:663–704, 1990.
140. Williams, R.A., Rode, J., Dhillon, A.P., Charlton, I.G., and McCartney, A. PGP9.5, S100 protein and neurone specific enolase in ocular melanomas. *J. Pathol.* 152:195A, 1987.
141. Winfield, J.B. Stress proteins: arthritis and autoimmunity. *Arthritis Rheum.* 32:1497–1504, 1989.
142. Woodruff, M.F. Cancer: The elusive enemy. *Proc. R. Soc. Lond. [B] 183*:87–104, 1973.
143. Yokoyama, T., Yoshie, O., Aso, H., Ebina, T., Ishida, N., and Mizuno, K. Role of natural killer cells in intraocular melanoma metastasis. *Invest. Ophthalmol. Vis. Sci.* 27:516–518, 1986.
144. Yonish-Rouach, E., Resnitzky, D., Lotem, J., Sachs, L., and Kimchi, A. Wild type P53 induces apoptosis of myeloid leukaemia cells that is inhibited by IL-6. *Nature* 352:345–347, 1991.

52
Vascular Diseases

Alec Garner
Institute of Ophthalmology, University of London, London, England

I. NORMAL BLOOD VESSELS

A. Development

The vascular system is a mesodermal structure with endothelium and, ultimately, definitive blood vessels arising from islands of primordial mesenchyme. Initially the emergent vessels are in the form of a capillary plexus (Fig. 1), as originally described by Aeby [5], and it is from such networks that there develops a recognizable system of arteries, capillaries, and veins by a process that involves atrophy of some vessels and hypertrophy of others. It has long been acknowledged that the earliest vascular development is under genetic control and that it involves the maturation of in situ foci of angioblastic mesoderm [452], although a subsidiary contribution by migrant angioblasts is also likely [408]. In this way solid cords of endothelium are created, these later linking with other cords to form a network of luminized capillaries. Subsequent growth is increasingly dependent on sprouting from these early vessels [404].

A major factor influencing the proliferation and maturation of the vasculature in the later stages of embryogenesis and fetal development is local metabolic demand, and it seems probable that this control persists throughout life. Other factors include hemodynamic forces, especially intraluminal pressure, and waning genetic influence. It is possible that genetic factors govern the development of the larger vessels more than they do the smaller channels, since the former can proceed for a time in the absence of blood flow [97]; the smaller vessels, however, are entirely dependent on an active circulation for their maturation.

Initial activity is concerned with cell proliferation and migration, functions facilitated by fibronectin secretion. There then follows a switch to laminin production, which induces further differentiation so that a lumen is formed [229] and cell-to-cell attachments develop. Anchorage of the developing endothelium to the extracellular matrix is vitally important [408], and production of heparan sulfate proteoglycan and the cell adhesion-promoting nidogen/entactin molecule encourages stability, type IV collagen serving to bind the various components and form a basement membrane on the abluminal side of the capillary. There are various possibilities concerning the emergence of a lumen, including the partial separation of adjacent cells and the formation of a transcellular channel within a single cell [183]. The addition of pericytes, smooth muscle cells, and fibroblasts to the outer aspect of the maturing vessels is less well understood but is believed to involve the perivascular mesenchyme [404].

These general principles are similarly observed in the embryogenesis of the ocular circulation, the latter having been studied most thoroughly in the retina, where a close meshwork of capillaries is laid down by in situ mesenchyme [182], possibly emanating from the adventitia of established vessels at the optic disk. Subsequently, some capillaries become acellular by a process of retraction or degeneration of the endothelial lining and are reduced to mere strands of basement membrane, whereas others hypertrophy and become recognizable arterioles and venules, depending on their relationship to the parent artery and vein [29]. The importance of tissue oxygenation in determining the density of the vascular bed in the retina is demonstrated by the wide capillary-free zone formed around the arterioles [90,387]; that surrounding the veins is considerably narrower (Fig. 2).

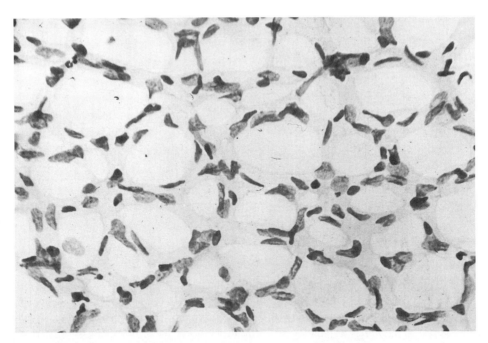

Figure 1 Embryonic development of peripheral vascular bed. Enzyme digest preparation of the developing vasculature in the retina of a 20-week-old fetus shows a network of endothelium-lined capillaries. Subsequent development involves the selective atrophy of some capillaries and the hypertrophy of others before the definitive circulation is established. (Hematoxylin and eosin, ×190). (Reproduced with permission from A. Garner, Ocular angiogenesis. *Int. Rev. Exp. Pathol. 28*:249–306, 1986).

B. Structure

The cardiovascular system is a continuum, and although it is clear that the regions responsible for conveying blood to the tissues, for allowing exchange of metabolites within the tissues, and for drainage have distinct properties, it is also clear that the transition from one to the next is a gradual process. Consequently, criteria for describing the various types of vessel within the system should not be interpreted too rigidly.

Arteries

Arteries have three coats: an inner intima provided by a single layer of endothelium resting on a collagenous zone in which smooth muscle cells and fibroblasts can be recognized, a media formed by smooth muscle, collagen, and elastic fibers, and an outer adventitia consisting of loose connective tissue. Between the coats of the larger vessels are elastic laminae, formed by condensation and cross-linkage of multiple elastic fibers, which completely encircle the wall.

The largest arteries, such as the aorta and its main branches, including the carotid vessels, must withstand the wide fluctuation in intraluminal tension that takes place between cardiac systole and diastole. The need is provided for by the presence of large amounts of elastic tissue within the medial coat, the recoil properties of which act as an energy reservoir and serve to propagate the onward movement of a pulse wave. The tensile properties of the collagen fibers, on the other hand, prevent overdistension during systole.

Arteries of smaller caliber, such as the ophthalmic artery and its branches, have rather less elastic tissue since they are required to withstand considerably smaller distending forces (intravascular pressure is proportional to the fourth power of the radius). Conversely, they have a greater proportion of muscular tissue, individual smooth muscle cells being wrapped around the intimal lining in a predominantly helical fashion, to facilitate the regulation of blood flow through the lumen.

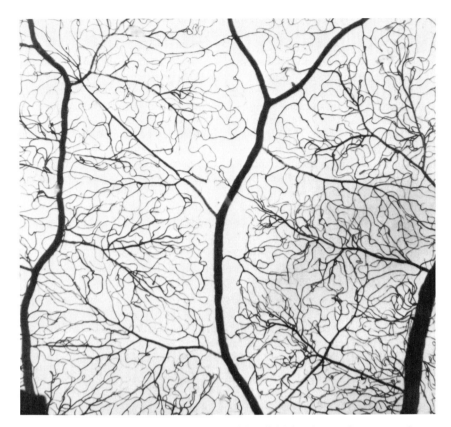

Figure 2   Flat preparation of a human retina injected with colloidal carbon to demonstrate the patent blood vessels. Next to the arteriole there is a zone free of perfused capillaries and considered a measure of the relatively high oxygen tension on the arterial side of the circulation since no such zone is adjacent to the venule. (×25)

Arterioles

As their name implies, arterioles are minute arteries and the distinction between a small artery and a large arteriole is inevitably somewhat arbitrary. Definitions have been based, variously, on internal diameter, absence of a continuous internal elastic lamina, and the number of smooth muscle cells in cross sections of the wall. Rhodin [457] makes a distinction between arterioles measuring between 50 and 100 μm with more than one layer of smooth muscle and a well-developed internal elastic lamina and terminal arterioles, with a caliber of 30–50 μm, a single layer of smooth muscle, and scanty or absent elastic tissue. As the capillary bed is approached, the elastic component diminishes and the muscle coat becomes discontinuous. The terminal or precapillary arterioles are the final arbiters of blood supply to the capillaries, and some, although not the retinal or uveal vessels of humans [273], have additional muscle fibers encircling the mouths of the capillaries to form sphincters. Selective perfusion regulated by sphincteric action does not appear to be a feature of the retinal circulation, the entire capillary bed being perfused at all times.

   It is within the small arteries and arterioles that the drop from an arterial pressure of around 100/70 mm Hg to nonpulsatile flow at approximately 25 mm Hg takes place, the rapid fall being attributable to the greatly increased surface area relative to blood volume and, hence, the frictional resistance to flow pertaining in vessels of small caliber.

Capillaries

Capillaries are distinguished from terminal arterioles by being entirely devoid of smooth muscle. They consist of a lumen lined by a single layer of endothelium resting on a basal lamina. In most capillaries, including those of ocular structures, a second type of cell lies external to the endothelium but still within the outer basal lamina. Now generally referred to as pericytes, such cells in the retinal circulation were originally called mural cells [338], but this term has tended to lapse since subsequent study has indicated their kinship with pericytes elsewhere.

Myofilaments have been described in the cytoplasm of both endothelial cells and pericytes, and both smooth muscle actin and myosin are present in pericytes [276]. Furthermore, it seems that the pericytes of bovine retinal capillaries possess receptors for the potent vasoconstrictor peptide endothelin-1 [449a,512] and that such receptors may be a general feature of the ocular circulation as a whole [204]. The extent to which this potential for caliber variation at the capillary level is involved in regulating ocular blood flow remains to be defined [95], but the possibility that endothelin-1 is fundamental to autoregulation is strong, especially because there is evidence that it is secreted in a paracrine fashion by the endothelial cells [554]. Endothelin-1 acts by initiating a sequence that results in prostaglandin E2 and thromboxane production [561]. The significance of the finding that the vasodilator prostacyclin can be synthesized by retinal capillary pericytes in culture is obscure [288].

The cells of the lining endothelium are generally linked by means of desmosomes, but those of the retinal circulation are characterized by tight encircling junctions (zonulae occludentes) to constitute an inner blood-retinal barrier. This effectively means that the movement of molecules in excess of a few hundred daltons between the lumen and the extravascular compartment must be transcellular. Induction of this type of junction appears to be a function of the retina per se, if comparisons with the cerebral circulation are valid, and to depend on the presence of astrocytes [297].

Venules

The only structural difference between the smallest venules and capillaries is one of caliber. Functionally, however, venules are more permeable, more susceptible to vasoactive amines, such as histamine, and more apt to become thrombosed than are capillary vessels. The larger venules have smooth muscle cells in their walls.

Veins

Veins have a narrow layer of smooth muscle in their walls and a little elastic tissue. Both are less conspicuous than in arteries of the same size, and in consequence, veins are relatively more distensible and are able to function as capacitance vessels.

C. Cellular and Other Vascular Components

Endothelium

Despite being continuous throughout the cardiovascular system, the lining endothelial cells vary in morphology and function to some degree according to the order of vessel size and the nature of the organ or tissue served. Even so, certain general properties can be identified [295,434]:

1. Preservation of vascular integrity with respect to maintaining uninterrupted blood flow by inducing platelet aggregation to plug injured sites and by triggering the extrinsic pathway of clotting.
2. Inhibition of inappropriate intravascular thrombosis and lysis of established clots.
3. Regulation of vascular permeability by virtue of active and passive transcellular transport and intercellular junctional complexes.
4. Participation in the control of vascular tone. Both vasodilator and vasoconstrictor substances are produced within the endothelium, nitric oxide (endothelium-derived relaxing factor) [420] being a potent mediator of the first of these functions and endothelin-1 [554] an equally effective mediator of the second.
5. Source of growth factors involved in angiogenesis and wound repair.
6. Inflammatory role in terms of leukocyte binding through the expression of specific adhesion molecules and subsequent egress. The endothelium can also express class II major histocompatibility complex antigens and function as an antigen-presenting tissue in immunological reactions.
7. Source of basement membrane constituents and other extracellular proteins, such as fibronectin.

Contractile filaments have been demonstrated in the cytoplasm of vascular endothelium, including that of the retina, by electron microscopy and immunofluorescence (Fig. 3) [448,556]. Filaments containing actin and myosin are particularly prominent in newly formed endothelium and may be related to the capacity of new vessels to infiltrate surrounding tissue.

The vascular endothelial cell is a manifestly complex cell with diverse functions, and it has a seminal role in the development of most vasculopathies, including those affecting the eye.

Smooth Muscle

Vascular smooth muscle cells are spindle shaped and measure from 20 to 50 μm in length. Their distinctive feature is a uniformly high density of contractile protein filaments, mostly in the form of a cell-specific actin, in the cytoplasm aligned parallel to the long axis of the cells. Contraction can be provoked by mechanical stretching, metabolic factors, and, in all but intraretinal vessels, adrenergic nerve stimulation.

Pericytes

Cells lying external to the endothelial lining are a feature of capillaries in all ocular tissues. Each cell has multiple pseudopodial processes that envelop the capillary and are sandwiched between layers of basement membrane; in the retina about 85% of the lining endothelium is covered in this way [196]. Other than a suggestion that they arise from the perivascular mesenchyme, their histogenesis is not clear. They are distinct from the endothelium, however, because they do not react with antibodies to factor VIII antigen or with the *Ulex europaeus* lectin. They also synthesize large quantities of heparan sulfate in vitro [508].

The location of the pericytes invites comparison with the smooth muscle of larger vessels, especially because they contain the smooth muscle isoforms of both actin and myosin [276]. Should the transmural pressure be increased, as occurs in shunt vessels, they will transform into muscle cells [38] and, as previously noted, have receptors for endothelin-1. Nevertheless, there is no good evidence that they exercise an appreciable contractile function under normal conditions, although it is feasible that the abnormal blood flow in diabetic microangiopathy is directly linked to pericyte dysfunction.

An in vitro inhibitory effect on endothelial cell proliferation, possibly mediated by transforming growth factor β [12], has also been described [417].

Basement Membrane

The endothelial lining of the cardiovascular system rests on an acellular membrane that is essentially amorphous, although electron microscopy may reveal occasional fine 4 nm filaments within the granular matrix. The basic component of vascular basement membranes, as with those elsewhere, is type IV collagen, which acts as a structural backbone and binds to the other membrane components; it also has an inhibitory effect on endothelial cell proliferation [462], such that basement membrane dissolution is obligatory before new vessel formation can take place [542]. Laminin is another major constituent relating primarily to cell attachment, whereas fibronectin has a wider range of binding capacity. The role of the entactin and nidogen molecules is less well defined but again may have to do with cell attachment and general binding activities. Proteoglycans, of which heparan sulfate proteoglycan is the overwhelming representative, are also present and, by virtue of their anionic charges, are crucial to the selective barrier function of the membranes. These and other properties of basement membranes are summarized in a number of reviews [1,382]. Additionally, particularly in disease situations associated with defective endothelium or increased transmural pressure, plasma-derived components may also accumulate [38,506].

The membranes covering the outer surfaces of the smaller blood vessels have a second layer in which fibrils of up to 10 nm diameter are observed. Such fibrils are probably contributed by adjacent connective tissue cells, including, possibly, pericytes. This second layer is likely to correspond to the argyrophilic network of fibers seen to surround the vessels of the retina in digest preparations (Fig. 4) [41].

D. Age-Related Changes

As with vessels in other parts of the cardiovascular system, those of the orbit and its contents are subject to degeneration with age. The extent to which aging per se is responsible for the observed changes, as opposed to the cumulative effects of continuous, and possibly increasing, hemodynamic stress, is debatable, especially as the changes are most obvious on the arterial side of the circulation.

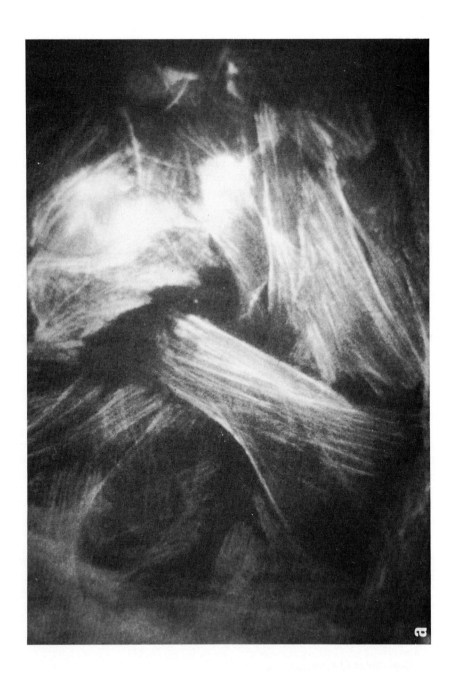

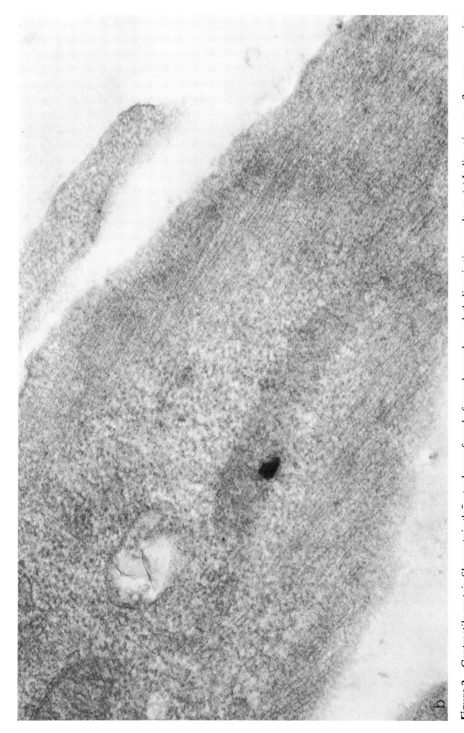

Figure 3 Contractile protein filaments in the cytoplasm of newly formed vascular endothelium in tissue culture. (a) Indirect immunofluorescence using antibody to actin shows bundles of myofilaments in the cytoplasm. (×1250) (b) Transmission electron microscopy shows numerous 4–7 nm diameter filaments aligned parallel to the long axis of the cell. (×66,000)

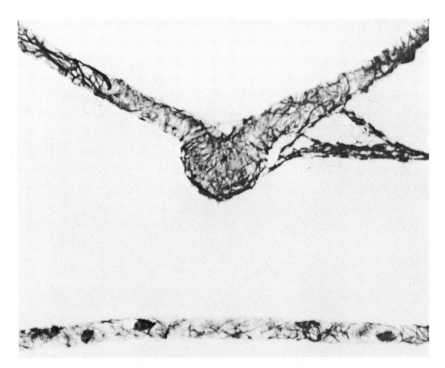

Figure 4   Retinal digest preparation stained to show a network of argyrophilic reticulin fibers surrounding the capillary blood vessels. Such fibers are considered collagenous and related to the vascular basement membranes. They are especially prominent in diabetic microangiopathy. (×490)

Arteries

From middle age onward, the smooth muscle cells of the media are slowly replaced by collagen, and the elastic tissue becomes progressively calcified and frayed. As a result there is loss of recoil capacity in response to the pulse wave, and the wall of the artery becomes fixed in a relatively dilated state to constitute senile arteriosclerosis. Some increase in intimal collagen is also usual, and commonly there is associated atherosclerosis. A progressive increase in interfibrillar cross-linkage of collagen fibers adds to the lack of distensibility and, morphologically, can be equated with increasing hyalinization of the media.

Arterioles

Arteriolar smooth muscle is likewise gradually replaced by collagen, but although the not uncommonly seen hyalinization may be due in part to maturation of the collagen, there is probably a second component to the mural hyaline change (Fig. 5). Thus, a study of arteriolar sclerosis in various sites, including the retina, indicated the importance of systemic hypertension in its pathogenesis [543], and it has been shown convincingly that leakage or insudation of plasma protein into the vessel wall is common in hypertensive states, even when the blood pressure elevation is fairly mild [201]. The mural thickening that results, allied to subendothelial collagen deposition, has the effect of reducing the caliber of the arteriole, whereas the reduced muscle content is paralleled in the retina by a reduced ability to autoregulate in response to changes in oxygen tension [450]. A further complication of mural thickening in retinal arterioles is compression of branch veins as they pass beneath the arteriole.

   The various degrees of mural thickening can cause different ophthalmoscopic appearances in the retina:

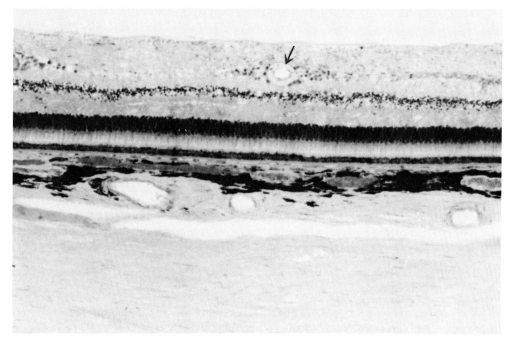

Figure 5   The wall of an arteriole in the retina of an individual with diabetes mellitus is thickened by the accumulation of a homogeneous eosinophilic (hyaline) material beneath the endothelium (arrow). (Hematoxylin and eosin, ×190)

1. Minor degrees are equated with an increased and widened light reflex, which probably represents some dilatation of the vessel.
2. Rather more thickening reduces the normal clear red appearance of the blood flowing through the lumen to a burnished copper color ("copper wiring").
3. Eventually, view of the bloodstream is obliterated and the arteriole presents a "silver wire" appearance.

Mural fibrosis also interferes with visualization of venous channels where they pass under the arteriole, and the apparent sheathing produces a variety of crossing defects.

Capillaries

Loss of endothelium followed by loss of pericytes to produce acellular capillaries is common at the retinal periphery [103] and is probably attributable to impaired perfusion through sclerosed arterioles. Capillary aneurysms may also develop in the periphery of the retina [510] and in some instances may be preceded by perivascular reticulin deposition with loop formation (see Sec. II.C). An analysis by Ashton [19], however, suggests that microaneurysms are more commonly a feature of concomitant vascular disease and are unusual as a function of aging alone.

Veins

Some increase in the collagenous content of venous channels is usual, and in the retina this can lead to loss of tone with dilatation and increased tortuosity.

II. GENERAL ASPECTS OF VASCULAR DISEASE IN THE EYE

A. Increased Permeability

Edema

Edema is the accumulation of inordinate quantities of fluid in the extravascular tissues. Both intracellular and extracellular edema is recognized, but in this section discussion is confined to extracellular fluid accumulation. The interstitial fluid may be in the form of an ultrafiltrate of the circulating blood and contain very little protein to constitute transudative edema, or it may include large amounts of protein, in which case it is properly described as exudative edema. In general there are two physiological mechanisms of importance in the regulation of fluid balance between the vascular and tissue compartments, exchange occurring predominantly through thin-walled capillaries:

1. Hydrostatic pressure: between the arterial and the venous sides of the capillary bed there is a steady fall in intravascular tension of about 20 mm Hg (from about 32 to 12 mm Hg in most extraocular tissues and from about 45 to 18 mm Hg within the globe).
2. Oncotic pressure: plasma proteins, especially albumin, exert an osmotic pressure of about 25 mm Hg and serve to keep the circulating fluid within the vessels.

Fluid exchange between the vascular and extravascular compartments depends on the interplay of these opposing factors and is such that fluid tends to leave the capillaries on the arterial side and return at the venous end. Edema results if this delicate balance is upset. Electrolyte ions pass unhindered across the capillary wall and are a factor in edema development only if there is an artificially increased sodium level or renal function is impaired, in which case there is overall retention of water to maintain isotonicity.

Transudates

Transudative edema usually reflects an increase in hydrostatic pressure within capillary blood vessels, and reduced oncotic pressure secondary to hypoproteinemia is of little consequence as far as the eye is concerned.

In the retinal context transudation is frequently a feature of hypertension and retinal vein occlusion, and increased hydrostatic pressure related to vascular dilatation may be a factor in the edema associated with acute inflammatory and allergic states throughout the eye and orbit. A net balance in favor of increased transudation into the tissues is also a feature of hypotony, being particularly marked in the uvea. A primary defect in the vascular endothelium resulting in increased permeability to small molecules is an early feature of the diabetic state. Transudation from superficial capillaries in the retina causes some haziness with diminished light reflexes and, in the neighborhood of the disk, is associated with separation of individual nerve fibers so that they are rendered unduly distinct. Deep retinal edema, however, is associated with a wet or shimmering appearance.

It is important to recognize that the differences between transudates and exudates is basically one of degree rather than of kind, the differences relating to the content of protein and lipid. Correspondingly, there is a range between these extremes, and it is a common observation that "true" retinal edema often leaves small residual "hard" exudates in its wake.

Exudates

Exudative edema in tissues of the eye and orbit occurring as a result of increased vascular permeability can be caused by the separation of adjacent endothelial cells. Such separation may accompany the dilatation provoked by vasoactive amine release in acute inflammation and hypersensitivity reactions. The retina is a special case because of the tight encircling junctions binding individual endothelial cells together, these serving to prevent significant plasma leakage in either hypertensive or inflammatory states [124]. As a rule, retinal exudates reflect structural damage to the endothelial lining, although observation of experimental and spontaneous hypertension in rats indicates that minor amounts of plasma protein might cross intact endothelium by means of increased pinocytosis [382]. In some instances retinal exudation is a measure of malformed vessels, as in the aneurysmal or telangiectatic capillary bed of Coats' disease (see Sec. III.F).

Once beyond the vessel wall, the exuded plasma spreads between the cellular components of the tissues along paths of least resistance, but because of the fibrinogen content, the exudates soon coagulate as a result of activation of the clotting process by contact with the tissues. The aqueous component is gradually reabsorbed, leaving a progressively inspissated residue, which because it contains exuded lipid as well as protein may appear waxy. In the retina such exudates also tend to have discrete edges and have a hard appearance (Fig. 6). Eventually, through fibrinolytic activity, the exudates begin to resolve, macrophages accumulating to take up and degrade residual material. Since lipid, especially cholesterol [433], is relatively less susceptible to biodegradation than protein, however, lipid residues tend to persist and may take months to disperse.

Retinal exudates are inclined to pool in the outer plexiform layer, where the tissue is most lax and where the absence of blood vessels may incur a reduced capacity for reabsorption: the natural movement of intraocular fluid toward the sclera [190] may also be a factor, large molecular complexes being held back by the intercellular junctional complexes of the ostensible outer limiting membrane. Exudates derived from vessels in the macular area are located between the radially disposed fibers of Henle's layer and assume a characteristic stellate pattern. Henle's layer consists of the axons of the foveal cones, which in the macular zone run in an almost horizontal direction, and corresponds to the outer plexiform layer of the surrounding retina. Where exudates are located a little farther away from the fovea, they are likely to be arranged in a ring or circinate fashion around the macula. A circinate distribution is also common around micro-aneurysms in diabetic retinopathy and around foci of capillary closure in retinal vascular occlusion. Rarely, a circinate retinopathy at the macula may present in the absence of any obvious underlying disorder, the affected subjects being mainly middle-aged females. The annular distribution of the exudates is likely to reflect centrifugal drainage from a focal origin, the initial fluid becoming progressively inspissated as the aqueous component drains unimpeded toward the choroid. Ultimately the solubility product of the residual protein and lipid is exceeded, and deposition forms a ring of recognizable hard exudates at some distance from the source.

Papilledema

Although the term "papilledema" was defined in the classic paper of Paton and Holmes [426] as passive edema due to raised intracranial pressure, to distinguish it from optic disk swelling associated with inflammatory processes, it has long been recognized that a number of conditions give rise to passive disk swelling in which there is no concomitant rise in cerebrospinal fluid pressure: a prime example of the latter is vascular hypertension. Edema of the optic disk can develop in a variety of situations that; although diverse in nature, are characterized by one or more of the following features, each of them likely to be of pathogenetic significance:

1. A shift in the hydrostatic pressure balance between the two sides of the lamina cribrosa (i.e., between the intraocular contents and the cerebrospinal fluid within the optic nerve sheath). A relative increase in pressure behind the disk is a feature of ocular hypotony and intracranial space-occupying lesions.
2. Mechanical distortion of the lamina cribrosa: posterior bowing in glaucoma and anterior bowing in ocular hypotony.
3. Impaired vascular perfusion of the disk region.

For many years it was believed that a major factor in the production of disk swelling was transudation as a result of impeded venous return, plasma exudation having a contributory role in vascular disturbances, such as malignant hypertension. However, although fluorescein angiography clearly shows that leakage occurs [549], histopathological studies provide only moderate evidence of increased interstitial volume, with the implication that other factors are involved.

Conversely, there is evidence of nerve fiber swelling, and it now appears that this is related to interference with axoplasmic flow. The movement of fluid along the axon with its complement of solutes and organelles is essential to the viability of the neuron [344] and, of necessity, is bidirectional [156,411,412]. Movement of axoplasm from cell nucleus to synapse (i.e., from retina to lateral geniculate body) is known as orthograde flow and occurs at two speeds:

1. Rapid: moving at about 15 mm/h, this concerns the movement of metabolites synthesized in the perikaryon. According to some investigators, such flow requires a continuous local provision of energy throughout the length of the axon and is therefore particularly vulnerable to ischemia (Fig. 7) [8].
2. Slow: the greater part of the axoplasmic transport, including mitochondria, occurs at the relatively slow speed of 1–2 mm/day [474]. The requisite energy source is uncertain, and there is particular doubt concerning its susceptibility to disruption by focal ischemia (see Sec. II.B).

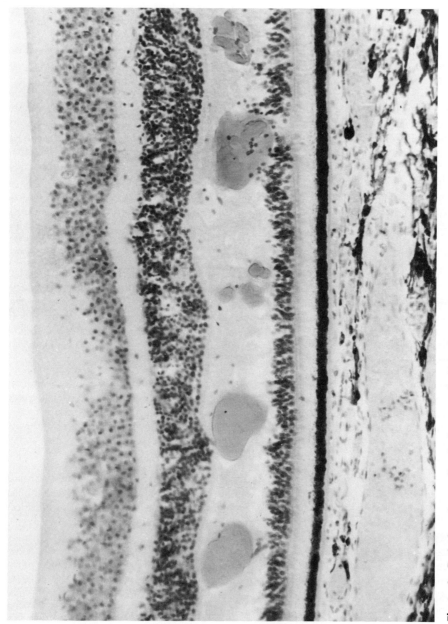

Figure 6 Retinal exudates collect in the outer plexiform layer, where they become inspissated to form eosinophilic masses with characteristically well-defined or "hard" borders. (Hematoxylin and eosin, ×190)

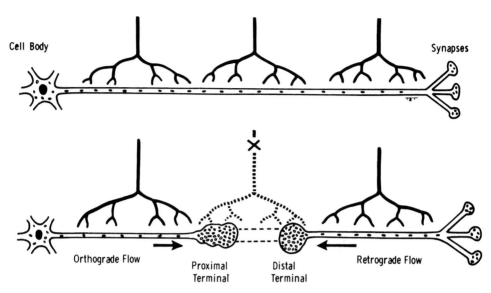

Figure 7 Axoplasmic transport. The bidirectional flow of axoplasm along the nerve fiber depends on local energy sources, and should focal ischemia develop, axoplasm is not transported across the affected segment of the nerve. Consequently, it accumulates at the edges of the ischemic zone. (Reproduced with permission from D. McLeod. Retinal ischaemia, disc swelling, and axoplasmic transport. *Trans. Opthalmol. Soc. UK* 96313–318, 1976.)

The return or retrograde flow of axoplasm is distinctly slower (2 mm/h) than the rapid phase of orthograde flow.

Of relevance to the pathogenesis of papilledema is the experimental evidence that ischemia initially interferes with rapid transport, both orthograde and retrograde, whereas slow axoplasmic flow is particularly vulnerable to moderate degrees of mechanical compression [8,391]. Clearly, however, prolonged ischemia results in axonal necrosis and cessation of all flow of whatever rate, as does compression if it is sufficient to crush the axon.

The nerve head swelling in both acute glaucoma and hypotony may be attributable in part to posterior and anterior bowing, respectively, of the lamina cribrosa. Such distortion is thought to constrict the available space for the nerve axons and thus interfere primarily with the slow orthograde phase of axoplasmic transport (both orthograde and retrograde in hypotony) [10,390]. Inadequate capillary perfusion due to primary vascular disease within the nerve head, however, may be important in the papilledema of hypertension [313] and giant cell arteritis.

The papilledema associated with raised intracranial pressure is mediated by increased cerebrospinal fluid pressure within the optic nerve sheath and appears to be due, in large part, to impaired slow orthograde axoplasmic transport [528] brought about by mechanical compression. The role of reduced blood flow in the region of the disk and lamina cribrosa, which undoubtedly occurs, is as yet undecided, however: it may be a purely secondary phenomenon due to compression by swollen nerve fibers within the rigid confines of the lamina cribrosa [258], or it may contribute to the axonal swelling by interfering with the rapid phase of axonal transport [370].

Interference with axoplasmic transport is almost certainly partial rather than complete, as tracer studies and the fairly minor impairment of visual acuity testify. Even so, some nerve fibers eventually succumb to unrelieved obstruction, the affected part becoming necrotic and the disrupted ends undergoing further distension due to the inflow of more axoplasm. Such swollen and disrupted axons constitute cytoid bodies (see p. 1634) and are identical to those seen in retinal cotton-wool spots [551].

Swelling of the disk occurs in both anterior and lateral directions, the latter causing blurring of the disk margins and sometimes producing tenting and limited detachment of the immediate peripapillary retina.

Hemorrhage

Although extrusion of erythrocytes through intact vessels by a process of diapedesis has been described in other tissues, there is no evidence that this occurs to any significant degree in the ocular circulation. For hemorrhage of appreciable extent to occur, there must be loss of structural integrity, this developing in a variety of circumstances:

1. Traumatic rupture, whether accidental or surgical.
2. Blood pressure elevation, both arterial and venous. Except in thin-walled aneurysms, the effect is likely to be indirect, resulting from associated necrosis as in systemic hypertension or obstruction and hypoxia as seen in venous occlusion.
3. Vasculitis.
4. Aneurysmal or telangiectatic vessels may bleed in the absence of blood pressure increase.
5. Angiomatous malformations, especially of the conjunctiva and orbit.
6. Neovascularization. Incompletely formed new vessel proliferations are prone to bleed, particularly when, as pertains within the vitreal cavity, they are poorly supported and subject to traction.
7. Hemorrhagic diatheses, most commonly those showing deficiency of platelets (e.g., leukemia), may give rise to ocular bleeding.

Hemorrhages from vessels in the inner retina tend to infiltrate between the axons of the nerve fiber layer and, consequently, assume a linear or flame-shaped distribution. Eventually, however, they also drain into the deeper layers of the retina, where there is no such alignment. Bleeding from capillaries in the outer retina tends to remain localized around the defective vessels.

Contact with the extravascular tissues activates the blood-clotting process, after which the clot is invaded by phagocytic cells that serve to remove the cellular and other debris. Autolysis is facilitated by proteolytic enzymes derived from both injured tissue and invading neutrophils. Subsequently the hematoma is infiltrated by fibroblasts (glia in the retina) and proliferating capillary blood vessels to leave a fibrous (or glial) scar in which most of the vessels eventually regress. Hematogenous pigment is converted to hemosiderin and may persist for months or even years in the tissues; the lipid content of the extravasated blood, especially free cholesterol, is similarly liable to persist and occasionally become the focus of a multinucleated giant cell reaction (Fig. 8).

Although this is the general response to hemorrhage in most tissues, including the retina, preretinal bleeding in the subhyaloid space may remain fluid with only a limited tendency toward organization and a correspondingly greater potential for autolysis and complete resolution. The lack of clot formation may be related to the absence of collagen fibers in this location, in contrast to the vitreous, where coagulation is usual [117]. The persistent fluidity of small anterior chamber hyphema may be due to dilution of clotting factors by the aqueous, but larger hemorrhages clot and ultimately fibrovascular adhesions are liable to form.

B. Ischemia

Reduced ocular blood flow can have very serious consequences, particularly in tissues with high metabolic requirements, such as the retina. At first the changes are reversible, but after a period determined by the degree of vascular insufficiency, the metabolic needs of the dependent tissues, and the availability of anastomotic compensation, irreversible changes ensue. In general the complications are a direct outcome of the metabolic deprivation, but there is also a risk of tissue damage following restoration of the circulation. Reperfusion can be associated with further damage, especially to the vessels themselves, as a result of free oxygen radicals formed by the activation of neutrophil granulocytes [511] or the formation of xanthine oxidase by the compromised endothelium [197]. In the rat retina the additional injury is manifested as increased edema [511].

Causes

Thrombosis.   There are three basic elements in the formation of a thrombus: changes in the vessel wall, changes in the circulating platelets, and activation of the coagulation cascade. Normally the endothelium insulates the bloodstream from the collagenous and other highly thrombogenic subendothelial structures, as well as secreting a number of antithrombotic factors, such as prostacyclin. Should the endothelium be

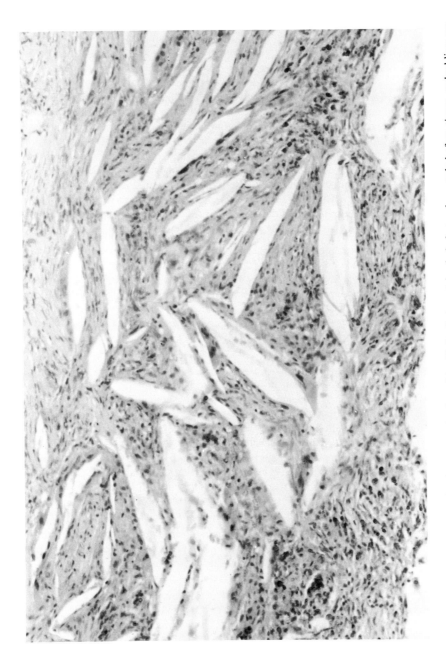

Figure 8 Part of an organizing hematoma in the orbit. Clefts that contained cholesterol crystals before tissue embedding are surrounded by multinucleated giant cells. Numerous macrophages with engulfed hemosiderin are also present. (Hematoxylin and eosin, ×190)

compromised, platelets adhere to the underlying tissues and are subject to an activation process involving the release of thromboxane A$_2$ and other agents that promote further platelet aggregation and trigger the clotting process. The latter culminates in the conversion of fibrinogen to fibrin and the formation of a definitive thrombus containing enmeshed blood cells.

Thrombosis as a pathological event is prone to occur under the following conditions:

1. Extensive or sustained endothelial damage. The chief causes are an underlying atheromatous plaque or vasculitis, but it is probable that other more subtle endothelial abnormalities may also predispose to thrombosis. It is possible, for instance, that patients with insulin-dependent diabetes have an enhanced risk of thrombosis because of impaired plasminogen activator secretion by the vascular endothelium [361].
2. Disturbance of smooth blood flow. Normally the forward movement of blood gives rise to a laminar flow, axial erythrocytes and leukocytes moving faster than the peripheral plasma zone. Between these are platelets that travel at an intermediate rate. Turbulence, which may develop over an atheromatous plaque or because of a localized narrowing of the vessel, disrupts such orderly flow and brings platelets into contact with the endothelium. Sluggish flow, which predominates on the venous side of the circulation, has a similar effect by allowing the cells, particularly the platelets, to settle out and lodge against the endothelium. Hyperviscosity states contribute to the risk of stasis [191,402].
3. Increased coagulability. This is a feature of several diverse conditions, such as disseminated cancer, the aftermath of severe trauma, and during and immediately after pregnancy, and is the basis of the disseminated intravascular coagulation syndrome.

Once formed the thrombus may propagate and occlude the affected vessel, fragments may break away and cause embolic ischemia downstream, and, ultimately, resolution or organization ensues. Resolution depends on activation of the fibrinolytic system by plasminogen activators, one of which, urokinaselike plasminogen, is present in the plasma; the other, tissue-type plasminogen activator (tPA), is a product of the endothelium and is activated only when attached to fibrin. Abnormalities of tPA secretion or its inhibitor may contribute to the pathogenesis of several vascular diseases associated with ischemic complications [421]. Organization is a feature of the larger thrombi or of situations involving impaired thrombolysis and involves capillary and fibroblast proliferation, which may lead to partial restoration of blood flow by a process of recanalization.

Embolism. Ocular ischemia can result from arterial emboli, the principal source of which is ulcerated atheromatous plaques. In amaurosis fugax, which is a complication in up to 40% of patients with occlusive carotid atherosclerosis [147], the emboli consist largely of cholesterol, but whitish emboli lodging in the retinal circulation for periods varying between a few minutes and several hours before breaking up are probably derived from platelet thrombi on the surface of the plaques [469]. Other sources of emboli include the mural thrombus from a fibrillating left atrium [560], infected vegetations from diseased cardiac valves [379], fat from fractured bones [306], and nitrogen bubbles in decompression sickness [472]. Fragments of endocardial myxoma [380], amniotic fluid [179], and radioopaque dyes used in arteriography [240,353] have also been reported as causing retinal embolism. Malignant tumor emboli also occur but are usually too small to produce significant ocular ischemia.

Spasm. Along with other muscular arteries, the central artery of the retina and its principal branches are susceptible to intense focal constriction. Spasm sufficient to obstruct flow can occasionally be responsible for visual loss in migraine [54,116] or may result from medication with ergot and its derivatives [252]. The spasm is usually short-lived, and irreversible damage to the dependent tissues is avoided, although rarely permanent visual disturbance has been reported.

Inadequacy of Perfusion. Organic narrowing or occlusion of the carotid arteries and their ophthalmic and orbital branches can impair ocular nutrition. Causes include atherosclerosis, Takayasu's arteritis, giant cell arteritis, and other forms of vasculitis.

The hypotension accompanying severe blood loss and apneic episodes in neonates constitute functional causes of ocular ischemia and hypoxia.

Ocular Complications

Globe: Chronic Ocular Ischemia. Ischemia of the whole eye involves occlusion of the ophthalmic artery and is usually a complication of carotid artery disease. Anterior segment findings [147] include protein-rich exudation into the aqueous as a result of blood-ocular barrier breakdown, atrophy of the iris and ciliary body, cataractous lens changes, and corneal edema as a sequel to the failure of energy-dependent endothelial cell function. Similar effects can be produced experimentally by interfering with the circulation to the anterior segment [435]. Iris neovascularization (rubeosis iridis) and peripheral anterior synechiae leading to secondary glaucoma may also develop, attributable to associated retinal hypoxia [147] or a direct response to the anterior segment ischemia [262]. The posterior segment damage involves panretinal atrophy [92] with peripheral hemorrhages and microaneurysms, optic disk neovascularization, and vitreous exudates, and trypsin digest preparations reveal widespread acellularity of the retinal capillaries [147].

Uvea.   Because uveal vessels, particularly those of the choroid, differ from those of the retina in having frequent anastomoses, ischemic damage is relatively less common. Major ciliary arteries, both anterior and posterior, can also be occluded without apparent harm because of anastomotic compensation. Nevertheless, uveal ischemia sometimes occurs, having been reported as a result of trauma (both accidental and surgical), hypertensive fibrinous necrosis, sickle cell disease, and various types of vasculitis. Advanced age-related arteriosclerosis and primary sclerosis of the choriocapillaris may also cause significant ischemia, and reduced choroidal blood flow is a prominent feature of severe glaucoma.

In the iris, acute ischemia produces an initial edema of the stroma, proceeding to dispersion, clumping and loss of the pigment epithelium, and eventual stromal thinning by necrosis. More gradual ischemia results in thinning by atrophy, with marked loss of cellular components.

Ciliary body infarction may attend acute ischemia, but less sudden deprivation of blood flow results in atrophy of the processes and selective degeneration of the nonpigmented epithelium.

In the choroid, arteriolar occlusion, such as might occur in accelerated hypertension, is associated with degeneration of the dependent pigment epithelium of the retina. This can manifest as focal depigmentation alone, but there may be an aggregate of dispersed pigment in the center (Elschnig's spots) or at the margins or, alternatively, strung along the length of the sclerosed vessel (Siegrist's streaks). More widespread ischemia is likely to cause the degeneration of the outer layers of the neuroretina as well as affect the pigment epithelium.

Retina.   *Central retinal artery occlusion.*   Central retinal artery occlusion is usually secondary to atherosclerosis, possibly as a result of hemorrhage within the plaque [129], and is often associated with systemic hypertension [13]. Embolism is a further cause [179], and occasionally an arteritis may be implicated. As a rule the obstruction occurs at or immediately behind the lamina cribosa, where the artery is at its narrowest.

Complete loss of vision is usually immediate and, if extrapolation of experimental data derived from monkeys is appropriate, irreversible neuronal changes are present after 2 h [245,271]. Initially, the retina becomes opaque and pale, due mainly to intracellular edema but also in part to necrosis of the inner layers. The outer layers of the retina (deep to the outer plexiform layer) are preserved, being dependent for their nutrition on the choroidal circulation, and this produces a cherry-red spot at the macula. Study of experimental occlusion of the central retinal artery in monkeys [336] shows early swelling of mitochondria with subsequent degeneration and imbibition of water by the neuronal cytoplasm. Such changes are ascribable to mitochondrial damage, reflecting breakdown of Na,K-ATPase-dependent electrolyte balance across cell membranes. It should be stressed, however, that reduction in blood flow need not be total before infarction occurs [214], and in some instances marginal flow can result in patchy necrosis. Eventually, the necrotic tissue is phagocytosed to leave an atrophic retina with no glial replacement since, possibly, astrocytes are also destroyed by the ischemia. The presence of cilioretinal circulation in about 25% of individuals means that the immediate peripapillary retina may be preserved, and ostensible clinical improvement in the first 2 weeks following central retinal artery occlusion is related to adaptation to the use of this rim of intact tissue. In view of the rapid rate at which irreversible retinal damage ensues, real improvement is rare and the therapuetic use of anticoagulant agents needs to be instituted within the first 4 h if any success is to be achieved [246]. Spontaneous fibrinolysis and dissolution may develop at a later stage, with restoration of retinal perfusion, but in other patients there is residual sclerosis of the main arteriolar branches. Where the initial occlusion is incomplete, a sluggish circulation may be produced that predisposes to central vein occlusion (stagnation thrombosis) [315]. Preretinal neovascularization is an unusual but well-substantiated complication, and iris neovascularization leading to angle-closure glaucoma is probably more common than is sometimes recognized [150,293a,431,552]. However, Hayreh and Podhajsky [266] presented evidence that in some patients the arterial occlusion follows rather than precedes the onset of neovascular glaucoma and suggest that the arterial occlusion is attributable to the combined effects of carotid artery disease with consequent low perfusion pressure and obstruction to inflow because of raised intraocular pressure. Partial obstruction of the central retinal artery is associated with the formation of multiple cotton-wool spots [414].

Branch retinal artery occlusion.   This is usually the result of embolism from atheromatous plaques and occurs mainly at vessel bifurcations. Direct thrombosis is unusual since the atherosclerotic process rarely extends beyond the optic disk. The effects on the dependent retina are identical to those described for central artery occlusion, although the risk of secondary iris neovascularization is slight [266].

Closure of the terminal precapillary arterioles is a prominent feature of hypertensive, sickle cell, and diabetic retinopathies (see later).

Cotton-wool spots.   Cotton-wool spots are discrete lesions in the nerve fiber layer of the retina associated with some elevation of the inner surface and characteristic fluffy whitish opacification. Lesions of this type predominate in the posterior part of the retina, where the nerve fiber layer is thickest, and are a feature of several vascular retinopathies as well as a frequent retinal finding in patients with the acquired immunodeficiency syndrome [537]. Cotton-wool spots appear to be a function of focal ischemia and can be regarded as microinfarcts (strictly there is some reason to classify them as preinfarcts since there is a limited capacity for recovery, but insistence on this point smacks of pedantry).

Histological examination shows focal aggregates of globular structures within the nerve fiber layer, which have been called cytoid bodies (Fig. 9), particularly because they commonly have a central weakly basophilic "nucleus." However, the absence of deoxyribonucleic acid, as evidenced by histochemical staining reactions, indicates that the central component is a pseudonucleus; teased preparations and electron microscopy have shown that cytoid bodies are the swollen ends of disrupted nerve axons [37,551]. Furthermore, the pseudonucleus is now known to consist of amorphous electron-dense material considered to have derived from the lipid-protein residues of degenerate cytoplasmic organelles [37]. Not all axons in the region of a cotton-wool spot are disrupted, those lying immediately beneath the inner limiting membrane in particular often being preserved [518]. Ganglion cells and parts of the inner nuclear layer in the involved region share in the necrosis, but cells in the deeper retinal layers normally remain viable.

Understanding of the pathogenesis of cotton-wool spots has come from experimental embolization of the retinal circulation combined with electron microscopy and tracer studies of axoplasmic transport. If artificial emboli are introduced into the cartoid circulation of a laboratory animal, some lodge in the smaller arterioles of the retina and are likely to be followed by the development of a cotton-wool spot [36]. Focal swelling related to fusiform expansion of nerve fibers in the territory supplied by the obstructed arteriole is present within 1 h and at this stage the swelling appears to be largely due to imbibition of water, since the distended region is unduly electron lucent, with few organelles and sparse neurofilaments (Fig. 10). Such intracellular edema is most readily explained by hypoxia and failure of the sodium pump mechanism, with additional damage caused by failure to remove the products of glycolysis and the development of intracellular acidosis. Thereafter, many of the distended axons become increasingly rich in mitochondria and other organelles (Fig. 11). This change is best seen toward the edges of the lesion, since the central part becomes necrotic with loss of axonal continuity. There is circumstantial evidence, now supported by tracer studies using [3H]leucine injected into the vitreous cavity of pigs with argon laser-induced cotton-wool spots [371], that much of this later nerve fiber swelling and mitochondrial increase is due to interference with axoplasmic transport [369]. Axoplasmic flow is normally bidirectional and requires local supply of energy from the surrounding tissue fluids along the entire length of the axon [411]. Consequently, focal vascular insufficiency results in axonal distension, because while axoplasm continues to be fed into the damaged region, there is no local source of energy necessary to pump it away (Fig. 12). Interruption of axoplasmic flow occurs on both the ganglion cell side of the ischemia or otherwise injured area (obstructed orthograde flow) and the side nearest the optic disk (obstructed retrograde flow). Whether all the mitochondrial increase in the distended and disrupted axons can be accounted for in this way is uncertain, there being the added possibility of in situ mitochondrial proliferation as part of a homeostatic mechanism designed to disperse the accumulated intracellular edema fluid [30,157]. Where there has been loss of axonal continuity, however, there is no prospect of a return to normal, and membranous whorls (myelin figures) develop, and after a few weeks, the residues of degenerate cytoplasmic organelles coalesce to form pseudonuclei.

Correlation of these findings with the clinical aspects of cotton-wool spot development suggests that

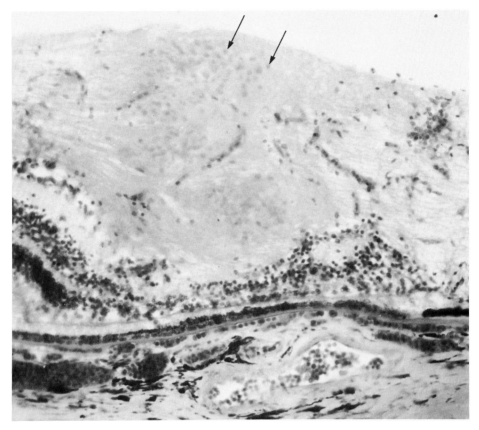

Figure 9   Retinal cotton-wool spots are made up of numerous cytoid bodies and, in the upper lesions, a central zone of necrosis. The cytoid bodies lie in the nerve fiber layer and represent the distended stumps of disrupted axons; the pseudonuclei (arrows) are formed by coalescence of the lipoprotein membranes of degenerate cytoplasmic organelles. (Hematoxylin and eosin, ×190)

the central grayish zone often seen in the larger lesions represents axonal land ganglion cell necrosis, and accumulation of axoplasm and edema fluid accounts for the rather more opaque whitish swelling at the margins. The width of the opaque whitish zone depends on the extent to which individual axons penetrate the ischemic area before axoplasmic flow is interrupted [372].

Fluorescein angiography not uncommonly shows preceding or associated vascular leakage at the site of a cotton-wool spot [212,283], but experimental embolization of the retinal circulation in animals indicates that this is not an essential or constant feature, and consequently, the term "soft exudate" has little or no justification. It is more probable that mural damage leading to leakage and occlusion leading to cotton-wool spot formation are simultaneous but separate products of the initiating vascular abnormality.

In the healing phase of cotton-wool spots, the necrotic debris is removed through autolysis and phagocytosis. Eventually a glial scar is formed, astrocytes apparently withstanding ischemia more successfully than nerve tissue. Although the nonperfused capillaries may reopen, there is no improvement in the focal scotoma or in the partial nerve fiber bundle defect caused by loss of axons passing through the ischemic zone.

Central retinal vein occlusion.   Central retinal vein occlusion is an acute event with a variable clinical expression and, possibly, variable pathogenesis. Common to all forms, however, are tortuous congested veins, hemorrhages, and angiographic evidence of vascular stasis caused by thrombotic occlusion of the vein at or behind the lamina cribrosa. Such occlusion can complicate any of a number of states, some of which have been substantiated but others merely postulated.

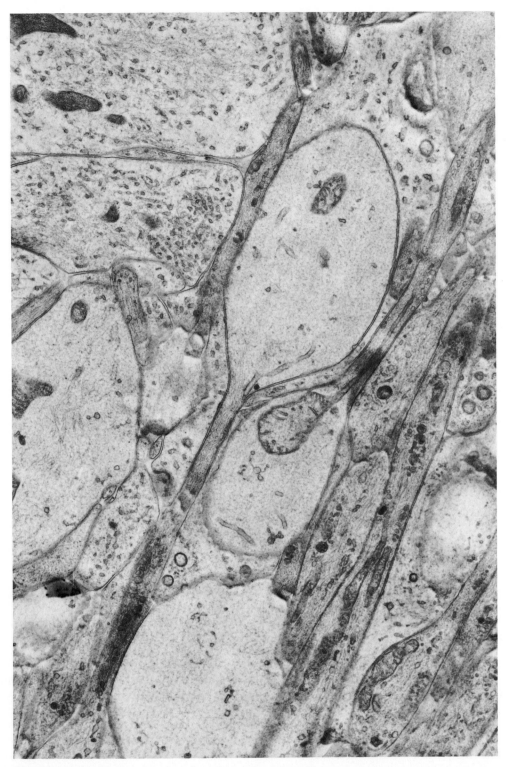

Figure 10 Electron micrograph of a cotton-wool spot at an early stage in its evolution. Individual axons in an area of retinal ischemia have become focally distended by the accumulation of relatively electron-lucent material containing few organelles. (From experimentally induced lesions in a pig retina 1 h after embolic occlusion of a terminal arteriole.) ($\times$16,500)

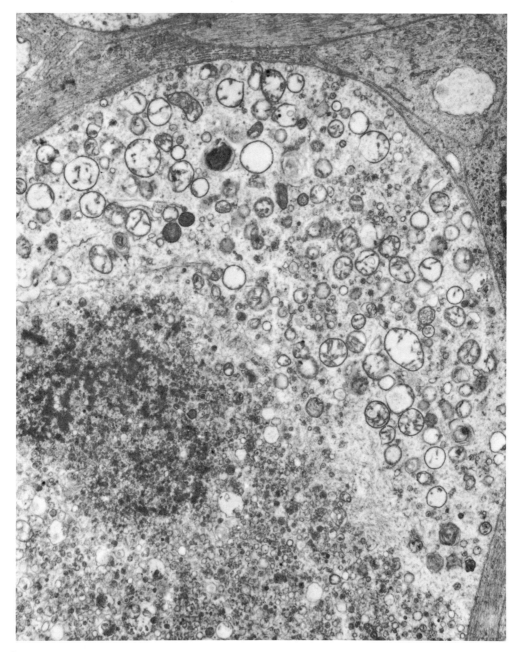

Figure 11 Cytoid body showing accumulated cytoplasmic organelles, mainly mitochondria, with a central electron-dense pseudonucleus formed by the residues of degenerate organelles. (×16,800)

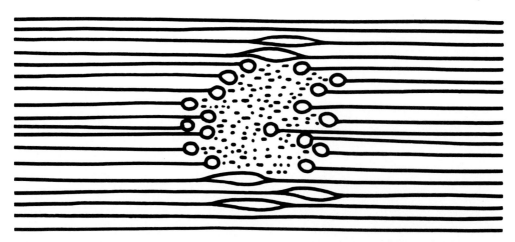

Figure 12   A large retinal cotton-wool spot. In the center, where the energy deprivation is most severe, axonal necrosis is liable to occur and nerve fiber swelling because of the disrupted flow of axoplasm develops at the edges of the infarcted zone. Clinically, the central necrotic zone may be relatively gray compared with the fluffy white edges.

Hyperviscosity states.   Whether the outcome of an increased number of cells in the circulating blood, as in polycythemia, abnormalities of the plasma proteins [525], or plasma lipids [139,303], increased viscosity is well documented in patients with retinal vein occlusions [366,460]. This promotes sluggish flow with a further increase in viscosity as the shear rate drops and complete cessation of flow in some situations.

Vasculitis.   Central retinal vein occlusion associated with perivascular leukocytic infiltration is sometimes seen in histological material and is said to be especially frequent in younger subjects [364]. The cause of the phlebitis is usually obscure, but on occasion it is attributable to sarcoidosis, Behçet's disease, or Eales disease. Nor is it always clear whether the leukocytic infiltration is the cause or result of the occlusion.

Reduced arterial perfusion.   It has been suggested on both clinical and experimental grounds that the characteristic retinal changes of central retinal vein occlusion represent a combination of obstructed venous outflow and reduced arterial inflow [259,264]. Impaired perfusion with a consequently reduced shear rate could be expected to engender thrombosis in the veins, where the circulation is in any case most sluggish, especially if there is an associated increase in intrinsic viscosity.

Turbulence.   In the region of the lamina cribrosa, the artery and the vein share the same adventitial sheath and any thickening and dilatation of the artery wall tends to impinge on and compress the vein within the rigid tunnel imposed by the lamina. Swelling of the venous endothelium has also been reported in association with atheromatous disease of the central retinal artery [315]. Compression by massive drusen of the optic nerve head has also been described in central retinal vein thrombosis [234]. Developments of this kind are expected to disturb the normal laminar flow and favor a thrombotic event. An unusual form of central retinal vein occlusion affecting persons under 40 years of age, although of obscure etiology, has speculatively been ascribed to turbulence resulting from a congenital anomaly of the vein at the level of the lamina cribrosa [536].

Obstructed outflow.   Apart from turbulence, interference with drainage secondary to raised intra-ocular pressure, raised intracranial pressure, or an adjacent neoplasm have also been associated with central retinal vein thrombosis [145].

Much of the earlier disagreement surrounding the interpretation of both clinical and experimental data advanced either to support or deny the importance of arterial disease in the pathogenesis of central retinal vein occlusion [202,257,368,424] has been dispelled by the recognition that there are two fairly distinct types of occlusive disease.

Ischemic form.   The ischemic form is much the more serious type but also the least common, accounting for between 20% [260] and 36% [446] of all central retinal vein occlusions. It is characterized by numerous hemorrhages (hence an alternative designation as hemorrhagic retinopathy) [260], cotton-wool spots and marked visual consequences. Fluorescein angiography frequently reveals microaneurysms and, eventually, areas of capillary closure. Circumstantial evidence of arterial disease is often forthcoming [259], and it is possible in these cases that a reduced inflow, which may be permanent as a consequence of atherosclerosis or, less often, transient as in migrainous subjects [191], precipitates a thrombotic event. It must be said, nevertheless, that despite the cogency of this reasoning, histopathological evidence of arterial insufficiency is sparse [234], and the argument that the reduced perfusion need not be permanent, as evidenced by experimental studies in monkeys [264], still begs the question of what the nature of any such temporary event may be in the clinical sphere. Spasm and hypotensive episodes are, as yet, unproven possibilities.

Nonischemic form.   The nonischemic form is a more benign condition claimed to represent the emergence of central retinal vein occlusion in the absence of detectable inflow deficiency [260]. This is not to say, however, that arterial disease is not a factor since transient functional reductions in perfusion pressure in a moderately compromised system could be enough to initiate the thrombotic process [260]. Hemorrhages are fewer than in the ischemic form, cotton-wool spots are rare, and, although there is circulatory stasis, there is no progression to permanent capillary closure. (It is unfortunate that the term "venous stasis retinopathy" is sometimes applied to the condition [260,265], given its earlier identification with the purportedly arterial insufficiency state described by Kearns and Hollenhorst [307].)

Up to half of patients with the nonischemic form of central retinal vein occlusion recover spontaneously, but others are prone to develop cystoid macular degeneration. Patients with the ischemic form suffer rather more severe macular degeneration, and a third are at risk of angle-closure glaucoma consequent to the formation of iris new vessels [267]. The risk is increased in patients with preexisting primary open-angle glaucoma [168a]. Less commonly vessels may develop over the optic disk [497], as, rarely, may preretinal neovascularization [376]. Release of substances with angiogenic properties from the hypoxic areas of the retina is the likely stimulus to these complications. There is no entirely satisfactory explanation for the overwhelming preponderance of irideal as opposed to retinal neovascularization in central retinal vein occlusion patients. Possibly it is related to the early onset of iris neovascularization in these patients ("100 days glaucoma"), this in some way preempting the emergence of posterior segment vascular proliferation [341]. Curiously, the regression of irideal new vessels promoted by retinal panphotocoagulation is followed in some eyes by retinal and disk neovascularization [399], but the proffered hypothesis that rubeosis iridis represents a response to more severe hypoxia than obtains in cases with posterior segment new vessels is hard to understand.

Branch retinal vein occlusion.   Occlusion produces visual defects appropriate to its drainage area and can be either an acute or a chronic process.

Acute occlusion presents with distension and tortuosity of the affected vein, with both superficial and deep retinal edema. Deep hemorrhages from capillaries or small venules are common, although superficial flame-shaped hemorrhages may be present if the obstruction takes place close to the disk. Cotton-wool spots may also develop in relation to peripapillary venous occlusions, and microaneurysms are common in the later stages.

More gradual occlusion occurs predominantly in patients with arterial hypertension and, although accounting for some otherwise unexplained visual loss in these individuals, may be obscured by the overlying arterial changes.

Occlusion occurs almost always at the site of arteriovenous crossing, particularly where the artery crosses in front of the vein [75,540]; here the artery and vein have a shared adventitial sheath, which is commonly thickened and responsible for some localized vascular narrowing [480]. Systemic hypertension was a feature in 93% of patients in a study reported by Kohner and Shilling [331]. Endothelial cell proliferation or swelling has also been described at these sites [480,544], but the possibility that such changes are secondary to obstructed flow, not the cause, is very real. Hyperviscosity may be a contributory factor in some patients [392].

The events that follow acute occlusion have been studied experimentally in the monkey [15,247,282]. Photocoagulation of a branch vein gives rise to an immediate reduction in arterial caliber and inflow, which may well represent an autoregulatory response to increased venous backpressure. Within the next few hours the capillaries and postcapillary venules in the drainage area become progressively distended so that transudative edema and plasma leakage develops, leakage initially appearing to be by increased pinocytosis across the endothelial lining [282]. Eventually some of the distended vessels rupture and bleed, but in many of those remaining intact, stagnation and thrombosis supervene. In consequence there is complete cessation of blood flow through the affected capillaries and venules, resulting, in some instances, in ischemia sufficient to provoke cotton-wool spot formation. The vessels themselves are liable to become acellular. In addition to interstitial edema, there is also intracellular swelling, which probably reflects tissue hypoxia, although Archer [15] concluded that oxygen deprivation is not likely to be a factor in the vascular injury, since concurrent occlusion of the feeding artery had no additional effect on the vessels of experimental animals. A collateral circulation is often established in monkeys with artificially induced branch vein obstruction within 2–3 days [16], and this may mitigate some of the tissue changes, but in the aging human population having varying degrees of arteriolosclerosis, this capacity is liable to be impaired, and collateral channels providing an alternative drainage route usually take weeks or months to develop. With the emergence of a collateral circulation the nonperfused vessels may regain their endothelial lining, but in some instances the capillaries remain closed, the lumina not infrequently being invaded by glial processes (Fig. 13) [282].

Persistence of capillary closure in the clinical situation is associated with a poor prognosis for visual recovery [341]. Iris neovascularizations and neovascular glaucoma are infrequent, possibly because there is inadequate stimulus [267]. Conversely, optic disk, particularly preretinal, neovascularization in relation to the ischemic tissue is considerably more common in patients with extensive branch vein occlusions than in those with central vein disorders [267]. Measurements of the oxygen levels in relation to the ischemic area in pigs with experimentally induced branch retinal vein occlusion have shown significant hypoxia in animals that later exhibit proliferative changes [444]. Other experiments in cats with similar venous occlusion have shown that vitrectomy can reduce the level of hypoxia over the ischemic area by allowing oxygen to diffuse more readily from other parts of the retina, with the inference that procedures of this sort may prevent subsequent preretinal angiogenesis [505].

Anterior Ischemic Optic Neuropathy.   The essential features of this condition are sudden onset of monocular blindness, usually in the absence of pain, in the presence of optic disk edema. Eventual involvement of the fellow eye is common. Two forms are generally recognized.

The *arteritic* form is the least common and is almost always attributable to occlusion of the posterior ciliary arteries by giant cell arteritis, although an instance of anterior ischemic optic neuropathy secondary to pulseless disease (Takayasu's arteritis) has been described [351]. A strong association between the arteritic form of anterior ischemic optic neuropathy and the finding of circulating anticardiolipin (antiphospholipid) antibodies has been described, but its significance is unclear [538].

In the *nonarteritic* form, vascular insufficiency caused by atherosclerosis is likely to be a principal factor, with an enhanced predisposition in diabetic and hypertensive individuals [64]. However, a convincing association with an absent or reduced physiological optic cup has been established [143], and it has been reasoned that because this implies a small scleral canal, the nerve fibers passing through the correspondingly restricted gap in Bruch's membrane at the disk are vulnerable to minor degrees of compression [53]. Thus, an otherwise inconsequential level of impaired arterial perfusion could provoke defective axoplasmic flow [371], with swelling that compresses the optic nerve capillaries and leads to further ischemic damage [53]. Nonarteritic ischemic optic neuropathy can also complicate severe hemorrhage, and although hypotension may be an adequate explanation in some cases, autoregulatory vasoconstriction has been suggested in others [261].

C. Aneurysms

Aneurysmal dilatation of the ocular and orbital vasculature can be congenital or acquired and, although sometimes seen in the orbit and conjunctiva, is most frequent and of greatest consequence in the retina.

Congenital

Leber's miliary aneurysms occur as telangiectasis or varicosity of circumscribed areas of the retinal capillary bed. By virtue of their excessive permeability, they are a cause of intra- and subretinal exudation, leading eventually to retinal detachment and Coats' disease. The affected vessels have thin walls at first, but gradually they become increasingly thickened by insudated plasma material, perhaps representing a primary focal defect in the blood-retina barrier [524].

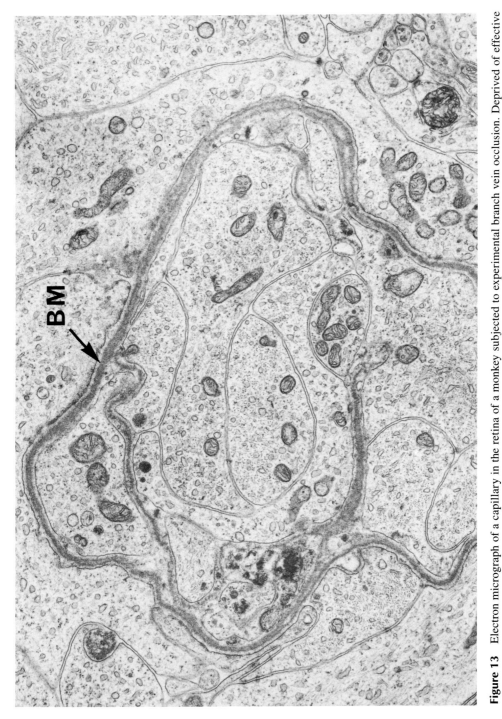

Figure 13 Electron micrograph of a capillary in the retina of a monkey subjected to experimental branch vein occlusion. Deprived of effective circulation, the endothelium and pericytes have sloughed off, leaving a basement membrane outline. The lumen of the defunct capillary is invaded by glial processes. BM, basement membrane. (×20,000) (Reproduced with permission from D.J. Hockley, R.C. Tripathi, and N. Ashton. Experimental retinal branch vein occlusion in the monkey: Histopathological and ultrastructural studies. *Trans. Opthalmol. Soc. UK 96*:202–209, 1976.)

Racemose retinal aneurysms are arteriovenous malformations presenting either as an isolated phenomenon or in conjunction with similar anomalies in the midbrain to constitute the Wyburn-Mason syndrome. They also occur in the orbit, where they are liable to cause proptosis.

Acquired

Microaneurysms.   Although capillary aneurysms are described in the conjunctiva, especially in diabetic subjects [119], they are most common and of greatest significance in retinal vasculopathy, being encountered in macroglobulinemia, sickle cell disease, and retinal vein occlusion, as well as diabetes mellitus. It was once thought that capillary microaneurysms do not develop in other tissues [20], but they have now been shown in both the kidney and heart of diabetics [170]. They occur chiefly, but not exclusively, on the venous side of the capillary bed, microaneurysms on the arterial side being especially associated with systemic hypertension. Sometimes developing in clusters, they are not uncommonly found encircling areas of capillary closure (Fig. 14).

The importance of microaneurysms is in their excessive permeability, which makes them a ready source of local serous exudation and hemorrhage. The wall of the aneurysms becomes thickened by accumulated plasma residues, which can be observed in flat mounts as a periodic acid–Schiff-positive cap covering the distended segment, and eventually many of them become coated on the internal aspect by fibrinous thrombus. Thrombotic occlusion of the aneurysm can manifest itself clinically as disappearance or apparent resolution (Fig. 15). The life of a microaneurysm can vary from months in hypertensive retinopathy to a year or more in diabetes mellitus.

Microaneurysms appear to originate in two different ways (Fig. 16): by focal dilatation of the wall or by the fusion of the two arms of a capillary loop [19,23]. Although several theories have been advanced to explain their origin, none is entirely satisfactory [205].

Ballantyne and Loewenstein [50] considered that they may be related to venous stasis, a view that finds support in the occurrence of microaneurysms in retinal vein occlusion and, possibly, hyperviscosity states, such as obtain in macroglobulinemia and diabetes mellitus. Others have sought an intrinsic defect in the capillary wall, and since changes in the basement membrane are an integral part of diabetic microangiopathy, several workers have looked to this structure for an explanation of aneurysm formation [284,442]. However, there is no good correlation between basement membrane changes, whether in the form of thickening or vacuolation, and the presence of microaneurysms. The finding of argyrophilic fibers (possible residual strands of the basement membranes of defunct capillaries) attached to the caps of some aneurysms has encouraged the notion that microaneurysms are the residual stumps of obliterated capillaries [555]. Focal pericyte degeneration as an explanation for microaneurysm formation [106] was originally based on the plausible assumption that this cell has a contractile function, but even if this is not the case, it is still conceivable that loss of passive support from a cell wrapped around the endothelial lining could weaken the wall sufficiently for focal distension to occur. A subsequent hypothesis [195] linking pericyte loss with microaneurysms takes their putative inhibitory affect on endothelial cell proliferation as an explanation for the frequently observed hypercellular aneurysms [23]. Should microaneurysms be formed in this way, they can be regarded as limited attempts at new vessel formation [195,555], additional support coming from the tendency for the aneurysmal sac to be oriented toward areas of capillary closure. However, why should the attempt be so abortive? It is relevant to note that were the dilatation produced by a different mechanism, this of itself would require an increase in endothelial cell numbers to line the enlarged surface area of the dilated sac. On the other hand, there is less than precise topographical correlation between degenerate pericytes, as evidenced by nuclear changes and the formation of "ghost" cells, and aneurysmal dilatation. If the importance of pericyte loss in the formation of microaneurysms is confirmed, it is likely to be as one of several developments in a multifactorial process.

Microaneurysms preceded by capillary loops may perhaps more readily be attributed to attempted revascularization of ischemic foci in the retina, the loops being associated with localized endothelial cell hyperplasia and capillary elongation. Nevertheless, loop aneurysms and neovascularization can each occur in the absence of the other [31], and the relationship is no more than speculative. Commonly, reticulin fibers that enmesh the outer surfaces of the capillaries can be observed straddling the base of a loop (Fig. 17) and may be an additional or alternative factor in the approximation of the arms of the loop. Increased amounts of perivascular reticulin are especially prominent in diabetic retinopathy [32].

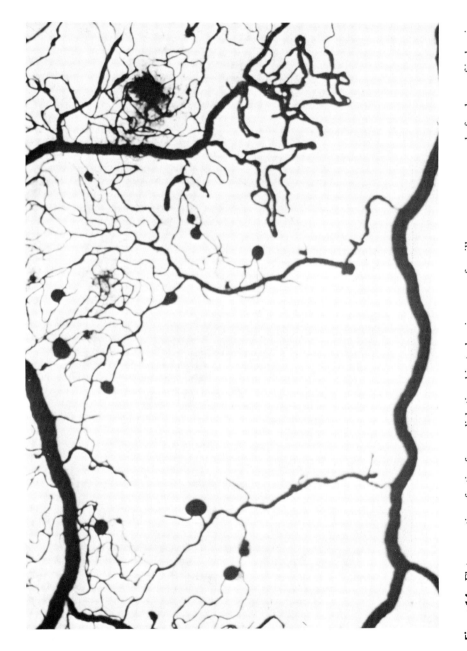

Figure 14 Flat preparation of retina from a diabetic subject, showing crops of capillary aneurysms around a focal area of ischemia. The patent vessels are perfused with colloidal carbon. (×55)

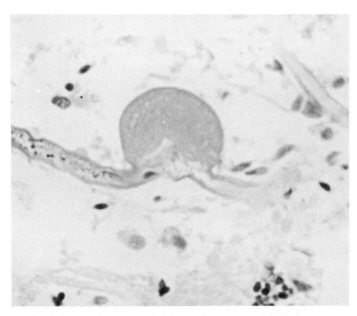

Figure 15 Retina from a diabetic individual sectioned parallel to the surface, showing a thrombosed micro-aneurysm. Such vessels appear normal in fluorescein angiograms and could lead to an erroneous clinical impression that the aneurysm has regressed. (Periodic acid–Schiff and hematoxylin, ×295)

Macroaneurysms.   Arteriolar aneurysms are much less common than their capillary counterparts and are found mainly on the second- or third-order branches. Structurally the aneurysms have been compared to those found on small intracerebral arteries, these showing a subendothelial accumulation of hyaline material and focal deficiency of the internal elastic lamina [108]. Moreover, like those in the brain [108,468], retinal macroaneurysms are usually a feature of aging and poorly controlled systemic hypertension [98,176], especially in women [345]. An association with retinal vein occlusion has also been noted [121,345]. The frequent occurrence of macroaneurysms at points of branching is suggestive of mechanical injury related to raised intraluminal pressure.

Some macroaneurysms are liable to leak [422] and, should they be present on vessels near the posterior pole, be a cause of macular edema and circinate exudates [98]. Others are asymptomatic.

D.   Neovascularization

The presence of blood vessels in most tissues is a condition of their survival and is wholly desirable, whereas their presence in tissues able to satisfy their metabolic needs by other means is not only superfluous but can have serious repercussions. Nowhere is this more true than in the eye, where the cornea and surfaces of the retina and iris are all vulnerable to symptomatic neovascularization [207].

Retina

Proliferation of blood vessels in postnatal life can be preretinal, intraretinal, or subretinal.

Preretinal Neovascularization.   New vessels in front of the retina usually take origin from or near the larger retinal veins [274]. Diabetes mellitus, branch retinal vein occlusion, retinopathy of prematurity, and sickle cell disease are well-recognized causes, but other less frequent conditions giving rise to proliferative retinopathy include various types of posterior segment inflammatory disease involving the retinal vasculature [228], such as sarcoidosis [144,227], Behcet's disease [298], Eales disease [24], malaria [309], toxoplasmosis [215], and dysproteinemia [11]. Preretinal vessels as an exceptional event have been reported in a considerable number of conditions, but the common denominator appears to be impaired retinal circulation (Fig. 18). The new vessels generally arise from the venous side of the capillary

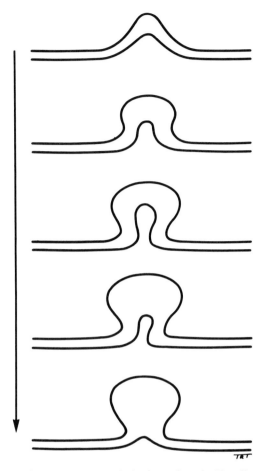

Figure 16   Sequence of events that appear to precede the formation of a "loop" capillary aneurysm. An initial focal proliferation of endothelial cells in the capillary wall produces dilatation and kinking of the vessel, which is tethered to the surrounding tissues by its surrounding network of reticulin fibers and glial attachments. Progressive proliferation leads to further dilatation and the development of a loop.

bed at the margins of the ischemic areas and are preceded by an increase in caliber of the parent vein. Origin from arterioles is exceptional, although it has been reported in both diabetic and sickle cell retinopathies. Two patterns of proliferation are recognized. One presents as budding of solid cords of endothelium from dilated segments of veins with subsequent canalization of capillaries, which although initially flat may form delicate fronds within the vitreous cavity. Commonly referred to as *rete mirabile*, this type of growth is frequently seen in diabetic and sickle cell retinopathies, the proliferating plexus of vessels in the latter condition often being further described as "sea fans" because of their resemblance to the sea fan coral *Gorgonia flabellum* found off the coast of Florida and the West Indies. This type of growth involves mitotic division of established and fully differentiated endothelium.

A second type of vasoproliferation that repeats the embryonic method of vessel growth has been described during the immediate neonatal period in retinopathy of prematurity and in later life in association with inflammation and preretinal hemorrhage [27]. Developing vessels are preceded by a band of undifferentiated cells (Fig. 19), which appear to be the source of the definitive endothelium, and fibroblasts. The immature endothelial cells fuse to form intercommunicating strands, these subsequently acquiring a lumen and becoming recognizable as capillaries continuous with the preexisting vessels from which the vasoformative mesenchyme arose [27]. This second type of proliferation is subject to extensive fibrous tissue deposition, but neither type is devoid of at least some surrounding fibrosis.

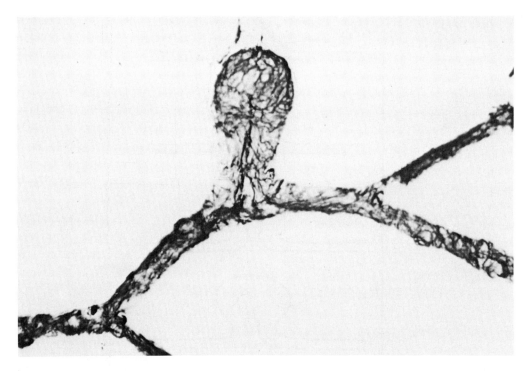

Figure 17   Retina in diabetic microangiopathy studied by trypsin digestion and reticulin staining. Perivascular reticulin fibers are prominent in many places and can be seen surrounding and straddling the base of a microaneurysm. (×490)

Subsequently, the newly formed tubes of endothelium secrete a basement membrane and acquire an outer covering of pericytes. The source of the pericytes is, as in the initial fetal development, not entirely clear, and although origin from the endothelium has been proposed [483], the associated connective tissue elements are a valid alternative. At one time it was considered usual for preretinal vessels to be devoid of pericytes, but later studies showed that this is not always the case [134,516]; the discrepancy may reflect the degree of vessel maturity. Electron microscopy has demonstrated tight encircling junctions between contiguous endothelial cells identical to those seen in the parent circulation [249,516], but at what stage they develop is uncertain. Fenestration of the new endothelium by unit membranes has also been reported [516] and may be a factor contributing to the tendency of preretinal vessels to leak and bleed.

In due course the new vessels may regress to leave a flat vitreoretinal scar, regression being most marked where there is least collagen deposition. Initially the redundant vessels are reduced to acellular basement tubes by a process that appears to involve the formation of platelet conglutinates and thrombotic occlusion [339]. The vasoproliferation observed in kittens with experimentally induced retinopathy of prematurity undergoes complete resolution because, it is presumed, the new vessels are completely free of surrounding fibrous tissue [43], and it is clinical experience that rete mirabile is more likely to regress than is fibrotic retinitis proliferans. Possibly the metabolic needs of the accompanying fibrous tissue are concerned in the perpetuation of a vasoformative stimulus.

The untoward effects of a preretinal neovascularization are related to the fragility of immature vessels and cicatrization of the accompanying fibrous tissue. Should the vitreous retract, capillaries bound to its posterior face are drawn forward to expose their fragility and encourage bleeding. There is also a direct risk of retinal tearing, and the possibility of detachment attributable to such tears is further increased by the concomitant perivascular fibrosis should it incur the formation of retinovitreal traction bands.

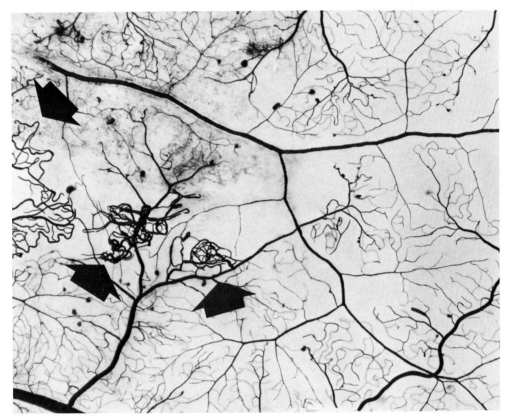

Figure 18 Flat mount of retina in proliferative diabetic retinopathy. The patent vessels have been perfused with colloidal carbon. Leashes of new capillaries on the surface of the retina (arrows) originated from venules at the edges of inadequately perfused foci in the underlying tissue. (×25)

Intraretinal Neovascularization. The proliferation of capillaries within the retina in the postnatal period represents revascularization of areas of failed perfusion. The presence of dilated tortuous vascular channels extending into areas of capillary closure has been recognized for many years, and fluorescein angiographic evidence suggests that they represent new capillaries [226,248]. Whether they are the result of remodeling preexisting defunct vessels or completely new formations cannot always be ascertained, and some observers have taken refuge in the noncommittal phrase "intraretinal microvascular abnormality" (IRMA) [133]. Where revascularization can be identified the process entails renewal of the endothelium along the residual basement membrane tubes [534], whereas presumed de novo capillaries have been observed within the interstices of glial scar tissue [15].

The anomalous intraretinal vessels differ in some respects from preretinal capillaries; they are wider than normal, with diameters of 20–50 μm, and do not leak significant amounts of fluorescein. The explanation of this difference is obscure, but Archer [15] suggested that it reflects a slower rate of growth and consequent greater maturity.

Subretinal Neovascularization. New vessels beneath the retina are usually of choroidal origin, reaching the retina either through gaps in Bruch's membrane or by passing around the edge of that membrane at the disk margin (see Chap. 20). Initially, such proliferation is between Bruch's membrane and the pigment epithelium, but eventually there is apt to be spread into the subretinal space proper. Neovascularization of this type is an essential characteristic of age-related diskiform macular degeneration.

Proliferation of retinal capillaries in the outer layer and on the deep surface of a detached retina has

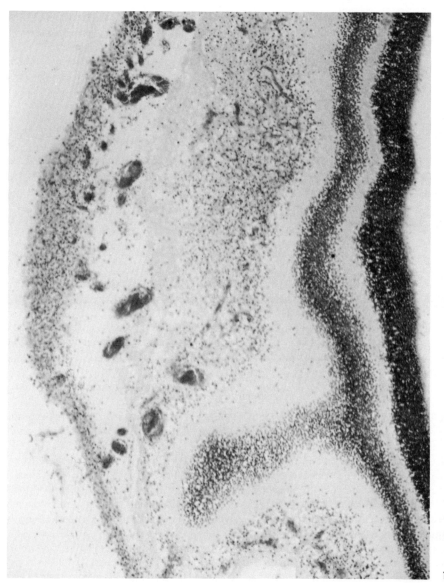

Figure 19 In the proliferative phase of retrolental fibroplasia a focus of preretinal vasoproliferation at the temporal periphery is preceded by a layer of primitive mesenchyme. Such tissue is the forerunner of definitive vessel formation and appears to reenact the embryonal process of vascular development. (Hematoxylin and eosin, ×190)

been observed in Coats' disease and retinopathy of prematurity, which suggests that it is a function of a relatively young vasculature. This concept is supported by the observation that subretinal neovascularization can be produced experimentally in response to detachment in kittens but not in the adult cat [34]. A retinal contribution to the vascularization of the fibrous plaque seen in the late stages of age-related macular diskiform degeneration may also occur [233,454].

Iris

Vascular proliferation on the front of the iris, so-called rubeosis iridis, generally originates from venules at the pupillary margin or near the iris root, where they are perhaps closest to the surface. Before there is manifest angiogenesis, the parent vessels dilate and show increased permeability [160]; the eventual new capillaries perpetuate the leakiness by having fenestrated endothelial cells joined by desmosomal junctions [514]. There is a variable degree of accompanying collagenous deposition, which experimental studies suggest may emanate from the iris stroma [409], and should the resultant fibrovascular membrane involve the peripheral iris, adhesion to the back of the cornea is probable, with obstruction to aqueous outflow proportional to the circumferential extent of the process. Ectropion uveae is also prone to develop as the fibrovascular tissue cicatrizes and pulls on the pigment epithelium of the iris at the pupil.

Predisposing conditions are numerous [213,287], many involving some impairment of the retinal circulation, especially the ischemic type of central retinal vein occlusion. Long-standing detachment of the retina, whether spontaneous or secondary to other intraocular disorders, may also underlie the formation of new vessels on the iris surface. Retinoblastoma is another potent cause of iris neovascularization, as is anterior uveitis.

Cornea

The clinical situations in which the cornea can be vascularized are many and varied, and the list of experimental means of achieving it runs to hundreds of causes [318]. Largely, however, they can be grouped under five headings: infection, trauma, allergy, toxicity, and metabolic disturbances. The new vessels originate from the perilimbal plexus of conjunctival venules and capillaries and may invade the cornea at any level.

Pannus.   Conditions giving rise to epithelial damage in the cornea from infection, trauma, or metabolic embarrassment are liable to be complicated by proliferation of blood vessels that spread between the epithelium and Bowman's layer. Adventitial fibroblasts accompany the vessels and form a pannus (Fig. 20), of which it is usual to describe two types:

1. Inflammatory pannus is associated with prominent leukocytic infiltration, which includes polymorphonuclear leukocytes in the active stages but is commonly made up of overwhelming numbers of lymphocytes and plasma cells by the time the pathologist sees it. Frequently there is some destruction of Bowman's layer, and the vessels wander in a rather wayward fashion through the anterior stroma.
2. Degenerative pannus has far fewer inflammatory cells, and eventually the vascular component, which may never have been very prominent, is liable to regress to leave a hyalinized, relatively acellular layer of fibrous tissue. This type of pannus is especially common in conditions, such as glaucoma, that give rise to chronic epithelial edema.

The vessels themselves are not of great clinical consequence and, once the stimulus is withdrawn, usually regress. The process of regression conforms to the general pattern in that it is preceded by thrombotic occlusion of redundant channels. Traces may persist as acellular ghost vessels, particularly within the stroma, but of greater significance is the presence of any collagenous tissue laid down by accompanying fibroblasts because this inevitably persists and may cause permanent corneal opacification.

Stromal Vascularization.   Vascularization of the corneal stroma is most common in inflammatory states in which there is interstitial edema. The vessels are characteristically straight, following the anatomical divisions of the corneal lamellae and branching in a brushlike manner.

Stromal vessels differ from their more superficial counterparts in being relatively free of collagen deposition and in this respect are associated with somewhat less risk of opacification. Conversely, their presence erodes much of the cornea's immunological privilege (see Chap. 4), so that grafted tissue is liable to be rejected. They also increase the capacity for lipid deposition in the stroma in later life.

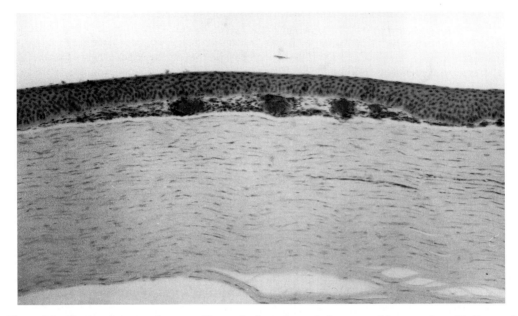

Figure 20   Neovascular corneal pannus. The newly formed vessels have spread between the epithelium and Bowman's layer of the substantia propria. (Hematoxylin and eosin, ×100)

Morphogenesis.   Arising from the conjunctival capillaries or venules [102], the new vessels begin as solid cords of endothelium and represent a budding type of growth [496]. Study of the neovascular process in the rat [319] indicates that there is an initial diapedesis of neutrophil leukocytes from dilated vessels at the limbus, followed by migration of existing endothelial cells through gaps in the basement membrane of the parent vessels. Subsequent mitotic activity pushes the dividing cells through the gap to form a column of cells, which eventually dispose to the formation of a lumen. Individual cords of proliferating endothelium have the potential to fuse with neighboring cords to create anastomosing loops, and eventually, as lumina develop and preferential patterns of blood flow are established, some of the new capillaries tend to dilate, whereas others atrophy. Evidence provided by in vitro cell culture suggests that the formation of lumens is induced in part by the keratocyte derived extracellular matrix [401a]. Pericytes are seen in established new vessels but are absent at first, and although metaplasia of stromal keratocytes has been postulated as a result of studies in rats [401], their origin, as in other situations, is in doubt.

The new capillaries allow easy egress of red cells and produce tiny hemorrhages; usually the cells escape through open interendothelial junctions but rarely have also been observed apparently passing directly through intact endothelium [290]. Regressed channels may leave acellular basement membrane residues equated with empty ghost vessels.

Pathogenesis of Neovascularization

The vascular endothelium is in constant need of renewal, cell loss occurring through hemodynamic damage and programmed cell death [461], and the angiogenic process under pathological conditions is to be seen as an extension of this physiological response. Control of the various stages of angiogenesis appears to be very finely tuned through the release or activation of either stimulatory or inhibitory factors as appropriate (Fig. 21).

Three key events are required before definitive capillary budding can occur: basement membrane lysis, endothelial cell proliferation, and migration.

Basement Membrane Lysis.   Degradation of the vascular basement membrane is a necessary precedent to the initiation of a capillary sprout or bud. In part this may be because of the physical constraints an intact membrane places on activated endothelium, but perhaps more important are its biochemical effects [475]. There is now clear evidence that cell-matrix interactions are a major influence in

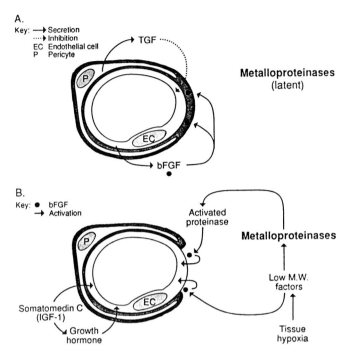

Figure 21   Early events in the stimulation of angiogenesis. (A) In the normal state basic fibroblast growth factor (bFGF) produced in an autocrine fashion by the endothelium is held in a bound, inactive form within the vascular basement membrane. Pericyte-derived transforming growth factor-β (TGF) also serves to restrain the proliferative potential of the endothelium. (B) In the initial stages of angiogenesis low-molecular-weight factors in the tissues, possibly liberated under hypoxic conditions, activate latent metalloproteinases, resulting in basement membrane lysis and activation of bFGF. Insulin-like growth factor (somatomedin C) is also likely to be involved.

the regulation of angiogenesis [188]. In part the effect may concern the ability of the proliferating endothelium to attach to the extracellular matrix [407], and whereas laminin and fibronectin are conducive to such anchorage, type IV collagen is not [462]. In addition it seems that basement membranes can bind angiogenic growth factors in an inactive state and that dissolution of the membranes is essential if the factors are to function. The mechanism of basement membrane lysis appears to involve neutral metalloproteinases [5] that are normally complexed with an inhibitor and need to be dissociated before the enzyme can be activated [367,413].

Endothelial Cell Proliferations.   The range of substances capable of supporting the growth of vascular endothelium is wide, indicating that the process is not only multifactorial but probably involves a complex sequence of events. Equally it is likely that the function of any one of the identified agents is dependent on its interaction with the milieu, and indeed, some factors can have either a positive or a negative influence according to the local circumstances [501] and concentration [171]. Correspondingly there is reason, as Glaser [220] proposes, to speak of modulating rather than growth factors. Some such factors of demonstrated relevance in an ocular context are considered here.

Fibroblast growth factors (FGF).   There are two structurally related forms of FGF, acid (14 kD) and basic (16 kD), and there is evidence that capillary endothelium, including that of the retina, can both bind and synthesize FGF [375,405]. Secreted basic FGF bound in an inactive form with heparin can be stored in the basement membrane [314] pending its release and activation should membrane lysis occur.

Low-molecular-weight angiogenic factors.   A number of agents, including substances as diverse as lactate, nucleotides and their derivatives, copper ions, and selenium, may function as intermediaries in the vascularization process [413]. Endothelial cell angiogenesis factor (ESAF) is a small molecule of unknown structure that not only releases the enzymes required for basement membrane lysis from their inhibitor but also potentiates the mitogenic activity of FGF on capillary endothelium [413]. This synergism may arise in part through the ability of ESAF to liberate the otherwise inactive metalloproteinases produced by the endothelium in response to FGF stimulation [367]. The role of copper ions [365] may also be within the context of collagenase activation [77,357].

Insulinlike growth factors (IGF). Previously referred to as somatomedins but now redesignated because of an amino acid sequence with some similarity to insulin, these factors are of widespread distribution and able to stimulate all phases of the angiogenic process. Production is both local, when they are probably concerned with autocrine and paracrine regulation of angiogenesis [477], and hepatic, with systemic distribution. They may act in concert with growth hormone, which serves to stimulate endothelial cell differentiation before mitosis [74a,477]. Of undoubted relevance in diabetic states, there is also evidence that IGF-I is involved in other proliferative retinopathies [230].

Transforming growth factor α (TGF-α) and epidermal growth factor. These are peptides with a range of specificities that include the ability to promote angiogenesis [476]. They have been demonstrated in bovine retina, but their relevance to vasoproliferative ocular disease is unknown [477].

Transforming growth factor β (TGF-β). Modulating factors of this type are potent chemoattractants for macrophages, which are subsequently stimulated to secrete TGF-α. Paradoxically, by virtue of an inhibitory effect on bFGF [62], they can also suppress endothelial cell division, and it may be that the stimulatory effect attributable to macrophage activation takes place at concentrations inimical to the inhibitory function [477]. Pericytes are a source of TGF-β, and this is possibly related to an in vitro description of the retraining effect of these cells on the capillary endothelium [418].

Angiogenin. This is a molecule of some similarity to pancreatic ribonuclease, but the mechanism of its in vivo vascularizing property is not known and may be indirect [175,184].

Inflammatory factors. Both humoral and cellular influences have been invoked in the pathogenesis of neovascularization and are considered further in the context of corneal angiogenesis, this being a circumstance in which they are especially relevant. It is also appropriate to note that macrophages in particular may be concerned in choroidal neovascularization [310] and, having been described in cultured explants of rabbit retinal vascular complexes [27], have more recently been ascribed a seminal role in the growth of comparable bovine retinal explants [189]. Furthermore, there is a possibility that many growth-modulating factors, although able to exert their effects in vitro in apparently immediate ways, may function in less direct fashion in vivo. Thus, the proliferative responses elicited by introducing a variety of growth factors into porous subcutaneous chambers in rats were generally preceded by leukocytic infiltration [502].

Inhibitory influences. The other side of the coin in the search for the mechanism of pathological angiogenesis is to consider the possibility that a natural inhibitor is deficient. There is no doubting the existence of biological substances with antiangiogenic properties, well-documented examples including heparin, platelet factor IV, and certain corticosteroids [123,377]. Conversely, there is no convincing evidence that neovascularization ever develops because of a primary lack of such factors. Antiangiogenic properties have been described in cartilage and aorta [161–163,397,499] and shown to reside in an extractable fraction with anticollagenase activity [397]. Vitreous also demonstrates a capacity for inhibition of vascularization [76], as can the RPE [221].

Endothelial Cell Migration. Activated cells freed from the constraints of the basement membrane move away from the parent vessel, and there is evidence that migration may precede mitotic activity [46]. A presumption that this is a chemotactic process governed by angiogenic factor concentrations is not as easily maintained given the evidence that the growing vessels may provide their own source of stimulation [63,478]. Possibly hypoxia per se, inflammatory factors, or some further disturbance engendered by the disease process prompting the neovascularization is involved in the directional growth pattern. Several of the agents associated with the proliferative response are also able to promote migration, and it appears that heparin, which may be bound to such factors as FGF, plays an integral part in the process [47]. The ability of heparin to stimulate endothelial cell migration depends on the presence of copper ions [449].

Retina. The pattern of events in the formation of preretinal new blood vessels parallels that described for neovascularization in general (Fig. 22). A usual feature of retinas exhibiting preretinal neovascularization is impaired perfusion of the capillary bed (Fig. 18). Presumed intraretinal vascular proliferation is similarly related to the margins of ischemic areas. Since circulatory inadequacy in the retina appears to antedate the emergence of new capillaries, it is reasonable to postulate a causal relationship [43,548]. Experimental support for this proposition is provided by the neovascularization that follows the occlusion of branch arterioles by glass microspheres in neonatal kittens [38] or branch veins using the argon

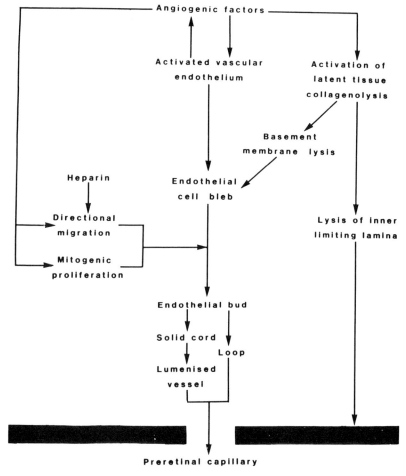

Figure 22 Some of the factors involved in the stimulation and modulation of angiogenesis. (Reproduced with permission from M.E. Boulton, D. McLeod, and A. Garner. Vasoproliferative retinopathies: Clinical, morpho-genetic and modulatory aspects. *Eye 2 (Suppl.)*:S124–139, 1988.

laser in monkeys [249]. The finding that the preretinal oxygen tension in diabetic patients with proliferative retinopathy is increased after panphotocoagulation may be the explanation for the beneficial effects of this form of treatment [504]. It is less common, however, for occlusion of the central retinal artery resulting in retinal infarction to provoke new vessel formation, which suggests that it is hypoxia, rather than anoxia, that is important. Subretinal neovascularization may also be dependent on tissue hypoxia, since it can develop at the base of retinochoroidal scars produced in monkeys by photocoagulation of the retinal vasculature [16]. Ashton [22] listed three prerequisites for retinal vasoproliferation: the presence of living tissue, low oxygen tension in the tissue, and poor venous drainage. The third element was included on the premise that a degree of stasis would increase the chance that effective levels of angiogenic factors released by the hypoxic tissue will be attained.

The nature of the link between retinal hypoxia and neovascularization has attracted a number of hypotheses.

Release of angiogenic factor by hypoxic tissue. The superimposition of neovascularization on deficient retinal perfusion has encouraged the idea that metabolically impoverished tissue releases a factor with vasoformative properties. Proliferation of new vessels in front of the retina might be explained were the postulated factor to have a molecular size small enough for it to diffuse from its origin in the retina into the vitreous cavity. Because of the largely stagnant nature of the vitreous, the vasoformative substance would accumulate there and exercise a chemotactic effect on vessels close to the retinal surface.

The presence of such substances in the context of retinal neovascularization, first suggested by Michaelson [386], is not now doubted. A succession of factors has been described, ranging from large molecules of 13–70 kD (130,131,451] to much smaller entities down to 300 D [168]. As with new vessel formation in general, retinal angiogenesis is a multifactorial process, and it would be wrong to impute any single agent in its pathogenesis, although evidence is accruing that basic FGF, modulated by TGF-β [62], proteinase activators and inhibitors, and other influences, is a key element. There is also evidence that retinal capillary endothelium can be its own source of FGF [63], with the possibility that pericytes, which have been claimed to exercise an inhibitory effect on vasoproliferative activity [417], achieve their effect through direct pericyte-endothelial cell contacts. Insulinlike growth factors may also be involved [230].

The link between angiogenic factor release and retinal ischemia has been demonstrated by showing that ESAF levels in the vitreous and retina of neonate kittens subjected to vasoobliterative amounts of oxygen were increased threefold over the levels in littermates [520,521].

Lactic acid accumulation.   In view of the connection between retinal ischemia and neovascularization, it is proper to examine the angiogenic potential of the metabolic products of hypoxic tissue. One consequence of a reduced oxygen supply, as well as being a feature of poorly controlled diabetes mellitus, is increased lactate formation. Enhanced activity of an isoenzyme of lactic dehydrogenase in experimental retinopathy of prematurity [231] is in keeping with this hypothesis, although subsequent direct measurement of lactate in animals with oxygen-induced retinal vasoobliteration and in drug-induced diabetic rats have not shown any difference from levels in intact animals [216,232]. Moreover, although Imre [289] succeeded in stimulating new vessel formation in a substantial number of kittens by giving them an intravitreal injection of lactic acid, there has not been any corroboration of these results by other workers. Odedra and Weiss [413] speculate that the role of lactate, if any, is likely to be greatest in inflammatory disease, since experiments have shown that macrophages can be stimulated to initiate angiogenic activity when incubated with lactate [299]. However, there is a possibility that macrophage-provoked angiogenesis may be a feature of retinal neovascularization in states other than inflammation [189]. Correspondingly, a contribution of lactate to retinal angiogenesis cannot be excluded.

Platelet activation.   Thrombotic vascular occlusion is a feature of a number of retinopathies giving rise to vasoproliferation, in which case it is reasonable to suppose that release of platelet-derived growth factors, deposition of fibrin, and activation of the plasminogen system could be involved in the angiogenic response.

Hemorrhage.   The formation of fibrovascular scar tissue as a complication of both preretinal and subretinal hemorrhage suggests that blood components are able to promote vasoproliferation. Apart from the platelet component, there is little to sustain this view, however. Rather it has been clinical experience that unless there is spread into the vitreous, where contact with vitreal collagen can initiate clotting [117, 118], preretinal hemorrhages remain fluid and are often dispersed without the formation of a residual scar. In situations in which intravitreal hemorrhage is followed by neovascularization, the predominant finding is fibroglial tissue proliferation, and it is possible that the stimulus to vasoproliferation is provided by the metabolic needs of the resulting scar. Evidence in support of this contention comes from the observation that collagen formation by autologous fibroblasts injected into the vitreous cavity of rabbit eyes is associated with vascular invasion of the implant and neovascularization on the retinal surface [7].

Inflammation and immunological factors.   In view of the well-documented association between inflammation and angiogenesis, it is proper to investigate the nature of the neovascularization prone to complicate such conditions as Eales disease and the retinal components of Behçet's syndrome and sarcoidosis.

Adequately documented examples of retinal inflammation in which the effects of associated thrombosis and tissue hypoxia can be excluded are very few [228], although Shorb and his colleagues [487] described disk neovascularization in five patients with chronic cyclitis and apparently normal retinal perfusion as revealed by fluorescein angiography. It would also, given the evidence that macrophages may be attracted by simple ischemia [189] and lowered oxygen levels [321,322], be illogical to deny them a part in obviously inflammatory retinal states. It would also be a mistake to dismiss the possibility that soluble mediators of inflammation contribute to the angiogenic stimulus even in apparently noninflammatory retinopathies, especially as levels of interleukin-6 have been found to correlate with proliferative activity in the vitreous of patients with diabetic retinopathy [163a].

Relevant experimental studies are equally sparse. On the basis of the vascular response to the intravitreal injection of insulin in hyperimmunized monkeys, it has been postulated that complexes of insulin and its antibody represent a stimulus to angiogenesis [482]. However, despite the presence of antibodies to exogenous insulin in the serum of many diabetic patients [109] and the demonstration of immune complexes of this type in the basement membranes of diabetic blood vessels, there is no evidence of vasculitis in diabetic retinopathy. It is therefore improbable that an immune reaction of the Arthus type is implicated in a direct way in the neovascularization complicating diabetes mellitus.

Failure of inhibition.   The avascularity of the normal vitreous is not so much due to the absence of angiogenic stimuli as to active suppression. Following experiments that demonstrated the ability of bovine vitreous extracts to prevent tumor-induced vascularization of the cornea [76], there have been several confirmatory reports involving both in vivo [174] and in vitro [363] test systems and including examination of human vitreous [294]. The character of the inhibitor(s) is uncertain. Raymond and Jacobson [451] described a molecule of G-2 kD that can inhibit smooth muscle cells and fibroblasts as well as vascular endothelium, and Singh and coworkers [488] refer to a moiety encountered in the vitreous after retinal panphotocoagulation, which, it is conjectured, might be TGF-β. There is no evidence, however, that preretinal neovascularization is a response to the failure of normal vasoinhibitory processes.

Iris.   Direct information bearing on the mechanism of iris neovascularization is sparse, but its frequent association with posterior segment disorders supports the concept of forward diffusion of angiogenic substances (Fig. 23).

Retina-derived angiogenesis factor.   Ashton [22] speculated that angiogenic factors released from the retina under hypoxic conditions drain anteriorly into the aqueous and stimulate vessels close to the iris surface. It is on this hypothesis that the practice of retinal panphotocoagulation to bring about regression of iris neovascularization is based, often with dramatic success [340,376]. Furthermore, there is evidence that developments that may be expected to facilitate such drainage, such as intracapsular lens extraction [439,458] and vitrectomy [378], are accompanied by an enhanced risk of iris neovascularization.

Experimental studies also point to the importance of retinal hypoxia with release of angiogenic factors. Rhegmatogenous detachment combined with lensectomy and vitrectomy in cats is followed by iris neovascularization [503], and the inhibitory effect of normal rabbit aqueous on in vitro endothelial cell proliferation is negated if aqueous from diabetic rabbits is added instead [415]. Conversely, aqueous from monkey subjected to experimental retinal vein occlusion culminating in iris neovascularization stimulates mitosis of cultured endothelial cells, whereas aqueous from unoperated control animals has no effect [239].

Iris hypoxia.   Whether direct ischemia of the iris is a factor in iris neovascularization is unresolved. Acute ischemia of the anterior segment is more commonly followed by infarction, and although new vessels on the iris surface are a well-recognized feature of chronic ocular ischemia resulting from carotid artery disease [266], this is usually explicable in terms of posterior segment hypoxia.

Tumor-derived angiogenesis factor.   Iris neovacularization is a frequent finding in children with retinoblastoma, and it is reasonable to suggest that this is the outcome of tumor-derived stimuli entering the anterior chamber, but direct evidence has yet to be provided.

Inflammation.   The association of iris new vessels and anterior uveitis may well be promoted by the inflammatory process, but here again there is a dearth of direct evidence.

Cornea.   In view of the variety of circumstances in which vascularization of the cornea can develop [318], it is not surprising that there should be more than one theory for its pathogenesis.

Tissue swelling.   A feature common to most, if not all, situations in which there is stromal vascularization is interstitial edema [33,101,102]. Consequently, vascular invasion of the stroma could be a sequel to loosening of the corneal lamellar structure, and as a corollary, it might be argued that the avascularity of the intact healthy cornea is largely due to the impenetrable nature of its densely compacted architecture [101]. The vascularization stimulated by experimental induction of stromal edema is in accord with this theory [33].

However, although interstitial edema may well facilitate stromal neovascularization, it is unlikely to be the full explanation, since the cornea can be edematous, as in the various types of endothelial dystrophy, without necessarily becoming vascularized.

Hypoxia.   Evidence that oxygen lack may be of importance comes from a number of sources. The vascularization linked with riboflavin deficiency in animals has been ascribed to interference with oxidative enzyme systems [67]; that seen as a complication of the prolonged wearing of contact lenses may be due to hindered gaseous interchange at the corneal surface [137].

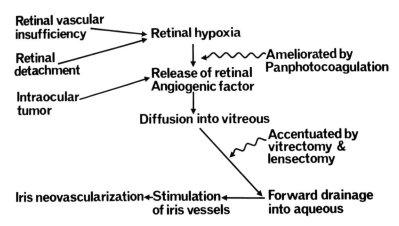

Figure 23 Postulated sequence of events in iris neovascularization. Factors released from the retina are presumed to reach the anterior chamber and activate the endothelium of vessels close to the iris surface. (Reproduced with permission from A. Garner, Ocular angiogenesis. *Int. Rev. Exp. Pathol.* 28:249–306, 1986.)

Langham [342] found the level of oxidation in the intact cornea to be less than optimal, and this led Ashton and Cook [33] to suggest that there is an inherent vasoformative stimulus that needs the concurrence of stromal swelling to have any effect. Lactate accumulation, which can be promoted in the cornea by interfering with the limbal circulation [352], is associated with vascularization, although as noted in the consideration of angiogenic mechanisms in general, its mode of action is likely to be indirect. Indeed, it is possible that the éffect of hypoxia as a whole is indirect and is mediated by secondary inflammation since the angiogenesis promoted by extended contact lens wearing in rabbits can be suppressed by antiinflammatory drug treatment [146].

Inflammation. There is persuasive evidence that the inflammatory process that accompanies the tissue response to injury can promote vascular proliferation [89,317]. Moreover, this function appears to be integral to the tissue response rather than to the exciting agent, since sepsis with the release of bacterial toxins retards healing. Substances that can promote the growth of fibroblasts were extracted from leukocytes many years ago by Carrel [93], with Ebeling [94], who called them trephones. Interest in the relevance of inflammatory factors to corneal vascularization was stimulated by Klintworth's discovery that corneas implanted in the cheek pouch of the hamster, should they be invaded by host blood vessels, always showed leukocytic infiltration [316]. Subsequently, Fromer and Klintworth [198] induced vascularization of the cornea in situ by a variety of means, ranging from chemical to physical trauma as well as immunological insults and dietary disturbance, and found that a pronounced leukocytic infiltrate generally preceded and accompanied the vascular ingrowth. The same workers then showed that by irradiating the experimental animal to destroy the hematopoietic bone marrow, they could prevent the corneal response to vasoproliferative stimuli (Fig. 24) [199]. They also concluded that an angiogenic principle was associated with the neutrophil polymorphonuclear leukocyte rather than with nonactivated cells of the lymphoid series [200].

Others, however, have presented evidence that, as in other situations [44,362], activated lymphocytes may be involved, in the cornea [169]. Macrophages activated by immune reactions and their secretory products have also been shown to be capable of inducing corneal vascularization [440], and endothelial proliferation is a feature of delayed cutaneous hypersensitivity reactions in guinea pigs [224,441]. The role of macrophages in the vascularizing process appears to depend on the milieu and the concentration of factors that both attract and are produced by the cells. Reference has already been made to the circumstances under which they may be attracted through the mediation of TGF-β and stimulated to release angiogenesis-promoting TGF-α. They are also a source of tumor necrosis factor α which acts in a bimodal fashion to stimulate angiogenesis at low concentration and then actively inhibit the process if the concentration rises above a certain level [171]. This dose-dependent nature of the angiogenic response has been noted in the specific context of the cornea [61,349].

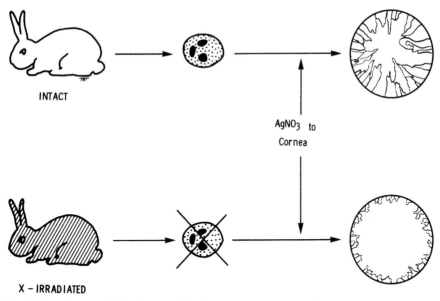

INTACT

AgNO$_3$ to
Cornea

X - IRRADIATED

Figure 24 Effect of neutrophil leukocyte depletion on corneal vascularization. Whereas the application of silver nitrate usually gives rise to vascular infiltration, whole-body x-irradiation destroys the myelocyte-forming bone marrow and is associated with a marked reduction in any such vasoproliferative response.

A further discovery by Fromer and Klintworth [199] was that corticosteroids inhibited leukocytic infiltration of the cornea and its subsequent vascularization, it having previously been shown that cortisone reduces the neovascularization response of the rabbit cornea to alloxan [35]. This may be due to the inhibition of vascular dilation and increase in permeability necessary for polymorphonuclear leukocyte emigration.

Whether leukocytes are essential for angiogenesis is not entirely clear, because others have found that corneal vascularization can be induced, albeit less markedly, even though the animals are depleted of leukocytes [164,165,485,486]. In the experiments of Sholley and colleagues [486], profound neutropenia was created by x irradiation combined with antineutrophil serum, and although the absence of leukocytic infiltration did not deter the vascular response to a corneal injury, the vessels were shorter than in controls. Despite the experimental evidence that corneal vascularization can proceed in the absence of cellular infiltrates, in practice this is unlikely. Klintworth has researched the matter extensively and has yet to find a naturally occurring situation in which inflammatory factors can definitely be excluded [318]. The demonstrated role of prostaglandins [277], interleukins [61], and other soluble mediators of inflammation in corneal vascular proliferation is extremely complex, and it is probably wrong to evaluate their role in isolation from the cells from which they emanate and with which they react. Indeed, evidence of interaction between the soluble and the cellular mediators of inflammation in the context of corneal angiogenesis is seen in a demonstration that prostaglandin E$_1$ serves to attract copper ions [559], which then stimulate polymorphonuclear leukocytes to produce collagenase [357]. Klintworth [318] considers the matter in his detailed review of corneal angiogenesis.

Failure of inhibition. Since the cornea is normally avascular, is vessel ingrowth due to failure of some natural inhibitor [385]? However, although the existence of such substances has been demonstrated in cartilage [337,397] and elsewhere, comparable inhibitors have not been described in the cornea apart from an unconfirmed report of an extractable proteinase inhibitor [337]. Nevertheless, looking at the matter from an opposite standpoint, it is possible that angiogenic factors are held within the normal cornea in a bound state and are activated only under pathological conditions. Thus, basic FGF, likely to have been formed by the endothelium [479] but inactivated through being complexed with heparan sulfate, has been detected in bovine Descemet's membrane [185]. Certain naturally occurring corticosteroids are able to inhibit vascularization, and, although this is commonly by virtue of their antiinflammatory effects [396], a minority appear to have a more direct influence [123], possibly mediated through interference with plasminogen activator activity [18]. The antiangiogenic properties of corticosteroids were initially described by Ashton and his coworkers [35], and since then evidence has accumulated that the more specifically angiostatic steroids are potentiated in the presence of heparin and some synthetic analogs [123,354].

III. SPECIFIC VASCULAR DISORDERS AND THEIR OCULAR EFFECTS

A. Atherosclerosis

Atherosclerosis is primarily a disease of large and medium-sized arteries and is characterized by focal intimal thickening, which, commencing with lipid accumulation, is ultimately associated with fibrous and smooth muscle cell proliferation. In the context of the orbit and its contents, atherosclerosis is seen chiefly in the ophthalmic artery, although potentiating factors, such as systemic hypertension and diabetes mellitus, can be associated with extension of the process into smaller vessels of central retinal and ciliary artery size. Contrary to some statements based on clinical appearance, however, involvement of intraocular vessels has not been substantiated by histological examination.

Nature

The archetypal lesion of atherosclerosis is a fibrolipid plaque in the intima consisting of a pool of extracellular lipid, mostly cholesterol and cholesteryl ester, lipid-laden foam cells, and cellular debris, covered on the luminal aspect by a fibrous cap of smooth muscle cells and macrophages embedded in a connective tissue matrix. There is evidence that plaque formation is preceded in many instances by fatty streaks that may be observed in infancy but such a progression is by no means inevitable.

Pathogenesis

The prevailing ideas concerning the evolution of atheromatous plaques hinge on primary damage to the arterial endothelium and subsequent imbibition of lipid by macrophages that accumulate within the intima [158,465]. In recent years there has been an increasing tendency to attach a pivotal role to the macrophage and to assign rather less importance to the muscle cells [14] than pertained previously [465].

Endothelial cell injury can be produced by hemodynamic stresses, and this almost certainly accounts for the tendency for plaques to form at forks and around the orifices of branch arteries [219]. More subtle mechanisms that fall short of frank denudation are also involved, taking the form of increased permeability in response to a range of risk factors, among which hypertension, cigarette smoking, diabetes, and, probably, hyperlipidemia are conspicuous [2,398,466].

As a result of the endothelial cell injury, platelets and circulating monocytes adhere to the damaged surface, where they are activated to promote migration of smooth muscle cells from the arterial media into the intima. There is some evidence that the process is self-perpetuating in that macrophage-derived cytokines can induce the expression of intercellular adhesion molecules (specifically, ICAM-1), which promote binding and subendothelial migration of further circulating blood monocytes [443]. Self-inducing processes of this sort, given a focal initiating event, go some way to explaining the tendency for atherosclerosis to form localized plaques. Mitogens derived from the platelets, transformed monocytes, and, possibly, the serum stimulate proliferation of the smooth muscle elements and the eventual synthesis of collagen, elastic fibers, and proteoglycans. The accumulation of lipid to form foam cells is believed to be primarily a function of monocyte-derived macrophages, these cells having a high affinity for oxidized low-density lipoprotein (LDL) [217]. Oxidized LDL is cytotoxic for macrophages [550], and it is possible that the macrophages themselves compound the problem by promoting LDL oxidation through the activity of cell-derived free radicals [447]. Such necrosis is likely to be an important element in the evolution of the developing plaque [455]. As a corollary, it has been shown that antioxidants inhibit the formation of atherosclerotic lesions in hypercholesterolemic rabbits [69]. Hyperlipidemia, especially the LDL component, is important not only because of its contribution to the plaque but because it may of itself increase endothelial cell permeability [218].

A somewhat different concept of atherosclerosis emphasizes the possibility that the prime event is relatively unregulated smooth muscle cell proliferation resulting from aberrant genetic mutation [58–60]. Cholesterol is regarded as a putative mutagen [58]. This theory, although much less widely held than the foregoing, takes account of the monotypic isoenzyme pattern encountered in smooth muscle cells of 75% of atheromatous plaques, which contrasts with the heterogeneous profile of normal arterial muscle.

Yet again, a viral pathogenesis has been proposed, the arguments being largely connected to the ability of herpesvirus in particular to induce abnormalities in cholesterol metabolism by virtue of gene modifications in the cells of the intima [244]. Allergic factors have also been implicated [253].

It is clear that whatever the reality of the situation, atherosclerosis is a multifactorial condition with regard to both cause and pathogenesis.

Complications

The clinical importance of atherosclerosis is its effect on downstream blood flow. As a rule serious interference with flow is due to massive secondary fibrinous thrombosis on the surface of a plaque or to embolism, the embolus representing fragments of a ruptured plaque or a disintegrating thrombus. Vascular stenosis by the plaque directly is not normally of significance unless the lumen is reduced by 90% or more, but lesser degrees can be important should left ventricular heart failure supervene.

Ocular Effects

Direct involvement of the ophthalmic artery close to its origin is not unusual, but atheroma of its branches is much less common. Thus, an autopsy study of diabetic subjects showed that although 34 of 60 eyes had ophthalmic artery atheroma, 13 with reduction of the orifice to less than half its normal caliber, only 3 eyes showed central retinal artery involvement, and this merely of a trivial degree [211]. The incidence of central retinal artery atheroma in the general population is probably even less. Nevertheless, the same study indicated that ophthalmic artery stenosis may contribute to the development of retinopathy in diabetic patients.

Moreover, the few subjects who incur central retinal artery involvement may occasionally succumb to thrombotic occlusion (see p. 1633). Retinal vein obstruction has also been attributed to atherosclerotic thickening of the adjacent artery. The relationship is unlikely to be straightforward, however, and may not be one of simple cause and effect. Thus, the hyperlipidemia so prominent in people with severe atherosclerosis can also increase viscosity and promote venous thrombosis.

Indirect involvement of the eye can be a feature of atheroma of the carotid artery in a number of ways. Occlusion or severe stenosis of the internal carotid artery can affect vision by reducing flow through the middle cerebral artery and interfering with occipital lobe function.

Reduction in ocular blood flow is conditioned by the capacity of the external carotid artery to provide a collateral condition, and should persistent loss of vision occur it is more commonly due to shedding of emboli and their lodgement in the central retinal artery [286]. Other less severely compromised patients may show compensatory dilatation of the retinal arteries and scattered cotton-wool spots associated with ophthalmodynamometric evidence of reduced arterial perfusion pressure.

Transient amaurosis may be a feature of shock or heart failure should the arterial supply to the eye be compromised by atherosclerotic narrowing, but a more frequent cause is embolism from a plaque close to the origin of the internal carotid artery [242,381,469]. Both cholesterol and platelet emboli have been described. Emboli to the retina usually break up after a few minutes and permanent visual loss is rare, but repeated attacks are not uncommon and may presage more serious embolization of the cerebral vessels. Presumably emboli also lodge in the uveal circulation, but because of the rich potential for anastomotic compensation, are not expected to cause significant functional disturbance.

B. Hypertension

The harmful effects of systemic hypertension are essentially a measure of the extent of the increase in blood pressure and of the rate at which it rises. Consequently, the terms "benign" and "malignant," which are commonly used in defining the severity of the hypertensive process, are relative only: benign hypertension can precipitate cardiac failure, accelerate arterial atherogenesis, and predispose to cerebral thrombosis; conversely, now that therapeutic measures have been improved, the malignant phase is not necessarily fatal. Indeed, because of the improved prognosis there is some reason to prefer the alternative designation "accelerated hypertension" to define the more severe grades, especially because this takes note of the increasing speed of the vascular degeneration.

Cause

Over 90% of clinical hypertension is idiopathic (essential), renal disease accounting for most of the remainder. Other rare causes include certain endocrine disorders, such as pheochromocytoma, toxemia of pregnancy, and coarctation of the aorta.

Systemic blood pressure is a function of the peripheral resistance and cardiac output. Hypertension attributable to increases in cardiac output may be a feature of the sodium retention and consequent rise in blood volume seen in some forms of renal disease. Otherwise hypertension is overwhelmingly the result of excessive arteriolar tone and peripheral resistance stimulated by various humoral, neurogenic, or local factors.

Circulating Humoral Factors.   The renin-angiotensin system is a major influence in several types of hypertension, especially malignant forms, the immediate stimulus to increased activity being reduced renal blood flow [492]. Studies involving the use of specific inhibitors of the renin-angiotensin system suggest that angiotensin acts both directly on systemic arterioles and indirectly by promoting aldosterone release from the adrenal cortex to cause sodium and water retention [82]. Sodium retention and hypervolemia are characteristic not only of secondary renal hypertension but are possibly features of essential hypertension, reflecting a primary genetic defect in the capacity of the renal tubular epithelium to excrete sodium [120]. Such inadequacy may be exposed by high dietary salt intake.

The role of prostaglandins and other circulating vasoactive substances is less clear [275].

Neurogenic Factors.   Increased sympathetic (α-adrenergic) activity is able to elevate sysemic blood pressure by increasing peripheral resistance and can be a response to stress.

Local Factors.   Both vasodilator substances, such as endothelium relaxing factor (in which the active principle appears to be nitric oxide) and a vasoconstrictor peptide (endothelin) [554], have been described as localized products of the vascular endothelium. Their contribution to the hypertensive process has yet to be assessed, but deficiency of local vasodilator capacity may be involved in essential hypertension [110].

Hypertensive Retinopathy

Benign Phase.   Retinopathy in the benign phase of systemic hypertension is unusual but, should it occur, is generally limited to tiny glistening whitish foci presumed to be serous exudates [438]. Exceptionally, small cotton-wool spots and isolated linear hemorrhages have been reported [51].

Nevertheless, although insufficient to cause retinal damage, changes in the arterioles of the retina are by no means uncommon, Bechgaard [52] having described abnormalities in just under half the patients he examined.

The larger arterioles surrounding the optic disk may exhibit sclerosis due to collagenous replacement of the muscle elements [543] and gradual accumulation of hematogenous insudate. The consequent loss of elasticity probably accounts for both the distension of these vessels seen in the later stages of benign hypertension [280] and the infrequency of malignant retinopathy in patients with long-standing mild hypertension and in those with age-related arteriolosclerosis, since the presence of increased collagen would protect against the disruptive effect of excessive elevation of blood pressure, "defense by sclerosis" [350].

Generalized narrowing of the smaller arterioles has been confirmed by measurement of fundus photographs [45], although casual ophthalmoscopy can give a misleading impression [507]. The narrowing is due to vasoconstriction, probably autoregulatory, and is most common in the early stages before sclerosis has developed.

Malignant (Accelerated) Phase.   The malignant phase is uncommon, affecting less than 5% of hypertensive patients, with a predilection for younger, male subjects and blacks. As a rule, elevation of the diastolic blood pressure to levels commensurate with vascular necrosis and the development of retinopathy occurs as a complicating event in patients with a previous history of benign hypertension. Situations in which the hypertension increases rapidly to diastolic levels in excess of 130 mm Hg de novo also include ischemic renal disorders and toxemia of pregnancy.

Retinopathy is a measure of arteriolar damage and is heralded by the emergence of linear hemorrhages and cotton-wool spots in the posterior fundus. Retinal edema quickly develops, and eventually serous exudates are observed; papilledema becomes apparent as the condition persists.

The retinal arteries may be narrowed [116,178,450], although overlying edema and congestion of the retinal veins can make subjective assessment deceptive [507], and a study of experimental renovascular hypertension in monkeys involving fluorescein angiography suggests that any narrowing is usually more apparent than real [270]. Information derived from histological [212] and angiographic [270] examination of hypertensive monkeys indicates that both constriction and dilatation occur. Potentially of greater importance in the pathogenesis of retinal damage are focal changes in the smaller, ophthalmoscopically unrecognizable terminal arterioles. The fundamental change is in the form of fibrinous necrosis, such as occurs elsewhere in the circulation, and represents the replacement of damaged smooth muscle fibers by fibrin and other plasma proteins leaking through defects in the endothelial lining of the affected vessels (Fig. 25).

   Pathogenesis.   It is reasonable to suppose that the ocular arterioles share the general response to whatever stimuli are initiating a rise in peripheral resistance, and although human data are wanting, there is evidence from animal experiments of muscle hypertrophy [481] and sensitivity to angiotensin [463]. To an extent any vasoconstriction can be regarded as an autoregulatory attempt to prevent overperfusion of the capillary bed, retinal and other ocular lesions developing should this attempt prove inadequate. In the benign phase of hypertension there is compensatory hypertrophy and hyperplasia of arteriolar smooth muscle to accommodate the process, but the malignant phase appears to be associated with a blood pressure rise sufficient to overcome the capacity for autoregulation.

   The regulatory arteriolar constriction can be marked before failure occurs, even to the point of virtual closure, according to findings in an electron microscope study of experimental renovascular hypertension in monkeys (Fig. 26) [40,212]. However, the extensive and detailed fluorescein angiographic analyses by Hayreh of a similar experimental model point to focal leakage (focal intraretinal periarteriolar transudates) as constituting the initial manifestation of retinopathy [263]. This suggests that the constriction, marked though it is, does not result in significant capillary closure and is not a likely cause of the subsequent cotton-wool spots. The leakage probably corresponds to the endothelial cell damage described in an electron microscope study of hypertensive primate retinas, the damage being in the form of holes or tears attributable to loss of support by a necrotic muscle wall (Fig. 27) [212].

   Cotton-wool spot formation is linked with foci of capillary nonperfusion [37] and is perhaps a sequel to structural, as opposed to functional, obliteration of the lumen of a damaged terminal arteriole. The cessation of blood flow may be a result of secondary thrombosis or the accumulation of fibrin and other plasma components in the vessel wall beneath the defective endothelium [212].

   In summary (Fig. 28), a possible sequence of events is as follows:

1.   An initial attempt at autoregulation involving conspicuous constriction of precapillary arterioles
2.   Eventual failure of autoregulatory capacity manifested by muscle necrosis and focal leakage
3.   Secondary closure of the necrotic arteriolar segment
4.   Capillary nonperfusion and cotton-wool spot formation

   It is possible that leakage may occur in ways other than endothelial cell disruption, studies of rats with both spontaneous and experimentally induced hypertension showing fairly widespread extravasation of a microperoxidase marker (2 kD) through a seemingly intact endothelium [356]. The mechanism of such blood-retina barrier failure is not clear, although an increase in active transport through pinocytosis has been postulated [557].

   Capillary microaneurysms may develop and are possibly more prominent on the arterial side of the retinal circulation, in contradistinction to the predominantly venous distribution in most other retinopathies. Possibly they reflect inadequate autoregulation and elevated perfusion pressure. Retinal hemorrhages may have a similar explanation: they originate predominantly from the radial peripapillary capillaries located in the nerve fiber layer, which gives them their characteristic linear or flame-shaped configuration [140,268].

Hypertensive Optic Neuropathy

The papilledema of hypertensive vascular disease involves both anterior and lateral swelling, the latter often causing displacement of the peripheral retina with the formation of a "neuritic roll." The swelling is associated with plasma leakage, as fluorescein angiography confirms [141], but the major factor in its pathogenesis appears to be swelling and disruption of the nerve fibers as they pass through the disk region. As with cotton-wool spots, this represents the effect of ischemia and consequent interference with

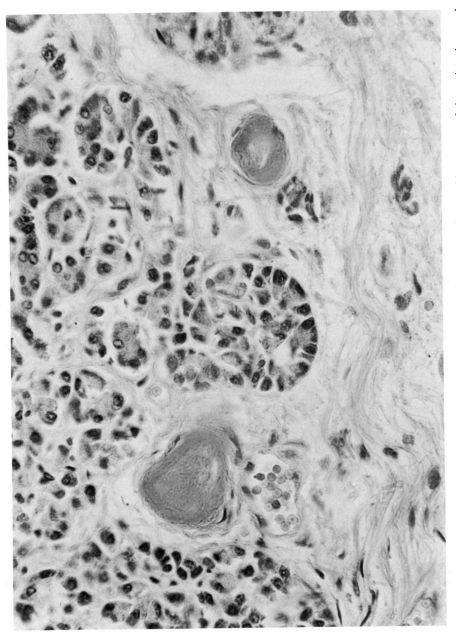

Figure 25   Arteriolar lesion in malignant hypertension. The "smudgy" appearance is caused by seepage of plasma into the vessel wall allied to necrosis of the smooth muscle cells. Such fibrinous necrosis increases the thickness of the wall of the arteriole, with consequent reduction in the lumen and blood flow. (Hematoxylin and eosin, ×470)

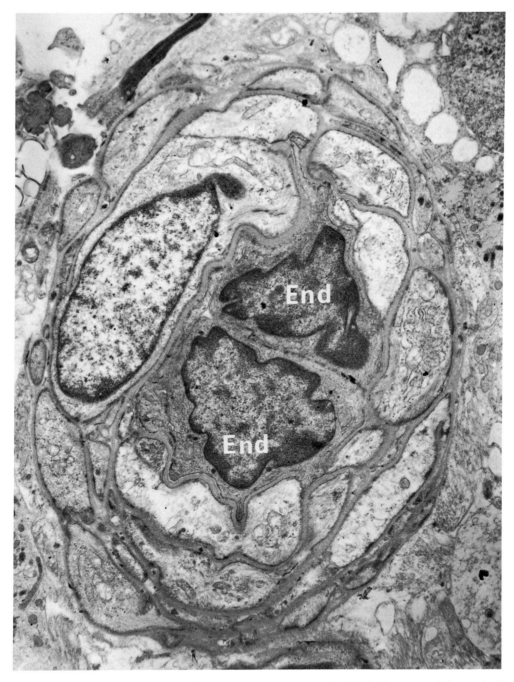

Figure 26   Experimentally induced hypertensive retinopathy in a monkey. Marked vasoconstriction resulted in obliteration of the arteriolar lumen. The endothelial lining (End) is compressed but otherwise normal, and although there is some increase in electron lucency in some cells, the smooth muscle coat shows no sign of necrosis. (×12,000)

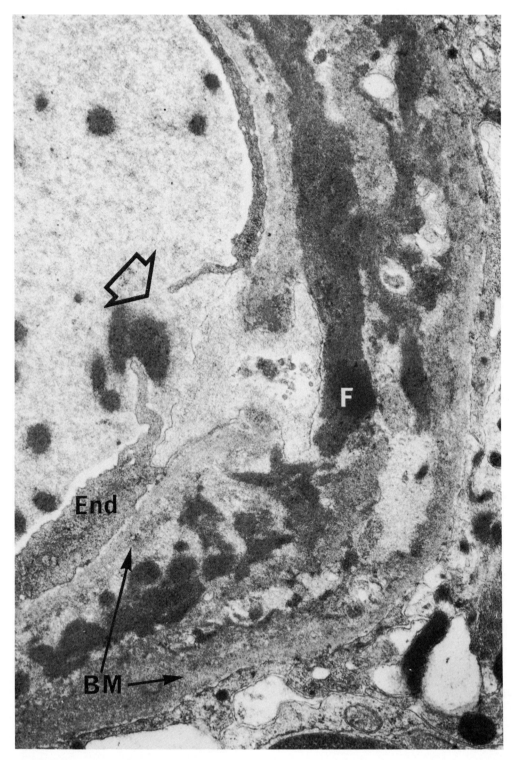

Figure 27 Electron micrograph of part of the wall of a precapillary retinal arteriole in an acutely hypertensive monkey. The endothelium (End) is attenuated and at one point is ruptured (arrow). The smooth muscle coat is degenerate and infiltrated with fibrin (F). BM, basement membrane. (×32,500)

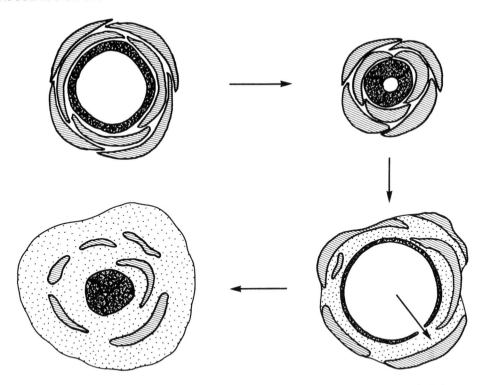

Figure 28   Postulated sequence of events in the pathogenesis of arteriolar fibrinous necrosis in hypertensive retinopathy. Initially, precapillary arterioles undergo extreme constriction, possibly as a result of an autoregulatory process. Subsequently, smooth muscle cell necrosis occurs in the face of persistently raised blood pressure, with resultant arteriolar dilatation and leakage of plasma into the degenerate wall through focal breaks in the unsupported lining endothelium. Ultimately, continued plasma insudation may produce a secondary reduction in the arteriolar lumen.

axoplasmic transport. Axolemmal swelling, both anterior and posterior to the lamina cribrosa, has been described in animal studies [313], and there is subsequent loss of axons with replacement gliosis. Both the exudation and the ischemia are the outcome of fibrinous necrosis of the smaller arterioles supplying the optic disk, although other factors, such as impeded venous outflow (as a result of raised intracranial pressure transmitted into the optic nerve sheath), may also be involved.

Hypertensive Choroidopathy

Choroidal involvement in malignant hypertension is a common histological finding [255,529] and clinically usually takes the form of Elschnig's spots. These are discrete serous exudates beneath the retinal pigment epithelium with secondary epithelial degeneration and, as with the retinal leakages, probably represent failed autoregulation culminating in fibrinous arteriolar necrosis [312,531]. Animal studies also indicate that extensive choroidal ischemia may supervene [269].

C.   Diabetes Mellitus

Diabetes mellitus is a chronic disorder affecting carbohydrate, fat, and protein metabolism. A predominant feature is hyperglycemia secondary to deficiency or resistance to insulin, the prime function of which is to promote glucose transport into certain types of cell. It can be a complication of certain pancreatic disorders, such as chronic pancreatitis and hemochromatosis, or other hormonal problems, but most cases are primary and of these two types are recognized.

   Type I diabetes (insulin dependent) is a consequence of pancreatic islet β cell loss and probably results from an autoimmune process precipitated by an environmental factor, usually in the form of one of a number of viral infections, in genetically susceptible persons. The genetic susceptibility is associated with aberrant expression of class II major histocompatibility products on the β cells [192] and is linked with the HLA-DR3, HLA-DR4, and certain HLA-DQ loci [56,523].

Type II diabetes (non–insulin dependent) is the more common type of primary diabetes, with a generally much later onset than the type I disease. Understanding of its pathogenesis is incomplete, although a relative deficiency of insulin allied to a target cell resistance to its transmembrane transport function has been established, the latter reflecting a relative lack of insulin receptors [86]. Genetic factors are even more important than in type I disease, but their mode of action is not clear.

Diabetic Vascular Disease

Few parts of the body are spared the vascular complications of the diabetic process, the incidence generally correlating with the duration of the metabolic defect. Circulatory disturbances are at the root of the renal complications, the neuropathy, and the tendency to gangrene, as well as the retinal problems. Largely because the vascular complications are far less responsive than the metabolic disorder to normoglycemic therapy, it was suggested that they are distinct aspects of the diabetic process under the control of related but separate genes [471,490]. This view is difficult to sustain, however, since angiopathy can also develop in diabetes secondary to pancreatic disease in which genetic factors are not involved [151,153], particularly tropical pancreatic diabetes, in which there is prolonged life expectancy [395]. It can also be produced in animals with artificially induced diabetes [70]. Moreover, microangiopathy develops after the onset of diabetes mellitus and may be delayed if the carbohydrate disturbance is kept under rigid control [87,111].

The metabolic consequences of diabetes are numerous, but there is good reason to implicate elevated blood glucose levels directly in the pathogenesis of the vascular complications.

One way in which hyperglycemia can affect the vasculature is by inducing nonenzymatic glycosylation of protein [81,235]. At first the changes are reversible, but ultimately stable complexes are formed, especially where collagen and other protein components of the vessel wall are concerned. There are then a number of ways in which the vessels and circulating blood can be adversely affected [80]:

1. The collagen-attached end products of glycosylation have an affinity for plasma protein, and this can interfere with transmural transport and possibly contribute to basement membrane thickening.
2. Cross-linkage of insoluble basement membrane components through their glycosylated units impairs their ability to bind to proteoglycans, and this in turn, by altering the ionic charge, leads to abnormal permeability.
3. The glycosylated elements may react with receptors on macrophages with subsequent release of interleukin-1 and tumor necrosis factor. These may then contribute to the endothelial cell changes integral to microangiopathy.
4. Glycosylation of hemoglobin (HbA_{1c}) increases its affinity for oxygen such that dissociation in the tissues is reduced [135], and although this may not be of a degree to cause significant hypoxia of itself, it may aggravate hypoxic tendencies attributable to diminished capillary perfusion. In addition, HbA_{1c}, by being intimately bound to the erythrocyte membrane, increases cell rigidity [430], and this can interfere with flow through the capillary bed.

A second way for hyperglycemia to damage the microvasculature is by causing increased utilization of the polyol route of glucose metabolism, resulting in its conversion to sorbitol under the influence of the aldose reductase enzyme. The accumulation of sorbitol not only causes an increase in osmolarity, but more importantly, it reduces the capacity for cellular uptake of myoinositol from the plasma. This in turn reduces the level of Na^+,K^+-ATPase activity, with consequent impairment of the ability of smooth muscle cells and pericytes to control vascular tone [539,547].

Capillary Changes. The hallmark of diabetic capillaropathy is a thickening of the basement membrane of up to five times the normal 80–120 nm width [489], a development that accompanies the metabolic disturbance and occurs in many tissues. It can be detected in renal glomeruli after 1.5–2.5 years of juvenile-onset diabetes [419] and appears to be secondary to the metabolic abnormality. Thus, it is a feature of secondary diabetes, it is retarded by therapeutic prevention of hyperglycemia, and that seen in the glomeruli of animals with experimentally induced diabetes can be reversed by grafting of pancreatic islet cells [348]. As with most developments in diabetes, it would be wrong to look to a single causative factor, but there is good evidence that hyperglycemia may have a direct effect. Thus it has been shown that the capillary basement membranes of eels with physiological hyperglycemia induced by keeping them in water at 4°C are several times thicker than those of eels swimming in warmer water [57]. Moreover, incorporation of proline and lysine by rat lens capsule can be enhanced in vitro by adding glucose to the incubation substrate [107]. On the other hand, synthesis of the noncollagenous basement membrane components appears to be reduced, any increase being attributed to enhanced sensitivity to insulin [347].

Reduced turnover as well as increased synthesis may also play a part in the thickening, possibly because of protein glycosylation [81], and may account for the lamination that is sometimes seen [203,284]. Binding of plasma protein constituents can be a further factor, particularly in glomerular capillaries, where there is high transmural flux.

Increased permeability develops in many tissues and, according to information derived from experimental situations [546], occurs at an early stage in the diabetic process. The defect is essentially functional and is possibly a consequence of polyol production, since it can be partially abolished in diabetic rats by using aldose reductase inhibitors [546].

Arteriolar Changes. It has long been recognized that hyaline arteriosclerosis of the type commonly identified with the benign phase of hypertension and senescence is particularly prominent in diabetes. The hyaline contains fibrin and lipid, and its composition suggests origin from the circulating plasma [152], leakage possibly being facilitated by alterations in the permeability of the endothelial lining and basement membrane integrity. In vivo measurements using labeled immunoglobulin and albumin markers have confirmed increased movement of protein across the blood vessels of the forearm and renal glomeruli [423] and support the contention that diabetic hyaline arteriosclerosis is largely a manifestation of plasmatic vasculosis. The process is accentuated in the presence of hypertension, which suggests a role for hydrostatic pressure in the increased endothelial permeability.

Hematological Abnormalities. Increased blood viscosity is common in diabetic patients and is a consequence of alterations to the erythrocytes and plasma. Reduced deformability of the circulating erythrocytes, increasing the possibility of obstructed flow through the smaller capillaries, is probably a direct effect of insulin deficiency, since the loss of deformability induced by adding diabetic plasma to normal red blood cells in vitro can be corrected by the further addition of insulin [530]. Plasma abnormalities also promote red cell aggregation [374]. The extent to which glycosylation of erythrocyte membranes contributes to reduced deformability [430] is uncertain but likely to be minimal in all but poorly controlled patients [509], and there is equal doubt about the contribution of HbA_{1c} to the tissue hypoxia incurred primarily by changes in the vessels.

Increases in plasma viscosity are well documented and probably multifactorial [373], with hyperlipidemia and hyperfibrinogenemia performing a key role [191].

Platelet abnormalities are also usual and have been shown to precede the onset of clinically recognizable vascular disease [296]. The abnormalities relate chiefly to the activating properties of adenosine diphosphate and epinephrine [138] and correlate with raised levels of von Willebrand's factor [296]. Increased thromboxane formation, reduced prostacyclin production, and increased platelet aggregation [112,305], together with associated endothelial cell changes, enhance the risk of thrombotic episodes.

Arterial Disease. Apart from microangiopathy, the larger arterial vessels are prone to develop excessively severe atherosclerosis such that all patients with diabetes of more than 10 years duration tend to have clinically significant plaque formation. Several factors are likely to be responsible for this accelerated atherogenesis, including associated hyperlipidemia, platelet abnormalities, and glycosylation of subendothelial and lipoprotein molecules. There is evidence that plaque formation at the origin of the ophthalmic artery sufficient to cause stenosis aggravates an established diabetic retinopathy (Fig. 29) [211].

Diabetic Retinopathy

Not all diabetics develop retinal disease, but the incidence rises with the duration of the metabolic defect, so that patients with juvenile-onset (type I) diabetes are at greatest risk. From an incidence of 12% after 0–5 years of diabetes, the figure in one series rose to 91% after 21 years [300]. Moreover, despite some doubts in the past, there is now widespread agreement that the risk of developing significant retinopathy is influenced by the quality of metabolic control. Visual impairment attributable to retinopathy sufficient to rate admission to the blind register affects just under 2% of the diabetic population in the United Kingdom, but this is likely to rise in view of a survey citing an incidence of type I diabetes of 13.5 per 100,000 in children under the age of 15 years in 1988 compared with 7.7 per 100,000 in 1973–1974 [384].

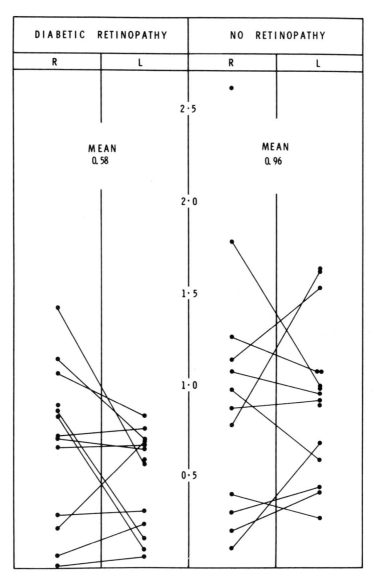

Figure 29 Comparison of the area (mm²) of the ophthalmic artery ostium at autopsy in diabetic subjects with and without retinopathy. Although the means of the areas were significantly different, the considerable overlap between the two groups and the variation in caliber between the right and left sides suggest that ophthalmic artery narrowing as a result of atherosclerosis is unlikely to be a major factor in diabetic retinopathy, although it may contribute.

From a clinical standpoint it is convenient to recognize four grades of diabetic retinopathy: background retinopathy (which rarely leads to blindness), macular edema, a preproliferative phase, and vitreoretinal disease. Inevitably, however, the biochemical complications of the diabetic state precede the clinical manifestations, and it is expected that premonitory functional disturbances constitute a pre-retinopathy phase.

Preretinopathy.   *Blood-retina barrier changes.*   Vitreous fluorophotometry points to limited breakdown of the blood-retina barriers at an early stage [125–127], and experimental studies suggest that this is likely to be a functional change since it is readily corrected by normoglycemic control [194] and can be prevented by dosing with aldose reductase inhibitors [128]. It is nevertheless salutary to note that no satisfactory evidence has yet been presented to show that such inhibitors have a beneficial effect in human diabetic retinopathy [195]. There is also clinical evidence from patients with early type I diabetes that leakage precedes neurosensory disturbance [55]. Animal studies indicate that both inner and outer blood-retina barriers may be affected, but the nature of the breakdown is uncertain. The permeability appears to be confined to small molecules initially, and leakage of protein, as judged by immunohistochemical examination of human retinas [533], does not occur until retinopathy is clinically evident. Morphological evidence is extremely sparse in humans or other species, but such as there is provides little reason to impute disruption of intercellular tight junctions [88,527]. Possibly there is increased cellular transport [88].

Retinal blood flow. Increased blood flow has been documented in the early and preretinopathy phases of diabetes [330], although information obtained by using more precise measurement techniques than were originally employed points to reduced velocity [17,65]. This implies a degree of vasodilatation, a contention supported by the observation that not only do in vitro cultures of vascular endothelium secrete reduced amounts of the vasoconstrictor substance endothelin when subjected to a hyperglycemic milieu [256], but pericytes are less responsive under such conditions [95]. Claims that flow is increased as a direct response to hyperglycemia, originally based on animal infusion experiments [279] and later supported by clinical observations in patients with background retinopathy [236,238], do not appear to hold in the macular circulation in human diabetics subjected to acute hyperglycemic episodes [172,173] or diabetic dogs free of retinal complications [495]. An alternative suggestion has been that the increased flow is a response to tissue hypoxia, a view supported by the demonstration that the increase can be partially negated if the patient is subjected to 100% oxygen breathing [237]. Formation of HbA_{1c} has been considered a factor in the underlying hypoxia [136,359].

Background Retinopathy: Clinical Features. The initial clinical manifestations of diabetic retinopathy are microaneurysms, exudates, punctate hemorrhages, and foci of capillary closure.

Microaneurysms. Aneurysmal dilatation of the retinal capillaries is a constant finding in background retinopathy and may be its presenting sign. Nevertheless, the propensity for microaneurysm formation is a feature not so much of diabetes as of the retinal capillaries, since on the one hand they occur in several other retinal disorders and, on the other, are rare in the capillaries of diabetic patients elsewhere in the body. They predominate on the venous side of the circulation in the posterior retina and are usually most frequent around foci of closed capillaries (Fig. 30).

The theories surrounding the pathogenesis of retinal microaneurysms were discussed earlier in this chapter, but it is worth emphasizing that aneurysms preceded by loop formation are particularly well documented in diabetic retinopathy.

Their importance lies in their excessive permeability and liability to rupture, resulting in focal serous exudation and hemorrhage. Accumulated thrombus within the aneurysmal sac causes many aneurysms to be obliterated, the life of individual lesions being of the order of several months [326]. When the thrombosis obliterates the sac but does not obstruct flow, fluorescein angiography may give a misleading impression of regression (Fig. 15).

Exudates. Serous exudation implies breakdown of the blood-retina barrier, and although endothelial cell degeneration and loss may be involved in leakage from microaneurysms and the later stages of the retinopathy, its occurrence in the earlier stages is probably a functional event. Animal experiments suggest that reversible dysfunction of the intercellular junctions may be involved [535]. Intravascular hypoxia occurring on the venous side of the circulation, by exaggerating any tendency to hyperviscosity and in this way raising the intraluminal pressure, may add to the risk of leakage [459]. Increased permeability of the thickened basement membranes may further promote exudation. Because the extravasated plasma is commonly rich in lipid, the exudates frequently have a glistening, waxy appearance and, by the same token, take a long time to resolve.

Hemorrhages. The extravasation of blood cells is contingent on a substantial endothelial cell deficit and is most often encountered in the vicinity of microaneurysms. An increase in venous pressure incurred by Valsalva-like maneuvers or a drop in intraocular pressure due to hypoglycemia have been thought to be contributory mechanisms [327].

Capillary Closure. Small foci in the posterior fundus in which the capillary vessels are not perfused are an early feature of background retinopathy. The vessels in these areas are devoid of both pericytes and endothelium and are represented merely by tubes of basement membrane [25,106]. The reason for the nonperfusion is uncertain, although there are several possibilities. One view, based on examination of

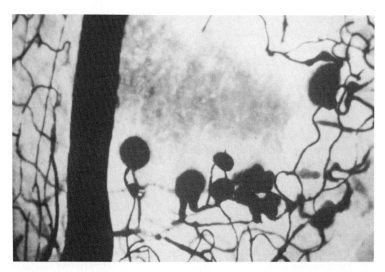

Figure 30 Diabetic retinopathy. Flat mount of retina perfused with colloidal carbon, showing a cluster of capillary aneurysms surrounding a zone of nonperfusion in which a cotton-wool spot developed.

digest preparations, is that it is a sequel to the formation of shunts, whereby blood is siphoned off into a few abnormally dilated vessels at the expense of neighboring capillaries [104]. The shunts in turn are presumed to be due to preferential loss of pericytes from selected capillaries. Fluorescein angiography provides little evidence to support this hypothesis, however, since blood flow through the "shunt" vessels is rarely increased to any appreciable extent, and in some instances the shunts follow rather than precede capillary closure [329]. It is more probable that such arteriolar-venular shunts are the surviving vessels in areas of closure [25]. Thrombotic occlusion of the feeding arteriole is a hypothesis that commands more support [21]. There is an added possibility that the capillaries are subject to external compression by surrounding tissue made edematous by ischemic hypoxia [31], as described in the brain [332].

The clinical significance of capillary closure is considerable because apart from scotomata caused by degeneration of nerve fibers and ganglion cells, it is in relation to such focal areas of ischemia that microaneurysms and neovascularization are prone to develop (Fig. 18). There is some evidence that limited attempts at revascularization may occur, possibly due to reendothelialization of residual basement membrane tubes where these have not been invaded by glial processes, but in general the areas of closure remain closed and may even increase in size.

Background Retinopathy: Underlying Vascular Pathology. The changes previously discussed in relation to diabetic microangiopathy in general are equally applicable in the retinal context [205,208]. There are certain peculiarities, however.

Endothelial cells. The retinal endothelium is associated with enhanced risk of thrombotic vascular occlusion caused not only by hypercoagulability of the circulating blood [467] but also by intrinsic abnormalities. Measurements of mRNA transcripts by solution hybridization have revealed increased capacity for forming an inhibitor of plasminogen activation in the retinas of type II diabetics [85], and an apparent reduction in tissue plasminogen activator has been described in the retinal arterioles of patients with type I diabetes [361].

With progression of the retinopathy, endothelial cell degeneration occurs predominantly but not exclusively in relation to areas of capillary closure.

Pericytes. An invariable feature of diabetic retinopathy is selective degeneration of capillary pericytes [106]. In retinal digest preparations stained with periodic acid–Schiff and hematoxylin, the nuclei of these cells fail to stain and have been termed ghost cells, but staining with hematoxylin and eosin produces an intense pink color (Fig. 31; see plate following p.1436) [25]. Eosinophilic degeneration of this sort is not peculiar to diabetic retinopathy, having been described in a variety of conditions, such as macroglobulinemia [39], multiple myelomatosis [26], and polycythemia [416], but in no other condition is it as marked. Eventually there is total degeneration of the pericyte nucleus and, presumably, of its cytoplasmic processes. Loss of pericytes is sometimes accompanied by loss of endothelium. A study of bovine capillaries suggests that both the endothelium and pericytes degenerate but that the former has a greater capacity for regeneration than the latter [484].

The cause of the degeneration is not clear, although there is some evidence that hyperglycemia is involved. Cultured pericytes multiply at a much reduced rate in the presence of supplemental glucose [355], and glucose inhibits ascorbate transport within these cells [308]. The metabolism of excessive blood glucose through the polyol pathway may be involved in the toxicity [311], aldose reductase inhibitors having a protective effect on the retinal pericytes of galactosemic dogs [302]. Even so, the finding that pericyte degeneration is apparently confined to the retinal circulation [4,416] indicates that other local factors are almost certainly involved.

The relevance of the observed pericyte changes to the retinopathy is only now beginning to be appreciated. Apart from a putative role in microaneurysm formation, as described earlier, the absence of pericytes may have a permissive effect on endothelial cell multiplication in the context of ensuing proliferative disease [417].

Basement membrane. The retinal capillaries share the basement membrane changes seen in other tissues (Fig. 32), the thickening possibly representing incorporation of plasma residues as well as increased synthesis [32]. An increase in perivascular reticulin is also usual [41]. Frank [195] speculated that the thickening serves to separate the cytoplasmic processes of the pericytes from contact with the underlying endothelial cells. This could impair the ability of the latter cell to restrict the proliferative tendencies of the endothelium and facilitate angiogenesis. He further suggested that the reduction in heparan sulfate proteoglycan, usual in the thickened membranes, reduces the capacity of the membranes to bind and therefore inactivate basic fibroblast growth factor [195].

Arterioles. Hyalinization of the retinal arterioles is usual and, like that in other tissues, is probably due to insudation of plasma and may well be related to the increased permeability of the retinal circulation. Arteriolar dilatation has also been described on the basis of clinical photographs [493]. Gradual reduction in the arteriolar lumen is one result of such insudation [21], occurring principally around the mouths of branch vessels. Eventual occlusion of these terminal arterioles due to presumed thrombus formation is the likely cause of the increasing number of foci of capillary closure. It seems that the occlusion in these circumstances is a relatively gradual process since it does not give rise to detectable tissue necrosis. On the other hand, occlusion of precapillary arterioles developing as a fairly rapid event would account for the cotton-wool spots seen in approximately a third of diabetic retinas [237].

Veins. Despite occasional statements to the contrary, most reports point to a mild increase in retinal vein caliber in a minority of patients, a figure of about 10% having been quoted as an average [493]. Initially the dilatation appears to be functional, since it may be reversed with improved control of the metabolic state [343] and may be a consequence of increased arterial flow in hypoxic conditions [330]. Eventually the abnormality is likely to become fixed as sclerotic changes take place within the wall. Conversely, age-related sclerosis could account for the reduced prevalence of venous abnormalities in older patients. Earlier concepts were based on venous stasis [122].

Maculopathy. Some diabetic patients have minimal background retinopathy but present with incapacitating visual loss attributable to changes at the macula. Commonly but not always accurately termed macular edema, such a pattern is most often associated with type II diabetes [71]. Histological examination reveals cystoid spaces presumed to represent edema fluid located mainly in the outer plexiform (Henle's) layer but also extending into the inner retinal layers [526]. Transudation and even exudation from perifoveal vessels may be a factor, although this is probably a minor consideration, and an ultrastructural analysis pointed to a primary swelling of Müller cells that only later rupture to spill their contents into the extracellular space and form cysts [177]. In view of the reduced circulation demonstrable in the maculae of affected patients, it may be more reasonable to look to ischemia for an explanation of the maculopathy, a conclusion supported by experimental models [526]. Defects of the retinal pigment epithelium in conjunction with capillary leakage have also been blamed [78]; others have drawn attention to a possible role of the vitreous, posterior detachment appearing to reduce the risk of macular edema [403].

Preproliferative Retinopathy. *Cotton-wool spots.* The emergence of cotton-wool spots is indicative of accelerating focal ischemia and as such is a harbinger of subsequent neovascularization [324,328]. They suggest that the causative arteriolar occlusions not only involve larger areas of the capillary bed but occur more rapidly.

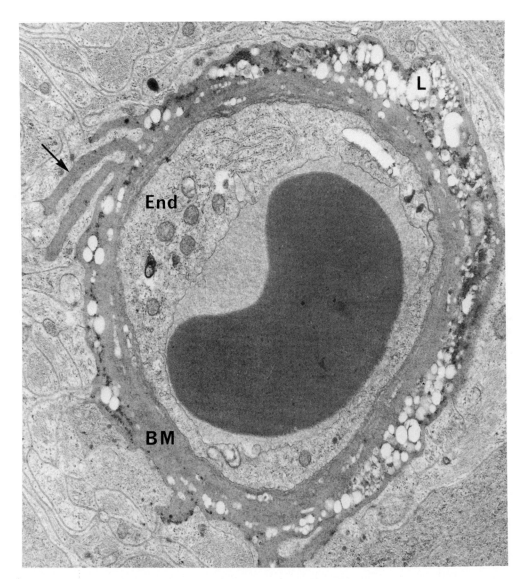

Figure 32   Retinal capillary in diabetic retinopathy, showing marked thickening of the basement membrane (BM). Globular spaces in the membrane probably represent lipid insudation, with much of the lipid (L) filling the site of a necrotic pericyte. Extension of the basement membrane material between adjacent neural tissue (arrow) is the likely counterpart of the argyrophilic membrane, which invests retinal capillaries and is particularly prominent in diabetes. End, endothelium. (×21,000) (Courtesy of N. Ashton.)

Intraretinal microvascular anomalies.   Dilated and elongated capillary loops, frequently forming bizarre hairpin or corkscrew patterns, are sometimes seen invading focal avascular zones of the retina. Such vessels, which are usually referred to as IRMA, are likely to be new endothelial cell proliferations in the form of either completely new capillaries or reendothelializations of previously defunct vessels. That revascularization of avascular areas can occur is undoubted [394] and to that extent are welcomed. Unfortunately they are also a sign that the potential for the background retinopathy to proceed to the proliferative phase is beginning to be realized.

Proliferative Retinopathy.   Proliferation of new blood vessels on the inner surface of the retina and within the vitreous is usually a late manifestation of diabetic retinopathy, with an incidence of around 60%

after 15–20 years of diabetes [325]. As a rule it is preceded by worsening background retinopathy and is associated with increasing areas of capillary closure. There is good reason, as with proliferative retinopathy in other disease states, to impute tissue hypoxia as the key pathogenetic factor.

A number of angiogenic factors have been implicated in the specific context of the diabetic retina, with, as in proliferative retinopathy in general, pride of place being given to bFGF [48,195,251,491]. The much smaller moiety described by Weiss and her colleagues [541] has also been shown to be present in the vitreous of patients with vitreoretinal proliferative disease [278,519]. Attention has similarly been drawn to the role of insulinlike growth factor I, levels of which are increased in both serum [383] and vitreous [230]. Moreover, it is to diabetes that the postulated permissive consequences of pericyte loss on endothelial cell proliferation [417] specifically refer. The presence of other inhibitory factors must also be considered, and it has been claimed that the retinal pigment epithelium behaves in this way [221], but the evidence is contradictory, other studies pointing to an angiogenic function [553].

The new vessels usually stem from the larger veins in relation to foci of capillary closure or near the optic disk. Initially they proliferate in the potential space between the inner limiting membrane and the posterior face of the vitreous, where they appear flat (Fig. 33), but eventually they can invade the vitreous, using condensations of the vitreal collagen as a support. Alternatively they may be dragged forward as a consequence of becoming bound to the posterior face of a retreating vitreous [132]. Vitreous syneresis and retraction is discussed elsewhere (see Chap. 22), but with specific reference to the diabetic state it is postulated that the risk is accentuated by non-enzymatic glycation and subsequent aggregation of the vitreal collagen [479a]. However, should the vitreous retract before such attachment has occurred, the vessels remain flat [74]. At first the proliferating capillaries are leaky, but this is largely corrected as the vessels mature and permanent intercellular junctions are formed [388]. Fenestrations of the endothelium are a rare finding [388,545]. Pericyte development and the formation of a fibrous adventitia also ensues, the responsible (myo)fibroblasts exerting traction in a way that incurs the risk of retinal detachment. It is at this stage that they are prone to bleed, since they are incompletely formed, poorly supported, and subject to traction by a retracting vitreous [132].

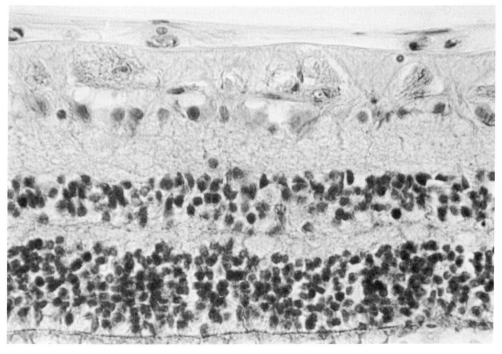

Figure 33 Section showing newly formed capillary blood vessels spreading between the inner limiting membrane of the retina and the posterior face of the vitreous. (Hematoxylin and eosin, ×450)

D. Sickle Cell Disease

Deformation of erythrocytes into a crescentic or sickle shape under hypoxic conditions is a feature of a group of familial disorders characterized by the presence of an abnormal hemoglobin variant.

Hemoglobin is a complex of four iron-containing molecules (heme) attached to a single protein molecule (globin). The globin moiety has four polypeptide chains, two having one type of amino acid composition and two another designated in the majority of normal adults as α and β, respectively. Minor variations determined by a mutant gene resulting in the substitution of a single amino acid within the β chain can modify the physicochemical properties of the hemoglobin molecule such that the function, shape, and viability of the erythrocytes are drastically impaired.

In sickle cell disease one glutamic acid radical at the 6 position of the β chain is replaced by valine, and this has the effect of promoting polymerization of the hemoglobin molecule, with a consequent drop in solubility in situations in which there is reduced oxygenation or acidosis: levels of deoxygenation that would halve the solubility of hemoglobin A (the normal adult hemoglobin) reduce the solubility of hemoglobin S (the hemoglobin of sickle cell disease) by a factor of 50 [432]. The insoluble hemoglobin in these situations forms slightly curved rod-shaped crystals (tactoids) that combine to give the red cell envelope a sickle or holly leaf configuration.

Factors governing the degree of sickling include the following:

1. The proportion of hemoglobin S (HbS) within the erythrocyte (25–45% in heterozygotes and virtually total in homozygotes).
2. The level of hypoxia.
3. Circulation time. The normal transit time through the tissue, including the eye, is insufficient for sickling to develop (a minimum of 15 s is required) but if the flow is sluggish there is an increased chance that some erythrocytes will succumb. This in turn increases viscosity and delays flow even more, so that a vicious spiral is created ("vicious cycle of erythrostasis"). Goldberg [225] reported prolongation of retinal transit time of up to 10 times the normal period.
4. Cellular hemoglobin concentration. Dehydration, by raising the mean cell concentration of HbS, increases the risk of polymerization.

Sickle cell disease results when an individual is homozygous for the HbS gene and virtually all the hemoglobin is abnormal. As the partial pressure of the blood oxygen drops during its passage through the tissues, there is a risk that sickling will occur, and this interferes with the pliability of the affected erythrocytes so that they do not easily pass through narrow capillaries. In consequence vasoocclusion readily occurs with untoward effects on the dependent tissues. Moreover, such cells are unduly fragile and give rise to hemolytic anemia.

The sickle cell trait represents the heterozygous carrier state and is usually asymptomatic. Nevertheless, the red cells contain 25–45% hemoglobin S and can be made to sickle in vitro; under exceptional circumstances, such as flying at high altitude in nonpressurized aircraft, sickling occurs in vivo.

Hemoglobin C, in which the glutamic acid at the 6 position of the β chain is replaced by lysine, can occur in combination with hemoglobin S in geographically defined communities where the genes for both abnormalities are rife. Patients with combined sickle cell and hemoglobin C disease usually have fewer occlusive and hemolytic complications but, perversely, the incidence of retinopathy is higher. Thus, proliferative retinopathy has been reported as involving 32.8% of patients with HbS-HbC disease compared with 2.6% of patients with pure HbS-HbS disease [114].

Sickle cell-β-thalassemia is another double heterozygous state that can be associated with retinal lesions. As much as 60–80% of the hemoglobin may be of the HbS type, and the symptoms of the disease resemble those of sickle cell disease more closely than those of thalassemia. (The defect in this hemoglobinopathy involves deficient synthesis of β-globin chains).

Sickle Cell Retinopathy

Although sludging of conjunctival capillaries [425] and occlusion of uveal vessels [115] are recorded, the ocular complications of serious proportions are confined to the retina. This is probably because alternative anastomotic sources of blood supply are considerably less.

The retinal manifestations of sickle cell disease and its variants resemble those of diabetes mellitus to a considerable degree, the principal difference relating to their distribution. Whereas the retinopathy of diabetes is essentially central (posterior), that due to sickling is mainly peripheral, although the macula is frequently involved in both. Typical features of sickle cell retinopathy are retinal and vitreal hemorrhages, neovascularization, and, in some instances, retinal detachment.

Pathogenesis. Much of our knowledge of the natural history and pathogenesis of sickle cell retinopathy has been gleaned by Goldberg and his associates [225,226]; the ensuing synopsis is based largely on their work, to which reference should be made for further information.

Arteriolar occlusion. The primary event is vasoocclusion, and although on theoretical grounds this is expected to predominate on the venous side of the retinal circulation, where the oxygen tension is lowest, clinical experience supported by fluorescein angiography and study of retinal digest preparations shows that arterioles, particularly the precapillary branches, are the elective sites. Correspondingly, the clinical picture of central and branch retinal vein occlusion is rare, whereas central retinal artery occlusion is not too uncommon. The reason for this is not clear, although a number of observations may be relevant:

1. The drop in pO_2 at precapillary level is sufficient to initiate sickling [254].
2. The precapillary arteriole has a very narrow lumen and is a potential bottleneck.
3. Even arterial blood is unusually viscous, because of the presence of erythrocytes that have undergone irreversible sickling [96].
4. Irreversibly sickled cells can act as microemboli [320].

Given these findings it is conceivable that irreversibly sickled cells arriving at the narrow precapillary arteriole become impacted and impede the passage of other erythrocytes so that they, too, begin to sickle. Furthermore, once started, a vicious cycle is established because stagnation and sickling are mutually stimulatory.

Occasionally the occluded arteriole reopens. Reopening within a few hours of the occlusion is probably due to breakup of the red cell aggregate, whereas reopening after a delay of weeks or months is a result of recanalization. Delayed reopening is associated with endothelial cell and pericyte loss in the dependent capillary bed, and although some limited revascularization from the recanalized arteriole may take place, the number of new closures outweighs the reopenings. As a result, the zone of ischemia enlarges and gradually spreads from the periphery of the retina toward the posterior pole. A similar pattern of closure develops around the terminal vessels at the macula, beginning at the horizontal raphe on the temporal side of the fovea.

The predilection of the peripheral and perimacular regions of the retina for occlusive lesions is unexplained but may be connected with the minimal capacity of the functional end vessels in these sites to establish collateral compensation.

A longitudinal study of Jamaican children with SS and SC disease has shown that the incidence of peripheral retinal closure increases with age from about 50% at 6 years to 90% at 13 years [513]. The relative protection during infancy is possibly due to the presence of fetal hemoglobin.

The effects of arteriolar occlusion are twofold, to cause hemorrhage and to stimulate neovascularization.

Retinal hemorrhage. Vascular necrosis at or adjacent to the site of occlusion predisposes to bleeding into the retina, and within a matter of days or weeks the hematoma assumes an orange-red color recognizable clinically as a "salmon patch." As histological study confirms [464], the hemorrhage at this stage is intraretinal, but eventually it may spill into the subhyaloid space and vitreous or dissect between the photoreceptor outer segments and pigment epithelium. Subretinal hemorrhage of the latter kind is usually associated with dispersion and hyperplasia of the retinal pigment epithelium to produce a so-called black sunburst effect. Alternatively, the hematoma may remain localized and ultimately be organized to leave a cavity or focal retinoschisis. Macrophages laden with hemosiderin may appear as irridescent granules on ophthalmic examination.

Neovascularization. When a precapillary arteriole is occluded, blood flow is diverted through proximal capillaries to the venous drainage channels. Such centripetal recession of the vascular arcades renders the preequatorial retina ischemic, and some 8–36 months later new capillary formations may commonly be seen arising from the sites of arteriolar-venular anastomosis. Initially, the new vessels lie on the surface of the retina, but gradually further proliferation results in delicate tufts of capillaries, each with a feeding arteriole and draining venule, projecting into the vitreous cavity. At first the tufts have little surrounding fibrous tissue and have been likened to sea fans.

The new capillaries are unduly permeable, and leakage of plasma into the vitreous, by virtue of its disruptive effect on gel stability [470], may be a factor in the commonly observed collapse of the vitreous body. Collapse and retraction of the vitreous stresses sea fans adherent to its posterior foci and predisposes to tearing and bleeding into the vitreal cavity. Traction on the subjacent retina may also develop and produce either crescentic tears or, where the region involved is ischemic, round holes. Both types of damage can give rise to rhegmatogenous detachment. Ultimately, a minority of the new vessels are themselves subject to occlusion and may regress. This pattern of events, first defined on the basis of direct observation and fluorescein angiography, has since been demonstrated histologically [464].

Proliferative retinopathy is rare in childhood [513] and should it develop in later life predominates in males and, as previously commented, is more common in SC than SS disease [193]. The reason for this is not immediately apparent, but the suggestion has been made that the moderate level of vascular occlusion seen in patients with SC disease would in time lead to a commensurate degree of proliferative retinopathy, whereas the higher risk of occlusion expected of homozygous sickle cell disease might relate to nascent as well as to established vessels and so abort most of the emergent neovascular tufts [193].

E. Retinopathy of Prematurity

The retinopathy of prematurity (ROP) occurs in retinas that are still undergoing active vascularization as part of normal fetal development and is characterized by the proliferation of fibrovascular tissue at the place where the vascularized and as yet unvascularized retina meet. Such tissue, by spreading onto the surface of the retina, is at risk of causing tractional retinal detachment, which in a minority of cases culminates in a retrolental mass.

Terry [522] was the first to define the clinical aspects of the condition, but it took a decade for its true nature to be recognized. A host of etiological factors was suggested, investigated, and discredited until eventually epidemiological evidence pointed to a link with the growing practice of nursing premature babies in oxygen-enriched incubators. One of the more intriguing pieces of evidence was the discovery that premature infants born in a private hospital in Melbourne, Australia had a lower incidence of retrolental fibroplasia than those born in a state-aided hospital; the essential difference in the nursing care was the much more sparing use of oxygen where cost was a consideration than where it came free [91]. The relationship was confirmed in a controlled clinical trial by Patz and colleagues [429] and subsequently shown to be causal by dint of experimental studies on laboratory animals [42,43,428]. Accordingly, the administration of oxygen in neonatal units came to be much more rigorously monitored, and the incidence of ROP dropped dramatically.

Even so, despite these measures, recent years have witnessed a minor resurgence of the condition, and although several factors may be concerned, this appears to be linked with the survival of increasing numbers of unusually small babies [83,436].

Clinicopathological Development

Irregular branching of the most recently formed retinal vessels with increased tortuosity of the more posteriorly located parent vessels may occur as a premonitory sign but is not specific. The pathognomonic changes of ROP commence at the margin or "brush border" of the developing vasculature and can be divided into five clinical stages [113,291] that correlate with the observed tissue changes [187,206]. The disease process may arrest spontaneously, however, especially in the early stages, and progression to the final cicatricial state is far from inevitable.

Stage 1. Demarcation Lines. Anterior to the fringes of the developing retinal vasculature there is normally a narrow rim of tissue made up of a vanguard of spindle-shaped cells and a rearguard of differentiating endothelium [186]. The early clinical phase of ROP is characterized by hyperplasia of both types of cell and, as a result, the usually inconspicuous demarcation between the vascularized and avascular zones becomes ophthalmoscopically apparent as an unmistakable white line. The nature of the spindle cells is in some doubt: they have long been regarded as primitive angioblasts [29], but there is an alternative suggestion that they are of glial origin [105]. An increase in gap junctions between individual spindle cells has been reported and construed as creating a physical obstacle to the further vascularization of the retina [334]. They may also be a source of angiogenic factors responsible for the subsequent preretinal proliferative developments [335].

Stage 2. Ridge.   Continued proliferation of the cells responsible for the demarcation line, particularly the endothelial cells in the rearguard, produces an elevation of the retinal surface to constitute a ridge. Initially white, the ridge becomes increasingly pink as definitive capillaries begin to form.

Stage 3. Ridge with Extraretinal Fibrovascular Proliferation.   The angiogenic tissue within the ridge is prone to break through the inner limiting lamina and erupt onto the retinal surface (Fig. 34). A glial component may also be recognized in the proliferating tissue [301].

Stage 4. Subtotal Retinal Detachment.   Further progression of the extraretinal tissue proliferation is associated with spread of the vessels into the vitreal cavity and attendant fibroblastic activity. Eventually this can predispose to tractional detachment of the underlying retina.

Stage 5. Total Retinal Detachment.   Depending on the degree and circumferential extent of the vitreoretinal proliferation, the retina is at risk of being completely detached and pulled into folds. The combined retina and extraretinal fibrovascular tissue may then be drawn forward and come to lie against the back of the lens (Fig. 35). This terminal cicatricial state is appropriately termed retrolental fibroplasia.

Since the obliterative effect of oxygen is in large measure a function of vascular maturity in the retina, the babies of lower birth weight are at most risk of developing the advanced cicatricial stages of ROP. In older babies nearing term, vessels at the retinal periphery alone are affected, and because the circulation on the temporal side is the last to be established, being farthest from the optic disk, the effects of oxygen toxicity at this stage are prone to provoke neovascularization in this region alone (Fig. 36). Subsequent cicatrization of such peripheral fibrovascular proliferation can cause temporal traction on the optic disk and displacement of the macula.

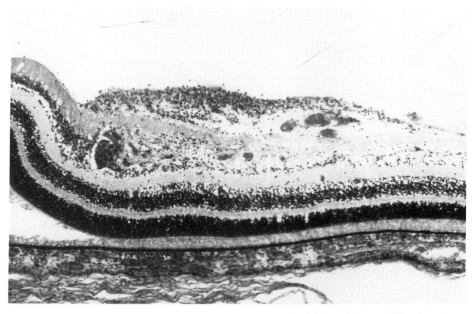

Figure 34   Retinopathy of prematurity, stage 3. The inner retina is thickened by a proliferation of vanguard (spindle) cells (V) and endothelial cell precursors (E) to constitute an elevated ridge. The cells lying on the surface of the retina represent a leash of developing new vessels that have broken through the inner limiting lamina in the region of the ridge. (Hematoxylin and eosin, ×105). (Reproduced with permission from A. Garner, The pathology of retinopathy of prematurity. In *Contemporary Issues in Fetal and Neonatal Medicine, 2. Retinopathy of Prematurity*, W.A. Silverman and J.T. Flynn (Eds.), Blackwell Scientific, Boston, pp. 19–52, 1986.)

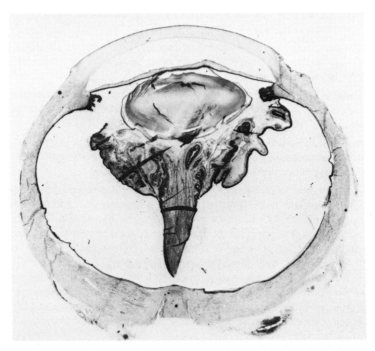

Figure 35   Retrolental fibroplasia. The retina is completely detached in conjunction with marked fibrovascular tissue proliferation on the anterior surface. (Hematoxylin and eosin, ×4) (Courtesy of N. Ashton.)

Pathogenesis

There is clear evidence from analysis of postmortem specimens and from experimental data that the vasoproliferative disease seen clinically is preceded by retinal ischemia (Fig. 37) [42,428]. This is attributable to endothelial cell necrosis and consequent obliteration of parts of the capillary bed, and as with the proliferative retinopathies as a whole, there is reason to interpret the relationship as causal, in which case an understanding of the pathogenesis of ROP requires knowledge of the factors giving rise to the initial ischemia.

   Hyperoxia.   Following the incrimination of hyperoxia on clinical grounds [429], experiments involving neonate kittens [42,43,210] and puppies [428] have provided further evidence that oxygen can be toxic to developing retinal capillary endothelium. Animal studies indicate an initial autoregulatory vasoconstriction in response to high levels of inspired oxygen [42,43] and provide evidence that this can be protective [181]. Eventually endothelial cell degeneration ensues, however, beginning with the most recently differentiated cells. Indeed, oxygen in high concentration is usually lethal to all cell types [49] by virtue of its tendency to form unstable free radicals, especially superoxide and hydroxyl ions [410]. The electrons needed to reduce these radicals are most readily stolen from lipid molecules present in intracellular membranes, and the consequent lipoperoxide formation damages the integrity of the cytoplasmic organelles with particular reference to mitochondrial function. Other effects include inhibition of enzyme systems involving sulfhydryl groups and oxidation of glutathione with secondary reduction in cellular energy production. Protection against atmospheric levels of oxygen depends on the presence of antioxidant enzymes, of which the best known is superoxide dismutase. The evidence that the toxic potential of oxygen is the major factor in the pathogenesis of ROP is overwhelming [209].

   Retinal Maturity.   The possibility that immaturity of the retina is important is emphasized by the preponderance of babies with birth weights under 1000 g in the most recently encountered cases. This observation grows in significance when it is recognized that the unduly large amounts of supplemental oxygen administered in the earlier epidemic are generally avoided in these babies. The link between retinal immaturity and ischemia is not altogether clear, but it is noteworthy that exposing neonate kittens to

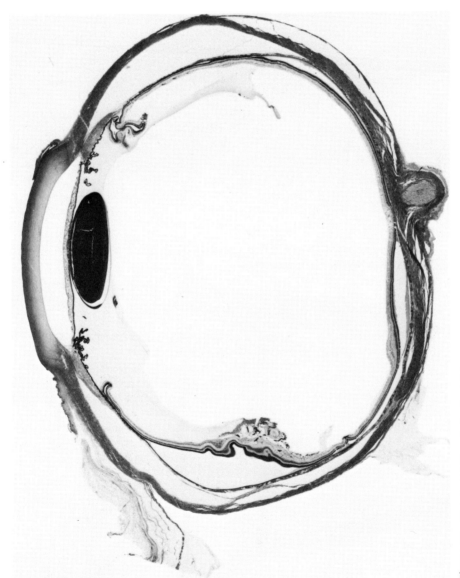

Figure 36 Retrolental fibroplasia of mild degree. Since the least mature retinal vessels are most vulnerable to oxygen excess and since the temporal periphery is the last part of the retina to be vascularized, in mild cases subsequent vasoproliferation may be confined to this zone. (Masson's trichrome, ×6)

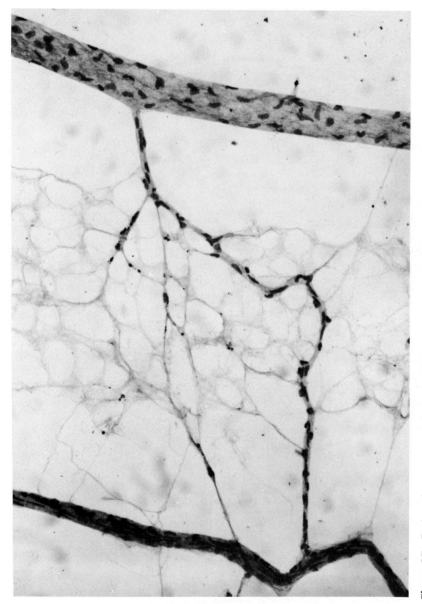

Figure 37 Retina of a premature infant subjected to excessive oxygen. There is marked obliteration of the capillary bed, leaving acellular basement membrane remnants. The main arterial and venous channels are also attenuated. (Periodic acid–Schiff and hematoxylin, ×200)

hyperoxia results in a decrease in superoxide dismutase, whereas levels of this enzyme are usually increased in such circumstances as part of an adaptive process [73]. Furthermore, there is in vitro evidence that developing endothelial cells are less well protected against free oxygen radicals in terms of superoxide activity than the cells of mature vessels [498]. Also, levels of vitamin E (tocopherol), another naturally occurring antioxidant, are also said to be low in the preterm state [437]. This could mean that the retina at this stage of development is inadequately prepared to cope with increased amounts of oxygen, even though the increases may be small. Indeed, a level of antioxidant activity appropriate to postnatal life is not expected before term since retinal metabolism in utero is predominantly provided by anerobic systems. There is even a suggestion that normal atmospheric oxygen concentrations may be harmful to the retinal capillaries in some extremely small babies [427].

Hypercapnia and Acidosis. In some instances abnormally high arterial levels of carbon dioxide are the most striking finding, blood oxygen figures being within accepted limits [72]. Hypercapnia is frequently a corollary of hypoxia, and it is entirely probable that occasional cases of ROP are the outcome of hypoxic damage to the retinal circulation [360] because it is the fact that the developing vessels have been destroyed that matters, insofar as the stimulus to preretinal vasoproliferation is concerned, rather than its cause. This cannot be the explanation in acidotic babies with normoxemia, however, particularly because there is no evidence that carbon dioxide per se is toxic to the vascular endothelium of premature infants. Nevertheless, animal experiments indicate that the arteriolar constriction occurring as an autoregulatory response to hyperoxia is prevented if there is simultaneous hypercapnia [180,389]. Such carbon dioxide-induced dilatation of the ocular circulation entails increased delivery of oxygen to the retina, even where the PaO_2 is not significantly elevated, with a potential for producing retinal vascular damage.

Light. Interest has been renewed in the potential for light to damage the retina in preterm infants. In one study infants protected by placing a neutral density filter over the incubators were shown to have a reduced incidence of ROP relative to a control group exposed to customary levels of illumination [222]. The putative mechanism of light-induced retinal vascular damage is unknown, but there is reason to think that formation of free oxygen radicals, on the one hand, allied to reduced oxygen consumption, on the other, may be involved [222,358].

Other Factors. A number of other factors have been incriminated, including sepsis [241,445], which may act by releasing toxic free radicals, and blood transfusion [241,558], which increases oxygen delivery to the tissues by replacing the original fetal hemoglobin (HbF) with adult hemoglobin (HbA). There is no evidence that these influences can themselves cause ROP, but they may contribute to the final disorder. One analysis of almost 50 potential risk factors suggests that xanthine, given to stimulate the respiratory center and relax the smooth muscle cells of the lung alveoli, is of significance in precipitating ROP [250]. The mechanism of the retinal damage is not known, although it may be relevant that xanthine oxidase activity, which is promoted by reperfusion of ischemic organs, leads to superoxide anion generation and tissue damage [197]. Additional sources of xanthine, especially in the context of an ischemic retina, could serve to exacerbate the problem.

F. Coats' Disease

As Coats himself recognized, the condition that bears his name may well have more than one cause [99,100], and correspondingly some prefer the term "Coats' lesion" [272] or "syndrome" [148] to Coats' disease.

Clinically, the condition is characterized by extensive creamy or yellowish exudates within and beneath the retina, with the addition in some cases of hemorrhages and glistening spots or patches in the detached retina. The lesion is usually unilateral, predominating on the temporal side [159], and although adult cases are described [272,500], it is essentially a disorder of childhood, with peak incidence around the age of 9 or 10 years. The majority of those affected are boys.

Pathology

The basic defect in the retina of a patient suffering from Coats' lesion rests with the capillary blood vessels and is manifested as a loss of integrity of the lining endothelium such that there is gradual leakage of plasma into the retinal tissue. Minor hemorrhage may also be seen. Phagocytic cells, which are likely to originate from circulating monocytes and the retinal pigment epithelium, then commence to engulf and remove the lipid and protein residues. Macrophage origin from the retinal pigment epithelium represents mitotic division and shedding of daughter cells into the subretinal space as free units [223]. Many of the phagocytes become engorged with lipid and qualify for description as bladder or balloon cells, and as the non-phagocytosed lipid increases in concentration, free cholesterol crystallizes and presents as iridescent particles liable to be a focus for a multinucleated giant cell response. Eventually new blood vessels may develop on the deep surface of the retina, possibly because of the relative hypoxia experienced by the detached outer layers of the retina. Organization of the exudate with partial replacement by fibrous tissue may be seen in the late stages; the retina becomes progressively degenerate and disorganized, the inner layers being the last to succumb.

Etiology

The nature of the underlying vascular defect is not always clear, and it is important to recognize that primary inflammatory states, of which toxocariasis is probably the most common [28], can produce the clinical picture of Coats' disease. A proportion of the cases described in the original report by Coats were related to the presence of angiomas as demonstrated by von Hippel [281], and it is now the accepted practice to consider this entity separately. Coats divided his remaining cases into those with and those without discernible vascular anomalies, the vascular disturbance taking the form of bizarre focal dilatation of capillaries to create congenital aneurysms [346] or areas of more generalized telangiectasis (Fig. 38) [453]. Electron microscopy of a case by Tripathi and Ashton [524] showed that the dilated capillaries were thickened by insudation of plasma, and they postulated that the primary event was a breakdown in the blood-retina barrier, with secondary damage to the capillary wall leading to irregular dilatation and aneurysm formation. The nature of the breakdown is unexplained, however, as is its focal distribution, although a genetic influence has been considered [494]. A familial tendency has been reported [393] but is exceptional, and in general there is no good evidence of genetic transmission. Retinal telangiectasia comparable to that occurring in typical Coats' disease has been described in cases of the autosomal dominant facioscapulohumeral muscular dystrophy [243], although the retinal exudation in this disorder does not proceed to detachment. It has also been suggested that Coats' disease without discernible vascular abnormality (type 2) represents an earlier phase of the same process before mural dilatation has the opportunity to develop [524]. Whether this is so remains to be seen, but certainly the presence of exuded plasma indicates that the lack of vascular abnormality in type 2 Coats' disease is apparent rather than real.

G. Eales Disease (Idiopathic Retinal Vasculitis)

The condition in which recurrent hemorrhages and perivascular sheathing by leukocytes develops in the periphery of the retinas of young adult males is associated with the name of Eales [154,155]. However, similar lesions can both occur in the central retina and present in older individuals. Thus, not only are there reports of central involvement, but in one case report [364] the disease was peripheral in one eye and central in the other. Again, there have been many instances of the disease first presenting in middle age and in women as well as in men [166,167]. Consequently, there is some reason to abandon the eponymous title in favor of "idiopathic retinal vasculitis" as a less restrictive term.

Pathology

Tissue studies are limited, but a detailed analysis by Donders [142] showed that although the histopathology is variable, a common feature is infiltration of retinal veins and perivascular cuffing by lymphocytes. Plasma cells may also be present, and occasionally there is a granulomatous reaction with multinucleated giant cells [24]. Less commonly the arterial side of the retinal vasculature is involved in the vasculitis. The sheathing of the vessels observed clinically in Eales disease is attributable to the surrounding mantle of leukocytes (Fig. 39) and can commonly be observed to spread from its origin at the retinal periphery to involve the more proximal vessels; rarely, spread in the reverse direction may be seen.

The retinal vasculitis may occur as an isolated lesion or be associated with uveal inflammation, and in some instances there is little or no sign of vasculitis, the vascular sheathing apparently being due to mural hyalinization and thickening. Nevertheless, there are many histologically confirmed descriptions of

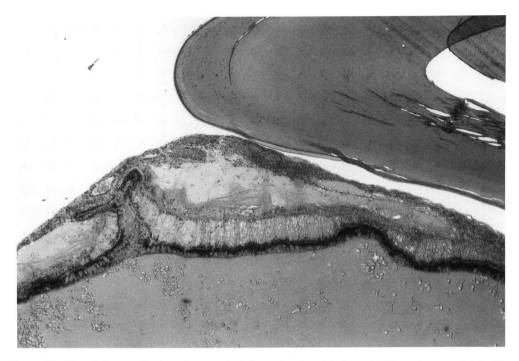

Figure 38 Coats' disease. Section of an enucleated eye showing detachment of the retina associated with a serous subretinal exudate. A zone of telangiectasia is seen in the retina (arrow) and appears to be the source of the exudation. (Hematoxylin and eosin, ×30)

vasculitis, and it is probable that the variable findings represent different stages of the disease process, mural hyaline thickening being a later phenomenon secondary to inflammation and increased endothelial cell permeability.

Complications attributable to vascular thrombosis and necrosis are common. Thrombotic branch vein occlusion with capillary closure and resultant tissue hypoxia is probably responsible for the preretinal neovascularization that may be seen. Aneurysmal dilatation and more extensive varicosities giving a beaded appearance to the venules and veins is also a product of inflammatory necrosis. Such weakened vessels, together with the intravitreal neovascular proliferations, are a source of recurrent hemorrhage. Intravitreal hemorrhage can develop even in the absence of preretinal vessels as an extension of intraretinal bleeding, a phenomenon that may be linked with damage to the inner limiting membrane in the vicinity of inflamed venous channels [549]. Frequently the inner limiting membrane is thickened, and although the cause is obscure there is a possibility of its being due to inspissation of proteinaceous exudates.

The fibrosis that accompanies the preretinal vasoproliferation can predispose eventually to retinal detachment and iris neovascularization with secondary angle closure glaucoma.

Etiology

The cause of Eales disease is not known but it is usual to put emphasis on a probable autoimmune process possibly triggered by an exogenous agent. The histological finding of a lymphocytic and occasionally granulomatous vasculitis is supportive of an immunological process without providing any etiological clues. Hematological abnormalities, especially as they affect the clotting mechanism and blood viscosity, are described [66], as are plasma protein irregularities [456], but as yet the significance of these findings, other than to enhance the risk of vascular occlusion, is obscure. A link with disease of the central nervous system has been alleged [51], but it is possible that a proportion of patients with neurological disturbance, diagnosed as suffering from Eales disease, are really in the early stages of multiple sclerosis [24,549].

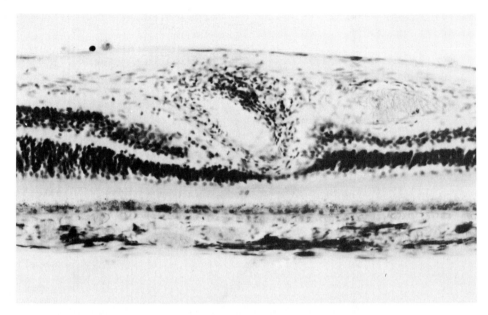

Figure 39 Eales disease. Section of retina showing a venule sheathed with lymphocytes and scanty plasma cells. (Hematoxylin and eosin, ×180)

H. Aortic Arch Syndrome

The aortic arch syndrome encompasses the sequelae of gradual stenosis and ultimate occlusion of the major arteries arising from the arch of the aorta. Cerebral and cardiac ischemia are the major manifestations of such a disturbance, but ocular involvement is by no means uncommon.

In the Western world, atherosclerosis is the predominant cause of the syndrome, syphilitic arteritis now being an uncommon condition, although exceptionally giant cell arteritis has been implicated. In Eastern Asia Takayasu's arteritis (pulseless disease) is a significant cause, particularly in young women. Little is known of the cause of the condition, although the presence of raised immunoglobulin levels and of antinuclear antibodies [400] is suggestive of an allergic factor operating, possibly on an autoimmune basis. The larger elastic arterioles only are affected, tissue examination revealing a panarteritis manifest as intimal hyperplasia and fibrosis, destruction of elastic tissue in the medial coat, and lymphocytic cuffing of the vasa vasorum in the adventitia [532]. The lesions are segmental and produce increasing reduction of the vessel lumen, complicated eventually by thrombotic occlusion.

The ocular manifestations of the aortic arch syndrome reflect stenosis and thrombosis of the carotid arteries. In the early stages symptoms may be precipitated by sudden movement of the head, by postural hypotension, or by exertion, when they usually take the form of transient blindness (amaurosis fugax), which is often bilateral. At this stage the eye may appear normal to clinical examination, although there is likely to be progressive reduction in the central retinal artery pressure. In time the retina becomes pale as a result of ischemic atrophy, the circulation time is prolonged [292], and the vessels that are dilated at first are liable to be occluded from the periphery. Arteriolovenular shunts, sometimes representing direct communications where the arterioles and veins cross, have been described in patients with Takayasu's arteritis [515]. Small hemorrhages and occasional cotton-wool spots may also develop, and preretinal neovascularization in the region of the optic disk sometimes ensues as a measure of retinal hypoxia. Optic disk atrophy has been described in association with absent posterior ciliary artery perfusion [293]. Anterior segment ischemia is also frequent, particularly in patients with severe bilateral carotid artery disease [323]. Mild enophthalmos is not uncommon [517] and is probably caused by ischemic atrophy of the orbital tissues surrounding the eye. Cataractous changes are occasionally observed in the lens [84] and are again likely to reflect arterial insufficiency, since carotid artery ligation has been shown to induce cataract formation in rats [333]. Not all individuals with the aortic arch syndrome develop ocular problems, and one clinicopathological study of a case was interpreted as providing evidence that intracranial steal of collateral blood flow is required in addition to carotid artery occlusion [304].

I. Arteriovenous Fistulas

Partly because of the unique anatomy of the retroorbital vasculature, whereby the internal carotid artery passes through the cavernous sinus of the intracranial venous system, and partly because of the fixity of the vessels in this region, a traumatic fracture involving the base of the skull is liable to be complicated by the development of an arteriovenous fistula. Less commonly the trauma is indirect and may represent contusion rather than fracture. Although the onset of symptoms is usually immediate, occasionally the establishment of a fistula may be preceded by focal weakening of the arterial wall and saccular aneurysm formation [473]. In some cases there is a preceding phase of aneurysmal dilatation, due to arterial disease secondary to arteriosclerosis or hypertension or to a congenital weakness [68]. Dural arteriovenous shunts in the region of the cavernous sinus are believed to account for most so-called spontaneous carotid-cavernous sinus fistulae [406].

Whatever the cause, once the fistula is established there is sudden increase in venous pressure with reversed blood flow, which spills into the ophthalmic veins. As a result, the orbital veins become markedly congested, and this in turn predisposes to interstitial edema and proptosis. These changes are accompanied by severe pain, and the proptosis is characteristically pulsatile because of transmission of the internal carotid artery pulse. Swelling of the eyelid is also common, and eventually periorbital and facial venous dilatation may be marked as alternative anastomotic drainage channels become established.

Simultaneous with the rise in venous pressure is a drop in ophthalmic artery pressure such that ocular ischemia is liable to develop [149,473]. As a consequence, the cornea is often edematous, and the retina may show superficial hemorrhages and microaneurysms, and eventually secondary neovascular glaucoma may occur. However, the retinal changes are almost certainly compounded by both diminished arterial perfusion and, perhaps more importantly, obstructed venous outflow [549].

REFERENCES

1. Abrahamson, D.R. Recent studies on the structure and pathology of basement membranes. *J. Pathol. 149*: 257–278, 1986.
2. Adams, C.W.M. *Vascular Histochemistry*, Lloyd-Luke (Medical Books), London, 1967.
3. Adams, C.W., Morgan, R.S., and Bayliss, C. The differential entry I^{125} albumin into mildly and severely atheromatous rabbit aortas. *J. Atheroscler. Res. 11*:119–124, 1970.
4. Addison, D.J., Garner, A., and Ashton, N. Degeneration of intramural pericytes in diabetic retinopathy. *Br. Med. J. 1*:264–266, 1970.
5. Aeby, C. Der Bau des menschlichen Körpers, F. Vogel, Leipzig, 1868.
6. Alexander, C.M., and Werb, Z. Proteinases and extracellular remodelling. *Curr. Opin. Cell Biol. 1*:974–982, 1990.
7. Algvere, P., and Kock, F. Experimental fibroplasia in the rabbit vitreous: Effects of hyaluronidase and implantation of autologous dermal tissue. *Graefes Arch. Ophthalmol. 199*:133–139, 1976.
8. Anderson, D.R. Axonal transport in the retina and optic nerve. In *Neuro-ophthalmology, Vol. 9*, J.S. Glaser (Ed.), C.V. Mosby, St. Louis, MO, pp. 140–153, 1977.
9. Anderson, D.R. Papilledema and axonal transport. In *Workshops in Neuro-ophthalmology: Five Topics in Neuro-ophthalmology*, H.S. Thompson (Ed.), Intercontinental Publications, Westport, CT, pp. 184–189, 1979.
10. Anderson, D.R., and Hendrickson, A.E. Effect of intraocular pressure on rapid axoplasmic transport in monkey optic nerve. *Invest. Ophthalmol. Vis. Sci. 13*:771–783, 1977.
11. Andersson, B., and Samuelson, A. A case of hyperglobulinemia with pronounced eye changes and acrocyanosis. *Acta Med. Scand. 117*:248–260, 1974.
12. Antonelli-Orlidge, A., Saunders, K.B., Smith, S.R., and D'Amore, P.A. An activated form of transforming growth factor beta is produced by co-cultures of endothelial cells and pericytes. *Proc. Natl. Acad. Sci. USA 86*:4544–4548, 1989.
13. Appen, R.E., Wray, S.H., and Cogan, D.G. Central retinal artery occlusion. *Am. J. Ophthalmol. 79*:374–381, 1975.
14. Agel, N.M., Ball, R.Y., Waldmann, H., and Mitchinson, M.J. Identification of macrophages and smooth muscle cells in human atherosclerosis using monoclonal antibodies. *J. Pathol. 146*:197–204, 1985.
15. Archer, D.B. Neovascularization of the retina. *Trans. Ophthalmol. Soc. UK 96*:471–493, 1976.
16. Archer, D.B., Ernest, J.T., and Maguire, C.J.F. Experimental branch vein obstruction. In *Vision and Circulation*,

Proceedings of the 3rd William Mackenzie Symposium, Glasgow, 1974, Henry Kimpton, London, pp. 226–242, 1976.

17. Arend, O., Wolf, S., Jung, F., Bertram, B., Postgens, H., Toonen, H., and Reim, R. Retinal microcirculation in patients with diabetes mellitus: Dynamic and morphological analysis of perifoveal capillary network. *Br. J. Ophthalmol. 75*:514–518, 1991.

18. Ashino-Fuse, H., Takano, Y., Oikawa, T., Shimamura, M., and Iwagichi, T. Medroxyprogesterone acetate, an anti-cancer and anti-angiogenic steroid, inhibits the plasminogen activator in bovine endothelial cells. *Int. J. Cancer 44*:859–864, 1989.

19. Ashton, N. Retinal microaneurysms in the non-diabetic subject. *Br. J. Ophthalmol. 35*:189–212, 1951.

20. Ashton, N. Discussion on diabetic retinopathy. *Proc. R. Soc. Med. 44*:747–753, 1951.

21. Ashton, N. Arteriolar involvement in diabetic retinopathy. *Br. J. Ophthalmol. 37*:282–292, 1953.

22. Ashton, N. Retinal vascularization in health and disease. *Am. J. Ophthalmol. 44*:7–17, 1957.

23. Ashton, N. Diabetic micro-angiopathy. *Adv. Ophthalmol. 8*(Bibl. Ophthalmol. Fasc. 52):1–84, 1958.

24. Ashton, N. Pathogenesis and aetiology of Eales's disease. In XIX International Congress of Ophthalmology, Acta. New Delhi, Y.K.C. Pandit, Bombay, pp. 828–840, 1962.

25. Ashton, N. Studies of the retinal capillaries in relation to diabetic and other retinopathies. *Br. J. Ophthalmol. 47*:521–538, 1963.

26. Ashton, N. Ocular changes in multiple myelomatosis. *Arch. Ophthalmol. 73*:487–494, 1965.

27. Ashton, N. Oxygen and the growth and development of retinal vessels: In vivo and in vitro studies. *Am. J. Ophthalmol. 62*:412–435, 1966.

28. Ashton, N. Toxocara canis and the eye. In *Corneo-Plastic Surgery: Proceedings of the Second International Corneo-Plastic Conference*, London 1967, P.V. Rycroft (Ed.), Pergamon Press, Oxford, pp. 579–591, 1969.

29. Ashton, N. Retinal angiogenesis in the human embryo. *Br. Med. Bull. 26*:103–106, 1970.

30. Ashton, N. Pathophysiology of retinal cotton-wool spots. *Br. Med. Bull. 26*:143–150, 1970.

31. Ashton, N. Diabetic retinopathy: Some current concepts. In *Proceedings of the International Symposium on Fluorescein Angiography*, Albi, 1969, Karger, Basel, pp. 334–345, 1971.

32. Ashton, N. Vascular basement membrane changes in diabetic retinopathy. *Br. J. Ophthalmol. 58*:344–366, 1974.

33. Ashton, N., and Cook, C. Mechanism of corneal vascularization. *Br. J. Ophthalmol. 37*:193–209, 1953.

34. Ashton, N., and Cook, C. Studies on developing retinal vessels. II. Influence of retinal detachment on oxygen vaso-obliteration. *Br. J. Ophthalmol. 39*:457–462, 1955.

35. Ashton, N., Cook, C., and Langham, M. Effect of cortisone on vascularization and opacification of the cornea induced by alloxan. *Br. J. Ophthalmol. 35*:718–724, 1951.

36. Ashton, N., Dollery, C.T., Henkind, P., Hill, D.W., Paterson, J.W., Ramalho, P.S., and Shakib, M. Focal retinal ischaemia: Opthalmoscopic, circulatory and ultrastructural changes. *Br. J. Ophthalmol. 50*:281–384, 1966.

37. Ashton, N., and Harry, J. The pathology of cotton-wool spots and cytoid bodies in hypertensive retinopathy and other diseases. *Trans. Ophthalmol. Soc. UK 83*:91–114, 1963.

38. Ashton, N., and Henkind, P. Experimental occlusion of retinal arterioles (using graded glass ballotini). *Br. J. Ophthalmol. 49*:225–234, 1965.

39. Ashton, N., Kok, D'A., and Foulds, W.S. Ocular pathology in macroglobulinaemia. *J. Pathol. Bacteriol. 86*:453–461, 1963.

40. Ashton, N., Peltier, S., and Garner, A. Experimental hypersensitive retinopathy in the monkey. *Trans. Am. Ophthlamol. Soc. UK 88*:167–186, 1968.

41. Ashton, N., and Tripathi, R.C. Perivascular and intervascular reticular fibres of the retina. *Am. J. Ophthalmol. 80*:337–359, 1975.

42. Ashton, N., Ward, B., and Serpell, G. Role of oxygen in the genesis of retrolental fibroplasia: Preliminary report. *Br. J. Ophthalmol. 37*:513–520, 1953.

43. Ashton, N., Ward, B., and Serpell, G. Effect of oxygen on developing retinal vessels with particular reference to the problem of retrolental fibroplasia. *Br. J. Ophthalmol. 38*:397–432, 1954.

44. Auerbach, R. Angiogenesis inducing factors: A review. In *Lymphokines: A Forum for Immunoregulatory Cell Products*, Vol. 4, E. Pick and M. Landy (Eds.), Academic Press, New York, pp. 69–88, 1981.

45. Aurell, E., and Tibblin, G. Hypertensive eye-ground changes in a Swedish population of middle-aged men. *Acta Ophthalmol. (Copenh.) 43*:355–361, 1965.

46. Ausprunk, D.H., and Folkman, J. Migration and proliferation of endothelial cells in preformed and newly formed blood vessels during tumor angiogenesis. *Microvasc. Res. 14*:53–65, 1977.

47. Azizkhan, R.G., Azizkhan, J.C., Zetter, B.R., and Folkman, J. Mast cell heparin stimulates migration of capillary endothelial cells in vitro. *J. Exp. Med. 152*:931–938, 1980.

48. Baird, A., Esch, F., Gospodarowicz, D., and Guillemin, R. Retina and eye-derived endothelial cell growth factors: Partial molecular characterization and identity with acidic and basic fibroblast growth factors. *Biochemistry 24*:7855–7860, 1985.

49. Balentine, J.D. *Pathology of Oxygen Toxicity*, Academic Press, London, 1982.

50. Ballantyne, A.J., and Loewenstein, A. Retinal microaneurysms and punctate haemorrhages. *Br. J. Ophthalmol. 28*:593–598, 1944.

51. Ballantyne, A.J., and Michaelson, I.C. *Textbook of the Fundus of the Eye*, 2nd ed. Livingstone, Edinburgh, pp. 167–184, 1970.

52. Bechgaard, P. The natural history of benign hypertension: One thousand hypertensive patients followed from 26 to 32 years. In *The Epidemiology of Hypertension: Proceedings of an International Symposium*, J. Stamler, R. Stamler, and T.N. Pullman (Eds.), Grune & Stratton, New York, pp. 357–370, 1967.

53. Beck, R.W., Servais, G.E., and Hayreh, S.S. Anterior ischemic optic neuropathy. IX. Cup-to-disc ratio and its role in pathogenesis. *Ophthalmology 94*:1503–1508, 1987.

54. Behrman, S. Amaurosis fugax et amaurosis fulminas. *Arch. Ophthalmol. 45*:458–467, 1951.

55. Bek, T., and Lund-Andersen, H. Localised blood-retinal barrier leakage and retinal light sensitivity in diabetic retinopathy. *Br. J. Ophthalmol. 74*:388–392, 1990.

56. Bell, G.I., Xiang, K., Horita, S., Sanz, N., and Karam, J.H. The molecular genetics of diabetes mellitus. *Ciba Found. Symp. 130*:167–183, 1987.

57. Bendayan, M., and Rasio, E.A. Hyperglycemia and microangiopathy in the eel. *Diabetes 30*:317–325, 1981.

58. Benditt, E.P. Implications of the monoclonal character of human atherosclerotic plaques. *Am. J. Pathol. 86*:693–702, 1977.

59. Benditt, E.P. Origins of human atherosclerotic plaque: The role of altered gene expression. *Arch. Pathol. Lab. Med. 112*:997–1001, 1988.

60. Benditt, E.P., and Benditt, J.M. Evidence for a monoclonal origin of human atherosclerotic plaques. *Proc. Natl. Acad. Sci. USA 70*:1753–1756, 1973.

61. BenEzra, D., Hemo, I., and Maftzir, G. In vivo angiogenic activity of interleukins. *Arch. Ophthalmol. 108*:573–576, 1990.

62. Bensaid, M., Malecaze, F., Bayard, F., and Tauber, J.P. Opposing effects of basic fibroblast growth factor and transforming growth factor-beta on the proliferation of cultured bovine retinal capillary endothelial (BREC) cells. *Exp. Eye Res. 48*:791–799, 1989.

63. Bensaid, M., Malecaze, F., Prats, H., Bayard, F., and Tauber, J.P. Autocrine regulation of bovine retinal capillary endothelial cell (BREC) proliferation by BREC-derived basic fibroblast growth factor. *Exp. Eye Res. 48*: 801–813, 1989.

64. Beri, M., Klugman, M.R., Kohler, J.A., and Hayreh, S.S. Anterior ischemic optic neuropathy. VII. Incidence of bilaterality and various influencing factors. *Ophthalmology 94*:1020–1028, 1987.

65. Bertram, B., Wolf, S., Fiehofer, S., Schulte, K., Arend, O., and Reim, M. Retinal circulation time in diabetes mellitus type I. *Br. J. Ophthalmol. 75*:462–465, 1991.

66. Bertram, B., Wolf, S., Hof, A., Jung, F., and Reim, M. Rheological findings in Eales disease (German). *Klin. Monatsbl. Augenheilk. 195*:254–256, 1989.

67. Bessey, O.A., and Wolbach, S.B. Vascularization of the cornea of the rat in riboflavin deficiency, with a note on corneal vascularization in vitamin A deficiency. *J. Exp. Med. 69*:1–12, 1939.

68. Bickerstaff, E.R. Mechanisms of presentation of caroticocavernous fistulae. *Br. J. Ophthalmol. 54*:186–190, 1970.

69. Björkhem, I., Henriksson-Freyschuss, A., Breuer, O., Diczfalusy, U., Berglund, L., and Henriksson, P. The antioxidant butylated hydroxytoluene protects against atherosclerosis. *Arterioscler. Thromb. 11*:15–22, 1991.

70. Bloodworth, J.M.B., and Molitor, D.L. Ultrastructural aspects of human and canine diabetic retinopathy. *Invest. Ophthalmol. 4*:1037–1048, 1965.

71. Bodansky, H.J., Cudwotrh, A.G., Whitelocke, R.A., and Dobree, J.H. Diabetic retinopathy and its relation to type of diabetes: Review of a retinal clinic population. *Br. J. Ophthalmol. 66*:496–499, 1982.

72. Bossi, E., and Koerner, F. Patterns of simultaneously measured PaO_2 and $PaCO_2$ levels in newborns developing retinopathy of prematurity. *Pediatr. Res. 19*:1128, 1985.

73. Bougle, D., Vert, P., Reichart, E., Hartemann, D., and Heng, E.L. Retinal superoxide dismutase activity in newborn kittens exposed to normobaric hyperoxia effect of vitamin E. *Pediatr. Res. 16*:400–402, 1982.

74. Boulton, M.E., McLeod, D., and Garner, A. Vasoproliferative retinopathies: Clinical, morphogenetic and modulatory aspects. *Eye (Suppl.) 2*:S124–139, 1988.

74a. Boulton, M., Patel, B., Khaliq, A., Moriarty, P., Jarvis-Evans, J., and McLeod, D. Modulators and milieu in preretinal neovascularisation. *Eye 6*:560–565, 1992.

75. Bowers, D.K., Finkelstein, D., Wolff, S.M., and Green, W.R. Branch retinal vein occlusion: A clinicopathologic case report. *Retina 7*:252–259, 1987.

76. Brem, S., Preis, I., Langer, R., Brem, H., Folkman, J., and Patz, A. Inhibition of neovascularization by an extract derived from vitreous. *Am. J. Ophthalmol. 84*:323–328, 1977.

77. Brem, S.S., Zagzag, D., Tsanaclis, A.M.C., Gately, S., Elkouby, M.-P., and Brien, S.E. Inhibition of angiogenesis and tumor growth in the brain: Suppression of endothelial cell turnover by penicillamine and the depletion of copper, an angiogenic cofactor. *Am. J. Pathol. 137*:1121–1142, 1990.

78. Bresnick, G.H. Diabetic maculopathy: A clinical review highlighting diffuse macular edema. *Ophthalmology 90*:1301–1317, 1983.

79. Brody, M.J., and Zimmerman, B.G. Peripheral circulation in arterial hypertension. *Prog. Cardiovasc. Dis. 18*:323–340, 1976.

80. Brownlee, M., Cerami, A., and Vlassara, H. Advanced glycosylation end products in tissue and the biochemical basis of diabetic complications. *N. Engl. J. Med.* *318*:1315–1321, 1988.

81. Brownlee, M., Vlassara, H., and Cerami, A. Nonenzymatic glycosylation and the pathogenesis of diabetic complications. *Ann. Intern. Med.* *101*:527–537, 1984.

82. Brunner, H.R., Gavras, H., and Laragh, J.H. Specific inhibition of the renin-angiotensin system: A key to understanding blood pressure regulation. *Prog. Cardiovasc. Res.* *17*:87–98, 1974.

83. Burgess, P., and Johnson, A. Ocular defects in infants of extremely low birth weight and low gestational age. *Br. J. Ophthalmol.* *75*:84–87, 1991.

84. Caccamise, W.C., and Okuda, K. Takayasu's or pulseless disease: Unusual syndrome with ocular manifestations. *Am. J. Ophthalmol.* *37*:784–786, 1954.

85. Cagliero, E., Grant, M.B., and Lorenzi, M. Measurement of gene expression in human retinal microvessels by solution hybridization. *Invest. Ophthalmol. Vis. Sci.* *32*:1439–1445, 1991.

86. Cahill, G.F. Beta cell deficiency, insulin resistance or both? *N. Engl. J. Med.* *318*:1268–1270, 1988.

87. Caird, F.I., Pirie, A., and Ramsell, T.G. *Diabetes and the Eye*, Blackwell, Oxford, 1969.

88. Caldwell, R.B., and Slapnick, S.M. Freeze-fracture and lanthanum studies of the retinal microvasculature in diabetic rats. *Invest. Ophthalmol. Vis. Sci.* *33*:1610–1619, 1992.

89. Cameron, G.R. *Pathology of the Cell*, Oliver & Boyd, Edinburgh, 1953.

90. Campbell, F.W. The influence of a low atmospheric pressure on the development of the retinal vessels in the rat. *Trans. Ophthalmol. Soc. UK* *71*:287–299, 1951.

91. Campbell, K. Intensive oxygen therapy as a possible cause of retrolental fibroplasia: A clinical approach. *Med. J. Aust.* *2*:48–50, 1951.

92. Carr, R.E., and Siegel, I.M. Electrophysiologic aspects of several retinal diseases. *Am. J. Ophthalmol.* *58*:95–107, 1964.

93. Carrel, A. Growth-promoting function of leukocytes. *J. Exp. Med.* *36*:385–391, 1922.

94. Carrel, A., and Ebeling, A.H. Tréphones embryonnaires. *C.R. Soc. Biol. (Paris)* *89*:1142–1144, 1923.

95. Chakravarthy, U., and Archer, D.B. Endothelin: A new vasoactive ocular peptide. *Br. J. Ophthalmol.* *76*:107–108, 1992.

96. Chien, S., Usami, S., and Bertles, J.F. Abnormal rheology of oxygenated blood in sickle cell anemia. *J. Clin. Invest.* *49*:623–634, 1970.

97. Clark, E.R. Studies on the growth of blood vessels in the tail of the frog larva—by observation and experiment on the living animal. *Am. J. Anat.* *23*:37–88, 1918.

98. Cleary, P.E., Kohner, E.M., Hamilton, A.M., and Bird, A.C. Retinal macroaneurysms. *Br. J. Ophthalmol.* *59*:355–361, 1975.

99. Coats, G. Forms of retinal disease with massive exudation. *R. Lond. Ophthalmol. Hosp. Rep.* *17*:440–525, 1908.

100. Coats, G. Über retinitis exsudativa (retinitis haemorrhagica externa). *Graefes Arch. Ophthalmol.* *81*:275–327, 1912.

101. Cogan, D.G. Vascularization of the cornea: Its experimental induction by small lesions and a new theory of its pathogenesis. *Arch. Ophthalmol.* *41*:406–416, 1949.

102. Cogan, D.G. Corneal vascularization. *Invest. Ophthalmol.* *1*:253–261, 1962.

103. Cogan, D.G. Development and senescence of the human retinal vasculature. *Trans. Ophthalmol. Soc. UK* *83*:465–489, 1963.

104. Cogan, D.G., and Kuwabara, T. Capillary shunts in the pathogenesis of diabetic retinopathy. *Diabetes* *12*:293–300, 1963.

105. Cogan, D.G., and Kuwabara, T. Accessory cells in vessels of the paranatal human retina. *Arch. Ophthalmol.* *104*:747–752, 1986.

106. Cogan, D.G., Toussaint, D. and Kuwabara, T. Retinal vascular patterns. IV. Diabetic retinopathy. *Arch. Ophthalmol.* *66*:366–378, 1961.

107. Cohen, M.P., Ciborowski, C.J., and Surma, M.L. Lens capsule basement membrane synthesis: Stimulation by glucose in vitro. *Diabetes* *31*:1084–1087, 1982.

108. Cole, F.M., and Yates, P.O. The occurence and significance of intracerebral microaneurysms. *J. Pathol. Bacteriol.* *93*:393–411, 1967.

109. Coleman, S.L., Becker, B., Canaan, S., and Rosenbaum, L. Fluorescent insulin staining of the diabetic eye. *Diabetes* *11*:375–377, 1962.

110. Collier, J., and Vallance, P. Physiological importance of nitric oxide: An endogenous vasodilator. *Br. J. Med.* *302*:1289–1230, 1991.

111. Colwell, J.A. Effect of diabetic control on retinopathy. *Diabetes* *15*:497–499, 1966.

112. Colwell, J.A., Winocour, P.D., and Haluzka, P.V. Do platelets have anything to do with diabetic microvascular disease? *Diabetes, 32* (Suppl.2):14–19, 1983.

113. Committee for the Classification of Retinopathy of Prematurity. An international classification of retinopathy of prematurity. *Arch. Ophthalmol.* *102*:1130–1134, 1984.

114. Condon, P.I., and Serjeant, G.R. Ocular findings in hemoglobin SC disease in Jamaica. *Am. J. Ophthalmol.* *74*:921–931, 1972.

115. Condon, P.I., Serjeant, G.R., and Ikeda, H. Unusual chorioretinal degeneration in sickle cell disease: Possible sequelae of posterior ciliary vessel occlusion. *Br. J. Ophthalmol. 57*:81–88, 1973.
116. Connor, R.C. Complicated migraine. A study of permanent neurological and visual defects caused by migraine. *Lancet 2*:1072–1075, 1962.
117. Constable, I.J. Pathology of vitreous membranes and the effect of haemorrhage and new vessels on the vitreous. *Trans. Ophthalmol. Soc. UK 95*:382–386, 1975.
118. Constable, I.J., Oguri, M., Chesney, C.M., Swann, D.A., and Colman, R.W. Platelet-induced vitreous membrane formation. *Invest. Ophthalmol. 12*:680–685, 1973.
119. Cook, C.A.G. The significance of conjunctival aneurysms in diabetes. In *XVII Congress of Ophthalmology*, Canada, USA. University of Toronto Press, Toronto, pp. 1878–1886, 1954.
120. Cotran, R.S., Kumar, V., and Robbins, S.L. *Robbins Pathologic Basis of Disease*, W.B. Saunders, Philadelphia, pp. 1062–1069, 1989.
121. Cousins, S.W., Flynn, H.W., Jr., and Clarkson, J.G. Macroaneurysms associated with retinal branch vein occlusion. *Am. J. Ophthalmol. 109*:567–570, 1990.
122. Cristini, G., and Tolomelli, E. Pathogenesis of diabetic retinopathy: A new concept. *Arch. Pathol. Clin. Med. 25*:271–291, 1947.
123. Crum, R., Szabo, S., and Folkman, J. A new class of steroids inhibits angiogenesis in the presence of heparin or a heparin fragment. *Science 230*:1375–1378, 1985.
124. Cunha Vaz, J.G. The blood-retinal barriers. *Doc. Ophthalmol. 41*:287–327, 1976.
125. Cunha-Vaz, J.G. Studies on the pathophysiology of diabetic retinopathy: The blood-retinal barrier in diabetes. *Diabetes 32*(Suppl. 2):20–27, 1983.
126. Cunha Vaz, J.G., Abreu, J.R., Campos, A.J., and Figo, G. Early breakdown of the blood-retinal barrier in diabetes. *Br. J. Ophthalmol. 59*:649–656, 1975.
127. Cunha Vaz, J.G., Fonseca, J.R., Abreu, J.F., and Ruas, M.A. A follow-up study by vitreous fluorophotometry of early retinal involvement in diabetes. *Am. J. Ophthalmol. 86*:467–473, 1978.
128. Cunha-Vaz, J.G., Mota, C.C., Leite, E.C., Abreu, J.R., and Ruas, M.A. Effect of sorbinil on blood-retinal barrier in early diabetic retinopathy. *Diabetes 35*:574–578, 1986.
129. Dahrling, B.E. The histopathology of early central retinal artery occlusion. *Arch. Ophthalmol. 73*:506–510, 1965.
130. D'Amore, P.A. Purification of an angiogenic factor from bovine retina. *Invest. Ophthalmol. Vis. Sci. 22(Suppl.)*:109, 1982.
131. D'Amore, P.A., Glaser, B.M., Brunson, S.K., and Fenselau, A.H. Angiogenic activity from bovine retina: Partial purification and characterization. *Proc. Natl. Acad. Sci. USA 78*:3068–3072, 1981.
132. Davis, M.D. Vitreous contraction in proliferative diabetic retinopathy. *Arch. Ophthalmol. 74*:741–751, 1965.
133. Davis, M.D., Norton, E.W.D., and Myers, F.L. The Airlie classification of diabetic retinopathy. In *Treatment of Diabetic Retinopathy*, M.F. Goldberg and S.L. Fine (Eds.), U.S. Public Health Ser. Publ. No. 1890, Washington, D.C., pp. 7–22, 1969.
134. Deruaz, J.P. Étude histo-pathologique de la vascularisation rétinienne par la méthode de la digestion enzymatique. *Doc. Ophthalmol. 25*:282–359, 1969.
135. Ditzel, J. Oxygen transport impairment in diabetes. *Diabetes 25*(Suppl. 2):832–838, 1976.
136. Ditzel, J. Affinity hypoxia as a pathogenetic factor of microangiopathy with particular reference to diabetic retinopathy. *Acta Endocrinol. (Copenh.) Suppl. 238*:39–45, 1980.
137. Dixon, J.M., and Lawaczek, E. Corneal vascularization due to contact lenses. *Arch. Ophthalmol. 69*:72–75, 1963.
138. Dobbie, J.G., Kwaan, H.C., Colwell, J.A., and Suwanela, N. The role of platelets in the pathogenesis of diabetic retinopathy. *Trans. Am. Acad. Ophthalmol. Otolaryngol. 77*:OP43–46, 1973.
139. Dodson, P.M., Galton, D.J., Hamilton, A.M., and Blach, R.K. Retinal vein occlusion and the prevalence of lipoprotein abnormalities. *Br. J. Ophthalmol. 66*:161–164, 1982.
140. Dollery, C.T., and Hodge, J.V. Hypertensive retinopathy studies with fluorescein. *Trans. Ophthalmol. Soc. UK 83*:115–123, 1963.
141. Dollery, C.T., Mailer, C.M., and Hodge, J.V. Studies by fluorescence photography of papilloedema in malignant hypertension. *J. Neurol. Neurosurg. Psychiatry 28*:241–246, 1965.
142. Donders, P.C. Eales' disease. *Doc. Ophthalmol. 12*:1–105, 1958.
143. Doro, S., and Lessell, S. Cup-disc ratio an ischemic optic neuropathy. *Arch. Ophthalmol. 103*:1143–1149, 1985.
144. Doxanas, M.T., Kelley, J.S., and Prout, T.E. Sarcoidosis with neovascularization of the optic nerve head. *Am. J. Ophthalmol. 90*:347–351, 1980.
145. Dryden, R.M. Central retinal vein occlusion and chronic simple glaucoma. *Arch. Ophthalmol. 73*:659–663, 1965.
146. Duffin, R.M., Weissman, B.A., Glasser, D.B., and Pettit, T.H. Flurbiprofen in the treatment of corneal neovascularization induced by contact lenses. *Am. J. Ophthalmol. 93*:607–614, 1982.
147. Dugan, J.D., and Green, W.R. Ophthalmic manifestations of carotid occlusive disease. *Eye 5*:226–237, 1991.
148. Duke-Elder, S., and Dobree, J.H. *Diseases of the Retina: System of Ophthalmology*, Vol. 10. Kimpton, London, 1967.

149. Duke-Elder, S., and MacFaul, P.A. *The Ocular Adnexa: System of Ophthalmology*, Vol. 13. Kimpton, London, 1974.
150. Duker, J.S., and Brown, G.C. Neovascularization of the optic disc associated with obstruction of the central retinal artery. *Ophthalmology 96*:87–91, 1989.
151. Duncan, L.J.P., Macfarlane, A., and Robson, J.S. Diabetic retinopathy and nephropathy in pancreatic diabetes. *Lancet 1*:822–826, 1958.
152. Dustin, P. Arteriolar hyalinosis. *Int. Rev. Exp. Pathol. 1*:73–138, 1962.
153. Dymock, I.W., Cassar, J., Pyke, D.A., Oakley, W.G., and Williams, R. Observations on the pathogenesis, complications, and treatment of diabetes in 115 cases of hemochromatosis. *Am. J. Med. 52*:203–210, 1972.
154. Eales, H. Cases of retinal haemorrhage associated with epistaxis and constipation. *Birmingham Med. Rev. 9*:262–272, 1880.
155. Eales, H. Primary retinal haemorrhage in young man. *Ophthalmol. Rev. 1*:41–46, 1882.
156. Editorial. Axonal transport and the eye. *Br. J. Ophthalmol. 60*:547–550, 1976.
157. Editorial. The retinal cotton-wool spot. *Br. J. Ophthalmol. 61*:161–163, 1977.
158. Editorial. Antibodies to oxidised LDL in atherosclerosis. *Lancet 339*:899–900, 1992.
159. Egerer, I., Tasman, W., and Tomer, T.L. Coat's disease. *Arch. Ophthalmol. 92*:109–112, 1974.
160. Ehrenberg, M., McCuen, B.W., II, Schindler, R.H., and Machemer, R. Rubeosis iridis: Preoperative fluorescein angiography and periocular steroids. *Ophthalmology 91*:321–325, 1984.
161. Eisenstein, R., Goven, S., Schumacher, B., and Choromokos, E. The inhibition of corneal vascularization with aortic extracts in rabbits. *Am. J. Ophthalmol. 88*:1005–1012, 1979.
162. Eisenstein, R., Kuettner, K.E., Neapolitan, C., Soble, L.W., and Sorgente, N. The resistance of certain tissues to invasion. III. Cartilage extracts inhibit the growth of fibroblasts and endothelial cells in culture. *Am. J. Pathol. 81*:337–348, 1975.
163. Eisenstein, R., Sorgente, N., Soble, L.W., Miller, A., and Kuettner, K.E. The resistance of certain tissues to invasion: penetrability of explanted tissues by vascularized mesenchyme. *Am. J. Pathol. 73*:765–774, 1973.
163a. El Asrar, A.M.A., Maimone, D., Morse, P.H., Gregory, S., and Reder, A.T. Cytokines in the vitreous of patients with proliferative diabetic retinopathy. *Am. J. Ophthalmol. 114*:731–736, 1992.
164. Eliason, J.A. Leukocytes and experimental corneal vascularization. *Invest. Ophthalmol. Vis. Sci. 17*:1087–1095, 1978.
165. Eliason, J.A. Angiogenic activity of the corneal epithelium. *Exp. Eye Res. 41*:721–731, 1985.
166. Elliot, A.J. Recurrent intraocular haemorrhage in young adults (Eales disease). *Trans. Am. Ophthalmol. Soc. 52*:811–875, 1954.
167. Elliot, A.J. 30-year observation of patients with Eales's disease. *Am. J. Ophthalmol. 80*:404–408, 1975.
168. Elstow, S.F., Schor, A.M., and Weiss, J.B. Bovine retinal angiogenesis factor is a small molecule (molecular mass <600). *Invest. Ophthalmol. Vis. Sci. 26*:74–79, 1985.
168a. Evans, K., Wishart, P.K., and McGalliard, J.N. Neovascular complications after central retinal vein occlusion. *Eye 7*:520–524, 1993.
169. Epstein, R.J., and Stulting, R.D. Corneal neovascularization induced by stimulated lymphocytes in inbred mice. *Invest. Ophthalmol. Vis. Sci. 28*:1505–1513, 1987.
170. Factor, S.M., Okun, E.M., and Minase, T. Capillary microaneurysms in the human diabetic heart. *N. Engl. J. Med. 302*:384–388, 1980.
171. Fajardo, L.F., Kwan, H.H., Kowalski, J., Prionas, S.D., and Allison, A.C. Dual role of tumor necrosis factor-α in angiogenesis. *Am. J. Pathol. 140*:539–544, 1992.
172. Fallon, T.J., Maxwell, D.L., and Kohner, E.M. Autoregulation of retinal blood flow in diabetic retinopathy measured by the blue-light entoptic technique. *Ophthalmology 94*:1410–1415, 1987.
173. Fallon, T.J., Sleightholm, M.A., Merrick, C., Chalal, P., and Kohner, E.M. The effect of acute hyperglycemia on flow velocity in the macular capillaries. *Invest. Ophthalmol. Vis. Sci. 28*:1027–1030, 1987.
174. Felton, S., Brown, G., Felberg, N.T., and Felton, S.M. Vitreous inhibition of tumor neovascularization. *Arch. Ophthalmol. 97*:1710–1713, 1979.
175. Fett, J.W., Strydom, D.J., Lobb, R.R., Aldeman, E.M., Bethune, J.L., Riordan, J.F., and Vallee, B.L. Isolation and characterization of angiogenin, an angiogenic protein from human carcinoma cells. *Biochemistry 24*:5480–5486, 1985.
176. Fichte, C., Streeten, B.W., and Friedman, A.H. A histopathologic study of retinal arterial aneurysms. *Am. J. Ophthalmol. 85*:509–518, 1978.
177. Fine, B.S., and Brucker, A.J. Macular edema and cystoid macular edema. *Am. J. Ophthalmol. 92*:466–481, 1981.
178. Finnerty, F.A. Hypertensive encephalopathy. *Am. J. Med. 52*:672–678, 1972.
179. Fischbein, F.I. Ischemic retinopathy following amniotic fluid embolization. *Am. J. Ophthalmol. 67*:351–357, 1969.
180. Flower, R.W. Perinatal retinal vascular physiology. In *Contemporary Issues in Fetal and Neonatal Medicine, 2. Retinopathy of Prematurity*, W.A. Silverman and J.T. Flynn (Eds.), Blackwell Scientific, Boston, pp. 97–120, 1985.
181. Flower, R.W., Blake, D.A., Wajer, S.D., Egner, P.G., McLeod, D.S., and Pitts, S.M. Retrolental fibroplasia:

Evidence for a role of the prostaglandin cascade in the pathogenesis of oxygen-induced retinopathy in the newborn beagle. *Pediatr. Res. 15*:1293–1302, 1981.

182. Flower, R.W., McLeod, D.S., Lutty, G.A., Goldberg, B., and Wajer, S.D. Postnatal retinal vascular development of the puppy. *Invest. Ophthalmol. Vis. Sci. 26*:957–968, 1985.

183. Folkman, J., and Haudenschild, C. Angiogenesis in vitro. *Nature 228*:551–556, 1980.

184. Folkman, J., and Klagsbrun, M. Angiogenic factors. *Science 235*:442–447, 1987.

185. Folkman, J., Klagsbrun, M., Sasse, J., Wadzinski, M., Ingber, D., and Vlodavsky, I. A heparin-binding angiogenic protein—basic fibroblast growth factor—is stored within basement membrane. *Am. J. Pathol. 130*:393–400, 1988.

186. Foos, R.Y. Acute retrolental fibroplasia. *Graefes Arch. Clin. Exp. Ophthalmol. 195*:87–100, 1975.

187. Foos, R.Y. Retinopathy of prematurity: Pathologic correlation of clinical stages. *Retina 7*:260–276, 1987.

188. Form, D.M., Pratt, B.M., and Madri, J.A. Endothelial cell proliferation during angiogenesis: In vitro modulation by basement membrane components. *Lab. Invest. 55*:521–530, 1986.

189. Forrester, J.V., Chapman, A., Kerr, C., Roberts, J., Lee, W.R., and Lackie, J.M. Bovine retinal explants cultured in collagen gels: A model system for the study of proliferative retinopathy. *Arch. Ophthalmol. 108*:415–420, 1990.

190. Foulds, W.S. Clinical significance of trans-scleral fluid transfer. *Trans. Ophthalmol. Soc. UK 96*:290–308, 1976.

191. Foulds, W.S. 'Blood is thicker than water': Some haemorheological aspects of ocular disease. *Eye 1*:343–363, 1987.

192. Foulis, A.K. The pathogenesis of beta cell destruction in type I (insulin-dependent) diabetes mellitus. *J. Pathol. 152*:141–148, 1987.

193. Fox, P.D., Dunn, D.T., Morris, J.S., and Serjeant, G.R. Risk factors for proliferative sickle retinopathy. *Br. J. Ophthalmol. 74*:172–176, 1990.

194. Frank, R.N. The mechanism of blood-retinal barrier breakdown in diabetes. *Arch. Ophthalmol. 103*:1303–1304, 1985.

195. Frank, R.N. On the pathogenesis of diabetic retinopathy: A 1990 update. *Ophthalmology 98*:586–593, 1991.

196. Frank, R.N., Turczyn, T.J., and Das, A. Pericyte coverage of retinal and cerebral capillaries. *Invest. Ophthalmol. Vis. Sci. 31*:999–1007, 1990.

197. Friedl, H.P., Smith, D.J., Till, G.O., Thomson, P.D., Louis, D.S., and Ward, P.A. Ischemia-reperfusion in humans: Appearance of xanthine oxidase activity. *Am. J. Pathol. 136*:491–495, 1990.

198. Fromer, C.H., and Klintworth, G.K. An evaluation of the role of leukocytes in the pathogenesis of experimentally-induced corneal vascularization. I. Comparison of experimental models of corneal vascularization. *Am. J. Pathol. 79*:537–554, 1975.

199. Fromer, C.H., and Klintworth, G.K. An evaluation of the role of leukocytes in the pathogenesis of experimentally-induced corneal vascularization. II. Studies on the effect of leukocyte elimination on corneal vascularization. *Am. J. Pathol. 81*:531–544, 1975.

200. Fromer, C.H., and Klintworth, G.K. An evaluation of the role of leukocytes in the pathogenesis of experimentally-induced corneal vascularization. III. Studies related to the vaso-proliferative capability of polymorphonuclear leukocytes and lymphocytes. *Am. J. Pathol. 82*:157–170, 1976.

201. Fuchs, U. Die Arteriosklerose des Menschen: Elektronen mikroskopische Befunde. *Zentralbl. Allg. Pathol. 113*:501–528, 1970.

202. Fujino, T., Curtin, V.T., and Norton, E.W.D. Experimental central retinal vein occlusion: A comparison of intraocular and extraocular occlusion. *Trans. Am. Ophthalmol. Soc. 66*:318–374, 1968.

203. Furness, P.N., Turner, D.R., and Cotton, R.E. Basement membrane charge in human glomerular disease. *J. Pathol. 150*:267–278, 1986.

204. Gardiner, T.A., Johnston, P.B., and Chakravarthy, U. Endothelin immunoreactivity and binding in human, rat and bovine retina and ocular vasculature. *Invest. Ophthalmol. Vis. Sci. 32(Suppl.)*:1302, 1991.

205. Garner, A. Pathology of diabetic retinopathy. *Br. Med. Bull. 26*:137–142, 1970.

206. Garner, A. The pathology of retinopathy of prematurity. In *Contemporary Issue in Fetal and Neonatal Medicine, 2. Retinopathy of Prematurity*, W.A. Silverman and J.T. Flynn (Eds.), Blackwell Scientific, Boston, pp. 19–52, 1985.

207. Garner, A. Ocular angiogenesis. *Int. Rev. Exp. Pathol. 28*:249–306, 1986.

208. Garner, A. Pathogenesis of diabetic retinopathy. *Semin. Ophthalmol. 2*:4–11, 1987.

209. Garner, A. The role of hyperoxia in the aetiology of retinopathy of prematurity. *Doc. Ophthalmol. 74*:187–193, 1990.

210. Garner, A., and Ashton, N. Vaso-obliteration and retrolental fibroplasia. *Proc. R. Soc. Med. 64*:774–777, 1971.

211. Garner, A., and Ashton, N. Ophthalmic artery stenosis and diabetic retinopathy. *Trans. Ophthalmol. Soc. UK 92*:101–110, 1972.

212. Garner, A., Ashton, N., Tripathi, R., Kohner, E.M., Bulpitt, C.J., and Dollery, C.T. Pathogenesis of hypertensive retinopathy: An experimental study in the monkey. *Br. J. Ophthalmol. 59*:3–44, 1975.

213. Gartner, S., and Henkind, P. Neovascularization of the iris (rubeosis iridis). *Surv. Ophthalmol. 22*:291–312, 1978.

214. Gass, J.D.M. A fluorescein angiographic study of macular dysfunction secondary to retinal vascular disease. I. Embolic retinal artery obstruction. *Arch. Ophthalmol. 80*:535–549, 1968.
215. Gaynon, M.W., Boldrey, E.E., Strahlman, E.R., and Fine, S.L. Retinal neovascularization and ocular toxoplasmosis. *Am. J. Ophthalmol. 98*:585–589, 1984.
216. Gerke, E., Spitznas, M., and Brodde, O.E. The role of lactic acid in retinal neovascularization. *Graefes Arch. Ophthalmol. 200*:79–84, 1976.
217. Gerrity, R.G. The role of the monocyte in atherogenesis. I. Transition of blood-borne monocytes into foam cells in fatty lesions. *Am. J. Pathol. 103*:181–190, 1981.
218. Gerrity, R.G. Vesicular transport and intimal accumulation of macromolecules in atherosclerosis-susceptible areas is augmented by hyperlipidemia. *Circulation 76*:295–299, 1987.
219. Glagov, S., Zarins, C., Giddens, D.P., and Ku, D.N. Hemodynamics and atherosclerosis: Insights and perspectives gained from study of human arteries. *Arch. Pathol. Lab. Clin. Med. 112*:1018–1031, 1988.
220. Glaser, B.M. Extracellular modulating factors and the control of neovascularization: an overview. *Arch. Ophthalmol. 106*:603–607, 1988.
221. Glaser, B.M., Campochiaro, P.A., Davis, J.L., Jr., and Sato, M. Retinal pigment epithelial cells release an inhibitor of neovascularization. *Arch. Ophthalmol. 103*:1870–1875, 1985.
222. Glass, P. Light and the developing retina. *Doc. Ophthalmol. 74*:195–203, 1990.
223. Gloor, B.P. Phagocytic activity of pigment epithelium after light-coagulation: The origin of macrophages in the retina. *Graefes Arch. Ophthalmol. 179*:105–117, 1969.
224. Gogi, R., Rahi, A.H.S., and Garner, A. The nature of retest reaction in delayed hypersensitivity. I. Light microscopic changes in the skin of the eyelid. *Histopathology 3*:51–67, 1979.
225. Goldberg, M.F. Retinal vaso-occlusion in sickling hemoglobinopathies. In *The Eye and Inborn Errors of Metabolism*, D. Bergsma, A.J. Bron, and E. Cotlier (Eds.), National Foundation—March of Dimes, Alan R. Liss, New York, pp. 475–515, 1976.
226. Goldberg, M.F. Retinal neovascularization in sickle cell retinopathy. *Trans. Am. Acad. Ophthalmol. Otolaryngol. 83*:OP409–431, 1977.
227. Goldberg, S., and Newell, M.F. Sarcoidosis with retinal involvement. *Arch. Ophthalmol. 32*:93–96, 1944.
228. Graham, E.M., Stanford, M.R., Shilling, J.S., and Sanders, M.D. Neovascularisation associated with posterior uveitis. *Br. J. Ophthalmol. 71*:826–833, 1987.
229. Grant, D.S., Tashiro, K.I., Bartolome, S.R., Yamada, Y., Martin, G.R., and Kleinman, H.K. Two different laminin domains mediate the differentiation of human endothelial cells into capillary-like structures in vitro. *Cell 58*:933–943, 1989.
230. Grant, M., Russell, B., Fitzgerald, C., and Merimee, T.J. Insulin-like growth factors in vitreous: Studies in control and diabetic subjects with neovascularization. *Diabetes 35*:416–420, 1986.
231. Graymore, C.N. Possible significance of the isoenzymes of lactic dehydrogenase in the retina of the rat. *Nature 201*:615–616, 1964.
232. Graymore, C.N. Biochemistry of the retina. In *Biochemistry of the Eye*, C.N. Graymore (Ed.), Academic Press, New York, pp. 645–735, 1970.
233. Green, W.R., and Gass, J.D.M. Senile disciform degeneration of the macula. *Arch. Ophthalmol. 86*:487–494, 1971.
234. Green, W.R., Chan, C.C., Hutchins, G.M., and Terry, J.M. Central retinal vein occlusion: A prospective histopathologic study of 29 eyes in 28 cases. *Trans. Am. Ophthalmol. Soc. 79*:371–421, 1981.
235. Greene, D.A., Lattimer, S.A., and Sima, A.A.F. Sorbitol, phosphoinositides and sodium potassium ATPase in the pathogenesis of diabetic complications. *N. Engl. J. Med. 316*:599–606, 1987.
236. Grunwald, J.E., Brucker, A.J., Schwartz, S.S., Braunstein, S.N., Baker, L., Petrig, B.L., and Riva, C.E. Diabetic glycemic control and retinal blood flow. *Diabetes 39*:602–607, 1990.
237. Grunwald, J.E., Riva, C.E., Baine, J., and Brucker, A.J. Total retinal volumetric blood flow rate in diabetic patients with poor glycemic control. *Invest. Ophthalmol. Vis. Sci. 33*:356–363, 1992.
238. Grunwald, J.E., Riva, C.E., Martin, D.B., Quint, A.R., and Epstein, P.A. Effect of an insulin-induced decrease in blood glucose on the human diabetic retinal circulation. *Ophthalmology 94*:1614–1620, 1987.
239. Gu, X.G., Fry, G.L., Lata, G.F., Packer, A.J., Servais, E.G., Hoak, J.C., and Hayreh, S.S. Ocular neovascularization: Tissue culture studies. *Arch. Ophthalmol. 103*:111–117, 1985.
240. Guerry, D., III, and Wiesinger, H. Ocular complications in carotid angiography. *Am. J. Ophthalmol. 55*:241–243, 1963.
241. Gunn, T.R., Easdown, J., Outerbridge, E.W., and Aranda, J.V. Risk factors in retrolental fibroplasia. *Pediatrics 65*:1096–1100, 1980.
242. Gunning, A.J., Pickering, G.W., Robb-Smith, A.H.T., and Ross, R. Mural thrombosis of the internal carotid artery and subsequent embolism. *Q.J. Med. 33*:155–195, 1964.
243. Gurwin, E.B., Fitzsimons, R.B., Sehmi, K.S., and Bird, A.C. Retinal telangiectasis in facioscapulohumeral muscular dystrophy with deafness. *Arch. Ophthalmol. 103*:1695–1700, 1985.
244. Hajjar, D.P. Viral pathogenesis of atherosclerosis: Impact of molecular mimicry and viral genes. *Am. J. Pathol. 139*:1195–1211, 1991.

245. Hamasaki, D.I., and Kroll, A.J. Experimental central retinal artery occlusion: An electro-physiological study. *Arch. Ophthalmol. 80*:243–248, 1968.
246. Hamilton, A.M., and Bird, A.C. Retinal vascular accidents. *Br. J. Hosp. Med. 13*:715–726, 1975.
247. Hamilton, A.M., Kohner, E.M., Bird, A.C., Marshall, J., Rosen, D.A., and Bowbyes, J.A. Experimental occlusion of retinal veins. *Trans. Ophthalmol. Soc. UK 96*:197, 1976.
248. Hamilton, A.M., Kohner, E.M., Rosen, D., and Bowbyes, J.A. Experimental venous occlusion. *Proc. R. Soc. Med. 67*:1045–1048, 1974.
249. Hamilton, A.M., Marshall, J., Kohner, E.M., and Bowbyes, J.A. Retinal new vessel formation following experimental venous occlusion. *Exp. Eye Res. 20*:493–497, 1975.
250. Hammer, M.E., Mullen, P.W., Ferguson, J.G., Pai, S., Cosby, C., and Jackson,K.L. Logistic analysis of risk factors in acute retinopathy of prematurity. *Am. J. Ophthalmol. 102*:1–6, 1986.
251. Hanneken, A., de Juan, E., Jr., Lutty, G.A., Fox, G.M., Schiffer, S., and Hjelmeland, L.M. Altered distribution of basic fibroblast growth factor in diabetic retinopathy. *Arch. Ophthalmol. 109*:1005–1011, 1991.
252. Hanselmayer, H., and Werner, W. Spasm of the retinal artery after oral overdose of dihydroergotamine (DHE). *Klin. Monatsbl. Augenheilkd. 162*:807–811, 1973.
253. Hardin, N.J., Minick, C.R., and Murphy, G.E. Experimental induction of atheroarteriosclerosis by the synergy of allergic injury to arteries and lipid-rich diet. *Am. J. Pathol. 73*:301–326, 1973.
254. Harris, J.W., Brewster, H.H., Ham, T.H., and Castle, W.B. Studies on the destruction of red blood cells. X. The biophysics and biology of sickle cell disease. *Arch. Intern. Med. 97*:145–168, 1956.
255. Harry, J., and Ashton, N. The pathology of hypertensive retinopathy. *Trans. Ophthalmol. Soc. UK 83*:71–90, 1963.
256. Hatori, Y., Kasai, K., Nakamura, T., Emoto, T., and Shimoda, S. Effect of glucose and insulin on immunireactive endothelin-1 release from cultured porcine aortic endothelial cells. *Metabolism 40*:165–169, 1991.
257. Hayreh, S.S. Occlusion of the central retinal vessels. *Br. J. Ophthalmol. 49*:626–645, 1965.
258. Hayreh, S.S. Pathogenesis of optic disc oedema in raised intracranial pressure. *Trans. Ophthalmol. Soc. UK 96*:404–407, 1976.
259. Hayreh, S.S. Central retinal vein occlusion. In *The Eye and Systemic Disease*, F.A. Mausolf (Ed.), C.V. Mosby, St. Louis, pp. 223–275, 1980.
260. Hayreh, S.S. Classification of central retinal vein occlusion. *Ophthalmology 90*:458–474, 1983.
261. Hayreh, S.S. Anterior ischemic optic neuropathy. VIII. Clinical features and pathogenesis of post-hemorrhagic amaurosis. *Ophthalmology 94*:1488–1502, 1987.
262. Hayreh, S.S. Chronic ocular ischemic syndrome in internal carotid artery occlusive disease: Controversy on "venous stasis retinopathy." In *Amaurosis Fugax*, E.F. Bernstein (Ed.), Springer-Verlag, New York, pp. 135–157, 1988.
263. Hayreh, S.S. Classification of hypertensive fundus changes and their order of appearance. *Ophthamologica 198*:247–260, 1989.
264. Hayreh, S.S., van Heuven, W.A.J., and Hayreh, M.S. Experimental retinal vascular occlusion. *Arch. Ophthalmol. 96*:311–323, 1978.
265. Hayreh, S.S., Klugman, M.R., Beri, M., Kimura, A.E., and Podhajsky, P. Differentiation of ischemic from non-ischemic central retinal vein occlusion during the early acute phase. *Graefes Arch. Clin. Exp. Ophthalmol. 228*:201–217, 1990.
266. Hayreh, S.S., and Podhajsky, P. Ocular neovascularization with retinal vascular occlusion. II. Occurrence in central and branch retinal artery occlusion. *Arch. Ophthalmol. 100*:1585–1596, 1982.
267. Hayreh, S.S., Rojas, P., Podhajsky, P., Montague, P., and Woolson, R.F. Ocular neovascularization with retinal vascular occlusion. III. Incidence of ocular neovascularization with retinal vein occlusion. *Ophthalmology 90*:488–506, 1983.
268. Hayreh, S.S., and Servais, G.E. Retinal hemorrhages in malignant arterial hypertension. *Int. Opthalmol. 12*:137–145, 1988.
269. Hayreh, S.S., Servais, G.E., and Virdi, P.S. Fundus lesions in malignant hypertension. VI. Hypertensive choroidopathy. *Ophthalmology 93*:1383–1400, 1986.
270. Hayreh, S.S., Servais, G.E., and Virdi, P.S. Retinal arteriolar changes in malignant arterial hypertension. *Ophthalmologica 198*:178–196, 1989.
271. Hayreh, S.S., and Weingeist, T.A. Experimental occlusion of the central retinal artery of the retina. IV. Retinal tolerance time to ischaemia. *Br. J. Ophthalmol. 64*:818–825, 1980.
272. Henkind, P., and Morgan, G. Peripheral retinal angioma with exudative retinopathy in adults (Coat's lesion). *Br. J. Ophthalmol. 50*:2–11, 1966.
273. Henkind, P., and Oliveira, L.N.F. de. Retinal arteriolar annuli. *Invest. Ophthalmol. 7*:584–591, 1968.
274. Henkind, P., and Wise, G.M. Retinal neovascularization, collaterals, and vascular shunts. *Br. J. Ophthalmol. 58*:413–422, 1974.
275. Herbaczynska-Cedro, H., and Vane, J.R. Contribution of intrarenal generation of prostaglandin to autoregulation of renal blood flow in the dog. *Circ. Res. 33*:428–436, 1973.
276. Herman, I.M., and D'Amore, P.A. Microvascular pericytes contain muscle and non-muscle actins. *J. Cell Biol. 101*:43–52, 1985.

277. Higgs, G.A., McCall, E., and Youlten, L.J.F. A chemotactic role for prostaglandins released from poly-morphonuclear leukocytes during phagocytosis. *Br. J. Pharmacol. 53*:539–546, 1975.
278. Hill, C.R., Kissun, R.D., Weiss, J.B., and Garner, A. Angiogenic factor in vitreous from diabetic retinopathy. *Experientia 39*:583–585, 1983.
279. Hill, D.W., and Atherton, H.A. Experimental studies of the retinal circulation relating to diabetic retinopathy. *Trans. Ophthalmol. Soc. UK 99*:4–7, 1979.
280. Hill, D.W., and Dollery, C.T. Calibre changes in retinal arterioles. *Trans. Ophthalmol. Soc. UK 83*:61–70, 1963.
281. von Hippel, E. Über eine sehr seltene Erkrankung der Netzhaut: Klinische Beobachtungen. *Graefes Arch. Ophthalmol. 59*:83–106, 1904.
282. Hockley, D.J., Tripathi, R.C., and Ashton, N. Experimental retinal branch vein occlusion in the monkey: Histopathological and ultrastructural studies. *Trans. Ophthalmol. Soc. UK 96*:202–209, 1976.
283. Hodge, J.V., and Dollery, C.T. Retinal soft exudates. *Q. J. Med. 33*:117–131, 1964.
284. Hogan, M.J., and Feeney, L. Ultrastructure of retinal blood vessels. II. The small vessels. *J. Ultrastruct. Res. 9*:29–46, 1963.
285. Hollenhorst, R.W. Ocular manifestations of insufficiency or thrombosis of the internal carotid artery. *Trans. Am. Ophthalmol. Soc. 56*:474–506, 1958.
286. Hollenhurst, R.W. The ocular manifestations of internal carotid thrombosis. *Med. Clin. North Am. 44*:897–908, 1960.
287. Hoskins, D. Neovascular glaucoma. *Trans. Am. Acad. Ophthalmol. Otolaryngol. 78*:330–333, 1974.
288. Hudes, G.R., Li, W., Rockey, J., and White, P. Prostacyclin is the major prostaglandin synthesized by bovine retinal capillary pericytes in culture. *Invest. Ophthalmol. Vis. Sci. 29*:1511–1516, 1988.
289. Imre, G. Studies on the mechanism of retinal neovascularization. *Br. J. Ophthalmol. 48*:75–82, 1964.
290. Inomata, H., Smelser, G.K., and Polack, F.M. Corneal vascularization in experimental uveitis and graft rejection: An electron microscopic study. *Invest. Ophthalmol. 10*:840–850, 1970.
291. International Committee for the Classification of Retinopathy of Prematurity. An international classification of retinopathy of prematurity: The classification of retinal detachment. *Arch. Ophthalmol. 105*:906–912, 1987.
292. Ito, M. Studies on the retinal circulation time and plasma fibrinogen level in Takayasu's disease. *Rinsho Ganka 29*:481–488, 1975.
293. Ito, M. Supplementary findings on an ophthalmological study of Takayasu's disease. II. Ischaemic optic neuropathy associated with Takayasu's disease. *Acta Soc. Ophthalmol. Jpn. 80*:353–360, 1976.
293a. Jacobs, N.A., and Trew, D.R. Occlusion of the central retinal artery and ocular neovascularisation: An indirect association? *Eye 6*:599–602, 1992.
294. Jacobson, B., Dorfman, T., Basu, P.K., and Hasany, S.M. Inhibition of vascular endothelial cell growth and trypsin activity by vitreous. *Exp. Eye Res. 41*:581–595, 1985.
295. Jaffe, E.A. Cell biology of endothelial cells. *Hum. Pathol. 18*:234–239, 1987.
296. Janka, H.U., Standl, E., Schramm, W., and Mehnert, H. Platelet enzyme activities in diabetes mellitus in relation to endothelial damage. *Diabetes 32*(Suppl. 2):47–51, 1983.
297. Janzer, R.C., and Raff, M.C. Astrocytes induce blood-brain properties in endothelial cells. *Nature 325*:253–257, 1987.
298. Jebejian, R., and Kalfayan, B. Le syndrome oculo-buccogénital. *Ann. Ocul. 179*:481–491, 1946.
299. Jensen, J.A., Hunt, T.K., Scheuenstuhl, H., and Banda, M.J. Effect of lactate, pyruvate, and pH on secretion of angiogenesis and mitogenesis factors by macrophages. *Lab. Invest. 54*:574–578, 1986.
300. Jerneld, B., and Algvere, P. Relationship of duration and onset of diabetes to prevalence of diabetic retinopathy. *Am. J. Ophthalmol. 102*:431–437, 1986.
301. de Juan, E., Gritz, D.C., and Machemer, R. Ultrastructural characteristics of proliferative tissue in retinopathy of prematurity. *Am. J. Ophthalmol. 104*:149–156, 1987.
302. Kador, P.F., Akagi, Y., Terubayashi, H., Wyman, M., and Kinoshita, J.H. Prevention of pericyte ghost formation in retinal capillaries of galactose-fed dogs by aldose reductase inhibitors. *Arch. Ophthalmol. 106*:1099–1102, 1988.
303. Kadoya, Y., Fujita, E., Shoji, E., Suchiya, H., and Obara, Y. Serum lipid level in retinal venous occlusion. *Folia Ophthalmol. Jpn. 41*:390–394, 1990.
304. Kahn, M., Knox, D.L., and Green, W.R. Clinicopathologic studies of a case of aortic arch syndrome. *Retina 6*:228–233, 1986.
305. Karpen, C.W., Cataland, S., O'Dorisio, T.M., and Panganamala, R.V. Interrelation of platelet vitamin E and thromboxane synthesis in type I diabetes mellitus. *Diabetes 33*:239–243, 1984.
306. Kearns, T.P. Fat embolism of the retina demonstrated by a flat retinal preparation. *Am. J. Ophthalmol. 41*:1–2, 1956.
307. Kearns, T.P., and Hollenhorst, R.W. Venous stasis retinopathy of occlusive disease of the carotid artery. *Mayo Clin. Proc. 38*:304–312, 1963.
308. Khatami, M., Li, W., and Rockey, J.H. Kinetics of ascorbate transport by cultured retinal capillary pericytes. *Invest. Ophthalmol. Vis. Sci. 27*:1665–1671, 1986.
309. Kiep, W.H. Ocular complications occuring in malaria. *Trans. Ophthalmol. Soc. UK 42*:394–398, 1922.

310. Killingsworth, M.C., Sarks, J.P., and Sarks, S.H. Macrophages related to Bruch's membrane in age-related macular degeneration. *Eye 4*:613–621, 1990.
311. Kinoshita, J.H. Aldose reductase in the diabetic eye. XLIII. Edward Jackson Memorial Lecture. *Am. J. Ophthalmol. 102*:685–692, 1986.
312. Kishi, S., Tso, M.O.M., and Hayreh, S.S. Fundus lesions in malignant hypertension. I. A pathologic study of experimental hypertensive optic choroidopathy. *Arch. Ophthalmol. 103*:1189–1197, 1985.
313. Kishi, S., Tso, M.O.M., and Hayreh, S.S. Fundus lesions in malignant hypertension. II. A pathologic study of experimental hypertensive optic neuropathy. *Arch. Ophthalmol. 103*:1198–1206, 1985.
314. Klagsbrun, M., and Vlodavsky, I. Biosynthesis and storage of basic fibroblast growth factor (bFGF) by endothelial cells: Implication for the mechanism of action of angiogenesis. In *Growth Factors and Other Aspects of Wound Healing: Biological and Clinical Implications*. T.K. Hunt (Ed.), Alan R. Liss, New York, pp. 55–61, 1988.
315. Klien, B.A. Occlusion of the central retinal vein: Clinical importance of certain histopathologic observations. *Am. J. Ophthalmol. 36*:316–324, 1953.
316. Klintworth, G.K. The hamster cheek pouch: An experimental model of corneal vascularization. *Am. J. Pathol. 73*:691–710, 1973.
317. Klintworth, G.K. The cornea—structure and macromolecules in health and disease: A review. *Am. J. Pathol. 89*:719–808, 1977.
318. Klintworth, G.K. *Corneal Angiogenesis; A Comprehensive Critical Review.* New York, Springer-Verlag, 1991.
319. Klintworth, G.K., and Burger, P.C. Neovascularization of the cornea: Current concepts of its pathogenesis. *Int. Ophthalmol. Clin. 23*:27–39, 1983.
320. Klug, P.P., Lessin, L.S., and Radice, P. Rheological aspects of sickle cell disease. *Arch. Intern. Med. 133*:577–590, 1974.
321. Knighton, D.R., Hunt, T.K., Scheuenstuhl, H., Halliday, B.J., Werb, Z., and Banda, M.J. Oxygen tension regulates the expression of angiogenesis factor by macrophages. *Science 221*:1283–1285, 1983.
322. Knighton, D.R., Silver, I.A., and Hunt, T.K. Regulation of wound healing angiogenesis—effect of oxygen gradients and inspired oxygen concentration. *Surgery 90*:262–270, 1981.
323. Knox, D.L. Ischemic ocular inflammation. *Am. J. Ophthalmol. 60*:995–1002, 1965.
324. Kohner, E.M. Dynamic changes in the microcirculation of diabetes as related to diabetic microangiopathy. *Acta Med. Scand. (Suppl.) 578*:41–47, 1975.
325. Kohner, E.M. The natural history of proliferative diabetic retinopathy. *Eye 5*:222–225, 1991.
326. Kohner, E.M., and Dollery, C.T. The rate of formation and disappearance of microaneurysms in diabetic retinopathy. *Trans. Ophthalmol. Soc. UK 90*:369–374, 1970.
327. Kohner, E.M., and Dollery, C.T. Diabetic retinopathy. In *Complications of Diabetes*, H. Keen and J. Jarrett (Eds.), Edward Arnold, London, pp. 7–98, 1975.
328. Kohner, E.M., Dollery, C.T., and Bulpitt, C.J. Cotton-wool spots in diabetic retinopathy. *Diabetes 18*:691–704, 1969.
329. Kohner, E.M., Dollery, C.T., Paterson, J.W., and Oakley, N.W. Arterial fluorescein studies in diabetic retinopathy. *Diabetes 16*:1–10, 1967.
330. Kohner, E.M., Hamilton, A.M., and Saunders, S.J. The retinal blood flow in diabetes. *Diabetologia 11*:27–33, 1975.
331. Kohner, E.M., and Shilling, J.S. Retinal vein occlusion. In *Medical Ophthalmology*, F.C. Rose (Ed.), Chapman & Hall, London, pp. 391–429, 1976.
332. Kowada, M., Ames, A., III, Majno, G., and Wright, R.L. Cerebral ischemia. I. An improved experimental method for study; cardiovascular effects and demonstration of an early vascular lesion in the rabbit. *J. Neurosurg. 28*:150–157, 1968.
333. Kremer, F., and Koch, H.R. Effect of x-rays and carotid ligature on lens transparency and on various biochemical parameters in rat lenses. *Interdiscip. Top. Gerontol. 12*:119–126, 1978.
334. Kretzer, F.L., Hittner, H.M., Johnson, A.J., Mehta, R.S., and Godio, L.B. Vitamin E and retrolental fibroplasia: Ultrastructural support of clinical efficacy. *Ann. NY Acad. Sci. 393*:145–166, 1982.
335. Kretzer, F.L., Mehta, R.S., Johnson, A.T., Hunter, D.G., Brown, E.S., and Hittner, H.M. Vitamin E protects against retinopathy of prematurity through action on spindle cells. *Nature 309*:793–795, 1984.
336. Kroll, A.J. Experimental central retinal artery occlusion. *Arch. Ophthalmol. 79*:453–469, 1968.
337. Kuettner, K.E., Croxen, R.L., Eisenstein, R., and Sorgente, N. Proteinase inhibitor activity in connective tissues. *Experientia 30*:595–597, 1974.
338. Kuwabara, T., and Cogan, D.G. Retinal vascular patterns. VI. Mural cells of the retinal capillaries. *Arch. Ophthalmol. 69*:492–502, 1963.
339. Kuwashima, L., Graeber, J., and Glaser, B.M. Stimulation of endothelial cell prostacyclin release by retina-derived factors. *Invest. Ophthalmol. Vis. Sci. 29*:1213–1220, 1988.
340. Laatikainen, L. Preliminary report on effect of retinal panphotocoagulation on rubeosis iridis and neovascular glaucoma. *Br. J. Ophthalmol. 61*:278–283, 1977.
341. Laatikainen, L., and Kohner, E.M. Fluorescein angiography and its prognostic significance in central retinal vein occlusion. *Br. J. Ophthalmol. 60*:411–418, 1976.

342. Langham, M. Utilization of oxygen by the component layers of the living cornea. *J. Physiol. (Lond.) 117*:461–470, 1952.
343. Larsen, H.W. Diabetic retinopathy. *Acta Ophthalmol. (Copenh.) Suppl. 60*:1–89, 1960.
344. Lasek, R.J. Protein transport in neurons. *Int. Rev. Neurobiol. 13*:289–324, 1970.
345. Lavin, M.J., Marsh, M.J., Peart, S., and Rehman, A. Retinal arterial macroaneurysms: A retrospective study of 40 patients. *Br. J. Ophthalmol. 71*:817–825, 1987.
346. Leber, T. Über eine durch Vorkommen multipler Miliaraneurysmen charakterisierte Form von Retinaldegeneration. *Graefes Arch. Ophthalmol. 81*:1–14, 1912.
347. Ledbetter, S.R., Wagner, C.W., Martin, G.R., Rohrbach, D.H., and Hassell, J.R. Response of diabetic membrane producing cells to glucose and insulin. *Diabetes 36*:1029–1034, 1987.
348. Lee, C.S., Mauer, S.M., Brown, D.M., Sutherland, D.E.R., Michael, A.F., and Najarian, J.S. Renal transplantation in diabetes mellitus in rats. *J. Exp. Med. 139*:793–800, 1974.
349. Leibovitch, S.J., Polverini, P.J., Shepard, H.M., Wiseman, D.M., Shively, V., and Nuseir, N. Macrophage-induced angiogenesis is mediated by tumor necrosis factor-α. *Nature 239*:630–632, 1987.
350. Leishman, R. The eye in general vascular disease: Hypertension and arteriosclerosis. *Br. J. Ophthalmol. 41*:641–701, 1957.
351. Leonard, T.J.K., and Sanders, M.D. Ischaemic optic neuropathy in pulseless disease. *Br. J. Ophthalmol. 67*:389–392, 1983.
352. Levene, R., Shapiro, A., and Baum, J. Experimental corneal vascularization. *Arch. Ophthalmol. 70*:242–249, 1963.
353. Levine, R.A., and Henry, M.D. Ischemic infarction of the retina following carotid angiography. *Am. J. Ophthalmol. 55*:365–367, 1963.
354. Li, W.W., Casey, R., Gonzalez, E.M., and Folkman, J. Angiostatic steroids potentiated by sulfated cyclodextrins inhibit corneal neovascularization. *Invest. Ophthalmol. Vis. Sci. 32*:2898–2905, 1991.
355. Li, W., Shen, S., Khatami, M., and Rockey, J.H. Stimulation of retinal capillary protein and collagen synthesis in culture by high glucose concentration. *Diabetes 33*:785–789, 1984.
356. Lightman, S., Rechthanh, E., Latker, C., Palestine, A., and Rapoport, S. Assessment of the permeability of the blood-retinal barrier in hypertensive rats. *Hypertension 10*:390–395, 1987.
357. Lin, M.T., and Chen, Y-L. Effect of copper ion on collagenase release: Its implication on corneal vascularization. *Invest. Ophthalmol. Vis. Sci. 33*:558–563, 1992.
358. Linsenmaier, R.A., and Yancey, C.M. Effects of hyperoxia on the oxygen distribution in the intact cat retina. *Invest. Ophthalmol. Vis. Sci. 30*:612–618, 1989.
359. Little, H.L. Pathogenesis. In *Diabetic Retinopathy, Clinical Evaluation and Management*, F.A. L'Esperance, Jr., and W.A. James, Jr. (Eds.), C.V. Mosby, St. Louis, pp. 58–88, 1981.
360. Lucey, J.F., Horbar, J.D., and Orishi, M.J. Cerebral and retinal hypoperfusion as a possible cause of retrolental fibroplasia: Hypothesis to explain non-oxygen-related RLF (abstract). *Pediatr. Res. 15*:670, 1981.
361. Lutty, G.A., Ikeda, K., Chandler, C., and McLeod, D.S. Immunolocalization of tissue plasminogen activator in the diabetic and nondiabetic retina and choroid. *Invest. Ophthalmol. Vis. Sci. 32*:237–245, 1991.
362. Lutty, G.A., Liu, S.H., and Prendergast, R.A. Angiogenic lymphokines of activated T-cell origin. *Invest. Ophthalmol. Vis. Sci. 24*:1595–1601, 1984.
363. Lutty, G.A., Thompson, D.C., Gallup, J.Y., Mello, R.J., Patz, A., and Fenselau, A. Vitreous: An inhibitor of retinal extract-induced neovascularization. *Invest. Ophthalmol. Vis. Sci. 24*:52–56, 1983.
364. Lyle, T.K., and Wybar, K.D. Retinal vasculitis. *Br. J. Ophthalmol. 45*:778–788, 1961.
365. McAuslan, B.R., and Reilly, W. Endothelial cell phagokinesis in response to specific metal ions. *Exp. Cell Res. 130*:147–157, 1980.
366. McGrath, M.A., Wechsler, F., Hunyor, A.B.L., and Penny, R. Systemic factors contributing to retinal vein occlusion. *Arch. Intern. Med. 138*:216–220, 1978.
367. McLaughlin, B., Cawston, T., and Weiss, J.B. Activation of the matrix metalloproteinase inhibitor complex by a low molecular weight angiogenic factor. *Biochim. Biophys. Acta 1073*:295–298, 1991.
368. McLeod, D. Cilio-retinal arterial circulation in central retinal vein occlusion. *Br. J. Ophthalmol. 59*:486–492, 1975.
369. McLeod, D. Ophthalmoscopic signs of obstructed axoplasmic transport after ocular vascular occlusions. *Br. J. Ophthalmol. 60*:551–556, 1976.
370. McLeod, D. Retinal ischaemia, disc swelling, and axoplasmic transport. *Trans. Ophthalmol. Soc. UK 96*:313–318, 1976.
371. McLeod, D., Marshall, J., and Kohner, E.M. Role of axoplasmic transport in the pathophysiology of ischaemic disc swelling. *Br. J. Ophthalmol. 64*:247–261, 1980.
372. McLeod, D., Marshall, J., Kohner, E.M., and Bird, A.C. The role of axoplasmic transport in the pathogenesis of retinal cotton-wool spots. *Br. J. Ophthalmol. 61*:177–191, 1977.
373. McMillan, D.E. Plasma protein changes, blood viscosity, and diabetic microangiopathy. *Diabetes 25*(Suppl. 2):858–864, 1976.
374. McMillan, D.E. The effect of diabetes on blood flow properties. *Diabetes 32*(Suppl. 2):56–63, 1983.
375. McNeil, P.L., Muthukrishnan, L., Warder, E., and D'Amore, P.A. Growth factors are released by mechanically wounded endothelial cells. *J. Cell. Biol. 109*:811–822, 1989.

376. Magargal, L.E., Brown, G.C., Augsburger, J.J., and Parrish, R.K. Neovascular glaucoma following central retinal vein occlusion. *Ophthalmology* 88:1095–1101, 1981.

377. Maione, T.E., Gray, G.S., Petro, J., Hunt, A.J., Donner, A.L., Bauer, S.I., Carson, H.F., and Sharpe, R.J. Inhibition of angiogenesis by recombinant human platelet factor-4 and related peptides. *Science* 247:77–79, 1990.

378. Mandelcorn, M.S., Blankenship, G., and Machemer, R. Pars plana vitrectomy for the management of severe diabetic retinopathy. *Am. J. Ophthalmol.* 81:561–570, 1976.

379. Manor, R.S., and Sachs, W. Visible retinal emboli in a case of subacute bacterial endocarditis. *Ophthalmologica* 166:10–15, 1973.

380. Manschot, W.A. Embolism of the central retinal artery. *Am. J. Ophthalmol.* 48:381–385, 1959.

381. Marshall, J. Cerebrovascular disease. In *Medical Ophthalmology*, F.C. Rose (Ed.), Chapman & Hall, London, pp. 355–362, 1976.

382. Martinez-Hernandez, A., and Amenta, P.S. The basement membrane in pathology. *Lab. Invest.* 48:656–677, 1983.

383. Merimee, T.J., Zapf, J., and Froesch, E.R. Insulin-like growth factor: Studies in diabetics with and without retinopathy. *N. Engl. J. Med.* 309:527–530, 1983.

384. Metcalfe, M.A., and Baum, J.D. Incidence of insulin dependent diabetes in children aged under 15 years in the British Isles during 1988. *Br. Med. J.* 302:443–447, 1991.

385. Meyer, K., and Chaffee, E. The mucopolysaccharide acid of the cornea and its enzymatic hydrolysis. *Am. J. Ophthalmol.* 23:1320–1325, 1940.

386. Michaelson, I.C. Mode of development of the vascular system of the retinal with some observations on its significance for certain retinal diseases. *Trans. Ophthalmol. Soc. UK* 68:137–180, 1948.

387. Michaelson, I.C. *Retinal Circulation in Man and Animals*. Thomas, Springfield, Illinois, 1954.

388. Miller, H., Miller, B., Zonis, S., and Nir, I. Diabetic neovascularization: Permeability and ultrastructure. *Invest. Ophthalmol. Vis. Sci.* 25:1338–1342, 1984.

389. Milley, J.R., Rosenberg, A.A., and Jones, M.D. Retinal and choroidal blood flow in hypoxic and hypercarbic newborn lambs. *Pediatr. Res.* 18:410–414, 1984.

390. Minckler, D.S., and Bunt, A.H. Axoplasmic transport in ocular hypotony and papilledema in the monkey. *Arch. Ophthalmol.* 95:1430–1436, 1977.

391. Minckler, D.S., Tso, M.O.M., and Zimmerman, L.E. A light microscopic, autoradiographic study of axoplasmic transport in the optic nerve head during ocular hypotony, increased intraocular pressure, and papilledema. *Am. J. Ophthalmol.* 82:741–757, 1976.

392. Miyashita, K., Tanahashi, N., and Akiya, S. Red blood cell aggregatability in branch retinal venous occlusion. *Acta Soc. Ophthalmol. Jpn.* 92:1569–1572, 1988.

393. Mizoguchi, T., Takagi, T., and Kajiwara, Y. Three familial cases with changes in the Coats' disease-like fundus. *Fol. Ophthalmol. Jpn.* 37:218–221, 1986.

394. Mohan, R., and Kohner, E.M. Retinal revascularization in diabetic retinopathy. *Br. J. Ophthalmol.* 70:114–117, 1986.

395. Mohan, R., Rajendran, B., Mohan, V., Ramachandran, A., Viswanathan, M., and Kohner, E.M. Retinopathy in tropical pancreatic diabetes. *Arch. Ophthalmol.* 103:1487–1489, 1985.

396. Mondino, B.J., Aizuss, D.H., and Farley, M.K. Steroids. In *Clinical Ophthalmic Pharmacology*, D.W. Lamberts and D.E. Potter (Eds.), Little, Brown, Boston, pp. 157–172, 1987.

397. Moses, M.A., Sudhalter, J., and Langer, R. Identification of an inhibitor of neovascularization from cartilage. *Science* 248:1408–1410, 1990.

398. Munro, J.M., and Cotran, J.S. The pathogenesis of atherosclerosis: Atherogenesis and inflammation. *Lab. Invest.* 58:249–261, 1988.

399. Murdoch, I.E., Rosen, P.H., and Shilling, J.S. Neovascular responses ischemic central retinal vein occlusion after panretinal photocoagulation. *Br. J. Ophthalmol.* 75:459–461, 1991.

400. Nakao, K., Ikeda, M., Kimata, S., Niitani, H., Miyahara, M., Ishimi, Z., Hashiba, K., Takeda, Y., Ozawa, T., Matsushita, S., and Kuramochi, M. Takayasu's arteritis: Clinical report of 84 cases and immunological studies of seven cases. *Circulation* 35:1141–1155, 1967.

401. Nakayasu, K. Origin of pericytes in neovascularization of rat cornea. *Jpn. J. Ophthalmol.* 32:105–112, 1988.

401a. Nakayasu, K., Hayashi, N., Okisaka, S., and Sato, N. Formation of capillary-like tubes by vascular endothelial cells cocultured with keratocytes. *Invest. Ophthalmol. Vis. Sci.* 33:3050–3057, 1992.

402. Nash, G.B. Blood rheology and ischaemia. *Eye* 5:151–158, 1991.

403. Nasrallah, F.P., Jalkh, A.H., van Coppenhollre, F., Kado, M., Trempe, C.L., McMeel, J.W., and Schepens, C.L. The role of the vitreous in diabetic macular edema. *Ophthalmology* 95:1335–1339, 1988.

404. Navaratnam, V. Organisation and reorganisation of blood vessels in embryonic development. *Eye* 5:147–150, 1991.

405. Neufeld, G., and Gospodarowicz, D. The identification and partial characterization of the fibroblast growth factor receptor of baby hamster kidney cells. *J. Biol. Chem.* 260:1386–1388, 1985.

406. Newton, T.H., and Hoyt, W.F. Dural arteriovenous shunts in the region of the cavernous sinus. *Neuroradiology* 1:71–81, 1970.

407. Nicosia, R.F., and Bonanno, E. Inhibition of angiogenesis in vitro by Arg-Gly-Asp-containing synthetic peptide. *Am. J. Pathol. 138*:829–833, 1991.
408. Noden, D.M. Origins and assembly of avian embryonic blood vessels. *Ann. NY Acad. Sci. 588*:236–249, 1990.
409. Nork, T.M., Tso, M.O.M., Duvall, J., and Hayreh, S.S. Cellular mechanisms of iris neovascularization secondary to retinal vein occlusion. *Arch. Ophthalmol. 107*:581–586, 1989.
410. Nunn, J.F. Oxygen—friend or foe? *J. R. Soc. Med. 78*:618–622, 1985.
411. Ochs, S. Local supply of energy to the fast axoplasmic transport mechanism. *Proc. Natl. Acad. Sci. USA 68*: 1279–1282, 1971.
412. Ochs, S. Trophic functions of the neuron. 3. Mechanisms of neutrophilic interactions. Systems of material transport in nerve fibers (axoplasmic transport) related to nerve function and control. *Ann. NY Acad. Sci. 228*:202–223, 1974.
413. Odedra, R., and Weiss, J.B. Low molecular weight angiogenesis factors. *Pharmacol. Ther. 49*:111–124, 1991.
414. Oji, E.O., and McLeod, D. Partial central retinal artery occlusion. *Trans. Ophthalmol. Soc. UK 98*:156–159, 1978.
415. Okamoto, T., Oikawa, S., and Toyota, T. Absence of angiogenesis-inhibitory activity in aqueous humor of diabetic rabbits. *Diabetes 39*:12–16, 1990.
416. de Oliveira, F. Pericytes in diabetic retinopathy. *Br. J. Ophthalmol. 50*:134–143, 1966.
417. Orlidge, A., and D'Amore, P.A. Inhibition of capillary endothelial cell growth by pericytes and smooth muscle cells. *J. Cell Biol. 105*:1455–1462, 1987.
418. Orlidge-Antonelli, A., Smith, S.R., and D'Amore, P.A. Influence on pericytes on capillary endothelial cell growth. *Am. Rev. Respir. Dis. 140*:1129–1131, 1989.
419. Osterby, R. Early phases in the development of diabetic glomerulopathy: A quantitative electron microscopic study. *Acta Med. Scand. (Suppl.) 574*:1–82, 1975.
420. Palmer, R.M.J., Ferrige, A.G., and Moncada, S. Nitric oxide release accounts for the biological activity of endothelium-derived relaxing factor. *Nature 327*:524–526, 1987.
421. Pandolfi, M., and Al-Rushood, A. The role of fibrinolytic factors in ischaemia. *Eye 5*:159–169, 1991.
422. Panton, R.W., Goldberg, M.F., and Farber, M.D. Retinal arterial macroaneurysms: Risk factors and natural history. *Br. J. Ophthalmol. 74*:595–600, 1990.
423. Parving, H.-H. Increased microvascular permeability to plasma proteins in short- and long-term juvenile diabetes. *Diabetes 25*(Suppl. 2):884–889, 1976.
424. Paton, A., Rubinstein, K., and Smith, V.H. Arterial insufficiency in retinal venous occlusion. *Trans. Ophthalmol. Soc. UK 84*:559–595, 1964.
425. Paton, D. The conjunctival sign of sickle-cell disease—further observations. *Arch. Ophthalmol. 68*:627–632, 1962.
426. Paton, L., and Holmes, G. The pathology of papilloedema: A histological study of sixty eyes. *Brain 33*:389–432, 1911.
427. Patz, A. Observations on the retinopathy of prematurity. *Am. J. Ophthalmol. 100*:164–168, 1985.
428. Patz, A., Eastham, A., Higginbotham, D.H., and Kleh, T. Oxygen studies in retrolental fibroplasia. II. The production of the microscopic changes of retrolental fibroplasia in experimental animals. *Am. J. Ophthalmol. 36*:1511–1522, 1953.
429. Patz, A., Hoeck, L.E., and LaCruz, E.de. Studies on the effect of high oxygen administration in retrolental fibroplasia. I. Nursery observations. *Am. J. Ophthalmol. 35*:1248–1252, 1952.
430. Paulsen, E.P., and Koury, M. Hemoglobin AI$_c$ levels in insulin-dependent and -independent diabetes mellitus. *Diabetes 25*(Suppl. 2):890–896, 1976.
431. Perraut, L.E., and Zimmerman, L.E. The occurrence of glaucoma after occlusion of the central retinal artery. *Arch. Ophthalmol. 61*:845–867, 1959.
432. Perutz, M.F., and Mitchison, J.M. State of haemoglobin in sickle-cell anaemia. *Nature 166*:677–679, 1950.
433. Peters, T.J., and deDuve, C. Lysosomes of the arterial wall. II. Subcellular fractionation of aortic cells from rabbits with experimental atheroma. *Exp. Mol. Pathol. 20*:228–256, 1974.
434. Petty, R.G., and Pearson, J.D. Endothelium—the axis of vascular health and disease. *J. R. Coll. Phys. Lond. 23*:92–102, 1989.
435. Pfister, R.R. The intraocular changes of anterior segment necrosis. *Eye 5*:214–221, 1991.
436. Phelps, D.L. Retinopathy of prematurity: An estimate of vision loss in the United States—1979. *Pediatrics 67*:924–925, 1981.
437. Phelps, D.L. Vitamin E and retinopathy of prematurity. In *Contemporary Issues in Fetal and Neonatal Medicine, 2. Retinopathy of Prematurity*, W.A. Silverman and J.T. Flynn (Eds.), Blackwell Scientific, Boston, pp. 181–205, 1985.
438. Pickering, G.W. *High Blood Pressure*, 2nd ed. Churchill, London, 1968.
439. Poliner, S., Christianson, D.J., Escoffery, R.F., Kolker, A.E., and Gordon, M.E. Neovascular glaucoma after intracapsular and extracapsular cataract extraction in diabetic patients. *Am. J. Ophthalmol. 100*:637–645, 1985.
440. Polverini, P.J., Cotran, R.S., Gimbrone, M.A., and Unanue, E.R. Activated macrophages induce vascular proliferation. *Nature 269*:804–806, 1977.

441. Polverini, P.J., Cotran, R.S., and Sholley, M.M. Endothelial proliferation in the delayed hypersensitivity reaction: An autoradiographic study. *J. Immunol.* *118*:529–532, 1977.
442. Pope, C.H., Jr. Retinal capillary microaneurysms: A concept of pathogenesis. *Diabetes 9*:9–13, 1960.
443. Poston, R.N., Haskard, C.O., Coucher, J.R., Gall, N.P., and Johnson-Tidey, R.R. Expression of intercellilar adhesion molecule-1 in atherosclerotic plaques. *Am. J. Pathol. 140*:665–673, 1992.
444. Pournaras, C.J., Tsacopoulos, M., Strommer, K., Gilodi, N., and Leuenberger, P.M. Experimental retinal branch vein occlusion in miniature pigs induces local tissue hypoxia and vasoproliferative retinopathy. *Ophthalmology 97*:1321–1328, 1990.
445. Prendiville, A., and Schulenberg, W.E. Clinical factors associated with retinopathy of prematurity. *Arch. Dis. Child. 63*:522–527, 1988.
446. Quinlan, P.M., Elman, M.J., Bhatt, M.K., Mardesich, P., and Enger, M.S. The natural course of central retinal vein occlusion. *Am. J. Ophthalmol. 110*:118–123, 1990.
447. Quinn, M.T., Parthasarathy, S., Fong, L.G., and Steinberg, D. Oxidatively modified low density lipoproteins: A potential role in recruitment and retention of monocyte/macrophages during atherogenesis. *Proc. Natl. Acad. Sci. USA 84*:2995–2998, 1987.
448. Rahi, A.H.S., and Ashton, N. Contractile proteins in retinal endothelium and other non-muscle tissues of the eye. *Br. J. Ophthalmol. 62*:627–643, 1978.
449. Raju, K.S., Alessandri, G., Ziche, M., and Gullino, P.M. Ceruloplasmin, copper ions, and angiogenesis. *J. Natl. Cancer Inst. 69*:1183–1188, 1982.
449a. Ramachandran, E., Frank, R.N., and Kennedy, A. Effects of endothelin on cultured bovine retinal microvascular pericytes. *Invest. Ophthalmol. Vis. Sci. 34*:586–595, 1993.
450. Ramalho, P., and Dollery, C.T. Hypertensive retinopathy: Calibre changes in retinal blood vessels following blood-pressure reduction and inhalation of oxygen. *Circulation 37*:580–588, 1968.
451. Raymond, L., and Jacobson, B. Isolation and identification of stimulatory and inhibitory factors in bovine vitreous. *Exp. Eye Res. 34*:267–286, 1982.
452. Reagan, F.R. Vascularisation phenomena on fragments of embryonic bodies completely isolated from yolk sac entoderm. *Am. J. Anat. 9*:329–341, 1915.
453. Reese, A.B. Telangiectasis of the retina and Coats' disease. *Am. J. Ophthalmol. 42*:1–8, 1956.
454. Reese, A.B., and Jones, I.S. Hematomas under the retinal pigment epithelium. *Am. J. Ophthalmol. 53*:897–910, 1962.
455. Reid, V.C., Brabbs, C.E., and Mitchinson, M.J. Cellular damage in mouse peritoneal macrophages exposed to cholesteryl linoleate. *Atherosclerosis 92*:251–260, 1992.
456. Rengarajan, K., Muthukkaruppan, V.R., and Namperumalsamy, P. Biochemical analysis of serum proteins from Eales's patients. *Curr. Eye Res. 8*:1259–1269, 1989.
457. Rhodin, J.A.G. The ultrastructure of mammalian arterioles and precapillary spinchters. *J. Ultrastruct. Res. 18*:181–223, 1967.
458. Rice, T.A., Michels, R.G., Maguire, M.G., and Rice, E.F. The effect of lensectomy on the incidence of iris neovascularization and neovascular glaucoma after vitrectomy for diabetic retinopathy. *Am. J. Ophthalmol. 95*: 1–11, 1983.
459. Rimmer, T., Fleming, J., and Kohner, E.M. Hypoxic viscosity and diabetic retinopathy. *Br. J. Ophthalmol. 74*:400–404, 1990.
460. Ring, C.P., Pearson, T.C., Sanders, M.D., and Wetherly-Mein, G. Viscosity and retinal vein thrombosis. *Br. J. Ophthalmol. 60*:397–410, 1976.
461. Robaye, B., Mosselmans, R., Fiers, W., Dumont, J.E., and Galand, P. Tumor necrosis factor induces apoptosis (programmed cell death) in normal endothelial cells in vitro. *Am. J. Pathol. 138*:447–453, 1991.
462. Roberts, J.M., and Forrester, J.V. Factors affecting the migration and growth of endothelial cells from microvessels of bovine retina. *Exp. Eye Res. 50*:165–172, 1990.
463. Rockwood, E.J., Fantes, F., Davis, E.B., and Anderson, D.R. The response of retinal vasculature to angiotensin. *Invest. Ophthalmol. Vis. Sci. 28*:676–682, 1987.
464. Romayananda, N., Goldberg, M.R., and Green, W.R. Histopathology of sickle cell retinopathy. *Trans. Am. Acad. Ophthalmol. Otolaryngol. 77*:652–676, 1973.
465. Ross, R. The pathogenesis of atherosclerosis: An update. *N. Engl. J. Med. 314*:488–500, 1986.
466. Ross, R., and Glomset, J.A. The pathogenesis of atherosclerosis. *N. Engl. J. Med. 295*:369–377, 420–425, 1976.
467. Roy, M.S., Podgor, M.J., and Rick, M.E. Plasma fibrinopeptide A, β-thromboglobulin, and platelet factor 4 in diabetic retinopathy. *Invest. Ophthalmol. Vis. Sci. 29*:856–860, 1988.
468. Russell, R.W.R. Observations on intracerebral aneurysms. *Brain 86*:422–425, 1963.
469. Russell, R.W.R. The source of retinal emboli. *Lancet 2*:789–792, 1968.
470. Ryan, S.J. Role of the vitreous in the haemoglobinopathies. *Trans. Ophthalmol. Soc. UK 95*:403–406, 1975.
471. Sabour, M.S., MacDonald, M.K., and Robson, J.S. An electron microscopic study of the human kidney in young diabetic patients with normal renal function. *Diabetes 11*:291–295, 1962.
472. Sachsenweger, R. Luftembolie und Auge. *Klin. Monatsbl. Augenheilkd. 130*:813–823, 1957.

473. Sanders, M.D., and Hoyt, W.F. Hypoxic ocular sequelae of carotid-cavernous fistulae. *Br. J. Ophthalmol. 53*: 82–97, 1969.

474. Schönbach, J., Schönbach, C.H., and Cuenod, M. Distribution of the transported proteins in the slow phase of axoplasmic flow. An electron microscopical autoradiographic study. *J. Comp. Neurol. 152*:1–16, 1973.

475. Schor, A.M., and Schor, L.S. Tumour angiogenesis. *J. Pathol. 141*:385–413, 1983.

476. Schreiber, A.B., Winkler, M.E., and Derynck, R. Transforming factor alpha: A more potent angiogenic factor than epidermal growth factor. *Science 232*:1250–1253, 1986.

477. Schultz, G.S., and Grant, M.B. Neovascular growth factors. *Eye 5*:170–180, 1991.

478. Schweigerer, L., Neufel, G., Friedman, J., Abraham, J.A., Fiddes, J.C., and Gospodarowicz, D. Capillary endothelial cells express basic fibroblast growth factor, a mitogen that promotes their own growth. *Nature 325*: 257–259, 1987.

479. Schweigerer, L., Ferrara, N., Haaparanta, T., Neufeld, G., and Gospodarowicz, D. Basic fibroblast growth factor: Expression in cultured cells derived from corneal endothelium and lens epithelium. *Exp. Eye Res. 46*:71–80, 1988.

479a. Sebag, J., Buckingham, B., Charles, M.A., and Reiser, K. Biochemical abnormalities in vitreous of humans with proliferative diabetic retinopathy. *Arch. Ophthalmol. 110*:1472–1476, 1992.

480. Seitz, R. *The Retinal Vessels* (translated by F. Blodi). C.V. Mosby, St. Louis, MO, 1964.

481. Sekino, T. Scanning and transmission electron microscopic studies on the retinal vessels of spontaneously hypertensive rats (SHR). *Acta Soc. Ophthalmol. Jpn. 79*:887–903, 1975.

482. Shabo, A.L., and Maxwell, D.S. Insulin-induced immunogenic retinopathy resembling the retinitis proliferans of diabetes. *Trans. Am. Acad. Ophthalmol. Otolaryngol. 81*:OP497–OP508, 1976.

483. Shakib, M., and de Oliveira, L.N.F. Studies on developing retinal vessels. X. Formation of the basement membrane and differentiation of intramural pericytes. *Br. J. Ophthalmol. 54*:124–133, 1966.

484. Sharma, N.K., Gardiner, T.A., and Archer, D.B. A morphologic and autoradiographic study of cell death and regeneration in the retinal microvasculature of normal and diabetic rats. *Am. J. Ophthalmol. 100*:51–60, 1985.

485. Sholley, M.M., and Cotran, R.S. Endothelial proliferation in inflammation. II. Autoradiographic studies in x-irradiated leukopenic rats after thermal injury of the skin. *Am. J. Pathol. 91*:229–242, 1978.

486. Sholley, M.M., Gimbrone, M.A., and Cotran, R.S. The effects of leukocyte depletion on corneal neovascularization. *Lab. Invest. 38*:32–40, 1978.

487. Shorb, R.S., Irvine, A.R., Kimura, S.J., and Morris, B.W. Optic disc neovascularization associated with chronic uveitis. *Am. J. Ophthalmol. 82*:175–178, 1976.

488. Singh, A., Boulton, M., Lane, C., Forrester, J., Gaal, J., and McLeod, D. Inhibition of microvascular endothelial cell proliferation by vitreous following retinal scatter photocoagulation. *Br. J. Ophthalmol. 74*:328–332, 1990.

489. Siperstein, M.D., Raskin, P., and Burns, H. Electron microscopic qualification of diabetic microangiopathy. *Diabetes 22*:514–524, 1973.

490. Siperstein, M.D., Unger, R.H., and Madison, L.L. Studies of muscle capillary basement membranes in normal subjects, diabetic and prediabetic patients. *J. Clin. Invest. 47*:1973–1999, 1968.

491. Sivalingam, A., Kenney, J., Brown, G.C., Benson, W.E., and Donoso, L. Basic fibroblast growth factors in the vitreous of patients with proliferative diabetic retinopathy. *Arch. Ophthalmol. 108*:869–872, 1990.

492. Skinner, S.L., McCubbin, J.W., and Page, I.H. Renal baroceptor control of renin secretion. *Science 141*:814–816, 1963.

493. Skovborg, F., Nielson, A.V., Lauritzen, E., and Hartkopp, O. Diameters of the retinal vessels in diabetic and normal subjects. *Diabetes 18*:292–298, 1969.

494. Small, R.G. Coats's disease and muscular dystrophy. *Trans. Am. Acad. Ophthalmol. Otolaryngol. 72*:255–231, 1968.

495. Small, K.W., Stefansson, E., and Hatchell, D.L. Retinal blood flow in normal and diabetic dogs. *Invest. Ophthalmol. Vis. Sci. 28*:672–675, 1987.

496. Smelser, G.K. Histology and experimental pathology of the cornea through electron microscopy. In *XXI Congress of Ophthalmology*, Mexico. Excerpta Medica, Amsterdam, pp. 621–644, 1970.

497. Smith, J.H.R. Thrombotic glaucoma: A clinico-pathological study. In *XVII Congress on Ophthalmology*, Canada, USA. University of Toronto Press, Toronto, pp. 1164–1175, 1954.

498. Smith, L.E.H., Sweet, E., Freedman, S., and D'Amore, P.A. Alterations in endothelial superoxide dismutase levels as a function of growth state in vitro. *Invest. Ophthalmol. Vis. Sci. 33*:36–41, 1992.

499. Sorgente, N., Kuettner, V.E., Soble, L.W., and Eisenstein, B. The resistance of certain tissues to invasion. II. Evidence for extractable factors in cartilage which inhibit invasion by vascularized mesenchyme. *Lab. Invest. 32*:217–222, 1975.

500. Spitznas, M., Joussen, F., Wessing, A., and Meyer-Schwickerath, G. Coats's disease: An epidemiological and fluorescein angiographic study. *Graefes Arch. Ophthalmol. 194*:73–85, 1975.

501. Sporn, M.B., and Roberts, A.B. Peptide growth factors are multifunctional. *Nature 332*:217–219, 1988.

502. Sprugel, K.H., McPherson, J.M., Clowes, A.W., and Ross, R. Effects of growth factors in vivo. I. Cell ingrowth into porous subcutaneous chambers. *Am. J. Pathol. 129*:601–613, 1987.

503. Stefansson, E., Landers, M.B., III, Wolbarsht, M.L., and Klintworth, G.K. Neovascularization of the iris: An experimental model in cats. *Invest. Ophthalmol. Vis. Sci. 25*:361–364, 1984.

504. Stefansson, E., Machemer, R., de Juan, E., Jr., McCuen, B.W., II, and Peterson, J. Retinal oxgenation and laser treatment in patients with diabetic retinopathy. *Am. J. Ophthalmol. 113*:36–38, 1992.

505. Stefansson, E., Novack, R.L., and Hatchell, D.L. Vitrectomy prevents retinal hypoxia in branch retinal vein occlusion. *Invest. Ophthalmol. Vis. Sci. 31*:284–289, 1990.

506. Steffes, M.W., Brown, D.M., and Mauer, S.M. Diabetic glomerulopathy following unilateral nephrectomy in the rat. *Diabetes 27*:35–41, 1978.

507. Stokoe, N.L. Fundus changes in hypertension: A longterm clinical study. In *William MacKenzie Centenary Symposium on the Ocular Circulation in Health and Disease*, Glasgow, 1968, J.S. Cant (Ed.), Kimpton, London, pp. 117–135, 1969.

508. Stramm, L.E., Li, W., Aguirre, G.D., and Rockey, J.H. Glycosaminoglycan synthesis and secretion by bovine retinal capillary pericytes in culture. *Exp. Eye Res. 44*:17–28, 1987.

509. Stuart, I., and Juhan-Vague, I. Erythrocyte rheology in diabetes mellitus. *Clin. Haemorheol. 7*:239–245, 1987.

510. Sugi, K. Studies on the pathological changes in the retinal vessels of human eyes using the trypsin digestion method. *Jpn. J. Ophthalmol. 10*:252–266, 1966.

511. Szabo, M.E., Droy-Lefaix, M.T., Doly, M., Carre, C., and Braquer, P. Ischemia and reperfusion-induced histologic changes in the rat retina. *Invest. Ophthalmol. Vis. Sci. 32*:1471–1478, 1991.

512. Takahashi, K., Brooks, R.A., Kanse, S.M., Ghatei, M.A., Kohner, E.M., and Bloom, S.R. Production of endothelin-1 by cultured bovine retinal endothelial cells and presence of endothelin receptors on associated pericytes. *Diabetes 38*:1200–1202, 1989.

513. Talbot, J.F., Bird, A.C., Maude, G.H., Acheson, R.W., Moriarty, B.J., and Serjeant, G.R. Sickle cell retinopathy in Jamaican children: Further observations from a cohort study. *Br. J. Ophthalmol. 72*:727–732, 1988.

514. Tamura, T. Electron microscopic study on the small blood vessels in rubeosis iridis diabetica. *Jpn. J. Ophthalmol. 13*:65–78, 1969.

515. Tanaka, T., and Shimizu, K. Retinal arteriovenous shunts in Takayasu disease. *Ophthalmology, 94*:1380–1388, 1987.

516. Taniguchi, Y., Saneshima, M., and Fukiyama, M. Electron microscopic study of newly formed blood vessels in diabetic retinopathy. *Acta Soc. Ophthalmol. Jpn. 77*:1383–1393, 1973.

517. Tarkkanen, A., Tala, P., Karjalainen, K., and Virkkula, L. Ocular manifestations of aortic arch syndrome. *Ann. Chir. Gynaecol. Fenn. 56*:141–143, 1967.

518. Tascopoulos, M., Beauchemin, M.L., Baker, R., and Babel, J. Studies of experimental retinal focal ischaemia in miniature pigs. In *Vision and Circulation, Proceedings of the 3rd William MacKenzie Memorial Symposium*, J.S. Cant (Ed.), Kimpton, London, pp. 93–103, 1976.

519. Taylor, C.M., Kissun, R.D., Schor, A.M., McLeod, D., Garner, A., and Weiss, J.B. Endothelial cell-stimulating angiogenesis factor in vitreous from extraretinal neovascularizations. *Invest. Ophthalmol. Vis. Sci. 30*:2174–2178, 1989.

520. Taylor, C.M., Weiss, J.B., Kissun, R.D., and Garner, A. Effect of oxygen tension on the quantities of procollagenase activating angiogenic factor present in the developing kitten retina. *Br. J. Ophthalmol. 70*:162–165, 1986.

521. Taylor, C.M., Weiss, J.B., McLaughlin, B., and Kissun, R.D. Increased procollagenase activating angiogenic factor in the vitreous humour of oxygen treated kittens. *Br. J. Ophthalmol. 72*:2–4, 1988.

522. Terry, T.L. Extreme prematurity and fibroblastic overgrowth of persistent vascular sheath behind each crystalline lens. I. Preliminary report. *Am. J. Ophthalmol. 25*:203–204, 1942.

523. Todd, J.A., Bell, J.I., and McDevitt, H.O. HLA-DQ B gene contributes to susceptibility and the resistance to insulin dependent diabetes mellitus. *Nature 329*:599–601, 1987.

524. Tripathi, R.C., and Ashton, N. Electron microscopical study of Coats's disease. *Br. J. Ophthalmol. 55*:289–301, 1971.

525. Trope, G.E., Lowe, G.D.O., McArdle, B.M., Douglas, J.T., Forbes, C.D., Prentice, C.M., and Foulds, W.S. Abnormal blood viscosity and haemostasis in long-standing retinal vein occlusion. *Br. J. Ophthalmol. 67*:137–142, 1983.

526. Tso, M.O.M. Pathological study of cystoid macular edema. *Trans. Opthalmol. Soc. UK 100*:408–413, 1980.

527. Tso, M.O.M., Cunha-Vaz, J.G., Shih, C.-Y., and Jones, C.W. Clinicopathologic study of blood-retinal barrier in experimental diabetes mellitus. *Arch. Ophthalmol. 98*:2032–2040, 1980.

528. Tso, M.O.M., and Hayreh, S.S. Optic disc edema in raised intracranial pressure. IV. Axoplasmic transport in experimental papilledema. *Arch. Ophthalmol. 95*:1458–1462, 1977.

529. Uyama, M. Histopathological studies on vascular changes, especially on involvement in the choroidal vessels, in hypertensive retinopathy. *Acta Soc. Ophthalmol. Jpn. 79*:357–370, 1975.

530. Vague, P., and Juhan, I. Red cell deformability, platelet aggregation, and insulin action. *Diabetes 32*(Suppl. 2):88–91, 1983.

531. de Venecia, G., Wallow, I., Houser, D., and Wahlstrom, M. The eye in accelerated hypertension. I. Elchnig's spots in nonhuman primates. *Arch. Ophthalmol. 98*:913–918, 1980.

532. Vinijchaikul, K. Primary arteritis of the aorta and its main branches (Takayasu's arteriopathy). *Am. J. Med. 43*:15–27, 1967.

533. Vinores, S.A., Gadegbeku, C., Campochiaro, P.A., and Green, W.R. Immunohistochemical localization of blood-retinal barrier breakdown in human diabetes. *Am. J. Pathol. 134*:231–235, 1989.

534. Vracko, R., and Benditt, E.P. Capillary basal lamina thickening: Its relationship to endothelial cell death and replacement. *J. Cell. Biol. 47*:281–285, 1970.

535. Wallow, I.H.L., and Engerman, R.L. Permeability and patency of retinal blood vessels in experimental diabetes. *Invest. Ophthalmol. Vis. Sci. 16*:447–461, 1977.

536. Walters, R.F., and Spalton, D.J. Central retinal vein occlusion in people aged 40 years or less: A review of 17 patients. *Br. J. Ophthalmol. 74*:30–35, 1990.

537. Ward, R.C., Weiner, M.J., and Albert, D.M. The eye. In *Pathology and Pathophysiology of AIDS and HIV-Related Diseases*, S.J. Harawi and C.J. O'Hara (Eds.), Chapman and Hall, London, pp. 363–377, 1989.

538. Watts, M.T., Greaves, M., Rennie, I.G., and Clearkin, L.G. Antiphospholipid antibodies in the aetiology of ischaemic optic neuropathy. *Eye 5*:75–79, 1991.

539. Webb, R.C., Lockette, W.E., Vanhoutte, P.M., and Bohr, D.H. Sodium potassium adenosine triphosphate and vasodilatation. In *Vasodilatation*, P.M. Vanhoutte and L. Leusen (Eds.), Raven Press, New York, pp. 319–330, 1981.

540. Weinberg, D., Dodwell, D.G., and Fern, S.A. Anatomy of arteriovenous crossings in branch retinal vein occlusion. *Am. J. Ophthalmol. 109*:298–302, 1990.

541. Weiss, J.B., Brown, R.A., Kumar, S., and Phillips, P. Tumour angiogenesis factor: A potent low molecular weight compound. *Br. J. Cancer 40*:493–496, 1979.

542. Weiss, J.B., Hill, C.R., and Schor, A. Low-molecular-mass tumour angiogenesis factor. *Biochem. Soc. Trans. 12*:260, 1984.

543. Wendland, J.P. Retinal arteriolosclerosis in age, essential hypertension and diabetes mellitus. *Ann. Ophthalmol. 2*:68–80, 1970.

544. Wetzig, P.C., and Thatcher, D.B. The treatment of acute and chronic central venous occlusion by light coagulation. *Mod. Probl. Ophthalmol. 12*:247–253, 1974.

545. Williams, J.M., de Juan, E., and Machemer, R. Ultrastructural characteristics of new vessels in proliferative diabetic retinopathy. *Am. J. Ophthalmol. 105*:491–499, 1988.

546. Williamson, J.R., Chang, K., Tilton, R.G., Prater, C., Jeffrey, J.R., Weigle, C., Sherman, W.R., Eades, D.M., and Kilo, C. Increased vascular permeability in spontaneously diabetic BB/W rats and in rats with mild versus severe streptozotocin-induced diabetes: Prevention by aldose reductase inhibitors and castration. *Diabetes 36*:813–821, 1987.

547. Winegrad, A.I. Does a common mechanism induce the diverse complications of diabetes? 1986 Banting Lecture. *Diabetes 36*:396–406, 1987.

548. Wise, G.N. Retinal neovascularization. *Trans. Am. Ophthalmol. Soc. 54*:729–826, 1956.

549. Wise, G.N., Dollery, C.T., and Henkind, P. *The Retinal Circulation*, Harper & Row, New York, 1971.

550. Witztum, J.L., and Steinberg, D. Role of oxidized low density lipoprotein in atherogenesis. *J. Clin. Invest. 88*:1785–1792, 1991.

551. Wolter, J.R. Pathology of a cotton-wool spot. *Am. J. Ophthalmol. 48*:473–485, 1959.

552. Wolter, J.R., and Ryan, R.W. Atheromatous embolism of the central retinal artery: Secondary hemorrhagic glaucoma. *Arch. Ophthalmol. 87*:301–304, 1972.

553. Wong, H.C., Boulton, M., McLeod, D., Bayly, M., Clark, P., and Marshall, J. Retinal pigment epithelial cells in culture produce retinal vascular mitogens. *Arch. Ophthalmol. 106*:1439–1443, 1988.

554. Yanagisawa, M., Kurihara, H., Kimura, S., Tomube, Y., Koboyashi, M., Mitsui, Y., Yazaki, Y., Goto, K., and Masaki, T. A novel potent vasoconstrictor peptide produced by vascular endothelial cells. *J. Clin. Invest. 84*:1373–1378, 1989.

555. Yanoff, M. Ocular pathology of diabetes mellitus. *Am. J. Ophthalmol. 67*:21–38, 1969.

556. Yoshimoto, H. Ultrastructural features of cytofilament with endothelial cell of the retinal arterioles: Observation on hypertensive rat and human eyes. *Acta Soc. Ophthalmol. Jpn. 79*:867–877, 1975.

557. Yoshimoto, H., and Irinoda, K. Study on permeability of the retinal vessels in spontaneously hypertensive rats. *Jpn. Heart J. 17*:365–366, 1976.

558. Yu, V.Y.H., Hookham, D.M., and Nave, J.R.M. Retrolental fibroplasia: Controlled study of 4 years experience in a neonatal intensive care unit. *Arch. Dis. Child. 57*:247–252, 1982.

559. Ziche, M., Jones, J., and Gullino, P.M. Role of prostaglandin E_1 and copper in angiogenesis. *J. Natl. Cancer Inst. 69*:475–482, 1982.

560. Zimmerman, L.E. Embolism of the central retinal artery. *Arch. Ophthalmol. 73*:822–826, 1965.

561. Zoja, C., Benigni, A., Renzi, D., Piccaneli, D., Perico, N., and Remussi, G. Endothelin and eicosanoid synthesis in cultured mesangial cells. *Kidney Int. 37*:927–933, 1990.

53

Ocular Involvement in Disorders of the Nervous System

Gordon K. Klintworth

Duke University Medical Center, Durham, North Carolina

I. INTRODUCTION

Vision, one of the most complex of all sensations interpreted by the nervous system, is dependent upon the integrity of pathways within the brain that comprise neurons and neuroglia, as well as blood vessels and other connective tissue elements.

Aside from the usual pathological processes, such as inflammation, developmental anomalies, vascular disorders, and neoplasia, that affect most tissues, the brain is prone to unique disorders that can be arbitrarily divided into diseases primarily of white matter (disorders of myelin) or gray matter (neuronal disorders). The optic nerve is involved in many conditions that affect the white matter of the central nervous system (CNS), and optic nerve demyelination, optic neuritis, and optic atrophy are features of numerous neurological disorders.

II. DISORDERS OF MYELIN

The myelin sheaths of axons within the optic nerve and other parts of the CNS are synthesized by oligodendrocytes and consist of this cell's external plasma membrane in the form of bimolecular lipid leaflets twisted in a spiral manner around the nerve axons. Oligodendrocytes express several specific antigens and enzymes (galactocerebroside, carbonic anhydrase, and 2',3'-cyclic nucleotide 3'-phospho-hydrolase) [230]. Myelin is composed of aggregates of lipid (such as monogalactosylceramide, ethanolamine phospholipid, long-chain fatty acids, galactosyl ceramides and cholesterol), proteins [myelin-associated glycoprotein and myelin basic proteins A_1, P_1, and P_2, small basic protein, prebasic proteins, intermediate protein, and proteolipid protein; (see Pelizaeus-Merzbacher Disease in Sec. II.E), Wolfgram protein, and peripheral myelin glycoprotein P_0, and glycosaminoglycans (GAG)] [114]. The metabolic turnover of most of these components is slow, but some proteins are metabolized more rapidly [269].

Disorders of myelin include conditions in which the myelin sheath becomes destroyed after it has formed (demyelinating diseases), as well as entities in which the myelin sheath does not form normally (leukodystrophies or dysmyelinating diseases). Myelin may be destroyed nonspecifically under natural circumstances as a result of viral infections, nutritional deficiencies, anoxic and toxic insults, and immunopathological reactions, as well as experimentally [8,96]. The phrase "demyelinating diseases" designates disorders with early myelin destruction often disproportionate to the injury noted in the axons, neurons, and neuroglia. Demyelinating diseases include multiple sclerosis (MS), neuromyelitis optica, subacute sclerosing panencephalitis (SSPE), progressive multifocal leukoencephalopathy (PML), and acute disseminated encephalomyelitis. Depending on the cause, axonal damage may be conspicuous. Since myelin represents the cell membrane of oligodendrocytes, degenerative changes in this cell type are usually prominent in demyelinating states. Microglia and blood-derived macrophages phagocytose degenerated myelin following its destruction. Loss of phospholipids, an increase in esterified cholesterol, proteolysis, and GAG breakdown accompany demyelination. Astrocytes later proliferate and impart a sclerotic texture to the lesions, but fibroblasts, because of their paucity within the CNS other than in the optic nerve, do not contribute significantly to this reaction.

A. Multiple Sclerosis

Multiple sclerosis, also called disseminated sclerosis, is the most common disease of the human CNS in which myelin is destroyed without damage to axons. The disease, with its characteristic pathological features, first became recognized as an entity slightly more than a century ago [59].

Clinical Features

This chronic relapsing and remitting disorder is typified by symptoms and signs pointing to multiple episodes of randomly located lesions in the CNS, which are disseminated in both time of onset and place. The term "multiple sclerosis" stresses the multitude of lesions, whereas "disseminated sclerosis" underscores their temporal and spatial dissemination. Poor health, fatigue, acute infections, trauma, allergic conditions, exposure to cold, and emotional upsets appear to provoke the acute episodes of MS, but how these factors operate is unknown. Classic MS (Charcot type) usually commences in early adulthood during the second to fourth decades of life. It rarely becomes symptomatic in childhood or in persons older than 50 years of age. The onset is generally rather abrupt, often within a period of hours or days, and may be manifest as visual or other neurological disturbances. As a rule this is followed within a few days or weeks by significant improvement with little functional deficit, probably when edema regresses and axonal conduction is restored. Nystagmus, intention tremor, and scanning speech (Charcot's triad) may be present in the early stages. At first the clinical diagnosis is difficult, a requirement being that various lesions appear at different times in different parts of the CNS. Occasionally the manifestations, such as a reduction in visual acuity, are accentuated by vigorous exercise (Uhthoff's syndrome) or by a hot bath.

The clinical picture of MS is highly variable not only with regard to the symptoms and signs, which depend on the location of the lesions, but also in the severity, time course, and progression of the disease. Most (90%) patients have spontaneous remissions and relapses in the early stages, with intervals of months or years preceding a relapse. MS is usually progressive with increasingly more severe episodes, each of which results in additional, permanent disability due to the accumulated incomplete recovery from each lesion. A slow, continuous deterioration in neurological status often becomes apparent late in the course of the disease, with fatality in 5–25 years or more. In some individuals, MS is inexorably progressive, giving rise to almost total disability and death within 1–2 years of onset. In most patients MS is more indolent; relapses develop at intervals of several years. Some patients experience only one or two attacks or appear to recover completely after each of a series of attacks. Rarely the disorder is asymptomatic, the only evidence of MS being old plaques found postmortem in brains of individuals with no history of neurological disease. In about one-third of patients, MS progresses so slowly, without serious disability, as not to reduce life span. In a series of 241 patients studied by McAlpine [178] and followed for a minimum of 10 years, approximately one-third were dead, one-third were disabled, and one-third had no physical restrictions or disabilities. As a rule, the longer the interval between the initial attack and the first relapse, the better is the prognosis. Younger patients occasionally experience a severe fulminating illness from the onset, whereas an onset in middle life is usually associated with a more indolent course.

Presumably some demyelinated axons transmit impulses, as vision may still be present in an eye that has a completely demyelinated optic nerve. Remission of symptoms can be accounted for on the assumption that demyelinated axons can transmit impulses [182]. Nerve conduction becomes temporarily impaired during acute demyelination, and permanent disability follows the axonal degeneration or interference with nerve conduction by poorly understood mechanisms.

Ocular Manifestations

The myelinated axons within the CNS that are concerned with visual function are commonly affected in MS. Ophthalmological findings include nystagmus from involvement of the vestibular system in the brain stem (about 70% of cases). Palsies of nerves that innervate the extraocular muscles, disturbances of conjugate gaze, and visual field defects occur as a result of plaques in the various parts of the visual pathways. Diplopia in most instances is of the type known as internuclear ophthalmoplegia (from involvement of the medial longitudinal fasciculus), and bilateral internuclear ophthalmoplegia is virtually pathognomonic of MS.

The optic nerve of one or both eyes is frequently affected in MS, particularly in Asia, where it is frequently bilateral and severe from the onset. The initial clinical manifestations of MS may be a sudden visual field differing in intensity and extent or a loss of central visual acuity. The maculopapillary fibers of the optic nerve appear to be preferentially involved. As with lesions elsewhere in the CNS, the first incident in the optic nerve frequently causes a transient loss of function (impaired central visual acuity and visual field defects) that persists for only several days or weeks before complete or almost total recovery; less often the lesion is serious and culminates in permanent visual loss. Succeeding incidents may affect the same or the contralateral eye. Acute optic neuritis or retrobulbar neuritis is the first clinical evidence of the disease in 15% of patients, and about 70% of patients hospitalized for MS eventually develop optic neuritis. Traub and Rucker [288] followed 87 patients 10–15 years after an initial bout of retrobulbar neuritis and found that 28 (32.2%) developed evidence of MS. Of these patients 26 were 20–40 years old at the time of the first bout, indicating that an individual in this age group who has an initial episode of retrobulbar neuritis has a 40–50% chance of developing other manifestations of MS within 10–15 years. When retrobulbar neuritis begins in persons older than 40 years, the chance of acquiring MS is remote [288]. Since this study by Traub and Rucker, however, others have found subsequent demyelinating episodes in 11.5–85% of cases of retrobulbar neuritis [48,151,179]. The risk of a patient with uncomplicated optic neuritis developing MS has been found in a prospective study to be about 35% [67].

During the course of the illness, visual impairment is a feature of 34% of cases in the United States, but in Japan, where MS is rare and differs clinically in several respects from that in the so-called Western countries, 70% of patients develop visual symptoms. In Japan, visual impairment is common at the onset, the optic nerves and the spinal cord are predominantly involved, and the disease tends to be severe and rapidly progressive [264].

In 1944 Rucker [247] drew attention to the frequent perivenous sheathing of retinal veins in patients with MS, an observation that has been confirmed repeatedly [205] (Fig. 1). Although this fundoscopic abnormality is also extremely common in patients with peripheral uveitis due to various causes, the small white clouds and sheaths about retinal veins in MS form without the usual visible accompaniments of uveitis, such as hemorrhage, cells in the vitreous, or pigment disturbance. Such lesions may remain unchanged for many months or years, and in some instances round dotlike opacities with the diameter of a medium-sized vein are visible in the vitreous close of the retina ("Rucker's bodies") [250]. In different

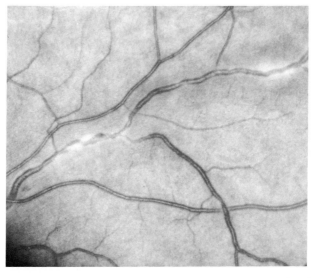

Figure 1 Periphlebitic venous sheathing in a patient with multiple sclerosis (Reproduced with permission from G.N. Wise, C.T. Dollery, and P. Henkind, *The Retinal Circulation*, Harper and Row, New York, p. 208, 1971.)

studies the incidence of perivenous sheathing in MS has ranged from 1.5 to 42% of cases [17,90,117, 249,250]. The sheathing of retinal veins in MS corresponds to a perivenous infiltrate of lymphocytes, sometimes with plasma cells (Fig. 2) [13,95,99,263,286]. Some histopathological studies of the retina in MS have disclosed an apparent rarefaction of the ganglion cells [107,286], and perhaps revelant to this is the finding of tissue-bound IgG on ganglion cells in several cases of MS, but not in controls [176].

Several authors have drawn attention to the higher incidence of peripheral uveitis (pars planitis or chronic cyclitis) in patients with MS compared with the general population [12,17,35,36,108]. In a study of 53 patients with MS, Breger and Leopold [35] detected a peripheral uveitis in 14 subjects (27%), and in 9 of these patients the disease was active but the other 5 were quiescent. The uveal disease may antecede the neurological involvement by several years [108], yet the significance of the association between uveitis and MS remains uncertain, and histological examinations of eyes in such cases have not been performed. The retinal arterioles appear unaffected [135,150,213,248,249,289,310], but the venous branches peripheral to the area of sheathing may become engorged and bleed. Yet, unlike the peripheral periphlebitis of Eales disease (see Chap. 52), hemorrhages are not associated with most of these mild perivascular lesions. Sheathing and progressive obliteration of peripheral retinal veins, peripheral and posterior uveitis, retinitis proliferans, retinal neovascularization, and retinal microaneurysms have been documented in patients with MS [12,36,192]. Although some of these nonspecific ocular manifestations (perivenous sheathing and peripheral uveitis) seem to be more frequent in subjects with MS than in the general population, others (microaneurysms and retinal neovascularization) have not been shown to be significantly more common in MS than one would expect by the chance association of coincidental diseases.

Histopathology

In patients dying with MS, specific lesions are restricted to the CNS, those occurring elsewhere being either unrelated to the disease or secondary to it, such as the muscle contractures that eventually develop in many cases. Peripheral nerves are not involved, and all other organs are normal in an uncomplicated case.

In classic MS numerous circumscribed areas of focal demyelination of different ages are found throughout the CNS, where any part can be affected. The lesions are usually readily apparent to the naked eye in cross sections of the brain, appearing in the gray and white matter as patches with sharply demarcated edges (Figs. 3 and 4). In the living patient MS plaques are readily visualized with magnetic resonance

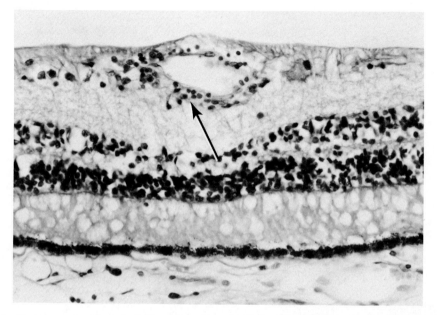

Figure 2 Perivenous lymphocytic infiltrate in retina of patient with multiple sclerosis. (Hematoxylin and eosin, ×300)

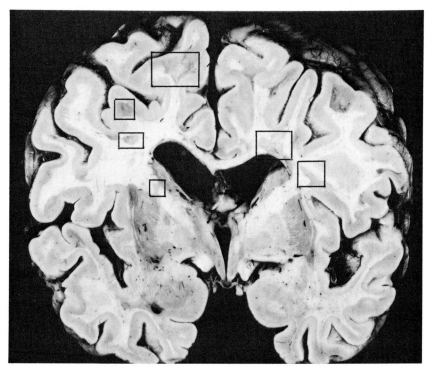

Figure 3 Coronal section through cerebral hemispheres showing plaques (boxes) in brain with multiple sclerosis.

imaging (Fig. 5). The larger areas of demyelination are usually irregular in shape with a lobulated outline. The abnormal regions vary in color; the recent ones tend to be pink, and the older ones, which are firm in the unfixed brain, are gray. Although the word *sclerosis* is descriptive of the firm texture of the numerous gliotic (sclerotic) foci, early lesions are softer in consistency than normal brain. Traditionally, the areas of myelin destruction have been termed plaques; however, they are not flat disks but are spherical or ovoid or have other three-dimensional configurations. The axons or nerve cell bodies are more or less uninvolved, but destruction of axons may be noted in some of the oldest lesions. Although, as mentioned, the distribution of the "plaques" varies considerably from case to case, they are commonly contiguous with the ventricles, especially the outer angles of the lateral ventricles, the floor of the sylvian aqueduct, and the fourth ventricle [99]. Demyelinated foci in the cerebral white matter tend to stop short of the cerebral cortex, leaving intact about 1 mm of subcortical myelin. In the spinal cord, a thin rim of subpial white matter is also frequently spared. In contrast to other neurological diseases, the myelin sheaths and axons distal to the lesions either do not undergo a series of morphological degenerative changes (Wallerian degeneration) or such alterations are minimal.

In tissue sections MS plaques are optimally visualized in preparations stained for myelin (such as luxol fast blue or Weil's stain). Dyes, like the Holzer stain, that accentuate glial tissue may be useful in disclosing older gliotic lesions. The dimensions, distribution, and age of MS plaques vary extensively from case to case. The preserved axons and cell bodies within the plaques of MS differentiate the lesions of MS from infarcts.

The histological appearance of the plaques in MS varies considerably with their age, but the loss of myelin, in the presence of unremarkable axons and nerve cell bodies, is a conspicuous feature. In long-standing plaques, as well as in some recent lesions, a loss of oligodendrocytes is conspicuous. However, in some recent plaques that are believed to be slightly older than the acute lesions, numerous cells of oligogendrocyte origin are abundant, presumably secondary to a reactive hyperplasia [230]. These cells, which appear on the basis of immunocytochemical markers to be phenotypically undifferentiated oligo-

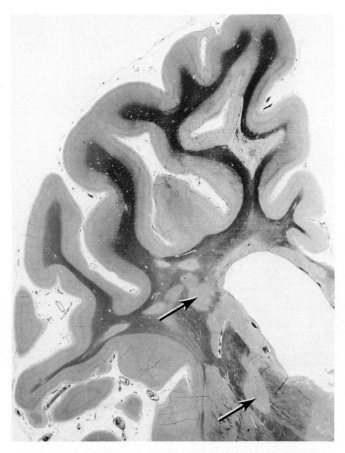

Figure 4 Higher magnification of multiple sclerosis plaques showing sharp line of demarcation between normal myelin and demyelinated area (arrows). (Hematoxylin and eosin–luxol fast blue, ×1.8)

dendrocytes, are thought to account for the extensive remyelination present in some plaques [229]. Some plaques do not entirely lack myelin ("shadow plaques"), and in long-standing plaques there is commonly a partial destruction of axons. Perivascular lymphocytic cuffing, usually modest in degree, commonly occurs within or around the lesions; this feature is often more prominent in older lesions. The plaques of MS are commonly surrounded by dense rings of macrophages or reactive microglia that express the human leukocyte antigen DR (HLA-DR) [33]. These cells expressing the major histocompatibility complex class II glycoprotein are believed to play a pivotal role in presenting antigen to T helper/inducer (CD4+) lymphocytes.

Aside from differences in the appearance of the plaques, which relate to the age of the lesion, there seems to be a continuous variation, from the typical, relatively indolent lesions to those that characterize the severe atypical clinical cases in which the tempo of the pathological processes is accelerated. In the latter patients, the lesions tend to be more destructive, and then axis cylinders and even nerve cell bodies are destroyed. The cellular reaction is also more intense, with an extensive perivascular infiltration of lymphocytes and lesser numbers of plasma cells.

The plaques of MS have been extensively investigated by transmission electron microscopy (TEM), and although many studies were concerned principally with descriptive morphology, others have disclosed structures resembling paramyxovirus nucleocapsids within some plaques [227,235,276,301], but as discussed elsewhere in this section, the significance of this observation remains unknown.

Thorough histopathological studies of the optic nerve during the initial stages of their involvement in MS have not been reported but are presumably identical to those elsewhere in the brain.

Variants of MS

Besides the classical form of MS (Charcot type) described earlier, other rare variants of the disease in which more destructive lesions are generally found are recognized in a younger age group.

Acute MS (Marburg type).　　Some patients die after an acute or subacute illness with lesions that are virtually all of recent onset and are necrotizing with a more florid inflammatory cellular reaction [218] than is customary in the Charcot type of the disease. As in the Schilder and Devic types of MS, this variant of the disease is common in younger patients and is often preceded by, or accompanied by, a febrile illness [218].

Neuromyelitis Optica (Devic Type).　　The designation "Devic's disease" refers to the combination of severe visual impairment and paraplegia occurring within several days or weeks of each other as a result of demyelinating lesions in the optic nerves and spinal cord [63,152,271]. Most cases are believed to be examples of acute MS, but the same clinical picture can arise from other causes, such as acute disseminated encephalomyelitis. Patients with Devic's disease seldom die as an immediate result of the illness and consequently knowledge about the histopathology of the more benign cases of Devic's disease is sparse [8]. Postmortem examinations in most lethal cases, however, have disclosed dispersed demyelinating lesions with attributes of acute MS, but frequently with considerable axonal degeneration. These lesions, which are of variable age, have a predisposition for the optic nerves and upper thoracic spinal cord but may also involve other parts of the CNS, such as the brain stem and cerebral hemispheres. Necrosis is often a conspicuous feature of the lesions in the spinal cord and optic chiasm, and this is believed to occur as a consequence of ischemia secondary to the acute edema that develops in these sites that possess a limited ability to undergo rapid expansion because of their constraining coverings. The necrosis frequently leads to cavitation, especially in the spinal cord, but also sometimes in the optic chiasm. The extent of the gliosis reflects the intensity of the necrosis and duration of survival.

Although the lesions in milder cases may be indistinguishable from the plaques of acute MS, severe cases have massive areas of central demyelination with destruction of axons and, occasionally, central liquefaction of the optic chiasm. Since tissue necrosis is not regarded as a feature of MS, some regard its presence as testimony of a different disease. However, the necrotic lesions in the optic nerve and spinal cord may be secondary to ischemia caused by severe edema, which sometimes accompanies acute lesions in MS. Indeed, the spinal cord is frequently explored surgically in Devic's syndrome and found to be swollen. Aside from the necrotic and demyelinated portions of the optic nerves and spinal cord, the remainder of the CNS is often normal apart from Wallerian degeneration.

Neuromyelitis optica clinically resembles subacute myeloopticoneuropathy, which occurs in Japan and Latin America and has been attributed to Entero-Vioform (Clioquinol, iodochlorhydroxyquin) [152]. From the late 1950s until 1972 it is estimated that more than 10,000 individuals with subacute myelo-opticoneuropathy were diagnosed in Japan. A herpesvirus related to avian infectious laryngotracheitis virus has been isolated from the feces and cerebrospinal fluid (CSF) of patients with subacute myelo-opticoneuropathy [128] and may be a causal agent of this entity. Neuromyelitis optica has been associated with pulmonary tuberculosis [18], raising the possibility that the disorder is a sequel to an immunological reaction.

Schilder Type.　　The Schilder type of MS has a more rapid course than the usual variety and a clinical picture dominated by progressive loss of intellectual function due to extensive, usually confluent, areas of demyelination in the cerebral hemispheres with or without small lesions elsewhere. In childhood the lesions are usually not associated with disseminated plaques, and the disease is typically characterized by an acute or subacute progressive course, with mental disturbances, blindness, and deafness. In acute cases, with large destructive lesions, there is often considerable cerebral edema, and a brain tumor or encephalitis is often suspected clinically. Should the affected tissue be biopsied, the pathologist may face a difficult diagnostic problem since the astrocytic proliferation may be prominent and some astrocytes may be enormous and multinucleated, suggestive of a glioma. When disseminated plaques are present, the age of onset and the clinical course are usually indistinguishable from the Charcot type of MS (discussed earlier), with extensive involvement of the cerebral white matter.

In the past the connotation "Schilder's disease" (diffuse sclerosis) was applied to a heterogeneous group of idiopathic neurological disorders primarily of childhood. Some of the Schilder's cases probably included adrenoleukodystrophy, subacute sclerosing panencephalitis, and other disorders with diffuse cerebral damage.

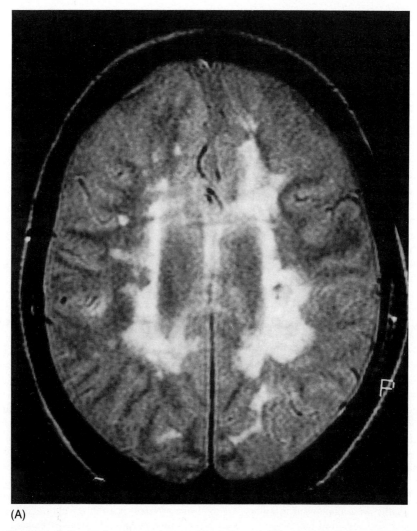

(A)

Figure 5 The plaques of multiple sclerosis appear white and are readily seen in the living patient with the aid of magnetic resonance imaging: (A) Horizontal section through head; (B) coronal section. (Courtesy of Orest B. Boyko, M.D., Ph.D.)

Concentric Sclerosis (Balo Type). This rare pathological curiosity is characterized by laminated concentric zones of demyelination separated by narrow bands of more or less intact myelin. Most cases have occurred in the second and third decades of life and have been typified clinically by a rapid, fulminant neurological illness [77].

Etiology and Pathogenesis

Ever since MS became recognized as an entity, this disease has challenged the minds of innumerable investigators and has remained without known cause and with a poorly understood pathogenesis. Morphological, epidemiological, and immunological observations on this disease have revealed information relevant to our understanding of the disease, but a similar disease is not known to occur naturally in animals, and a comparable condition has not been produced experimentally.

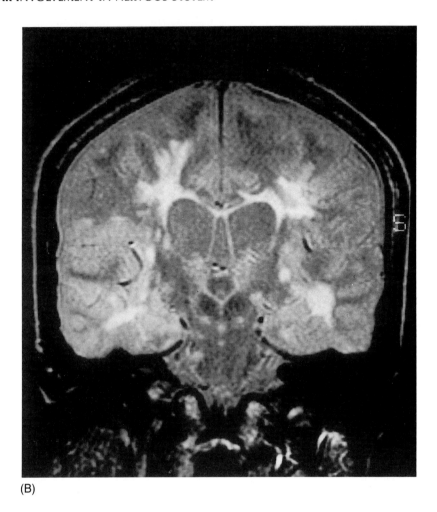

(B)

Morphological Clues to Pathogenesis

The basic morphological lesion is the destruction of myelin within the CNS. This is followed by its phagocytosis by macrophages and subsequently by an astrocytic proliferation with a production of glial fibrils. The perivenous location of small multiple sclerotic plaques [92,97,98], as well as their frequent periventricular distribution, suggests a myelinolytic substance that diffuses from the blood or CSF, or both. The existence of such a substance is underscored by the observation that sera from patients with MS can destroy myelin in tissue culture [30,234]. A humoral immune process seems to be operative, since complement and immunoglobulins have been demonstrated in the active plaques [177,285], but whether cellular hypersensitivity plays a role in MS remains unclear [25]. Trypan blue, which does not normally cross the blood-brain barrier, leaks from the cerebral veins in MS plaques following perfusion of the brain with this dye [41]. The role of this breakdown in blood-brain barrier in the genesis of the lesion is also unclear.

Contribution of Epidemiology

Epidemiological investigations indicate that the incidence of MS varies considerably in different geographical areas and that critical environmental factors influence the appearance of the disease. A high-frequency band occurs in the northern temperate zones of Europe and North America and in southern Australia and

New Zealand; MS is uncommon in Asia [155] and rare in the tropics [1]. The disease is nonexistent or extremely rare among African blacks. Currently half a million people are estimated to have MS in the United States. Women are affected slightly more often than men, and whites more often than blacks. Interestingly, MS preferentially affects people of relatively high socioeconomic backgrounds [156].

Studies of migrant populations suggest that the risk of an individual developing MS depends on where the individual lived during the first 15–20 years of life. Residence in high-risk regions during that age period retain a high incidence of MS [84,154]. Thus, an emigrant from a high- to a low-risk area retains the high risk, or vice versa.

Genetic Aspects

There is evidence to suggest that the genetic constitution of the host plays an important role in the predisposition to MS [194]. Numerous familial cases of the disease are documented [180], and there is an increased prevalence of MS in families suffering from the condition [255]. This can be accounted for either by exposure to the same pathogen and/or a genetic susceptibility to the disease. The latter possibility is supported by studies with histocompatibility antigens [22,133,195,279,306], which are thought to be markers of immune response genes. Certain inherited histocompatibility antigens are more frequent in patients with MS than in the population at large. However, the specific histocompatibility genes that are found with an increased incidence in MS vary from country to country. In the United States and Europe, individuals with the antigens HLA-A3 and HLA-B7 have at least twice the risk of developing MS than individuals with other histocompatibility antigens [26,134,157,195]. Not only is there a high incidence of the histocompatibility antigen LD7 on the surface of lymphocytes in MS, but this histocompatibility antigen tends to be related to the severity of the disease [133]. Twin siblings, however, have not shown concordance rates compatible with a strong inherited predisposition [28,153].

Immunological Aspects

The immune competence of patients with MS has been studied extensively [10,132,172,200,201, 212,235,273], and the following observations have been made: reduced T cell responsiveness to mitogens, apparently linked to histocompatibility type [132,200,212]; a reduction in circulating T cells with preservation of normal numbers of B cells [172,201,238]; and borderline suppressor T cell activity in young but not elderly patients with inactive MS but not in patients with recent exacerbations [10]. The question remains unanswered whether the underrepresented circulating population of T lymphocytes reflects the genetic endowment of patients with MS or an acquired loss of T cells. In patients with MS the lymphocyte reactivity to measles, parainfluenza, and vaccinia viruses does not differ significantly from that in controls until the subject becomes disabled. This suggests that the deficient cellular response to certain viruses is a consequence of the disease rather than a causal factor [273]. Mutant T cell clones isolated from the peripheral blood of MS patients have been found to proliferate in response to myelin basic protein (MBP), an antigen envisaged to partake in the induction of MS, even without prior exposure to this antigen [6]. T cells that are reactive to MBP use the gene for the variable region of the T cell receptor β (TCR Vβ) chain for the recognition of MBP. MBP has two immunodominant regions: residues MBP(84–102) and MBP(143–168). Individuals with MS have a higher frequency of T cells reactive with MBP(84–102) in their blood than controls, and reactivity with MBP(84–102) is associated with the DR2 allele of the HLA region; MBP(143–168) is associated with the DRw11 allele [309]. An analysis of the TCR Vβ genes used by T cell lines from both MS and healthy individuals has disclosed that Vβ17 is selectively involved in the recognition of the immunodominant MBP(84–102). This finding is of potential value in the immunotherapy of MS because 60% of patients with MS are DR2+ [309].

Humoral immunity in MS has also attracted attention. The CSF immunoglobin G (IgG) is usually elevated [137,171,284], and the IgM is often elevated as well [305]. The elevated immunoglobulin is oligoclonal in type, and there is evidence for its synthesis within the CNS [171]. That the antibody is formed locally in the CNS rather than from other sources points to the presence of antigenic stimulation within the neural tissue. Antibodies to myelin are present in serum of most patients and correlate with the active phases of the disease [177]. Immunofluorescent studies have disclosed antimyelin antibodies, particularly of the IgG type, together with complement at the edges of demyelinated plaques [177].

Evidence for an Infectious Agent

An infectious agent has long been suspected, but nobody has isolated a pathogen that would produce MS when injected into experimental animals [228]. Sabin and Messare [251] reported specific immunofluorescence for herpes simplex in the tissues of several patients with MS. Others have noted a slightly elevated titer of antimeasles antibodies in the serum and CSF in a high proportion of these patients [2,40,228] compared with control subjects. However, in contrast to SSPE (see Sec. II.B), not all patients with MS have elevated levels of measles antibody. It is noteworthy that an antigenic similarity between measles virus and the most active constituent of brain extracts capable of inducing experimental allergic encephalomyelitis (encephalitogenic factor) of central myelin has been claimed [181]. It seems unlikely that the measles virus is the causative agent of MS because its geographical distribution is difficult to reconcile with the worldwide presence of measles. Moreover, antibodies to various other common viruses, including herpes simplex, influenza, mumps, parainfluenza, poliomyelitis, and vaccinia, are also often elevated in the serum and CSF in patients with MS [38,142,244]. Structures resembling paramyxovirus nucleocapsids have been identified by TEM in mononuclear cells of plaques [227,235,276,301]. However, viruses cannot be identified unequivocally by morphology alone, and similar virus-like structures have been seen in a variety of unrelated conditions [159,227]. More significantly a parainfluenza type I virus, 6/94, has been isolated by cocultivation of brain tissue from two patients with MS [280].

Current Concept of MS

Some viral infections are characterized by long incubation periods, often many years preceding the overt disease [148]. Since the recognition of such "slow viruses," a pathogen of this nature has been suspected in MS [97]. A persistent (latent) virus disease analogous to SSPE (discussed later) or an immunological disorder resulting from an infection akin to postinfective encephalomyelitis [265] are both possible.

The aforementioned epidemiological, morphological, genetic, and immunological observations, taken together, are consistent with the hypothesis that MS is due to a common viral infection that usually causes trivial symptoms and a lifelong immunity. Alternatively and rarely, perhaps because of a genetic susceptibility, an individual who seems unable to develop immunity to certain antigens and infectious agents develops MS.

B. Subacute Sclerosing Panencephalitis

Clinical Features

Historically subacute sclerosing panencephalitis has been known as Dawson's disease, Van Bogaert's disease, subacute sclerosing leukoencephalitis, nodular panencephalitis, subacute inclusion body encephalitis, encephalitis of Pette-Döring, and diffuse encephalitis with sclerosing inflammation of the hemisphere white matter [314]. Several clinical features enable the diagnosis of this rare viral infection to be suspected during life. Typically it presents with an insidious onset of a slowly progressive intellectual and personality deterioration, followed over a variable period by involuntary myoclonic movements of the face, fingers, or limbs or rapid torsional spasms of the trunk [102,202]. The movements tend to occur at regular intervals, often once every 5–10 s and can last for many days at a time. A large proportion of cases develop a pathognomonic electroencephalogram with periodic successions of high-voltage complexes that are synchronous with the involuntary movements. The CSF usually contains a few lymphocytes and a normal glucose level; although the total protein is often normal or moderately raised, the gammaglobulin is characteristically elevated, and this is reflected in the paretic (first zone) colloidal gold curve of the older literature. An elevated titer of measles antibodies is also consistently present in the CSF.

Most reported cases have occurred between the ages of 4 and 20 years; the mean onset is at about 7 years. Although SSPE mainly affects children and young adults, on rare occasions adults in the third to sixth decade of life have been the victim [80,139,187,239,277]. A noteworthy sex predisposition exists, males being affected about three times more frequently than females [131].

Unfortunately, the disease characteristically progresses insidiously to a lethal termination in 6 weeks to 2 years [102], usually after a period of profound dementia and decerebrate rigidity. Some cases have had a relatively prolonged course of 5–9 years, however, occasionally with remissions and exacerbations [64,91,161,175]. A rare patient has survived the illness [240].

Ophthalmological Manifestations

During the course of the illness, approximately 50% of individuals with SSPE develop ophthalmic abnormalities [163], which include cortical blindness, nystagmus, and visual impairment due to involvement of the brain and/or a focal chorioretinitis [65,101,111,162,163,196,240,295]. Visual failure usually begins after the onset of the neurological disorder, but occasionally it antedates other signs of the disease by several weeks [111,162,163,196,274]. In one case the ocular lesions antedated the neurological illness by 22 months [111]. For this reason, SSPE must be considered in the clinical differential diagnosis of all maculopathies in children and young adults. A measles retinopathy can follow immunosuppressive therapy for malignant neoplasms [118]. The most striking ocular lesion is a focal retinitis [196,206,240,283] with patchy areas of inflammatory edema (Fig. 6). There is a striking predilection for the macular or perimacular area [9,101,111,138,162,196,253]. Usually a single discrete lesion is apparent, but multiple foci may be seen, and in about 30% of cases, the juvenile macular degeneration is bilateral [138]. The retinopathy is not usually associated with hemorrhage or apparent vitreous reactions and is not consistently related to the retinal vasculature, although hemorrhagic detachment of the macula can develop [158]. A profound loss of vision may follow retinal vasculitis [253].

The precise incidence of retinal lesions in SSPE is unknown. The retina has not been examined carefully in many patients with this disease, either during life or postmortem. The retinopathy is probably much more common than the literature suggests, however. Since the presence of antimeasles antibodies in the CSF is virtually diagnostic of SSPE, this serological test should be carried out in all individuals with obscure retinal lesions.

Histopathology

The major pathological changes in SSPE generally involve the white matter of the CNS to a greater degree than the gray matter. Intranuclear and intracytoplasmic inclusion bodies, in the absence of cytomegaly, are the morphological hallmark of SSPE. The inclusions occur in neurons and oligodendrocytes and are most numerous in cases that pursue a rapid clinical course [96]. The most noticeable inclusion is a large, discrete eosinophilic, intranuclear mass surrounded by a prominent halo (Cowdry's type A inclusion; Fig. 7) [82], which appears in neurons often accompanied by the diagnostically important intracytoplasmic inclusions. Inclusions within the nuclei of oligodendrocytes [161,183] appear as an amphophilic homogenized zone. In

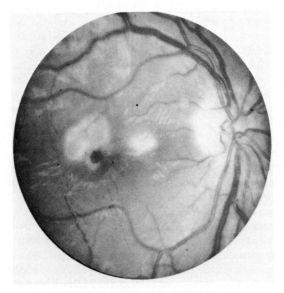

Figure 6 Fundoscopic appearance of macular lesion in subacute sclerosing panencephalitis. [Reproduced with permission from M.B. Landers, III, and G.K. Klintworth, Subacute sclerosing panencephalitis (SSPE). *Arch. Ophthalmol.* 86:156–163, 1971. Copyright 1971, American Medical Association.]

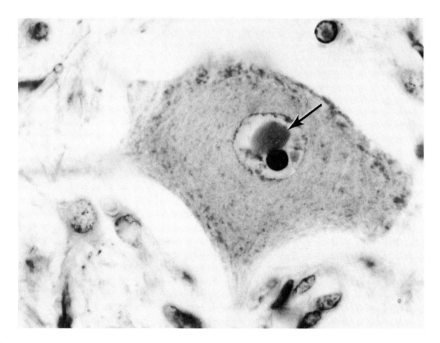

Figure 7   Large intranuclear eosinophilic inclusion body (arrow) adjacent to nucleolus in neuron in subacute sclerosing panencephalitis. (Hematoxylin and eosin–luxol fast blue, ×1000)

some cases inclusion bodies are not prominent, but inflammation and gliosis of the white matter is the conspicuous finding. Inclusion bodies have been found in cerebral biopsies before death, but not in subsequent postmortem examinations [119,256]. In severely affected areas of the cerebral cortex, a focal increase in microglia and astrocytes, as well as loss of neurons with neuronophagia, is common, and Alzheimer's neurofibrillary degeneration of neurons has been reported [75,183]. A perivascular infiltration by lymphocytes and plasma cells and a slight leptomeningeal infiltration of mononuclear cells are frequently present. Myelin loss commonly occurs in focal inflammatory lesions in the white matter as part of a necrotizing process that ultimately results in the loss of all cellular elements. When necrosis is less pronounced, gliosis tends to be more conspicuous than myelin destruction [292]. Areas of more complete demyelination probably reflect the involvement of oligodendrocytes [7,100]. Atypical morphological features may occur [210,259], and the spinal cord, dorsal root ganglia, spinal nerve roots, and peripheral nerves are sometimes involved [34,210,232,293].

When viewed by TEM, tubular structures (18–20 nm in diameter) have been observed in cortical neurons and neuroglia of affected tissue [303]. These measles virus nucleocapsids occur in the nucleus and the cytoplasm and are occasionally seen in the neuronal processes (Fig. 8) [130].

Retina.   Tissue examinations of the retina in SSPE have disclosed a retinopathy with atrophic areas that is not associated with a prominent cellular infiltrate; choroidal involvement is generally minimal. Intranuclear inclusion bodies have been observed within retinal cells [101,162,196] and in the optic nerve [101]. The region of the macula may develop a mottled pigmentation, and multinucleated giant cells have even been observed in the atrophic retina [101]. By TEM, filamentous microtubular structures identical to those in the CNS have been identified in affected retinal cells (neurons and glial cells) [101,118,162]. Measles antigen has been demonstrated in infected retinal cells by immunofluorescent techniques [101,118].

Etiology and Pathogenesis

The character of the encephalitis combined with the presence of inclusion bodies prompted Dawson to suggest a viral pathogen in 1933 [81]. The presence of large, discrete, eosinophilic intranuclear inclusions

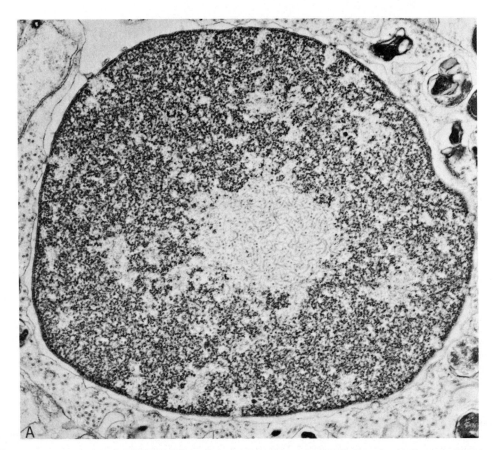

Figure 8 A. Filamentous microtubules within nucleus in subacute sclerosing panencephalitis. (×12,000). B. Tubular intranuclear viral particles in subacute sclerosing panencephalitis at higher magnification than Figure 8A. (×100,000)

surrounded by a prominent halo (Cowdry type A inclusions) led early investigators to suspect herpes simplex despite the morphological evidence against this possibility (cytoplasmic inclusions bodies are not an attribute of herpes simplex-infected cells) [291]. Three decades later structures resembling myxovirus- or paramyxoviruslike particles were identified in affected brain tissue by many investigators using TEM (Fig. 8) [31,83,103,216,217,261,262,278,315]. These particles were morphologically identical to those seen in tissue cultures inoculated with measles virus. Their identity as the nucleocapsids of the measles virus was reinforced by Connolly and colleagues [72,73], who found markedly elevated titers of measles antibodies in the serum and CSF of affected individuals. Also, rising measles antibody titers were observed during the course of the disease [3,83,167,281]. Additional evidence was provided by immunofluorescent microscopy, which localized measles antigen in the neurons and neuroglia of brain biopsy specimens from patients with SSPE [72,103,165]. Other investigators confirmed and expanded these observations [119,210,278,314], and measles virus antigen was also found by fluorescent antibody techniques in cells in the CSF from patients with SSPE [124].

That an infectious agent was involved was greatly strengthened by the occurrence in ferrets and, later, weanling hamsters [52,235] of a chronic encephalitis [141] following intracerebral inoculation of brain tissue from patients with SSPE.

Despite this evidence, which implicated a measles or measleslike virus, the infectious agent could not be isolated until cell cultures were established from fresh brain explants of patients with SSPE. During the process of subculturing serial passages of the cell lines, many cells developed syncytia and giant cells in a

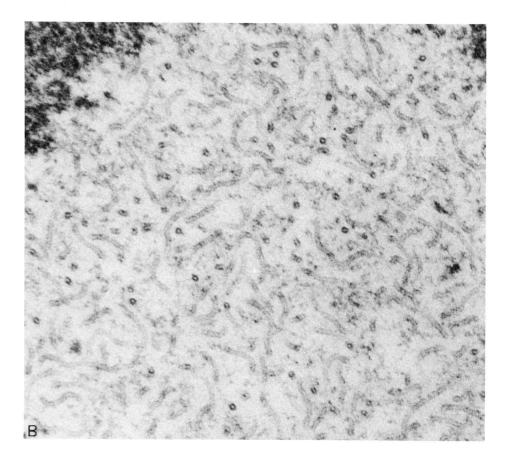

manner simulating cells infected by measles virus. Measles antigen was demonstrated in such cells [23] and structures resembling paramyxovirus nucleocapsids were recognized [140], but it was only after such cells were cocultivated or fused with human or simian cells that infectious virus was isolated [139]. In 1969 the measles virus was recovered from several cases of SSPE by independent investigators [62,124, 140,214]. Measles virus matrix protein gene expression has been demonstrated in the brain in SSPE using cDNA hybridization and immunohistochemistry [43]. Measles virus genomic sequences have also been detected in brains with SSPE by the polymerase chain reaction [109]. Aside from being located in the brain, the measles virus has been isolated from peripheral blood mononuclear cells in SSPE [258]. By in situ hybridization using a probe to the measles virus RNA and immunocytochemical studies to localize measles antigen, evidence of the virus has been found in several tissues (spleen, thymus, kidney, lung, pancreas, adrenal glands, and pituitary gland) in individuals with SSPE [42]. An additional piece of evidence implicating the measles virus in SSPE is the recognition that SSPE has become rare following widespread measles vaccination [58,203].

Once this firm link between the measles virus and SSPE became established, the manner in which the organism initiates the disease required explanation. Clearly, the disease differs in several respects from the usual infection produced by the measles virus. Also, the levels of serum antibody to measles virus in SSPE are not only much higher than those found after primary measles infection but increase during the illness. Furthermore, in contrast to the classic measles infection, a high titer of antibody to virus occurs in the CSF.

For several years the precise relationship of the pathogen of SSPE to the measles virus remained ill defined [93,207], as did the possible role of the paramyxovirus group in other demyelinating diseases [227]. Several explanations [227] were considered. These included defective measles virus maturation, a nonmeasles virus, and an impaired immune responsiveness. The first view was supported by the observation that the nucleocapsids of the naturally occurring measles virus acquire a fuzzy coat of protein during replication before budding from the cell, but neither alignment nor budding of virus from plasma membrane has been observed in SSPE [160]. Conceptually, an absent or reduced surface expression of viral antigens would render infected cells more resistant to immunological injury, and maturation of such a defective measles virus could account for the several differences between measles and SSPE. This seemed unlikely, however, since the markedly elevated antibody levels were difficult to reconcile with a concept of reduced viral antigenicity. Although the viruses of SSPE and measles resemble each other, numerous differences have also been detected [139]. The measles virus genome encodes for six structural proteins: three complexed with RNA and the rest associated with the viral envelope (M, H, and F proteins). A mutation in the structure of the matrix genes has been detected in viral isolates from individuals with SSPE [16,56,57,307]. Measles isolates from brains with SSPE also appear to manifest a reduced expression of viral envelope proteins, and this may account for the lack of viral budding that allows the virus to persist and elude the immune surveillance [55,56]. Some measles virus subpopulations are resistant to interferon, and such interferon-resistant viruses may account for viral persistence in SSPE [54]. It is noteworthy that the carboxyl-terminal domains of the hemagglutinin glycoprotein of both measles and SSPE viruses have considerable amino acid sequence similarities with the active domain of long neurotoxins that specifically bind to the nicotinic acetylcholine receptor [313]. This may account at least in part for the adverse neural effects of the measles virus.

Both lymphoid cells and sera from patients with SSPE are capable of destroying cells infected with measles virus in vitro [150,204]; however, the capacity of peripheral blood lymphocytes to generate measles virus-specific cytotoxic T lymphocytes is reduced in SSPE [85]. IgM and IgG antibodies to measles are both normally high in the serum and CSF in SSPE [74]. The measles virus-specific antibodies in patients with SSPE are found mainly in the IgG_1 subclass irrespective of the clinical stage and duration of the disease [188]. Measles-specific IgD activity is also significantly increased in SSPE [211]. The abnormally high titers of antimeasles antibodies, especially in the CSF, suggest that repeated antigenic stimulation occurs over prolonged periods of time and that immunoglobulins are synthesized in the CNS [86]. The possibility that SSPE is a persistent infection by the measles virus in a patient with an abnormal immunological response has been raised [70]. Interestingly, measles usually occurs at an extremely early age in patients who later develop SSPE (ordinarily during the first 2 years of life), and in about 15% of cases a history of clinical measles is absent [131]. This high incidence of inapparent or early-onset measles may reflect an initial exposure to measles before complete loss of passive immunity derived from the mother [39]. Perhaps the existence of some passive immunity inhibits the development of full active immunity, the latter being sufficient to protect the individual from further episodes of clinical measles but insufficient to prevent the persistence of the measles virus in certain cells.

The pathogenesis of the retinal lesions, in particular their temporal relationship to the encephalitis and the pathway of virus spread to the eye, remains unknown. Conceptually, the virus may reach the eye by a hematogenous dissemination at the time of primary measles exposure. The presence of viral nucleocapsids in the retina indicates a direct invasion of this tissue by the same pathogenic agent that affects the CNS. The production of retinal lesions in suckling and weanling hamsters by the intracerebral inoculation by several strains of measles virus has provided support for the hematogenous spread of the pathogen to the retina [143,209]. Experiments in ferrets have demonstrated that cell-associated SSPE virus reaches the brain after intracardiac inoculation [282].

C. Progressive Multifocal Leukoencephalopathy

Progressive multifocal leukoencephalopathy (PML) is a subacute progressive demyelinating disease of the human CNS characterized by multiple foci of demyelination and abnormal oligodendrocytes that contain large numbers of intranuclear papovavirus virions [4,136]. The demyelination appears to follow the devastation of oligodendrocytes by this unique opportunistic papovavirus. PML can potentially involve the optic nerve, but severe visual loss has followed involvement of the occipital lobe [11]. Tumors of the CNS develop in some brains with PML. The condition develops in patients in whom cell-mediated immunity is suppressed. Most affected individuals are adults with lymphoproliferative disorders, but the disease also occurs in persons with AIDS and following immunosuppression for organ transplantation [298]. It has also rarely been reported with sarcoidosis [127].

PML, which can strike at any age, is produced by an ubiquitous papovavirus that was isolated from diseased tissue in 1971 [208]. The pathogen contains early and late genes, as well as genes for T antigen and other viral structural proteins. It infects oligodendrocytes and was designated JC virus, the initials of the first patient from whom the virus was first isolated. This unfortunate connotation has led to confusion with the totally unrelated causal agent of Creutzfeldt-Jakob disease.

The direct inoculation of JC virus into mice fails to evoke a perceptible disorder, but transgenic mice encompassing the early region of the JC virus genome under the control of JC virus promoter/enhancer elements develop a marked tremor on motion and seizures by 3 weeks of age, before expiring at the age of 4–6 weeks [268]. These mice lack normal myelin sheaths in the CNS, but not in the peripheral nervous system. This dysmyelination, which is not attended by prominent myelin phagocytosis, is combined with the expression of JC virus T antigen in the brain, especially in oligodendrocytes [254].

Other viruses (BKV and simian virus 40, SV40) have been implicated in some cases of PML, but a recent analysis of affected tissue in two cases previously attributed to SV40 casts serious doubt on the notion that SV40 can cause PML. This investigation, using specific biotinylated DNA probes and monoclonal antibodies, indicated the presence of JC virus, not SV40 as originally believed [272]. The genes for the early regions of BKV, which was isolated from the urine of a patient with PML undergoing chemotherapy, evoked tumors following their introduction into transgenic mice (primary renal, hepatic, and lung carcinomas) [268].

D. Acute Disseminated Encephalomyelitis

Acute disseminated encephalomyelitis is characterized by an acute onset of multiple lesions throughout the CNS, including the optic nerve and other visual pathways. In contrast to MS, the specific lesions are smaller (a few millimeters in diameter) but more extensive, with a striking perivenous distribution in both gray and white matter (hence the older connotation "acute perivenous encephalomyelitis"). There is an intense lymphocytic and plasma cell inflammatory response. The ultimate outcome is variable, and although sometimes fatal, a good recuperation may ensue.

Acute disseminated encephalomyelitis may follow a specific infection (particularly measles and vaccinia, but also smallpox, varicella, and influenza; postinfectious encephalomyelitis) or vaccination (such as antirabies vaccination with emulsions of nervous tissue; postvaccinial encephalomyelitis). Sometimes the entity develops in the apparent absence of an antecedent vaccination or infection (spontaneous acute disseminated encephalomyelitis). An unusually fulminant variety of encephalomyelitis that affects mainly young men is typified by vessel wall necrosis, hemorrhage, and a prominent polymorphonuclear leukocytic infiltrate (acute hemorrhagic leukoencephalitis).

The human disease closely resembles experimental allergic encephalomyelitis (induced by injecting foreign peripheral nerve tissue with Freund's adjuvant) [297]. Guinea pigs sensitized with isogenic spinal cord emulsified with Freund's adjuvant develop acute allergic optic neuritis with clinical features of "retrobulbar optic neuritis" and "neuroretinitis" and with histopathological features of experimental acute disseminated encephalomyelitis [236]. Such animals develop multiple foci of a mononuclear cell infiltrate in the retrobulbar portion of the optic nerve and chiasm with associated demyelination.

E. The Leukodystrophies

A heterogeneous group of clinically distinct neurological disorders is characterized by defective myelination of the CNS, a loss of sensory, motor, and intellectual functions, and eventual death. These so-called leukodystrophies include metachromatic leukodystrophy (see Chap. 29), globoid (Krabbe's) leukodystrophy (see Chap. 29), the adrenoleukodystrophies, Canavan's disease, Pelizaeus-Merzbacher disease, Cockayne's syndrome, and Alexander's disease.

The Adrenoleukodystrophies

The adrenoleukodystrophies are rare disorders characterized by mental and neurological deterioration due to a diffuse paucity of myelin within the CNS and atrophic, hypofunctional adrenal glands (low plasma cortisol levels that do not increase after corticotropin administration). Very long chain fatty acids (VLCFA) accumulate within various tissues, the serum, and other body fluids because of their impaired oxidation [189,193]. In the past many cases of adrenoleukodystrophy were designated Schilder's disease (bronze Schilder's disease).

Clinical Features.   Bronzing of the skin and other clinical features of Addison's disease may or may be evident [225], and adrenocortical disease may precede evidence of neurological disease. Three clinical variants of the disorder are recognized: neonatal adrenoleukodystrophy, childhood adrenoleukodystrophy, and adrenomyeloneuropathy. The pathological changes are comparable in these variants [115], and the biochemical alterations have similarities but are due to defects in different genes involved in VLCFA metabolism. In childhood adrenoleukodystrophy VLCFA acyl-CoA synthetase is defective [15]. A progressive visual loss secondary to bilateral optic atrophy or cortical blindness develops early in the neonatal and childhood variants of the adrenoleukodystrophies and proceeds within months to no light perception.

Neonatal adrenoleukodystrophy.   The neonatal variant of adrenoleukodystrophy affects both sexes and has an autosomal recessive mode of inheritance. Dolichocephaly, a prominent high forehead, epicanthal folds, broad nasal bridge, and low-set ears typify the external appearance of the head in neonatal adrenoleukodystrophy. Mental retardation is severe, and seizures are common. Nystagmus and a pigmentary retinopathy are early manifestations of neonatal adrenoleukodystrophy [68,185].

Childhood adrenoleukodystrophy.   The childhood X-linked form of adrenoleukodystrophy is the most common variant. Gaze nystagmus and sluggish pupillary responses may precede the cortical blindness and optic atrophy [68,308]. Severe loss of nerve fibers occurs in the optic nerve head.

Adrenomyeloneuropathy.   In X-linked adrenomyeloneuropathy, young adult males develop progressive spastic paraparesis and a distal symmetrical polyneuropathy in addition to adrenal gland dysfunction [115]. Individuals with this variant of adrenoleukodystrophy may have affected male kindred with the childhood variant, and both childhood adrenoleukodystrophy and adrenomyeloneuropathy are linked to the long arm of the X chromosome (Xq28), indicating that nonneonatal adrenoleukodystrophy and adrenomyeloneuropathy are caused by a mutation in the same gene [304]. Moreover, the phenotypic difference between nonneonatal adrenoleukodystrophy and adrenomyeloneuropathy is not necessarily a consequence of allelic heterogeneity due to different mutations in the same gene. Some individuals with either adrenomyeloneuropathy or childhood adrenoleukodystrophy have abnormal color vision. This is readily accounted for by the fact that red-green visual pigment genes are located in the same part of the X chromosome [15]. In at least one family adrenomyeloneuropathy has been associated with cataracts [147].

Histopathology.   The white matter of the CNS contains confluent areas of active demyelination surrounding inflammatory zones that contain necrotic axons. This inflammatory reaction, which includes macrophages and reactive astrocytes, as well as T lymphocytes of the T4 and CD45R subsets, distinguishes the adrenoleukodystrophies from other leukodystrophies. B lymphocytes and plasma cells are uncommon [224]. Birefringent intracytoplasmic crystals accumulate within the brain, adrenal gland, and other affected tissues. By TEM the crystals appear lamellar.

The eyes from several individuals with the childhood [68,308] and neonatal forms of adrenoleukodystrophy [68] have been studied by light microscopy late in the course of the disease. Extensive atrophy of the nerve fiber and ganglion cell layers of the retina and a diffuse optic atrophy with narrowing of the nerve fiber bundles, glial hypercellularity, and partial demyelination have been features. Marked axonal loss and numerous intracytoplasmic inclusions, including dense lipofuscin granules and macrophages, have been prominent in affected regions. The optic atrophy appears to be secondary to CNS and optic nerve lesions (descending optic atrophy), as well to retinal neuronal destruction (ascending optic atrophy) [68]. Swelling of the optic nerve head may occur, probably as a sequel to elevated intracranial pressure [68]. The photoreceptors degenerate, and cells in the outer retina may contain pigment in a configuration reminiscent of retinitis pigmentosa [68]. TEM has disclosed a marked decrease in myelin and axonal degeneration. Advanced demyelination of the optic chiasm with loss of oligondendroglia and an increased number of astrocytes occurs, and numerous macrophages accumulate. The typical intracytoplasmic inclusions that gather in the brain and other tissues have not been identified in the optic nerve or optic chiasm, implying that the process in these parts of the visual pathway are involved secondarily rather than by the primary metabolic defect.

Metabolic Defect and Pathogenesis of Lesions.   At one time adrenoleukodystrophy was thought to be a genetically determined lipid storage disease caused by an error in membrane sterol metabolism [49,223]. It is now recognized that these disorders are due to an inherited deficiency of a peroxisomal enzyme known as very long chain fatty acid acyl-CoA synthetase (lignoceroyl-CoA ligase). The deficiency results in defective β oxidation of very long chain fatty acids, which accumulate largely in the brain and adrenal gland. These predominantly saturated VLCFA are toxic and are thought to account for the destruction of numerous cell types, including adrenocortical cells, the testicular interstitial cells of Leydig, and Schwann cells. An inherent myelin instability, together with the cytotoxic effect of VLCFA on myelin and oligodendroglia, are believed to cause myelin breakdown. The characteristic inflammatory response around areas of demyelination seems to be a natural immune response to demyelination, rather than the cause of it [224].

Pelizaeus-Merzbacher Disease

Pelizaeus-Merzbacher disease is a rare, clinically heterogeneous, X-linked recessive, slowly progressive sudanophilic leukodystrophy, with severe psychomotor retardation, dwarfism in childhood, and premature aging. Neurological manifestations are secondary to a failure of oligodendrocyte differentiation and defective myelination due to point mutations in, or deletions of, the gene encoding the main integral protein of myelin (myelin proteolipid protein, PLP) [88,126,219,237], which is found on the short arm of the X chromosome (Xp22) [290]. The mutations include a valine to phenylalanine point mutation in the putative extracellular loop of myelin proteolipid [219] and a C to T transition in exon 4 of the PLP gene (changes amino acid 155 from threonine to isoleucine within the hydrophobic intramembrane domain) [226]. Ocular manifestations include demyelination and atrophy of optic nerve axons, loss of retinal ganglion cells and gliosis, "salt and pepper" retinopathy, anterior segment pigment dispersion, cataracts, corneal ulceration and opacification, and pupillary aberrances [233]. Death usually occurs in the second or third decade.

The disorder is not limited to humans. Mutations have been identified in the PLP gene in several animal models with X chromosome-linked disorders of myelin (jimpy mouse, msd mouse, myelin-deficient (md) rat, and shaking pup) [302].

Cockayne's Syndrome

Cockayne's syndrome is characterized by an onset in childhood of developmental and mental retardation leading to dwarfism, a distinctive facies with prognathism and birdlike features, loss of subcutaneous fat, partial deafness, and a photosensitive dermatitis. In common with Pelizaeus-Merzbacher disease premature aging is a feature, and affected individuals usually also die within the second or third decade.

The ocular manifestations of this autosomal recessive condition include cataracts, demyelination and atrophy of optic nerve axons with gliosis, a degenerative retinopathy (with a loss of retinal ganglion cells and atrophy of the photoreceptors and outer nuclear layer), irregular hypo- and hyperpigmentation of the retinal pigment epithelium (giving the retinal fundus a "salt and pepper" appearance on ophthalmoscopy), anterior segment pigment dispersion, ulceration and other abnormalities of the cornea, nystagmus, and an unresponsiveness of the pupils to mydriatics [37,66,120,169,215,246,312]. Exposure and inadequate moistening of the corneal surface secondary to anhidrosis, failure of Bell's phenomenon (movement of eyes up and backward on forced closure), and loss of blinking are thought to be major reasons for the corneal lesions.

In Cockayne's syndrome the possibility of an abnormality in DNA repair has been raised [231,257] on the basis of abnormal responses to ultraviolet light by cultured fibroblasts and lymphocytes from affected individuals. The predicted 1493 amino acid protein product of the gene for Cockayne's syndrome, which is located on the long arm of chromosome 10 (10q11-21), contains seven consecutive motifs conserved among RNA and DNA helicases and a putative nucleotide binding domain. cDNA that encodes a putative DNA helicase corrects the DNA repair defect from cells cultured from persons with Cockayne's syndrome [289a].

Canavan's Disease

Canavan's disease is a rare autosomal recessive lethal disorder of infancy characterized by a spongy state of the white matter in the brain and defective myelination. This condition, which is associated with elevated levels of N-acetylaspartic acid in the plasma and urine due to a deficiency of aspartoacylase (EC 3.5.1.15), is considered in Chapter 31.

Alexander's Disease

A rare leukodystrophy, which was first described in an infant by Alexander in 1949 [5], is characterized by megalocephaly, progressive mental retardation, a heavy brain, and an abundance of homogeneous, eosinophilic carrot-shaped bodies. These so-called Rosenthal fibers are located in the white matter, including that of the optic nerve and visual pathways, especially around blood vessels. These structures consist of αB-crystallin, and brain tissue from patients with Alexander's disease contain abundant phosphorylated αB-crystallin B [184]. They are sparse in the retrobulbar optic nerve and do not accumulate in Müller cells of the retina [287]. Identical structures are sometimes conspicuous in optic nerve astrocytomas (see Chap. 50). Alexander's disease has been subdivided into infantile, juvenile, and adult varieties depending upon the age of onset, the clinical manifestations, and the extent of the abnormalities [69,296].

III. DISEASES OF NEURONS

The nervous system contains a wide variety of distinct neuronal populations that are not only situated in different parts of the brain but have specific characteristics [121]. Many diseases of the CNS involve specific neuronal populations.

A. Degenerative Diseases Due to Prions

Studies of certain neurodegenerative diseases in both humans and animals have led to the highly significant discovery of minute infectious pathogens that resist physical and chemical inactivation (including ionizing and ultraviolet irradiation, formaldehyde, and chlorine dioxide) [106,270]. These unconventional infectious agents, called prions, produce disease after a long latent period and have as yet not been shown to induce a detectable immune reaction. Prions cause at least three distinct human diseases (Creutzfeldt-Jakob disease, the Gerstmann-Straussler-Streinker syndrome, and kuru), as well as several animal diseases (scrapie, bovine spongiform encephalopathy, and transmissible mink encephalopathy) [270]. Some of these diseases are transmissible as autosomal dominant inherited disorders. In contrast to orthodox pathogens, prions lack nucleic acids and are impervious to maneuvers that alter or demolish nucleic acids. They require protein for infectivity, and a component of the infectious particle has been found to be a host-derived protein designated PrP^{SC} [270]. The manner by which prions replicate remains as mysterious as the infectious agents themselves.

Creutzfeldt-Jakob Disease

Creutzfeldt-Jakob disease is characterized by progressive dementia and other neurological manifestations and, usually, death within 6 months. The abnormal prion protein has been demonstrated in brains with Creutzfeldt-Jakob disease by immunohistochemical methods in association with synaptic structures, but the tissue processing needs special fixatives to yield positive results [145]. The disorder is important to ophthalmologists not only because of the visual field defects that frequently accompany the cerebral disease but also because of the risk of transmitting the disease by corneal grafting [94]. Despite the apparent transmission of Creutzfeldt-Jakob disease by keratoplasty in a human patient [94], the pathogen has not been identified in or isolated from human corneal tissue [47]. It has been detected in corneas of guinea pigs with experimental Creutzfeldt-Jakob disease, however [47]. Histological studies of eyes from persons dying from Creutzfeldt-Jakob disease have disclosed either no abnormalities [245] or a questionable mild optic atrophy [168].

Although most authorities accept the notion that prions cause Creutzfeldt-Jakob disease, unusual intracellular spiral inclusions have been identified in the brains of several patients with this disease [20,241]. These structures bear a morphological resemblance to the spiroplasma, a wall-free prokaryote known to produce disease in plants and cataracts in suckling mice (suckling mouse cataract; see Chap. 17). When inoculated intracerebrally into suckling mice, at least one strain of *Spiroplasma melliferum* readily replicates in the brain for up to 9 months, and the *Spiroplasma* is apparently well tolerated, causing minimal lesions and symptoms. Progressive spongiform encephalopathy has not been produced, however [60]. The fibril protein isolated from *Spiroplasma mirum* seems to be serologically similar to a protein (scrapie-associated fibril protein) found in another spongioform encephalopathy (scrapie, discussed later) [21].

Nevertheless, available evidence indicates spiroplasmas are probably not involved in Creutzfeldt-Jakob disease. *Spiroplasma* has not been isolated from the brains of numerous affected individuals [164], and not all investigators have identified spiroplasmalike bodies within brains of patients with Creutzfeldt-Jakob disease [71]. Others have noted crystalline artifacts that have been erroneously interpreted as spiroplasma fragments in brains of patients with Creutzfeldt-Jakob disease [112].

Scrapie

Scrapie, a naturally occurring spongiform encephalopathy of sheep and goats, is also caused by a prion. Dark retinal patches and spots have been observed ophthalmoscopically in affected sheep [19], and degenerative changes have been reported in the outer retina of hamsters following intracerebral inoculation of the scrapie agent [50,51,123].

B. Mitochondrial Disorders

The brain, retina, striated muscle, and many other tissues derive their main source of energy from the generation of adenosine triphosphate (ATP) by oxidative phosphorylation within mitochondria. The complex generation of this energy, which is under the control of both nuclear DNA (nDNA) and mitochondrial DNA (mtDNA) genes (see Chap. 24) [299], involves five multiple-subunit enzyme complexes (designated complex I–V) in addition to the adenine nucleotide translator (all situated within the mitochondrial inner membrane). Complexes I–IV make up the electron transport chain. In complex I reduced nicotinamide adenine dinucleotide (NADH) is oxidized by NADH dehydrogenase to nicotinamide adenine dinucleotide (NAD^+). This complex consists of more than 30 polypeptides. In complex II, which involves 4 nDNA-encoded polypeptides, succinate dehydrogenase oxidizes succinate to fumarate, and electrons are transferred to ubiquinone (coenzyme Q, CoQ) to yield ubiquinol (reduced CoQ). Electrons are then transferred to cytochrome c by way of complex III (ubiquinol: cytochrome c oxireductase), which consists of 10 polypeptides, and finally to oxygen in the 13 polypeptide-containing complex IV (cytochrome c oxidase). Complex V (ATP synthetase), which embraces 12 polypeptides, forms ATP by condensing adenosine diphosphate (ADP) and inorganic phosphate (P_i).

A heterogeneous group of disorders of oxidative phosphorylation within mitochondria affect the CNS, skeletal muscle, and many other organs. The so-called mitochondrial encephalomyopathies comprise several distinct syndromes: Leigh syndrome, Alper's syndrome, Kearns-Sayre syndrome, myoclonus epilepsy with "ragged-red fibers" (MERRF), and MELAS (mitochondrial myopathy, encephalopathy, lactic acidosis, and strokelike episodes; see Chap. 54).

Leber's Hereditary Optic Neuropathy

Leber's hereditary optic atrophy (LHON) is a maternally inherited disorder characterized by a retinal peripapillary telangiectatic microangiopathy and by the sudden onset of severe bilateral visual loss due to optic neuropathy [197–199]. The severity of the disease varies within pedigrees [53], and an asymptomatic peripapillary microangiopathy characterized by unusually tortuous dilated vessels seems to be the mildest expression of the disorder [198,199].

A total of 11 mutations in parts of mtDNA that encode for the subunits of the electron transport chain complexes I, III, and IV have been associated with LHON (Table 1) [44]. Some individuals have more than one mutation [44,45], and these mutations interact synergistically, with each increasing the probability of blindness. The most common mutation involves nt11778 of mtDNA in the gene of subunit ND4 of the respiratory complex I and converts arginine[340] to histidine[340] [129,174,267,300]. It accounts for about half the LHON patients worldwide [44,267].

LHON may result from the additive effects of various genetic and environmental insults to oxidative phosphorylation, each of which increases the probability of blindness [44]. Based on the genetic mutation in mtDNA, individuals are classified according to the risk of developing LHON and becoming blind. Class I (high-risk) mutations appear to be primary genetic causes of LHON; class II (low-risk) mutations seem to cause LHON only if accompanied by class I or other class II mutations. Although relatively uncommon, the np 7444 and np 3394 mutations have features intermediate between those of class I and class II (class I/II, intermediate risk) and cause significant changes in electron transport chain polypeptides [44]. Data suggests that the np 7444 mutation results in partial respiratory deficiency and thus contributes to the onset of LHON [46]. Different LHON pedigrees can harbor different combinations of class I, II, and I/II mtDNA mutations [44].

Table 1 Mitochondrial Mutations in Leber's Hereditary Optic Neuropathy (LHON)[a]

Mutation	Class	Gene	Nucleotide change	Amino acid change	Estimated frequency in all cases of LHON (%)
3460	I	ND1	G to A	Ala to Thr	15
4160	I	ND1	T to C	Leu to Pro	<1
11778	I	ND4	G to A	Arg to His	50
15257	I	Cytb	G to A	Asp to Asn	9
3394	I/II	ND1	T to C	Tyr to His	?
7444	I/II	CO1	G to A	Term to Lys	5
4216	II	ND1	T to C	Tyr to His	—
4917	II	ND2	G to A	Asp to Asn	—
5244	II	ND2	G to A	Gly to Ser	—
13708	II	ND5	G to A	Ala to Thr	—
15812	II	Cytb	G to A	Val to Met	—

[a]Abbreviations: A, adenine; Ala, alanine; Arg, arginine; Asn, asparagine; Asp, aspartic acid; C, cytosine; CO1 = cytochrome c oxidase subunit 1; Cytb = cytochrome b; G, guanine; Gly, glycine; His, histidine; Leu, leucine; Lys, lysine; Met, methionine; NADH, nicotamide adenine dinucleotide dehydrogenase; ND1, ND1 subunit of NADH; ND2, ND2 subunit of NADH; ND4, ND4 subunit of NADH; Pro, proline; Ser, serine; Term, termination codon; Thr, threonine; Tyr, tyrosine; U, uracil; Val, valine.
Source: Modified from Brown and colleagues [44].

The involvement of both mitochondrial complex I and complex III mutations in LHON suggests that the manifestations of this disease result from a decrease in mitochondrial energy production rather than from a defect in a specific mitochondrial enzyme.

Males are affected four times as often as females [44], but unlike X-linked disorders males never transmit the disease. To explain the high preponderance of males, which is not accounted for by a single mtDNA mutation, an interaction between an X-linked gene and a mitochondrial DNA defect has been proposed, but a conspicuous linkage between LHON and numerous markers on the X chromosome has not been detected [61].

Despite clinical findings related mainly to optic nerve dysfunction and the peripapillary retina, LHON is not a tissue-specific disorder. Electroencephalographic abnormalities are common [199], and phosphorus 31 magnetic resonance spectroscopy can detect altered energy metabolism in muscle during exercise. The brain has been found to manifest decreased energy reserve with this technique [76]. Moreover, abnormal myelin has been detected in the brain by magnetic resonance imaging, and some cases have manifested delayed psychomotor development or autistic features [79]. Minor neurological abnormalities have been noted in some LHON pedigrees [44]. Cardiac palpitations due to arrthymias occur in some patients with LHON [32,199], and young affected males and their maternal relatives may be at risk of sudden death [32]. Muscle biopsies and biochemical assays of mitochondrial enzymes in muscle and platelet are normal.

Subacute Necrotizing Encephalomyelopathy (Leigh Syndrome or Disease, Infantile Wernicke's Disease)

The progressive, degenerative neurological condition described by Leigh [166] usually has an insidious onset and typically affects infants and children between the ages of 2 months and 6 years. The condition occasionally occurs in adults [27,105,242]. Although sometimes occuring sporadically, this familial disorder probably has an autosomal recessive mode of inheritance and parental consanguinity is common [29,125].

This mitochondrial disorder of oxidative metabolism is characterized by markedly elevated blood and CSF lactate and pyruvate concentrations. An intravenous pyruvate loading test can aid in the diagnosis of mitochondrial (encephalo)myopathies [294]. This entity may result from a defect in one of several mitochondrial enzymes involved in the respiratory chain (enzyme complex I [104,243] or enzyme complexes IV [14,87,146,173,190,191) or a deficiency of the pyruvate dehydrogenase complex or NADH dehydrogenase [149,266], as well as from biotinidase deficiency with decreased carboxylase activities (propionyl-CoA carboxylase, 3-methylcrotonyl-CoA carboxylase, or pyruvate carboxylase) [24]. An inhibitor of the conversion of thiamine pyrophosphate to thiamine triphosphate is present in the blood, urine, and CSF of some patients with Leigh syndrome [220–222]. The enzymatic defects can be detected in assays of many tissues, as well as cultured skin fibroblasts. Values of hepatic cytochrome c oxidase activity have varied immensely.

The clinical features of Leigh syndrome vary considerably and include alterations in the state of consciousness, intention tremor, truncal ataxia, hypoactive tendon reflexes, a disordered central regulation of respiration, recurrent vomiting, difficulty in swallowing, failure to thrive, dysfunction of multiple cranial nerves secondary to necrosis of the nerve nuclei, progressive psychomotor retardation and deterioration, a nonspecific generalized weakness, proximal hypotonia and paresis, bilateral pyramidal signs, and peripheral neuropathy.

Diagnostic imaging displays the lesions conspicuously in the living patient. The T2-weighted magnetic resonance imaging [113,186,311] and computed tomography (CT) [113,186,275] display the images remarkably well. Bilateral symmetrically distributed low attenuation areas on CT that are suggestive of necrosis can be readily detected in the tectum of the midbrain, caudate nucleus, putamen, globin pallidum, and substantia nigra, but in contrast to Wernicke's encephalopathy, the mammillary body and red nucleus are spared. Ultrasonography is also useful in detecting early intracranial lesions in Leigh syndrome because of the hyperechoic nature of the major lesions during the preclinical stage [311]. The abnormal images, especially in the putamen, which appears to be invariably involved, are not only of diagnostic value to the clinician but enable the evolution of the lesions within the brain to be documented serially.

Disordered skeletal and cardiac muscle function is conspicuous (see Chap. 54), and progressive general muscle weakness and hypotonia from infancy are followed by an inability to sit, stand, or walk. Respiratory difficulties commonly ensue and usually culminate in death after several weeks to 15 years.

The peripheral nerves have thin hypomyelinated sheaths. Numerous vacuoles account for characteristic spongy lesions in the central gray matter of the CNS, but white matter is also affected. The vacuolar abnormalities seem to form as a consequence of myelin splitting [144]. Many tissues (including striated muscle, leptomeningeal and intracerebral endothelial and vascular smooth muscle cells, choroid plexus epithelia, ependymal cells, and astrocytes or some neurons) contain numerous abnormal mitochondria (without crystalline inclusions) that may be deformed and bizarre. The damaged areas may contain an increased number of astrocytes (reactive gliosis).

Other histopathological abnormalities include intracytoplasmic ovoid to round proteinaceous inclusions that cross-react with antisera to tropomyosin [170] and the loss of immunohistochemically detectable cytochrome c oxidase subunits [191].

Abnormalities in the brain and extraocular muscles, as well as optic atrophy, account for the ophthalmological manifestations [125,260]. The tissue of few eyes have been studied after death, and reported abnormalities include loss of retinal ganglion cells (especially in the macular area), thinning of the nerve fiber layer, and loss of myelin and axons, with some sparing of peripheral axonal bundles in the optic nerve [89,116,125]. Retinal mitochondria manifest destruction of the cristae and accumulations of intramitochondrial electron-dense material.

The optic tracts and chiasm may also be demyelinated, with axonal loss. Lesions of the optic nerves, brain stem, and extraocular muscles account for abnormal visual evoked responses and other bilateral ophthalmic manifestations. The latter include strabismus, ocular motility disorders, optic nerve abnormalities, diminished pupillary response to light, ptosis, ocular innervation, external and internuclear impaired ophthalmoplegia, diplopia, episodic downward gaze with limitation of horizontal eye movement, wandering eye movements, and nystagmus [29].

The neuropathological features of Pelizaeus-Merzbacher disease have accompanied at least one case of subacute necrotizing encephalopathy [78].

Potential causes of the metabolic defect in Leigh syndrome include a deficiency of cytochrome c oxidase due to mutations of either the nuclear [190] or the mitochondrial DNA encoding for different subunits of the enzyme, or large deletions of mtDNA. It is noteworthy that cytochrome c oxidase defects may accompany syndromes other than Leigh syndrome, presumably because of the selective or more widespread involvement of specific organ systems. This delicate status of oxidative metabolism probably accounts for the apparent predisposition of individuals with Leigh syndrome to significant risks of general anesthesia [110].

C. Alzheimer's Disease

Alzheimer's disease is an extremely common degenerative disease of the CNS with a considerable morbidity. This important cause of dementia is characterized histopathologically by cerebral atrophy in association with distinctive neuronal degenerative changes (neurofibrillary tangles and deposits of amyloid within the affected cerebral tissue ("senile plaques"). Although visual abnormalities are not a feature in the vast majority of cases, optic atrophy has been reported in some cases [122,252]. In view of the rarity of conspicuous abnormalities in the optic nerve in Alzheimer's disease, the question of whether the reported abnormalities in the optic nerve are a sequel to Alzheimer's disease or a nonspecific reaction to other common cerebral disorders associated with aging, such as arteriolar sclerosis, remains to be determined.

REFERENCES

1. Acheson, E.D. The epidemiology of multiple sclerosis. In *Multiple Sclerosis: A Reappraisal*, 2nd ed., D. McAlpine, C.E. Lumsden, and E.D. Acheson (Eds.), Williams and Wilkins, Baltimore, Chaps. 1 and 2, pp. 3–80, 1972.
2. Adams, J.M., and Imagawa, D.T. Measles antibodies in multiple sclerosis. *Proc. Soc. Exp. Biol. Med. 111*: 562–566, 1962.
3. Adels, B.R., Gajdusek, D.C., Gibbs, C.J., Jr., Albrecht, P., and Rogers, N.C. Attempts to transmit subacute sclerosing panencephalitis and isolate a measles related agent, with a study of the immune response in patients and experimental animals. *Neurology 18*:30–35, 1968.
4. Aksamit, A.J., Major, E.O., Ghatak, N.R., Sidhu, G.S., Parisi, J.E., and Guccion, J.C. Diagnosis of progressive multifocal leukoencephalopathy by brain biopsy with biotin labelled DNA: DNA in situ hybridization. *J. Neuropathol. Exp. Neurol. 46*:556–566, 1987.
5. Alexander, W.S. Progressive fibrinoid degeneration of fibrillary astrocytes associated with mental retardation in a hydrocephalic infant. *Brain 72*:373–381, 1949.
6. Allegretta, M., Nicklas, J.A., Sriram, S., and Albertini, R.J. T cells responsive to myelin basic protein in patients with multiple sclerosis. *Science 247*:718–721, 1990.
7. Allen, I.V. Pathological findings in subacute sclerosing panencephalitis. In *Virus Diseases and the Nervous System*, C.W.M. Whitty, J.T. Hughes, and F.O. MacCallum (Eds.), Blackwell Scientific, Oxford, pp. 157–162, 1969.
8. Allen, I.V., and Kirk, J. Demyelinating diseases. In *Greenfield's Neuropathology*, 5th ed, J.H. Adams and L.W. Duchen (Eds.), John Wiley and Sons, New York, Chap. 9. pp. 447–520, 1992.
9. Andriola, M., and Karlsberg, R.O. Maculopathy in subacute sclerosing panencephalitis. *Am. J. Dis. Child. 124*:187–189, 1972.
10. Antel, J.P., Weinrich, M., and Arnason, B.G.W. Mitogen responsiveness and suppressive cell function in multiple sclerosis. *Neurology 28*:999–1003, 1978.
11. Appen, R.E., Roth, H., ZuRhein, G.M., and Varakis, J.N. Progressive multifocal leukoencephalopathy: A cause of visual loss. *Arch. Ophthalmol. 95*:656–659, 1977.
12. Archambeau, P.L., Hollenhorst, R.W., and Rucker, C.W. Posterior uveitis as a manifestation of multiple sclerosis. *Mayo Clin. Proc. 40*:544–551, 1965.
13. Arnold, A.C., Pepose, J.S., Helper, R.S., and Foos, R.Y. Retinal periphlebitis and retinitis in multiple sclerosis. I. Pathologic characteristics. *Ophthalmology 91*:255–262, 1984.
14. Arts, W.F., Scholte, H.R., Loonen, M.C., Przyrembel, H., Fernandes, J., Trijbels, J.M., and Luyt-Houwen, I.E. Cytochrome c oxidase deficiency in subacute necrotizing encephalomyelopathy. *J. Neurol. Sci. 77*:103–115, 1987.
15. Aubourg, P., Feil, R., Guidoux, S., Kaplan, J.-C., Moser, H., Kahn, A., and Mandel, J.-L. The red-green visual pigment gene region in adrenoleukodystrophy. *Am. J. Hum. Gent. 46*:459–469, 1990.
16. Baczko, K., Brinckmann, U., Pardowitz, I., Rima, B.K., and ter Meulen, V. Nucleotide sequence of the genes encoding the matrix protein of two wild-type measles virus strains. *J. Gen. Virol. 72*:2279–2282, 1991.
17. Bamford, C.R., Ganley, J.P., Sibley, W.A., and Laguna, J.F. Uveitis, perivenous sheathing and multiple sclerosis. *Neurology 28*:119–124, 1978.
18. Barbizet, J., Degos, J.-D., and Meyrignac, C. Neuromyélite optique aiguë associée a une tuberculose pulmonaire aiguë. *Rev. Neurol. (Paris) 136*:303–309, 1980.
19. Barnett, K.C., and Palmer, A.C. Retinopathy in sheep affected with natural scrapie. *Res. Vet. Sci. 12*:383–385, 1971.
20. Bastian, F.O. Spiroplasma-like inclusions in Creutzfeldt-Jakob disease. *Arch. Pathol. Lab. Med. 103*:665–669, 1979.

21. Bastian, F.O., Jennings, R.A., and Gardner, W.A. Antiserum to scrapie-associated fibril protein cross-reacts with *Spiroplasma mirum* fibril proteins. *J. Clin. Microbiol.* 25:2430–2431, 1987.

22. Batchelor, J.R., Compston, A., and McDonald, W.I. The significance of the association between HLA and multiple sclerosis. *Br. Med. Bull.* 34:279–284, 1978.

23. Baublis, J.V., and Payne, R.E. Measles antigen and syncytium formation in brain cell cultures from subacute sclerosing panencephalitis (SSPE). *Proc. Soc. Exp. Biol. Med.* 129:543–597, 1968.

24. Baumgartner, E.R., Suormala, T.M., Wick, H., Probst, A., Blauenstein, U., Bachmann, C., and Vest, M. Biotinidase deficiency: A cause of subacute necrotizing encephalomyelopathy (Leigh syndrome). Report of a case with lethal outcome. *Pediatr. Res.* 26:260–266, 1989.

25. Behan, P.O., Behan, W.M.H., Feldman, R.G., and Kies, M.W. Cell-mediated hypersensitivity to neural antigens: Occurrence in humans and non-human primates with neurological diseases. *Arch. Neurol. Psychiatry* 27:145–152, 1972.

26. Bertrams, J., and Kuwert, E. HL-A antigen frequencies in multiple sclerosis. *Eur. Neurol.* 7:74–78, 1972.

27. Bianco, F., Floris, R., Pozzessere, G., and Rizzo, P.A. Subacute necrotizing encephalomyelopathy (Leigh's disease): Clinical correlations with computerized tomography in the diagnosis of the juvenile and adult forms. *Acta Neurol. Scand.* 75:214–217, 1987.

28. Bobowick, A.R., Kurtzke, J.F., Brody, J.A., Hrubec, Z., and Gillespie, M. Twin study of multiple sclerosis: An epidemiologic inquiry. *Neurology* 28:978–987, 1978.

29. Borit, A. Leigh's necrotizing encephalomyelopathy: Neuro-ophthalmological abnormalities. *Arch. Ophthalmol.* 85:438–442, 1971.

30. Bornstein, M.B. A tissue-culture approach to demyelinative disorders. *Natl. Cancer Inst. Monogr.* 11:197–214, 1963.

31. Bouteille, M., Fontaine, C., Vedrenne, C., and Delarue, J. Sur un cas d'encéphalite subaiguë à inclusions: Étude anatomo-clinique et ultrastructurale. *Rev. Neurol.* 113:454–458, 1965.

32. Bower, S.P., Hawley, I., and Mackey, D.A. Cardiac arrhythmia and Leber's hereditary optic neuropathy (letter). *Lancet* 339:1427–1428, 1992.

33. Boyle, E.A., and McGeer, P.L. Cellular immune response in multiple sclerosis plaques. *Am. J. Pathol.* 137:575–584, 1990.

34. Brain, W.R., Greenfield, J.G., and Russell, D.S. Subacute inclusion encephalitis (Dawson type). *Brain* 71:365–385, 1948.

35. Breger, B.C., and Leopold, I.H. The incidence of uveitis in multiple sclerosis. *Am. J. Ophthalmol.* 62:540–545, 1966.

36. Brockhurst, R.J., Schepens, C.L., and Okamura, I.D. Peripheral uveitis: Clinical description, complications and differential diagnosis. *Am. J. Ophthalmol.* 49:1257–1266, 1960.

37. Brodrick, J.D., and Dark, A.J. Corneal dystrophy in Cockayne's syndrome. *Br. J. Ophthalmol.* 57:391–399, 1973.

38. Brody, J.A. Epidemiology of multiple sclerosis and a possible virus aetiology. *Lancet* 2:173–176, 1972.

39. Brody, J.A., and Detels, R. Subacute sclerosing panencephalitis: A zoonosis, following aberrant measles. *Lancet* 2:500–501, 1970.

40. Brody, J.A., Sever, J.L., Edgar, A., and McNew, J. Measles antibody titers of multiple sclerosis patients and their siblings. *Neurology* 22:492–499, 1972.

41. Broman, T. Supravital analysis of disorders in the cerebral vascular permeability. II. Two cases of multiple sclerosis. *Acta Psychiat. Neurol. Scand. Suppl.* 46:58–71, 1947.

42. Brown, H.R., Goller, N.L., Rudelli, R.D., Dymecki, J., and Wisniewski, H.M. Postmortem detection of measles virus in non-neural tissues in subacute sclerosing panencephalitis. *Ann. Neurol.* 26:263–268, 1989.

43. Brown, H.R., Goller, N.L., Thormar, H., Rudelli, R., Tourtellotte, W.W., Shapshak, P., Boostanfar, R., and Wisniewski, H.M. Measles virus matrix protein gene expression in a subacute sclerosing panencephalitis patient brain and virus isolate demonstrated by cDNA hybridization and immunocytochemistry. *Acta Neuropathol. (Berl.)* 75:123–130, 1987.

44. Brown, M.D., Voljavec, A.S., Lott, M.T., MacDonald, I., and Wallace D.C. Leber's hereditary optic neuropathy: A model for mitochondrial neurodegenerative diseases. *FASEB J.* 6:2791–2799, 1992.

45. Brown, M.D., Voljavec, A.S., Lott, M.T., Torroni, A., Yang, C.C., and Wallace, D.C. Mitochondrial DNA complex I and III mutations associated with Leber's hereditary optic neuropathy. *Genetics* 130:163–173, 1992.

46. Brown, M.D., Yang, C.C., Trounce, I., Torroni, A., Lott, M.T., and Wallace, D.C. A mitochondrial DNA variant, identified in Leber hereditary optic neuropathy patients, which extends the amino acid sequence of cytochrome c oxidase subunit I. *Am. J. Hum. Genet.* 51:378–385, 1992.

47. Brown, P. An epidemiologic critique of Creutzfeldt-Jakob disease. *Epidemiol. Rev.* 2:113–135, 1980.

48. Burde, R.M. Retrobulbar neuritis revisited. *Am. J. Ophthalmol.* 79:695–697, 1975.

49. Burton, B.K., and Nadler, H.L. Schilder's disease: Abnormal cholesterol retention and accumulation in cultivated fibroblasts. *Pediatr. Res.* 8:170–175, 1974.

50. Buyukmichci, N., Marsh, R.F., Albert, D.M., and Zelinski, K. Ocular effects of scrapie agent in hamsters: Preliminary observations. *Invest. Ophthalmol. Vis. Sci.* 16:319–324, 1977.

51. Buyukmichci, N., Rorvik, M., and Marsh, F.F. Replication of the scrapie agent in ocular neural tissues. *Proc. Natl. Acad. Sci. USA* 77:1169–1171, 1980.

52. Byington, D.P., and Johnson, K.P. Experimental subacute sclerosing panencephalitis in the hamster: Correlation of age with chronic inclusion-cell encephalitis. *J. Infect. Dis. 126*:18–26, 1972.

53. Carducci, C., Leuzzi, V., Scuderi, M., De Negri, A.M., Gabrieli, C.B., Antonozzi, I., and Pontecorvi, A. Mitochondrial DNA mutation in an Italian family with Leber hereditary optic neuropathy. *Hum. Genet. 87*:725–727, 1991.

54. Carrigan, D.R., and Knox, K.K. Identification of interferon-resistant subpopulations in several strains of measles virus: Positive selection by growth of the virus in brain tissue. *J. Virol. 64*:1606–1615, 1990.

55. Cattaneo, R., Rebmann, G., Baczko, K., ter Meulen, V., and Billeter, M.A. Altered ratios of measles virus transcripts in diseased human brains. *Virology 160*:523–526, 1987.

56. Cattaneo, R., Schmid, A., Billeter, M.A., Sheppard, R.D., and Udem, S.A. Multiple viral mutations rather than host factors cause defective measles virus gene expression in a subacute sclerosing panencephalitis cell line. *J. Virol. 62*:1388–1397, 1988.

57. Cattaneo, R., Schmid, A., Spielhofer, P., Kaelin, K., Baczko, K., ter Meulen, V., Pardowitz, J., Flanagan, S., Rima, B.K., Udem, S.A., and Billeter, M.A. Mutated and hypermutated genes of persistent measles viruses which caused lethal human brain diseases. *Virology 173*:415–425, 1989.

58. Cernescu, C., Popescu-Tismana, G., Alaicescu, M., Popescu, L., and Cajal, N. The continuous decrease in the number of SSPE annual cases ten years after compulsory anti-measles immunization. *Rev. Roumaine Virol. 41*:13–18, 1990.

59. Charcot, J.M. *Lectures on the Disease of the Nervous System*, first series (translated by G. Sigerson), delivered 1868, Lecture 6, New Sydenham Society, London, 1877.

60. Chastel, C., Le Goff, F., and Humphery-Smith, I. Multiplication and persistence of *Spiroplasma melliferum* strain A56 in experimentally infected suckling mice. *Res. Microbiol. 142*:411–417, 1991.

61. Chen, J.D., and Denton, M.J. X-chromosomal gene in Leber hereditary optic neuroretinopathy (letter; comment). *Am. J. Hum. Genet. 49*:692–693, 1991.

62. Chenn, T.T., Watanabe, I., Zeman, W., and Mealey, J., Jr. Subacute sclerosing panencephalitis: Propagation of measles virus from brain biopsy in tissue culture. *Science 163*:1193–1194, 1969.

63. Cloys, D.E., and Netsky, M.G. Neuromyelitis optica. In *Handbook of Clinical Neurology*, Vol. 9, P.J. Vinken and G.W. Bruyn (Eds.), North Holland, Amsterdam, Chap. 14, pp. 426–436, 1970.

64. Cobb, W.A., and Morgan-Hughes, J.A. Nonfatal subacute sclerosing leucoencephalitis. *J. Neurol. Neurosurg. Psychiatry 31*:115–123, 1968.

65. Cochereau-Massin, I., Prost, F., Bron, A.J., Delbosc, B., Zazoun, L., Wolff, M., Royer, F., and Rousselie, F. Rétinite révélatrice de panencéphalite sclérosante subaiguë. *Bull. Soc. Ophtalmol. Fr. 90*:479–481, 1990.

66. Cockayne, E.A. Dwalfism with retinal atrophy and deafness. *Arch. Dis. Child. 11*:1–8, 1936.

67. Cohen, M.M., Lessel, S., and Wolf, P.A. A prospective study of the risk of developing multiple sclerosis in uncomplicated optic neuritis. *Neurology 29*:208–213, 1979.

68. Cohen, S.M.Z., Green, W.R., De la Cruz, Z.C., Brown, F.R., III, Moser, H.W., Luckenbach, M.W., Dove, D.J., and Maumenee, I.H. Ocular histopathologic studies of neonatal childhood adrenoleukodystrophy. *Am. J. Ophthalmol. 95*:82–96, 1983.

69. Cole, G., DeVilliers, F., Proctor, N.S.F., Freiman, I., and Bill, P. Alexander's disease: Case report including histopathological and electron microscopic features. *J. Neurol. Neurosurg. Psychiatry 42*:619–624, 1979.

70. Connolly, J.H. Subacute sclerosing panencephalitis. *Postgrad. Med. J. 48*:342–345, 1972.

71. Connolly, J.H., Allen, I.V., and Dermott, E. Transmissible agent in the amyotrophic form of Creutzfeldt-Jakob disease (letter). *J. Neurol. Neurosurg. Psychiatry 51*:1459–1460, 1988.

72. Connolly, J.H., Allen, I.V., Hurwitz, L.J., and Millar, J.H.D. Measles-virus antibody and antigen in subacute sclerosing panencephalitis. *Lancet 1*:542–544, 1967.

73. Connolly, J.H., Allen, I.V., Hurtwitz, L.J., and Millar, J.H.D. Subacute sclerosing panencephalitis: Clinical, pathological, epidemiological, and virological findings in three patients. *Q. J. Med. 37*:625–644, 1968.

74. Connolly, J.H., Haire, M., and Hadden, D.S.M. Measles immunoglobulins in subacute sclerosing panencephalitis. *Br. Med. J. 1*:23–25, 1971.

75. Corsellis, J.A.N. Sub-acute sclerosing leucoencephalitis: A clinical and pathological report of two cases. *J. Ment. Sci. 97*:570–583, 1951.

76. Cortelli, P., Montagna, P., Avoni, P., Sangiorgi, S., Bresolin, N., Moggio, M., Zaniol, P., Mantovani, V., Barboni, P., Barbiroli, B., and Lusaresi, I. Leber's hereditary optic neuropathy: Genetic, biochemical, and phosphorus magnetic resonance spectroscopy study in an Italian family. *Neurology 41*:1211–1215, 1991.

77. Courville, C.B. Concentric sclerosis. In *Handbook of Clinical Neurology*, Vol. 9, P.J. Vinken and G.W. Bruyn (Eds.), North Holland, Amsterdam, pp. 437–451, 1970.

78. Cruz-Sanchez, F.F., Cervos-Navarro, J., Rossi, M.L., and Lafuente, J.V. Pelizaeus-Merzbacher disease with thiamine deficiency or Leigh disease with extensive involvement of white matter? Case report. *Clin. Neurol. Neurosurg. 91*:261–263, 1989.

79. Curless, R.G., Flynn, J.T., Olsen, K.R., and Post, M.J. Leber congenital amaurosis in siblings with diffuse dysmyelination. *Pediatr. Neurol. 7*:223–235, 1991.

80. David, P., Elia, M., Mariotti, P., and Macchi, G. Adult onset of subacute sclerosing panencephalitis: A case report. *Rivista Di Neurol. 60*:83–87, 1990.
81. Dawson, J.R., Jr. Cellular inclusions in cerebral lesions of lethargic encephalitis. *Am. J. Pathol. 9*:7–16, 1933.
82. Dawson, J.R., Jr. Cellular inclusions in cerebral lesions of epidemic encephalitis. *Arch. Neurol. Psychiatry 31*:685–700, 1934.
83. Dayan, A.D., Gostling, J.V.T., Greaves, J.L., Stevens, D.W., and Woodhouse, M.A. Evidence of a pseudomyxovirus in the brain in subacute sclerosing leucoencephalitis. *Lancet 1*:980–981, 1967.
84. Dean, G., and Kurtzke, J.F. On the risk of multiple sclerosis according to age at immigration to South Africa. *Br. Med. J. 3*:725–729, 1971.
85. Dhib-Jalbut, S., Jacobson, S., McFarlin, D.E., and McFarland, H.F. Impaired human leukocyte antigen-restricted measles virus-specific cytotoxic T-cell response in subacute sclerosing panencephalitis. *Ann. Neurol. 25*:272–280, 1989.
86. Dick, G. Sub-acute sclerosing panencephalitis. In *Virus Diseases and the Nervous System: A Symposium*, C.W.M. Whitty, J.T. Hughes, and F.O. MacCallum (Eds.), Blackwell Scientific, Oxford, pp. 149–155, 1969.
87. DiMauro, S., Servidei, S., Zeviani, M., DiRocco, M., DeVivo, D.C., DiDonato, S., Uziel, G., Berry, K., Hoganson, G., Johnsen, S.D., and Johnson, P.C. Cytochrome c oxidase deficiency in Leigh syndrome. *Ann. Neurol. 22*:498–506, 1987.
88. Doll, R., Natowicz, M.R., Schiffman, R., and Smith, F.I. Molecular diagnostics for myelin proteolipid protein gene mutations in Pelizaeus-Merzbacher disease. *Am. J. Hum. Genet. 51*:161–169, 1992.
89. Dooling, E.C., and Richardson, E.P., Jr. Ophthalmoplegia and Ondine's curse. *Arch. Ophthalmol. 95*:1790–1793, 1977.
90. Donders, P.C. Eales' disease. *Doc. Ophthalmol. 12*:1–105, 1958.
91. Donner, M., Waltimo, O., Porras, J., Forsius, H., and Saukkonen, A.L. Subacute sclerosing panencephalitis as a cause of chronic dementia and relapsing brain disorder. *J. Neurol. Neurosurg. Psychiatry 35*:180–185, 1972.
92. Dow, R.S., and Berglund, G. Vascular pattern of lesions of multiple sclerosis. *Arch. Neurol. Psychiatry 47*:1–18, 1942.
93. Dubois-Dalcq, M., Barbosa, L.H., Hamilton, R., and Sever, J.L. Comparison between productive and latent subacute sclerosing panencephalitis viral infection in vitro: An electron microscopic and immunoperoxidase study. *Lab. Invest. 30*:241–250, 1974.
94. Duffy, P., Wolf, J., Collins, G., DeVoe, A.G., Streeten, B., and Cowen, D. Possible person-to-person transmission of Creutzfeldt-Jakob disease. *N. Engl. J. Med. 290*:692, 1974.
95. Engell, T., Jenson, O.A., and Klinken, L. Periphlebitis retinae in multiple sclerosis: A histopathological study of two cases. *Acta Ophthalmol. (Copenh.) 63*:83–88, 1985.
96. Esiri, M.M., and Kennedy, P.G.E. Virus diseases. In *Greenfield's Neuropathology*, 5th ed. J.H. Adams and L.W. Duchen (Eds.), John Wiley and Sons, New York, Chap. 7, pp. 335–399, 1992.
97. Field, E.J. Slow virus infections of the nervous system. *Int. Rev. Exp. Pathol. 8*:129–239, 1969.
98. Fog, T. The topographic distribution of plaques in the spinal cord in multiple sclerosis. *Arch. Neurol. Psychiatry 63*:382–414, 1950.
99. Fog, T. The topography of plaques in multiple sclerosis. *Acta Neurol. Scand. (Suppl. 15) 41*:1–161, 1965.
100. Foley, J., and Williams, D. Inclusion encephalitis and its relation to subacute sclerosing leucoencephalitis. *Q. J. Med. 22*:157–194, 1953.
101. Font, R.L., Jenis, E.H., and Tuck, K.D. Measles maculopathy associated with subacute sclerosing panencephalitis: Immunofluorescent and immunoultrastructural study. *Arch. Pathol. 96*:168–174, 1973.
102. Freeman, J.M. The clinical spectrum and early diagnosis of Dawson's encephalitis. *J. Pediatr. 75*:590–603, 1969.
103. Freeman, J.M., Magoffin, R.L., Lennette, E.H., and Herndon, R.M. Additional evidence of the relation between subacute inclusion-body encephalitis and measles virus. *Lancet 2*:129–131, 1967.
104. Fujii, T., Ito, M., Okuno, T., Mutoh, K., Nishikomori, R., and Mikawa, H. Complex I (reduced nicotinamide-adenine dinucleotide-coenzyme Q reductase) deficiency in two patients with probable Leigh syndrome. *J. Pediatr. 116*:84–87, 1990.
105. Fulham, M., Lawrence, C., and Harper, C. Diagnostic clues in an adult case of Leigh's disease. *Med. J. Aust. 149*:320–322, 1988.
106. Gajdusek, D.C. Unconventional viruses and the origin and disappearance of Kuru. *Science 197*:943–960, 1977.
107. Gartner, S. Optic neuropathy in multiple sclerosis: Optic neuritis. *Arch. Ophthalmol. 50*:718–726, 1953.
108. Giles, C.L. Peripheral uveitis in patients with multiple sclerosis. *Am. J. Ophthalmol. 70*:17–19, 1970.
109. Godec, M.S., Asher, D.M., Swoveland, P.T., Eldadah, Z.A., Feinstone, S.M., Goldfarb, L.G., Gibbs, C.J., Jr., and Gajdusek, D.C. Detection of measles virus genomic sequences in SSPE brain tissue by the polymerase chain reaction. *J. Med. Virol. 30*:237–244, 1990.
110. Grattan-Smith, P.J., Shield, L.K., Hopkins, I.J., and Collins, K.J. Acute respiratory failure precipitated by general anesthesia in Leigh's syndrome. *J. Child Neurol. 5*:137–141, 1990.
111. Gravina, R.F., Nakanishi, A.S., and Faden, A. Subacute sclerosing panencephalitis. *Am. J. Ophthalmol. 86*:106–109, 1978.
112. Gray, A., Francis, R.J., and Scholtz, C.L. Spiroplasma and Creutzfelt-Jakob disease (letter to editor). *Lancet 2*:152, 1980.

113. Greenberg, S.B., Faerber, E.N., Riviello, J.J., de Leon, G., and Capitanio, M.A. Subacute necrotizing encephalomyelopathy (Leigh disease): CT and MRI appearances. *Pediatr. Radiol. 21*:5–8, 1990.
114. Gregson, N.A. The molecular biology of myelin. In *Multiple Sclerosis: Pathology, Diagnosis and Management*, J.F. Hallpike, C.W.M. Adams, and W.W. Tourtellotte (Eds.), Williams and Wilkins, Baltimore, Chap. 1, pp. 1–28, 1983.
115. Griffin, J.W., Goren, E., Schaumburg, H., Engel, W.H., and Loriaux, L. Adrenomyeloneuropathy: A probable variant of adrenoleukodystrophy. *Neurology 27*:1107–1113, 1977.
116. Grover, W.D., Green, W.R., and Pileggi, A.J. Ocular findings in subacute necrotizing encephalomyelitis. *Am. J. Ophthalmol. 70*:599–603, 1970.
117. Haarr, M. Periphlebitis retinae in association with multiple sclerosis. *Acta Psychiatr. Neurol. Scand. 28*:175–190, 1953.
118. Haltia, M., Tarkkanen, A., Vaheri, A., Paetau, A., Kaakinen, K., and Erkkilä, H. Measles retinopathy during immunosuppression. *Br. J. Ophthalmol. 62*:356–360, 1978.
119. Herndon, R.M., and Rubinstein, L.J. Light and electron microscopy observations on the development of viral particles in the inclusions of Dawson's encephalitis (subacute sclerosing panencephalitis). *Neurology 18*:8–18, 1968.
120. Hijikata, F., Hirooka, M., and Ohno, T. Cockayne's syndrome: A histopathological study of the ocular tissues. *Rinsho Ganka 23*:187–194, 1969.
121. Hinton, D.R., Henderson, V.W., Blanks, J.C., Rudnicka, M., and Miller, C.A. Monoclonal antibodies react with neuronal subpopulations in the human nervous system. *J. Comp. Neurol. 267*:398–408, 1988.
122. Hinton, D.R., Sadun, A., Blanks, J.C., and Miller, C.A. Optic nerve degeneration in Alzheimer's disease. *N. Engl. J. Med. 315*:485–487, 1986.
123. Hogan, R.N., Baringer, J.R., and Prusiner, S.B. Progressive retinal degeneration in scrapie-infected hamsters. *Lab. Invest. 44*:34–42, 1981.
124. Horta-Barbosa, L., Fuccillo, D.A., Sever, J.L., and Zeman, W. Subacute sclerosing panencephalitis: Isolation of measles virus from a brain biopsy. *Nature 221*:974, 1969.
125. Howard, R.O., and Albert, D.M. Ocular manifestations of subacute necrotizing encephalomyelopathy (Leigh's disease). *Am. J. Ophthalmol. 74*:386–393, 1972.
126. Hudson, L.D., Puckett, C., Berndt, J., Chan, J., and Genic, S. Mutation of the proteolipid protein gene PLP in human X chromosome-linked myelin disorder. *Proc. Natl. Acad. Sci. USA 86*:8128–8131, 1989.
127. Iannarella, G., Makdassi, R., Schmit, J.L., Gontier, M.F., Legars, D., Deramond, H., Duverlie, G., Rosa, A., and Fournier, A. Association d'une leucoencephalite multifocale progressive et d'une sarcoidose. *Ann. Med. Intern. 143*:71–74, 1992.
128. Inoue, Y.K. An avian-related new herpesvirus infection in man: Subacute myelo-optico-neuropathy (SMON). *Prog. Med. Virol. 21*:35–42, 1975.
129. Isashiki, Y., Ohba, N., Uto, M., Nakagawa, M., Nakano, T., Kitahara, K., Hotta, A., Okamura, R., Ozaki, M., Futami, Y., and Sawada, A. Nonfamilial and unusual cases of Leber's hereditary optic neuropathy identified by mitochondrial DNA analysis. *Jpn. J. Ophthalmol. 36*:197–204, 1992.
130. Iwasaki, Y., and Koprowski, H. Cell to cell transmission of virus in the central nervous system. I. Subacute sclerosing panencephalitis. *Lab. Invest. 31*:187–196, 1974.
131. Jabbour, J.T., Duenas, D.A., Sever, J.L., Krebs, H.M., and Horta-Barbosa, L. Epidemiology of subacute sclerosing panencephalitis (SSPE): A report of the SSPE registry. *JAMA 220*:959–962, 1972.
132. Jensen, M.K. Lymphocyte transformation in multiple sclerosis. *Acta Neurol. Scand. 44*:200–206, 1968.
133. Jersild, C., Hansen, G.S., Svejgaard, A., Fog, T., Thomsen, M., and Dupont, B. Histocompatibility determinants in multiple sclerosis, with special reference to clinical course. *Lancet 2*:1221–1225, 1973.
134. Jersild, C., Svejgaard, A., Fog, T., and Ammitzboll, T. HL-A antigens and diseases. I. Multiple sclerosis. *Tissue Antigens 3*:243–250, 1973.
135. Johnson, H.C. Retinal venous sheathing in multiple sclerosis. *Am. J. Ophthalmol. 29*:1150–1151, 1946.
136. Johnson, R.T. Evidence for polymaviruses in human neurological diseases. In *Polyomaviruses and Neurological Disease*, J.L. Sever and D.L. Maddend (Eds.), Alan R. Liss, New York, pp. 183–190, 1983.
137. Kabat, E.A., Freedman, D.A., Murray, J.P., and Knaub, V. A study of a crystalline albumin, gamma globulin and total protein in the cerebrospinal fluid of 100 cases of multiple sclerosis and in other diseases. *Am. J. Med. Sci. 219*:55–64, 1950.
138. Karlsberg, R.C., and Andriola, M. Funduscopy in subacute sclerosing panencephalitis. *J. Fla. Med. Assoc. 59*:25–29, 1972.
139. Katz, M. Subacute sclerosing panencephalitis. In *Slow Virus Infections of the Central Nervous System: Investigational Approaches to Etiology and Pathogenesis of These Diseases*, V. ter Meulen and M. Katz (Eds.), Springer-Verlag, New York, pp. 106–114, 1977.
140. Katz, M., Oyanagi, S., and Koprowski, H. Subacute sclerosing panencephalitis: Structures resembling myxovirus nucleocapsids in cells cultured from brains. *Nature 222*:888–890, 1969.
141. Katz, M.L., Rorke, L.B., Masland, W.S., Koprowski, H., and Tucker, S.H. Transmission of an encephalitogenic agent from brains of patients with subacute sclerosing panencephalitis to ferrets: Preliminary report. *N. Engl. J. Med. 279*:793–798, 1968.

142. Kempe, C.H., Takabayashi, K., Miyamato, H., McIntosh, K., Tourtellotte, W.W., and Adams, J.M. Elevated cerebrospinal fluid antibodies in multiple sclerosis. *Arch. Neurol. 28*:278–297, 1973.

143. Khalifa, M.A., Rodrigues, M.M., Rajagopalan, S., and Swoveland, P. Eye pathology associated with measles encephalitis in hamsters. *Arch. Virol. 119*:165–173, 1991.

144. Kimura, S., Kobayashi, T., and Amemiya, F. Myelin splitting in the spongy lesion in Leigh encephalopathy. *Pediatr. Neurol. 7*:56–58, 1991.

145. Kitamoto, T., Shin, R-W., Doh-ura, K., Tomokane, N., Miyazono, M., Muramoto, T., and Tateishi, J. Abnormal isoform of prion proteins accumulates in the synaptic structures of the central nervous system in patients with Creutzfelt-Jakob disease. *Am. J. Pathol. 140*:1285–1294, 1992.

146. Koga, Y., Nonaka, I., Nakao, M., Yoshino, M., Tanaka, M., Ozawa, T., Nakase, H., and DiMauro, S. Progressive cytochrome c oxidase deficiency in a case of Leigh's encephalomyelopathy. *J. Neurol. Sci. 95*:63–76, 1990.

147. Komori, T., Nagashima, T., Hirose, K., Tanabe, H., and Tsubaki, T. Adrenomyeloneuropathy associated with congenital cataract: Report of a family with MRI study (Japanese). *Rinsho Shinkeigaku [Clin. Neurol.] 28*:532–535, 1988.

148. Kreth, W.H., Käckell, M.Y., and ter Meulen, V. Demonstration of in vitro lymphocyte-mediated cytotoxicity against measles virus in SSPE. *J. Immunol. 114*:1042–1046, 1975.

149. Kretzschmar, H.A., DeArmond, S.J., Koch, T.K., Patel, M.S., Newth, C.J., Schmidt, K.A., and Packman, S. Pyruvate dehydrogenase complex deficiency as a cause of subacute necrotizing encephalopathy (Leigh disease). *Pediatrics 79*:370–373, 1987.

150. Kuhl, W. Seltene "Begleit"-Bilder bei periphlebitis retinae. *Acta Ophthalmol. (Copenh.) 46*:1105–1112, 1968.

151. Kurland, L.T., Beebe, E.W., Kurtzke, J.F., Nagler, B., Auth, T.L., Lessell, S., and Nefzger, M.D. Studies on the natural history of multiple sclerosis. 2. Optic neuritis as a prelude to multiple sclerosis. *Acta Neurol. Scand. 42*(Suppl. 19):157–176, 1966.

152. Kuroiwa, Y. Neuromyelitis optica (Devic's disease, Devic's syndrome). In *Handbook of Clinical Neurology*, Vol. 47 (revised series), P.J. Vinken and G.W. Bruyn (Eds.), North Holland, Amsterdam, Chap. 13, pp. 397–408, 1985.

153. Kurtzke, J.F. Familial incidence and geography in multiple sclerosis. *Acta Neurol. Scand. 41*:127–139, 1965.

154. Kurtzke, J.F. On the time of onset in multiple sclerosis. *Acta Neurol. Scand. 41*:140–153, 1965.

155. Kurtzke, J.F. A reassessment of the distribution of multiple sclerosis, parts one and two. *Acta Neurol. Scand. 51*:110–136, 137–157, 1975.

156. Kurtzke, J.F., and Kurland, L.T. Multiple sclerosis in the epidemiology of neurologic disease. In *Clinical Neurology*, Vol. 3, A.B. Baker and L.H. Baker (Eds.), Harper and Row, Chap. 48, pp. 22–30, 1976.

157. Kuwert, E.K., and Bertrams, H.J. Genetic aspects of multiple sclerosis. In *Slow Virus Infections of the Central Nervous System*, V. ter Meulen and M. Katz (Eds.), Springer-Verlag, New York, pp. 186–199, 1975.

158. Lakhanpal, V., Schocket, S.S., Nirankari, V.S., and Hameroff, S.B. Hemorrhagic detachment of the macula in subacute sclerosing encephalitis. *South Med. J. 71*:1025, 1978.

159. Lampert, F., and Lampert, P.W. Multiple sclerosis: Morphologic evidence of intranuclear paramyxovirus or altered chromatin fibers. *Arch. Neurol. 32*:425–427, 1975.

160. Lampert, P.W., Joseph, B.S., and Oldstone, M.B.A. Morphological changes of cells infected with measles or related viruses. In *Progress in Neuropathology*, Vol. 3, H.M. Zimmerman (Ed.), Grune and Stratton, New York, pp. 51–68, 1976.

161. Landau, W.M., and Luse, S.A. Relapsing inclusion encephalitis (Dawson type) of eight years duration. *Neurology 8*:669–676, 1958.

162. Landers, M.B., III, and Klintworth, G.K. Subacute sclerosing panencephalitis (SSPE): A clinicopathologic study of the retinal lesions. *Arch. Ophthalmol. 86*:156–163, 1971.

163. La Piana, F.G., Tso, M.O.M., and Jenis, E.H. The retinal lesions of subacute sclerosing panencephalitis. *Ann. Ophthalmol. 6*:603–610, 1974.

164. Leach, R.H., Matthews, W.B., and Will, R. Creutzfelt-Jakob disease: Failure to detect spiroplasmas by cultivation and serological tests. *J. Neurol. Sci. 59*:349–353, 1983.

165. Legg, N.J. Virus antibodies in subacute sclerosing panencephalitis. *Br. Med. J. 3*:350–352, 1967.

166. Leigh, D. Subacute necrotizing encephalopathy in an infant. *J. Neurol. Neurosurg. Psychiatry 14*:216–221, 1951.

167. Lennette, E.H., Magoffin, R.L., and Freeman, J.M. Immunologic evidence of measles virus as an etiologic agent in subacute sclerosing panencephalitis. *Neurology 18*:21–27, 1968.

168. Lesser, R.L., Albert, D.M., Bobowick, A.R., and O'Brien, F.H. Creutzfeldt-Jakob disease and optic atrophy. *Am. J. Ophthalmol. 87*:317–321, 1979.

169. Levin, P.S., Green, W.R., Victor, D.I., and MacLean, A.L. Histopathology of the eye in Cockayne's syndrome. *Arch. Ophthalmol. 101*:1093–1097, 1983.

170. Lew, E.O., Rozdilsky, B., Munoz, D.G., and Perry, G. A new type of neuronal cytoplasmic inclusion: Histological, ultrastructural, and immunocytochemical studies. *Acta Neuropathol. (Berl.) 77*:599–604, 1989.

171. Link, H., and Tibbling, G. Principles of albumin and IgG analyses in neurological disorders. III. Evaluation of IgG synthesis within the central nervous system in multiple sclerosis. *Scand. J. Clin. Invest. 37*:397–401, 1977.

172. Lisak, R.P. Multiple sclerosis: Evidence for immunopathogenesis. *Neurology 39*:99–105, 1980.
173. Lombes, A., Nakase, H., Tritschler, H.J., Kadenbach, B., Bonilla, E., DeVivo, D.C., Schon, E.A., and DiMauro, S. Biochemical and molecular analysis of cytochrome c oxidase deficiency in Leigh's syndrome. *Neurology 41*:491–498, 1991.
174. Lott, M.T., Voljavec, A.S., and Wallace, D.C. Variable genotype of Leber's hereditary optic neuropathy. *Am. J. Ophthalmol. 109*:625–631, 1990.
175. Lowenthal, A., Moya, G., Poire, R., Macken, J., and De Smedt, R. Subacute sclerosing panencephalitis: A clinical and biological reappraisal. *J. Neurol. Sci. 15*:267–270, 1972.
176. Lucarelli, M.J., Pepose, J.S., Arnold, A.V., and Foos, R.Y. Immunopathologic features of retinal lesions in multiple sclerosis. *Ophthalmology 98*:1652–1656, 1991.
177. Lumsden, C.E. The immunogenesis of the multiple sclerosis plaque. *Brain Res. 28*:365–390, 1971.
178. McAlpine, D. The benign form of multiple sclerosis. *Brain 84*:186–203, 1961.
179. McAlpine, D. The benign form of multiple sclerosis: Results of a long term study. *Br. Med. J. 2*:1029–1032, 1964.
180. McAlpine, D., Lumsden, C.E., and Acheson, E.D. *Multiple Sclerosis: A Reappraisal*, 2nd ed., Churchill Livingstone, Edinburgh, 1972.
181. McDermott, J.R., Field, E.J., and Caspary, E.A. Relation of measles virus to encephalitogenic factor, with reference to the aetiopathogenesis of multiple sclerosis. *J. Neurol. Neurosurg. Psychiatry 37*:282–287, 1974.
182. McDonald, W.I. Pathophysiology in multiple sclerosis. *Brain 97*:179–196, 1974.
183. Malamud, N., Haymaker, W., and Pinkerton, H. Inclusion encephalitis with a clinicopathologic report of three cases. *Am. J. Pathol. 26*:133–153, 1950.
184. Mann, E., McDermott, M.J., Goldman, J., Chiesa, R., and Spector, A. Phosphorylation of alpha-crystallin B in Alexander's disease brain. *FEBS Lett. 294*:133–136, 1991.
185. Manz, H.J., Schuelein, M., McCullough, D.C., Kishimoto, Y., and Eiben, R.M. New phenotype variant of adrenoleukodystrophy: Pathologic, ultrastructural and biochemical study in two brothers. *J. Neurol. Sci. 45*:245–260, 1980.
186. Martin, J.J., Van de Vyver, F.L., Scholte, H.R., Roodhooft, A.M., Ceuterick, C., Martin, L., and Luyt-Houwen, I.E. Defect in succinate oxidation by isolated muscle mitochondria in a patient with symmetrical lesions in the basal ganglia. *J. Neurol. Sci. 84*:189–200, 1988.
187. Mattinson, P.J. Suspected SSPE: A delayed psychiatric presentation. *Br. J. Psychiatr. 154*:116–118, 1989.
188. Mehta, P.D., Patrick, B.A., Sobczyk, W., Kulczycki, J., Woyciechowska-Camenga, J., Camenga, D., and Thormar, H. Immunoglobulin G subclass antibodies to measles virus in patients with subacute sclerosing panencephalitis or multiple sclerosis. *J. Clin. Microbiol. 27*:62–65, 1989.
189. Menkes, J.H., and Corbo, L.M. Adrenoleukodystrophy: Accumulation of cholesterol esters with very long-chain fatty acids. *Neurology 27*:928–932, 1977.
190. Miranda, A.F., Ishii, S., DiMauro, S., and Shay, J.W. Cytochrome c oxidase deficiency in Leigh's syndrome: Genetic evidence for a nuclear DNA-encoded mutation. *Neurology 39*:697–702, 1989.
191. Miyabayashi, S., Ito, T., Abukawa, D., Narisawa, K., Tada, K., Tanaka, M., Ozawa, T., Droste, M., and Kadenbach, B. Immunochemical study in three patients with cytochrome c oxidase deficiency presenting Leigh's encephalomyelopathy. *J. Inherit. Metab. Dis. 10*:289–292, 1987.
192. Morse, P.H. Retinal venous sheathing and neovascularization in disseminated sclerosis. *Ann. Ophthalmol. 7*:949–952, 1975.
193. Moser, H.W., Moser, A.B., Frayer, K.K., Chen, W., Schulman, J.D., O'Neill, B.P., and Kishimoto, Y. Adrenoleukodystrophy: Increased plasma content of saturated very long-chain fatty acids. *Neurology 31*:1241–1249, 1981.
194. Myrianthopoulos, N.C. Genetic aspects of multiple sclerosis. In *Handbook of Clinical Neurology*, Vol. 9, P.J. Vinken and G.W. Bruyn (Eds.), North Holland, Amsterdam, pp. 85–106, 1970.
195. Naito, S., Namerow, N., Mickey, M.R., and Terasaki, P.I. Multiple sclerosis: Association with HL-A3. *Tissue Antigens 2*:1–4, 1972.
196. Nelson, D.A., Weiner, A., Yanoff, M., and de Perlta, J. Retinal lesions in subacute sclerosing panencephalitis. *Arch. Ophthalmol. 84*:613–621, 1970.
197. Newman, N.J. Leber's hereditary optic neuropathy. *Ophthalmol. Clin. North Am. 4*:431–447, 1991.
198. Nikoskelainen, E.K., Hoyt, W.F., and Nummelin, K. Ophthalmologic findings in Leber's hereditary optic neuropathy. I. Fundus findings in asymptomatic family members. *Arch. Ophthalmol. 100*:1597–1602, 1987.
199. Nikoskelainen, E.K., Savontaus, M.-L., Wanne, O.P., Katila, M.J., and Nummelin, K.U. Leber's hereditary optic neuropathy, a maternally inherited disease. *Arch. Ophthalmol. 105*:665–671, 1987.
200. Offner, H., Konat, G., and Clausen, J. Effect of phytohemagglutinin, basic protein and measles antigen on myo-(2-³H)inositol incorporation into phosphatidylinositol of lymphocytes from patients with multiple sclerosis. *Acta Neurol. Scand. 50*:791–800, 1974.
201. Oger, J.F., Arnason, B.G.W., Wray, S.H., and Kistler, J.P. A study of B and T cells in multiple sclerosis. *Neurology 25*:444–447, 1975.
202. Ohya, T., Martinez, A.J., Jabbour, J.T., Lemmi, H., and Duenas, D.A. Subacute sclerosing panencephalitis: Correlation of clinical, neurophysiologic and neuropathologic findings. *Neurology 24*:211–218, 1974.

203. Okuno, Y., Nakao, T., Ishida, N., Konno, T., Mizutani, H., Fukuyama, Y., Sato, T., Isomura, S., Ueda, S., Kitamura, I., and Kaji, M. Incidence of subacute sclerosing panencephalitis following measles and measles vaccination in Japan. *Int. J. Epidemiol.* 18:684–689, 1989.
204. Oldstone, M.B.A., Bokisch, V.A., Dixon, F.J., Barbosa, L.H., Fuccillo, D., and Sever, J.L. Subacute sclerosing panencephalitis: Destruction of human brain cells by antibody and complement in an autologous system. *Clin. Immunol. Immunopathol.* 4:52–58, 1975.
205. Orban, T. Beiträge zu den Augenhintergrund sveränderungen bei Sclerosis multiplex. *Ophthalmologica* 130:387–396, 1955.
206. Osetowska, E., and Torck, P. Subacute sclerosing leukoencephalitis: Analysis of complementary features. *World Neurol.* 3:566–579, 1962.
207. Oyanagi, S., ter Muelen, V., Katz, M., and Koprowski, H. Comparison of subacute sclerosing panencephalitis and measles viruses: An electron microscope study. *J. Virol.* 7:176–187, 1971.
208. Padgett, B.L., Walker, D.L., ZuRhein, G.M., Eckroade, R.J., and Dessel, B.H. Cultivation of papova-like virus from human brain with progressive multifocal leukoencephalopathy. *Lancet* 1:1257–1260, 1971.
209. Parhad, I.M., Johnson, K.P., Wolinsky, J.S., and Swoveland, P. Measles retinopathy: A hamster model of acute and chronic lesions. *Lab. Invest.* 43:52–60, 1980.
210. Parker, J.C., Klintworth, G.K., Graham, D.G., and Griffith, J.F. Uncommon morphologic features in subacute sclerosing panencephalitis (SSPE). *Am. J. Pathol.* 61:275–284, 1970.
211. Patrick, B.A., Mehta, P.D., Sobczyk, W., Kulczycki, J., Woyciechowska-Camenga, J., Camenga, D., and Thormar, H. Measles virus-specific immunoglobulin D antibody in cerebrospinal fluid and serum from patients with subacute sclerosing panencephalitis and multiple sclerosis. *J. Neuroimmunol.* 26:69–74, 1990.
212. Paty, D.W., Cousin, H.K., and Stiller, C.R. HLA antigens and mitogen responsiveness in multiple sclerosis. *Transplant. Proc. Suppl.* 19:187–189, 1977.
213. Paufique, L., and Étienne, R. Un signe peu connu de la sclérose en plaque: La périphlébite des veines rétiniennes. *Ann. Oculist* 188:701–707, 1955.
214. Payne, F.E., Baublis, J.V., and Itabashi, H.H. Isolation of measles virus from cell cultures of brain from a patient with subacute sclerosing panencephalitis. *N. Engl. J. Med.* 281:585–589, 1969.
215. Pearce, W.G. Ocular and genetic features of Cockayne's syndrome. *Can. J. Ophthalmol.* 7:435–443, 1972.
216. Périer, O., and Vanderhaeghen, J.J. Indications étiologigues approtées par la microscopie électronique dans certaines encéphalites humaines. *Rev. Neurol.* 115:250–254, 1966.
217. Périer, O., Vanderhaeghen, J.J., and Pele, S. Subacute sclerosing leukoencephalitis. *Acta Neuropathol.* 8:362–380, 1967.
218. Peters, G. Multiple Sklerose. In *Hundbuch der speziellen pathologischen Anatomie und Histologie*, Vol. 13/2A, O. Lubarsch, F. Henke, and R. Rossle (Eds.), Springer-Verlag, Berlin, pp. 519–602, 1958.
219. Pham-Dinh, D., Popot, J.L., Boespflug-Tanguy, O., Landrieu, P., Deleuze, J.F., Boue, J., Jolles, P., and Dautigny, A. Pelizaeus-Merzbacher disease: A valine to phenylalanine point mutation in a putative extracellular loop of myelin proteolipid. *Proc. Natl. Acad. Sci. USA* 88:7562–7566, 1991.
220. Pincus, J.H., Cooper, J.R., Itokawa, Y., and Gumbinas, M. Subacute necrotizing encephalomyelopathy: Effects of thiamine and thiamine propyl disulfide. *Arch. Neurol.* 24:511–517, 1971.
221. Pincus, J.H., Cooper, J.R., Piros, K., and Turner, V. Specificity of the urine inhibitor test for Leigh's disease. *Neurology* 19:885–890, 1974.
222. Pincus, J.H., Itokawa, Y., and Cooper, J.R. Enzyme-inhibiting factor in subacute necrotizing encephalomyelopathy. *Neurology* 19:841–845, 1969.
223. Powell, H., Tindall, R., Schultz, P., Paa, D., O'Brien, J., and Lampert, P. Adrenoleukodystrophy: Electron microscopic findings. *Arch. Neurol.* 32:250–260, 1975.
224. Powers, J.M., Liu, Y., Moser, A.B., and Moser, H.W. The inflammatory myelinopathy of adreno-leukodystrophy: Cells, effector molecules, and pathogenetic implications. *J. Neuropathol. Exp. Neurol.* 51:630–643, 1992.
225. Powers, J.M., and Schaumburg, H.H. The adrenal cortex in adrenoleukodystrophy. *Arch. Pathol.* 96:304–310, 1973.
226. Pratt, V.M., Troffater, J.A., Schinzel, A., Dlouhy, S.R., Conneally, P.M., and Hodes, M.E. A new mutation in the proteolipid protein (PLP) gene in a German family with Pelizaeus-Merzbacher disease. *Am. J. Med. Genet.* 38:136–139, 1991.
227. Prineas, J. Pathology of the early lesion in multiple sclerosis. *Hum. Pathol.* 6:531–554, 1975.
228. Prineas, J.W. The neuropathology of multiple sclerosis. In *Handbook of Clinical Neurology*, Vol. 47 (revised series), P.J. Vinken and G.W. Bruyn (Eds.), North Holland, Amsterdam, Chap. 8, pp. 213–257, 1985.
229. Prineas, J.W., Kwon, E.E., Goldenberg, P.Z., Cho, E.-S., and Sharer, L.R. Interaction of astrocytes and newly formed oligodendrocytes in resolving multiple sclerosis lesions. *Lab. Invest.* 61:489–503, 1989.
230. Prineas, J.W., Kwon, E.E., Goldenberg, P.Z., Ilyas, A.A., Quarles, R.H., Benjamins, J.A., and Sprinkle, T.J. Multiple sclerosis: Oligodendrocyte proliferation and differentiation in fresh lesions. *Lab. Invest.* 61:489–503, 1989.
231. Proops, R., Taylor, A.M.R., and Insley, J. A clinical study of a family with Cockayne's syndrome. *J. Med. Genet.* 18:288–293, 1981.

232. Radcrmcckcr, J. Leucoencéphalite subaiguë sclérosant avec lesions des ganglions rachidiens et des nerfs. *Rev. Neurol.* 81:1009–1017, 1949.
233. Rahn, E.K., Yanoff, M., and Tucker, S. Neuro-ocular considerations in the Pelizaeus Merzbacher syndrome: A clinicopathologic study. *Am. J. Ophthalmol.* 66:1143–1151, 1968.
234. Raine, C.S., Hummelgard, A., Swanson, E., and Bornstein, M.B. Multiple sclerosis: Serum-induced demyelination in vitro. *J. Neurol. Sci.* 20:127–148, 1973.
235. Raine, C.S., Powers, J.M., and Suzuki, I. Acute multiple sclerosis: Confirmation of "paramyxovirus-like" intranuclear inclusions. *Arch. Neurol.* 30:39–46, 1974.
236. Rao, N.A., Tso, M.O.M., and Zimmerman, L.E. Experimental allergic optic neuritis in guinea pigs: Preliminary report. *Invest. Ophthalmol. Vis. Sci.* 16:338–342, 1977.
237. Raskind, W.H., Williams, C.A., Hudson, L.D., and Bird, T.D. Complete deletion of the proteolipid protein gene (PLP) in a family with X-linked Pelizaeus-Merzbacher disease. *Am. J. Hum. Genet.* 49:1355–1360, 1991.
238. Reddy, M.M., and Goh, R.O. B and T lymphocytes in man. III. B, T, and "null" lymphocytes in multiple sclerosis. *Neurology* 26:997–999, 1976.
239. Reinikainen, K., Saksa, M., Murros, K., Kulju, T., Partanen, J., Paljärvi, L., and Riekkinen, P. Aikuispolitaan subakuutti sklerosoiva panenkefaliitti. *Duodecim* 104:1712–1717, 1988.
240. Resnick, J.S., Engel, W.K., and Sever, J.L. Subacute sclerosing panencephalitis spontaneous improvement in a patient with elevated measles antibody in blood and spinal fluid. *N. Engl. J. Med.* 279:126–129, 1968.
241. Reyes, J.M., and Hoenig, E.M. Intracellular spiral inclusions in cerebral cell processes in Creutzfeldt-Jakob disease. *J. Neuropathol. Exp. Neurol.* 40:1–8, 1981.
242. Reynaud, P., Loiseau, H., Coquet, M., Vital, C., and Loiseau, P. Un cas adulte d'encephalomyelopathie necrosante subaiguë de Leigh. *Rev. Neurol.* 144:259–265, 1988.
243. Robinson, B.H., De Meirleir, L., Glerum, M., Sherwood, G., and Becker, L. Clinical presentation of mitochondrial respiratory chain defects in NADH-coenzyme Q reductase and cytochrome oxidase: clues to pathogenesis of Leigh disease. *J. Pediatr.* 110:216–222, 1987.
244. Ross, C.A.C., Lenman, J.A.R., and Melville, I.D. Virus antibody levels in multiple sclerosis. *Br. Med. J.* 3:512–513, 1969.
245. Roth, A.M., Keltner, J.L., Ellis, W.G., and Martins-Green, M. Virus-simulating structures in the optic nerve head in Creutzfeldt-Jakob disease. *Am. J. Ophthalmol.* 87:827–823, 1979.
246. Rowlatt, U. Cockayne's syndrome: Report of case with necropsy findings. *Acta Neuropathol. (Berl).* 14:52–61, 1969.
247. Rucker, C.W. Sheathing of the retinal veins in multiple sclerosis. *Mayo Clin. Proc.* 19:176–178, 1944.
248. Rucker, C.W. Sheathing of the retinal veins in multiple sclerosis. *JAMA* 127:970–973, 1945.
249. Rucker, C.W. Retinopathy of multiple sclerosis. *Trans. Am. Ophthalmol. Soc.* 45:564–570, 1947.
250. Rucker, C.W. Sheathing of the retinal veins in multiple sclerosis. *Mayo Clin. Proc.* 47:335–340, 1972.
251. Sabin, A.B., and Messare, G. Fluorescent antibody technique in the study of fixed tissues from patients with encephalitis. In *Encephalitides: Proceedings of a Symposium on the Neuropathology, Electroencephalography and Biochemistry of Encephalitides*, Antwerp, 1959, L. Van Bogaert, J. Radermecker, J. Hozay, and A. Lowenthal (Eds.), Elsevier, Amsterdam, pp. 621–626, 1961.
252. Sadun, A.A., Borchert, M., DeVita, E., Hinton, D., and Bassi, C. Assessment of visual impairments in patients with Alzheimer's disease. *Am. J. Ophthalmol.* 104:113–120, 1987.
253. Salmon, J.F., Pan, E.L., and Murray, A.D. Visual loss with dancing extremities and mental disturbances. *Surv. Ophthalmol.* 35:299–306, 1991.
254. Scangos, G., and Bieberich, C. Gene transfer into mice. *Adv. Genet.* 24:285–322, 1987.
255. Schapira, K., Poskanzer, D.C., and Miller, H. Familial and conjugal multiple sclerosis. *Brain* 86:315–332, 1963.
256. Schiott, C.R. On the significance of inclusion bodies in subacute encephalitis. In *Encephalitides: Proceedings of a Symposium on the Neuropathology, Electroencephalography and Biochemistry of Encephalitides*, Antwerp, 1959, L. Van Bogaert, J. Radermecker, J. Hozay, and A. Lowenthal (Eds.), Elsevier, Amsterdam, pp. 410–413, 1961.
257. Schmickel, R.D., Chu, E.H.Y., Trosko, J.E., and Chang, C.C. Cockayne syndrome: A cellular sensitivity to ultraviolet light. *Pediatrics* 60:135–139, 1977.
258. Schneider-Schaulies, S., Kreth, H.W., Hofmann, G., Billeter, M., and ter Meulen, V. Expression of measles virus RNA in peripheral blood mononuclear cells of patients with measles, SSPE, and autoimmune diseases. *Virology* 182:703–711, 1991.
259. Schubert, P. Atypischer Fall einer subakuten sklerosierenden Leukoencephalitis (van Bogaert). *Acta Neuropathol. (Berl.)* 6:93–97, 1966.
260. Sedwick, L.A., Burde, R.M., and Hodges, F.J. Leigh's subacute nectrotizing encephalopathy presenting as spasmus nutans. *Arch. Ophthalmol.* 102:1046–1048, 1984.
261. Shaw, C.M. Electron microscopic observations in subacute sclerosing panencephalitis: A supplementary report. *Neurology* 18:144–145, 1968.
262. Shaw, C.M., Buchan, G.C., and Carlson, C.B. Myxovirus as a possible etiologic agent in subacute inclusion-body encephalitis. *N. Engl. J. Med.* 277:511–515, 1967.

263. Shaw, P.J., Smith, N.M., Ince, P.G., and Bates, D. Chronic periphlebitis retinae in multiple sclerosis: A histopathological study. *J. Neurol. Sci.* 77:147–152, 1987.
264. Shibasaki, H., Okirhiro, M.M., and Kuroiwa, Y. Multiple sclerosis among Orientals and Caucasians in Hawaii: A reappraisal. *Neurology* 28:109–112, 1978.
265. Sibley, W.A., and Foley, J.M. Infection and immunization in multiple sclerosis. *Ann. Acad. Sci.* 122:457–468, 1965.
266. Siemes, H., Goebel, H.H., Sengers, R.C.A., Ruitenbeek, W., and Trijbels, J.M.F. Subakute nekrotisierende Encephalomyelopathie Leigh infolge verminderter Aktivatat des Pyruvat-Dehydrogenase-Komplexes. *Monatsschr. Kinderheilkd.* 135:821–826, 1987.
267. Singh, G., Lott, M.T., and Wallace, D.C. A mitochondrial DNA mutation as a cause of Leber's hereditary optic neuropathy. *N. Engl. J. Med.* 320:1300–1305, 1989.
268. Small, J.A., Scangos, G.A., Cork, L., Jay, G., and Khoury, G. The early region of human papovavirus JC induces dysmyelination in transgenic mice. *Cell* 46:13–18, 1986.
269. Smith, M.E. The turnover of myelin proteins. *Neurobiology* 2:35–40, 1972.
270. Stahl, N., and Prusiner, S.B. Prions and prion proteins. *FASEB J.* 5:2799–2812, 1991.
271. Stansbury, F.C. Neuromyelitis optica (Dévic's disease). *Arch. Ophthalmol.* 42:292–335, 465–501, 1949.
272. Stoner, G.L., and Ryschkewitsch, C.F. Evidence for JC virus in two progressive multifocal leukoencephalopathy (PML) brains previously reported to be infected with SV 40. *J. Neuropathol. Exp. Neurol.* 50:342, 1991.
273. Symington, G.R., and Mackay, I.R. Cell-mediated immunity to measles virus in multiple sclerosis: Correlation with disability. *Neurology* 28:109–112, 1978.
274. Szreterowa, M., and Karkowska, B. Zaburzenia widzenia i zmiany na dnie oczu jako pierwsze objawy podostrego, stwardniającego zapalenia mózgu u dzieci dzieci. *Klin. Oczna* 90:329–330, 1988.
275. Taccone, A., Di Rocco, M., Fondelli, P., and Cottafava, F. Leigh disease: Value of CT in presymptomatic patients and variability of the lesions with time. *J. Comput. Assist. Tomogr.* 13:207–210, 1989.
276. Tanaka, R., Iwasaki, Y., and Koprowski, A. Unusual intranuclear filament in multiple sclerosis brain. *Lancet* 1:1236–1237, 1974.
277. Tanaka, J., Nakamura, H., and Fukada, T. Adult-onset subacute sclerosing panencephalitis: Immunocytochemical and electron microscopic demonstration of the viral antigen. *Clin. Neuropathol.* 6:30–37, 1987.
278. Tellez-Nagel, I., and Harter, D.H. Subacute sclerosing leukoencephalitis: Ultrastructure of intranuclear and intracytoplasmic inclusions. *Science* 154:899–901, 1966.
279. Terasak, P.I., Park, M.S., Opelz, G.G., and Ting, A. Multiple sclerosis and high incidence of a B lymphocyte antigen. *Science* 193:1245–1237, 1976.
280. Ter Meulen, B., Koprowski, H., Iwasaki, Y., Kackell, Y.M., and Müller, D. Fusion of cultured multiple sclerosis brain cells: Presence of nucleocapsids and virions and isolation of parainfluenza-type virus. *Lancet* 2:1–5, 1972.
281. Thiry, L., Dachy, A., and Lowenthal, A. Measles antibodies in patients with various types of measles infection. *Arch. Ges. Virusforsch.* 28:278–284, 1969.
282. Thormar, H., Brown, H.R., Goller, N.L., Barshatzky, M.R., and Wisniewski, H.M. Transmission of measles virus encephalitis to ferrets by intracardiac inoculation of a cell-associated SSPE virus strain. *Acta Pathol. Microbiol. Immunol. Scand.* 96:1125–1128, 1988.
283. Timm, G. Histologische Retina-Befunde bei der subakuten sklerosierenden Leukoencephalitis van Bogaert. *Confin. Neurol.* 25:147–155, 1965.
284. Tourtellotte, W.W. Cerebrospinal fluid in multiple sclerosis. In *Handbook of Clinical Neurology*, Vol. 47, P.J. Vinken and G.W. Bruyn (Eds.), North Holland, Amsterdam, Chap. 4, pp. 79–130, 1985.
285. Tourtellotte, W.W. Cerebrospinal fluid immunoglobulins and the central nervous system as an immunological organ particularly in multiple sclerosis and subacute sclerosing panencephalitis. *Res. Publ. Assoc. Res. Nerv. Ment. Dis.* 49:112–155, 1971.
286. Toussaint, D., Perier, O., Verstappen, A., and Bervoets, S. Clinicopathological study of the visual pathways, eyes, and cerebral hemispheres in 32 cases of disseminated sclerosis. *J. Clin. Neuro Ophthalmol.* 63:211–220, 1983.
287. Towfighi, J., Young, R., Sassani, J., and Horoupian, D.S. Alexander's disease: Further light-, and electron-microscopic observations. *Acta Neuropathol. (Berl.)* 61:36–42, 1983.
288. Traub, R.G., and Rucker, C.W. The relationship of retrobulbar neuritis to multiple sclerosis. *Am. J. Ophthalmol.* 37:494–497, 1954.
289. Treusch, J.V., and Rucker, C.W. Incidence of changes in the retinal veins in multiple sclerosis. *Proc. Mayo Clin.* 19:253–254, 1944.
289a. Troelstra, A., van Gool, J., de Wit, J., Vermeulen, W., Bootsma, D., and Hoeijmakers, J.H.J. ERCC6, a member of a subfamily of putative helicases, is involved in Cockayne's syndrome and preferential repair of active genes. *Cell* 71:939–953, 1992.
290. Troffatter, J.A., Dlouhy, S.R., DeMeyer, W., Conneally, P.M., and Hodes, M.E. Pelizaeus-Merzbacher disease: Tight linkage to proteolipid protein gene exon variant. *Proc. Natl. Acad. Sci. USA* 86:9427–9430, 1989.
291. Ulrich, J., and Kidd, M. Subacute inclusion body encephalitis: A histological and electron microscopical study. *Acta Neuropathol. (Berl.)* 6:359–370, 1966.

292. Van Bogaert, L. Die klinischc Einheit und die pathologische Variationsbreite der "subakuten sklerosierenden Leukoenzephalitis." *Wien. Z. Nervenheilkd. 13*:185–203, 1957.
293. van Buren, J.M. A case of subacute inclusion encephalitis studied by the metallic methods. *J. Neuropathol. Exp. Neurol. 13*:230–247, 1954.
294. van Erven, P.M.M. Gabreëls, F.J., Wevers, R.A., Doesburg, W.H., Ruitenbeek, W., Renier, W.O., and Lamers, K.J. Intravenous pyruvate loading test in Leigh syndrome. *J. Neurol. Sci. 77*:217–227, 1987.
295. Vignaendra, V., Lim, C.L., and Chen, S.T. Subacute sclerosing panencephalitis with unusual ocular movements: Polygraphic studies. *Neurology 28*:1052–1056, 1978.
296. Vogel, F.S., and Hallervorden, J. Leukodystrophy with diffuse Rosenthal fiber formation. *Acta Neuropathol. (Berl.) 2*:126–143, 1962.
297. Waksman, B.H., and Adams, R.D. Allergic neuritis: An experimental disease of rabbits induced by the injection of peripheral nervous tissue and adjuvants. *J. Exp. Med. 102*:231–235, 1955.
298. Walker, D.L. Progressive multifocal leukoencephalopathy. In *Handbook of Clinical Neurology*, Vol. 47, P.J. Vinken and G.W. Bruyn (Eds.), North Holland, Amsterdam, Chap. 18, pp. 503–524, 1985.
299. Wallace, D.C. Mitochondrial genetics: A paradigm for aging and degenerative disease? *Science 256*:628–632, 1992.
300. Wallace, D.C., Gurparkash, S., Lott, M.T., Hodge, J.A., Schurr, T.C., Lezza, A.M.S., Elsas, L.J., and Nikoskelinen, E.K. Mitochondrial DNA mutation associated with Leber's hereditary optic neuropathy. *Science 242*:1427–1430, 1988.
301. Watanabe, I., and Okazaki, H. Virus-like structure in multiple sclerosis. *Lancet 2*:569–570, 1973.
302. Weimbs, T., Dick, T., Stoffel, W., and Boltshauser, E. A point mutation at the X-chromosomal proteolipid locus in Pelizaeus-Merzbacher disease leads to disruption of myelinogenesis. *Biol. Chem. Hoppe Seyler 371*:1175–1183, 1990.
303. Wiener, L.P., Johnson, R.T., and Herndon, R.M. Viral infections and demyelinating diseases. *N. Engl. J. Med. 288*:1103–1110, 1973.
304. Willems, P.J., Vits, L., Wanders, R.J., Coucke, P.J., van der Auwera, B.J., van Elsen, A.F., Raeymaekers, P., van Broeckhoven, C., Schutgens, R.B., Dacremont, G., Leroy, J.G., Martin, J.J., and Dumon, J.E. Linkage of DNA markers at Xq28 to adrenoleukodystrophy and adrenomyeloneuropathy present within the same family. *Arch. Neurol. 47*:665–669, 1990.
305. Williams, A.C., Mingioli, E.S., McFarland, H.F., Tourtellotte, W.W., and McFarlin, D.E. Increased CSF IgM in multiple sclerosis. *Neurology 28*:996–998, 1978.
306. Winchester, R.J., Ebers, G., Fu, S.M., Espinosa, L., Zabriskie, J., and Kunkel, H.G. B-cell alloantigen Ag 7a in multiple sclerosis. *Lancet 2*:814, 1975.
307. Wong, T.C., Ayata, M., Hirano, A., Yoshikawa, Y., Tsuruoka, H., and Yamanouchi, K. Generalized and localized biased hypermutation affecting the matrix gene of a measles virus strain that causes subacute sclerosing panencephalitis. *J. Virol. 63*:5464–5468, 1989.
308. Wray, S.H., Cogan, D.G., Kuwabara, T., Schaumburg, H.H., and Powers, J.M. Adrenoleukodystrophy with disease of the eye and optic nerve. *Am. J. Ophthalmol. 82*:480–485, 1976.
309. Wucherpfennig, K.W., Ota, K., Endo, N., Seidman, J.G., Rosenzweig, A., Weiner, H.L., and Hafler, D.A. Shared human T cell receptor Vβ usage to immunodominant regions of myelin basic protein. *Science 248*:1016–1019, 1990.
310. Wybar, K.C. The ocular manifestations of disseminated sclerosis. *Proc. R. Soc. Med. 45*:315–320, 1952.
311. Yamagata, T., Yano, S., Okabe, I., Miyao, M., Momoi, M.Y., Yanagisawa, M., Hirata, H., and Komatsu, K. Ultrasonography and magnetic resonance imaging in Leigh disease. *Pediatr. Neurol. 6*:326–329, 1990.
312. Yamaguchi, K., Okabe, H., and Tamai, M. Corneal perforation in a patient with Cockayne's syndrome. *Cornea 10*:79–80, 1991.
313. Yoshikawa, Y., Yamanouchi, K., Takasu, T., Rauf, S., and Ahmed, A. Structural homology between hemagglutinin (HA) of measles virus and the active site of long neurotoxins. *Virus Genes 5*:57–67, 1991.
314. Zeman, W., and Kolar, O. Reflections on the etiology and pathogenesis of subacute sclerosing panencephalitis. *Neurology 18*:1–7, 1968.
315. Zu Rhein, G.M., and Chou, S.M. Subacute sclerosing panencephalitis: Ultrastructural study of a brain biopsy. *Neurology 18*:146–158, 1968.

54
Muscular Disorders

Edward H. Bossen
Duke University Medical Center, Durham, North Carolina

I. INTRODUCTION

Most evaluations of muscle disease have been derived from the study of extremity muscles, which differ from extraocular muscles. Before discussing muscle diseases that affect the eye, the structure of both extremity (limb) muscle and extraocular muscles is considered so that the differences can be pointed out.

II. NORMAL LIMB MUSCLES

A skeletal muscle, such as the biceps, consists of bundles (fasciculi) of individual muscle fibers with connective tissue surrounding each fasciculus (perimysium) and individual muscle fibers (endomysium; Fig. 1). The contractile element of the muscle fiber is the myofibril, which is composed of essentially parallel arrays of actin and myosin filaments. Skeletal muscle is called striated muscle because of its banded microscopic appearance from the A (anisotropic), I (isotropic), and Z (*Zwischenscheibe*) bands. The I band, which is pale when stained with hematoxylin and eosin, contains the actin filaments (5–8 nm in diameter), which are anchored at the thin, dense Z band. The dark A band contains the thicker (15 nm in diameter) myosin filaments, as well as actin filaments, which slide between the myosin filaments during contraction. The basic contractile unit of skeletal muscle is the sarcomere, which extends from Z band to Z band (Fig. 2).

In addition to myofibrils, the muscle fibers contain mitochondria, which contribute energy; sarcoplasmic reticulum, believed to be important in the release and uptake of calcium essential for muscle contraction and relaxation; transverse tubules, believed to aid in transmission of the action potential from the periphery to the interior of the cells; and other cytoplasmic components, including glycogen, ribosomes, and rare lysosomes (Fig. 3).

The concept of the motor unit—a neuron, its axon, and the muscle fibers it innervates—is important for understanding the histopathology of muscle disease. The muscle fibers contract when stimulated by the axon at a specialized portion of the fiber, the motor end plate. The action potential travels along the surface of the muscle fiber and into the interior of the fibers via the transverse tubules. A portion of the sarcoplasmic reticulum, known as junctional sarcoplasmic reticulum, abuts the plasmalemma at the transverse tubule and the periphery of the fiber [8]. Calcium bound within the junctional sarcoplasmic reticulum is released, in an unknown fashion, by the action potential, allowing contraction. Relaxation occurs when calcium is taken up by the free sarcoplasmic reticulum, which lacks the granules of the junctional sarcoplasmic reticulum.

Reference should be made to specialized texts for more detailed information on the structure and physiology of muscle [154,116].

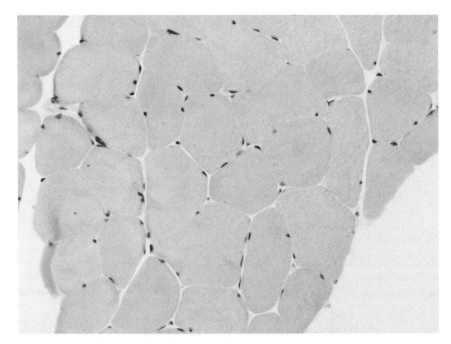

Figure 1   Normal muscle. (Hematoxylin and eosin, ×250)

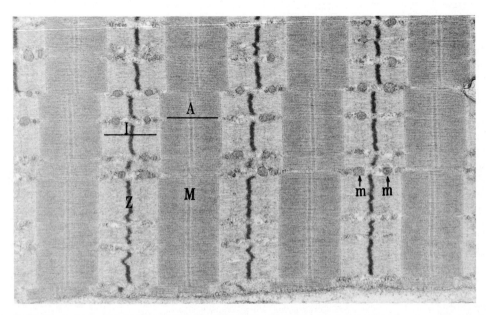

Figure 2   Normal muscle. A, A band; I, I band; M, M line (middle of A band); Z, Z line; m, mitochondria.
(×12,500)

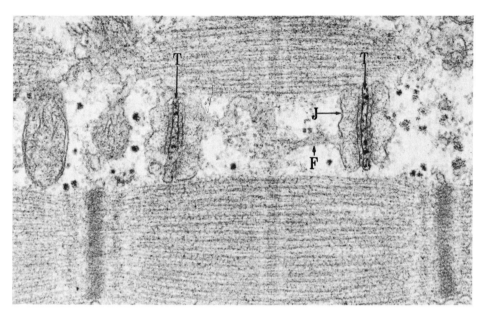

Figure 3 Normal muscle. T, transverse tubular system; J, junctional sarcoplasmic reticulum; F, free sarcoplasmic reticulum. (×50,000)

III. GENERAL CONCEPTS OF MUSCLE PATHOLOGY

Abnormalities of any of the components of the motor unit may lead to neuromuscular disease, of which there are two main categories: myopathies and neurogenic disorders. The characteristic histological features of a myopathy, as defined in limb muscle, are variation in fiber size, rounding of fibers (normally polygonal), both hypertrophic and atrophic fibers, central nuclei in more than 3% of fibers, fiber regeneration and degeneration, myophagocytosis (macrophages within degenerating muscle fibers), endomysial fibrosis (increase in connective tissue around individual fibers), and fiber splitting (Fig. 4). Polymyositis, an inflammatory myopathy, has an infiltrate of lymphocytes, plasma cells, and sometimes eosinophils in addition to the aforementioned features of a myopathy. Some experts exclude fiber hypertrophy from the list of features of polymyositis. Neurogenic atrophy is characterized by group fiber atrophy (Fig. 5) with angulation of the atrophic fibers (Fig. 6). Central nuclei and endomysial fibrosis are not basic features of neurogenic atrophy but can be seen together with degenerating, regenerating, and hypertrophic fibers in long-standing denervation. This pattern is referred to as myopathic change secondary to chronic denervation.

Enzyme histochemistry is a considerable aid in the diagnosis of neuromuscular disorders, its usefulness being based on the fact that all muscle fibers do not have the same distribution of cytoplasmic components. For diagnostic purposes, human skeletal muscle fibers can be divided into two major groups: type 1 and type 2. In general, type 1 fibers are slow-twitch fibers with predominantly aerobic metabolism reflected by the presence of numerous mitochondria. Type 2 fibers are fast twitch and mainly anaerobic and have fewer mitochondria than type 1 fibers. Fiber characteristics are largely determined by neurogenic influence and can be altered by cross-innervation [84,300]. In humans, muscles are composed of both type 1 and 2 fibers, arranged in a checkerboard pattern (Figs. 7 and 8). This pattern is demonstrated by a variety of histochemical techniques, but muscle fiber typing is based primarily on the distribution of myosin adenosine triphosphatase. Type 1 fibers stain poorly for this enzyme, whereas type 2 fibers stain intensely (Fig. 7 and Table 1). Further subdivisions can be based on other staining procedures [86].

Histochemistry is particularly helpful in the diagnosis of denervation. In denervating diseases, some fibers lose their nerve supply and atrophy, but others are reinnervated by sprouting of axons normally supplying adjacent muscle fibers. When this occurs, the reinnervated fibers assume the histochemical staining of the neighboring fibers normally supplied by that axon. This results in a pattern termed "fiber

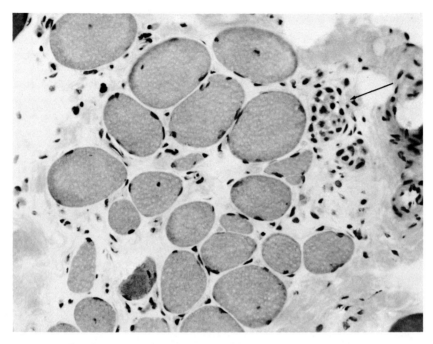

Figure 4   Myopathy. Note the rounded fibers, internal nuclei, increased connective tissue around fibers, and myophagocytosis (arrow). (Metatoxylin and eosin, ×250)

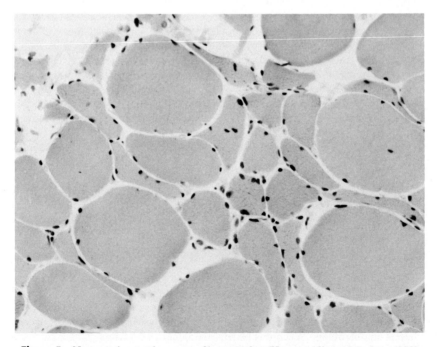

Figure 5   Neurogenic atrophy, group fiber atrophy. (Hematoxylin and eosin, ×250)

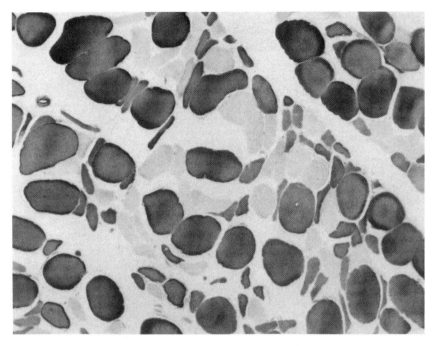

Figure 6 Denervation. Angulated, atrophic fibers that are both type 1 (pale) and type 2 (dark) are seen. (Myosin adenosine triphosphatase stain, ×100)

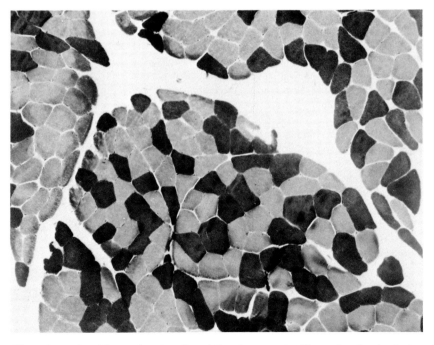

Figure 7 Normal muscle with myosin adenosine triphosphatase stain, illustrating the checkerboard pattern with pale type 1 and dark type 2 fibers. (×110)

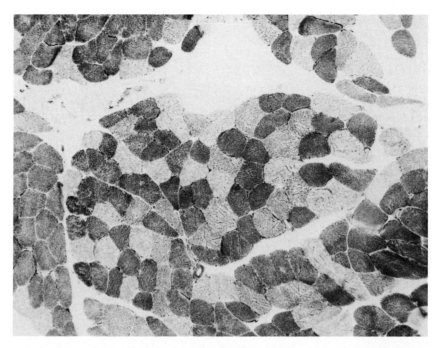

Figure 8 Normal muscle illustrating dark type 1 and pale type 2 fibers. Compare with Figure 7, which is the same field but slightly rotated. (Nicotinamide adenine dinucleotide tetrazolium reductase stain, ×100)

type grouping" rather than the normal checkerboard pattern (Fig. 9). Such fibers may be of normal size and configuration and thus are not recognized in the absence of histochemical enzyme staining. Eventually the neuron or axon supplying this group of fibers may itself become involved in the disease process, resulting in the classic feature of denervation, group fiber atrophy (Fig. 5). In denervation, atrophic fibers are both type 1 and 2 (Fig. 6), whereas in disuse atrophy, or steroid myopathy the atrophic fibers are type 2.

    Another characteristic of denervation best seen with histochemical stains is that of the "target" fiber (Fig. 10). In denervation there is segmental central disruption of the myofibrils, with loss of membranous structures, including mitochondria, in this central zone and aggregation of mitochondria at the periphery of the disrupted area. Staining of a cross section of muscle for nicotinamide adenine dinucleotide tetrazolium reductase, which demonstrates mitochondria, reveals a central clear zone (no mitochondria) surrounded by an intensely staining zone (aggregates of mitochondria), the remainder of the fiber assuming normal staining characteristics. Not all denervated muscle manifest this change, but when it is seen, it is strongly suggestive of denervation.

Table 1 Muscle Fiber Types: Limb Muscles

	Muscle type	
Attribute	Type 1	Type 2
Myosin adenosine triphosphatase stain	Pale	Dark
Succinic dehydrogenase stain	Dark	Pale
Mitochondria	More	Fewer
Twitch type	Slow	Fast

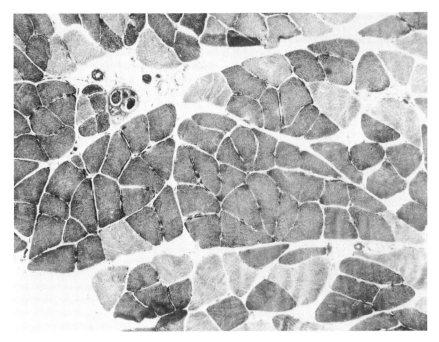

Figure 9 Denervation. The normal checkerboard pattern is lost, with almost entire fasciculi of one type, a change referred to as type grouping. In this instance the dark fibers are type 1. (Nicotinamide adenine dinucleotide tetrazolium reductase stain, ×100)

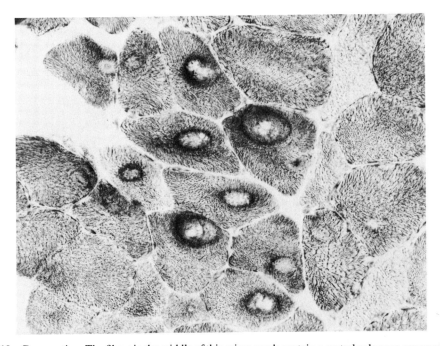

Figure 10 Denervation. The fibers in the middle of this micrograph contain a central pale zone surrounded by a dark rim. These are target fibers. (Nicotinamide adenine dinucleotide tetrazolium reductase stain, ×250)

IV. NORMAL EXTRAOCULAR MUSCLES

Extraocular muscles differ from limb muscles. They are rounder, smaller (10–38 μm in diameter versus 40–60 μm) [52], have more internal nuclei, and have more endomysial tissue than limb muscle [59]. Variation in fiber size is normal for extraocular muscle fibers, larger fibers tending to be in the center of muscles and smaller fibers at the periphery (Fig. 11). These features, normal in extraocular muscle, are considered myopathic in limb muscle. *Ringbinden* (ringed fibers; see Sec. V.B) can also be seen in normal extraocular muscle [214].

The number of fiber types in extraocular muscle and their classification is controversial [40]. A number of subdivisions of extraocular muscles have been suggested [38,52,89,229,262,269,296], but basically there are three principal fiber types: fine, granular, and coarse (Table 2). The fine and granular fibers are referred to as *Fibrillenstruktur* and the coarse as *Felderstruktur* in the older literature [89,230]. In the levator palpebrae superioris, the three types are arranged randomly, but in the extraocular oblique and rectus muscles peripheral (orbital), intermediate, and central (global) zones are discernible [52,89,229, 296,310]. In the levator palpebrae superioris 75–80% of the fibers are coarse, the remainder being granular. In the oblique and rectus muscles the peripheral and intermediate zones consist of 80% coarse and 20% fine fibers, whereas the granular fibers comprise 75% of the central zone, the remainder being composed of equal portions of fine and coarse fibers.

Histochemical staining of extraocular muscles reveals that the fine fibers resemble limb muscle fiber type 1 in having minimal myosin adenosine triphosphatase activity, but in contrast to type 1 limb muscle fibers they have less succinic dehydrogenase and other oxidative enzyme activity. The granular fibers resemble type 2 limb muscle fibers, staining intensely for myosin adenosine triphosphatase and weakly for succinic dehydrogenase. The coarse fibers have properties of both type 1 and type 2 fibers, staining strongly for both myosin adenosine triphosphatase and succinic dehydrogenase [89,296].

Striated muscle has *en plaque* (plaquelike) and *en grappe* (grapelike) nerve endings [75,310]. Extraocular coarse fibers possess *en grappe* nerve endings; the fine and granular fibers have *en plaque* nerve

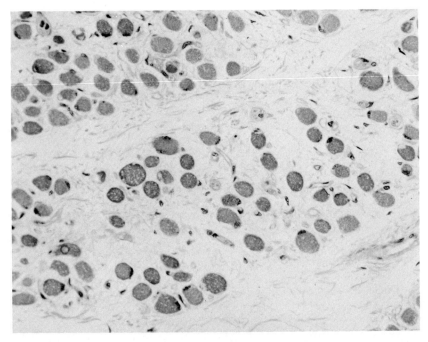

Figure 11 Normal extraocular muscle. Note the variation in fiber size, rounding of fibers, and abundant connective tissue. The fiber size is not directly comparable with illustrations of skeletal muscle since this is of fixed tissue and the skeletal muscle illustrations are of frozen tissue, except as indicated. (Hematoxylin and eosin, ×250)

Table 2 Muscle Fiber Types: Extraocular

| | Muscle type | | |
Attribute	Coarse	Fine	Granular
Myosin adenosine triphosphatase stain	Dark	Pale	Dark
Succinic dehydrogenase stain	Dark	Intermediate	Pale
Nerve endings	En grappe	En plaque	En plaque

Source: Modified from Durston, J.H.J., Histochemistry of primate extraocular muscles and the changes of denervation. Br. J. Ophthalmol. 58:193–216, 1974.

endings. Mammalian limb muscles are of the *en plaque* type, but slow tonic fibers in lower animals have the *en grappe* type of endings [89,296]. For this reason several authors have suggested that coarse fibers are related to slow tonic muscles [229,230,310], although histochemical differences exist [89,296]. Based on the histochemical findings and nerve endings, Durston [89] concluded that the coarse fibers were recruited primarily for fixation movements and the granular fibers for brief, eccentric movements. He did not assign a specific role to the fine fibers. The extraocular fibers with *en grappe* neuromuscular junctions have multiple neuromuscular junctions and may be supplied by more than one nerve. The *en grappe* neuromuscular junctions lack the secondary junctional folds of singly innervated extremity end plates, which may be a factor in the susceptibility of these fibers to myasthenia gravis [38].

The importance of these studies of normal extraocular muscles lies in the interpretation of myopathic as opposed to neurogenic changes in these muscles, the criteria for which were developed with respect to limb muscles. Do these rules also apply to extraocular muscles? Drachman and colleagues [81] studied the extraocular muscles of dogs following intracranial avulsion or crushing of the oculomotor nerve. They found the most striking changes 2 weeks to 1 month following denervation, with a gradual restoration of normal morphology thereafter. During the period of maximum change they noted infiltrates of inflammatory cells (predominantly lymphocytes), central nuclei in 20% of the fibers (their normal for extraocular muscles being 3–5%), fiber degeneration, myophagocytosis, basophilic fibers with plump vesicular nuclei (probably regenerating fibers), occasional fiber splitting, and increased connective tissue around individual fibers (endomysial fibrosis) and about muscle fasciculi (perimysial fibrosis). These findings indicate a myopathy in limb muscle. The one feature these authors noted that was not typical of a myopathy was loss of nerve fibers in the denervated animals. Large groups of atrophic fibers [89,246,296] were not seen in experimental denervation of extraocular muscles, presumably because the motor unit is much smaller in these muscles than those of the limbs. However, Minoda [230] reports group atrophy in neurogenic extraocular paralysis in humans.

Durston studied denervated extraocular muscles in baboons [89] with histochemical techniques and noted type grouping 6 months after denervation. The grouped fibers were predominantly of the fine type, which is most comparable to the principal fiber type involved in type grouping after denervation of limb muscle (limb type 1 fibers).

Ringel and colleagues [296] did not find type grouping in their studies of extraocular denervation in rhesus monkeys and had difficulty establishing the diagnosis of denervation by the morphological criteria used in limb muscle. Employing α-bungarotoxin, they were able to demonstrate extrajunctional binding, a characteristic of experimental denervation in limb muscle. This phenomenon is not diagnostic of denervation; moreover, only a minority of fine and granular fibers gave a positive response, and none did after 12 weeks.

Another component of limb muscle is the muscle spindle. The muscle fibers of the spindle, referred to as intrafusal muscle fibers, are divided into "nuclear chain" and "nuclear bag" fibers. As in limb muscles, muscle spindles also occur in human extraocular muscle, but the muscle fibers of the spindle (intrafusal fibers) cannot be differentiated into nuclear chain or nuclear bag types. Muscle spindles are not present in the baboon extraocular muscle [89].

When viewed by transmission electron microscopy extraocular muscles basically resemble limb skeletal muscle, but Z band alterations, abnormal mitochondria, and leptomeres (zebra bodies) have been reported in otherwise normal extraocular muscles [214]. The proportion of cytoplasm containing mitochondria is greater in extraocular muscles than in limb muscles [52]. Singly innervated orbital muscle fibers are the most oxidative [354].

Readers desiring more details of extraocular muscle structure and function are referred to the reviews of Ruff and colleagues [310] and Carry and Ringel [52].

V. NEUROMUSCULAR DISORDERS

A. Myasthenia Gravis

Clinical Features

Myasthenia gravis is a neuromuscular disorder characterized clinically by increasing weakness with repetitive muscle use but improved by anticholinesterase drugs. Estimates of the incidence for myasthenia gravis range from 2 to 10 per 100,000, 20% of the cases beginning in patients under 20 years old [329]. It is most commonly a generalized disease, 69–90% of the patients having extraocular muscle involvement, but in 13–14% of the cases there is only ptosis and/or ophthalmoplegia [136,212]. In approximately one-half of patients ocular myasthenia becomes generalized within 2 years [204]. Individuals who have pure ocular myasthenia who develop generalized myasthenia gravis do so within 3 years after onset of their ocular diseases [127,136,148,261]. Chinese have a higher percentage of pure ocular myasthenia [56].

The best diagnostic tool is the presence of serum anti-acetylcholine receptor (anti-ACR) antibodies; approximately 10% of patients with clinical myasthenia lack these antibodies [203], and 30–50% of those with pure ocular myasthenia lack anti-ACR antibodies [157,249].

In adults generalized myasthenia gravis affects females twice as often as males. The onset, usually between the ages of 20 and 35 years, may be gradual or sudden and may be precipitated by an illness or emotional disturbance. The course is variable, with most deaths during the first year and rarely after having the disease for 10 years. In a large study in Italy, 4% of patients died of myasthenia gravis [212]. Although any muscle may be affected, the extraocular muscles are most commonly involved, the neck muscles being the next most frequently affected. An abnormal facial expression, dysphagia, and dysarthria may be present, but sensory changes are uncommon [344].

Involvement of the extraocular muscles is manifest by ptosis and external ophthalmoplegia, which may be alternating and recurrent [28,125,261]. Pure ocular myasthenia is slightly more common in males, but the female-male ratio in patients under 20 years of age is 2:1. The extraocular muscles may be particularly vulnerable because of a lower safety factor for neuromuscular transmission due to the rapidity of firing and the simplified end plates normally present in these muscles [252]. The fetal isoforms of ACR present in the multiterminal fibers of extraocular muscles may make the eye muscles more susceptible [174,252]. Myasthenia gravis may be mistaken for progressive external ophthalmoplegia [43] or a focal lesion of the medial longitudinal fasciculus [129,227]. Internal ophthalmoplegia, characterized by dilated unequal pupils that respond to anticholinesterase agents, is very rare [18,153].

Approximately 10–20% of cases of myasthenia gravis occur in association with other autoimmune diseases, including rheumatoid arthritis [1,261,377], Sjögren's syndrome [148], systemic lupus erythematosus [261,377,408], polymyositis [189], scleroderma [261,272], hyperthyroidism [261], and Hashimoto's thyroiditis [260,377]. Patients over the age of 40 years are most likely to have other autoimmune diseases [61]. Patients treated with d-penicillamine for rheumatoid arthritis [324] or Wilson's disease may also develop myasthenia gravis [217]. From the standpoint of ophthalmologists, the association with thyroid disease is particularly important, since both myasthenia gravis and hyperthyroidism affect the extraocular muscles.

An inherited predisposition to myasthenia gravis may exist, and 3–5% of cases are familial. Studies on the association with human transplantation antigens (HLA; see Chap. 3) have shown an increase frequency of HLA-8 [249]. Pirskanen reported 72% of female myasthenics under 35 years old are HLA-8 (controls 17.5%) [279]. More than 70% of myasthenics with thymic hyperplasia are also HLA-8, whereas only 6–10% of those with thymoma are HLA-8 [120]. However, myasthenics with thymomas have a higher frequency of HLA-2 and a lower incidence of HLA-1 than controls or myasthenics without thymoma. The myasthenic patients with thymoma generally possess antibodies to skeletal muscle striations, whereas only 11% of those without thymoma have these antimuscle antibodies [257]. Pure ocular myasthenia gravis does not correlate with specific HLA antigens [279]. Fritze and colleagues [120] suggested that there are two forms of adult myasthenia gravis: a form occurring in females under 40 years old with thymic hyperplasia and low antimuscle antibody titers who are HLA-8, and non-HLA-8 patients, usually males over 40 years of age, with thymomas and high antimuscle antibody titers. The antibodies referred to here are those detected at muscle striations, not anti-ACR, which are discussed later. Compston and colleagues [61] found the highest anti-ACR antibody titers in patients with thymomas and the lowest in males over 40 years of age.

In myasthenia gravis electromyography discloses a diminished muscle action potential with repetitive nerve stimulation and reduced miniature end-plate potential amplitude. Miniature end-plate potentials are normal and produced by spontaneous release of small quantities of acetylcholine. Their amplitude is usually well below the threshold required to produce muscle contraction. The pharmacological tests for myasthenia gravis include improvement with anticholinesterase drugs, such as edrophonium or neostigmine, and increased sensitivity to curare. Extraocular muscles may not respond to neostigmine but are curare sensitive [43].

Morphological Features

In myasthenia gravis morphological abnormalities occur principally in skeletal muscle and the thymus. The muscle changes consist of a denervation pattern [41], with group fiber atrophy, angulated fibers, type grouping (Fig. 8), and focal infiltrates of lymphocytes ("lymphorrhages"). Maselli and colleagues [215] demonstrated monocytes or macrophages at the neuromuscular junction. In an analysis of 61 muscle biopsies from 46 myasthenics, Oosterhuis and Bethlem [257] found 17 examples of neurogenic atrophy and 26 lymphorrhages. Of 17 patients with thymoma 9 had lymphorrhages, but the denervation pattern did not correlate with the presence of thymoma. The question of denervation in myasthenia gravis is controversial despite morphological evidence of its presence [21]. Coërs and Telerman-Toppet point out that myasthenic patients characteristically have enlarged, elongated motor endings, whereas denervation is characterized by collateral branching of motor endings. However, they found evidence of denervation in 7 of 45 patients, all 7 being over 50 years old [57].

Of all myasthenic individuals 75% have thymic hyperplasia (85%) or a thymoma (15%) [247]. Chinese have a higher incidence of thymoma, 13 of 27 patients in one study, approximately two to three times the level in Western countries [372].

Of all patients with myasthenia gravis, 95% between the ages of 20 and 30 have thymic hyperplasia, which is defined as the presence of germinal centers in the thymus [249]. Berrih-Aknin and colleagues [24] point out that germinal centers may also occur in the thymus in other autoimmune diseases. Thymectomy is advocated early in the course of the disease for young patients [117,317], who usually have thymic hyperplasia (thymoma is rare in persons under 20 years of age) [117,311]. Following thymectomy, improvement is gradual, increasing from 10–12% remission in the first postoperative year to 30–37% in the fifth year, but eventually improvement occurs in 90% of thymectomized myasthenic patients with thymic hyperplasia. The presence of germinal centers in the thymus may be of prognostic significance, and those patients who lack germinal centers, or only have rare ones, improve more quickly than those with many germinal centers [128,267]; 10 years after thymectomy the improvement rate is equal regardless of the number of germinal centers [275]. Moran and colleagues [235] found no correlation between numbers of germinal centers and clinical improvement, but they found that the mean cross-sectional area, perimeter, and diameter were less in those who improved than in those who did not after thymectomy (excluding thymoma). Patients with thymoma do not respond as well following thymectomy, the first year remission and improvement rates being 6.5 and 18.8%, respectively, although patients who survive 2 years reportedly have a 33% remission rate if male and 13% if female [267]. Thymectomy is not used for pure ocular myasthenia [127]. Durelli and colleagues [88] found that patients operated on within 1 year after onset who did not require additional immunosuppressive therapy had a stable remission rate within 2 years after thymectomy of 44% versus 26% for other postthymectomy patients. They found improved remission rates after transsternal extended thymectomy but not after cervical thymectomy.

The thymus is a source of anti-ACR antibody production [122,319], thymic plasma cells being a major producer [404]. Thymectomy not only reduces a source of antibody but it also removes a source of antigen that maintains the autoimmune response [203]. There is a steady decrease in anti-ACR antibody titers between 6 weeks and 1 year after thymectomy [193]. The source may be thymic myoid cells or a source within the epithelial compartment of the thymus [24].

Etiology and Pathogenesis

The concept that myasthenia gravis is a presynaptic defect held sway until recently. Elmqvist and colleagues [90] demonstrated reduced miniature end-plate potential amplitude in myasthenia gravis, which was interpreted as a difficulty in packaging acetylcholine. Electron microscopy disclosed normal cholinergic vesicles, however, and a decreased surface area of the postsynaptic membrane with simplification of the postsynaptic area (specifically loss of secondary clefts), suggesting a postsynaptic defect [94,313]. Ito and colleagues [165] demonstrated normal acetylcholine release and increased acetylcholine in the intercostal muscle of myasthenic patients. Thornell and colleagues [378] suggested that degeneration of the postsynaptic folds with subsequent increased distance between pre- and postsynaptic areas may account for the diminished miniature end-plate potential and explain previous interpretations of a presynaptic defect in myasthenia gravis.

The discovery that α-bungarotoxin in snake venom binds irreversibly to ACR has enabled investigators to study these receptors, which are located principally on the terminal portions of the postsynaptic folds [98], where there are estimated to be 20,000–25,000 mm^{-2} [283]. The number of receptors is markedly reduced in myasthenia gravis (11–30% of controls) [106] and correlates with the patient's clinical status and the amplitude of the miniature end-plate potential [98]. Currently, myasthenia gravis is believed to be produced by antibodies to the ACR at the motor end plate [82].

The possibility of a humoral factor or toxin [50] in the pathogenesis of myasthenia gravis was suggested in the nineteenth century, when similarities between myasthenia and the effects of curare were noted. Other factors also pointed to a humoral factor: the transient myasthenia in infants of mothers with myasthenia gravis, the improvement in myasthenic patients after hemodialysis [150,360] or thoracic duct drainage [23,379], and the recurrence of myasthenia gravis with retransfusion of cell-free lymph from myasthenic individuals [23].

The association of myasthenia gravis with autoimmune diseases and the frequent occurrence of thymic abnormalities suggests an immunological role in myasthenia gravis. A major advance was the discovery that 70–90% of myasthenic patients had antibodies against the ACR [12,13,202]. The anti-ACR antibody titer cannot be used to predict severity when comparing groups of patients, but the decline in titer in patients with transient infantile myasthenia gravis [180] or undergoing plasma exchange [248] correlates with the clinical improvement in particular patients. The lowest titers occur in pure ocular myasthenia gravis [202]. The antibody to ACR does not correlate with a second type of antibody in myasthenia gravis, which is directed toward muscle striations [198], and the binding site of anti-ACR is not the same as the bungarotoxin binding site, since it only incompletely blocks toxin binding [181,202]. There is more than one type of antibody to the ACR [415]. Anti-ACR antibodies are polyclonal and are mostly directly against the main immunogenic region of the receptor [385]. Blocking, binding, and modulating antibodies exist [157].

Toyka et al. [382] demonstrated decreased miniature end-plate potential amplitude and fewer ACR in mice after repeated injections with human serum from myasthenic patients and identified the active fraction as IgG. This explains infantile transient myasthenic gravis, since IgG can cross the placenta. In experimental autoimmune myasthenia gravis of neonatal rats (see later), anti-ACR is passed through milk [314].

There is also morphological evidence for the role of immunoglobulins in myasthenia gravis. Rash and colleagues [291] described particles suggestive of antibodies on the surface of junctional folds in myasthenic muscle. A key link in the chain of evidence for the role of immunoglobulin in myasthenia gravis was the demonstration of IgG and the third component of complement (C3) at the motor end plate in patients with myasthenia at the sites of ACR [100]. Similar findings develop in experimental autoimmune myasthenia gravis, in which the amplitude of the miniature end-plate potential correlates with the length of the postsynaptic membrane containing IgG and C3 [313]. Experimental autoimmune myasthenia gravis induced in various mammals by injection of purified ACR from electric eels [268,314,370,378] is characterized morphologically by an inflammatory infiltrate at the end plate 7–11 days after the injection of ACR. The postsynaptic region of the end plate degenerates, but in most animals it gradually regenerates, although some animals suffer a relapse with severe degeneration, as in the human disease [99].

Antibodies against ACR may produce their effect by causing end-plate degeneration mediated by complement, by accelerated degeneration of ACR, or by blocking the ACR [16,83].

The basic reason ACR antibodies develop remains unknown, but speculation centers on the concept that myasthenia gravis is an autoimmune disease [345] and on the role of the thymus in myasthenia gravis and other autoimmune diseases [131]. Autoantibodies until recently were thought to be "forbidden," but increasingly sensitive tests have shown them to be normal [332]. Why they proliferate to damaging levels in some individuals is not known. The antibodies are a T cell-mediated, major histocompatibility complex-restricted process in humans [333] and probably develop in response to an endogenous source, such as extrajunctional receptors in denervated muscle [403], thymic myoid cells [175,323], or the epithelial component of the thymus [24]. Epithelial and myoid cells of the thymus may arise from primitive pericapillary desmin-positive mesenchymal cells in the medulla of the thymus [414].

"Myoid" cells have been identified in the thymus, and some authors report that skeletal muscle with ACR can be grown in culture from dissociated rat and human thymus [175]. α-bungarotoxin binds to thymic epithelial cells of myasthenic patients [101], suggesting the presence of ACR. The presence of these cells has led to the belief that the changes in skeletal muscle are due to cross-reactivity between skeletal muscle and thymic myoid cells. Indeed, Aharonov and colleagues [6] have demonstrated cross-reactivity between calf thymus and eel ACR and thymuses from patients with myasthenia gravis have epitopes of the ACR [185].

Of all myasthenic patients 90% have antithymic antibodies [158], and it is conceivable that a viral infection of the thymus affecting thymic myoid cells leads to the production of antibodies against myoid cells, such antibodies cross-reacting with skeletal muscle. One theory postulates that exposure to viruses and bacteria leads to the formation of antibodies against ACR because of shared epitopes between the organisms and the receptors or because of shared epitopes in the antibodies against the microorganisms and the ACR. Numerous microorganisms have been identified as possible culprits [74]. Schwimmbeck and colleagues [334] demonstrated cross-reactivity between a subunit of ACR and herpes simplex virus. Increased B cells and decreased T cells have also been noted in the thymus in myasthenia gravis [205], suggesting that decreased T suppressor cells permit the synthesis of autoantibodies. Anti-ACR production by the thymus, as well as T lymphocytes, has been shown [390], but the favorable therapeutic effect of thymectomy may result from the removal of sources of both antibody production and antigen, the thymic myoid cell.

Thymomas do not have myoid cells, but there is evidence that they have genomic loci with a very restricted nucleotide sequence similarity to the acetylcholine receptor α subunit gene [128a].

Patients without measurable antibodies to ACR are of interest because they do not fit the standard model of myasthenia gravis as an autoimmune response to the ACR. Some respond to immunosuppression, and the disease can be passively transferred, indicating an immune mechanism. The explanations include an antibody against another portion of the motor end plate, complete binding of the ACR antibody [249], inadequate assay, or the possibility that some of these cases are not autoimmune [30]. They have decreased ACR [16].

Childhood Forms of Myasthenia Gravis

Several forms of childhood myasthenia gravis are recognized [111].

Juvenile Myasthenia Gravis. Juvenile myasthenia gravis is similar to the adult disease, but with onset after the first year of life. Of all the cases 75% involve children over 10 years of age. Complete spontaneous remissions occur in approximately 20% of patients, including almost all with symptoms restricted to extraocular and facial muscles.

Transitory Neonatal Myasthenia Gravis. Although all infants of mothers with myasthenia gravis have anti-ACR antibodies, only 12% of children born to myasthenic mothers develop a transitory myasthenic syndrome [245], usually beginning on the first day of life and persisting for a few weeks, but sometimes for as long as 5 months. The level of anti-ACR antibodies correlates better with the severity of the transitory infantile myasthenia gravis than with adult myasthenia gravis [105]. The reason is not known, but there is no difference in antibodies [384].

Familial Limb-Girdle Myasthenia Gravis. Patients with familial limb-girdle myasthenia gravis are usually adolescents. They manifest an abrupt onset of symmetrical weakness of the proximal limb muscles without ocular involvement [169,223].

Other apparently non–immune-mediated forms of congenital myasthenia are recognized [93].

Congenital Myasthenia Gravis. Congenital myasthenia gravis also begins shortly after birth, but the mother is not myasthenic, although the siblings may be, and extraocular involvement is the predominant feature [126].

Familial Infantile Myasthenia Gravis. Infants with familial infantile myasthenia gravis have severe respiratory and feeding difficulties with little or no extraocular involvement. The siblings, but not the mother, may have myasthenia gravis. Spontaneous remissions can occur, but apnea may reappear with infection [62,135].

Congenital Acetylcholinesterase Deficiency. The only patient reported with congenital acetylcholinesterase deficiency had small nerve terminals, reduced acetylcholine release, and reduced acetylcholinesterase in the muscle [97,352].

Slow-Channel Syndrome. There is involvement of the cervical, scapular, and finger extensor muscles as well as ocular weakness in slow-channel syndrome. There are degenerative changes at the neuromuscular junction. Engel [93] speculates that a mutation in the ACR hinders the closure of the ACR ion channel.

B. Myotonic Dystrophy

Clinical Features

Myotonic dystrophy, first described by Steinert in 1909 [357], is an autosomal dominant multisystemic disease. It is said to have an incidence of 1 per 7500 [142]. The estimated prevalence in Italy of 69–90 per 1,000,000 population, makes it the most common neuromuscular disease in that country [239]. Roses [302], based on his experience with large pedigrees, found that less than 20% of heterozygotes were known to be clinically affected, indicating that the prevalence of the dystrophia myotonia gene is greatly underestimated. He believes it to be the most common dystrophy. Shaw and Harper [337] believe it to be the most common dystrophy in adults.

The mean ages of onset and death are 20–25 years [143] and 50.6 years [188], respectively. Ptosis, cataracts, facial weakness, cardiac conduction defects, atrophy of the distal limb musculature, mental impairment, and, in males, frontal baldness and testicular atrophy are the most common findings in this disease. Myotonia, which is prolonged contraction of muscle after stimulation or a delay in muscle relaxation after a strong contraction, is a key feature. An abnormal glucose tolerance and decreased IgG levels are present in some affected individuals [298]. The phenotype varies considerably, some patients having any combination of the foregoing features, whereas others manifest no apparent clinical characteristics and are recognized only by biochemical abnormalities or because they are obligate heterozygotes [306].

Myotonic dystrophy may manifest itself in childhood [7], and almost all reported cases of infantile myotonic dystrophy have been transmitted by an affected mother, for which there is no good explanation, although a maternal environmental factor has been suggested. Not all siblings are affected [144]. Partial myotonic dystrophy has been reported in children with affected fathers, which makes it less likely that a maternal environmental factor plays the key role in the development of childhood infantile myotonic dystrophy [284]. Megacolon, constipation, or spruelike symptoms may occur in childhood [200]. Profound hypotonia, clubfeet, and cerebral abnormalities have been noted, and involvement of respiratory muscles may cause apnea in children and adults [36,51,55]. Patients who survive infancy show facial diplegia and delay in motor development. With age, hypotonia decreases but myotonia becomes manifest [306]. Cataracts are rare in childhood myotonic dystrophy. Lotz and Van der Meyden reported cataracts in a 27 year old with congenital myotonic dystrophy [207].

Morphological Features

Limb Muscle. The principal histological findings in skeletal muscle are fiber atrophy, particularly of type 1 fibers [287], fiber hypertrophy, long chains of internal nuclei, ringed fibers (ringbinden), and pale-staining peripheral portions of fibers (sarcoplasmic pads; Fig. 12) [407].

Fiber differentiation may be poor in infants. With histochemical techniques oxidative enzymes are evident in the center of the muscle fiber but not at their periphery, resulting in a halo effect (Fig. 13) [109].

When ringbinden are present, a fiber seen in cross section has myofibrils running at oblique angles to other myofibrils, usually at the periphery of a fiber but sometimes associated with a more peripheral sarcoplasmic pad (Figs. 13 and 14). Ringbinden have been described in numerous normal and abnormal muscles, including extraocular muscles [26], and are probably a nonspecific response to muscle fiber injury [171].

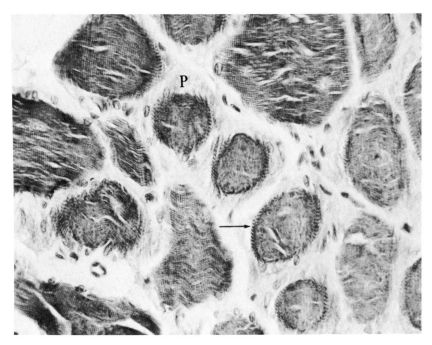

Figure 12   Myotonic dystrophy (adult). Several fibers contain ringbinden (arrow) and sarcoplasmic pads (P). (Hematoxylin and eosin, formalin fixed, ×400)

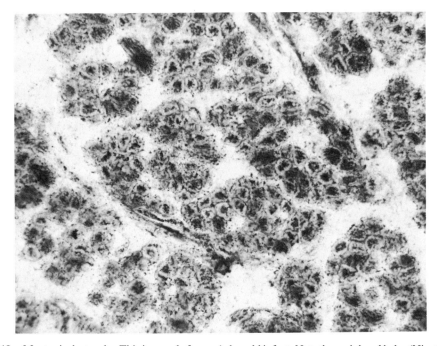

Figure 13   Myotonic dystrophy. This is muscle from a 1-day-old infant. Note the peripheral halo. (Nicotinamide adenine dinucleotide tetrazolium reductase stain, ×400)

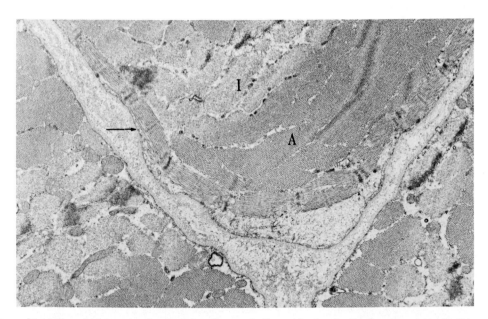

Figure 14 Myotonic dystrophy. Cross section of a muscle fiber with a longitudinally oriented myofibril (arrow) at the periphery. A, A band; I, I band. (×12,500)

Ultrastructural studies have shown the sarcoplasmic pads to consist of disorganized cytoplasmic components, including myofibrils, sarcoplasmic reticulum, glycogen, lipid, and lysosomes [108,187, 191,243]. Fiber degeneration and regeneration are occasionally seen, and endomysial fibrosis may be present in advanced cases. Ultrastructural abnormalities of the myofibrils in myotonic dystrophy have led some authors to suggest a defect in the synthesis of myofibrils [5]. The sarcoplasmic reticulum, important in muscle contraction and relaxation, has been suspected of being important in myotonic dystrophy, but the morphological changes, such as dilatation and multiple terminal cisternae, are nonspecific.

Intramuscular nerves exhibit extensive sprouting of subterminal axons, an increase in end-plate size, and multiple end plates in single fibers (more than in denervation) [10,58]. However, denervation has been reported in myotonic dystrophy [412].

In myotonic dystrophy the muscle fibers of the muscle spindles (intrafusal fibers) resemble those outside the muscle spindles (extrafusal fibers) [219], but the intrafusal fibers are considerably increased in number, being more than 100 (normal 5–14) [362–364]. Histochemical stains disclose most of the intrafusal fibers in myotonic dystrophy as type 1, instead of both type 1 and type 2 [151]. This may indicate type grouping, a feature of the reinnervation phase of denervation, or it could result from an increased need for oxidative activity because of chronic overloading of the spindle by myotonia. Studies of motor innervation to the spindle have shown an increased number of motor axon sprouts [362], many of which do not appear to terminate on the simplified end plates. The question of whether the abnormal innervation leads to the splitting of intrafusal fibers or constitutes an attempt to innervate previously split fibers remains unanswered. Currently, the latter view is favored [219,364].

Ocular Muscles.   Extraocular weakness is uncommon [201], occurring in only 7% of patients [207]. Histological studies of the extraocular muscles, including the levator palpebrae superioris, have shown various degrees of fiber atrophy and hypertrophy and centrally placed nuclei, sometimes in chains, as well as increased connective tissues and fat [70,173,273,407]. Ultrastructural observations have included only nonspecific changes, including disorganization and loss of myofibrils, clusters of sarcoplasmic reticulum and transverse tubules, and abnormal Z lines [194,195]. Increased numbers of inner cristae of mitochondria with concentrically arranged cristae are sometimes noted [195]. Similar alternations have been observed in the extraocular muscles of rats fed diazacholesterol [263]. Neuromuscular junctions are said to be normal except for few synaptic vesicles and swollen mitochondria [194].

Ocular Hypotonia

Ocular hypotonia is common in myotonic dystrophy [289,335,398]. Junge [173] found the intraocular pressure to be low in 84 of 101 eyes from 51 patients with myotonic dystrophy (control mean 16.3 mm Hg; myotonic mean 8.8 mm Hg), and in a few instances the intraocular pressure was lower than normal in asymptomatic blood relatives of myotonic patients. Junge [173] speculated that the ocular hypotonia may in part be due to degeneration of the ciliary muscle, which has been described in myotonic dystrophy. Atrophy [228], hyaline degeneration, and vacuole formation in ciliary muscles have been reported several times [47,211,383], but the vacuolar change has been found in individuals without myotonic dystrophy. Burns [47] reported a fibrotic sphincter pupillae and sparse muscle fibers in the dilator pupillae.

Cataracts

Opacities form in the lens in almost all adults with myotonic dystrophy [149,188], but rarely in childhood. The clinical features of myotonic cataracts have been well characterized since the first report more than 50 years ago [115]. They pass through three stages of development [87]: (1) dustlike irregularly shaped opacities intermingled with iridescent crystals of varying red and green hue appear in the anterior and posterior lens cortex just beneath the capsule [392]; (2) the opacities become more diffuse, increase in density, and assume a stellate shape [115]; (3) finally, vacuoles and lamellar separations develop [11,87].

Histological studies have shown nucleated fibers in the vicinity of vacuoles and lacunae [383,396], which may contain crystalline material [318]. The suggestion that lipids, particularly cholesterol, cause the iridescence of the lens in myotonic dystrophy [45] has not been confirmed histochemically. Electron microscope studies [68,102], show the iridescent particles corresponded to vacuoles containing whorls of multilaminated membranes. Filaments (8–12 nm in diameter) appearing as hollow tubes on cross sections have also been described. They are also seen in the aging lens [68].

Decreased lenticular glutathione is associated with cataract formation, and increased gamma-glutamyltranspeptidase, which aids in the catabolism of glutathione, has been found to be increased in the serum of victims of myotonic dystrophy [388]. Horrobin and Morgan [155] suggested zinc could play a role in cataract development because zinc deficiency not only has some similarities to myotonic dystrophy but also causes cataracts in trout [182] and in humans with acrodermatitis enteropathica [285].

Changes in the Iris and Ciliary Body

The vasculature of the iris is said to be abnormal in myotonic dystrophy and to be characterized by a slow circulation, leakage, and peripupillary tufting [216,359]. All the myotonic patients with tufts described by Mason [216] were latent diabetics, and it should be noted that non-myotonic diabetics may also have tufts. Meyer and colleagues [228] described vacuolization of the epithelium of the iris. Depigmentation of the ciliary processes has also been noted [149].

Retina

Hayasaka and colleagues [149] described patterned dystrophy and peripheral yellow flecks in the retina that they believed to be in the deep retinal pigment epithelium (RPE) or Bruch's membrane. Raitta and Karli [289] described fundic lesions that they interpreted as fundic scars. Pinto and colleagues [278] reported abnormal visual evoked potentials, pattern stimulation electroretinograms, and electrooculograms, which were attributed to involvement of the proximal retinal layers and retrodiasmatic pathways. Retinal degeneration is common, and degenerated photoreceptors, increased pigment cells, and cystic changes have been noted in tissue sections of the retina [156,211]. Of all patients with myotonic dystrophy 85% have abnormal electroretinograms [46,173].

Cornea

Studies of the cornea in myotonic dystrophy have been few [103,173], and lesions seen have been attributed to disordered function of the eyelids or deficient tear secretion.

The relationship between the ocular and the other manifestations of myotonic dystrophy is not clear. They do not seem to be related to defects in carbohydrate metabolism, although cataracts are more common in myotonics with diabetes mellitus [306,343]. An abnormal lipid metabolism has been suspected in the evolution of the cataract, in part because hypocholesterolemic drugs can produce cataracts and myotonia

[184,405]. Thomas and Harper [374], however, failed to detect abnormalities of lipid composition in membranes of erythrocytes or cultured skin fibroblasts of patients with myotonic dystrophy.

Heart

Cardiac abnormalities, principally electrocardiographic, occur in 68% of patients [112]. Although conduction defects with the consequent possibility of sudden death [276] are the most common cardiac abnormality, the conduction system has rarely been evaluated completely [376]. Fatty infiltration and fibrosis of the cardiac muscle are common [25,44,369,375,386].

Nervous System

Mental deficiency may be prominent [54,307,375] in myotonic dystrophy. Recently eosinophilic cytoplasmic inclusions were described in the thalamus of myotonic dystrophy victims. Culebras and colleagues [65] consider these inclusions to represent premature senescence in myotonic dystrophy since increasing numbers of similar inclusions occur with normal aging.

Although electromyographic studies suggest peripheral nerve involvement [220,234,266], morphological changes are seldom seen in peripheral nerves [34,282], except at the nerve endings. A quantitative study of the spinal cord reported no decrease in the number of motor neurons [400].

The few anatomic studies of the autonomic nervous system have been generally negative [25,407], although degenerative changes in portions of the sympathetic nervous system have been noted [402].

Endocrine and Metabolic Dysfunction

Interest in the endocrine glands in myotonic dystrophy dates from 1917, when Naegeli [244] suggested that the primary defect in the disease resided in them. The most common pathological change is testicular atrophy, but abnormal ovaries have also been reported [25]. Plasma follicle-stimulating and luteinizing hormones are increased; testosterone is decreased, supporting the concept of a primary gonadal disorder rather than a pituitary defect [146,312]. The pituitary gland is morphologically normal in three-fourths of cases [25,110], but nonspecific changes may occur in the pituitary and other endocrine glands [306].

Diabetes mellitus is present in 7% of patients with myotonic dystrophy [306]. Of all patients with myotonic dystrophy 40–60% manifest hyperinsulinemia in the presence of glucose loading and other insulin stimulators [240,373], for reasons that are not known. Circulating monocytes obtained during glucose tolerance tests disclosed no difference in insulin binding between controls and myotonic patients [190].

Pathogenesis

A defect in the cell membrane could explain the widespread manifestations of myotonic dystrophy [303–305]. Studies on erythrocytes have shown alterations in protein conformation or organization in myotonic dystrophy but not in myotonia congenita [48]. Membrane fluidity is increased in myotonic dystrophy and myotonia congenita. Other abnormalities of erythrocytes in myotonic dystrophy include altered calcium transport and impaired protein phosphorylation [281].

Brumback and colleagues [42], observing that myotonic patients treated with tricyclic antidepressants had decreased myotonia and improved gastrointestinal function, postulated that myotonic dystrophy is a generalized disorder of aminergic and peptidergic receptors since tricyclic agents increase amine neurotransmission.

Tanaka [368] suggested that bile acid plays a role in the pathogenesis of myotonic dystrophy, noting that serum deoxycholic acid, which is toxic to cells, is elevated in all mothers of children with congenital myotonic dystrophy.

The greatest advance in understanding this disease has been the identification of a defective gene (DM) localized to the long arm of chromosome 19 (19q13.3) [142]. There is evidence that the DM gene increases in length with succeeding generations [49]. Attempts to detect preclinical cases of myotonic dystrophy have utilized products of genes linked to the DM gene. These include the genes for the ABH secretor locus [145], apolipoprotein E [351], and apolipoprotein C-II [139]. Apolipoprotein C-II, about 4 centimorgans from the DM locus [338], is useful as a prenatal marker of myotonic dystrophy. Myotonic dystrophy was one of the first human diseases for which linkage to a genetic marker (secretor) was utilized [225].

C. Ocular Myopathies

This section considers those disorders that primarily involve the muscles of the eye that produce ptosis and external ophthalmoplegia. Myopathies that are primarily systemic, such as centronuclear myopathy, which may affect the ocular muscle, are discussed separately.

Ocular myopathies can be divided into progressive external ophthalmoplegia (oculocraniosomatic syndromes, OCSS) and oculopharyngeal muscular dystrophy (OPMD). The major morphological distinction between these two groups is the association of abnormal mitochondria with OCSS [411], but not with OPMD.

Progressive External Ophthalmoplegia

Von Graefe [393,394] is usually credited with the first clinical description of progressive external ophthalmoplegia, but Hutchinson [161] introduced the term "ophthalmoplegia externa" for what he thought was of syphilitic origin. The brain of one of Hutchinson's cases had changes in the oculomotor, trochlear, and abducent nerves and their nuclei [134]. This led to the concept that external ophthalmoplegia was of nuclear origin [29]; Möbius [233] thought it was congenital and heredofamilial, a view bolstered by family studies [20].

Histological studies [121,183,315,330,342] challenged the neurogenic nature of progressive external ophthalmoplegia by demonstrating normal oculomotor, trochlear, and abducent nerve nuclei [330] and what were interpreted as myopathic changes [183]. Involvement of muscles in the limbs, pharynx, larynx, face, and neck in some patients gave further support to progressive external ophthalmoplegia being a form of muscular dystrophy, hence the terms "ocular myopathy," "ocular dystrophy," and "oculopharyngeal muscular dystrophy" [170,242,297,371,389].

The aforementioned histopathological reports, however, did not end the controversy over the pathogenesis of progressive external ophthalmoplegia. Some patients have degenerative neurological diseases, such as Friedreich's ataxia, Charcot-Marie-Tooth disease [358], Kugelberg-Welander disease [2], cerebellar ataxia [176], and spastic quadriplegia [9]. Also, studies of experimental denervation in extraocular muscle (see Sec. IV) [81] are noteworthy in this regard, because they show that denervation of extraocular muscles produces morphological changes comparable to myopathies in limb muscle, thus invalidating previous conclusions of the myopathic origin of progressive external ophthalmoplegia based on the "myopathic" changes in extraocular muscles.

Paralysis of the ocular muscles clearly has many causes, and classification of these disorders remains controversial [79,80,308]. The primary abnormality may involve the oculomotor, trochlear, and abducent nerves, their nuclei, or central connections in the cerebral cortex or midbrain, as well as the myoneural junction or the extraocular muscles themselves. The nature of the insults includes trauma, toxins, degenerative disorders, infectious agents, metabolic disorders, and neoplasms. Ophthalmoplegia may be associated with other disease processes or injury (Table 3). Moreover, the association of ophthalmoplegia with other clinical or laboratory features suggests distinct entities. This problem is addressed elsewhere [22,79,308].

Clinical Features. The ophthalmoplegia is frequently associated with and preceded by ptosis. Weakness of facial, neck, and limb muscles is common but may occur years after the onset of ophthalmoplegia [63]. A wide variety of clinical abnormalities have accompanied progressive ophthalmoplegia (Table 3), some sufficiently often to warrant the designation of a syndrome. Detailed clinical discussions can be found in the reviews on the subject [19,380]. Some findings associated with ophthalmoplegia are listed in Table 3.

Basically, progressive external ophthalmoplegia can be subdivided into the following clinical groups:

1. Progressive external ophthalmoplegia alone (ocular myopathy, ocular muscular dystrophy).
2. Progressive external ophthalmoplegia with minor involvement of the orbicularis oculi, other facial muscles, and sometimes of limb muscles (descending ocular myopathy).
3. Kearns-Sayre (Kearns-Shy, Kearns-Sayre-Daroff) syndrome [22,179]: sporadic cases of progressive external ophthalmoplegia, associated with pigmentary retinopathy, cardiopathy (usually conduction defects and proneness to sudden death), and sometimes cerebellar disorders, deafness, short stature,

Table 3   Some Associations with Ophthalmoplegia

Clinical and laboratory findings
  Ocular
    Cataracts [274]
    Optic atrophy [79]
    Proptosis [79,341]
    Pigmentary retinopathy [79,237,256,301]
  Ear, nose, and throat
    Hearing loss [67,79,178]
    Dysphonia [79]
  Nervous system
    Absent tendon jerks [176,237]
    Ataxia [63,79,176,301]
    Abnormal electroencephalogram [79,178,253,256]
    Cerebellar atrophy [176]
    Elevated CSF protein [67,178,256,326]
    Mental retardation [79,176,253,301]
    Peripheral neuropathy [63]
    Seizures [237,301]
  Musculoskeletal
    Dysarthria [176,253,301]
    Dystonia [301]
    Extremity weakness [63,67,79,178,237,301,341]
    Facial weakness [63,67,79,237]
    Myotonia [196]
    Myopathic electromyogram [67,178,256,347]
    Neck flexor weakness [53,63,256,341]
    Short stature [176,178,179,326]
  Cardiac
    Abnormal electrocardiogram (heart block commonly)
[69,178,326]
  Gastrointestinal
    Diarrhea [340]
    Dysphagia [63,79,253,301]
    Masticatory weakness [178]
  Genital
    Genital hypoplasia [172,179,209]
Associated disorders
  Bassen-Kornzweig syndrome [301]
  Dermatomyositis [361]
  Diabetes mellitus [196]
  Hypoparathyroidism [381]
  Infantile spinal muscular atrophy [301]
  Juvenile spinal muscular atrophy [2]
  Marfan syndrome [137]
  Möbius' syndrome [183,231,232]
  Primary biliary cirrhosis [292]
  Syphilis [161]
  Wernicke's encephalopathy [391]
Associated physical and chemical agents
  Drugs and toxins (coal gas, diphenylhydantoin, primadone) [258]
  Trauma [336]

and mental retardation; onset is before the end of the second decade of life, and the CSF protein is elevated.
4.   Progressive external ophthalmoplegia associated with other disorders (Table 3).

Because these conditions can be considered a spectrum ranging from isolated chronic progressive ophthalmoplegia to the more generalized disorders, they are discussed here as a single morphological entity.

Histopathology.   Because there are relatively few detailed morphological studies in individuals with external ophthalmoplegia and because of the uncertainty of many earlier studies, the histopathology of all cases is discussed together except when stated otherwise. Readers interested in an extensive historical account should consult specific publications [63,178].

Extraocular muscles and levator palpebrae superioris.   Variation in fiber size, fiber degeneration, and/or atrophy (not fiber group atrophy) and increased fat and connective tissue are frequently observed in biopsies of extraocular muscles in progressive external ophthalmoplegia [63,81,121,315,342]. Ring fibers (see Sec. V.B) may occur [63], but intramuscular nerves at motor end plates are unremarkable [53,63].

Transmission electron microscopy has disclosed loss of myofibrils and irregularities of the sarcoplasmic reticulum and transverse tubular system in addition to an accumulation of mitochondria, many of which contain concentric cristae and crystalloids [53,326,413] and excess glycogen [322].

Skeletal muscle.   Skeletal muscle abnormalities have been interpreted as myopathic [67,297,301, 389], but frequently the limb muscles are normal [39,330] or contain only rare atrophic or degenerated fibers in hematoxylin and eosin–stained microscopic sections [140,163,250,367]. However, in many cases staining with a modified Gomori's trichrome reveals abnormal fibers with accumulations of red-staining material, particularly beneath the sarcolemma [163,238,367,381]. The appellation "ragged-red fibers" has been applied to these abnormal fibers [256], which usually constitute fewer than 5% of the fibers [176,255,347], although 20–60% of the fibers may be of this type [162,320]. The red-staining areas react positively with histochemical methods for oxidative enzymes (nicotinamide adenine dinucleotide tetrazolium reductase and succinic dehydrogenase; Fig. 15) and may also contain increased amounts of stainable glycogen and lipids. These abnormalities affect the type 1 fibers (based on myosin adenosine triphosphatase activity) much more frequently than type 2 fibers [53,163,176,238,253,347].

Transmission electron microscopy of these abnormal zones reveals accumulations of unusual mitochondria (extremely large mitochondria, mitochondria with concentric cristae, and mitochondria distended with granular material, with and without electron-dense bodies, and crystalloids; Figs. 16 and 17). Lipid deposits and glycogen may be prominent in the mitochondrial aggregates [76,349], presumably secondary to defective mitochondrial metabolism. Other ultrastructural changes include nonspecific Z band streaming and myofibril degeneration.

Patients with progressive external ophthalmoplegia frequently have ragged-red fibers, but these are not specific for that condition. Rarely they are observed in hypothyroidism, glycogen storage disease type II (Pompe's disease; see Chap. 27), myotonic dystrophy, polymyositis, regenerating muscle, mitochondrial myopathy [159,340], Luft's disease (a hypermetabolic mitochondrial disease) [76,208], Leigh syndrome [64] (see Chap. 53), and other disorders. All patients with Kearns-Sayre syndrome whose muscles have been examined by transmission electron microscopy have had abnormal mitochondria [22]. A personal study of four patients with ocular myopathy disclosed ragged-red fibers with crystalloids, concentric lamellae, and large electron-dense spherical deposits in mitochondria within biopsied skeletal muscle in all cases [35].

Ragged-red fibers and their mitochondrial abnormalities, with and without ophthalmoplegia, are associated with loose coupling of oxidative phosphorylation (defective respiratory control and normal phosphorylative ability) [31,33,76,159,320,328]. Some or a few ragged-red fibers are produced when uncouplers of oxidative phosphorylation (2,4-dinitrophenocarbonylcyanide-*m*-chlorophenylhydrazine and oleic acid) are introduced into the hind limbs of rats [224]. However, these mitochondrial inclusions are not identical to the crystalloids of human ragged-red fibers, perhaps because the human diseases are chronic. Korman and colleagues [192] suggest that the paracrystalline array most likely forms in the nonenergized configuration of mitochondria (which presumably develops in the uncoupled state).

The significance of ragged-red fibers in progressive extraocular ophthalmoplegia remains unclear, but it is unlikely that they cause the muscle weakness. In Luft's disease most mitochondria are abnormal, yet muscle weakness may be negligible [208]. Moreover, fewer than 5% of mitochondria in the ragged-red fibers of progressive external ophthalmoplegia are usually morphologically abnormal. In all likelihood the

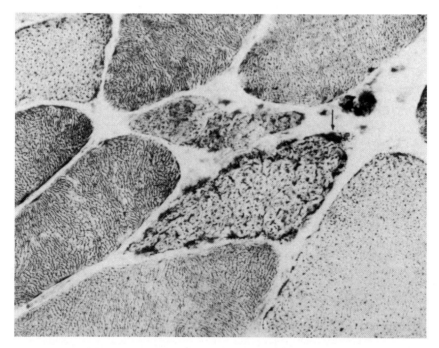

Figure 15 Progressive external ophthalmoplegia, with accumulation of dense material in a fiber (arrow). (Nicotinamide adenine dinucleotide tetrazolium reductase stain, ×400)

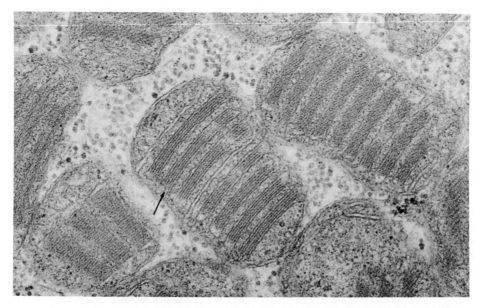

Figure 16 Progressive external ophthalmoplegia. Crystalline array (arrow) between cristae of mitochondria. (×75,000)

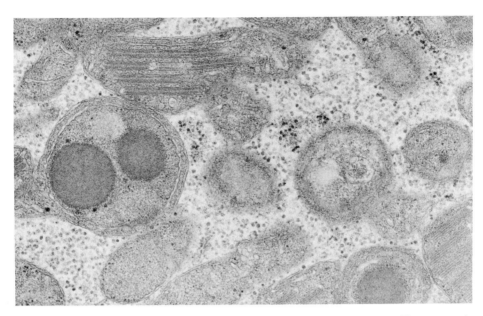

Figure 17 Progressive external ophthalmoplegia. Electron micrograph showing crystalline arrays, electron-dense material, and concentric cristae. (×50,000)

ragged-red fibers and ocular changes are both manifestations of an as yet to be determined common mechanism.

Nervous system. Changes in the CNS are central to the question of whether the cause of progressive external ophthalmoplegia is neurogenic or myogenic. Unfortunately, available data do not provide a clear-cut answer. The nerves supplying the extraocular muscles and their nuclei are described as normal by some authors [63,179] but abnormal by others [167,197,330]. Croft and coworkers [63] reported neuronal loss and astrocytic hyperplasia in subthalamic nuclei and foci of neuronal degeneration with gliosis in the substantia nigra. Crystalloids in the mitochondria of Purkinje's and granular cells of the cerebellum, loss of neurons and siderosis in the lateral portion of the substantia nigra and vestibular nuclei, and increased astrocytes in the substantia nigra have also been described [326], as has siderosis of the globus pallidum, vestibular nuclei, and substantia nigra [179].

The neuronal cell bodies of the oculomotor, trochlear, and abducent nerves are reported as reduced in number [69,197], smaller and rounder with fewer dendrites than normal [330], and with abnormal variations in size and shape [197].

Vacuoles have been described in the brain [69,179], being so diffuse in one case [69] that spongiform encephalopathy was diagnosed. Such alterations are common artifacts, so there is questionable significance to them.

A normal spinal cord has been reported in one case [60], but spinal cord and peripheral nerve abnormalities have been observed in other patients. Croft and colleagues [63] observed demyelination of the posterior columns, loss of ganglion cells, hypertrophied capsular cells of dorsal root ganglia, nodules of cells with hyperchromatic nuclei and scant cytoplasm in the lower lumbar posterior roots, and loss of myelinated fibers in the peroneal nerve. A hypertrophic interstitial neuropathy has been documented [79]. "Zebra" bodies similar to those seen in the mucopolysaccharidoses have been observed in Schwann cells of a peripheral nerve [132].

Other tissues. A pigmentary retinopathy (Table 3; see also Chap. 41) has been noted. A loss of retinal pigment epithelium (RPE) may accompany circinate atrophic areas in a pseudorosette pattern in Giemsa-stained flat retinal preparations [178,179]. A pigmentary retinopathy accompanies many of the same disorders as progressive external ophthalmoplegia (e.g., cardiac conduction defects, auditory disorders, and cerebellar anomalies) [37].

Heart block is a common electrocardiographic abnormality [133], but the heart, including its conducting system, may be normal [69]. A normal heart has been reported in a patient with heart block [168], but specific mention of the conduction system was not made. Cardiac hypertrophy, subendocardial fibrosis, and a thickened epicardium have also been described [178].

Radiography and motility studies suggest that the smooth muscle in the lower esophagus is abnormal, but histological abnormalities have not been reported [297].

In progressive external ophthalmoplegia the mitochondrial abnormalities are not restricted to muscle and have been noted in the liver [253] and sweat glands [176].

Nature of Progressive External Ophthalmoplegia (the Oculocraniosomatic Syndromes) Progressive external ophthalmoplegia may be considered a mitochondrial disorder, but biochemical abnormalities are not always detected and they are not consistent. A detailed discussion of these mitochondrial disorders is beyond the scope of this chapter. For additional information, the reader should consult Chapter 52 and reviews on the subject [77,78,237].

Briefly, the mitochondrial disorders of muscle include three syndromes: Kearns-Sayre syndrome, myoclonic epilepsy with red-ragged fibers (MERRF), and mitochondrial myopathy, encephalopathy, lactic acidosis, and strokelike episodes (MELAS). The only group of interest here is Kearns-Sayre syndrome.

The metabolic pathways in the mitochondria involve transport of metabolites and substrates, substrate utilization, Krebs' cycle, oxidative phosphorylation, and the respiratory chain.

Disorders of the respiratory chain of interest to ophthalmologists, include Kearns-Sayre syndrome (associated with combined complex I and III deficiencies) and Leber's optic atrophy (associated with defects of complex I), are reported to manifest type atrophy in the muscle [321]. The complexes are discussed in Chapter 52.

Harding and Holt [141] noted that in 40% of 71 cases of mitochondrial myopathy up to one-half of the mitochondrial DNA was deleted and that all these cases manifested progressive external ophthalmoplegia, but a specific biochemical deletion did not correlate with chronic external ophthalmoplegia. Of 43 patients with chronic external ophthalmoplegia 12 had no apparent deletion of mitochondrial DNA.

Oculopharyngeal Muscular Dystrophy

Oculopharyngeal muscular dystrophy is inherited as an autosomal dominant trait, and patients develop ptosis and dysphagia in middle age. The condition is most common in French-Canadians but has been reported in several other ethnic groups [380]. It is rare in blacks [309].

External ophthalmoplegia occurs but is rarely complete [380]. Progression to the facial muscles takes place, and late in the disease, the proximal limb muscles may be involved. Distal muscle involvement has been reported in Japan [123] and in an elderly German who was subsequently autopsied and found to have some anterior horn cell loss [325]. Cardiac abnormalities are unusual, but a few cases with bundle branch block have been reported.

Abnormalities detected by skeletal muscle biopsy include variation in fiber size, fibrosis, increased muscle fibers with internal nuclei, and rarely, necrosis and inflammation. Angulated atrophic fibers may be seen, but this could be an aging change. Autopsies, except for the elderly patient described by Schmitt and Krause [325], have not suggested a neurogenic origin [206]. Ragged-red fibers are not a feature of this disorder. Vacuoles with a basophilic edge (rimmed vacuoles) may be seen in skeletal muscle [85]. The key morphological abnormality is the presence of intranuclear filaments (approximately 8 nm in diameter; Fig. 18), which frequently palisade. These are considered unique to oculopharyngeal muscular dystrophy, but they must be distinguished from intranuclear filaments found in other disorders, such as inclusion body myositis (Fig. 19). The filaments in the latter disease are approximately 18–23 nm in diameter and occur in cytoplasmic vacuoles as well as within the nucleus. Interestingly, Fukuhara and colleagues [123] described a patient with oculopharyngeal muscular dystrophy and distal muscle weakness whose rimmed vacuoles contained filaments similar to those of inclusion body myositis. Coquet and colleagues report similar findings [62a].

D. Miscellaneous Syndromes with External Ophthalmoplegia

Möbius' Syndrome

Möbius' syndrome, also referred to as facial diplegia, congenital oculofacial paralysis, or infantile nuclear aplasia, is characterized by paralysis of lateral gaze and varying degrees of facial paresis [152,280,

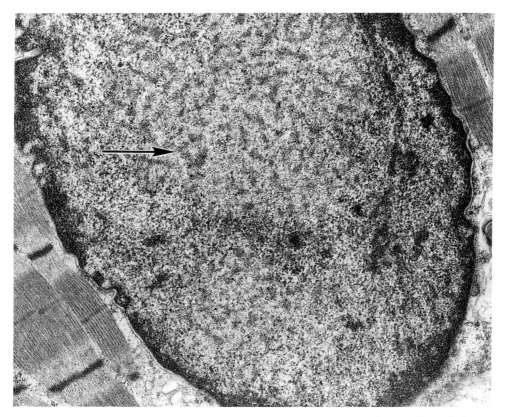

Figure 18 Short filaments (arrow) within the nucleus of a muscle cell of a patient with oculopharyngeal dystrophy. (×18,000)

356,395]. Clubfeet, micrognathia, absent portions of the extremities, peripheral neuropathy, hypogonadism, and other anomalies may also be present [4,152,255,299]. Möbius [231,233] thought the disorder was degenerative; currently, some consider the basic defect to be in the central nervous system (CNS), whereas others believe that it involves the mesoderm, or mesoectoderm, and that the neurological changes are secondary. The few documented morphological studies [280,353] show abnormalities in the brain stem, such as diminished numbers of cell bodies in cranial nerves, particularly the abducent nerves. These findings thus support a primary defect in the CNS, as do electromyographic observations and a morphologically normal biopsied external rectus muscle [387]. Proponents of a mesodermal origin of the disorder [104,294,399] argue that there is no obvious direct link between the neurological and the musculoskeletal abnormalities. They contend that the decreased number of neurons in the brain stem is secondary to a defective development of mesodermal structures forming toward the end of the second fetal month [104,399]. Pitner and colleagues [280] performed a meticulous anatomical study of this disorder, and although they found abnormalities of the cerebellum, the cranial nerves and their nuclei were normal. These investigators reported extensive fatty and fibrous replacement of facial muscles and interpreted their findings as due to a primary failure of muscle development. They suggested, however, that like arthrogryposis multiplex congenita, Möbius' syndrome may be produced by multiple factors. Interestingly, at least one patient with arthrogryposis also had Möbius' syndrome [356].

Arthrogryposis Multiplex Congenita

Arthrogryposis multiplex congenita is a syndrome characterized by fixation of multiple joints at birth. It may be caused by anything that decreases fetal movement but most commonly is associated with

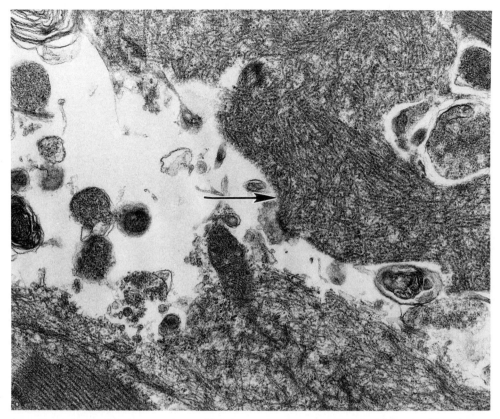

Figure 19 Intracytoplasmic filaments (approximately the size of myosin filaments) are present within the striated muscle of a patient with inclusion body myositis. Similar filaments may be found in nuclei. These filaments are approximately three times the diameter of those seen in oculopharygeal muscular dystrophy. (×23,500)

neurogenic features. Reported associations include external ophthalmoplegia, a decreased corneal blinking reflex and deteriorated visual evoked responses [265], trichiasis of the upper eyelid [213], and optic atrophy [118], as well as cataracts and glaucoma [366].

Centronuclear Myopathy

First reported by Spiro and colleagues [355], centronuclear myopathy is named for its histological appearance. In this disease most striated muscle fibers have central nuclei, in contrast to normal muscle, in which fewer than 3% of the fibers have nuclei in this location [339]. Because the muscle in this disorder resembles the myotubular phase of developing muscle, the term "myotubular myopathy" is sometimes used [27].

The condition is characterized by a nonprogressive or slowly progressive weakness and wasting of many muscle groups and with ptosis and/or external ophthalmoplegia present in over one-half the cases [27,339]. Facial weakness is also common [27,259,271,327]. Severe distal muscle deficits may also be evident [107]. The age of onset is variable, although most patients are floppy infants [290,327]. Ptosis is less frequent when the disease is diagnosed in adults, and the adult and childhood forms may be different diseases [130].

The cause of this ailment, which can be familial [222,293], remains unknown. Histochemical stains disclose both type 1 and 2 fibers in limb muscles, although type 1 may predominate [271,286]. When viewed in the transmission electron microscope, a zone devoid of myofibrils is evident adjacent to the centralized nuclei [259]. The muscle differs from true embryonic fibers since this myotubular zone (clear zone) does not occupy the full length of the fiber and because fiber differentiation is present [286]; hence the term "myotubular myopathy" is misleading.

A case of centronuclear myopathy in a patient with Marfan syndrome, who also had "fingerprint" inclusions in his muscle biopsy, has been reported. The patient had bilateral ptosis, alternate divergent strabismus, myopia, bilateral cataracts, subluxed lenses, and reduced pupillary reflexes to convergence [166].

Multicore Disease

Multicore disease, first described by Engel and Gomez in 1966 [95], is a congenital, nonprogressive myopathy characterized morphologically by multiple focal areas of myofibrillar degeneration in many striated muscle fibers. The condition is of uncertain origin, although a mitochondrial abnormality has been suggested [96,114]. Sporadic as well as familial cases have been reported. The clinical presentation is variable but includes proximal muscle weakness, marfanoid features, weakness of the orbicularis oris [95], ptosis, and external ophthalmoplegia [96,164,365].

Congenital Ophthalmoplegia

A few cases of congenital ophthalmoplegia are associated with hypotonia [183] and amino aciduria [160], as well as syndromes, such as Möbius' syndrome.

Spinal Muscular Atrophy

External ophthalmoplegia has been reported in infantile spinal muscular atrophy (Werdnig-Hoffman) [264,301], juvenile spinal muscular atrophy (Kugelberg-Welander) [2], and in a Japanese family with progressive spinal muscular atrophy [218].

Celiac Disease

Sandyk and Brennan [316] reported a 12-year-old girl with celiac disease who had diplopia due to medial rectus weakness. Treatment of the celiac disease eliminated the diplopia.

E. Other Neuromuscular Diseases Affecting the Eye

Inflammatory Myopathies

The inflammatory myopathies can be subdivided into polymyositis, dermatomyositis, and inclusion body myositis (Fig. 20) [66].

Polymyositis.   Polymyositis uncomplicated by involvement of the skin is a cell-mediated auto-immune disease. Lymphocytes from patients with this disease are cytotoxic to fetal muscle in culture, whereas the serum is not [71,72]. Furthermore, experimental allergic myositis, which can be induced by injecting muscle components in Freund's adjuvant into animals [236,401], can be transferred by lymphocytes but not serum [236]. Although antibodies are produced in experimental allergic myositis, they do not correlate with the degree of muscle involvement and therefore are believed to be a secondary phenomenon [401].

Dermatomyositis.   Dermatomyositis is an inflammatory myopathy that also has skin abnormalities, including a blue-purple rash on the face and upper eyelids (heliotropic rash) and a scaly eruption on the knuckles (Gottron's sign).

The childhood form of dermatomyositis may have other systemic manifestations, such as gastrointestinal hemorrhages [17,199,406], presumably because of the vascular involvement. Microangiopathy with subsequent muscle necrosis is characteristic of dermatomyositis [186].

In dermatomyositis the principal ocular abnormality is a retinopathy generally attributed to vascular disease. It is characterized by exudates and hemorrhage, which may resolve or leave areas of depigmentation and sometimes optic atrophy [73,147,241]. Extraocular muscle involvement is rare [270], but nystagmus [397], external ophthalmoplegia [361], incomplete eyelid closure [32], and diplopia [251] have been reported.

Inclusion Body Myositis.   The third form of inflammatory myopathy is inclusion body myositis. It most commonly presents in males over the age of 50 years and involves skeletal muscle of both the distal as well as proximal portions of limbs. It is frequently slowly progressive over several years. Morphologically it is characterized by a myositis with cytoplasmic and intranuclear filaments (Fig. 19). Ocular muscle involvement is unusual. The disease does not respond to immunosuppressive therapy [66].

Miscellaneous Diseases of Muscle

Schwartz-Jampel Syndrome.   Schwartz-Jampel syndrome is characterized by blepharophimosis, dwarfism, skeletal and facial anomalies, and myotonia [3,119,331] and in most cases hypertrophied muscle [119]. Normal [3] or scattered atrophic fibers [331] are seen by light microscopy [3], but transmission electron microscopy has disclosed intermyofibrillar vacuoles [3] and perinuclear lamellar dense bodies [226]. Features of arthrogryposis multiplex congenita and Schwartz-Jampel syndrome may be present in the same patient [113].

   Duchenne (Pseudohypertrophic) Muscular Dystrophy.   Duchenne (pseudohypertrophic) muscular dystrophy, which is associated with a deficiency of the cytoskeletal protein dystrophin [348], is a sex-linked disorder [190a] that usually becomes symptomatic by the age of 3–5 years, progressing to death in the late teens. Rarely it is associated with abnormalities in ocular motility, but a retinopathy has been documented [221]. Deutan color blindness has been reported in some individuals with Duchenne and Becker's muscular dystrophy (similar to Duchenne muscular dystrophy but with later onset and slower course) [91,92,277].

   Local Anesthetic Myopathy.   Postoperative diplopia and ptosis have been described in some patients following exposure of the rectus muscles to local anesthetics [288]. Some local anesthetics induce myotoxic effects experimentally in extraocular muscles [51a,254].

   Gunn's Syndrome.   Marcus Gunn in 1883 [138] described a 15 year old with ptosis of the left eyelid, which would involuntarily jerk upward while eating or speaking. Gunn found that the elevation of the levator palpebral was produced by movement of the jaw to the right, which involves the action of the left external pterygoid. Many theories have been proposed concerning this phenomenon, sometimes referred to as the "winking jaw" phenomenon [400a]. Lyness and colleagues [210a] have studied the levator

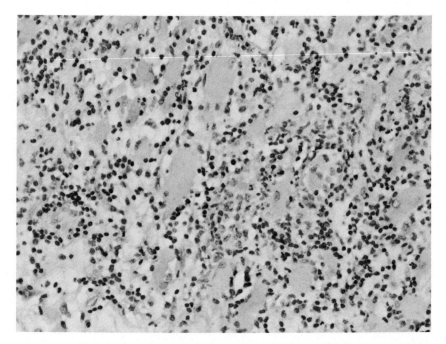

Figure 20   Ocular myositis. An infiltrate of mononuclear cells and neutrophils is associated with degenerating muscle fibers. (Hematoxylin and eosin, formalin fixed, ×250)

palpebrae superioris muscle and demonstrated neurogenic atrophy in the affected eyelid, as well as in some clinically unaffected eyelids from the same patients. They postulate a pathological process in the brain stem.

Other Disorders of Muscle. The literature contains a report of four siblings with Coats' disease, muscular dystrophy, mental retardation, and deafness [350].

Acute and chronic forms of ocular myositis [295,410] may present as proptosis, sometimes alternating from one orbit to the other [177]. Morphologically, lymphocytes and other inflammatory cells infiltrate between the muscle fibers, and perivascular muscle degeneration and fibrosis may be present (Fig. 20). An inflammatory myopathy has been reported in scleroderma [14].

A study of 21 individuals with gyrate atrophy of the choroid and retina (see Chap. 31) [346] disclosed type 2 fiber atrophy in all cases and tubular aggregates in 13 patients. Tubular aggregation in muscle are nonspecific, but their frequency in gyrate atrophy is unusual.

Several reports document unspecified myopathies with visual impairment or ocular abnormalities (visual loss, cataracts, retinopathy, and corneal crystals), sometimes associated with anomalies in other tissues [15,124,140,210,409,411].

REFERENCES

1. Aarli, J.A., Milde, E.J., and Thunold, S. Arthritis in myasthenia gravis. *J. Neurol. Neurosurg. Psychiatry* 38:1048–1105, 1975.
2. Aberfeld, D.C., and Namba, T. Progressive ophthalmoplegia in Kugelberg-Welander disease: Report of a case. *Arch. Neurol. 20*:253–256, 1969.
3. Aberfeld, D.C., Namba, T., Vye, M.V., and Grob, D. Chondrodystrophic myotonia: Report of two cases, myotonia, dwarfism, diffuse bone disease, and unusual ocular and facial abnormalities. *Arch. Neurol. 22*:455–462, 1970.
4. Abid, F., Hall, R., Hudgson, P., and Weiser, R. Moebius syndrome peripheral neuropathy, and hypo-gonadotrophic hypogonadism. *J. Neurol. Sci. 35*:309–315, 1978.
5. Adams, R.D., and Rebeiz, J.J. Histopathologie der myotonischen Erkrankungen. In *Progressive Muskel-dystrophie, Myotonie, Myasthenie*, E. Kuhn (Ed.), Springer-Verlag, Berlin, pp. 191–203, 1966.
6. Aharonov, A., Tarrab-Hazdai, R., Abramsky, O., and Fuchs, S. Immunological relationship between acetylcholine receptor and thymus: A possible significance in myasthenia gravis. *Proc. Natl. Acad. Sci. USA 72*:1456–1459, 1975.
7. Aicardi, J., Conti, D., and Goutieres, F. Les formes néo-natales de la dystrophie myotonique de Steinert. *J. Neurol. Sci. 22*:149–164, 1974.
8. Alexander, C.B., and Bossen, E.H. Peripheral couplings in human skeletal muscle. *Lab. Invest. 39*:17–20, 1978.
9. Alfano, J.E., and Berger, J.P. Retinitis pigmentosa, ophthalmoplegia, and spastic quadriplegia. *Am. J. Ophthalmol. 43*:231–240, 1957.
10. Allen, D.E., Johnson, A.G., and Woolf, A.L. The intramuscular nerve endings in dystrophia myotonica: A biopsy study by vital staining and electron microscopy. *J. Anat. 105*:1–26, 1969.
11. Allen, J.H., and Barer, C.G. Cataract of dystrophia myotonica. *Arch. Ophthalmol. 24*:867–884, 1940.
12. Almon, R.R., and Appel, S.H. Serum acetylcholine receptor antibodies in myasthenia gravis. *Ann. N.Y. Acad. Sci. 274*:235–243, 1976.
13. Appel, S.H., Almon, R.R., and Levy, N. Acetylcholine receptor antibodies in myasthenia gravis. *N. Engl. J. Med. 293*:760–761, 1975.
14. Arnett, F.C., and Michels, R.G. Inflammatory ocular myopathy in systemic sclerosis scleroderma, a case report and review of the literature. *Arch. Intern. Med. 132*:740–743, 1973.
15. Arnold, R.W., Stickler, G.B., Bourne, W.M., and Mellinger, J.F. Corneal crystals, myopathy and nephropathy: A new syndrome? *J. Pediatr. Ophthalmol. Strabismus 24*:151–155, 1987.
16. Ashizawa, T., and Appel, S.H. Immunopathologic events at the endplate in myasthenia gravis. *Springer Semin. Immunopathol. 8*:177–196, 1985.
17. Banker, B.Q., and Victor, M. Dermatomyositis systemic angiopathy of childhood. *Medicine (Baltimore) 45*:261–289, 1966.
18. Baptista, A.G., and Souza, H.S. Pupillary abnormalities in myasthenia gravis, report of a case. *Neurology 11*:210–213, 1961.
19. Bastiaensen, L.A.K. Chronic progressive external ophthalmoplegia. *Bull. Soc. Belge Ophtalmol. 237*:381–423, 1989.
20. Beaumont, W.M. Family tendency to ophthalmoplegia externa. *Trans. Ophthalmol. Soc. UK 20*:258–264, 1900.
21. Bender, A.N., Ringel, S.P., Engel, W.K., Vogel, Z., and Daniels, M.P. Immunoperoxidase localization of alpha bungarotoxin: A new approach to myasthenia gravis. *Ann. N.Y. Acad. Sci. 274*:20–30, 1976.

22. Berenberg, R.A., Pellock, J.M., DiMauro, S., Schotland, D.L., Bonilla, E., Eastwood, A., Hays, A., Vicale, C.T., Behrens, M., Chutorian, A., and Rowland, L.P. Lumping or splitting? "Ophthalmoplegia plus" or Kearns-Sayre syndrome. *Ann. Neurol. 1*:37–54, 1977.

23. Bergström, K., Franksson, C., Matell, G., and von Reis, G. The effect of thoracic duct lymph drainage in myasthenia gravis. *Eur. Neurol. 9*:157–167, 1973.

24. Berrih-Aknin, S., Morel, E., Raimond, F., Safar, D., Gaud, C., Binet, J.P., Levasseur, P., and Bach, J.F. The role of the thymus in myasthenia gravis: Immunohistological and immunological studies in 115 cases. *Ann. N.Y. Acad. Sci. 505*:50–70, 1987.

25. Berthold, H. Zur pathologischen Anatomie der Dystrophia myotonica Curschmann-Steinert. *Dtsch. Z. Nervenheilkd. 178*:394–412, 1958.

26. Bethlem, J., and van Wijngaarden, G.K. The incidence of ringed fibers and sarcoplasmic masses in normal and diseased muscle. *J. Neurol. Neurosurg. Psychiatry 26*:326–332, 1963.

27. Bethlem, J., van Wijngaarden, G.K., Mumenthaler, M., and Meijer, A.E.F. Centronuclear myopathy with type 1 fiber atrophy and "myotubes." *Arch. Neurol. 23*:70–73, 1970.

28. Bielschowsky, A. Bietrag zur Kenntnis der rezidivierenden und alternierenden Ophthalmoplegia exterior. *Graefes Arch. Ophthalmol. 90*:433–451, 1915.

29. Birdsall, W.R. Progressive paralysis of the external ocular muscle, or ophthalmoplegia externa. *J. Nerv. Ment. Dis. 14*:65–77, 1887.

30. Birmanns, B., Brenner, T., Abramsky, O., and Steiner, I. Seronegative myasthenia gravis: Clinical features, response to therapy, synthesis of acetylcholine receptor antibodies in vitro. *J. Neurol. Sci. 102*:184–189, 1991.

31. Black, J.T., Judge, D., Demers, L., and Gordon, S. Ragged-red fibers, a biochemical and morphological study. *J. Neurol. Sci. 26*:479–488, 1975.

32. Bogousslavsky, J., Perentes, D., Regli, F., and Deruaz, J.P. Polymyositis with severe facial involvement. *J. Neurol. Sci. 228*:277–281, 1982.

33. Bonilla, E., Schotland, D.L., DiMauro, S., and Lee, C.-P. Luft's disease: An electron cytochemical study. *J. Ultrastruct. Res. 58*:1–9, 1977.

34. Borenstein, S., Noel, P., Jacquy, J., and Flament-Durand, J. Myotonic dystrophy with nerve hypertrophy: Report of a case with electrophysiological and ultrastructural study of the sural nerve. *J. Neurol. Sci. 34*:87–99, 1977.

35. Bossen, E.H. Unpublished observations, 1981.

36. Bossen, E.H., Shelburne, J.D., and Verkauf, B.S. Respiratory muscle involvement in infantile myotonic dystrophy. *Arch. Pathol. 97*:250–252, 1974.

37. Botermans, C.H.G. Primary retinal degeneration and its association with neurological diseases. In *Handbook of Clinical Neurology, Neuroretinal Degeneration*, Vol. 13, P.J. Vinken and G.W. Bruyn (Eds.), American Elsevier, New York, pp. 148–379, 1972.

38. Brandt, D.E., and Leeson, C.R. Structural differences of fast and slow fibers in human extraocular muscle. *Am. J. Ophthalmol. 62*:478–487, 1966.

39. Bray, G.M., Kaarsoo, M., and Ross, R.T. Ocular myopathy with dysphagia. *Neurology 15*:678–684, 1965.

40. Breinin, G.M. The structure and function of extraocular muscle—an appraisal of the duality concept. *Am. J. Ophthalmol. 72*:1–9, 1971.

41. Brownell, B., Oppenheimer, D.R., and Spalding, J.M.K. Neurogenic muscle atrophy in myasthenia gravis. *J. Neurol. Neurosurg. Psychiatry 35*:311–322, 1972.

42. Brumback, R.A., Carlson, K.M., Wilson, H., and Staton, R.D. Myotonic dystrophy as a disease of abnormal membrane receptors: An hypothesis of pathophysiology and a new approach to treatment. *Med. Hypotheses 7*:1059–1066, 1981.

43. Brust, J.C.-M., List, T.A., Catalano, L.W., and Lovelace, R. Ocular myasthenia gravis mimicking progressive external ophthalmoplegia, rare case of myasthenia associated with peripheral neuropathy and spastic paraparesis. *Neurology 24*:755–760, 1974.

44. Bulloch, R.T., Davis, J.L., and Hara, M. Dystrophia myotonica with heart block. *Arch. Pathol. 84*:130–140, 1967.

45. Bunge, E. Der cholestesingehalt normaler und getrübter menschlicher Linsen. *Graefes Arch. Ophthalmol. 139*:50–61, 1938.

46. Burian, H.M., and Burns, C.A. Ocular changes in myotonic dystrophy. *Trans. Am. Ophthalmol. Soc. 64*:250–273, 1966.

47. Burns, C.A. Ocular histopathology of myotonic dystrophy: A clinicopathologic case report. *Am. J. Ophthalmol. 68*:416–422, 1969.

48. Butterfield, D.A. Electron spin resonance investigations of membrane proteins in erythrocytes in muscle diseases. Duchenne and myotonic muscular dystrophy and congenital myotonia. *Biochim. Biophys. Acta 470*:1–7, 1977.

49. Buxton, J., Shelbourne, P., Davies, J., Jones, C., Van Tongeren, T., Aslanidis, C., de Jong, P., Jansen, G., Anvret, M., Riley, B., Williamson, R., and Johnson, K. Detection of an unstable fragment of DNA specific to individuals with myotonic dystrophy. *Nature 355*:547–548, 1992.

50. Campbell, H., and Branwell, E. Myasthenia gravis. *Brain 23*:277–336, 1900.

51. Cannon, P.J. The heart and lungs in myotonic muscular dystrophy. *Am. J. Med. 32*:765–775, 1962.

51a. Carlson, B.M., Emerick, S., Komorowski, T.E., Rainin, E.A., and Shepard, B.M. Extraocular muscle regeneration in primates. Local anesthetic-induced lesions. *Ophthalmology 99*:582–589, 1992.
52. Carry, M.R., and Ringel, S.P. Structure and histochemistry of human extraocular muscle. *Bull. Soc. Belge Ophtalmol. 237*:303–319, 1989.
53. Castaigne, P., Laplane, D., Fardeau, M., Dordain, G., Autret, A., and Hirt, L. Myopathie avec anomalies mitochondriales localisées aux fibres de type 1. *Rev. Neurol. 126*:81–96, 1972.
54. Caughey, J.E., and Myrianthopoulos, N.C. *Dystrophia Myotonica and Related Disorders.* Charles C. Thomas, Springfield, IL, pp. 119–123, 1963.
55. Caughey, J.E., and Pachomov, N. The diaphragm in dystrophia myotonica. *J. Neurol. Neurosurg. Psychiatry 22*:311–313, 1956.
56. Chiu, H.-C., Vincent, A., Newsom-Davis, J., Hsieh, K.-H., and Hung, T.-P. Myasthenia gravis: Population differences by disease expression and acetylcholine receptor antibody titers between Chinese and caucasians. *Neurology 37*:1954–1957, 1987.
57. Coërs, C., and Telerman-Toppet, N. Morphological and histochemical changes of motor units in myasthenia. *Ann. N.Y. Acad. Sci. 274*:6–19, 1976.
58. Coërs, C., and Woolf, A.L. *The Innervation of Muscle*, Charles C. Thomas, Springfield, IL, pp. 107–112, 1959.
59. Cogan, D.G. Extraocular muscles and their diseases. In *Neurophthalmology*, Vol. 3, J.L. Smith (Ed.), C.V. Mosby, St. Louis, pp. 16–34, 1967.
60. Cogan, D.G., Kuwabara, T., and Richardson, E.P.G. Pathology of abiotrophic ophthalmoplegia externa. *Bull. Johns Hopkins Hosp. 111*:42–56, 1962.
61. Compston, D.A.S., Vincent, A., Newsom-Davis, J., and Batchelor, J.R. Clinical, pathological, HLA antigen and immunological evidence for disease heterogeneity in myasthenia gravis. *Brain 103*:579–601, 1980.
62. Conomy, J.P., Levinsohn, M., and Fanaroff, A. Familial infantile myasthenia gravis: A case of sudden death in young children. *J. Pediatr. 87*:428–430, 1975.
62a. Coquet, M., Vital, C., and Julian, J. Presence of inclusion body myositis-like filaments in oculopharyngeal muscular dystrophy: Ultrastructural study of 10 cases. *Neuropathol. Appl. Neurobiol. 16*:393–400, 1990.
63. Croft, P.B., Cutting, J.C., Jewesbury, E.C.O., Blackwood, W., and Mair, W.G.P. Ocular myopathy progressive external ophthalmoplegia with neuropathic complications. *Acta Neurol. Scand. 55*:169–197, 1977.
64. Crosby, T.W., and Chou, S.M. "Ragged-red" fibers in Leigh's disease. *Neurology 24*:49–54, 1974.
65. Culebras, A., Feldman, R.G., and Merk, F. Cytoplasmic inclusion bodies within neurons of the thalamus in myotonic dystrophy: A light and electron microscopic study. *J. Neurol. Sci. 19*:319–329, 1973.
66. Dalakas, M.C. Polymyositis, dermatomyositis, and inclusion-body myositis. *N. Engl. J. Med. 325*:1487–1498, 1991.
67. Danta, G., Hilton, R.C., and Lynch, P.G. Progressive external ophthalmoplegia. *Trans. Am. Neurol. Assoc. 99*:28–34, 1974.
68. Dark, A.J., and Streeten, B.W. Ultrastructural study of cataract in myotonia dystrophica. *Am. J. Ophthalmol. 84*:666–674, 1977.
69. Daroff, R.B., Solitare, G.B., Pincus, J.H., and Glaser, G.H. Spongiform encephalopathy with chronic progressive external ophthalmoplegia. *Neurology 16*:161–169, 1966.
70. Davidson, S.I. The eye in dystrophia myotonica, with a report on electromyography of the extra-ocular muscles. *Br. J. Ophthalmol. 45*:183–196, 1961.
71. Dawkins, R.L. Experimental autoallergic myositis, polymyositis and myasthenia gravis, autoimmune muscle disease associated with immunodeficiency and neoplasia. *Clin. Exp. Immunol. 21*:185–201, 1975.
72. Dawkins, R.L., and Mastaglia, F.L. Cell-mediated cytoxicity to muscle in polymyositis. *N. Engl. J. Med. 288*:434–438, 1973.
73. DeVries, S. Retinopathy in dermatomyositis. *Arch. Ophthalmol. 46*:432–435, 1951.
74. Dieperink, M.E., and Stefansson, K. Molecular mimicry and microorganisms: A role in the pathogenesis of myasthenia gravis. *Curr. Topics Microbiol. Immunol. 145*:57–65, 1989.
75. Dietert, S.E. The demonstration of different types of muscle fibers in human extraocular muscle by electron microscopy and cholinesterase staining. *Invest. Ophthalmol. 4*:51–63, 1965.
76. DiMauro, S., Schotland, D.L., Bonilla, E., Lee, C.-P., Gambetti, P., and Rowland, L.P. Progressive ophthalmoplegia, glycogen storage, and abnormal mitochondria. *Arch. Neurol. 29*:170–179, 1973.
77. DiMauro, S., Bonilla, E., Zeviani, M., Nakagawa, M., and De Vivo, D.C. Mitochondrial myopathies. *Ann. Neurol. 17*:521–538, 1985.
78. DiMauro, S., Bonilla, E., Lombes, A., Shanske, S., Minetti, C., and Moraes, C.T. Mitochondrial encephalomyopathies. *Neurol. Clin. 8*:483–506, 1990.
79. Drachman, D.A. Ophthalmoplegia plus: The neurodegenerative disorders associated with progressive external ophthalmoplegia. *Arch. Neurol. 18*:654–674, 1968.
80. Drachman, D.A. Ophthalmoplegia plus; a classification of the disorders associated with progressive external ophthalmoplegia. In *Handbook of Clinical Neurology*, Vol. 22, Part 2, *Systems Disorders and Atrophies*, P.J. Vinken and G.W. Bruyn (Eds.), American Elsevier, New York, pp. 203–216, 1975.
81. Drachman, D.A., Wetzel, N., Wasserman, M., and Naito, H. Experimental denervation of ocular muscles, a critique of the concept of "ocular myopathy." *Arch. Neurol. 21*:170–183, 1969.

82. Drachman, D.B. Myasthenia gravis. *N. Engl. J. Med.* 298:136–142; 186–192, 1978.
83. Drachman, D.B., De Silva, S., Ramsay, D., and Pestronk, A. Humoral pathogenesis of myasthenia gravis. *Ann. N.Y. Acad. Sci.* 505:90–105, 1987.
84. Dubowitz, V. Cross-innervated mammalian skeletal muscles: Histochemical physiological and biochemical observations. *J. Physiol. (Lond.)* 193:481–496, 1967.
85. Dubowitz, V. *Muscle Biopsy. A Practical Approach*, 2nd ed. Baillière, Tindall, Philadelphia, pp. 398–404, 1985.
86. Dubowitz, V. *Muscle Biopsy: A Modern Approach*, 2nd ed. W.B. Saunders, Philadelphia, pp. 28–30, 1985.
87. Duke-Elder, S. *Diseases of the Lens and Vitreous; Glaucoma and Hypotony: System of Ophthalmology*, Vol. 1. Kimpton, London, pp. 183–189, 1969.
88. Durelli, L., Maggi, G., Casadio, C., Ferri, R., Rendine, S., and Bergamini, L. Actuarial analysis of the occurrence of remissions following thymectomy for myasthenia gravis in 400 patients. *J. Neurol. Neurosurg. Psychiatry* 54:406–411, 1991.
89. Durston, J.H.J. Histochemistry of primate extraocular muscles and the changes of denervation. *Br. J. Ophthalmol.* 58:193–216, 1974.
90. Elmqvist, D., Hofmann, W.W., Kugelberg, J., and Quastel, D.M.J. An electrophysiological investigation of neuromuscular transmission in myasthenia gravis. *J. Physiol. (Lond.)* 174:417–434, 1964.
91. Emery, A.E.H. Genetic linkage between the loci for colour blindness and Duchenne type muscular dystrophy. *J. Med. Genet.* 3:92–95, 1966.
92. Emery, A.E.H., Smith, C.A.B., and Sanger, R. The linkage relations of the loci for benign Becker type X-borne muscular dystrophy, colour blindness and the Xg blood groups. *Ann. Hum. Genet.* 32:261–269, 1969.
93. Engel, A.G. Congenital disorders of neuromuscular transmission. *Semin. Neurol.* 10:12–26, 1990.
94. Engel, A.G., and Santa, T. Histometric analysis of the ultrastructure of the neuromuscular junction in myasthenia gravis and in the myasthenic syndrome. *Ann. N.Y. Acad. Sci.* 183:46–63, 1971.
95. Engel, A.G., and Gomez, M.R. Congenital myopathy associated with multifocal degeneration of muscle fibers. *Trans. Am. Neurol. Assoc.* 91:222–223, 1966.
96. Engel, A.G., Gomez, M.R., and Groover, R.V. Multicore disease: A recently recognized congenital myopathy associated with multifocal degeneration of muscle fibers. *Mayo Clin. Proc.* 46:666–681, 1971.
97. Engel, A.G., Lambert, E.H., and Gomez, M.R. A new myasthenic syndrome with end-plate acetylcholinesterase deficiency, small nerve terminals, and reduced acetylcholine release. *Ann. Neurol.* 1:315–330, 1977.
98. Engel, A.G., Lindstrom, J.M., Lambert, E.H., and Lennon, V.A. Ultrastructural localization of the acetylcholine receptor in myasthenia gravis and in its experimental autoimmune model. *Neurology* 27:307–315, 1977.
99. Engel, A.G., Tsujihata, M., Lindstrom, J.M., and Lennon, V.A. The motor end plate in myasthenia gravis and in experimental autoimmune myasthenia gravis: A quantitative ultrastructural study. *Ann. N.Y. Acad. Sci.* 274:60–79, 1976.
100. Engel, A., Lambert, E.H., and Howard, F.M., Jr. Immune complexes IgG and C3 and the motor end-plate in myasthenia gravis. *Mayo Clin. Proc.* 52:267–280, 1977.
101. Engel, W.K., Trotter, J.L., McFarlin, D.F., and McIntosh, C.L. Thymic epithelial cells contain acetylcholine receptor. *Lancet* 1:1310–1311, 1977.
102. Eshaghian, J., March, W.F., Goossens, W., and Rafferty, N.S. Ultrastructure of cataract in myotonic dystrophy. *Invest. Ophthalmol. Vis. Sci.* 17:289–293, 1978.
103. Eustace, P. Corneal lesions in myotonic dystrophy. *Br. J. Ophthalmol.* 53:633–637, 1969.
104. Evans, P.R. Nuclear agenesis, Möbius' syndrome: The congenital facial diplegia syndrome. *Arch. Dis. Child.* 30:237–243, 1955.
105. Eymard, B., Vernet-der Garabedian, B., Berrih-Aknin, S., Pannier, C., Bach, J.-F., and Morel, E. Anti-acetylcholine receptor antibodies in neonatal myasthenia gravis: Heterogeneity and pathogenic significance. *J. Autoimmun.* 4:185–195, 1991.
106. Fambrough, D.M., Drachman, D.B., and Satyamurti, S. Neuromuscular junction in myasthenia gravis: Decreased acetylcholine receptors. *Science* 182:293–295, 1975.
107. Fardeau, M. Some orthodox or non-orthodox considerations on congenital myopathies. *EEG (Suppl.)* 39:85–90, 1987.
108. Fardeau, M., Lapresle, I., and Milhaud, M. Contribution à l'étude des lèsions élémentaires du muscle squelettique: Ultrastructure des masses sarcoplasmiques latérales (observées dans un cas de dystrophie myotonique). *C.R. Soc. Biol. Paris* 159:15–17, 1965.
109. Farkas, E., Tome, F.M.S., Fardeau, M., Arsenio-Nunes, M.L., Dreyfus, P., and Diebler, M.F. Histochemical and ultrastructural study of muscle biopsies in 3 cases of dystrophia myotonica in the newborn child. *J. Neurol. Sci.* 21:273–288, 1974.
110. Febres, F., Scaglia, H., Lisker, R., Espinosa, J., Morato, T., Shkurovich, M., and Perez-Palacios, G. Hypothalamic-pituitary-gonadal function in patients with myotonic dystrophy. *J. Clin. Endocrinol. Metab.* 41:833–840, 1975.

111. Fenichel, G.M. Clinical syndromes of myasthenia in infancy and childhood, a review. *Arch. Neurol.* 35:97–103, 1978.
112. Fisch, C. The heart in myotonica atrophia. *Am. Heart J.* 41:525–538, 1951.
113. Fitch, N., Karpati, G., and Pinsky, L. Congenital blepharophimosis, joint contractures, and muscular hypotonia. *Neurology* 21:1214–1220, 1971.
114. Fitzsimons, R.B., and Tyer, H.D.D. A study of a myopathy presenting as idiopathic scoliosis: Multicore disease of mitochondrial myopathy. *J. Neurol. Sci.* 46:33–48, 1980.
115. Fleischer, B. Uber myotonische Dystrophie mit Katarakt. *Graefes Arch. Ophthalmol.* 96:91–133, 1918.
116. Fleischer, S., and Inui, M. Biochemistry and biophysics of excitation-contraction coupling. *Annu. Rev. Biophys. Chem.* 18:333–364, 1989.
117. Fonkalsrud, E.W., Herrmann, C., Jr., and Mulder, D.G. Thymectomy for myasthenia gravis in children. *J. Pediatr. Surg.* 5:157–165, 1970.
118. Fowler, M. Case of arthrogryposis multiplex congenita with lesions in the nervous system. *Arch. Dis. Child.* 34:505–510, 1959.
119. Fowler, W.M., Jr., Layzer, R.B., Taylor, R.G., Eberle, E.D., Sims, G.E., Munsat, T.L., Philippart, M., and Wilson, B.W. The Schwartz-Jampel syndrome. *J. Neurol. Sci.* 22:127–146, 1974.
120. Fritze, D., Herrmann, C., Jr., Naeim, F., Smith, G.S., Zeller, E., and Walford, R.L. The biologic significance of HL-A antigen markers in myasthenia gravis. *Ann. N.Y. Acad. Sci.* 274:440–450, 1976.
121. Fuchs, E. Ueber isolirte doppelseitige Ptosis. *Graefes Arch. Ophthalmol.* 36:234–259, 1890.
122. Fujii, Y., Hashimoto, J., Mondeu, Y., Ito, T., Nakahase, K., and Kawashima, Y. Specific activation of lymphocytes against acetylcholine receptor in the thymus in myasthenia gravis. *J. Immunol.* 136:887–891, 1986.
123. Fukuhara, N., Kumamato, T., Tsubaki, T., Mayuzumi, T., and Nitta, H. Oculopharyngeal muscular dystrophy and distal myopathy: Intrafamilial difference in the onset and distribution of muscular involvement. *Acta Neurol. Scand.* 65:458–467, 1982.
124. Furukawa, T., Takagi, A., Nakao, K., Sugita, H., Tsukagoshi, H., and Tsubaki, T. Hereditary muscular atrophy with ataxia retinitis pigmentosa, and diabetes mellitus, a clinical report of a family. *Neurology* 18:942–947, 1968.
125. Garcin, R., Fardeau, M., and Godet-Guillain, Mme. A clinical and pathological study of a case of alternating and recurrent external ophthalmoplegia with amyotrophy of the limbs observed for forty-five years: Discussion of the relationship of this condition with myasthenia gravis. *Brain* 88:739–752, 1965.
126. Gath, I., Kayan, A., Leegaard, J., and Sjaastad, O. Myasthenia congenita: Electromyographic findings. *Acta Neurol. Scand.* 46:323–330, 1970.
127. Genkins, G.L., Kornfeld, P., Papatestas, A.E., Bender, A.N., and Matta, R.J. Clinical experience in more than 2000 patients with myasthenia gravis. *Ann. N.Y. Acad. Sci.* 505:500–516, 1987.
128. Genkins, G., Papatestas, A.E., Horowitz, S.H., and Kornfeld, P. Studies in myasthenia gravis: Early thymectomy, electrophysiologic, and pathologic correlations. *Am. J. Med.* 58:517–524, 1975.
128a. Geuder, K.I., Marx, A., Witzemann, V., Schalke, B., Kirchner, T., and Müller-Hermelink, H.K. Genomic organization and lack of transcription of the nicotinic acetylcholine receptor subunit genes in myasthenia gravis-associated thymoma. *Lab. Invest.* 66:452–458, 1992.
129. Glaser, J.S. Myasthenic pseudo-internuclear ophthalmoplegia. *Arch. Ophthalmol.* 75:363–366, 1966.
130. Goebel, H.H., Meinck, H.M., Reinecke, M., Schimrigk, K., and Mielke, U. Centronuclear myopathy with special consideration of the adult form. *Eur. Neurol.* 23:425–434, 1984.
131. Goldstein, A.L., Thurman, G.B., Cohen, G.H., and Rossio, J.L. The endocrine thymus: Potential role for thymosin in the treatment of autoimmune disease. *Ann. N.Y. Acad. Sci.* 274:390–401, 1976.
132. Gonatas, N.K. A generalized disorder of nervous system, skeletal muscle, and heart resembling Refsum's disease and Hurler's syndrome. Part II. Ultrastructure. *Am. J. Med.* 42:169–178, 1967.
133. Goto, I., Kanazawa, Y., Kobayashi, T., Murai, Y., and Kuroiwa, Y. Oculopharyngeal myopathy with distal and cardiomyopathy. *J. Neurol. Neurosurg. Psychiatry* 40:600–607, 1977.
134. Gowers, W.R. *A Manual of Diseases of the Nervous System* V. 2, 2nd ed. Blakiston, Philadelphia, pp. 196–197, 1897.
135. Greer, M., and Schotland, M. Myasthenia gravis in the newborn. *Pediatrics* 26:101–108, 1960.
136. Grob, D., Arsura E.L., Brunner, N.G., and Namba, T. The course of myasthenia gravis and therapies affecting outcome. *Ann. N.Y. Acad. Sci.* 505:472–499, 1987.
137. Gross, M.L.P.,Teoh, R., Legg, N.J., and Pallis, C. Ocular myopathy and Marfan's syndrome. *J. Neurol. Sci.* 46:105–112, 1980.
138. Gunn, M. Congenital ptosis with peculiar associated movements of the affected lid. *Trans. Ophthalmol. Soc. UK* 3:283–287, 1883.
139. Haan, E.A., Mulley, J.C., Gedeon, A.K., Sheffield, L.J., and Sutherland, G.R. Presymptomatic testing for myotonic dystrophy by means of the linked DNA marker APOC. *Med. J. Aust.* 149:326–329, 1988.
140. Hanson, P.A., Mastrianni, A.F., and Post, L. Neonatal ophthalmoplegia with microfibers. *Neurology* 27:974–980, 1977.
141. Harding, A.E., and Holt, I.J. Mitochondrial myopathies. *Br. Med. Bull.* 45:760–771, 1989.

142. Harley, H.G., Brook, J.D., Rundle, S.A., Crow, S., Reardon, W., Buckler, A.J., Harper, P.S., Housman, D.E., and Shaw, D.J. Expansion of an unstable DNA region and phenotypic variation in myotonic dystrophy. *Nature* 355:545–546, 1992.

143. Harper, P.S. *Myotonic Dystrophy.* Saunders, London, pp. 28–30, 1989.

144. Harper, P.S., and Dyken, P.R. Early-onset dystrophia myotonica, evidence supporting a maternal environmental factor. *Lancet* 2:53–55, 1972.

145. Harper, P.S., Bias, W.B., Hutchinson, J.R., and McKusick, V.A. ABH secretor status of the fetus: A genetic marker identifiable by amniocentesis. *J. Med. Genet.* 8:438–440, 1971.

146. Harper, P., Penny, R., Roley, T.P., Jr., Migeon, C.J., and Blizzard, R.M. Gonadal function in males with myotonic dystrophy. *J. Clin. Endocrinol. Metab.* 35:852–856, 1972.

147. Harrison, S.M., Frenkel, M., Grossman, B.J., and Matalon, R. Retinopathy in childhood dermatomyositis. *Am. J. Ophthalmol.* 76:786–790, 1973.

148. Havard, C.W.H. Progress in myasthenia gravis. *Br. Med. J.* 2:1008–1011, 1977.

149. Hayasaka, S., Kiyosawa, M., Katsumata, S., Honda, M., Takase, S., and Mizuno, K. Ciliary and retinal changes in myotonic dystrophy. *Arch. Ophthalmol.* 102:88–93, 1984.

150. Hedger, R.W., Davis, F.A., Schwartz, F.P., and Ing, T.S. Improvement of myasthenia gravis by hemodialysis in a patient with chronic renal failure. *Ann. Intern. Med.* 75:749–752, 1971.

151. Heene, R. Histological and histochemical findings in muscle spindles in dystrophia myotonica. *J. Neurol. Sci.* 18:369–372, 1973.

152. Henderson, J.L. The congenital facial diplegia syndrome: Clinical features, pathology, and aetiology. *Brain* 62:381–403, 1939.

153. Herishanu, Y., and Lavy, S. Internal "ophthalmoplegia" in myasthenia gravis. *Ophthalmologica* 163:302–305, 1971.

154. Herrmann, H. The unification of muscle structure and function: A semicentennial anniversary. *Perspect. Biol. Med.* 33:1–11, 1989.

155. Horrobin, D.F., and Morgan, R.O. Myotonic dystrophy: A disease caused by functional zinc deficiency due to an abnormal zinc-binding ligand? *Med. Hypotheses* 6:375–388, 1980.

156. Houber, J.P., and Babel, J. Les lésions uvéorétiniennes de la dystrophie myotonique. *Ann. Ocul.* 203:1067–1076, 1970.

157. Howard, F.M., Jr., Lennon, V.A., Finley, J., Matsumoto, J., and Elveback, L.R. Clinical correlations of antibodies that bind, block, or modulate human acetylcholine receptors in myasthenia gravis. *Ann. N.Y. Acad. Sci.* 505:526–538, 1987.

158. Huang, S.-O.W., Rose, J.W., and Mayer, R.F. Assessment of cellular and humoral immunity of myasthenics. *J. Neurol. Neurosurg. Psychiatry* 40:1053–1059, 1977.

159. Hudgson, P., Bradley, W.G., and Jenkison, M. Familial "mitochondrial" myopathy, a myopathy associated with disordered oxidative metabolism in muscle fibers. Part I. Clinical, electrophysiological, and pathological findings. *J. Neurol. Sci.* 16:343–370, 1972.

160. Hurwitz, L.J., Carson, N.A.J., Allen, I.V., and Chopra, J.S. Congenital ophthalmoplegia, floppy baby syndrome, myopathy, and aminoaciduria. *J. Neurol. Neurosurg. Psychiatry* 32:495–508, 1969.

161. Hutchinson, J. On ophthalmoplegia externa or symmetrical immobility (partial) of the eyes, with ptosis. *Med. Chir. Trans. Lond.* 62:307–329, 1879.

162. Hyman, B.N., Patten, B.M., and Dodson, R.F. Mitochondrial abnormalities in progressive external ophthalmoplegia. *Am. J. Ophthalmol.* 83:362–371, 1977.

163. Iannaccone, S.T., Griggs, R.C., Markesbery, W.R., and Joynt, R.J. Familial progressive external ophthalmoplegia and ragged-red fibers. *Neurology* 24:1033–1038, 1974.

164. Isaacs, H., and Badenhorst, M. Multicore disease. *S. Afr. Med. J.* 57:543–546, 1980.

165. Ito, Y., Miledi, R., Molenaar, P.C., Vincent, A., Polak, R.L, van Elder, M., and Davis, J.N. Acetylcholine in human muscle. *Proc. R. Soc. Lond. [Biol.]* 192:475–480, 1976.

166. Jadro-Santel, D., Grcevic, N., Dogan, S., Franjic, J., and Benc, H. Centronuclear myopathy with type I fibre hypotrophy and "fingerprint inclusions" associated with Marfan's syndrome. *J. Neurol. Sci.* 45:43–56, 1980.

167. Jedlowski, P. Sulla oftalmoplegia esterna nucleare cronica progressiva. *Riv. Oto-Neuro-Oftalmol.* 20:203–239, 1943.

168. Jeger, B.V., Fred, H.L., Butler, R.B., and Carnes, W.H. Occurrence of retinal pigmentation, ophthalmoplegia, ataxia, deafness and heart block: Report of a case, with findings at autopsy. *Am. J. Med.* 29:888–893, 1960.

169. Johns, T.R., Campa, J.F., and Crowley, W.J. Familial myasthenic myopathy. *Neurology* 21:449, 1971.

170. Johnson, C.C., and Kuwabara, T. Oculopharyngeal muscular dystrophy. *Am. J. Ophthalmol.* 77:872–879, 1974.

171. Jonecko, A. Die Ringbinden als eine allgemeine unspezifische Reaktion der quergestreiften Muskulatur. *Experientia* 18:166–167, 1962.

172. Julien, J., Vital, C., Vallat, J.M., Roger, P., Lunel, G., and Vallat, M. Myopathie oculaire avec hypogonadisme primare: Anomalies mitochondriales en ultrastructure. *Rev. Neurol.* 128:365–377, 1973.

173. Junge, J. Ocular changes in dystrophia myotonica, paramyotonia, and myotonia congenita. *Doc. Ophthalmol.* 21:1–115, 1966.

174. Kaminski, H.J., Maas, E., Spiegel, P., and Ruff, R.L. Why are eye muscles frequently involved in myasthenia gravis. *Neurology 40*:1663–1669, 1990.
175. Kao, I., and Drachman, D.B. Thymic muscle cells bear acetylcholine receptors: Possible relation to myasthenia gravis. *Science 195*:74–75, 1977.
176. Karpati, G., Carpenter, S., Larbrisseau, A., and Lafontaine, R. The Kearns-Shy syndrome, a multisystem disease with mitochondrial abnormality demonstrated in skeletal muscle and skin. *J. Neurol. Sci. 19*:133–151, 1973.
177. Keane, J.R. Alternating proptosis, a case report of acute orbital myositis defined by the computerized tomographic scan. *Arch. Neurol. 34*:642–643, 1977.
178. Kearns, T.P. External ophthalmoplegia, pigmentary degeneration of the retina, and cardiomyopathy: A newly recognized syndrome. *Trans. Am. Ophthalmol. Soc. 63*:559–625, 1965.
179. Kearns, T.P., and Sayre, G.P. Retinitis pigmentosa, External ophthalmoplegia and complete heart block, unusual syndrome with histologic study in one of two cases. *Arch. Ophthalmol. 60*:280–289, 1958.
180. Keesey, J., Lindstrom, J., Cokely, H., and Herrmann, C., Jr. Antiacetylcholine receptor antibody in neonatal myasthenia gravis. *N. Engl. J. Med. 296*:55, 1977
181. Keesey, J., Shaikh, I., Wolfgram, F., and Chao, L.-P. Studies on the ability of acetylcholine receptors to bind alpha-bungarotoxin after exposure to myasthenic serum. *Ann. N.Y. Acad. Sci. 274*:244–253, 1976.
182. Ketola, H.G. Influence of dietary zinc on cataracts in rainbow trout (*Salmo gairdneri*). *J. Nutr. 109*:965–969, 1979.
183. Kiloh, L.G., and Nevin, S. Progressive dystrophy of the external ocular muscles (ocular myopathy). *Brain 74*:115–143, 1951.
184. Kirby, T.J., Achoc, R.W.P., Perry, H.O., and Winkelmann, R.K. Cataract formation after triparanol therapy. *Arch. Ophthalmol. 68*:486–489, 1962.
185. Kirchner, T., Tzartos, S., Hoppe, F., Schalko, B., Wekerle, H., and Müller-Hermelink, H.K. Pathogenesis of myasthenia gravis, acetylcholine receptor-related antigenic determinants in tumor-free thymuses and thymic epithelial tumors. *Am. J. Pathol. 130*:268–280, 1988.
186. Kissel, J.T., Mendell, J.R., and Rammohan, K.W. Microvascular deposition of complement membrane attack complex in dermatomyositis. *N. Engl. J. Med. 314*:329–334, 1986.
187. Kito, S., Yamamoto, M., Fujimori, N., Itoga, E., and Kosaka, K. Studies on myotonic dystrophy. Part I. Ultrastructural lesions of the muscle and the nerve in myotonic dystrophy. In *Basic Research in Myology*, B. Takulas (Ed.), Excerpta Medica, Amsterdam, pp. 651–673, 1973.
188. Klein, D. La dystrophie myotonique Steinert et la myotonie congénitale Thomsen en suisse. Etude clinique, génétique et démographique. *J. Genet. Hum. (Suppl.) 7*:1–328, 1958.
189. Klein, J.J., Gottlieb, A.J., Mones, R.J., Appel, S.H., and Osserman, K.E. Thymoma and polymyositis: Onset of myasthenia gravis after thymectomy. Report of two cases. *Arch. Intern. Med. 113*:142–152, 1964.
190. Kobayashi, M., Meek, J.C., and Streib, P. The insulin receptor in myotonic dystrophy. *J. Clin. Endocrinol. Metabol. 45*:821–824, 1977.
190a. Koenig, M., Hoffman, E.P., Bertelson, C.J., Monaco, A.P., Feener, C., and Kunkel, L.M. Complete cloning of the Duchenne muscular dystrophy (DMD) gene in normal and affected individuals. *Cell 50*:509–517, 1987.
191. Korenyi-Both, A., Lapis, K., Gallai, M., and Szobor, A. Fine structural alterations of muscle fibers in diseases accompanied by myotonia. *Beitr. Pathol. 156*:241–256, 1975.
192. Korman, E.F., Harris, R.A., Williams, C.H., Wakabayashi, T., Green, D.E., and Valdivia, E. Paracrystalline arrays in mitochondria. *Bioenergetics 1*:387–404, 1970.
193. Kuks, J.B.M., Oosterhuis, H.J.G.H., Limburg, P.C., and The, T.H. Anti-acetylcholine receptor antibodies decrease after thymectomy in patients with myasthenia gravis. Clinical correlations. *J. Autoimmun. 4*:197–211, 1991.
194. Kuwabara, T., and Lessell, S. Electron microscopic study of extraocular muscles in myotonic dystrophy. *Am. J. Ophthalmol. 82*:303–309, 1976.
195. Lagoutte, F., Coquet, M., and Vital, C. Étude ultrastructurale de la musculature oculaire dans deux cas familiaux de maladie de Steinert. *Arch. Ophtalmol. Paris 36*:565–574, 1976.
196. Lakin, M., and Locke, S. Progressive ocular myopathy with ovarian insufficiency and diabetes mellitus: Report of a case. *Diabetes 10*:228–231, 1961.
197. Langdon, H.M., and Cadwalader, W.B. Chronic progressive external ophthalmoplegia: Report of a case with necropsy. *Brain 51*:321–333, 1928.
198. Lefvert, A.K., and Matell, G. Antibodies against human cholinergic receptor proteins in patients with myasthenia gravis: Studies during immunosuppressive treatment. *Acta Med. Scand. 20*:181–182, 1977.
199. Lell, M.E., and Swerdlow, M.L. Dermatomyositis of childhood. *Pediatr. Ann. 6*:203–212, 1977.
200. Lenard, H.G., Goebel, H.H., and Weigel, W. Smooth muscle involvement in congenital myotonic dystrophy. *Neuropediatrics 8*:42–52, 1977.
201. Lessell, S., Coppeto, S., and Samet, S. Ophthalmoplegia in myotonic dystrophy. *Am. J. Ophthalmol. 71*:1231–1235, 1971.
202. Lindstrom, J.M., Seybold, M.E., Lennon, V.A., Whittingham, S., and Duane, D.D. Antibody to acetylcholine receptor in myasthenia gravis. *Neurology 26*:1054–1059, 1976.

203. Lindstrom, J., Shelton, D., and Fujii, Y. Myasthenia gravis. *Adv. Immunol.* 42:233–284, 1988.
204. Linton, D.M., and Philcox, D. Myasthenia gravis. *Dis. Mon.* 36:595–637, 1990.
205. Lisak, R.P., Abdou, N.I., Zweiman, B., Zmijewski, C., and Penn, A. Aspects of lymphocyte function in myasthenia gravis. *Ann. N.Y. Acad. Sci.* 274:402–410, 1976.
206. Little, B.W., and Perl, D.P. Oculopharyngeal muscular dystrophy: An autopsied case from the French-Canadian kindred. *J. Neurol. Sci.* 53:145–158, 1982.
207. Lotz, B.P., and Van der Meyden, C.H. Myotonic dystrophy. Part II. A clinical study of 96 patients. *S. Afr. Med. J.* 67:815–817, 1985.
208. Luft, R., Ikkos, D., Palmierl, G., Ernster, L., and Afzelius, B. A case of severe hypermetabolism of non-thyroid origin with a defect in maintenance of mitochondrial respiratory control: A correlated clinical, biochemical, and morphological study. *J. Clin. Invest.* 41:1776–1804, 1962.
209. Lundberg, P.O. Ocular myopathy with hypogonadism. *Acta Neurol. Scand.* 38:142–155, 1962.
210. Lundberg, P.O. Hereditary myopathy, oligophrenia, cataract, skeletal abnormalities, and hypergonadotrophic hypgonadism: A new syndrome. *Eur. Neurol.* 10:261–280, 1973.
210a. Lyness, R.W., Collin, J.R.O., Alexander, R.A., and Garner, A. Histological appearances of the levator palpebrae superioris muscle in the Marcus Gunn phenomenon. *Br. J. Ophthalmol.* 72:104–109, 1988.
211. Manschot, W.A. Histological findings in a case of dystrophia myotonica. *Opthalmologica* 155:294–296, 1968.
212. Mantegazza, R., Beghi, E., Pareyson, D., Antozzi, C., Peluchetti, D., Sghirlanzoni, A., Cosi, V., Lombardi, M., Piccolo, G., Tonali, P., Evoli, A., Ricci, E., Batocchi, A.P., Angelini, C., Micaglio, G.F., Marconi, G., Tailuti, R., Bergamini, L., Durelli, L., and Cornelio, F. A multicentre follow-up study of 1152 patients with myasthenia gravis in Italy. *J. Neurol.* 237:339–344, 1990.
213. Margolis, S., and Luginbuehl, B. Eye abnormalities associated with arthrogryposis multiplex congenita. *J. Pediatr. Ophthalmol.* 12:57–60, 1975.
214. Martinez, A.I., Hay, S., and McNeer, K.W. Extraocular muscles, light microscopy and ultrastructural features. *Acta Neuropathol. (Berl.)* 34:237–253, 1976.
215. Maselli, R.A., Richman, D.P., and Wollmann, R.L. Inflammation at the neuromuscular junction in myasthenia gravis. *Neurology* 41:1497–1504, 1991.
216. Mason, G.I. Iris neovascular tufts: Relationship to rubeosis, insulin, and hypotony. *Arch. Ophthalmol.* 97:2346–2352, 1979.
217. Masters, C.L., Dawkins, R.L., Zilko, P.J., Simpson, J.A., Leedman, R.J., and Lindstrom, J. Penicillamine-associated myasthenia gravis, antiacetylcholine receptor, and antistriational antibodies. *Am. J. Med.* 63:689–694, 1977.
218. Matsunaga, M., Inokuchi, T., Ohnishi, A., and Kuroiwa, Y. Oculopharyngeal involvement in familial neurogenic muscular atrophy. *J. Neurol. Neurosurg. Psychiatry* 36:104–111, 1973.
219. Maynard, J.A., Cooper, R.R., and Ionaescu, V.V. An ultrastructure investigation of intrafusal muscle fibers in myotonic dystrophy. *Virchows Arch. [A]* 373:1–13, 1977.
220. McComas, A.J., Campbell, M.J., and Sica, R.E.P. Electrophysiological study of dystrophia myotonica. *J. Neurol. Neurosurg. Psychiatry* 34:132–139, 1971.
221. McCormack, W.M., and Spatter, H.F. Muscular dystrophy, alveolar hypoventilation, and papilledema. *JAMA* 197:957–960, 1966.
222. McLeod, J.G., Baker, W.D., Lethlean, A.K., and Shorye, C.D. Centronuclear myopathy with autosomal dominant inheritance. *J. Neurol. Sci.* 15:375–387, 1972.
223. McQuillen, M.P. Familial limb-girdle myasthenia. *Brain* 89:121–165, 1966.
224. Melmed, C., Karpati, G., and Carpenter, S. Experimental mitochondrial myopathy produced in vivo uncoupling of oxidative phosphorylation. *J. Neurol. Sci.* 26:305–318, 1975.
225. Meredith, A.L., Huson, S.M., Lunt, P.W., Sarfarazi, M., Harley, H.G., Brook, J.D., Shaw, D.J., and Harper, P.S. Application of a closely linked polymorphism of restriction fragment length to counseling and prenatal testing in families with myotonic dystrophy. *Br. Med. J.* 293:1353–1356, 1986.
226. Mereu, T.R., Porter, I.H., and Hug, G. Myotonia, shortness of stature, and hip dysplasia, Schwartz-Jampel syndrome. *Am. J. Dis. Child.* 117:470–478, 1969.
227. Metz, H.S. Myasthenia gravis presenting as internuclear ophthalmoplegia. *J. Pediatr. Ophthalmol.* 14:23–24, 1977.
228. Meyer, E., Navon, D., Auslender, L., and Zonis, S. Myotonic dystrophy: Pathological study of the eyes. *Ophthalmologica (Basel)* 181:215–220, 1980.
229. Miller, J.E. Cellular organization of rhesus extraocular muscle. *Invest. Ophthalmol.* 6:18–39, 1967.
230. Minoda, K. Histochemical and electron microscopic studies of extraocular muscles. Part IV. Fine structure or neuropathic extraocular muscles. *Acta Soc. Ophthalmol. Jpn.* 75:1184–1195, 1971.
231. Möbius, P.J. Über infantilen Kernschwund. *Muench. Med. Wochenschr.* 39:17–21, 41–43, 55–58, 1892.
232. Möbius, P.J. Ueber angeborenedoppelseitige Abducens-Facialis-Lähmung. *Muench. Med. Wochenschr.* 35:91–94, 1888.
233. Möbius P.J. Über periodische oculomotoriuslähmung. *Dtsch. Z. Nervenheilkd.* 17:294–305, 1900.
234. Mongia, S.K., and Lundervold, A. Electrophysiological abnormalities in cases of dystrophia myotonica. *Eur. Neurol.* 13:360–376, 1975.

235. Moran, C.A., Suster, S., and Jagirdar, J. Morphometric analysis of germinal centers in nonthymomatous patients with myasthenia gravis. *Arch. Pathol. Lab. Med. 114*:689–691, 1990.

236. Morgan, G., Peter, J.B., and Newbould, B.B. Experimental allergic myositis in rats. *Arthritis Rheum. 14*:599–609, 1971.

237. Morgan-Hughes, J.A., and Mair, W.G,P. A typical muscle mitochondria in oculoskeletal myopathy. *Brain 96*:215–224, 1973.

238. Morgan-Hughes, J.A., Cooper, J.M., Schapira, A.H.V., Hayes, D.J., and Clark, J.B. The mitochondrial myopathies: Defects of the mitochondrial respiratory chain and oxidative phosphorylation system. *EEG (Suppl.) 39*:103–114, 1987.

239. Mostacciuolo, M.L., Barujani, G., Armani, M., Danieli, G.A., and Angelini, C. Genetic epidemiology of myotonic dystrophy. *Genet. Epidemiol. 4*:289–298, 1987.

240. Moxley, R.T. Metabolic studies in muscular dystrophy: A role for insulin. *Adv. Neurol. 17*:161–173, 1977.

241. Munro, S. Fundus appearances in a case of acute dermatomyositis. *Br. J. Ophthalmol. 43*:548–558, 1959.

242. Murphy, S.F., and Drachman, D.B. The oculopharyngeal syndrome. *JAMA 203*:1003–1008, 1968.

243. Mussini, I.D., Mauro, S., and Angelini, C. Early ultrastructural and biochemical changes in muscle in dystrophia myotonica. *J. Neurol. Sci. 10*:585–604, 1970.

244. Naegeli, W. Über Myotonica atrophica, speziell über die Symptome und die Pathogenese der Krankheit nach 22 eigenen Fällen. *Muench. Med. Wochenschr. 64*:1631–1632, 1917.

245. Namba, T., Brown, S.B., and Grob, D. Neonatal myasthenia gravis: Report of two cases and review of the literature. *Pediatrics 45*:488–504, 1970.

246. Namba, T., Nakamura, T., and Grob, D. Motor nerve endings in human extraocular muscle. *Neurology 18*:403–407, 1968.

247. Namba, T., Nakata, Y., and Grob, D. The role of humoral and cellular immune factors in neuromuscular block in myasthenia gravis. *Ann. N.Y. Acad. Sci. 274*:493–515, 1976.

248. Newsom-Davis, J., Pinching, A.J., Vincent, A., and Wilson, S.G. Function of circulating antibody to acetylcholine receptor in myasthenia gravis: Investigation by plasma exchange. *Neurology 28*:266–272, 1978.

249. Newsom-Davis, J., Willcox, N., Schluep, M., Harcourt, G., Vincent, A., Mossman, S., Wray, D., and Burges, J. Immunological heterogenity and cellular mechanisms in myasthenia. *Ann. N.Y. Acad. Sci. 505*:12–38, 1987.

250. Nicolaissen, B., and Brodal, A. Chronic progressive external ophthalmoplegia. *Arch. Ophthalmol. 61*:202–210, 1959.

251. O'Leary, P.A., and Waisman, M. Dermatomyositis: A study of forty cases. *Arch. Dermatol. Syphilol. 41*:1001–1019, 1940.

252. Oda, K. Motor innervation and acetylcholine receptor distribution of human extraocular muscle fibres. *J. Neurol. Sci. 74*:125–133, 1986.

253. Okamura, K., Santa, T., Nage, K., and Omae, T. Congenital oculoskeletal myopathy with abnormal muscle and liver mitochondria. *J. Neurol. Sci. 27*:79–91, 1976.

254. Oklund, S., Komorowski, T.E., and Carlson, B.M. Ultrastructure of mepivacaine-induced damage and regeneration in rat extraocular muscle. *Invest. Ophthamol. Vis. Sci. 20*:1643–1651, 1989.

255. Olsen, W.K., Bardin, C.W., Walsh, O., and Engel, W.K. Moebius syndrome: Lower motor neuron involvement and hypogonadotrophic hypogonadism. *Neurology 20*:1002–1008, 1970.

256. Olson, W., Engel, W.K., Walsh, G.O., and Einaugler, R. Oculocraniosomatic neuromuscular disease with "ragged-red" fibers. *Arch. Neurol. 26*:193–211, 1972.

257. Oosterhuis, H. and Bethlem, J. Neurogenic muscle involvement in myasthenia gravis, a clinical and histopathological study. *J. Neurol. Neurosurg. Psychiatry 36*:224–254, 1973.

258. Orth, D.N., Almeida, H., Walsh, F.B., and Henda, M. Ophthalmoplegia resulting from diphenylhydantoin and primidone intoxication: Report of four cases. *JAMA 201*:225–227, 1967.

259. Ortiz deZarate, J.C., and Maruffo, A. The descending ocular myopathy of early childhood: Myotubular or centronuclear myopathy. *Eur. Neurol. 3*:1–12, 1970.

260. Osher, R.H., and Smith, J.L. Ocular myasthenia gravis and Hashimoto's thyroiditis. *Am. J. Ophthalmol. 79*:1038–1043, 1975.

261. Osserman, K.E., and Genkins, G. Studies in myasthenia gravis: Review of a twenty year experience in over 1200 patients. *Mt. Sinai J. Med. 38*:497–537, 1971.

262. Pachter, B.R., Davidowitz, J., and Breinin, G.M. Light and electron microscopic serial analysis of mouse extraocular muscle: Morphology, innervation, and topographical organization of component fiber populations. *Tissue Cell 8*:547–560, 1976.

263. Pachter, B.R., Eberstein, A., and Breinin, G.M. Electromyographic and electron microscopic findings in the central extraocular muscles of the myotonic rat. *Exp. Neurol. 57*:971–983, 1977.

264. Pachter, B.R., Pearson, J., Davidowitz, J., Reuben, R., Boal, D., Carr, R., and Breinin, G.M. Congenital total external ophthalmoplegia associated with infantile spinal muscular atrophy: Fine structure of extraocular muscle. *Invest. Ophthalmol. 15*:320–324, 1976.

265. Paez, J.H., Tuulonen, A., Yarom, R., Arad, H., Zelikovitch, A., and Ben Ezra, D. Ocular findings in arthrogryposis multiplex congenita. *J. Pediatr. Ophthalmol. Strabismus 19*:75–79, 1982.

266. Panayiotopoulos, C.P., and Scarpalezos, S. Dystrophia myotonica, a model of combined neural and myopathic muscle atrophy. *J. Neurol. Sci.* *31*:261–268, 1977.
267. Papatestas, A.E., Genkins, G., Horowitz, S.H., and Kornfeld, P. Thymectomy in myasthenia gravis: Pathologic, clinical, and electrophysiologic correlations. *Ann. N.Y. Acad. Sci.* *274*:555–573, 1976.
268. Patrick, J., and Lindstrom, J. Autoimmune response to acetylcholine receptor. *Science* *180*:871–872, 1973.
269. Peachey, L. The structure of the extraocular muscle fibers of mammals. In *The Control of Eye Movements*, P. Bach-Y-Rita and C.C. Collins (Eds.), Academic Press, New York, pp. 47–66, 1971.
270. Pearson, C.M. Polymyositis. *Annu. Rev. Med.* *17*:63–82, 1966.
271. PeBenito, R., Sher, J.H., and Cracco, J.B. Centronuclear myopathy: Clinical and pathologic features. *Clin. Pediatr.* *17*:259–265, 1978.
272. Peck, S.M., Osserman, K.E., Weiner, L.B., Lefkovits, A., and Osserman, R.S. Studies in bullous diseases: Immunofluorescent serologic tests. *N. Engl. J. Med.* *279*:951–958, 1968.
273. Pendefunda, G., Cernea, P., and Dobrescu,G. Manifestarile oculare in miotonia atrofica Steinert. *Oftalmologia* *8*:219–224, 1964.
274. Pepin, B., Mikol. J., Goldstein, B., Aron, J.J., and Lebuisson, D.A. Familial mitochondrial myopathy with cataract. *J. Neurol. Sci.* *45*:191–203, 1980.
275. Perlo, V.P., Arnason, B., Poskanzer, D., Castleman, B., Schwab, R.S., Osserman, K.E., Papatestis, A., Alpert, L., and Kark, A. The role of thymectomy in the treatment of myasthenia gravis. *Ann. N.Y. Acad. Sci.* *183*: 308–317, 1971.
276. Petkovich, N.J., Dunn, M., and Reed, W. Myotonia dystrophica with A-V dissociation and Stokes-Adams attacks. *Am. Heart J.* *68*:391–396, 1964.
277. Philip, U., Walton, J.N., and Smith, C.A.B. Colour blindness and the Duchenne-type muscular dystrophy. *Ann. Hum. Genet.* *21*:155–158, 1956.
278. Pinto, F., Amantini, A., de Scisciolo, G., Scaioli, V., Frosini, R., Pizzi, A., and Marconi, G. Electrophysiological studies of the visual system in myotonic dystrophy. *Acta Neurol. Scand.* *76*:351–358, 1987.
279. Pirskanen, R. On the significance of HL-A and LD antigens in myasthenia gravis. *Ann. N.Y. Acad. Sci.* *274*:451–460, 1976.
280. Pitner, S.E., Edwards, J.E., and McCormick, W.F. Observations on the pathology of the Moebius syndrome. *J. Neurol. Neurosurg. Psychiatry* *28*:362–374, 1965.
281. Plishker, G.A., Gitelman, H.J., and Appel, S.H. Myotonic muscular dystrophy: Altered calcium transport in erythrocytes. *Science* *200*:323–325, 1978.
282. Pollock, M., and Dyck, P.J. Peripheral nerve morphometry in myotonic dystrophy. *Arch. Neurol.* *33*:33–39, 1976.
283. Porter, C.W., and Barnard, E.A. Ultrastructural studies on the acetylcholine receptor at motor end plates of normal and pathologic muscles. *Ann. N.Y. Acad. Sci.* *274*:85–107, 1976.
284. Pryse-Phillips, W., Johnson, G.J., and Larsen, B. Incomplete manifestations of myotonic dystrophy in a large kinship in Labrador. *Ann. Neurol.* *11*:582–591, 1982.
285. Racz, P., Kovacs, B., Varga, L., Ujlaki, E., Zombai, E., and Karbuczky, S. Bilateral cataract in acrodermatitis enteropathica. *J. Pediatr. Ophthalmol. Strabismus* *16*:180–182, 1979.
286. Radu, H., Killyen, I., Ionescu, V., and Radu, A. Myotubular centronuclear neuromyopathy. I. Clinical, genetical, and morphological studies. *Eur. Neurol.* *15*:285–300, 1977.
287. Radu, H., Pendefunda, G., Blucher, G., Radu, A., Darko, Z., and Godri, I. Comparative and correlative study of the myotonias. In *Muscle Diseases*, J.N. Walton, N. Canal, and G. Scarlato (Eds.), Excerpta Medica, Amsterdam, pp. 332–336, 1970.
288. Rainin, E.A., and Carlson, B.M. Postoperative diplopia and ptosis: A clinical hypothesis bases on the myotoxicity of local anesthestics. *Arch. Ophthalmol.* *103*:1337–1339, 1985.
289. Raitta, C., and Karli, P. Ocular findings in myotonic dystrophy. *Ann. Ophthalmol.* *14*:646–650, 1982.
290. Raju, T.N.K., Vidyasagar, D., Reyes, M.G., and Chokroverty, S. Centronuclear myopathy in the newborn period causing severe respiratory distress. *Pediatrics* *59*:29–34, 1977.
291. Rash, J.E., Albuquerque, E.X., Hudson, C.S., Mayer, R.F., and Satterfield, J.R. Studies of human myasthenia gravis: Electrophysiological and ultrastructural evidence compatible with antibody attachment to acetylcholine receptor complex. *Proc. Natl. Acad. Sci. USA* *73*:4584–4588, 1976.
292. Remacle, J.-P., Pellissier, J.-F., Chamlian, A., Benkoèl, L., Aubert, L., and Monges, H. Progressive ophthalmoplegia associated with asymptomatic primary biliary cirrhosis. *Hum. Pathol. (Suppl.)* *11*:540–548, 1980.
293. Reske-Nielsen, E., Hein-Sorensen, O., and Vorre, P., Familial centronuclear myopathy: A clinical and pathological study. *Acta Neurol. Scand.* *76*:115–122, 1987.
294. Richards, R.N. The Möbius syndrome. *J. Bone Joint Surg. [Am.]* *35*:437–444, 1953.
295. Ricker, K., and Pohlenz, S. Ocular myositis and neuromyositis. *Eur. Neurol.* *1*:41–49, 1968.
296. Ringel, S.P., Engel, W.K., Bender, A.N., Peters, N.D., and Yee, R.D. Histochemistry and acetylcholine receptor distribution in normal and denervated monkey extraocular muscle. *Neurology* *28*:55–63, 1978.
297. Roberts, A.H., and Bamforth, J. The pharynx and esophagus in ocular muscular dystrophy. *Neurology* *18*:645–652, 1968.

298. Roberts, D.F., and Bradley, W.G. Immunoglobulin levels in dystrophia myotonica. *J. Med. Genet. 14*:16–19, 1977.
299. Rogers, E.L., Hatch, G.F., Jr., and Gray, I. Möbius syndrome and limb abnormalities. *J. Pediatr. Ophthalmol. 14*:134–138, 1977.
300. Romanul, F.C.A., and van der Meulen, J.P. Slow and fast muscles after cross-innervation, enzymatic, and physiological changes. *Arch. Neurol. 17*:387–402, 1967.
301. Rosenberg, R.N., Schotland, D.L., Lovelace, R.E., and Rowland, L.P. Progressive ophthalmoplegia. *Arch. Neurol. 19*:362–376, 1968.
302. Roses, A.D. Myotonic muscular dystrophy: From clinical description to molecular genetics. *Arch. Intern. Med. 145*:1487–1492, 1985.
303. Roses, A.D., and Appel, S.H. Protein kinase activity in erythrocyte ghosts of patients with myotonic muscular dystrophy. *Proc. Natl. Acad. Sci. USA 70*:1855–1859, 1973.
304. Roses, A.D., and Appel, S.H. Muscle membrane protein kinase in myotonic muscular dystrophy. *Nature 250*:245–247, 1974.
305. Roses, A.D., and Appel, S.H. Phosphorylation of a component of the human erythrocyte membrane in myotonic muscular dystrophy. *J. Membr. Biol. 20*:51–58, 1975.
306. Roses, A.D., Harper, P.S., and Bossen, E.H. Myotonic muscular dystrophy. In *Handbook of Clinical Neurology*, Vol. 40, Part 1, P.J. Vinken and F.W. Bruyn (Eds.), American Elsevier, New York, pp. 485–532, 1979.
307. Rosman, N.P., and Kakulas, B.A. Mental deficiency associated with muscular dystrophy: A neuropathological study. *Brain 89*:769–788, 1966.
308. Rowland, L.P. Progressive external ophthalmoplegia. In *Handbook of Clinical Neurology*, Vol. 22, *Systems Disorders and Atrophies*, Part 2, P.J. Vinken and G.W. Bruyn (Eds.), American Elsevier, New York, pp. 177–202, 1975.
309. Rubin, F.H., and Cross, S.A. Oculopharyngeal dystrophy. *Arch. Intern. Med. 141*:1103, 1981.
310. Ruff, R., Kaminski, H., Maas, E., and Spiegel, P. Ocular muscles: Physiology and structure-function correlations. *Bull. Soc. Belge Ophtalmol. 237*:321–352, 1989.
311. Ryniewicz, B., and Badurska, B. Follow-up study of myasthenic children after thymectomy. *J. Neurol. 217*:133–138, 1977.
312. Sagel, J., Distiller, L.A., Morley, J.E., and Isaacs, H. Myotonia dystrophica: Studies on gonadal function using luteinizing hormone-releasing hormone LRH. *J. Clin. Endocrinol. Metab. 40*:1110–1113, 1975.
313. Sahashi, K., Engel, A.G., Lindstrom, J.M., Lambert, E.H., and Lennon, W.A. Ultrastructural localization of immune complexes IgG and C3 at the end-plate in experimental autoimmune myasthenia gravis. *J. Neuropathol. Exp. Neurol. 37*:212–223, 1978.
314. Sanders, D.B., Cobb, E.E., and Winfield, J.B. Neonatal experimental autoimmune myasthenia gravis. *Muscle Nerve 1*:146–150, 1978.
315. Sandifer, P.H. Chronic progressive ophthalmoplegia of myopathic origin. *J. Neurol. Neurosurg. Psychiatry 9*:81–83, 1946.
316. Sandyk, R., and Brennan, M.J.W. Isolated ocular myopathy and celiac disease in childhood. *Neurology 33*:792, 1983.
317. Sarnat, H.B., McGarry, J.D., and Lewis, J.E. Effective treatment of infantile myasthenia gravis by combined prednisone and thymectomy. *Neurology 27*:550–553, 1977.
318. Sautter, H. Myotonie und cataracta myotonica. *Graefes Arch. Ophthalmol. 143*:1–26, 1941.
319. Scadding, G.K., Vincent, A., Newsom-Davis, J., and Henry, K. Acetylcholine receptor antibody synthesis by thymic lymphocytes: Correlation with thymic histology. *Neurology 31*:935–943, 1981.
320. Scarlato, G., and Spinnler, H. Histochemical evidence of muscular neurogenic involvement associated with hereditary optic atrophy. *Med. J. Aust. 1*:282–283, 1974.
321. Scarlato, G., Pellegrini, G., and Veicsteinas, A. Morphologic and metabolic studies in a case of oculo-craniosomatic neuromuscular disease. *J. Neuropathol. Exp. Neurol. 37*:1–12, 1978.
322. Scelsi, R., Marchetti, C., Faggi, L., Sandrini, G., and Rocchelli, B. An ocular myopathy with glycogen storage and abnormal mitochondria in muscle fibers: Histochemical and ultrastructural findings. *Eur. Neurol. 20*:440–444, 1981.
323. Schluep, M., Willco, N., Vincent, A., Dhoot, G.K., and Newsom-Davis, J. Acetylcholine receptors in human thymic myoid cells in an immunohistological study. *Ann. Neurol. 22*:212–222, 1987.
324. Schmidt, D., and Kommerell, G. Okuläre myasthenie durch D-penicillamin-Behandlung. *Klin. Msbl. Augenheilkd. 168*:409–413, 1976.
325. Schmitt, H.P., and Krause, K.-H. An autopsy study of a familial oculopharyngeal muscular dystrophy OPMD with distal spread and neurogenic involvement. *Muscle Nerve 4*:296–305, 1981.
326. Schneck, L., Adachi, M., Briet, P., Wolintz, A., and Volk, B.W. Ophthalmoplegia plus with morphological and chemical studies of cerebellar and muscle tissue. *J. Neurol. Sci. 19*:37–44, 1973.
327. Schochet, S.S., Jr., Zellweger, H., Ionasescu, V., and McCormick, W.F. Centronuclear myopathy: Disease entity or a syndrome? Light and electron-microscopic study of two cases and review of the literature. *J. Neurol. Sci. 16*:215–228, 1972.

328. Schotland, D.L., DiMauro, S., Bonilla, E., Scarpa, A., and Lee, C.-P. Neuromuscular disorder associated with a defect in mitochondrial energy supply. *Arch. Neurol. 33*:475–479, 1976.

329. Schönbeck, S., Chrestal, S., and Hohlfeld, R. Myasthenia gravis: Prototype of the antireceptor diseases. *Int. Rev. Neurobiol. 32*:175–200, 1990.

330. Schwartz, G.-A., and Liu, C.-N. Chronic progressive external ophthalmoplegia, a clinical and neuropathologic report. *Arch. Neurol. Psychiatry 71*:31–53, 1954.

331. Schwartz, O., and Jampel, R.S. Congenital blepharophimosis associated with a unique generalized myopathy. *Arch. Ophthalmol. 68*:82–87, 1962.

332. Schwartz, R. Some speculations on the origins of autoantibodies. *Ann. N.Y. Acad. Sci. 505*:8–11, 1987.

333. Schwartz, R.H. T-lymphocyte recognition of antigen in association with gene products of the major histocompatibility complex. *Annu. Rev. Immunol. 3*:237–261, 1985.

334. Schwimmbeck, P.L., Dyrberg, T., Drachman, D.B., and Oldstone, M.B.A. Molecular mimicry and myasthenia gravis: An autoantigenic site of the acetylcholine receptor alpha-subunit that has biologic activity and reacts immunoochemically with herpes simplex virus. *J. Clin. Invest. 89*:1174–1179, 1989.

335. Segal, B.S. The retinopathy of dystrophia myotonia Steinert. *Metab. Pediatr. Ophthalmol. 9*:585–588, 1986.

336. Senita, G.R., and Fisher, E.R. Progressive dystrophic external ophthalmoplegia following trauma. *Arch. Ophthalmol. 60*:422–426, 1958.

337. Shaw, D.J., and Harper, P.S. Myotonic dystrophy: Developments in molecular genetics. *Br. Med. Bull. 45*:745–755, 1989.

338. Shaw, D.J., Meredith, A.L., Sarfarazi, M., Huson, S.M., Brook, J.D., Myklebost, O., and Harper, P.S. The apolipoprotein C2 gene: Subchromosomal localization and linkage to the myotonic dystrophy locus. *Hum. Genet. 70*:271–273, 1985.

339. Sher, J.H., Rimalovski, A.B., Athanassiades, T.J., and Aronson, S.M. Familial centronuclear myopathy: A clinical and pathological study. *Neurology 17*:727–742, 1967.

340. Shy, G.M., and Gonatas, N.K. Human myopathy with giant abnormal mitochondria. *Science 145*:493–496, 1964.

341. Shy, G.M., Silberberg, D.H., Appel, S.H., Mishkin, M.M., and Godfrey, E.H. A generalized disorder of nervous system, skeletal muscle, and heart resembling Refsum's disease and Hurler's syndrome. I. Clinical, pathologic, and biochemical characteristics. *Am. J. Med. 42*:163–168, 1967.

342. Silex, P. Progressive paralysis of the levator. *Arch. Ophthalmol. 28*:430–440, 1899.

343. Simon, K.A. Diabetes and lens changes in myotonic dystrophy. *Arch. Ophthalmol. 67*:312–315, 1962.

344. Simpson, J.A. Myasthenia and related disorders. In *Disorders of Voluntary Muscle*, 5th ed., J.N. Walton (Ed.), Churchill, Edinburgh, pp. 628–665, 1988.

345. Simpson, J.A., Behan, P.O., and Dick, H.M. Studies on the nature of autoimmunity in myasthenia gravis: Evidence for an immunodeficiency type. *Ann. N.Y. Acad. Sci. 274*:382–389, 1976.

346. Sipila, I., Simell, O., Rapola, J., Sainio, K., and Tuuteri, L. Gyrate atrophy of the choroid and retina with hyperornithinemia: Tubular aggregates and type 2 fiber atrophy in muscle. *Neurology 29*:996–1005, 1979.

347. Slaiman, W.R., Doyle, D., Johnson, R.H., and Jennett, S. Myopathy with mitochondrial inclusion bodies: Histological and metabolic studies. *J. Neurol. Neurosurg. Psychiatry 37*:1236–1246, 1974.

348. Slater, C.R. Muscle proteins and muscle dystrophy. *Curr. Opin. Cell Biol. 1*:110–114, 1989.

349. Sluga, E., and Moser, K. Myopathy with glycogen storage and giant mitochondria ultrastructural and biochemical findings. In *Muscle Diseases*, J.N. Walton, N. Canal, and G. Scarlato (Eds.), Excerpta Medica, Amsterdam, pp. 116–119, 1969.

350. Small, R.G. Coats' disease and muscular dystrophy. *Trans. Am. Acad. Ophthalmol. Otolaryngol. 72*:225–231, 1968.

351. Smeets, B., Poddighe, J., Brunner, H., Ropers, H.-H., and Wieringa, B. Tight linkage between myotonic dystrophy and apolipoprotein E genes revealed with allele specific oligonucleotides. *Hum. Genet. 80*:49–52, 1988.

352. Smit, L.M.E., Veldman, H., Jennekens, F.G.I., Molenaar, P.C., and Oen, B.S. A congenital myasthenic disorder with paucity of secondary synaptic clefts: Deficiency and altered distribution of acetylcholine receptors. *Ann. N.Y. Acad. Sci. 505*:346–356, 1987.

353. Spatz, H., and Ullrich, O. Klinischer und anatomischer Beitrag zu den angeborenen Beweglichkeits-defekten in Hirnnervenbereich. *Z. Kinderheilkd. 51*:579–597, 1931.

354. Spencer, R.F., and McNeer, K.W. Morphology of the extraocular muscles in relation to the clinical manifestation of strabismus. In *Strabismus and Amblyopia. Experimental Basis for Advances in Clinical Management*, G. Lennerstrand, G.K. von Noorden, and E.C. Campos (Eds.), Plenum, New York, pp. 37–41, 1988.

355. Spiro, A.J., Shy, G.M., and Gonatas, N.K. Myotubular myopathy. *Arch. Neurol. 14*:1–14, 1966.

356. Sprofkin, B.E., and Hillman, J.W. Moebius's syndrome—congenital oculofacial paralysis. *Neurology 6*:50–54, 1956.

357. Steinert, H. Über das Klinische und anatomische Bild des Muskelschwunds der Myotoniker. *Dtsch. Z. Nervenheilkd. 37*:59–104, 1909.

358. Stephens, J., Hoover, M.L., and Denst, J. On familial ataxia, neural amyotrophy, and their association with progressive external ophthalmoplegia. *Brain 81*:556–566, 1958.

359. Stern, L.Z., Cross, H.E., and Crebo, A.R. Abnormal iris vasculature in myotonic dystrophy. *Arch. Neurol.* 35:224–227, 1978.

360. Stricker, E., Thölen, H., Massini, M.-A., and Staub, H. The effect of haemodialysis in myasthenia gravis. *J. Neurol. Neurosurg. Psychiatry* 23:291–294, 1960.

361. Susac, J.O., Garcia-Mullin, R., and Glaser, J.S. Ophthalmoplegia in dermatomyositis. *Neurology* 23:305–310, 1973.

362. Swash, M. The morphology and innervation of the muscle fibers in dystrophia myotonica. *Brain* 95:357–368, 1972.

363. Swash, M., and Fox, K.P. Abnormal intrafusal muscle fibers in myotonic dystrophy: A study using serial sections. *J. Neurol. Neurosurg. Psychiatry* 38:91–99, 1975.

364. Swash, M., and Fox, K.P. The fine structure of the spindle abnormality in myotonic dystrophy. *Neuropathol. Appl. Neurobiol.* 1:171–187, 1975.

365. Swash, M., and Schwartz, M.S. Familial multicore disease with focal loss of cross-striations and ophthalmoplegia. *J. Neurol. Sci.* 52:1–10, 1981.

366. Swinyard, C.A., and Mayer, V. Multiple congenital contractures. Public health considerations of arthrogryposis multiplex congenita. *JAMA* 183:23–27, 1963.

367. Tamuna, K., Santa, T., and Kuroiwa, Y. Familial oculocranioskeletal neuromuscular disease with abnormal muscle mitochondria. *Brain* 97:665–672, 1974.

368. Tanaka, K. Myotonic dystrophy. *Med. Hypotheses* 17:415–425, 1985.

369. Tanaka, N., Nanaka, H., Takeda, M., Niimura, T., Kanehisa, T., and Terashi, S. Cardiomyopathy in myotonic dystrophy: A light and electron microscopic study of the myocardium. *Jpn. Heart J.* 14:202–212, 1973.

370. Tarrab-Hazdai, R., Aharonov, A., Silman, I., Fuchs, S., and Abramsky, O. Experimental autoimmune myasthenia induced in monkeys by purified acetylcholine receptor. *Nature* 256:128–130, 1975.

371. Taylor, E.W. Progressive vagus-glossopharyngeal paralysis with ptosis: A contribution to the group of family diseases. *J. Nerve. Ment. Dis.* 42:129–139, 1915.

372. Teoh, R., McGuire, L., Wong, K., and Chin, D. Increased incidence of thymoma in Chinese myasthenia gravis: Possible relationship with Epstein-Barr virus. *Acta Neurol. Scand.* 80:221–225, 1989.

373. Tevaarwerk, G.J.M., and Hudson, A.J. Carbohydrate metabolism and insulin resistance in myotonia dystrophica. *J. Clin. Endocrinol. Metab.* 44:491–498, 1977.

374. Thomas, N.S.T., and Harper, P.S. Myotonic dystrophy: Studies on the lipid composition and metabolism of erythrocytes and skin fibroblasts. *Clin. Chim. Acta* 83:13–23, 1978.

375. Thomasen, E. *Myotonia in Thomsen's Disease, Paramyotonia Dystrophia Myotonica. A Clinical and Heredobiologic Investigation*, Munksgaard, Copenhagen, pp. 121–124, 128–132, 1948.

376. Thomson, A.M.P. Dystrophia cordis myotonica studied by serial histology of the pacemaker and conducting system. *J. Pathol. Bacteriol.* 96:285–295, 1968.

377. Thoriacius, S., Aarli, J.A., Riise, T., Matre, R., and Johnsen, H.J. Associated disorders in myasthenia gravis: Autoimmune diseases and their relation to thymectomy. *Acta Neurol. Scand.* 80:290–295, 1989.

378. Thornell, L.E., Sjöstrom, M., Mattson, C.H., and Heilbronn, E. Morphological observations on motor endplates in rabbits with experimental myasthenia. *J. Neurol. Sci.* 29:389–410, 1976.

379. Tindall, S.C., Peters, B.H., Caverly, J.R., Sarles, H.E., and Fish, J.C. Thoracic duct lymphocyte depletion in myasthenia gravis. *Arch. Neurol.* 29:202–203, 1973.

380. Tome, F.M.S., and Fardeau, M. Ocular myopathies. In *Myology*, Vol. 2 A.G. Engel and B.Q. Banker (Eds.), McGraw-Hill, New York, pp. 1327–1347, 1986.

381. Toppet, M., Telerman-Toppet, N., Szliwowski, H.B., Vainsel, M., and Coers, C. Oculocraniosomatic neuromuscular disease with hypoparathyroidism. *Am. J. Dis. Child.* 131:437–441, 1977.

382. Toyka, K.V., Drachman, D.B., Griffin, D.E., Pestronk, A., Winkelstein, J.A., Fischbeck, J.H., Jr., and Kao, I. Myasthenia, gravis: Study of humoral immune mechanisms by passive transfer to mice. *N. Engl. J. Med.* 296:125–131, 1977.

383. Trelles, J.P., Gutierrez, C., Aranibar, A., and Palomino, L. Estudio anatomoclínico de la enfermedad de Steinert. *Riv. Neuro-Psiquiat.* 19:139–204, 1956.

384. Tzartos, S.J., Efthimiadis, A., Morel, E., Eymard, B., and Bach, J.-F. Neonatal myasthenia gravis: Antigenic specificities of antibodies in sera from mothers and their infants. *Clin. Exp. Immunol.* 80:376–380, 1990.

385. Tzartos, S.J., Seybold, M.E., and Lindstrom, J.M. Specificities of antibodies to acetylcholine receptors in sera from myasthenia gravis patients measured by monoclonal antibodies. *Proc. Natl. Acad. Sci. USA* 79:188–192, 1982.

386. Uemura, N., Tanaka, H., Niimura, T., Hashiguchi, H., Yoshimura, M., Terushi, S., and Kenehisa, T. Electrophysiological and histological abnormalities of the heart in myotonic dystrophy. *Am. Heart J.* 96:616–624, 1973.

387. Van Allen, M.W., and Blodi, F.C. Neurologic aspects of the Möbius syndrome. *Neurology* 10:249–259, 1960.

388. Vassilopoulos, D., Alevizos, B., and Spengos, M. Cataract and γ-glutamyl cycle in myotonic dystrophy. *Ophthalmologica* 174:167–169, 1976.

389. Victor, M., Hayes, R., and Adams, R.D. Oculopharyngeal muscular dystrophy: A familial disease of late life characterized by dysphagia and progressive ptosis of the eyelids. *N. Engl. J. Med.* 267:1267–1272, 1962.

390. Vincent, A., Thomas, H.C., Scadding, G.K., and Newsom-Davis, J. In vitro synthesis of anti-acetylcholine receptor antibody by thymic lymphocytes in myasthenia gravis. *Lancet 1*:305–307, 1978.

391. Vogel, R.M., and Lee, R.V. Bilateral ptosis in Wernicke's disease. *Neurology 17*:85–86, 1967.

392. Vogt, A. Die Cataract bei myotonischer Dystrophie. *Schweiz. Med. Wochenschr. 51*:669–674, 1921.

393. Von Graefe, A. Notizen vermischten lnhalts. *Arch. Ophthalmol. 2*:299–329, 1856.

394. Von Graefe, A. VI. Verhandlungen ärzlicher Gesellschaften. *Berl. Klin. Wochenschr. 5*:126–127, 1868.

395. Von Graefe, A. Diagnostic der Augen muskellähmungen. §42. In *Handbuch der gesammten Augenheilkunde*, Vol. 6, A. Graefe and T. Saemisch (Eds.), Engelmann, Leipzig, pp. 59–61, 1880.

396. Vos, T.A. 25 years dystrophia myotonica (D.M.). *Ophthalmologica 141*:37–44, 1961.

397. Wagner, E. Fall einer seltnen Muskel krankheit. *Arch. Heilk. Lpz. 4*:282–283, 1863.

398. Walker, S.P., Brubaker, R.F., and Magataki, S. Hypotony and aqueous humor dynamics in myotonic dystrophy. *Invest. Ophthalmol. Vis. Sci. 22*:744–751, 1982.

399. Wallis, P.G. Creatinuria in Möbius' syndrome. *Arch. Dis. Child. 35*:393–395, 1960.

400. Walton, J.N., Irving, D., and Tomlinson, B.E. Spinal cord limb motor neurons in dystrophia myotonica. *J. Neurol. Sci. 34*:199–211, 1977.

400a. Wartenberg, R. Winking-jaw phenomenon. *Arch. Neurol. Psychiatry 59*:734–753, 1948.

401. Webb, J.N. Experimental immune myositis in guinea pigs. *J. Reticuloendothel. Soc. 7*:305–316, 1970.

402. Weil, A., and Keschner, M. Ein Beitrag zur Klinik und Pathologie der Dystrophia myotonica. *Z. Ges. Neurol. Pschiat. 108*:687–702, 1927.

403. Weinberg, C.B., and Hall, Z.W. Antibodies from patients with myasthenia gravis recognize determinants unique to extrajunctional acetylcholine receptors. *Proc. Natl. Acad. Sci. USA 76*:504–508, 1979.

404. Willcox, H.N.A., Newsom-Davis, J., and Calder, L.R. Cell types required for anti-acetylcholine receptor antibody synthesis by cultured thymocytes and blood lymphocytes in myasthenia gravis. *Clin. Exp. Immunol. 58*:97–106, 1984.

405. Winer, N., Klachko, D.M., Baer, R.D., Langley, P.L., and Burns, T.W. Myotonic response induced by inhibitors of cholesterol biosynthesis. *Science 153*:312–313, 1966.

406. Winfield, J. Juvenile dermatomyositis with complications. *Proc. R. Soc. Med. 70*:548–551, 1977.

407. Wohlfart, G. Dystrophia myotonica and myotonica congenita, histopathologic studies with special reference to changes in the muscles. *J. Neuropathol. Exp. Neurol. 10*:109–124, 1951.

408. Wolf, S.M., and Barrows, H.S. Myasthenia gravis, and systemic lupus erythematosus. *Arch. Neurol. 14*:254–258, 1966.

409. Wolf, S.M., Davidson, S., Grossman, R., Barrows, H.S., and Wagner, J.H. Myopathy, tremor, emotional illness, and visual loss in a large family. *Bull. L.A. Neurol. Soc. 33*:197–208, 1968.

410. Wolter, J.R., Hoy, J.E., and Schmidt, D.M. Chronic orbital myositis, its diagnostic difficulties and pathology. *Am. J. Ophthalmol. 62*:292–298, 1966.

411. Yong, S.L., Lowry, R.B., and Jan, J.E. Syndrome of myopathy, short stature, seizures, retinitis pigmentosa, and cleft lip. *Birth Defects 13*:210–215, 1977.

412. Zacks, S. *The Motor Endplate*. Krieger, Huntington, NY, pp. 363–366, 1973.

413. Zintz, R., and Villiger, W. Elektronmikroskopische befunde bei 3 Fällen von chronisch progressive okulärer Muskeldystrophie. *Ophthalmologica 153*:439–459, 1967.

414. Zoltowska, A. Myoid and epithelial cell differentiation in myasthenic thymuses. *Thymus 17*:237–248, 1991.

415. Zurn, A.P., and Fulpius, B.W. Study of two different subpopulations of antiacetylcholine receptor antibodies in a rabbit with experimental autoimmune myasthenia gravis. *Eur. J. Immunol. 8*:529–532, 1977.

Index

hyaluronate-binding proteoglycan, **859**

hyaluronic acid (hyaluronate) 615, 619,667,701,705,707,708, 710,718,719,720,730,731, 856,857,859,880,882,1054, 1058,1059,1130,1409

hydatid disease, 356

hydranencephaly, 1317,1320,1325

hydrocephalus (hydrocephaly), 868,812,871,1290,1318, 1323,1365

hydrogen bond formation, 1034

hydrogen peroxide, 438,439,534, 547,548,549,1105,1153, 1164,1165,1166,1169
  detoxification 439,548,566
  toxicity 548

hydrops, acute 759

hydroxyapatite, 420,510,755,1137, 1138
  cornea 1138

hydroxyl radical, 554,1111,1164, 1165

hyperammonemia II, 828

hypercalcemia, 510,754,755,757, 815,821,**1137-1138**,1155

hypercapnia, 1690

hypercholesterolemia, 729,817, 824,1101,1102,1112,1113, 1114,1116,1231,1667

hyperfibrinogenemia, 1676

hypergammaglobulinemia, 955, 984,985,985-990

hyperglycemia, 565,1092,1093, 1094,1674,1675,1676,1680

hyperhidrosis, 812

hyperinsulinemia 1763

hyperlacticacidemia, 850

hyperlipemia, 850,1093,1112, 1113,1667,1668,1676

hyperlipidemia, familial combined 824

hyperlipoproteinemia, 816,817,824

hyperlysinemia, 513,801,822,**960**

hypermetropia, 447,1207

hypernephroma, 1357

hyperopia, 418,419,729,814,1224, 1295,1296,1304,1430

hyperornithinemia, 762,801, 816,822,**957-960**

hyperoxaluria, 665,815,828

hyperoxia, 483,1687,1156,1690

hyperparathyroidism, 754,755

hyperplasia, 1414,1415,1417
  reactive with dysplasia 1370

hypersensitivity,
  anaphylactic 152
  basophil 82,111
  cellular 1720
  cold 994
  cutaneous 1619,1665
    delayed 1438,1665
  delayed, 105,108,120,947,

[hypersensitivity]
  1612,1614,1665
  drug 1163
  IgE-mediated, 80
  immediate (see hypersensitivity type I)
  reaction 122,131,1635
  T cell 728
  type I 81,122,151,152
  type II **123-127**,153,159
  type III **127-130**,153,164, 166,167
  type IV **130-131**,153,172

hypertelorism, 830,831,832,833, 1309,1330,1331,1332
  choroidopathy 1674

hypertension, ocular acute 506
  optic neuropathy **1670-1674**

hypertension, systemic 632,652, 729,812,991,1007,1042, 1093,1107,1109,1152,1180, 1214,1633,1635,1636,1638, 1639,1642,1648,1649,1651, 1653,1667,**1668-1674**,1676, 1694
  vascular disease 1670

hypertensive retinopathy, 1643, 1651,**1669-1670**,1672,1674

hyperthermia, 1180

hyperthyroidism, 1106,1123, 1126,1128,1755

hypertrichosis, 831,1332

hypertriglyceridemia, 816,824, 1101,1102

hyperuricemia, 850

hyperviscosity syndrome, 984

hypervitaminosis A, 1152,1290

hypervitaminosis D, 1137

hypervolemia, 1669

hyphema, 389,390,391,411,412, 413,417,418,425,506,720, 731,1135,1172,1446,1457, 1460,1639

hypocalcemia, 485,490,1138

hypocholesterolemia, 824,1107, 1762

Hypoderma bovis, 381

Hypoderma tarandi, 381

hypogammaglobulinemia, 947,990

hypogenitalism, 830

hypoglycemia, 485,850,1315,1678

hypogonadism, 813,831,1770

hypoinsulinism, 849

hypomelanosis, congenital heritable 942

hypoparathroidism, 485,490,1138, 1765

hypophosphatasia, 485,754, 755,820,828,1137

hypophosphatemia, 757

hypopigmentation, oculocerebral 942,947

hypopigmentation-microphthalmos syndrome, 942,947 (see

[hypopigmentation-microphthalmos syndrome]
  also syndrome,Cross-McKusick-Breen)

hypoplasia,
  adrenal gland congenital 949
  congenital 1332

hypoproteinemia, 1635

hypopyon, 210,212,388,404,413, 421,506,519

hypospadias, 830,831

hypotelorism, 831,832,833

hypotension,
  eye 402,412
  postural 812,1693
  vascular 1641,1648

hypothermia, 424

hypothyroidism, 762,1100, 1109,1128,1766

hypotonia, 813,830,831,832,833, 900,960,1141,1290,1734, 1759,1772
  eye 402,412,417,418,419,420, 425,457,478,652,656,757, 1442,1635,1636,1638,1762

hypotrichosis, 1332

hypoxia, 983,1299,1639,1649,1661, 1662,1675,1678,1682,1692
  posterior segment 1664
  relative 1691
  tissue 1657,1663,1676,1682, 1692

I

I-cell disease, 815,841,843,844, 845,846,847,923,924,**933-936**

ICAM-1, 104,121,981,982,1616, 1667

ICAM-2 981

ICE syndrome, 459,**777-779**

ichthyosis, 483,485,819,820,829, 859,1304

IgA, secretory 145 (see also immunoglobulin, A)
  serum 1582

IgD (see immunoglobulin, D)

IgE (see immunoglobulin, E)

IgG, serum decreased 1759 (see also immunoglobulin, G)

IgG_1, 1727

IgH locus, 1579

IgM, (see immunoglobulin, M)

ileum, carcinoid tumor 1589

immotile cilia syndrome, 11

immune adherence, 66,125,126

immune complex, 127,495,1610

immune complex disease, 128,129

immune deficiency, 949,1143
  acquired (see AIDS) 1577,1614
  congenital 1614
  humoral 1364
  with albinism 942,947,950

[phagocytosis]
1227,1237,1644,1720,1728
defect 634,636
phagolysosome, 634,635,841
phagosome, 78,633,634,635,1212,
1227,1236,1238
phakodonesis, 622
phakoma, 1356
phakomatosis, 825,**1356-1367**
phalanx, hypoplasia 832,948
pharyngoconjunctival fever, 234
Phaseolus vulgaris erythroagglutinin
765
phenol, 951,1178,1179
phénomène de Mizou inverse, 1207
phenylalanine, metabolism disorders
939-953
phenylalanine hydroxylase, deficiency 817
phenylketonuria, 486,817,828
pheochromocytoma, 994,1356,
1357,1669
pheomelanin, 939
pheomelanosome, 945,946
phi body, 33,35
Philly mouse cataract, **503**,568
philtrum,
hypoplasia 1290
long 830,831,832
prominent pillars 832
phlebitis, 172,656,720,1647
phlyctenulosis, **168**
phocomelia, 1289
phosphatase, inhibition 569
phosphate, impaired excretion 1138
phosphaturia, 955
phosphodiesterase,
gene mutation 1233
mutation **1233**
phospholipase, 68,69,70,71,73,75,
80,84,122,123,495,542,
839,928
inhibitor 84
phospholipase C, agonist 542
phospholipid, 541,542,564,,633,
928,932,1009,1012,1104,
1105,1106,1107,1108,1109,
1156,1166,1226,1231,1713
antibody 1649
peroxidation 1164
photocoagulation, 424,696,1357,
1451
laser 425,649,657,1357
xenon arc 424
photolysis, 553,554,573
photooxidation, 553,554,556,569,
573,1153
photoreceptor, 12,27,801,864,881,
915,947,959,961,991,992,
1059,1149,1211,1221,1226,
1229,1230,1231,1235,1236,
1317,1318,1323,1414
abnormal 640
atrophy 690,693,1142,1730

[photoreceptor]
cation channel 1209
cilium, 1211,1226
congenital defect **1223-1226**
damage 1230
degeneration 424,664,**688**,802,
807,865,1172,1215,1229,
1230,1231,1238,1729
differentiation, 1263,1265,1617
disorders 666,**1205-1245**
dystrophies **1205-1223**
function 1239
interaction with retinal pigment
epithelium 1226,**1236-1238**
loss 663,664,1142
mutation 801
outer segment 633,1155,1226,
1227,1236
outer-segment degeneration **688**
primitive 1267
photosensitization, 553,554,556,
557,561
phototoxic reaction, 1178
phototoxicity, riboflavin 554
phototoxin, 1231
phototransduction, 1233,1239
Phthirus, 383
Phthirus capitis, 383
Phthirus pubis, 383,384
phthisis bulbi, 383,389,398,402,
404,418,420,425,735,752,
754,811,812,1152,1390,
1357,1416
Phycomycetes, 322
phycomycosis, 322,324
cerebrorhinoorbital 323
physaliphorous cell 1556
phytanate, 1110,1111
phytanic acid, 1110,1229
α-hydroxylase deficiency, 825,
1110-1111
oxidation, 1229
phytol, 1110
phytosterolemia, 1116
Picocornaviridae, 232
picornavirus, 228,234,**251**
piebaldism, 942,948
Pierre Robin syndrome, 485,1323
Pierre-Marie hereditary ataxia,
1223
pigment, 598
age 918
black 940
brown 940
cone (see cone pigment) 623
dispersion anterior segment 1730
disturbance peripapillary 1324
endogenous 1394
fluorescent 560,561
formation 561
granule anterior chamber 596
green cone 802
hematogenous 1639
melanin 597

[pigment]
mercury 506
yellow 940,1153
yellow-orange 1432
pigment dispersion syndrome 450,
453,597
pigment gene, red-green visual 803
pigmentary retinopathy, 370,485,
495,656,762,827,845,863,
864,868,869,956,1110,1138,
1172,1225,1729,1764,1765,
1768 (see also retinitis
pigmentosa)
atypical 1110
mottled 956
peripheral 915
pigmentation, 553,561,947,950,
951,1141,1166,1168,1169,
1170,1173,1724,1178,1179,
1390,1394,1416,1417,1425,
1429,1448
excessive mucous membrane
1417
fundus mosaic pattern 950
melanin decreased 939
melanin disorder 825
mucous membranes excessive
1416
regulation 939
pigmented ciliary epithelium, hyperplasia 1445
pilocarpine, 484,1168,1180
pilomatrixoma, 1381
pineal gland, 950,951,992
pinealitis, 992
pinealoblastoma, 803
tumor 1504
pinguecula, 620,621,**743-745**,
747,750,753,896,951,1013,
1014,1389
pinocytosis, 36,1648,1670
endothelium vascular 1636
pit, preauricular 830
pituitary gland, 551,1763
absence 1327
ascorbic acid 1155
subacute sclerosing
pityrosporiosis, 322
placenta, 546
basement membrane, 1041
collagen 1036
plagiocephaly, 486
plaglobin, 980
plaque,
anchoring 1042
atheromatous 1107
diskiform 663
plasma,
albumin 1105
cortisol low 1728
insudation 1674,1680,1691
lipid 1099,1229,1647
protein 991
retinol binding protein 1230

About the Editors

ALEC GARNER is Professor and Director of the Department of Pathology at the Institute of Ophthalmology, University of London, England. The author of over 200 scientific articles that reflect his research interests in vascular retinopathy, ocular angiogenesis, ocular onchocerciasis, and tumor immunology, he is a Fellow of the Royal College of Physicians, the Royal College of Pathologists, the Royal College of Ophthalmologists, and the Royal Society of Medicine. Dr. Garner received the M.B.Ch.B. (1960) and the M.D. (1966) degrees from the University of Manchester, England, and the Ph.D. degree (1972) in pathology from the University of London, England.

GORDON K. KLINTWORTH is Professor of Pathology and Joseph A. C. Research Professor of Ophthalmology at Duke University Medical Center and Director of Research at the Duke University Eye Center, Durham, North Carolina. A charter member and immediate past President of the American Association of Ophthalmologists, the Founder and past President of the International Society for Ophthalmic Pathology and a former member of the Visual Science Study Section A of the National Institutes of Health, his research focuses on diseases of the cornea, experimental ophthalmic pathology, and inherited eye diseases. Dr. Klintworth, certified by the American Board of Pathology in anatomic pathology and neuropathology, received his medical degree (1957) and the Ph.D. degree (1966) in anatomy from the University of the Witwatersrand, Johannesburg, South Africa.